The Complete Reference Guide to MEDICINE AND HEALTH

EDITED BY
Richard J. Wagman, M.D., F.A.C.P.
Assistant Clinical Professor of Medicine
Downstate Medical Center
New York, New York

Volume One

FACTS ON FILE/NEW YORK

ISBN 0-8160-6144-0 (hardcover)

Printed in the United States of America

Contributors to The New Complete Medical and Health Encyclopedia

Consultant in Surgery

N. Henry Moss, M.D., F.A.C.S.
Associate Clinical Professor of Surgery
Temple University Health Sciences Center and Albert Einstein Medical Center;
Past President, American Medical Writers Association;
Past President, New York Academy of Sciences

Consultant in Gynecology

Douglass S. Thompson, M.D.
Clinical Professor of Obstetrics and Gynecology and Clinical Associate Professor of Community Medicine
University of Pittsburgh School of Medicine

Consultant in Pediatrics

Charles H. Bauer, M.D.
Clinical Associate Professor of Pediatrics and Chief of Pediatric Gastroenterology
The New York Hospital-Cornell Medical Center
New York, New York

Consultants in Psychiatry

Julian J. Clark, M.D.
Assistant Professor of Psychiatry

and

Rita W. Clark, M.D.
Clinical Assistant Professor of Psychiatry
Downstate Medical Center

Consulting Editor

Kenneth N. Anderson
Formerly Editor
Today's Health

Bruce O. Berg, M.D.
Associate Professor
Departments of Neurology and Pediatrics
Director, Child Neurology
University of California
San Francisco, California

D. Jeanne Collins
Assistant Professor
College of Allied Health Professions
University of Kentucky
Lexington, Kentucky

Anthony A. Davis
Vice President and Education Consultant
Metropolitan X-Ray and Medical Sales, Inc.
Olney, Maryland

Peter A. Dickinson
Editor Emeritus
Harvest Years/Retirement Living

Gordon K. Farley, M.D.
Associate Professor of Child Psychiatry
Director, Day Care Center
University of Colorado Medical Center

Arthur Fisher
Group Editor
Science and Engineering
Popular Science

Edmund H. Harvey, Jr.
Editor
Science World

Helene MacLean
Medical writer

Ben Patrusky
Science writer

Stanley E. Weiss, M.D.
Assistant Attending Physician, Renal Service
Beth Israel Hospital and Medical Center, New York

Jeffrey S. Willner, M.D.
Attending Radiologist
Southampton Hospital
Southampton, New York

Editor
Richard J. Wagman, M.D., F.A.C.P.
Assistant Clinical Professor of Medicine
Downstate Medical Center
New York, New York

Contents

Volume II

Volume III

Volume IV

INTRODUCTION

Beyond following a well-balanced diet and exercising regularly, the best thing you can do to improve your health is to educate yourself. THE NEW COMPLETE MEDICAL AND HEALTH ENCYCLOPEDIA provides you and your family with an excellent resource for learning about and understanding the human body and what it needs to remain healthy. Beginning with a basic guide to the body and all its functioning parts, THE NEW COMPLETE MEDICAL AND HEALTH ENCYCLOPEDIA then covers every stage of life in terms of health care—from newborns to toddlers to teenagers to adults and seniors. Each section contains valuable information on everything from teething pain to mammograms. Special attention is given to the health concerns unique to women and men, including in-depth coverage of crucial developments in cancer research and treatments.

Within these pages you will find up-to-date information on health care, medicine, and the treatment of illnesses and diseases. Articles feature easy-to-understand descriptions and definitions, clear and concise summaries of symptoms and treatments, as well as preventive measures. Medically-accurate illustrations and diagrams enhance your understanding by providing further detail, so that if and when the time comes, you can comfortably ask your doctor the important questions.

THE NEW COMPLETE MEDICAL AND HEALTH ENCYCLOPEDIA also helps you make your home as safe as possible. Tips on child-proofing your home are included, as are ways to make it emergency-free by eliminating the potential for danger. A special Medical Emergency section, edged in color for speedy use in an emergency, guides you through the steps in administering first aid for injuries.

In addition to featuring lengthy discussions of particular disorders and diseases, THE NEW COMPLETE MEDICAL AND HEALTH ENCYCLOPEDIA details common aches and pains and simple remedies for them, describes a typical physical examination and other diagnostic procedures which physicians routinely use, covers drug and alcohol abuse, and lists voluntary health agencies you can contact for further information on specific areas from diabetes to mental health to family planning to sexually transmitted diseases.

Your health is your most valuable asset. To help protect that asset, THE NEW COMPLETE MEDICAL AND HEALTH ENCYCLOPEDIA educates you about the latest accepted treatments and procedures, giving you a good start on providing a safe, healthy, and happy life for you and those you love.

It is important to note, that while THE NEW COMPLETE MEDICAL AND HEALTH ENCYCLOPEDIA attempts to provide the most current health care information, it is no substitute for actual conversation and consultation with your family physician.

1

Your Body

The Skeleton

Say "skeleton" to children and you probably conjure up in their minds a rickety structure of rigid sticks, or, to the more fanciful child, a clickety-clacketing collection of rattling bones cavorting under a Halloween moon. A look at almost any anatomical drawing of the human skeletal system bears out the child's image: dry sticks of bones, stripped of skin and flesh, muscle and tendon—a grotesque caricature of a living human being.

Our living bones are something quite different. They are rigid, yes, but not entirely so: they also may bend a little and grow and repair themselves; and they are shaped and fitted so that—rather than the herky-jerky motions of a wooden puppet—they permit the smooth grace and coordination power displayed by an accomplished athlete or a prima ballerina.

Our bones do not do just one thing but many things. Some bones, like the collarbone or *clavicle,* mainly give support to other body structures. Others, like the skull and ribs, encase and protect vulnerable organs. Still others, like the *metacarpi* and *phalanges* that make up our hands and fingers, give us mechanical advantages—leverage and movement. There are even bones, the tiny *ossicles* in the middle ear, whose vibrations enable us to hear.

Finally, to think of bone simply as a structural member, like a solid steel girder in a skyscraper, ignores the fact that bone is living tissue. It is one of the busiest tissues in our bodies, a chemical factory that is continually receiving, processing and shipping a wide variety of mineral salts, blood components, and a host of other vital materials.

How the Bones of the Skeletal System Fit and Work Together

Medical textbooks name a total of 206 bones making up the skeletal system of the normal, adult human being. The words "normal" and "adult" are significant. A newborn baby normally has 33 vertebrae making up its backbone (also called *spinal column* or simply *spine*); but by the time a person reaches adulthood, the number of individual vertebrae has shrunk to 26.

The Human Skeleton

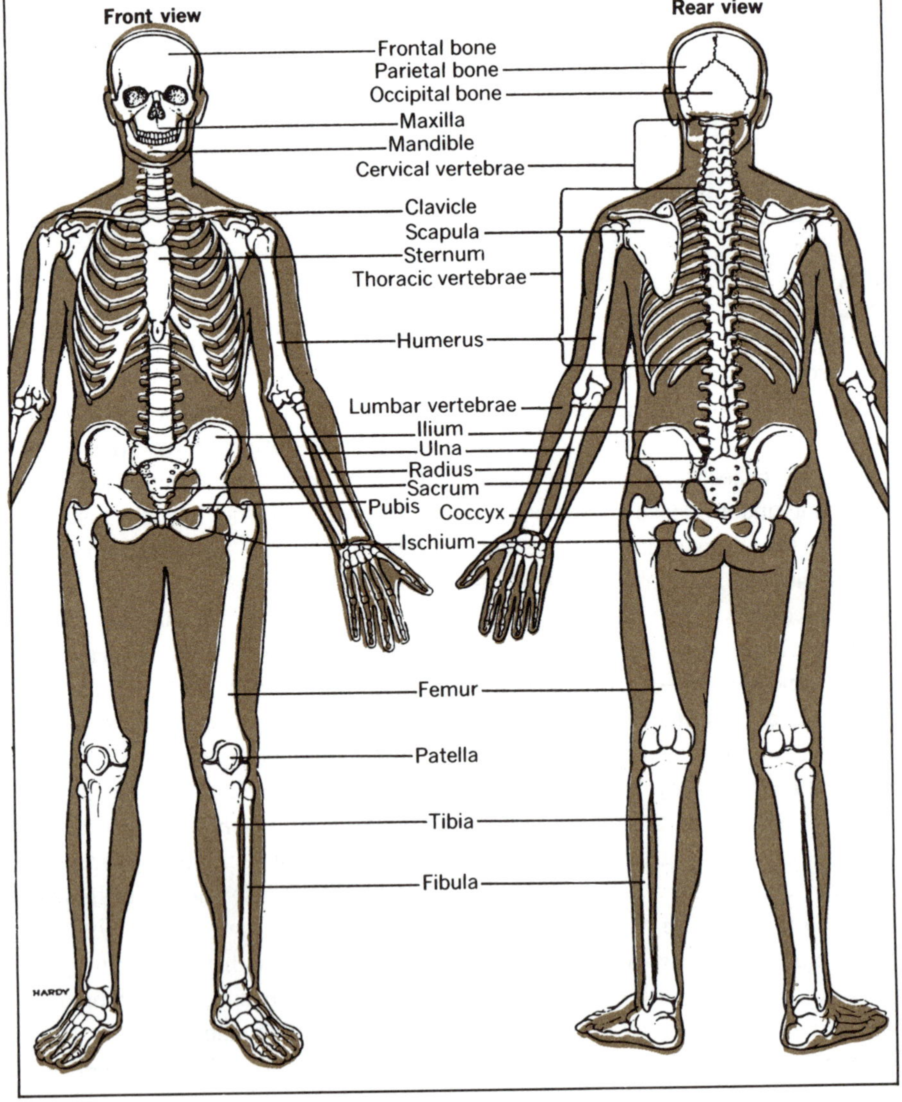

The explanation: during the growth process, the nine bottom vertebrae fuse naturally into just two. In like fashion, we "lose" some 60 bones as we grow up. Some otherwise perfectly normal adults have "extra" bones or "missing" bones. For example, although the normal number of ribs is 12 pairs, some adults may have 11; others may have 13 pairs.

Even a practicing physician might be hard-pressed to identify each of our 200-plus bones and describe its function. An easier way to gain a general understanding of the various functions, capabilities—and weaknesses, too—of our bones is to visualize the skeletal system as a standing coatrack, say, about six feet high.

Call the central pole the backbone. About ten inches down from its top (the top of your skull) is a horizontal crossbar (your shoulders—collarbones and shoulder blades), approximately a foot-and-a-half across. Sixteen or so inches below the bottom of the top crossbar is another, shorter crossbar, broader and thicker—the*pelvic girdle.* The coatrack with its two crossbars is now a crude model of the bones of the head and trunk, collectively called the *axial skeleton.* Its basic unit is the backbone, to which are attached the skull at the top, then the bones of the shoulder girdle, the ribs, and at the bottom, the bones of the pelvic girdle.

By hanging down (or appending) members from the two ends of the top crossbar, and doing the same at the lower crossbar, we would simulate what is called the *appendicular skeleton*—arms and hands, legs and feet.

Now, make the coatrack stand on its new legs, cut off the central pole just below the lower bar (if you wish, calling it man's lost tail), and you have the two main components of the skeletal system, joined together before you. Let us look at each more closely.

The Axial Skeleton

Within the framework of the axial skeleton lie all the most vital organs of the body. People have gone on living with the loss of a hand or a leg—indeed, with the loss of any or all of their limbs. But nobody can live without a brain, a heart, a liver, or lungs—all of which are carried within the framework of the axial skeleton.

The Skull

The bones of the skull have as their most important function the protection of the brain and some sense organs. There are also, of course, the jawbones that support the teeth and gums and which enable us to bite and chew our food.

Most of the skull appears to consist of a single bone—a hard, unbroken dome. Actually, the brain cage or *cranium* consists of eight individual platelike bones which have fused together in the process of growth. At birth, these bones are separated, causing the soft spots or *fontanelles* we can readily feel on a baby's head. As the baby's brain enlarges, the bones grow along their edges to fill in the fontanelles, finally knitting together in what are called *suture lines,* somewhat resembling inexpertly mended clothes seams. Along the suture lines, the skull bones continue to grow until the individual's mature skull size is reached.

Teeth

The hardest substance in the human body is the *enamel* that covers the exposed surface of a tooth. Below the gum, the tooth's outside surface is composed of somewhat softer *cementum.* Beneath enamel and cementum is a bonelike substance, called *dentin,* which covers the soft interior of the tooth, called *pulp.* Pulp is serviced by blood vessels and nerves through the root or roots of the tooth. The passageway of nerves and blood vessels that lead up through the tooth from the gum sockets is called a *root canal.* Tooth and gum are stuck to each other by a tough, adhesive tissue called *periodontal* (or peridental—"surrounding the tooth") *membrane.* See Ch. 22, *The Teeth and Gums,* for further information on teeth.

The Backbone

At the base of the skull, the backbone begins. The skull is supported by the topmost *cervical* (neck) vertebra. The curious thing about a backbone is that the word has come to suggest something solid, straight, and unbending. The backbone, however, just isn't like that: it consists of 26 knobby, hollowed-out bones—*vertebrae,* rather improbably held together by muscles, ligaments, and tendons. It is not straight when we stand, but has definite backward and forward curvatures; and even some of its most important structures (the disks between the vertebrae) aren't made of bone, but of cartilage.

All in all, however, the backbone is a fairly well designed structure in terms of the several different functions it serves—but with some built-in weaknesses. For a discussion of backache, see Ch. 23, *Aches, Pains, Nuisances, Worries.*

The Vertebrae

Although they will have features in common, no two of our 26 vertebrae are exactly alike in shape, size, or function. This is hardly surprising if we consider, for example, that the cervical vertebrae do not support ribs, while the *thoracic* vertebrae (upper trunk, or chest) do support them.

But for a sample vertebra, let us pick a rib-carrying vertebra, if for no other reason than that it lies about midway along the backbone. If viewed from above or below, a thoracic vertebra, like most of the others, would look like a roundish piece of bone with roughly scalloped edges on the side facing inward toward the chest and on the side facing outward toward the surface of the back, and would reveal several bony projections. These knobby portions of a vertebra—some of which you can feel as bumps along your backbone—are called *processes.* They serve as the vertebra's points of connection to muscles and tendons, to ribs, and to the other vertebrae above and below.

A further conspicuous feature is a hole, more or less in the middle of the typical vertebra, through which passes the master nerve bundle of our bodies, the spinal cord, running from the base of the skull to the top of the pelvis. Thus, one of the important functions of the backbone is to provide flexible, protective tubing for the spinal cord.

Between the bones of one vertebra and the next is a piece of more resilient cartilage that acts as a cushion or shock absorber to prevent two vertebrae from scraping or bumping each other if the backbone gets a sudden jolt, or as the backbone twists and turns and bends. These pieces of cartilage are the intervertebral disks—infamous for pain and misery if they become ruptured or slipped disks.

Regions of the Backbone

The backbone can be divided into five regions, starting with the uppermost, or *cervical* region, which normally has seven vertebrae. Next down is the *thoracic* (chest) section, normally with 12 vertebrae. From each vertebra a rib extends to curl protectively around the chest area. Usually, the top ten ribs come all the way around the trunk and attach to the breastbone (or *sternum*); but the bottom two ribs do not reach the breastbone and are thus called floating ribs. The thoracic section also must support the shoulder girdle, consisting of the collarbones (*clavicles*) and shoulder blades (*scapulas*). At the end of each shoulder blade is a shoulder joint—actually three distinct joints working together—where the arm connects to the axial skeleton.

Below the thoracic vertebrae come the five vertebrae of the *lumbar* section. This area gets a good deal of blame for back miseries: lower back pain often occurs around the area where the bottom thoracic vertebra joins the top lumbar vertebra. Furthermore, the lumbar region or small of the back is also a well-known site of back pain; indeed, from the word "lumbar" comes *lumbago,* medically an imprecise term, but popularly used to describe very real back pain.

Below the lumbar region are two vertebrae so completely different from the 24 above them—and even from each other—that it seems strange they are called vertebrae at all: the *sacrum* and the *coccyx.* These two vertebrae are both made up of several distinct vertebrae that are present at birth. The sacrum is a large bone that was once five vertebrae. The coccyx was originally four vertebrae—and, incidentally, is all that remains of man's tail in his evolution from the primates.

The Pelvic Girdle

The sacrum is the more important of these two strange-looking vertebrae. It is the backbone's connection to the *pelvic girdle,* or pelvis. On each side of the sacrum, connected by the sacroiliac joint, is a very large, curving bone called the *ilium,* tilting (when we stand) slightly forward and downward from the sacrum toward the front of the groin. We feel the top of the ilium as the top of the hip—a place mothers and fathers often find convenient for toting a toddler.

Fused at each side of the ilium and slanting toward the back is the *ischium,* the bone we sit on. The two *pubis* bones, also fused to the ilium, meet in front to complete the pelvic girdle. All the bones of the pelvis—ilium, ischium, and pubis—fuse together so as to form the hip joint (*acetabulum*), a deep socket into which the "ball" or upper end of the thighbone fits.

The Appendicular Skeleton

The bones of the appendages—arms, hands, and fingers; legs, feet, and toes—allow human beings to perform an astonishing array of complex movements, from pushing themselves through the physical rigors of the Olympic decathlon to creating an elaborate piece of needlework. The key points in the appendicular skeleton, as indeed, in the axial skeleton, are where the ends or edges of bones lie close together and must work with or against one another in order to achieve coordinated movement. These key points are the *joints*—not really bones at all but the non-bony spaces between bones.

The Joints

A typical joint consists of several different structures. First, there are the bones themselves—two, three, four, or more almost touching in the area of the joint—with their ends or edges shaped to fit in their respective niches. Between the bones of an appendage joint (as between the vertebrae of the back) is the smooth, resilient material called *cartilage* that allows the bones to move over one another without scraping or catching. At the joint, the bones, with their layer of cartilage between them, are held together by tough bonds of muscle. *Bursas,* tiny sacs containing a lubricating fluid, are also found at joints; they help to reduce the friction between a joint's moving parts.

The Hip and Knee

The hip joint must not only support the weight of the head and trunk, but must allow for movement of the leg and also play a part in the constant balancing required to maintain upright posture. Similar stresses and strains, often literally tending to tear the joint apart, are placed on every joint in the body.

The notoriety of athletes' bad knees attests to the forces battering at the knee joint, the largest in the human body. Sports involving leaping or sudden changes in direction, such as basketball, are especially hard on the knee. However, the fact that there are not more disabled sports heroes speaks well for the design of the knee joint. The same can be said of the ankle joint and the joints of the foot and toes.

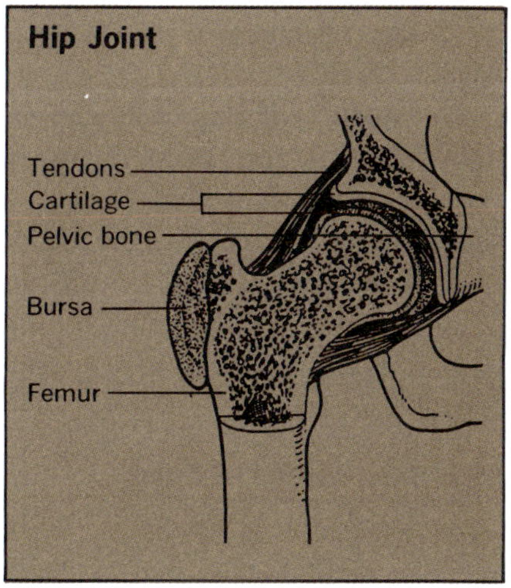

The Shoulder, Elbow, and Wrist

The counterpart of the hip joint in the upper trunk is the shoulder joint. Free of weight-bearing responsibilities, the shoulder has a system of three interconnected joints that allow it and the arm far more versatile movements than the hip and leg.

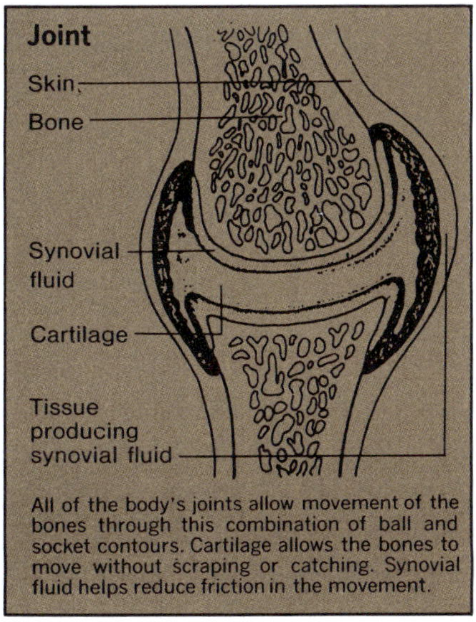

All of the body's joints allow movement of the bones through this combination of ball and socket contours. Cartilage allows the bones to move without scraping or catching. Synovial fluid helps reduce friction in the movement.

The elbow connects the upper arm bone (*humerus*) with the two bones of the lower arm (*radius* and *ulna*). Like the knee, it is basically a hinge joint, which allows the lower arm to be raised and lowered. The elbow is also constructed to allow some rotation by the hand; likewise, the knee joint allows us to waggle the foot.

Of all our body parts, the wrist, hand, and fingers are perhaps the most elegantly and finely jointed—witness the performance of a concert pianist—and our ankles, feet, and toes probably the most subject to everyday misery.

Bone as Living Tissue

Our bones, like all our tissues, change as we grow up, mature, and finally grow old. There are changes in the chemical activity and composition of bone representative of each stage of life.

In young children, the ends and edges of bones are mainly cartilage, forming a growing surface on the bone that is gradually replaced by hard bone as full size is attained. The bones of a child are more pliable and less likely to break than those of a full-grown adult.

Similarly, as an adult ages, the bones turn from a resilient hardness to a more brittle hardness. This accounts for the much greater danger of broken bones in older people.

These changes with age are an indication of the great amount of chemical activity going on within bone. We sometimes forget that our bones are amply supplied and penetrated by blood vessels. There is a constant building up and breaking down, an interchange of materials between blood and bone.

The Composition of Bone

A living bone does not have a single uniform composition, but instead is composed of several different kinds of tissue. To begin with, there are actually two types of bone tissue in the same bone: compact and spongy. In addition, bone is sheathed in a tough membranous tissue called the *periosteum,* interlaced with blood vessels. Finally, within most of the larger and longer bones of the body, as well as in the interior of the skull bones and vertebrae, are two more kinds of tissue: red marrow and yellow marrow.

Bones of the Hand and Foot

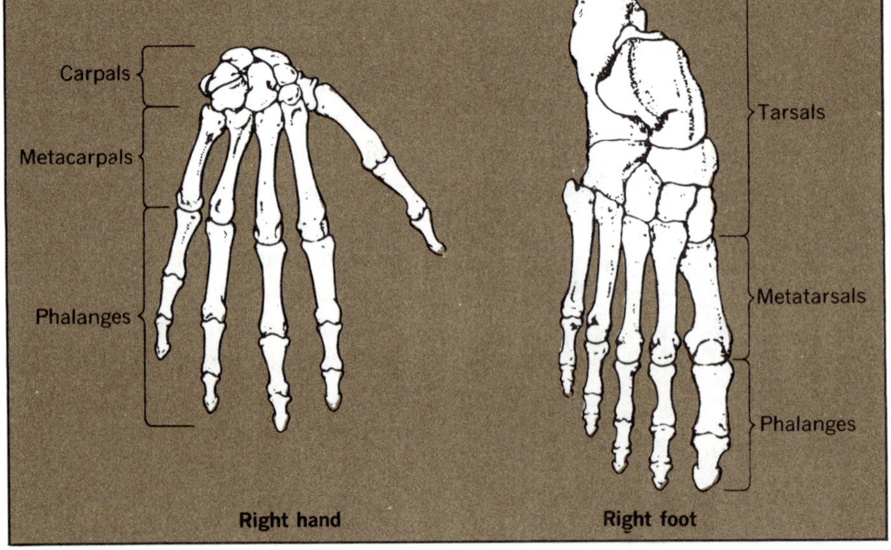

Marrow

Within the spongy bone areas, *red marrow* produces enormous numbers of red blood cells, at a rate of millions per minute. These are needed for growth as well as for replacement of red cells, which also die in enormous numbers. Children's bones contain greater proportions of red marrow than adults'. With age, *yellow marrow,* composed mainly of fat cells, begins to fill the interior bone cavities formerly occupied by red marrow.

Calcium

Bone also serves as a storage and distribution center for one of the most important elements in our body. Calcium, in the form of calcium phosphate, is the basic chemical of bone tissue, but this element also must always be present in the bloodstream at a certain level to ensure normal heartbeat, blood clotting, and muscle contraction. When the calcium level in the blood is deficient, the bones release some calcium into the bloodstream; when the blood has a surplus of calcium, the bones reabsorb it.

Fractures

Like most other tissues, broken bone can repair itself, and it is a remarkable process to observe. It is a process, however, that will proceed even if the ends are not aligned or set—an important reason why any suspected fracture should be checked by a physician.

A break in a bone causes a sticky material to be deposited by the blood around the broken ends. This material begins the formation of a kind of protective, lumpy sleeve, called a *callus,* around the broken ends. Mainly cartilage, the callus hardens into spongy bone, normally within a month or two. Then, the spongy bone begins to be reduced in size by bone-dissolving cells produced in the marrow, while at the same time the spongy bone in the area of the break is beginning to be replaced by hard bone.

Depending on the particular bone involved and the severity of the fracture, the broken bone can be completely healed within four to ten months.

Potential Trouble Spots

Essentially there are two kinds of things that can go wrong with the skeletal system and cause trouble.

Mechanical Difficulties

A healthy bone's main mechanical functions—support, movement, protection—can be impaired. This can happen as a result of a physical injury resulting in a fracture or dislocation.

The stack of vertebrae called the backbone is vulnerable to a number of painful conditions from top to bottom, especially in the region of the lower back. Unfortunately, man seems to have evolved relatively quickly from a four-footed creature, and his backbone is not ideally suited for standing and walking on two feet. Back troubles become increasingly common with age.

Areas where bones interact are also very susceptible to injury because of the stresses and strains they undergo even in people who are not especially active. Normal wear and tear also takes its toll on our bones and joints; for example, the bones' structure or their alignment at a joint may be altered slightly with age, making one bone or another prone to slipping out of the joint causing a dislocation. In any case, it is not advisable to make the same demands on our skeletal system at 40 as we did at 20. Joints are also the site of arthritis.

Disease

Second, and generally more serious if untreated, the interior bone tissues themselves may become infected and diseased. This can lead as a secondary effect to impairment of the bones' mechanical functions. *Osteomyelitis,* for example, an infection of bony tissues, can destroy large portions of bone unless antibiotics are started at once.

Fortunately, disorders of the skeletal system generally reveal themselves early and clearly by pain. Any severe or lingering pain of the joints or bones should be reported to a physician. For example, some people may feel that aching feet are unavoidable—and a little undignified. But a foot is not meant to hurt, nor is any part of the skeletal system. Consulting a physician could prevent much present and future misery. See also Ch. 7, *Diseases of the Skeletal System.*

The Muscles

Some 600 muscles of all sizes and shapes are attached to the framework of the skeletal system. Altogether these muscles make up nearly half of a normal adult's weight. They hold the skeleton together and, on signals originating in the brain, empower its various parts to move. Everywhere throughout the skeletal system, muscles work together with bones to protect the body's vital organs and to support and move its parts.

Skeletal Muscle

Such muscles are called, collectively, *skeletal muscle.* They are also called *voluntary muscles* because, for the most part, we can choose when we want them to act and what we want them to do—drive a car, kick a football, turn a page, jump a brook, ride a bicycle. Skeletal muscle also goes by two other names, based on its appearance under a microscope—striped and striated.

Skeletal, voluntary, striped, striated—all refer to the same general type of muscle. To avoid confusion, the term used throughout this section is skeletal muscle.

Muscles of the Abdomen and Thorax

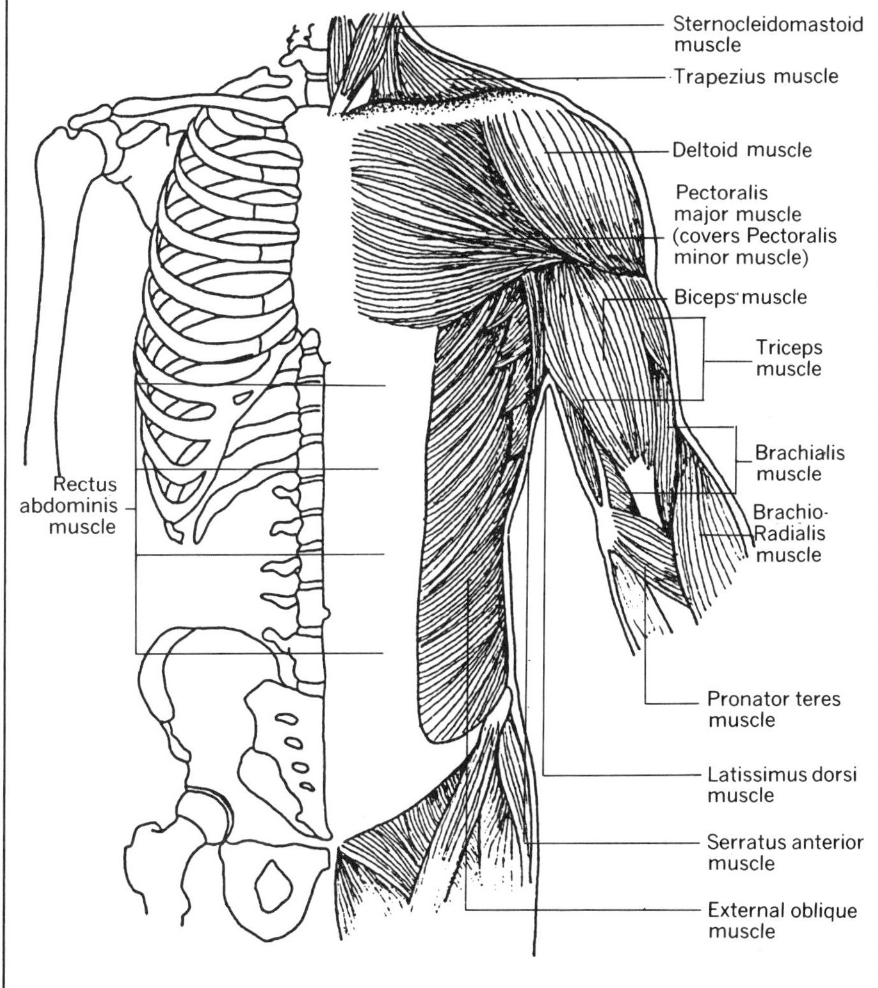

Smooth Muscle

There are two other general types of muscle. One is called *smooth muscle* because, under the microscope, it lacks the clearly defined stripes of skeletal muscle. Smooth muscle has another name, *involuntary muscle*, so called because the brain does not voluntarily control its actions. Smooth muscle is responsible for movements such as the muscular action that moves food and waste along the digestive tract, or the contraction and dilation of the pupil of the eye, as well as countless other involuntary movements of the sense and internal organs—with the exception of the heart.

Muscles of the Back

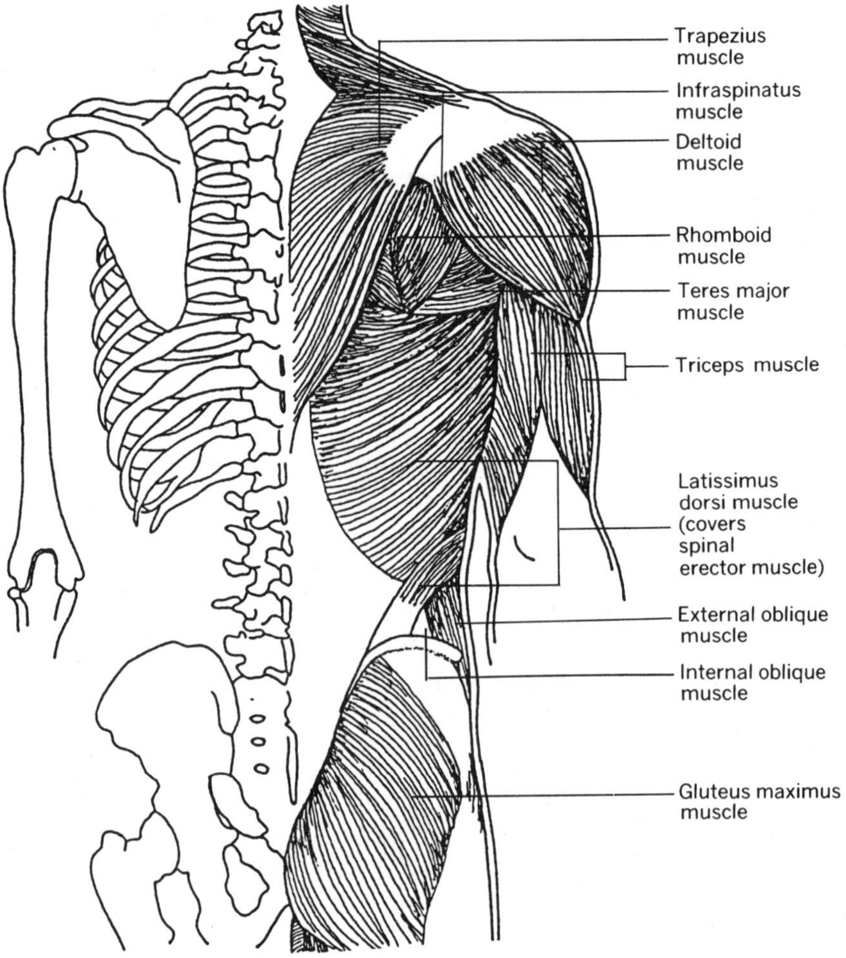

Cardiac Muscle

The third and last general type of muscle is confined to the heart area, and is called *cardiac muscle.* (Cardiac means having to do with the heart.) It is involved in the rhythmic beating and contractions of the heart, which are not under conscious control, and cardiac muscle is therefore termed involuntary.

Structure of the Muscles

Each of the three kinds of muscle shares certain structural similarities with one or both of the others. All are made up of bundles of varying numbers of hair-thin fibers. In skeletal and smooth muscles, these fibers are lined up side by side in the bundle, while in cardiac muscle the fibers tend more to crisscross over one another. Skeletal muscle and cardiac muscle

Muscles, Their Locations, and Exercises that Strengthen Them

Muscle	Location	Movement
Trapezius	Upper back and each side of neck	Shoulder-shrugging and upward-pulling movements
Deltoids	Shoulders	Arm raising and overhead pressing
Pectorals	Chest	Horizontal pressing and drawing arms across body
Latissimus dorsi	Wide back muscle stretching over back up to rear Deltoids	Pulling and rowing movements
Serratus	Jagged sawtooth muscles between Pectorals and lattissimus Dorsi	Pullover and Serratus leverage movements
Spinal erectors	Lower length of spinal column	Raising upper body from a bent-over position
Biceps	Front portion of upper arm	Arm bending and twisting
Forearms	Between wrist and elbow	Reverse-grip arm bending
Triceps	Back of upper arm	Pushing and straightening movements of upper arms
Rectus abdominals	Muscular area between sternum and pelvis	Sit-up, leg-raising, knee-in movements
Intercostals	Sides of waist, running diagonally to Serratus	Waist twisting
External oblique abdominals	Lower sides of waist	Waist twisting and bending
Buttocks	Muscular area covering seat	Lunging, stooping, leg raising
Leg biceps	Back of thighs	Raising lower leg to buttocks, bending forward and stretching
Frontal thighs	Front of thighs	Extending lower leg and knee bending
Calves	Lower leg between ankle and knee	Raising and lowering on toes

are both striped, that is, they show darker and lighter bands crossing over a group of adjacent fibers, while smooth muscle lacks these distinct cross-bands.

Both involuntary muscle types, smooth and cardiac, are controlled by signals carried by the autonomic nervous system. Signals that result in movements of the skeletal muscles are carried by a different nerve network, the central nervous system. The individual fibers in a muscle bundle with a particular function all react simultaneously to a signal from the nervous system; there is no apparent time lag from fiber to fiber.

How the Skeletal Muscles Work

The great range and variety of functions served by skeletal muscles can be suggested by naming just four: the diaphragm, used in breathing; the muscles that make the eye wink; the deltoid muscle that gives the shoulder its shape; and the tongue.

As with the bones, the body tends to make its greatest demands on muscle tissue in the area of the joints and the backbone. A smoothly functioning joint requires that bone, cartilage, and muscle all be sound and able to work together effectively.

Tendons and Ligaments

We often hear the words tendon and ligament used in the description of the knee or another joint. These are actually two types of skeletal muscles, distinguished as to their function.

A *tendon* can be described as a tight cord of muscle tissue that attaches other skeletal muscle to bone. For example, the Achilles tendon running down the back of the calf, the strongest tendon in the body, connects the muscles of the calf with the bone of the heel. A *ligament* is a somewhat more elastic band of muscle fibers that attaches bone to bone.

A tendon is not always evident in the connection of muscle to bone. Various groups and shapes of muscle fibers may be similarly employed, forming connective tissue without the formation of tendon.

Various associated tissues between or around skeletal muscles serve to reduce the wear and tear of

Tendon

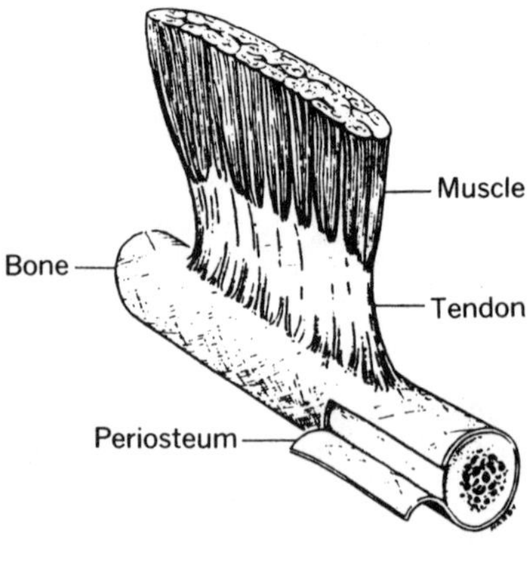

The muscle is attached to the bone by a tendon. The fibers of the tendon interlace with the fibers of the periosteum, forming a strong bond.

Structure of the Femur

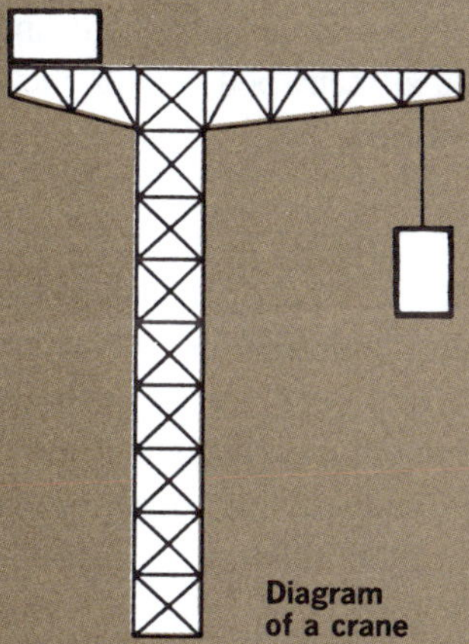

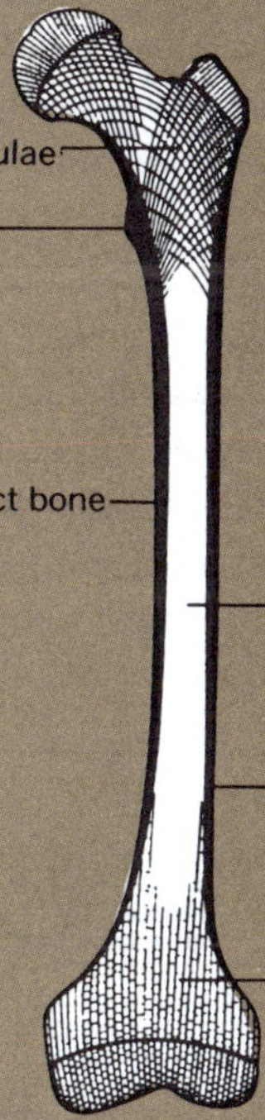

The femur, the large bone of the upper leg, combines strength and lightness better than all but the strongest materials. The minimum of substance is used by having the bone shaft hollow, like the girders of a crane. This is feasible because most of the stress on a long structure occurs at the outside. Within the head of the femur are *trabeculae* (strands of connective tissue) that crisscross roughly at right angles. They correspond to the main lines of the compression and tension when a bone is bearing weight. A similar device is used in the crisscross girders of the crane. Ridges provide areas for muscle attachment and reinforce bones against the pull of muscles.

friction in areas such as a joint, where muscle, bone, and cartilage may rub against one another. For example, the tendons that pass along the back of the hand from the wrist to the fingertips, as well as many other muscle groups throughout the body, are enclosed in lubricated sheaths. The muscle-sheathed *bursas,* lined inside with lubricating fluid, are also found in areas subject to friction, such as where a tendon passes closely over a bone.

Man's upright posture and two-legged locomotion subject the backbone to heavy stresses. It is buttressed, however, with scores of tightly packed bundles of muscle attached to either side of the spinal column.

Flexors and Extensors

Most of us probably first used the word "muscle" when, as children, we watched an older child or adult flex an arm and proudly display the bump of muscle between the crook of elbow and shoulder. This biceps muscle works together with the triceps muscle on the underside of the arm. The arm is bent at the elbow by contraction of the biceps, which makes this muscle get shorter and thicker; in this position, called *flexion,* the triceps muscle is relaxed. To return the arm to its normal straight position, called *extension,* the biceps relaxes and the triceps contracts. In this bit of muscle teamwork, the biceps, which bends the arm at the elbow joint, is called the *flexor,* while the triceps straightens the arm and is called the *extensor.* Similar flexor–extensor action can be observed at many body joints, including the fingers.

Smooth Muscle

Beginning about midway down the esophagus, layers of smooth muscle line the walls of the 25 feet of digestive tract, extending into the stomach and through the intestines. These muscles keep the stomach and intestinal walls continually in motion, constricting and relaxing to push food along. Smooth muscle also effects the opening and closing of important valves, called *sphincters,* along the digestive tract.

Muscular Contraction

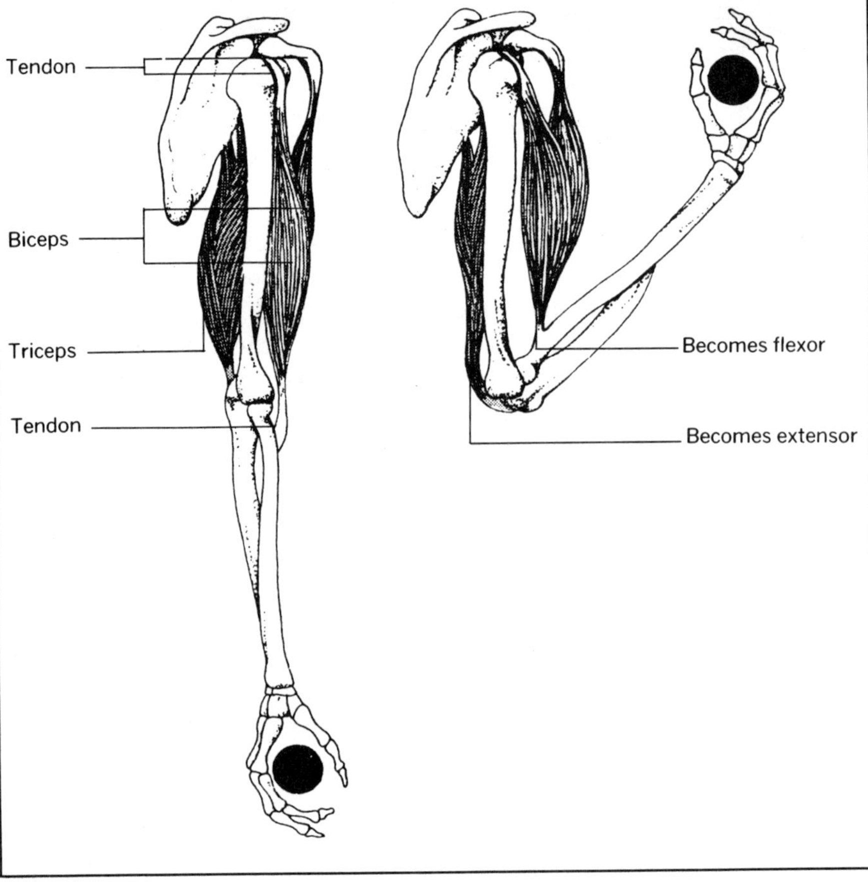

How Muscles Reduce Stress on Bones

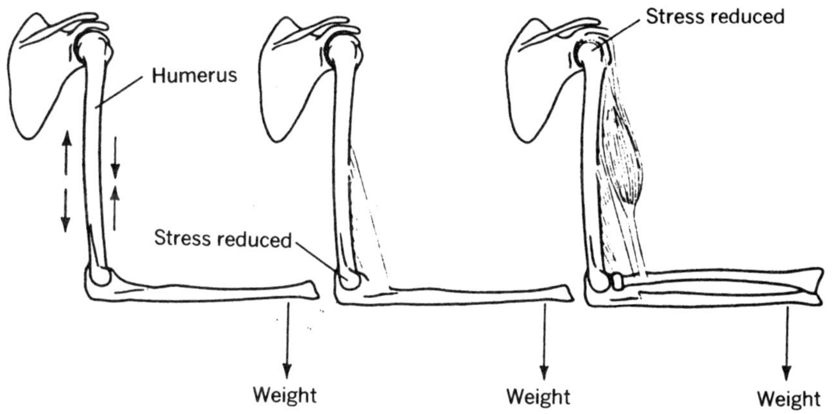

Bones are prevented from bending under normal stress by a system of braces, in which ligaments play an important role. But the main braces are the muscles. The diagrams above show the arm attached to the shoulder blade with the hand supporting a weight. Without muscles *(left)*, the weight would pull unevenly on the humerus, which would bend, thus compressing one side of the bone and stretching the other side. *(Middle)* Addition of a single-jointed muscle (as the brachialis) reduces the stress on the lower end of the humerus. *(Right)* Addition of a two-jointed muscle (as the biceps) also reduces the stress on the upper part of the humerus. There is now no shearing stress that is liable to break the bone, only a compression.

Trouble Spots

The functions and failures of the skeletal muscles are closely allied to those of the skeletal system. The same areas are vulnerable—joints and back—and the same rule holds: severe or persistent muscle pain is a cause to consult your physician.

Hernia

One type of disorder associated exclusively with a weakness or abnormality of muscle is a rupture or *hernia*. This is the protrusion of part of another organ through a gap in the protective muscle. A likely area for a hernia to appear is in the muscles lining the abdomen, although hernias may occur in any other part of the body where there is pressure against

Muscle Action in Forearm Movement

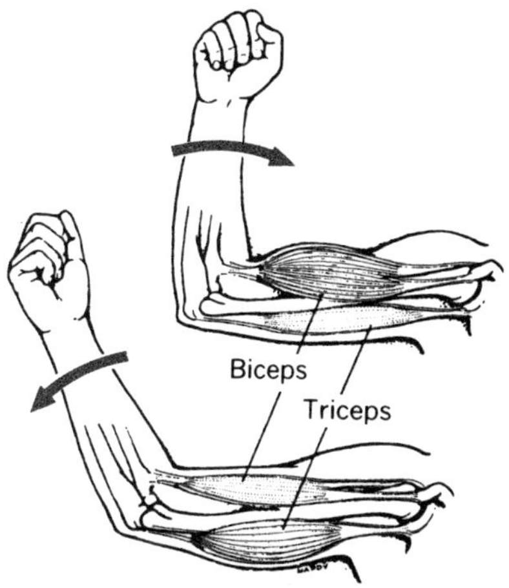

Muscles usually work in pairs to produce movement of a part of the body. Contraction of the biceps bends, or flexes, the arm. The biceps is a flexor muscle. Contraction of the triceps extends the arm. The triceps is an extensor muscle.

a muscle wall that is not as strong as it should be. Weight control and a sensible program of exercise—abdominal muscles being particularly liable to slackness—are good preventive measures against hernia.

All our muscles, in fact, benefit from regular exercise; but you don't have to exhaust yourself physically every day to reach and maintain the desirable plateau physicians describe as good muscle tone.

Atrophy of Muscle Tissue

Muscle tissues are likely to *atrophy* (shrink and weaken) if they are not used for too long a time. Thus, illness or injuries that cause paralysis or an extended period of immobility for the body or a part of it must be followed by a medically supervised program of physical therapy to rebuild the weakened muscles. See also Ch. 8, *Diseases of the Muscles and Nervous System.*

Skin, Hair, and Nails

Perhaps no other organ of the human body receives so much attention both from its owner and the eyes of others as the skin and its associated structures—hair and nails.

Vanity is hardly the issue. The simple facts are that skin is the last frontier of our internal selves, the final boundary between our inside and outside, and our principal first line of defense against the dangers of the outside world. It shows, not always clearly, evidence of some internal disorders; and it shows, often quite clearly, the evidence of external affronts—a bump, a cut, a chafe, an insect bite, or an angry reaction to the attack of germs.

In personal encounters, the unclothed portion of our skin is one of the first things other people observe, and—if we happen to have some unsightly scratch, rash, or blemish—the last thing by which we wish to be remembered. Of all our organs, the skin is the most likely candidate for a program of self-improvement.

The Organ Called Skin

It is always a little surprising to hear, for the first time, the skin referred to as a single organ. This is not to say it is a simple organ; on the contrary, it is an exceedingly complex and varied one. However, despite variations in appearance from part to part of the body, our entire outer wrapper (the

Anatomy of the Skin

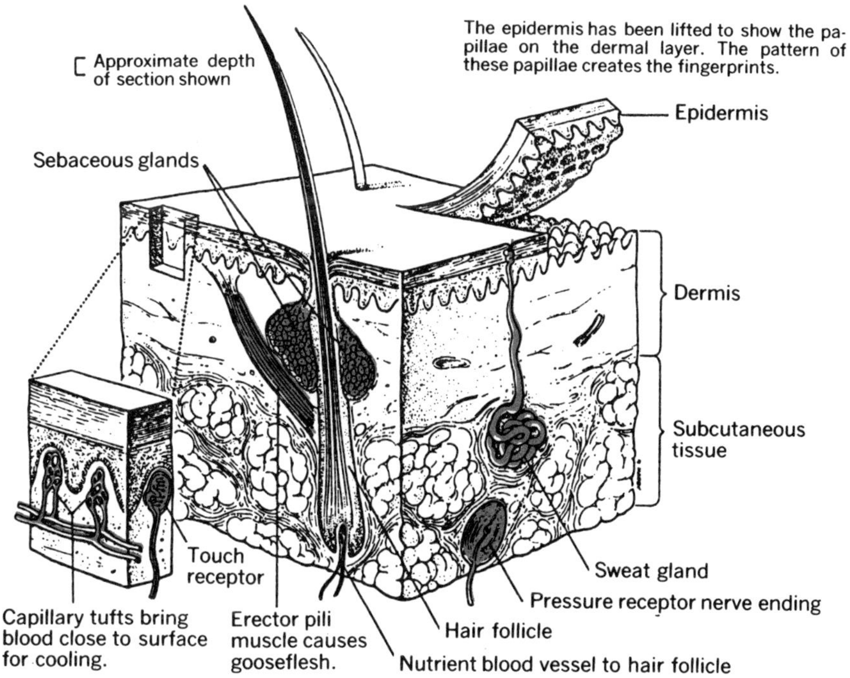

more technical word is *integument*) is similarly constructed.

One might object: "But my nails and hair certainly look different from the skin on my nose!" This is perfectly true, but nails and hair are extensions of the skin, and wherever they occur are composed of similar tissues: the nail on a little toe is made of the same material as the hair.

Functions of the Skin

The skin has three main functions, and its different outward appearance on different parts of the body reflects to some extent which of these functions a certain area of skin primarily serves. The three main functions are protection (from germs or blows), temperature control (e.g., through perspiration, to aid in keeping the body's internal organs near our normal internal temperature of 98.6° F.), and perception. Nerve endings in the skin give us our sensations of touch, pain, heat, and cold. Associated with the skin's important role in temperature regulation is its function as an organ of excretion—the elimination, via perspiration, and subsequent evaporation of water and other substances. Skin is also the site of the body's natural production of vitamin D, stimulated by exposure to sunlight.

Anatomy of the Skin

Skin has three more or less distinct layers. The outermost is called the *epidermis;* the middle, the *dermis;* and the innermost, *subcutaneous* (underskin) tissue. The epidermis may also be called *cuticle;* and the dermis either *corium* or *true skin.*

The Subcutaneous Layer

The subcutaneous layer is really a rather vague border zone between muscle and bone tissues on one side, and the dermis on the other, a kind of springy, fatty padding that gives bounce and a look of firmness to the skin above it. With age, the fatty cells of the subcutaneous layer are not continually replaced as they die, and this layer tends to thin out. The result is wrinkles, which form where the outer layers of skin lose their subcutaneous support, much like the slipcover of a cushion that has lost some of its stuffing.

The Dermis

The dermis is serviced by the multitude of tiny blood vessels and nerve fibers that reach it through the subcutaneous tissue. In addition, many special structures and tissues that enable the skin to perform its various functions are found in the dermis: *sebaceous* (skin oil) glands and sweat glands; minuscule muscles; and the roots of hairs encased in narrow pits called *follicles.*

The topmost layer of the dermis, interconnecting with the epidermis above it, resembles, under a microscope, nothing so much as a rugged, ridge-crossed landscape carved with valleys, caves, and tunnels. The basic forms of this microscopic terrain are cone-shaped hills called *papillae;* between 100 and 200 million of them are found in the dermis of an adult human being.

Because the dermal papillae serve as the bedrock for the surface layer of skin, the epidermis, we can understand why there is really no such thing as smooth skin; even the smoothest patch of a baby's skin appears ridged and cratered under a magnifying glass.

The distribution of papillae in the skin falls into certain distinctive patterns that are particularly conspicuous on the soles of babies' feet and on the fingertips, and give each of us our unique finger, toe, and footprints. The mathematical possibility of one person having the same fingerprints as another is thought to be about one in 25 billion. The papillae ridges on the fingertips also make it easier for us to pick up and handle such things as needles or pencils or buttons.

Finally, because there are relatively more papillae concentrated at the fingertips than on most other areas of the body, and because papillae are often associated with dense concentrations of nerve endings, the fingertips tend to be more responsive to touch sensations than other parts of the body.

The Epidermis

The bottom layer of the epidermis, its papillae fitted into the pockets of the layers of the dermis beneath it, is occupied by new young cells. These cells gradually mature and move upward. As they near the surface of the skin, they die, becoming tough, horny, lifeless tissue. This is the outmost layer of the epidermis, called the *stratum corneum* (horny layer), which we are continually shedding, usually unnoticed, as when we towel off after a bath, but sometimes very noticeably, as when we peel after a sunburn.

A suntan, incidentally, is caused by the presence of tiny grains of pigment, called *melanin,* in the bottom layers of epidermis. Sunlight stimulates the production of melanin, giving the skin a darker color. A suntan fades as the melanin granules move to the surface and are shed with dead skin cells.

Fingerprint

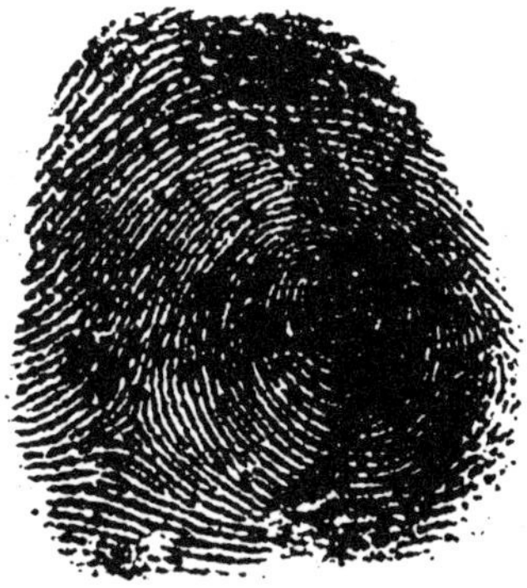

The pattern of ridges in a fingerprint reflects the contours of the papillae (conelike bumps) of the upper layer of the dermis, just below the epidermis.

Hair and Nails

Certainly the most noticeable of the specialized forms of skin are our hair and nails. What we see of them is really a dead tissue, called *keratin,* similar to the dead skin cells that are continually being shed by our bodies, but much more firmly packed together. However, hair and nails both originate in cells that are very much alive—as anyone who has plucked a group of hairs or suffered the pain of a torn-out nail knows very well. Growth occurs in this living region, with new cells pushing the dead, hard hair and nail stalks upward, then dying themselves and being replaced from below.

The bottom end or root of a hair is lodged, as noted above, in a *follicle,* a hollow resembling a rounded bottle with a long, narrow neck slanting toward the skin's surface. Each follicle is supported by the little hummock of a papilla, and is serviced by tiny oil glands that lubricate the shaft (or neck) through which the hair pushes toward the surface.

The follicles of the long hairs of the scalp, groin, and armpits may be found deep in the subcutaneous layers of the skin; others are no deeper than the top layers of dermis. Attached to a follicle are microscopic muscle fibers that, if stimulated by cold or emotional factors, can contract around the follicle; the result is gooseflesh or sometimes even the sensation that our hair is standing on end.

A nail's living, growing part is found beneath the whitish half moon, or *lunula,* at its base. The lunula is sometimes obscured because a layer of epidermis (cuticle) has grown over it. Except at its very top (the part we can trim without pain), the nail is firmly attached to the ridged upper layer of the dermis, a region richly laced with tiny blood vessels.

Oil Glands

The skin's oil-producing (or *sebaceous*) glands are almost always associated with hair follicles, into which they seep their oils (or *sebum*). The oily substance works its way up toward the surface, lubricating both the hair and outer layers of epidermis, which need continual lubrication in order to stay soft and flexible. Also, skin oils serve as a kind of protective coat against painful drying and chapping.

Sweat Glands and Blood Vessels

While everybody is aware that the amount we perspire is related to the temperature around us, not everybody is aware that the countless tiny blood vessels in our skin—some 15 feet of them coursing beneath every square inch of skin—also react to changes in outside temperatures. Working together, and both controlled by an automatic "thermostat" in our brain, sweat glands and blood vessels have the all-important role of keeping our internal organs near their normal 98.6° Fahrenheit temperature.

The trick in maintaining an internal body temperature near normal is to conserve body heat when it is colder outside and to lose heat when it is warmer. Blood circulating near the surface of the skin is warmed (gains heat) or cooled (loses heat) according to the outside temperature.

The skin's myriad blood vessels constrict when the outside temperature is colder. This means that less blood can come into contact with the colder outside air, and therefore the overall temperature level of the blood remains warmer than if the blood vessels had not become constricted. On the other hand, when the body needs to lose heat—for example, during and after a vigorous tennis match—the skin's blood vessels dilate. This accounts for the "heat flush" or reddening of skin that light-skinned people exhibit when very heated.

Sweat glands aid in temperature regulation by secreting moisture, which, evaporating on the skin's surface, cools the skin and therefore the blood flowing beneath it. Moisture that does not evaporate but remains as liquid on the skin or runs off in rivulets is not efficient in cooling. Humid air tends to prevent evaporation, while moving air or wind aids it. Sweat that evaporates as soon as it reaches the skin's surface usually goes unnoticed. Fresh sweat has no odor; but if it remains without evaporating, bacteria begin to give it the odor known medically as *bromhidrosis.*

There are some two million sweat glands in the skin. Each consists of a coiled, corkscrewlike tube that tunnels its way up to the surface of the skin from the dermis or from the deeper subcutaneous layer.

Potential Trouble Spots

All of us are very conscious of the condition of our skin and worry when something seems to be wrong with it. The temptations to worry too much, to overtreat, to take the advice of a well-meaning friend, to use the wrong (but heavily advertised) product are very great. Knowing about the properties of the skin and what medical knowledge has to say about skin problems can help to avoid mistakes in caring for it. See Ch. 21, *Skin and Hair.* For a discussion of adolescent skin problems, see also Ch. 3, *The Teens.*

The Nervous System and the Brain

Most of us have heard often enough that the brain, acting as control center for a communication network we call our nervous system, is an incredible computer, weighing a mere three pounds. Its form and functions, however, are often described as being so much more intricate and complex than any existing or imagined computer that thorough knowledge of the brain seems very remote. This is certainly true. But it doesn't prevent us from knowing some general things about the brain and nervous system, or what its most significant parts are and how they work.

Basically, the nervous system has just two functions: first, getting information (impulses, signals, messages) from outside or inside the body to where it can be acted upon, usually in the brain; and secondly, feeding back information (for example, to the muscles) so that the indicated action can be taken. Thus, nerves can be divided by their function into two general types, each following a separate pathway. Those that receive information—for example, from our senses—and pass it along are called *sensory,* or *afferent* (inward-traveling). Those that relay information back, with a directive for action, are called *motor,* or *efferent* (outward-traveling).

The brain and the spinal cord can be considered as the basic unit of the *central nervous system.* All sensory and motor information comes or goes from this central core. The spinal cord is the master nerve tract (or nerve trunk) in our body and consists of millions of nerve fibers bundled together, somewhat like many small threads making up a large rope.

Like the spinal cord, all the lesser nerves, shown as single cords in a typical anatomical drawing, are made up of hundreds of thousands of individual fibers. Each fiber is part of a single nerve cell, or *neuron.* Neurons—there are 12 to 15 billion of them in our brain alone—are the basic structural units of the brain and nervous system, the tubes and transistors and circuits of which our personal computer is built.

The Brain

The appearance of the brain within the skull has been described as a huge gray walnut and a cauliflower. The inelegance of such descriptions is the least of many good reasons why we should be happy our brains are not exposed to public view.

Brain tissue—pinkish gray and

The Brain

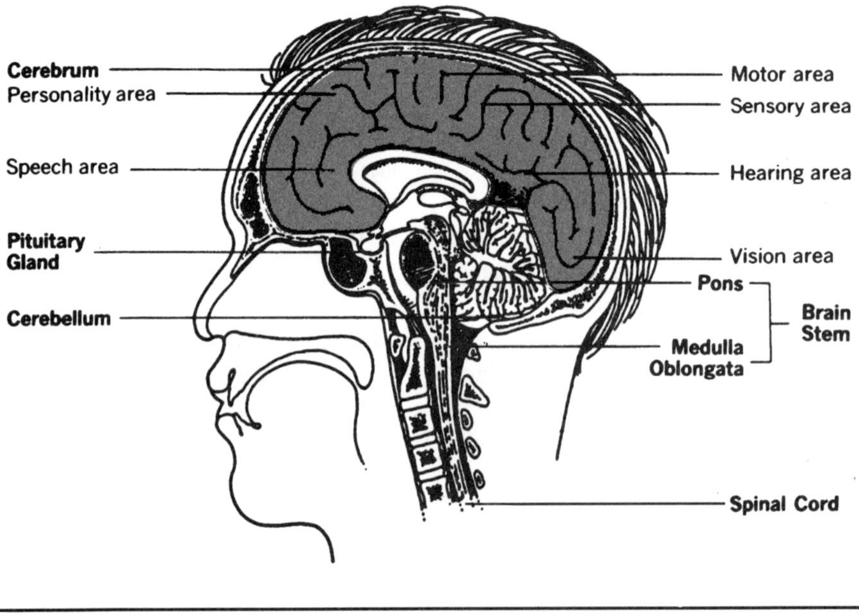

white—is among the most delicate in our body, and the destruction of even a small part may mean lasting impairment or death. Its protection is vital and begins (if we are so fortunate) with a mat of hair on the top, back, and sides of our skull. Next comes the resilient layer of padding we call the scalp, and then the main line of defense—the rounded, bony helmet of skull.

The brain's armor does not stop with bone. Beneath are three strong, fibrous membranes called *meninges* that encase the brain in protective envelopes. Meninges also overlie the tissue of the spinal cord; infection or inflammation of these membranes by bacteria or viruses is called *cerebrospinal meningitis.*

Between two of the meninges is a region laced with veins and arteries and filled with *cerebrospinal fluid.* This fluid-filled space cushions the brain against sudden blows and collisions. The cerebrospinal fluid circulates not only about the brain but through the entire central nervous system. Incidentally, chemical analysis of this fluid, withdrawn by inserting a hypodermic needle between vertebrae of the spinal column (a spinal tap), can provide clues to the nature of brain and nervous system disorders.

The Cerebrum

What we usually mean by "brain" is that part of the brain called the *cerebrum.* It is the cerebrum that permits us all our distinctly human activities—thinking, speaking, reading, writing. Only in man does the cerebrum reach such size, occupying the interior of our entire dome above the level of the eyes.

The surface of the cerebrum is

The Brain and the Cranial Nerves

Cranial nerves

1. Olfactory: smell
2. Optic: vision
3. Oculomotor: muscle of eyes
4. Trochlear: muscle of eyes
5. Trigeminal: sense of touch in face
6. Abducens: muscle of eyes
7. Facial: muscles of face
8. Acoustic: hearing and balance
9. Glossopharyngeal: taste
10. Vagus: heart, lungs, abdomen
11. Hypoglossal: tongue muscles
12. Accessory: neck muscles, eyeball

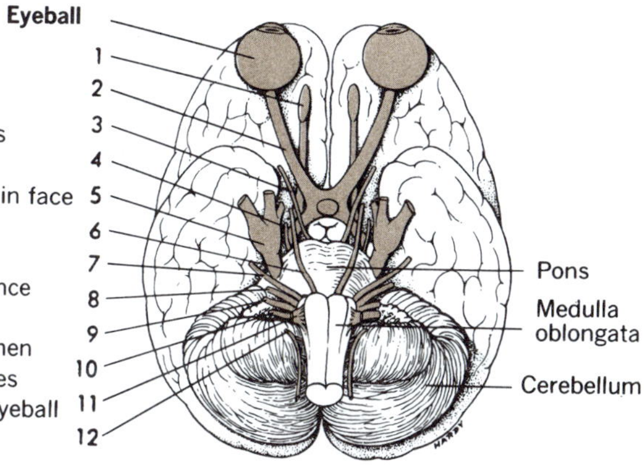

View of the underside of the brain

wrinkled, furrowed, folded and infolded, convoluted, fissured—anything but smooth. This lavishly wrinkled outer layer of the cerebrum, about an eighth of an inch thick, is called the *cerebral cortex.* From its grayish color comes the term "gray matter" for brain tissue. There is a pattern among its wrinkles, marked out by wider, or deeper fissures, or furrows, running through the brain tissue. The most conspicuous fissure runs down the middle, front to back, dividing the cerebrum into two halves, the left hemisphere and the right hemisphere. The nerves from the left half of the body are served by the right hemisphere, and the right half of the body by the left hemisphere, so that damage to one side of the brain affects the other side of the body.

The Lobes of the Cerebrum

Smaller fissures crisscross the cerebrum and mark out various specific areas of function called *lobes.* The frontal lobes, one on the left hemisphere and one on the right in back of our eyes and extending upward behind the forehead, are perhaps the most talked about and the least understood by medical researchers. The specific functions of most other lobes in the cerebrum, such as the two occipital lobes (centers for seeing), and the temporal lobes (centers for hearing) are much better known.

The Brain Stem

The cerebrum, like a large flower obscuring part of its stalk, droops down around the *brain stem.* Thus, while the brain stem originates just about in the middle of our skull, it does not emerge completely from the folds of the cerebral hemispheres until it reaches the back of the neck. Then it soon merges into the spinal cord.

Associated with this portion of the brain—roughly speaking, between the cerebrum and the spinal cord—are centers that take care of the countless necessary details involved in just plain existing, and structures (such as the *medulla oblongata* and the *pons*) that serve also as traffic control points for the billions of nerve impulses traveling to and from the cerebrum. The largest of these "lesser brains" is the *cerebellum,* whose two hemispheres straddle the brain stem at the back of the head.

The Cerebellum

The cerebellum is the site of balance and body and muscle coordination, allowing us, for example, to "rub the tummy and pat the head" simultaneously, or tap the foot and strum a guitar, or steer a car and operate the foot pedals. Such muscle-coordinated movements, though sometimes learned only by long repetition and practice, can become almost automatic—such as reaching for and flicking on the light switch as we move into a darkened room.

But many other activities and kinds of behavior regulated by the part of the brain below the cerebrum are more fully automatic: the control of eye movement and focusing, for example, as well as the timing of heartbeat, sleep, appetite, and metabolism; the arousal and decline of sexual drives; body temperature; the dilation and constriction of blood vessels; swallowing; and breathing. All these are mainly functions of the *autonomic nervous system,* as opposed to the more voluntary actions controlled by the *central nervous system.*

The Body's Nervous Systems

Simply speaking, the human body has only one nervous system, and that is all the nerve cells, nerve cords, nerve centers (both voluntary and involuntary) in the body. It is helpful, however, though quite arbitrary, to divide our nerves into the central and autonomic nervous systems. This division tends to obscure the countless interconnections and interplay between the two systems. For example, where do you place the control of breathing or blinking? Such actions are automatic except when we choose to regulate them.

The Central Nervous System

The central nervous system, as noted above, includes the brain and the spinal cord. It also includes all the nerves of conscious response and voluntary action that link up with the brain and spinal cord.

Twelve pairs of *cranial nerves* originate within the brain and emerge at its base. These include the very important nerves that connect with our sense organs, nerve bundles that control the facial and neck muscles, and the *vagus* (or tenth cranial nerve) that serves the heart, lungs, stomach, intestines, esophagus, larynx, liver, kidneys, spleen, and pancreas. The vagus nerve, although anatomically part of the central nervous system, controls bodily functions that are mainly automatic.

Spinal nerves branch out from the spinal cord as it snakes its way through the vertebrae of the spinal column. All the major nerve cords that wrap around the trunk and reach the arms and hands, legs and feet, originate from spinal nerves.

The cranial nerves and the spinal nerves, together with all those nerves lying outside the confines of the brain and spinal cord, are sometimes referred to as the *peripheral nervous system.* This term can be confusing, however, because it is also used to include all the nerves of the autonomic nervous system, next discussed.

The Autonomic Nervous System

The muscles served by the central nervous system are all of one general type (striated), while the muscles served by the autonomic system are called involuntary or smooth. The autonomic nerves regulate body activity without our conscious control—for example, as we sleep. They are rather elegantly divided into two categories: *sympathetic* and *parasympathetic* nervous systems. These are distinguishable primarily by their op-

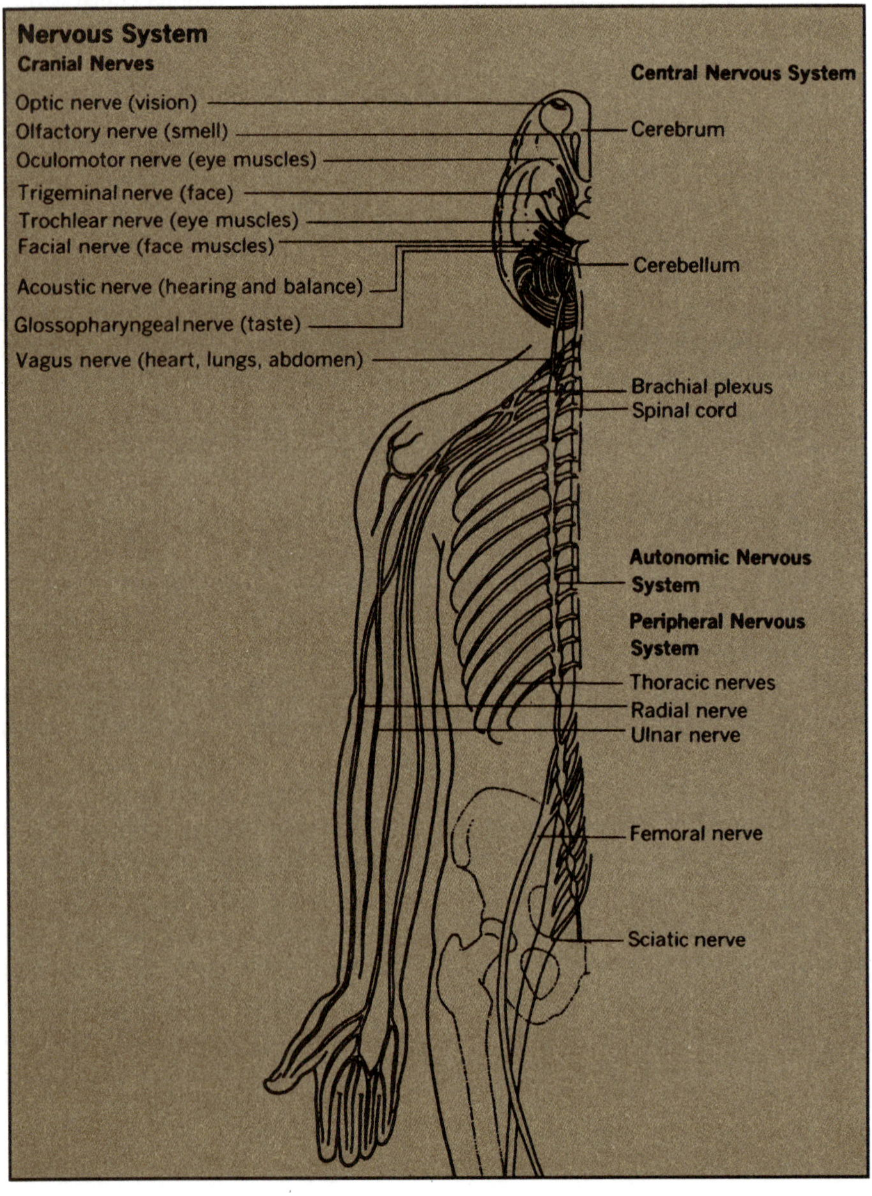

posite effects on the body organs. For example, impulses along parasympathetic nerve trunks dilate blood vessels, slow the heartbeat rate, and increase stomach secretions, while the sympathetic system constricts blood vessels, increases rate of heartbeat, and inhibits stomach secretions.

The Neuron—What Nerves Are Made Of

A nerve cell is a grayish blob of tissue from which protrude several short gray fibers, *dendrites,* and one longer whitish fiber, an *axon.* Both the dendrites and the axon resemble ropes with their ends splayed and frayed. Dendrites register impulses coming into the central blob of the neuron (perhaps from a neighboring neuron's axon); an axon picks up the incoming impulses and carries them away.

Both units are equally important for normal nerve functioning, but the axon is far more showy as an anatomical structure. All nerve cords are made up of the single strands of many axons, which may reach lengths of several feet. In other words, if we could stretch out certain neurons in our body—for example, those making

THE NEURON

Sensory, or afferent ("carrying in"), neurons respond to external stimuli and conduct impulses to the central nervous system—the brain and spinal column—where the message is interpreted.

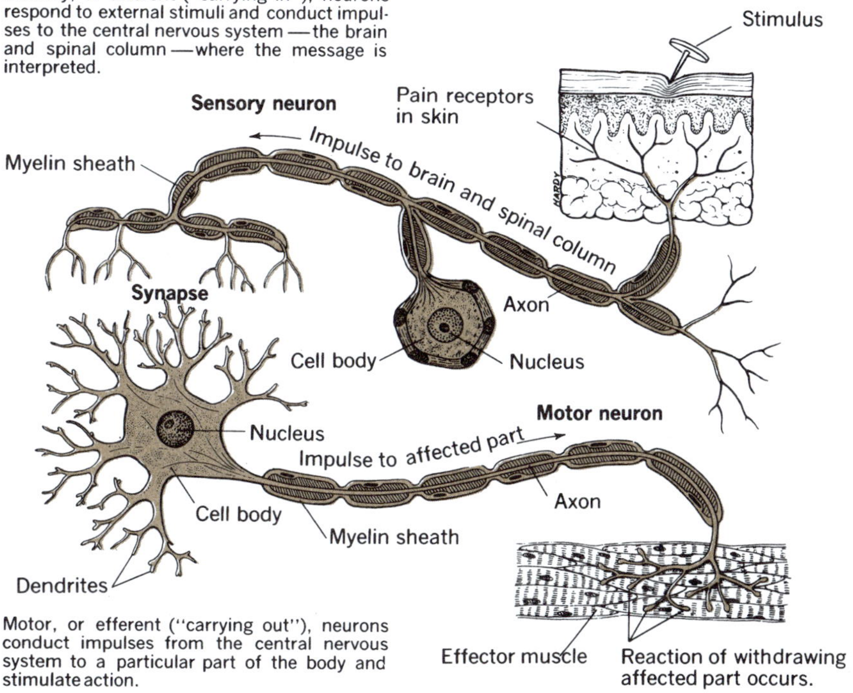

Motor, or efferent ("carrying out"), neurons conduct impulses from the central nervous system to a particular part of the body and stimulate action.

up the sciatic nerve that runs from the small of the back to the toes—their axon "tails" would make them three or four feet long.

Myelin

A normal axon usually has a fatty coating of insulation called *myelin.* An axon severed into two pieces cannot grow together again; but if the myelin sheath is pretty much intact, a surgeon can sometimes restore nerve function by sewing the two ends together, or replace the nerve with one from another part of the body. The part of the severed axon connecting to the central portion usually remains alive in any case—which is why a person can often retain the sensation of feeling in an amputated part.

Certain serious and progressively disabling diseases involve the gradual loss (*demyelination*) of this coating, causing paralysis, numbness, or other loss of function in an organ; a demyelinated nerve fiber is not able to carry impulses to and from the brain. Two such diseases are multiple sclerosis and "Lou Gehrig's disease" (amyotrophic lateral sclerosis).

Effects of Aging

Once we reach maturity, the number of our nerve cells begins to decrease, because our bodies do not regularly manufacture new neurons to replace the ones that die in the normal process of living. (Other kinds of tissue are continually replenished with new cells.) This has some relation to senility, but the loss of a few million out of many billions of brain and nerve cells has little effect on mental powers unless the losses are concentrated in one area.

Synapse, Ganglion, and Plexus

When a nerve impulse, traveling away from the neuron's central part, reaches the ends of an axon, it meets a gap that it must jump to get to the tentaclelike dendrites of the next neuron. This gap is called a *synapse.*

At certain points in the body a great many nerve cell bodies and branches are packed closely together, with a resulting profusion of interwoven axons, dendrites, and synapses. Such a concentration of nervous tissue is called a *ganglion,* or *plexus.* A blow or jolt to such an area can be extremely painful and even stupefying—affecting as it does a whole network of nerves—as anyone who has been hit in the solar plexus or learned the pressure points of karate knows.

The Movement of Impulses along Nerve Fibers

There is really no exact counterpart in the mechanical world for how an impulse moves along a nerve fiber and then jumps across a synapse to the next nerve. Nor is this movement completely understood by scientists. Suffice it to say that it is somewhat like an electrical current moving along in a chemical environment that allows the impulse to travel, in discreet little jumps, at a speed of about 200 miles per hour—quite slowly when we compare it to the speed of light or electricity: 186,000 miles per second. This speed serves us quite well in most situations, but there are times when we wish human beings' nerves could act more quickly—on the highway, for example, or when a cherished vase starts to topple off the mantelpiece.

One of the simplest and quickest kinds of reactions to an outside stimulus is one that bypasses the brain. We don't really think to pull our hand away from a piping hot radiator. This is called a *spinal reflex*. What happens is that the sensory nerve endings in the finger pick up the "too hot" impulse from the radiator; the impulse then travels to the spinal cord where it activates the motor nerve pathway back to the burned finger, carrying the message, "Jerk your finger away!"

When to Suspect Trouble

Our entire existence as human beings depends so much on the normal functioning of our brain and nervous system that any real brain or nervous disorder or disease is a very serious matter. A sprained joint or cut foot can spell doom for an animal that depends on speed and mobility for survival; but the same injury is often not much more than a painful inconvenience to us. Impairment of our brain or nervous system is far more of a threat to our survival.

Multiple sclerosis and meningitis have been mentioned as serious disorders affecting the nerves, others are Parkinsonism, shingles, encephalitis, and brain tumors. The possible presence of one of these disorders is reason enough not to shrug off any of the following signs and symptoms: recurrent headaches, intense pain of unknown cause, tremors, numbness, loss of coordination, dizziness, blackouts, tics, cramps, visual difficulties, and loss of bowel and bladder control. Also, any person who has remained unconscious for more than a few minutes should be taken to a physician as soon as possible. This applies even when the person has regained consciousness and says he feels fine.

Our complex emotions, of course, are linked to the functioning of our brain and nervous system. A mind free of undue anxiety, guilt, and frustration functions better than a mind racked with worries and conflicts, and is a much more efficient and reliable leader of the body. See also Ch. 8, *Diseases of the Muscles and Nervous System*. For a discussion of mental and emotional health, see Ch. 36.

The Circulatory System, the Heart, and Blood

When a person's heart stops beating (stops pumping blood) for longer than a couple of minutes, the individual stops living. But the heart, fortunately, is extremely sturdy. It is also simple in construction, capable of operating at a great many different speeds, in many cases self-repairing if damaged, and probably the one continuously operating automatic pump that we could, with any confidence, expect to last 70 years or longer.

These simple facts tend to be forgotten today, in what is probably the most heart-conscious era in history. True, heart disease, along with cancer, is statistically one of today's major killers. But we should remember two circumstances: not until about 50 years ago did deaths from heart disease begin to be accurately recognized and reported; second, with longer and longer life spans, it becomes more likely that a nonstop vital organ like the heart will simply wear out. Heart transplants, open heart surgery, and artificial heart parts—often reported sensationally in the public media—have also conditioned us to think of our hearts as terribly vulnerable, rather delicate, a bit inadequate to their tasks, and quite open to improvement.

Advances in heart surgery do, indeed, hold greater promise for persons whose hearts had been considered, until now, irreversibly damaged or diseased. But the great attention accorded such miracles of medicine tends to obscure the humdrum, day-in-day-out, low-key drama performed for a lifetime by a healthy, uncomplaining heart.

The Heart and Circulatory Network

Perhaps the best way to learn about the heart is to study it in relation to the body's circulatory system. This hollow, fist-sized lump of sinewy tissue is located behind the breastbone, centered just about at the vertical midline of our chest. It is connected into a closed system of flexible tubes, called blood vessels, ranging down from finger-thick to microscopically slender, that reach into every cavern, crevice, and outpost of our body—a network of some 70,000 miles.

The heart has essentially one function—to push blood, by pumping action, through this enormous network of blood vessels. We have about six quarts of blood in our body, pumped at the rate of about five ounces every time the heart beats (normally about 72 times a minute for an adult), which we feel as our pulse. The blood circulates and recirculates through the blood vessels, pushed along by the pumping of the heart.

Arteries and Veins

The blood vessels are generally described as *arterial,* referring to the *arteries* that carry blood away from the heart; or *venous,* referring to the

The Circulatory System

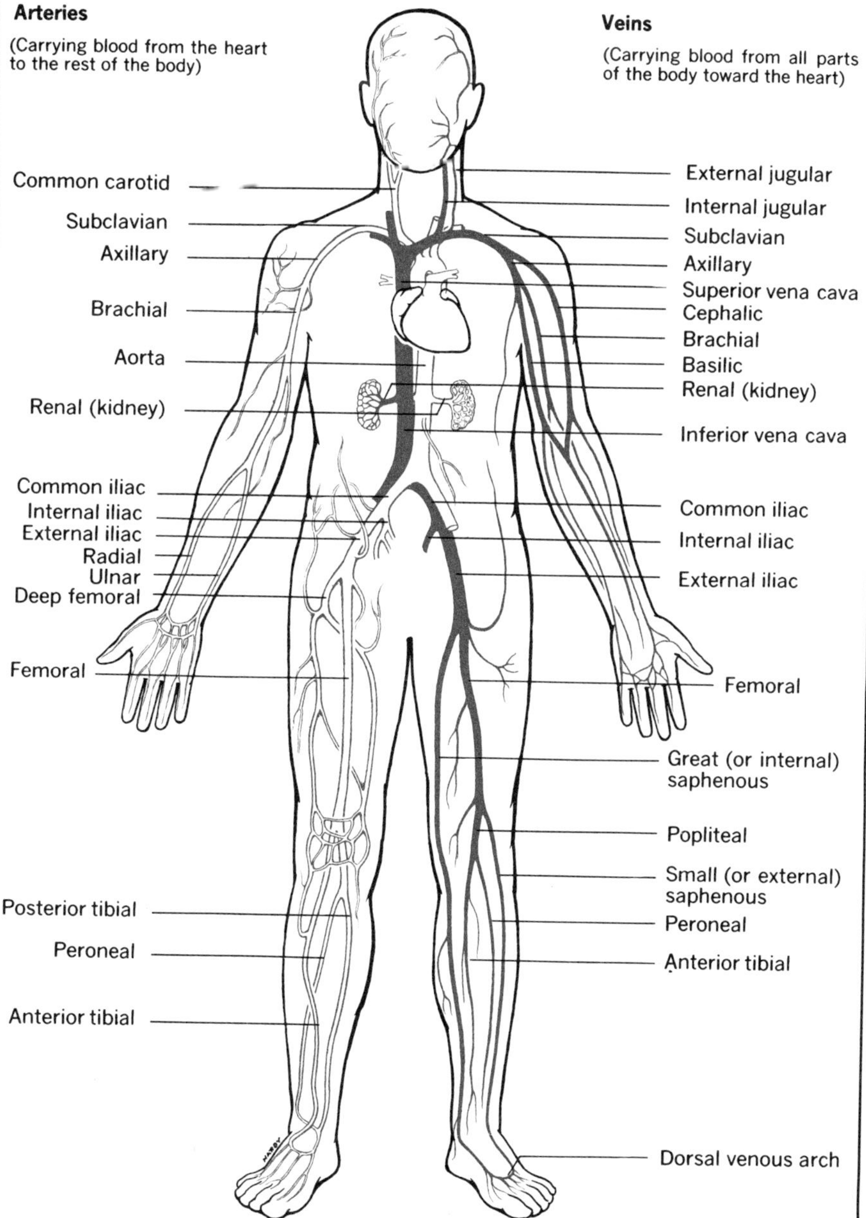

veins through which blood seeps and flows back toward the heart to be re-pumped. A large artery such as the *aorta* branches into smaller arteries, and these eventually into still smaller vessels called *arterioles,* and the arterioles, finally, into the smallest blood vessels, the *capillaries.* These in turn open onto other capillaries, which are the starting point for the return of blood to the heart.

The microscopic capillaries typically form a kind of cat's cradle connection, sometimes called a capillary bed, at the transition zone where arterial blood becomes venous blood. The returning blood moves from the capillaries to small veins called *venules* (the counterparts of arterioles) and through successively larger veins back to the heart.

Diagram of Artery–Capillary–Vein Sequence

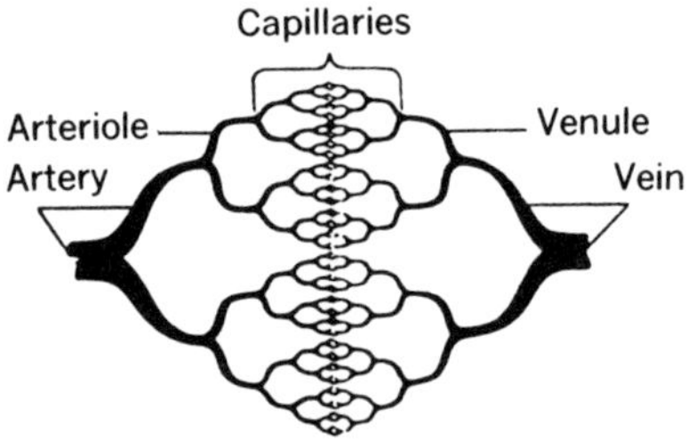

Blood and Our Internal Fluid Environment

What makes this fairly rudimentary collection of plumbing so absolutely indispensable to life is the fluid it pumps—blood. If any part of the body—cell, tissue, or major organ—is denied circulating blood and the substances it carries with it for longer than a few minutes, that part will fail. It is the job of the heart and the blood vessels to get blood to all the body's far-flung tissues, where it both picks up and deposits substances.

Blood is really a kind of fluid tissue. About 80 percent of its volume is water, and blood's indispensable, life-sustaining power is owed in great part to its watery base, which permits it both to flow and to take up and carry materials in solution. All our tissues and organs have a kind of give-and-take arrangement with the circulating blood.

Carrier of Oxygen

Perhaps the most critical of these give-and-take transactions occurs in the lungs; it is this transaction that if interrupted by heartbeat stoppage for more than a few minutes causes death by oxygen starvation of vital tissues. Before a unit of blood is pumped out by the heart to the body, it picks up in the lungs the oxygen that we have inhaled and which every cell in the body needs to function. The blood then transports the oxygen, delivering it to other parts of the body. By the time a given unit of blood has made a tour of the blood vessels and returned to the lungs, it has given up most of its oxygen and is laden instead with carbon dioxide, the principal waste product of living processes. The venous blood releases its carbon dioxide, to be exhaled by the lungs.

Distributor of Nutrients

Food, or more accurately the nutrient molecules needed by cells, are also transported throughout the body by the blood. In the digestive tract, food is broken down into tiny submicroscopic pieces that can pass through the tract's walls (mainly along the small intestine) and be picked up by the blood for distribution around the body.

One of the specialized, small-volume transportation jobs handled by the blood is to pick up hormones from the endocrine glands and present these chemical messengers to the organs they affect.

Composition of Blood

Blood is a distinctive and recognizable type of tissue, but this does not mean it is a stable, uniform substance with a fixed proportion of ingredients. Quite the opposite is true; its composition is ever changing in response to the demands of other body systems. Other organs are constantly pouring substances into the blood, or removing things from it. Blood in one part of the body at a given moment may be vastly different in chemical makeup from blood in another part of the body.

Despite its changing makeup, blood does have certain basic components. A sample of blood left to stand for an hour or so separates into a clear, watery fluid with a yellowish tinge and a darker, more solid clump. The clear yellow liquid is called *plasma,* and accounts for about 55 percent of the volume of normal blood. The darker clump is made up mainly of the blood's most conspicuous and populous inhabitants, the red cells that give blood its color.

Plasma

It is the plasma that enables our blood to carry out most of the transportation tasks assigned it. Being over 90 percent water, the plasma has water's property of being able to carry substances both in solution and in suspension. (A substance in solution is one, like salt, that must be removed from water by chemical or physical action, such as boiling; while a substance in suspension—such as red blood cells within whole blood in a standing test tube—separates out more readily, particularly when its watery carrier has been contained and its flow stilled.)

Red Blood Cells

Red blood cells (or *erythrocytes*) numbering in the trillions are carried in suspension by the plasma. In turn, the red blood cells carry the single most important substance needed by the body's cells—oxygen. For such an important task, the red blood cell looks hardly adequate. As it matures, this cell loses its nucleus. Lacking a nucleus, it is sometimes not even called a cell but a red blood *corpuscle.* What gives red blood cells their special oxygen-carrying ability, and also their color, is their possession of a complex iron-protein substance called *hemoglobin.*

Hemoglobin

Molecules of hemoglobin have the property of loosely combining with oxygen where it is plentiful, as in the lungs. They can then hold on to oxygen until they reach an area where oxygen has been depleted by the demands of living processes. There—usually in the fine tubes of the capillaries—hemoglobin's hold on oxygen is challenged by the demands of other cells, and the red cells give up their oxygen. The hemoglobin of red cells develops an immediate affinity for carbon dioxide, the waste product of cell metabolism, and the red blood cells then carry this carbon dioxide back to the lungs for exhalation.

Hemoglobin's ability to carry oxygen is not unique. Water, and therefore plasma, also have this ability. Hemoglobin's specialness lies in how much oxygen it can carry. Hemoglobin increases by more than 50 times the oxygen-carrying capacity of our blood.

White Blood Cells

White blood cells have many different shapes and sizes, all going under the general scientific name of *leukocytes.* They are typically larger than red blood cells, but far less numerous. If we accept an estimate of 25 trillion as the number of living red blood cells in our body, then the number of white blood cells might be generously estimated at around 40 billion, a ratio of one white cell to about 600–700 reds.

According to their shape, size, and other characteristics, white blood cells have been divided into various categories such as lymphocytes, monocytes, and granulocytes. But as a group these blood cells are distinguished by their common propensity for attacking foreign bodies that invade our tissues, whether these invaders be sizable splinters or microscopic bacteria. White blood cells move in force to the site of an infection, do battle with the intruding agents, and frequently strew the area with the wreckage of the encounter—a collection of dismantled alien bacteria and dead white cells, which we know as pus.

Platelets

Platelets, also called *thrombocytes,* initiate some of the first steps in the complex biochemical process that leads to the clotting of blood. They thus help to spare us from bleeding to death from a slight injury. Platelets are the most rudimentary and diminutive of the major blood components. Like mature red blood cells, they lack nuclei, but are only one-quarter as big. By no stretch of the imagination can they be called blood cells. Rather, they are blood elements—bits of cell substance with a recognizable size and shape, circulating with the blood.

The Proportions of Blood Cells

All the several types of blood cells and subcells in a healthy body occur in proportions that, though never precisely fixed and unchanging, are recognized as having normal upper and lower limits. If a particular type of cell shows a sudden increase or decrease in population, so that its proportion relative to other blood cells shows a variation markedly outside its normal range, some infection, disease, or disorder must be suspected.

In addition to occurring in certain normal-range proportions, each type of cellular blood component has a typical shape, appearance, and set of chemical and physical properties. Variations from these norms occur in many diseases.

The analysis of blood samples (usually taken from the finger or arm) and their inspection under a microscope have proved invaluable in diagnosing illness and disease, often before a person feels any symptoms whatsoever. This is why a thorough medical checkup should always include taking a sample of your blood. It is then up to the physician to decide which of the dozens of tests should be made on your blood in the medical laboratory. One common test is a *blood count,* in which the number of a certain type of cell in a given unit of your blood can be estimated, and then compared to the normal number in the same amount of blood.

Blood Groups and Rh Factors

The identification of *blood groups* and *Rh factors* is another aspect of blood analysis. The four most common blood groups are called A, B, AB, and O, classifications based on chemical differences that may be incompatible if one group is mixed with another. Thus, it is absolutely essential before a person receives a blood transfusion to know both his own blood type and the type of the blood he is to be given. Blood group O is considered the safety for transfusion, and people with type O blood are sometimes called "universal donors." It is a wise practice to carry, along with your other important cards, a card giving your own blood type. The blood of a donor, however, is always *cross-matched* (checked for compatibility) with the blood of the person who is to receive it in order to avoid transfusion reactions.

Blood Cell Manufacture and Turnover

Most types of blood cells, both red and white, are manufactured in the red marrow of bones. The rate and quantity of total production is staggering; estimates range from one to five million red blood cells per second. This prodigious output is necessary because blood cells are disintegrating, having served their useful lives, in the same enormous numbers every second. The normal life span of a red blood cell is about four months, which means that four months from now every blood cell in your body will have died and been replaced with new cells.

The Liver As a Producer of Red Blood Cells

The red bone marrow is backed up by several other tissues that can, if called upon, turn out blood cells in quantity or serve as specialized producers of certain blood cells and blood elements. One such organ is the liver, which, before and after birth and into childhood, is a site of red blood cell production. In an emergency, such as severe internal hemorrhage, the liver sometimes reverts to its earlier function of manufacturing red cells. The liver also serves as a kind of salvage yard for the iron from dead red cells. It stores the iron for later combination into hemoglobin and passes off the rest of the red blood cell fragments as part of the bile pigments that empty into the duodenum of the small intestine.

The Spleen As a Producer of Blood Cells

Certain white blood cells, in particular the lymphocytes, are produced at a variety of locations in the body—for example, by the lymph nodes, by little clumps of tissue called *Peyer's patches* in the intestinal tract, and by the spleen.

The spleen plays a number of interesting secondary roles in blood cell production. Like the liver, it can be pressed into service as a manufacturer of red blood cells and serve as a salvage yard for iron reclaimed from worn-out red blood cells. A newborn baby is almost totally dependent on its spleen for the production of red blood cells, with a little help from the liver. In an adult, however, a damaged or diseased spleen can be surgically removed, with little or no apparent effect on the health or life span of the person, provided the patient's bone marrow is in good functioning order.

Movement of Blood Cells through the Capillaries

A blood cell must be able to slip through the microscopic, twisting and turning tunnels of the capillaries that mark the turn-about point in the blood cell's round-trip voyage from the heart. Blood cells, therefore, must be small (the point of a pin could hold dozens of red blood cells), and they must be jellylike in order to navigate the tight tortuous, capillary channels without either blocking the channel or breaking apart themselves. A red blood cell is further adapted to sneaking through the capillaries by its concave-disk shape, which allows it to bend and fold around itself. Nevertheless, so narrow are the passageways within some of the capillaries that blood cells must move through them in single file. If a substantial number of the cells are misshapen, as in sickle-cell anemia, they tend to move sluggishly or clog up the passageway—a condition that can have serious consequences. See also Ch. 9, *Diseases of the Circulatory System.*

Lymph and the Lymphatic System

Of all our body systems, perhaps the most ignored is the lymphatic system, although it forms a network throughout our body comparable to the blood vessels of our circulatory system.

Lymph is a whitish fluid that is derived from blood plasma. As plasma circulates through the body, some of it seeps through the walls of capillaries and other blood vessels. This leakage is of the utmost importance, because the leaked fluid, lymph, supplies the liquid environment around and between individual cells and tissues that is essential for their survival.

The presence of lymph requires a drainage system to keep the fluid moving. If there were no drainage system, two things could happen: the dammed-up lymph could create areas swollen with water in which cells would literally drown, or stagnant pools of lymph could become breeding grounds for infection.

As it moves through the vessels of the lymphatic system, lymph carries away from the tissues the bits and pieces of cells that have died and disintegrated, and also potentially harmful bacteria and viruses.

Lymph and Lymphocytes

Confusion often arises about the connection between the white blood cells called *lymphocytes* and the lymph itself. Lymph is not made up of lymphocytes, although it often carries them; lymph is simply a watery vehicle moving through the lymphatic network. At certain points along this network, the vessels enlarge into clumpy structures called *lymph nodes* (or, misleadingly, lymph glands). Lymph nodes are major manufacturing sites for lymphocytes.

Lymph Nodes

Swollen glands are actually swollen lymph nodes, where a small army of lymphocytes is doing battle against invading bacteria or other harmful microscopic organisms. The lymph nodes, more than a hundred of them distributed around the body, serve as defense outposts against germs approaching the interior of the body. Those in the neck, groin, and armpits most frequently exhibit the pain and swelling that may accompany germ-fighting.

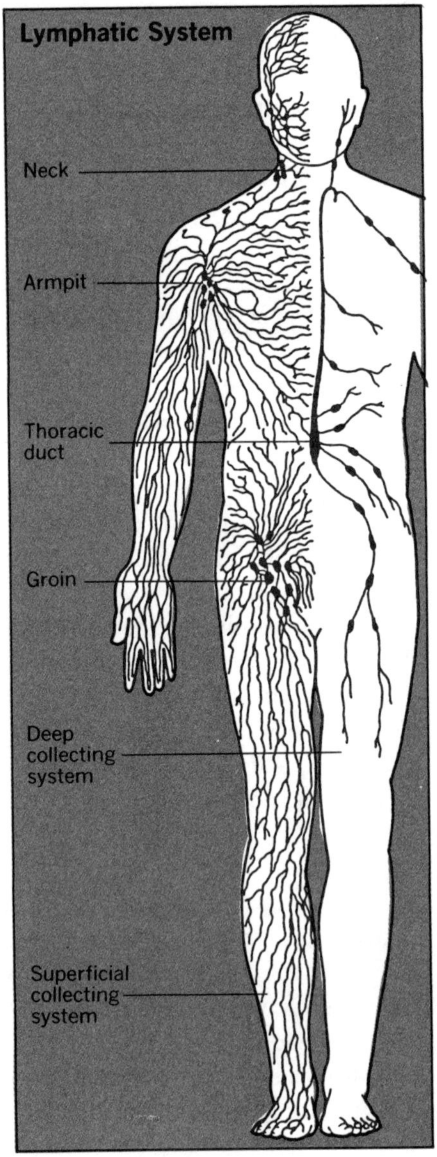

Circulation of Lymph

Lymph circulates without any help from the heart. From the spaces between cells, it diffuses into lymph capillaries which, like the venous capillaries, merge into larger and larger vessels moving inward toward the heart. The lymph moves—even upward from the legs and lower part of the body—because the muscles and movements of the body are constantly kneading and squeezing the lymph vessels. These vessels are equipped with valves that prevent back-flow. This is not so very different from the way venous blood makes its way back to the heart.

Eventually, master lymph vessels from the head, abdomen, and torso join in the thoracic lymph duct, which then empties into large neck veins that carry lymph and venous blood, mixed together, back to the heart.

The Heart at Work

The structure and performance of the heart, at first glance rather complicated, assume a magnificent simplicity once we observe that this pulsating knot of hollow, intertwining muscle uses only one beat to perform two distinct pumping jobs.

The heart has a right side (your right) and a left side (your left), divided by a tough wall of muscle called a *septum.* Each side has two chambers, an upper one called an *atrium* (or *auricle*), and a lower one called a *ventricle.*

How the Heart Pumps the Blood

Venous blood from the body flows into the right atrium via two large veins called the *superior vena cava* (bringing blood from the upper body) and the *inferior vena cava* (bringing blood from the lower part of the body). Where the blood enters the right atrium are valves that close when the atrium chamber is full.

Then, through a kind of trapdoor valve, blood is released from the right atrium into the right ventricle. When the right ventricle is full, and its outlet valve opens, the heart as a whole contracts—that is, pumps.

To the Lungs

The blood from the right ventricle is pumped to the lungs through the pulmonary artery to pick up oxygen. The trapdoor valve between the right atrium and ventricle has meanwhile closed, and venous blood again fills the right atrium.

Having picked up oxygen in the lungs, blood enters the left atrium through the right and left pulmonary veins. (They are called veins despite the fact that they carry the most oxygen-rich blood, because they lead *to* the heart; just as the pulmonary artery carries the oxygen-poorest blood away from the heart, to the lungs.) Like the right atrium, the left atrium serves as a holding reservoir and, when full, releases its contents into the left ventricle. A valve between left atrium and ventricle closes, and the heart pumps.

How Blood Circulates through the Heart

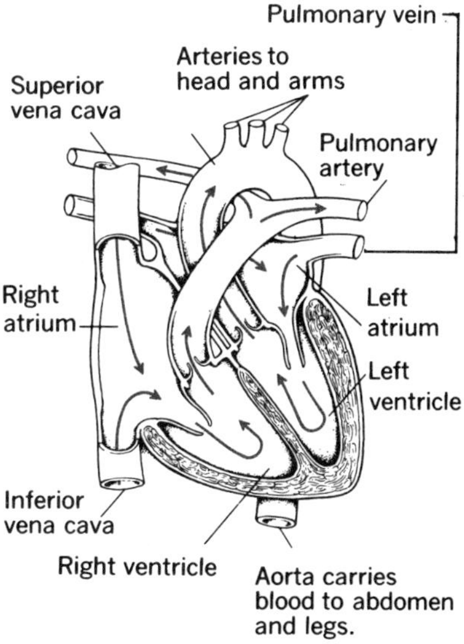

Blood from the head and arms enters the right atrium from the superior (i.e., upper) vena cava. Blood from the torso and legs enters from the inferior (i.e., lower) vena cava. The blood, controlled by a valve, passes to the right ventricle. It is then pumped into the pulmonary artery, which divides into two vessels, one leading to each lung. After being enriched with oxygen, the blood is brought back to the left atrium via the pulmonary veins, is admitted by a valve into the left ventricle, and is pumped through the aorta to be distributed to all parts of the body.

Both atria contract at the same time, forcing blood into the ventricles. Then both ventricles contract (while the atria relax), forcing blood into the great arteries. This period of contraction is called systole, and is followed by a period of relaxation called diastole.

To the Body

Blood surges through an opening valve of the left ventricle into the aorta, the major artery that marks the beginning of blood's circulation throughout the body. The left ventricle, because it has the job of pumping blood to the entire body rather than just to the lungs, is slightly larger and more muscular than the right ventricle. It is for this reason, incidentally, that the heart is commonly considered to be on our left. The organ as a whole, as noted earlier, is located at the center of the chest.

The Heart's Own Circulatory System

Heart tissue, like that of every other organ in the body, must be continually supplied with fresh, oxygen-rich blood, and used blood must be returned to the lungs for reoxygenation. The blood inside the heart cannot serve these needs. Thus the heart has its own circulation network, called *coronary arteries* and *veins,* to nourish its muscular tissues. There are two

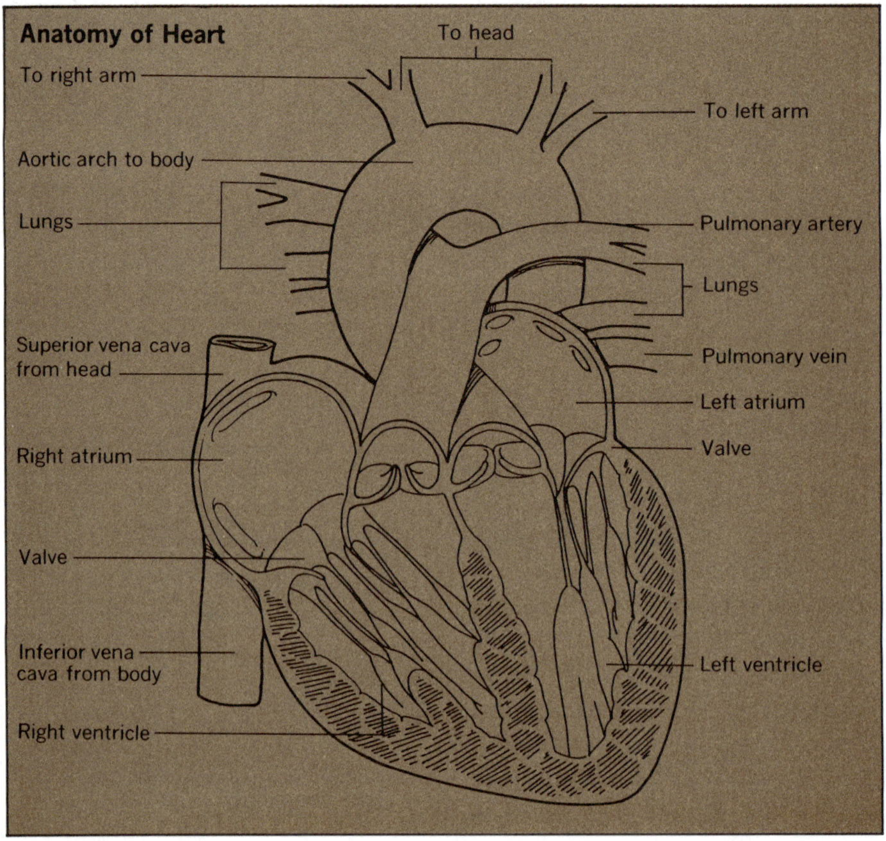

major arteries on the surface of the heart, branching and rebranching eventually into capillaries. Coronary veins then take blood back to the right atrium.

Structure of the Heart

The musculature of the heart is called cardiac muscle because it is different in appearance from the two other major types of muscle. The heart muscle is sometimes considered as one anatomical unit, called the *myocardium.* A tough outer layer of membranous tissue, called the *pericardium,* surrounds the myocardium. Lining the internal chambers and valves of the heart, on the walls of the atria and ventricles, is a tissue called the *endocardium.*

These tissues, like any others, are subject to infections and other disorders. An infection of the endocardium by bacteria is called *bacterial endocarditis.* (Disease of the valves is also called *endocarditis,* although it is a misnomer.) An interruption of the blood supply to the heart muscle is called a *myocardial infarction,* which results in the weakening or death of the portion of the myocardium whose blood supply is blocked. Fortunately, in many cases, other blood vessels may eventually take over the job of supplying the blood-starved area of heart muscle.

Heartbeat

The rate at which the heart beats is controlled by both the autonomic nervous system and by hormones of the endocrine system. The precise means by which the chambers and valves of the heart are made to work in perfect coordination are not fully understood. It is known, however, that the heart has one or more natural cardiac pacemakers that send electrical waves through the heart, causing the opening and closing of valves and muscular contraction, or pumping, of the ventricles near the normal adult rate of about 72 times per minute.

One particular electrical impulse (there may be others) originates in a small area in the upper part of the right atrium called the *sinus node.* Because it is definitely known that the contraction of the heart is electrically activated, tiny battery-powered devices called *artificial pacemakers* have been developed that can take the place of a natural pacemaker whose function has been impaired by heart injury or disease. Through electrodes implanted in heart tissue, such devices supply the correct beat for a defective heart. The bulk of the device is usually worn outside the body or is implanted just under the skin.

The fact that both ventricles give their push at the same time is very significant. It allows the entire heart muscle to rest between contractions—a rest period that adds up to a little more than half of a person's lifetime. Without this rest period, it is more than likely that our hearts would wear out considerably sooner than they do.

Blood Pressure

A physician's taking of blood pressure is based upon the difference between the heart's action at its period of momentary rest and at the moment of maximum work (the contraction or push). The split-second of maximum work, at the peak of the ventricles' contraction, is called the *systole.* The split-second of peak relaxation, when blood from the atria is draining into and filling up the ventricles, is called the *diastole.*

Blood pressure measures the force with which blood is passing through a major artery, such as one in the arm, and this pressure varies between a higher *systolic* pressure, corresponding to the heart's systole, and a lower *diastolic* pressure, reflecting the heart's diastole, or resting phase. The device with which a physician takes your blood pressure, called a *sphygmomanometer,* registers these higher and lower figures in numbers

Interaction between Heart and Lungs

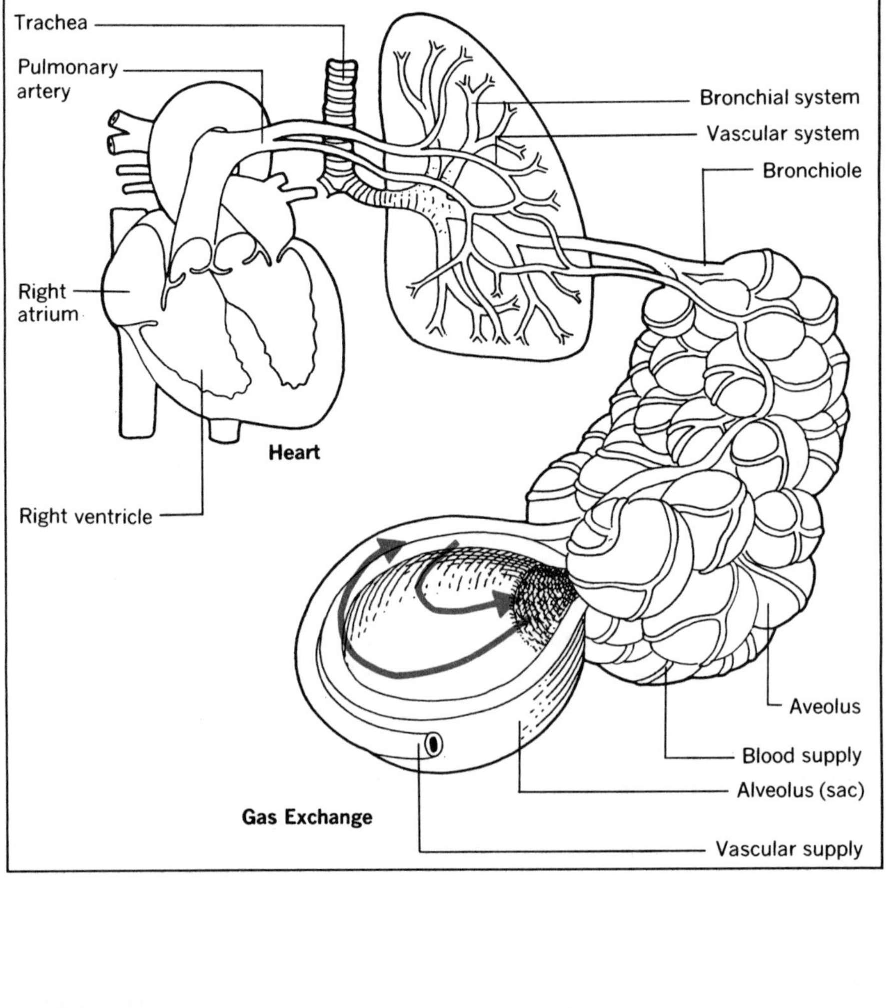

equivalent to the number of millimeters the force of your arterial blood would raise a column of mercury. The higher systolic force (pressure) is given first, then the diastolic figure. For example, a reading of less than 120/80 is within the normal range of blood pressure. A reading of 120 to 139 over 80 to 89 is considered *prehypertensive.* Readings that are above the prehypertensive range—and stay elevated over a period of time—indicate a person has high blood pressure, or *hypertension.* Hypertension has no direct connection with nervous tension, although the two may be associated in the same person. What it does indicate is that a heart is working harder than the average heart to push blood through the system. See also Ch. 9, *Diseases of the Circulatory System* and Ch. 10, *Heart Disease.*

The Digestive System and the Liver

A physician once remarked that a great many people seem to spend about half their time getting food into their digestive tracts and the other half worrying about how that food is doing on its travels. The physician was exaggerating, but he made his point.

The digestive tract has essentially one purpose: to break down food, both solid and fluid, into a form that can be used by the body. The food is used as energy to fuel daily activities or to nourish the various tissues that are always in the process of wearing out and needing replacement.

A normally functioning digestive tract, dealing with a reasonable variety and quantity of food, is designed to extract the maximum benefit from what we eat. Urine and feces are the waste products—things from which our body has selected everything that is of use.

Our digestive system's efficiency and economy in getting food into our bodies, to be utilized in all our living processes, can be attributed basically to three facts.

First, although the straight-line distance from the mouth to the bottom of the trunk is only two or three feet, the distance along the intestinal tract is about 10 times as great—25-30 feet—a winding, twisting, looping passageway that has more than enough footage to accommodate a number of ingeniously constructed way stations, checkpoints, and traffic-control devices.

Second, from the moment food enters the mouth, it is subjected to both chemical and mechanical actions that begin to break it apart, leading eventually to its reduction to submicroscopic molecules that can be absorbed through the intestinal walls into the circulatory system.

Finally, each of the three main types of food—carbohydrates, fats, and proteins—receives special treatment that results in the body deriving maximum benefit from each.

Sensing the Right Kind of Food

Lips, eyes, and nose are generally given scant notice in discussions of the digestive process. But if we consider digestion to include selection of food and rejection of substances that might do us harm, then all three play very important roles.

The sensitive skin of our lips represents one of our first warning station that food may be harmful if taken into the mouth. It may tell us if a forkful of food is too hot or warn us of a concealed fishbone.

Our eyes, too, are important selection-rejection monitors for food. What else keeps us from sitting down

The Digestive System

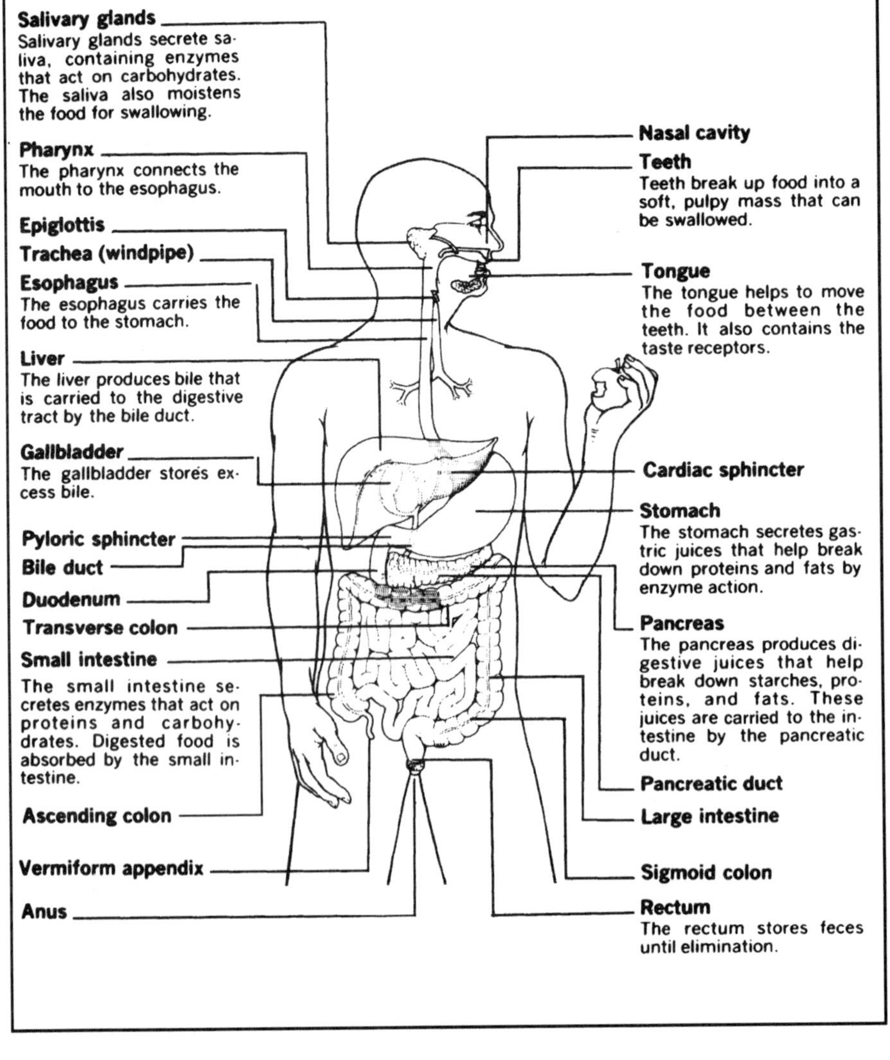

to a crisp salad of poison ivy, or, less facetiously, popping a moldy piece of cake into our mouth?

As mammals' noses go, man's is a very inferior and insensitive organ. Nevertheless, we make good use of our sense of smell in the selection and enjoyment of foods. The nose adds to our enjoyment of favorite food and drink not only before they enter the mouth, but also after, because stimulation of the olfactory cells in the nasal passages combines with the stimulation of the taste cells on the tongue to produce the sensation-and-discrimination gradations of taste.

The Mouth: Saliva, Teeth, and Tongue

By the time food leaves the mouth and is pushed down into the gullet (or esophagus), it has already received a sampling of all the kinds of punishment and prodding that will be provided by the 30-foot tube that lies ahead of it. The chances are slim that any piece of food will end that journey in the same condition it started, but if it did it would have traveled those 30 tortuous feet at the rate of something less than two feet per hour. Normally, the elapsed time is between 17 and 25 hours.

As in the rest of the digestive tract, the mouth puts both chemical and mechanical apparatus to work on a bite of food. Saliva supplies the chemical action. Teeth and tongue, backed up by powerful sets of muscles, are the mashers, crushers, and prodders.

Saliva

The mere presence of food in our mouth—or even the smell, memory, or anticipation of it—sends signals to our brain, and our brain in turn sends messages back to a system of six salivary glands: one pair, called the *sublingual glands,* located under the tongue toward the front of the mouth; another pair, the *submaxillary* (or *submandibular*) glands, a bit behind and below them; and the largest, the *parotid glands,* tucked in the region where jaw meets neck behind the ear lobes.

Saliva is mainly composed of water, and water alone begins to soften up food so that it can pass more smoothly down the esophagus toward encounters with more powerful chemical agents.

Salivary Glands

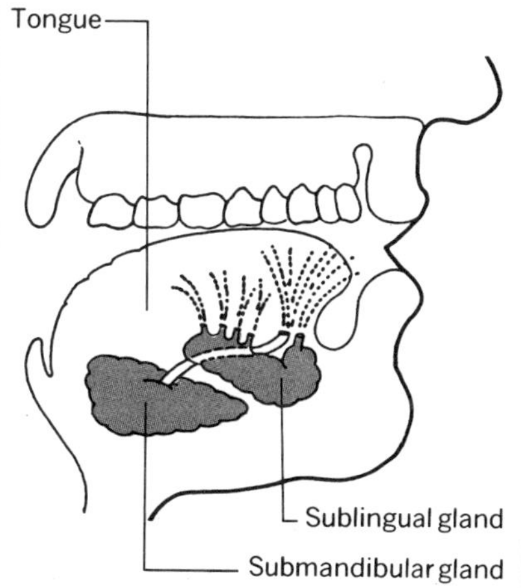

There is also a very special substance in saliva, an enzyme called *ptyalin,* whose specific job is to begin the breakdown of one of the toughest kinds of food our digestive system has to handle—starches. Starch is a kind of carbohydrate, the group of foods from which we principally derive energy; but in order for the body to utilize carbohydrate, it must be broken down into simpler forms, which are called simple sugars. Ptyalin, then, begins the simplification of carbohydrate starch into carbohydrate sugar.

Saliva also does a favor or two for the dominating structures of the mouth—the tongue and teeth. Without its bathing action, the tongue's taste cells could not function up to par; and because it has a mild germicidal effect in addition to a simple rinsing action, saliva helps protect our mouth and teeth from bacterial infection.

Teeth

The role of the teeth in digestion can be summed up in one word: destruction. What the wrecker's ball is to a standing building, our teeth are to a lump of solid food. They do the first, dramatic demolishing, leaving smaller fragments to be dealt with and disposed of in other ways.

Starting from the center of the mouth, we have two incisors on either side, top and bottom, followed by a canine, a couple of premolars, and three molars, the most backward of which (it never appears in some people) is the curiously named "wisdom" tooth, so called because it commonly appears as physical maturity is reached, at about 20 years of age.

Our teeth equip us for destroying chunks of food by a gamut of mechanical actions ranging from gripping and puncturing to grinding and pulverizing. The teeth in front—canines and incisors—do most of the gripping, ripping, and tearing, while the premolars and molars at the back of the jaws do the grinding.

The Tongue

The surface of the tongue is not smooth, but has a finely corrugated look and feel. This slightly sandpapery surface results from the presence of thousands of tiny papillae, little pyramid-shaped bumps. When we are young, the walls of a single papilla may contain up to 300 taste cells, or buds. As we get older, the maximum number of taste buds per papilla may decline to under 100.

There are four kinds of taste cells, distinguished by the type of taste message each sends to the brain: salty, sweet, sour, and bitter. Each of the four types is a narrow specialist in one type of taste. However, simultaneous or successive stimulation of all four types (combined almost always with information picked up by our sense of smell) can produce a tremendous variety of recognizable tastes—although perhaps not so many as some gourmets or wine-tasters might have us believe.

All four types of taste buds—salty, sweet, sour, and bitter—are found associated with papillae in all areas on the surface of the tongue; but there tend to be denser populations of one or the other kinds of taste cells in certain places. For example, salty and sweet cells predominate at the tip of the tongue and about halfway back along its sides; sour cells are more numerous all the way back along the sides; bitter buds are densest at the back of the tongue.

In addition to its tasting abilities, the tongue is a very versatile, flexible, and admirably shaped bundle of muscle. Not only can it flick out to moisten dry lips and ferret out and dislodge food particles in the oral cavity, but it also performs the first mechanical step in the all-important act of swallowing.

Swallowing

Swallow. You'll find that you feel the top of your tongue pressing up against the roof of your mouth (hard palate). You may never have thought about it consciously, but the pressing of the tongue against the hard palate prevents food from slipping to the front of your mouth—and also gives the food a good shove up and to the back of your mouth. At this point, the *soft palate* (from which the teardrop-shaped piece of tissue called the

The Transition from Breathing to Swallowing

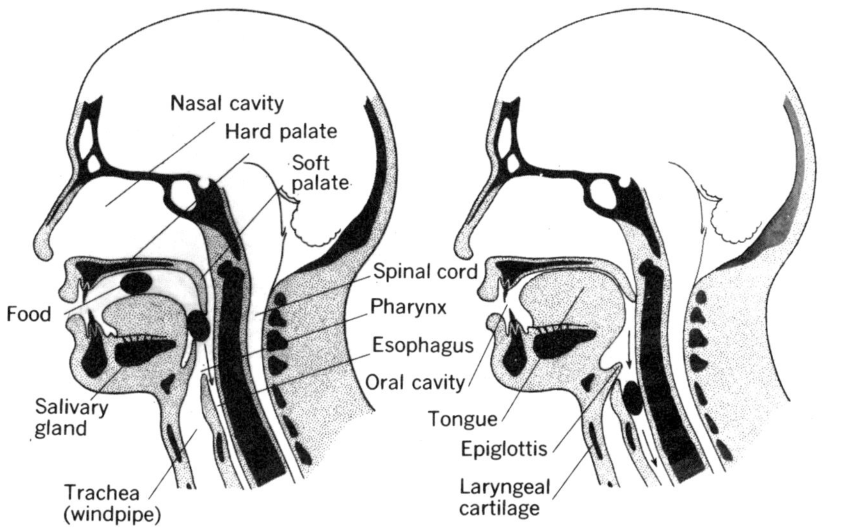

(Left) The soft palate begins to move upward to close off the nasal cavity, and the epiglottis to move downward to close off the trachea. (Right) By the time the food has passed into the esophagus, the trachea and the nasal cavity are completely shut off.

uvula hangs down) slips up to cover the passageway between mouth (oral cavity) and nasal cavity, nicely preventing the food from being misdirected toward your nose.

Once past the soft palate, the food is in the *pharynx,* a kind of anatomical traffic circle with two roads entering at the top, those from the mouth and nasal cavity, and two roads leading away from the bottom, the *trachea* (windpipe) and the *esophagus* or food tube.

The Epiglottis

A wedge of cartilage called the *epiglottis* protrudes from the trachea side, the side toward the front of the neck. When we are breathing, the epiglottis is flattened up against the front wall of the pharynx, allowing free movement of air up and down the trachea. Simultaneously, the epiglottis helps to close off the entrance to the esophagus; a good part of the esophagus-closing work is done by a bundle of sinewy, elastic tissue we associate primarily with speech—the tissue of the vocal cords, otherwise known as the voice box or *larynx.* The laryngeal tissue is connected to the epiglottis above it, and supplies the epiglottis with most of its muscle for movement.

During the movement of a swallow, the larynx exerts an upward force against the epiglottis that serves to block off the trachea. At the same time, the larynx relaxes some of its pressure on the esophagus. Result: food enters the esophagus, where it is meant to go, and not the windpipe, which as we all know from having had something "go down the wrong way," produces an immediate fit of coughing.

Once we have swallowed, we lose almost completely the conscious ability to control the passage of food along the intestinal tract. Only when wastes reach the point of elimination do we begin to reassert some conscious control.

Peristalsis

The mechanical action called *peristalsis,* affected by muscles in the walls of all the organs of the gastrointestinal tract, first comes into play in the esophagus. Two layers of muscles intermesh in the intestinal walls: the inner layer encircles the esophagus in a series of rings; the outer layer stretches lengthwise along the tube. These two sets of muscles work in tandem to produce the basic action of persistalsis, called a *peristaltic wave.*

The alternative contraction and relaxation of the muscles—closing behind swallowed food and opening in front of it—combine to move both liquid and solid food (medical term, *bolus*) along the digestive tract. Gravity, in a sense, is left behind once food enters the esophagus. Because of peristalsis, we can swallow lying down or even standing on our heads; and astronauts are able to eat in near zero-gravity or under weightless conditions.

Peristalsis has another important function besides moving food through the body. The constricting and relaxing muscles serve also to knead, churn, and pummel the solid remains of the food left after our teeth have done their best.

Digestive Sphincters

If you think about it, the gastrointestinal tract has to be equipped with a number of gates that can open or shut, depending on the amount of food that is passing through. Otherwise, the food might push through so fast that little nourishment could be extracted from it: we would feel hungry one minute and glutted the next. The gastrointestinal tract is thus equipped at critical junctures with a number of muscular valves, or *sphincters,* which, usually under the direction of the autonomic nervous system, can regulate the movement of food through the digestive tube. Another function of a sphincter is to prevent backflow of partially digested food.

The muscles of a sphincter are often described as "pursestring muscles" because the way they draw together the sides of the digestive tube is roughly similar to drawing up the strings of a purse. The first of these pursestring valves occurs at the *cardia,* the opening where the esophagus meets the stomach, and is called the *cardiac sphincter,* from its location almost directly in front of the heart. (But there is no physical connection.)

Another important muscle ring is the *pyloric sphincter,* at the opening called the *pylorus,* located at the other end of the stomach, at the connection between stomach and small intestine. The release of waste from the rectum is controlled, partly voluntarily, by an *anal sphincter,* located at the *anus,* which marks the end of the tract.

The Stomach

About ten inches down the esophagus, the food we swallow must pass the cardiac sphincter. Then the food, by now fairly well diced and mashed, passes into the stomach.

Inelegant as it sounds, the stomach is best described as a rough, leather-skinned balloon. When empty, its skin shrivels around itself like a deflated balloon; but when "pumped up" by a hearty meal, the stomach becomes a plump, J-shaped bag about a foot long and six inches wide, holding about two quarts of food and drink.

The Passage of Food through the Stomach

Although its food-processing function tends to get more attention, the stomach's role as a storage reservoir is equally important. A moderate, well-rounded meal with a good blend of carbohydrates, proteins, and fats takes usually a minimum of three hours to pass out of the pyloric sphincter into the small intestine—more if the meal is heavy in fats and

The Passage of Food through the Alimentary Canal

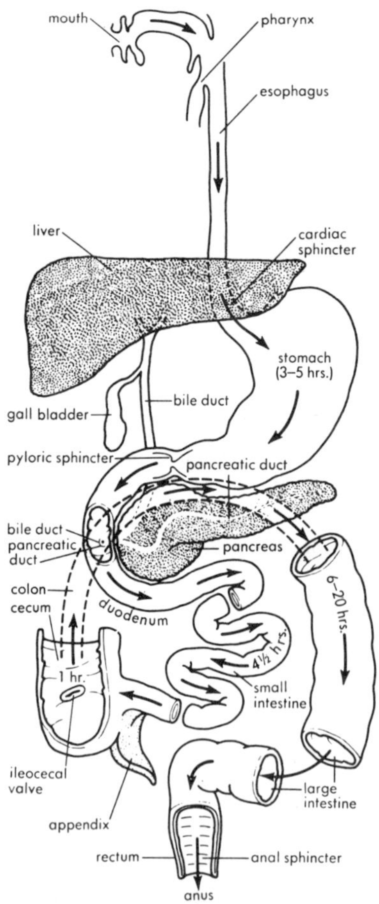

This drawing indicates the duration of each digestive process. Food enters the mouth and is passed through the pharynx and esophagus into the stomach, where it is partly digested. The small intestine completes digestion and absorbs digested food. The large intestine absorbs excess water. Indigestible residue collects in the rectum for later disposal.

rich foods. Thus, a meal that might take us 15 minutes to eat, may take up to 20 times as long to pass from the stomach into the small intestine. This decelerating of food's rate of passage has two very significant results: first, it allows time for the food-processing activities within the stomach; and second, it releases food (in a mushy form called *chyme*) in small, well-spaced amounts that can be efficiently handled by the small intestine.

Although the stomach is not an absolutely essential organ—a person can live a full life with part or even all of it removed—it is a tremendous convenience. Without a stomach, frequent, carefully selected, well-chewed small feedings rather than "three square meals a day" are necessary so as not to overburden the small intestine, which can handle only a small quantity of food, well-mashed, at one time. If too much food goes directly to the small intestine, only so much nourishment (carbohydrates, proteins, fats) per meal can be supplied to the body, with the result that we would be weak from hunger after going a few hours without eating.

It will come as no surprise to know that the food processing done in the stomach is both mechanical and chemical. The three layers of crisscrossing muscles in the stomach walls are rarely still. They contract and relax continually, squeezing, pummeling, and mixing the stomach's contents into chyme. So active and relentless is the stomach's muscular activity that it actually "chews up" pieces of food that have been swallowed too hastily.

Stomach Chemicals

The various chemicals found in the stomach are produced and secreted into the stomach cavity by some 40 million gland cells that line the interior stomach walls. The constant wiggling and jouncing of the stomach helps to mix these chemicals thoroughly into the food. Each of the chemicals is secreted by a special type of cell and has a specific function. They include the digestive enzymes pepsin, rennin, and lipase; hydrochloric acid; and watery mucus.

A look at the special assignments of rennin, pepsin, hydrochloric acid, and mucus—and how they interact with and depend upon one another—provides a good glimpse into the elegant and complex chemical events that occur when the stomach encounters a swallow of food.

Rennin and Pepsin

Rennin, well known to cheesemakers, has essentially one task: to turn milk into milk curds. But the curds are not ready to pass on to the small intestine until they are further dismantled by *pepsin.* Pepsin has other duties as well: one of them is to begin the breakdown of proteins. But pepsin can only begin to split up protein foods after they have been worked on by *hydrochloric acid.*

Hydrochloric Acid

Hydrochloric acid is a corrosive substance and, except in very dilute strengths, could quite literally eat away the lining of the stomach. (This is apparently what happens in cases of gastric ulcers.) Mucus secretions, with the help of fluids in the food itself, dilute the hydrochloric acid to a point where (in a normal stomach) it is rendered harmless. Even so, the normal, healthy condition inside our stomach is slightly acid. The slight acidity of the stomach serves to inhibit the growth of organisms such as bacteria.

The Small Intestine

By the time food-turned-chyme gets through the pyloric sphincter, it has already traveled about two-and-a-half feet: about 6 inches from lips to epiglottis; 10 or 12 inches down the esophagus; and about a foot through the stomach. But at this point it has actually traveled less than one-tenth of the gastrointestinal (GI) tract, and the longest stretch lies just ahead: the 20-plus feet of the small intestine, so named because of its relatively small one-to-two inch diameter. The preparation of food particles to pass through the walls of the GI tract is completed in the small intestine—almost completed, in fact, before the chyme has traveled the first foot of the small intestine. By the time it leaves the small intestine, chyme has given up virtually all its nutrients. In other words, the process called *absorption* or *assimilation* has taken place: the nutrients have left the GI tract for other parts of the body via the circulating blood and lymph. What passes on to the large intestine is principally waste and water.

The small intestine is somewhat arbitrarily divided into three sections: the *duodenum,* the *jejunum,* and the *ileum.*

The Duodenum

Within this horseshoe loop, eight to ten inches long and about two inches in diameter, more chemical interactions are concentrated than in any other section of the GI tract. One of the first jobs in the duodenum is to neutralize the acidity of the chyme. The final steps of digestion, and the absorption of food through the intestinal lining, proceed best in a slightly alkaline environment.

The alkaline juices needed to neutralize the acidity of the chyme come mainly from the liver in the form of bile. Bile produced by the liver but not needed immediately in the duodenum is stored in concentrated form in the gallbladder, a pouchlike, three-inch-long organ. On signal from the autonomic nervous system, the membranous muscular walls of the gallbladder contract, squeezing concentrated, highly alkaline bile into a short duct that leads to the duodenum. Bile components are indispensable for the digestion and absorption of stubborn fatty materials.

Through a duct from the pancreas, a host of pancreatic enzymes, capable of splitting apart large, tough molecules of carbohydrate, protein, and fat, enters the duodenum. These digestive enzymes manufactured by the pancreas are the most powerful in the GI tract.

What triggers the production of bile and pancreatic juice for the duodenum? Apparently, it is a two-step process involving hormones. When the stomach walls secrete hydrochloric acid on the arrival of food, hormones are released; they travel to the liver and pancreas with instructions to step up their production of digestive juices.

Still other strong enzymes are secreted by the walls of the duodenum and join the bile and pancreatic enzymes in the duodenum.

Thus, in the not quite foot-long tube of the duodenum, the final breakdown of food—digestion—reaches a dramatic climax. The nutrients in the food eaten some hours ago have almost all been reduced to molecules small enough to be absorbed through the intestinal walls into the bloodstream. Carbohydrates are reduced to simpler sugars; proteins to amino acids; and fats to fatty acids and glycerol.

Some absorption of these nutrients occurs in the duodenum, but the far greater proportion takes place in the next two, longer sections of the small intestine: the eight- to ten-foot jejunum and the twelve-foot ileum. Likewise, some oversize food molecules that get past the duodenum may be digested further along in their passage through the small intestine.

The Jejunum

As peristalsis pushes the nutrient broth out of the duodenum and into the first reaches of the jejunum, a gradual change in the appearance of the intestinal lining is evident. Greater and greater number of *villi*—microscopic, hairlike structures—sprout from the already bumpy walls of the intestinal lining into the GI tube.

The Villi

The villi (singular, *villus*) have the primary responsibility for absorbing amino acids (from protein), sugars (from carbohydrates), and fatty acids and glycerol (from fats) from the digested contents of the small intestine, and starting them on their way to other parts of the body. What the villi do not remove from the chyme—such as the cellulose fragments of fruits and vegetables—passes on to the large intestine in a thin, watery soup almost completely lacking in nutritional value.

Gland cells near the bottom of a villus secrete various enzymes, mucus, and other substances that perform digestive "mop-up operations" along the whole length of the small intestine.

The Ileum

In this third and final 12-foot section of the small intestine, villi line the walls in such profusion that the intestinal lining resembles, under moderate magnification, nothing so much as a plush, velvety carpet. The greatest numbers of the estimated five or six million villi in the small intestine are found along the lining of the ileum, making it the primary absorption site of the GI tract.

Also adding to the ileum's absorption efficiency is its gradually narrowing diameter (just one inch at its junction with the large intestine), which helps to keep the chyme always in close contact with the swishing villi. The end of the ileum is marked by the *ileocecal valve,* beyond which lies the first bulge of the large intestine, the *cecum.*

Principally because of vigorous peristaltic contractions and relaxations, the walls of the small intestine are always moving like the walls within some spasmodically flexing, nightmarish tunnel. Attached to the intestinal walls, the villi, too, are always in restless motion: waving and thrashing, protracting and retracting, even growing thinner or fatter.

Although the entire distance through the small intestine, from the pyloric sphincter to the ileocecal valve at the junction with the large intestine, is only a bit over 20 feet, the villi give the small intestine's internal lining a relatively gigantic surface area—over 100 square feet. This is about five times the surface area of our body's skin. Of course, the greatly enlarged surface area gives the small intestine lining that much more space in which to absorb nutrients.

The small intestine is supported in the abdomen by a fan-shaped web of tissues called the *mesentery.* Attached at the back of the abdomen, the mesentery connects to the small intestine at various points, and yet allows it some freedom to squirm and sway—much like the V network of ropes that attaches either end of a hammock to a tree. Nerve fibers and blood vessels also reach the small intestine via the mesentery.

The Liver, Gallbladder, and Pancreas

These three organs all share a common function—sending digestive substances to the duodenum—although, except in the case of the gallbladder, it is not their only function. Lying outside the GI tract proper, they nevertheless are indispensable in the processes of digestion and absorption. Digestive fluids from all three converge like tributaries of a river at the common bile duct, and their flow from there into the duodenum is controlled by a sphincter muscle-ring separating the duodenum and common bile duct.

From the liver, bile drips into the *hepatic duct,* which soon meets the *cystic duct* arriving from the gallbladder. Converging, they form one duct, the *common bile duct,* which meets the *pancreatic duct,* carrying enzymatic fluid from the pancreas. Like a smaller river meeting a larger one, the pancreatic duct loses its own name at this confluence and becomes part of the common bile duct, which empties on demand into the duodenum. When the sphincter of the bile duct is closed, bile from the liver is forced to back up into the cystic duct, and eventually into the gallbladder. There it is stored and concentrated until needed, when it flows back down the cystic duct.

The Liver

Four pounds of highly efficient chemical-processing tissues, the liver is the largest solid organ in the body. You can locate it by placing your left hand over your right, lowermost ribs; your hand then just about covers the area of the liver. More than any other organ, the liver enables our bodies to benefit from the food we eat. Without it, digestion would be impossible, and the conversion of food into living cells and energy practically nonexistent. Insofar as they affect our body's handling of food—all the many processes that go by the collective name of nutrition—the liver's functions can be roughly divided into those that break down food molecules and those that build up or reconstitute these nutrients into a form that the body can use or store efficiently.

Breaking Down Food Molecules

Bile, as we have seen, assists in the destruction of large food molecules in the small intestine, enabling absorption of nutrients by the villi. Bile acts to increase alkalinity, breaking down big fat molecules; stimulates peristalsis; and prevents food from putrefying within the digestive tract. Unusable portions of the bile, destined to be eliminated as waste, include excess cholesterol, fats, and various components of dead disintegrated cells. Pigments from dead cells in bile give feces its normal, dark, yellow-brown color. Other cell fragments in bile, especially iron from disintegrated red blood cells, are reclaimed from the intestines and eventually make their way via the bloodstream to other parts of the body, where they are built into new cells.

Reconstituting Nutrients

Oddly enough, the liver rebuilds some of the proteins and carbohydrates that the bile has just so effectively helped to break down in the digestive tract. But this is really not so strange as it sounds. The types of proteins and carbohydrates that can be used by man for cell-rebuilding and energy are usually somewhat different in fine structure from those in food. Thus, the liver receives the basic building blocks of proteins and carbohydrates—amino acids and sugars—and with them builds up molecules and cells that can be utilized by the human body. The amino acids and sugars reach the liver through the *portal vein,* which is the great collection tube for nutrient-carrying blood returning from capillaries along the stomach and small intestine.

Glycogen and Glucose

In the liver, sugars from the small intestine are converted into a special substance called *glycogen;* amino acids are made available as needed for building new cells to replace the cells that are always naturally dying in a healthy normal body. Glycogen, simply speaking, is the liver's solution to a difficult space and storage problem. The form of carbohydrate the body can use best is a sugar called *glucose,* but the liver isn't large enough to store the necessary amount of glucose. The answer is glycogen, a tidy, compact sugar molecule that the liver can store in great quantities. When a call comes from any part of the body for glucose, the liver quickly converts some glycogen to glucose and releases it into the bloodstream. By this mechanism, healthy blood sugar levels are maintained.

The liver also builds up human fats from fatty acids and glycerol, packs them off to storage, then reverses the process when necessary by breaking down body fats into forms that can serve as fuel to be burned by the body for energy.

Other Functions

In addition to its functions closely related to digestion and nutrition, the liver also serves as a storehouse and processor of vitamins and minerals—it is, in fact, the manufacturer of vitamin A. It can remove many toxic substances from the blood and render their poisons harmless. It picks up spent red blood cells from the circulation and dismantles them; and it continually manufactures new blood elements.

The liver is also a manufacturing site for *cholesterol,* a substance belonging to the class of body chemicals called steroids. Above-normal levels of cholesterol in the blood have been linked to hardening of the arteries and heart disease; but cholesterol in the proper amounts is needed by almost every tissue in the body. Some brain and spinal tissues, for example, have cholesterol as one of their main structural components.

With all these vital chemical activities and more, the liver might be expected to be a most delicate and fragile organ. In a sense it is: minor liver damage from one cause or another is thought to be fairly common. But what saves our lives (and us) is that we have a great deal more of it than we need for a normal healthy life. Before symptoms of a liver deficiency appear, more than 50 percent of the liver cells may be destroyed. Furthermore, the liver has a great capacity for regeneration, rebuilding diseased tissues with new liver cells.

The Gallbladder

Bile stored in the gallbladder is much more concentrated and thicker than bile that is fresh from the liver. This allows the three-inch gallbladder to store a great deal of bile components. But the thickening process can also create problems in the form of extremely painful gallstones, which are dried, crystallized bile. Fortunately, the entire gallbladder can be removed with little or no lasting ill effect. All that is missing is a small storage sac for bile.

The Pancreas

This manufacturer of powerful digestive enzymes, only six inches long, resembles a branchlet heavily laden with ripe berries. Its important role in digestion is often overshadowed by the fact that it also manufactures the hormone *insulin.* The pancreas cells that manufacture digestive enzymes are completely different from those that manufacture insulin. The latter are grouped into little clusters called the *islets of Langerhans,* which are discussed under *The Endocrine Glands* in this chapter.

The Large Intestine

The large intestine, also called the large bowel, is shaped like a great, lumpy, drooping question mark—arching, from its beginning at the ileocecal valve, over the folds of the small intestine, then curving down and descending past more coiled small intestine to the anus, which marks the end of the GI tract. From ileocecal valve to anus, the large intestine is five to six feet in length.

The junction between the ileum and the *cecum,* the first section of the large intestine, occurs very low in the abdomen, normally on the right-hand side. The cecum is a bowl-like receptacle at the bottom of the colon, the longest section of the large intestine.

Just below the entrance of the ileum, a dead-end tube dangles down from the cecum. This is the *appendix vermiformis* (Latin, "worm-shaped appendage") commonly known as the appendix. Three to six inches long and one-third inch in diameter, the appendix may get jammed with stray pieces of solid food, become infected, swell, and rupture, spewing infection into the abdominal cavity. This is why early diagnosis of *appendicitis* and removal (*appendectomy*) are critically important.

Sections of the Colon

The colon is divided into three sections by pronounced *flexures,* or bends, where the colon makes almost right-angle changes of direction. Above the bowl of the cecum, the *ascending colon* rises almost vertically for about a foot and a half.

Then there is a flexure in the colon, after which the *transverse colon* travels horizontally for a couple of feet along a line at navel height. At another flexure, the colon turns vertically down again, giving the name of *descending colon* to this approximately two feet of large intestine. At the end of the descending colon, the large intestine executes an S-shaped curve, the *sigmoid flexure,* after which the remaining several inches of large intestine are known as the *rectum.*

Some people confuse the terms rectum and anus: the rectum refers specifically to the last section of the large intestinal tube, between sigmoid flexure and the anal sphincters, while the anus refers only to the opening controlled by the outlet valves of the large intestine. These valves consist of two ringlike voluntary muscles called anal sphincters.

Any solid materials that pass into the large intestine through the ileocecal valve (which prevents backflow into the small intestine) are usually indigestible, such as cellulose, or substances that have been broken down in the body and blood in the normal process of cell death and renewal, such as some bile components. But what the cecum mainly receives is water.

Functions of the Large Intestine

The principal activity of the large intestine—other than as a channel for elimination of body wastes—is as a temporary storage area for water, which is then reabsorbed into the circulation through the walls of the colon. Villi are absent in the large intestine, and peristalsis is much less vigorous than in the small intestine.

As water is absorbed, the contents of the large intestine turn from a watery soup into the semisolid feces. Meanwhile, bacteria—which colonize the normal colon in countless millions—have begun to work on and decompose the remaining solid materials. These bacteria do no harm as long as they remain inside the large intestine, and the eliminated feces is heavily populated with them. Nerve endings in the large intestine signal the brain that it is time for a bowel movement.

The Peritoneum

Lining the entire abdominal cavity, as well as the digestive and other abdominal organs, is a thin, tough, lubricated membrane called the *peritoneum.* In addition to protecting and supporting the abdominal organs, the peritoneum permits these organs to slip and slide against each other without any harm from friction. The peritoneum also contains blood and lymph vessels that serve the digestive organs. See Ch. 11, *Diseases of the Digestive System.*

The Respiratory System and the Lungs

The heart, by its construction and shape, tells us a great deal about the lungs and respiration.

Interaction between Heart and Lungs

The heart is divided vertically by a wall called a septum into right (your right) and left parts. The right part is smaller than the left: its muscles only have to pump blood a few inches to the lungs, while the muscles of the left half have to pump blood to the whole body.

The function of the right half of our heart is to receive oxygen-poor blood from the veins of the body. Venous blood empties into the top-right chamber, or right atrium, of the heart, and the right ventricle pumps that oxygen-poor blood (via the pulmonary artery) to the lungs, where the blood, passing through minute capillaries, picks up oxygen.

From the lungs, the oxygen-rich blood flows back into the heart's left atrium via the pulmonary veins; and from the left atrium, the oxygen-rich blood drains into the left ventricle, from whence it is pumped via the aorta to the body.

The blood pumped to the lungs by the right ventricle is oxygen-poor blood; it has given up its oxygen to the cells that need it around the body. But this "used blood" is rich in something else—carbon dioxide. As the body's cells have taken oxygen, they

Interaction between Heart and Lungs

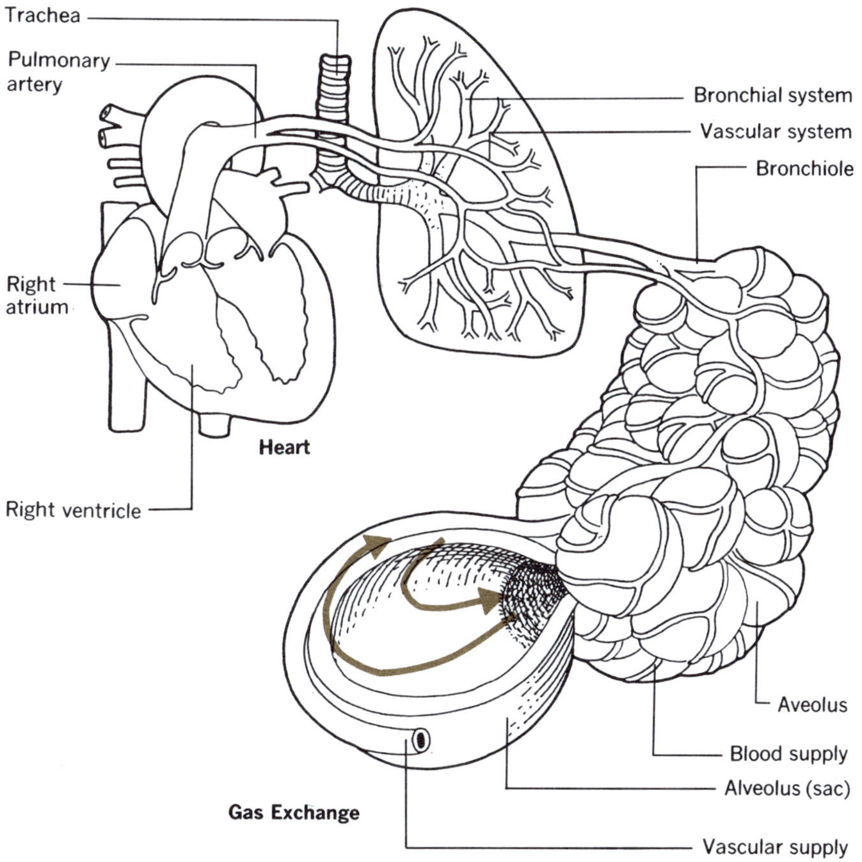

have given up carbon dioxide to the circulating blood. For both oxygen and carbon dioxide, the "carrier" has been *hemoglobin,* a complex iron-protein substance that is part of our red blood cells.

Capillaries and Alveoli

The pulmonary artery carrying this lung-bound blood soon branches into smaller and smaller vessels, and eventually into microscopic capillaries that reach into every crook and crevice of the lungs.

In the lungs, the walls of the capillaries touch the walls of equally microscopic structures called *alveoli* (singular, *alveolus*). The alveoli are the smallest air sacs of the lungs. These tiny, expandable air cells are the destination of every breath of air we take. Estimates of the total number of alveoli in both our lungs vary between 300 million and a billion—in any case, we normally have several hundred million of them.

The Alveoli

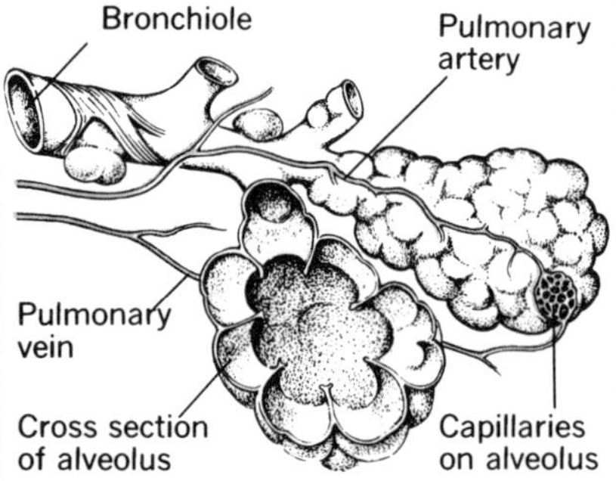

The branches of the pulmonary tree terminate in the alveoli, grapelike clusters of air sacs covered by capillaries, where the gaseous exchange occurs.

Carbon Dioxide and Oxygen Exchange

Where they meet, the membranous walls of both a capillary and an alveolus are both about as thin as any living tissue can be—a thickness that is only the width of one cell. Under such conditions, the carbon dioxide carried by the hemoglobin in our blood to the lungs diffuses (as tiny gaseous "bubbles") across both the wall of a capillary and the wall of an alveolus.

Once inside the sac of the alveolus, carbon dioxide is ready to be exhaled from the body by "breathing out." One indication of just how well this system works is the fact that the air we exhale has roughly 100 times more carbon dioxide than the air we breathe in.

At the same time that hemoglobin dumps carbon dioxide at the interface of the capillary and alveolus walls, it picks up the oxygen made available from inhaled fresh air that has reached the alveoli. The molecular oxygen bubbles cross the membranes in the same way—but in the opposite direction—as the carbon dioxide.

Hemoglobin in the capillaries picks up the oxygen and carries it via veins leading away from the lungs, to the left atrium of the heart.

Essential Role of Moisture

The alveolar membranes are supplied with a thin film of moisture that is absolutely indispensable to the exchange of gases in the lungs. As in so many of our body's reactions, our evolutionary descent from water-dwelling ancestors is revealed by the wet environment demanded if our lungs are to supply our body with oxygen.

Respiration at the One-Cell Level

Oxygen molecules, then, are carried to the body's cells by the hemoglobin of the arterial blood pumped by the heart's left ventricle. But how does a cell take oxygen from the blood and use it?

Exchange of Gases

The transfer of oxygen from blood to cell is accomplished in much the same way as the exchanges that take place in the lungs. The circulating arterial blood has a surplus of oxygen; the cells have a surplus of carbon dioxide. When the oxygen-rich blood reaches the finest capillaries, only the very thinnest membranous walls (of cell and capillary) separate it from the carbon-dioxide-rich cells. As in the lungs, both these gases (dissolved in water) diffuse through these thinnest of membranes: the oxygen into the cell, the carbon dioxide into the blood for eventual deposit in the alveoli, and exhalation.

Within the cell, the oxygen is needed so that food, the body's fuel, can be burned to produce energy. At the cellular level, the most convenient and common food is a fairly simple carbohydrate molecule called glucose.

Conversion of Carbohydrates into Energy

Energy is locked into a carbohydrate molecule such as glucose in the form of chemical bonds between its atoms. If one of these bonds is broken—say, a bond holding together a carbon and a hydrogen atom—a bit of pent-up energy is released as if, in a stalemated tug of war, the rope suddenly broke and both teams went hurtling off a few feet in opposite directions. This is precisely the effect of respiration within a cell: the cell "breaks the ropes" holding together a carbohydrate molecule. The result is the release of energy—either as body heat or to power other activities within the cell.

It is useful—but a somewhat misleading oversimplification—to consider cellular respiration as a type of burning, or combustion. When a typical cell burns food, a carbohydrate molecule (glucose) together with molecules of oxygen are changed into carbon dioxide and water. During this change, chemical energy is released—energy that has been trapped, as we have seen, in the carbohydrate molecule. That complex, energy-rich molecule has been dismantled into the simpler molecules of carbon dioxide (CO_2) and water (H_2O). Oxygen is necessary here just as it is in fiery combustion. But the energy released here, instead of rushing out as heat and flame, is used to power the living activities of the cell.

This description of cellular respiration is all right in principle, but the trouble is this: if it all happened at once—if carbohydrate was so abruptly dismantled, split up at one stroke to water and carbon dioxide—such a great amount of energy would be released that the cell would simply burn itself up. As one biologist has said, the cell would be in exactly the same position as a wood furnace built of wood.

What protects the cell is its army of enzymes. These remarkable protein molecules combine briefly with energy-containing food molecules, causing them to break down bit by bit, so that energy is released gradually rather than all at once.

Carbon Dioxide–Precious Waste

In most of our minds, oxygen tends to be the hero of respiration and carbon dioxide the villain or at least the undesirable waste gas. This isn't really a fair picture. While it is true that too much carbon dioxide would act as a poison in our body, it is also true that we must always have a certain amount of the gas dissolved in our tissues. If we did not, two potentially fatal events could occur. First, our blood chemistry, especially its delicate acid-alkali balance, would get completely out of control. Second—and something of a paradox—the body's whole automatic system of regulating breathing would be knocked out.

It is the level of carbon dioxide in the bloodstream that controls our breathing. This level is continuously being monitored by the autonomic nervous system, specifically by the lower brain's "breathing center" in the medulla at the top of the spinal cord. When the level of carbon dioxide in our body goes above a certain level, signals from the medulla force us to breathe. Almost everybody has played, "How long can you hold your breath?" and knows that, past a certain point, it becomes impossible *not* to breathe. When you are holding your breath, the unexhaled carbon dioxide rapidly builds up in your system until the breathing center is besieged with signals that say "Breathe!" And you do.

Our Big Breathing Muscle: The Diaphragm

What gets air into and out of our lungs? The answer may seem as obvious as breathing in and out. But except for those rare instances when we consciously regulate our breathing pattern—which physicians call "force breathing"—we do not decide when to inhale and when to exhale. And even when we do force-breathe, it is not primarily the action of opening the mouth and gulping in air, then blowing it out, that gets air down the windpipe and into the alveoli of the lungs. The main work of inhaling and exhaling is done by the contraction and relaxation of the big helmet-shaped muscle on which the lungs rest and which marks the "floor" of the chest or thoracic cavity and the "ceiling" of the abdominal cavity. This muscle is the *diaphragm.*

It is the diaphragm that causes the lungs to swell and fill with fresh air, then partially collapse to expel used gases. The muscles and tendons of the sinewy diaphragm are attached at the back to the spinal column, at the front to the breastbone (*sternum*), and at the lower sides to the lower ribs.

The diaphragm contracts and relaxes on orders from the brain's breathing center, orders that are carried along the pathways of the autonomic nervous system. When the medulla sends messages to the breathing muscles to contract, the diaphragm is pulled downward, en-

Diaphragm

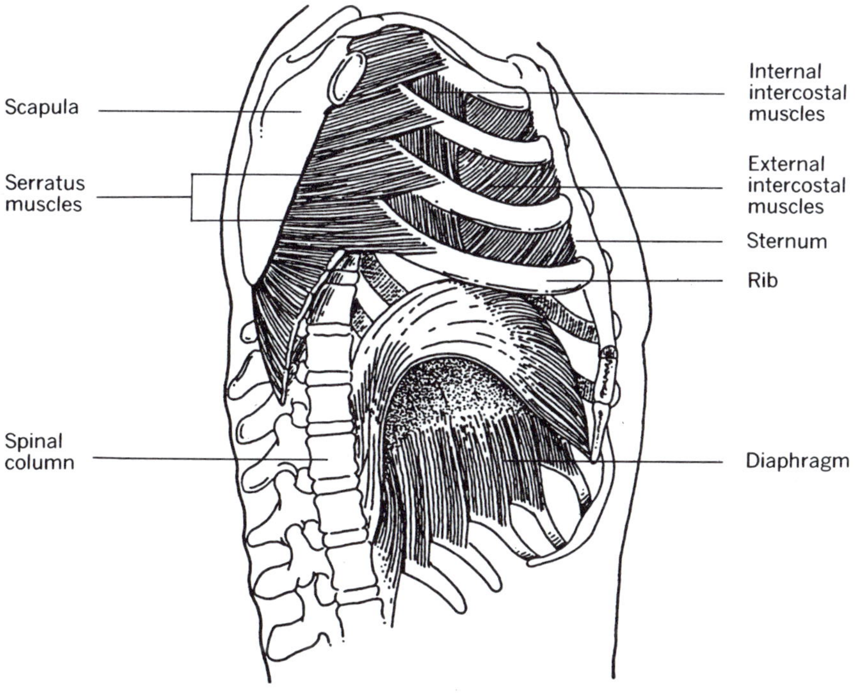

larging the space filled by the lungs. This creates a temporary partial vacuum, into which air rushes, inflating and expanding the lungs. When the diaphragm relaxes, the lung space is reduced, pushing air out.

Other Breathing Muscles

The diaphragm muscle's leading role in breathing is supported by several other muscles that play minor parts. Among these are the *intercostal muscles* between the ribs that give the rib cage a slight push upward and outward, enlarging the thoracic cavity, and the *serratus muscles,* which are mainly muscular sheaths along the ribs, to which other muscles are attached.

The Trachea and the Lungs

The right lung (your right) is somewhat bigger than the left. The lungs hang in the chest attached to the windpipe or *trachea.*

The Trachea

The trachea itself branches off at the back of the throat, or *pharynx,* where the epiglottis prevents food from entering the trachea and channels swallowed food along its proper route, the esophagus. The top part of the trachea forms the voice box or *larynx,* made up of vocal cords—actually two flaps of cartilage, muscle, and membranous tissue that protrude into the windpipe—whose vibrations in response to air exhaled from the lungs give us our voice.

Below the larynx, the trachea descends five or six inches to a spot just about directly behind your breastbone, where the first of many thousands of branchings into *bronchi, bronchioles,* and alveoli occurs. C-shaped rings of cartilage give the trachea both support and flexibility. Running your finger down the front of your neck, you can feel the bumps made by the cartilage rings.

Above the base of the trachea in midchest the lungs arch on either side like giant butterfly wings, then fall to fill out the bottom of each side of the thoracic cavity.

The Pleural Membranes

Both lungs are encased in moist, clinging, tissue-thin membrane called the *pleura,* which also lines the inside of the thoracic cavity where it comes into contact with the pleural coating of the lungs. The slippery pleural membranes hold tightly to each other, because there is an air lock or vacuum between them, but at the same time are free to slide over each other. The principle is the same as that illustrated by moistening the surfaces of two pieces of plate glass and placing the moistened surfaces together: the two pieces of glass will slide over each other but will resist being pried apart, because a partial vacuum exists between them.

The Pleural Cavity

The vacuum space between the pleura of the lung and the pleura of the thoracic cavity—although it is normally not a space at all—is called the *pleural cavity.* Each lung has its own pleural membrane: that of one lung does not interconnect with the other, so that one pleura may be injured without affecting the other.

It is extremely fortunate for us that the pleural linings both stick fast and can slide along each other's surfaces. Although the lungs are virtually without muscle, they are extremely elastic and in their natural condition are stretched fairly taut, held to the sides of the thoracic cavity by the suction of the pleura.

Collapsed Lung

Should this suction be broken and the pleural linings pull apart, the lung would shrink up like a deflated balloon. Such a condition, caused by the rush of outside air into the pleural cavity, is known medically as *pneumothorax* and causes a lung collapse. Violent injuries such as gun and stab wounds, various lung diseases, and obstructions of the breathing tubes can cause a lung or portion of a lung to collapse.

In the surgical procedure called *artificial pneumothorax,* a physician deliberately injects air between the pleural linings to collapse a portion of a lung. This is done to rest a lung in severe diseases such as tuberculosis, or to control heavy bleeding within the thoracic cavity.

Pleurisy

The intense chest pains called *pleurisy* are caused by inflammation of the pleura. The pleural linings lose their slipperiness and the increased friction stimulates pain receptors in the pleural lining of the chest. There are, however, no pain receptors in the lungs' pleural linings nor in the lungs themselves: this is why pain is not an early warning signal of lung cancer.

The Bronchi

Just behind the breastbone and just in front of the heart, the trachea divides into the right bronchus and the left bronchus, leading respectively to the right and left lungs. These are the primary two *bronchi* or *bronchial tubes.* Each is the main trunk of a bronchial tree that serves its respective lung.

Soon after leaving the trachea, each bronchus branches repeatedly into smaller tubes called *bronchioles,* which in turn branch into alveolar ducts, which terminate finally with the hundreds of millions of microscopic air sacs called alveoli, discussed at the beginning of this section. The alveoli are the site of the all-important exchange of carbon dioxide and oxygen.

Lobes and Segments

The larger right lung has three distinctive sections, or *lobes*—upper, middle, and lower. The left lung has only an upper and lower lobe. The lobes themselves are divided into smaller segments. Medically, these lobes and segments are important because they are somewhat independent of each other and can be damaged or removed surgically, as in operations for lung cancer, usually without damaging the function of adjacent, healthy segments or lobes.

The fact that a lung segment, lobe, or even an entire lung can be removed implies that we have plenty of reserve lung tissue, and this is indeed the case. When we are at rest, we use only about one-tenth of our total lung capacity. The total surface area exposed within our lungs to outside air is, amazingly, 600 square feet. This compares to a mere 20 square feet of skin surface. To appreciate the incredibly intricate, lacelike finery of the lungs' structure, we need only know that those 600 square feet of surface area are contained within two organs that together weigh only two-and-a-half pounds.

Oxygen Requirements

How much air do we breathe, and how much oxygen do we absorb into our body from the air? A normal, moderately active person breathes in and out (a complete respiration or breath cycle) about 18 times a minute; that is, the diaphragm contracts and relaxes 18 times a minute, or something over 25,000 times every day. At about four-fifths of a pint of air per breath cycle, this means that we inhale and exhale about 20,000 pints, or 10,000 quarts, or 2,500 gallons of air every day.

Only a very small proportion of this volume is oxygen that finds its way into our bloodstream: about a pint every minute in normal, quiet breathing, a little over 1,400 pints, or 700 quarts, or 175 gallons of oxygen every day. The amount of oxygen our lungs are capable of delivering to our body, however, varies tremendously: during sleep a person may need only a half-pint of oxygen per minute, half the average, while the lungs of a hard-driving athlete striving to break the mile record can deliver up to five quarts to the bloodstream—ten times the average.

At any given time, there are about two quarts of oxygen circulating in our blood. This is why a stoppage of breathing has an upper time limit of about four minutes before it causes irreversible damage or death. With our body needing about a pint of oxygen every minute for normal functioning, we have about four minutes before we use up the oxygen dissolved in our blood and other tissues.

Pollution Control–Filters, Cleaners, and Traps

Air pollution being what it is these days, it is fortunate that we have several natural devices that serve to filter out and wash away most of the impurities in the air we inhale.

Air gets into the lungs from outside about equally well via the nose or mouth. The mouth offers the advantage of getting more air in at a faster rate—absolutely a must if we have to push our body physically. But the nose has more and better equipment for cleaning air before it reaches the trachea. Via the mouth, air must only pass over a few mucous membranes and the tonsils, which can collect only so many germs and impurities.

Nose Filter System

Air taken in through the nose, however, first meets the "guard hairs" (*vibrissae*) of the nostrils, and then must circulate through the nasal cavity, a kind of cavern framed by elaborate scroll-shaped bones called *turbinates,* and lined with mucus-secreting membranes and waving, hairlike fibers called *cilia.* Foreign particles are caught by the cilia and carried away by the mucus, which drains slowly down the back of the throat.

It would be nice to be able to ascribe an important function to the eight *paranasal sinuses,* four on either side of the nose: the headache and discomfort of sinusitis might then be more bearable. But these "holes in the head" seem to exist simply to cause us trouble; for example—swelling to close the nasal air passages, making it impossible to breathe, as recommended, through the nose.

Filter System beyond the Nose

The cleansing and filtering action started in the nose and mouth does not stop there, but is repeated wherever air travels along the air passages of the lungs. Cilia project inward from the walls of even the tiniest bronchioles of the lungs, and impurities are carried from the alveoli on films of mucus that move ever back toward the trachea for expulsion—as when we cough. See also Ch. 12, *Diseases of the Respiratory System* and Ch. 13, *Lung Disease.*

The Endocrine Glands

Technically speaking, a gland is any cell or organ in our bodies that secretes some substance. In this broad sense, our liver is a gland, because one of its many functions is to secrete bile. So too, is the placenta that encloses a developing baby and supplies it with chemicals that assure normal growth. Even the brain has been shown by modern research to secrete special substances. But lymph glands are not considered true glands and are more correctly called lymph nodes.

Physicians divide the glands into two categories. *Endocrine glands* are

Endocrine Glands

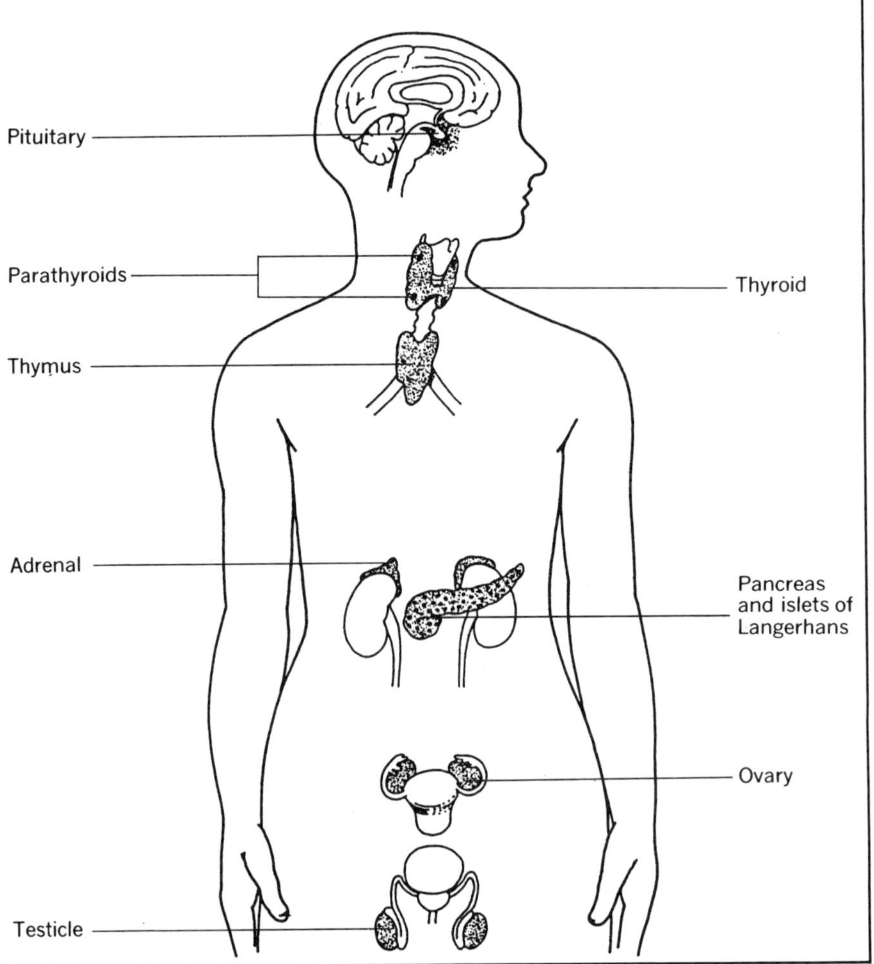

also known as *ductless glands,* because they release their secretions directly into the bloodstream. *Exocrine glands,* by contrast, usually release their substances through a duct or tube. Exocrine glands include the sebaceous and sweat glands of the skin; the mammary or milk glands; the mucous glands, some of which moisten the digestive and respiratory tract; and the salivary glands, whose secretions soften food after it enters the mouth. The pancreas has both an endocrine and an exocrine function and structure.

Role of the Endocrine Glands

The *endocrine glands* have the all-important role of regulating our body's internal chemistry. The substances they secrete are complex compounds called *hormones,* or chemical messengers.

Together with the brain and nerves, the system of endocrine glands controls the body's activities. The nervous system, however, is tuned for rapid responses, enabling the body to make speedy adjustments to changing circumstances, internal and external. The endocrine glands, with some exceptions, like the adrenal, are more concerned with the body's reactions over a longer period of time—from season to season, as it were. They regulate such processes as growth, levels of metabolism, fertility, and pregnancy.

For a group of tissues that exercise awesome power over our body's well-being, the endocrine glands are surprisingly small and inconspicuous—all of them together would weigh less than half a pound. Nor are they placed with any particular prominence in our body. They tend to be little lumps of tissue attached to or tucked behind grander bodily structures. Their power comes from the hormones they release into the bloodstream.

Scientists have discovered the exact chemical makeup of a number of these complex substances, have extracted several in pure form from living tissue, and have succeeded in making a few synthetically in the laboratory. This avenue of research, called *endocrinology,* has enabled physicians to treat persons suffering from certain endocrine gland disorders.

Hormones have been aptly described as chemical messengers. Their action, while still not completely understood, is that of catalysts. This means that the presence of a hormone (the name comes from a Greek word meaning "arouse to activity"), even in very small quantities, can affect the rate at which a chemical change occurs or otherwise stimulate a reaction, and without itself being affected. The hormone is a promoter, either of a positive or negative sort; it speeds up a process or slows it down.

The endocrine glands form an interdependent family. The functioning or malfunctioning of one can affect all the others.

The Pituitary–Master Gland

The *pituitary* is often called the master gland because the hormones it secretes play an active part in controlling the activities of all the other endocrine glands. This impressive power is wielded from two little bumps at the base of the brain, about midway between the ears at eye level. The two parts, or lobes, are connected by a tiny bridge of tissue, the three structures together being about the size of a small acorn. The lobe lying toward the front of the head is the *anterior lobe;* the one at the back, the *posterior lobe.* Each lobe is really an independent gland in itself, with its own quite distinct activities.

The Pituitary Gland

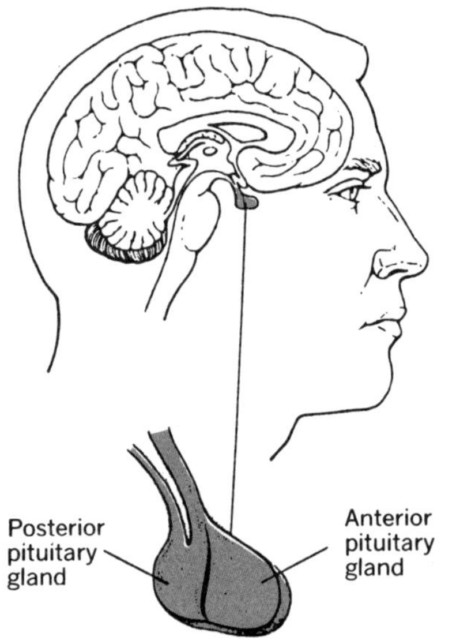

The Posterior Lobe and the Hypothalamus

The posterior lobe, so far as is known, does not make any of its own hormones, but serves as a storehouse for two hormones manufactured by the *hypothalamus.* The hypothalamus, apart from having a role in controlling the body's autonomic nervous system, also functions as an endocrine gland, secreting its own hormones, and as a connecting link between the brain's cerebral cortex and the pituitary gland.

The posterior lobe of the pituitary releases the two hormones it receives from the hypothalamus, called *vasopressin* and *oxytocin,* into the bloodstream. Vasopressin plays a role in the fluid balance of the body; oxytocin is thought to pace the onset and progress of labor during childbirth.

The Anterior Lobe

The anterior lobe secretes no fewer than six known hormones, five of which act as stimulators of hormone production by other endocrine glands. The sixth, identified as *somatotrophin* in medical textbooks, is more popularly known as the *growth-stimulating hormone* or simply as the growth hormone. It controls the rate of growth and multiplication of all the cells and tissues in our bodies—muscle, bone, and all our specialized organs.

Gigantism

In rare instances, during childhood, the pituitary releases too much or too little somatotrophin. If too much is secreted, the result is an overstimulation of growth processes, causing a disorder known as *gigantism.* Victims of this disorder have been known to grow nine feet tall and weigh 500 pounds.

Dwarfism

If too little somatotrophin is secreted, *dwarfism* results. This pituitary-type dwarf, of which Tom Thumb was one, is different from a dwarf suffering from a disorder of the thyroid (another endocrine gland, discussed below). The pituitary dwarf is usually well proportioned despite a miniature size, while the thyroid dwarf typically has short, deformed limbs.

Neither pituitary gigantism nor dwarfism affects basic intelligence. If oversecretion of somatotrophin occurs after full size has been reached—as, for example, because of a tumor affecting the pituitary, the condition known as *acromegaly* occurs. The bones enlarge abnormally, especially those of the hands, feet, and face.

Pituitary Gland

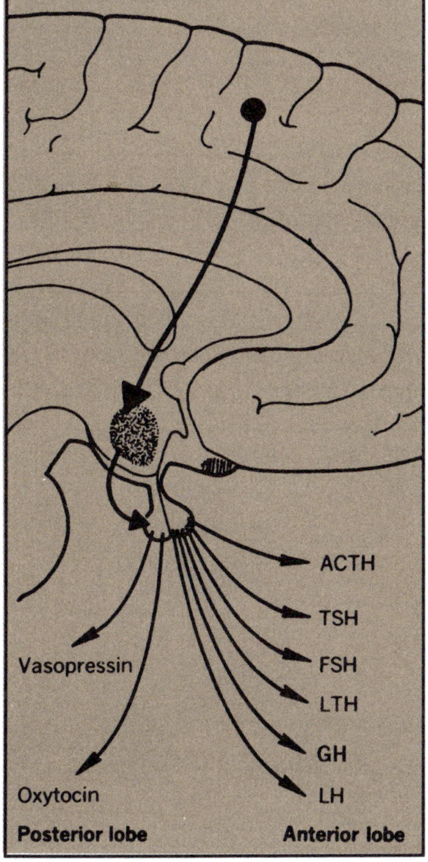

Anterior Pituitary Hormones

Of the five anterior pituitary hormones that regulate other endocrine glands, one affects the adrenal glands, one the thyroid, and the remaining three the sex glands or gonads (the testicles in men and the ovaries in women). Each is identified by a set of initials derived from its full name, as follows:

- *ACTH,* the *a*drenocor*t*icotrophic *h*ormone, affects the production of hormones by the outer "bark" of the adrenal glands, called the *adrenal cortex.*

- *TSH,* the *t*hyroid-*s*timulating *h*ormone, also known as *thyrotrophin,* causes the thyroid gland to step up production of its hormone, *thyroxin.*

- *FSH,* the *f*ollicle-*s*timulating *h*ormone, spurs production in women of estrogen, a sex hormone produced by the ovaries; and in men, of sperm by the testicles. Follicle here refers to the *Graafian follicles* in the ovary, which contain developing female egg cells whose growth is also stimulated by FSH. Graafian follicles have approximate counterparts in the male—tiny pouches (seminal vesicles) on either side of the prostate gland that store mature sperm cells.
- *LH,* the *l*uteinizing *h*ormone, transforms a Graafian follicle, after the follicle has released a ripened egg cell, into a kind of tissue called *corpus luteum.* The corpus luteum, in turn, produces *progesterone,* a hormone that prepares the mucous membrane lining the uterus (the endometrium) to receive a fertilized egg.
- *LTH,* the *lact*ogenic *h*ormone, or *luteotrophin,* stimulates the mother's mammary glands to produce milk; LTH also joins with LH in promoting the production of progesterone by the sex glands.

The last three hormones mentioned—follicle-stimulating, luteinizing, and lactogenic—are sometimes called the *gonadotrophic* hormones because they all stimulate activity of the gonads.

The Adrenal Glands

Resting like skull caps on the top of both kidneys are the two identical *adrenal glands.* Each has two distinct parts, secreting different hormones.

Adrenaline

The central internal portion of an adrenal gland is called the *medulla.* Its most potent contribution to our body is the hormone *adrenaline* (also called *epinephrine*). This is the hormone that, almost instantaneously, pours into our bloodstream when we face a situation that calls for extraordinary physical reaction—or keeps us going past what we think to be our normal limit of endurance.

A surge of adrenaline into the bloodstream stimulates our body to a whole array of alarm reactions—accelerating the conversion of stored foods into quick energy; raising the blood pressure; speeding up breathing; dilating the pupils of the eyes for more sensitive vision; and constrict-

Adrenal Glands

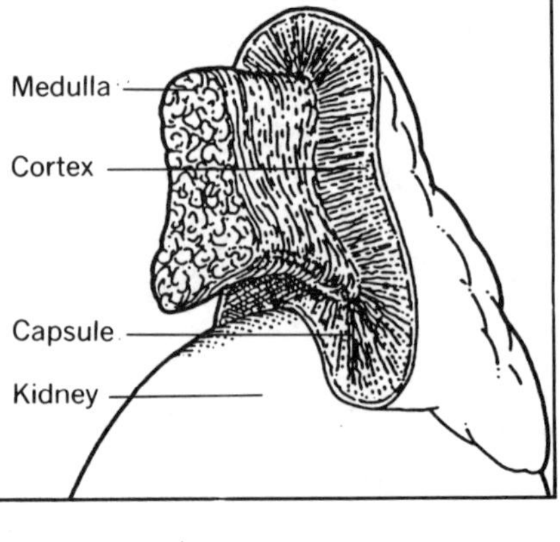

ing the blood vessels, making them less vulnerable to bleeding.

Adrenaline provides a good example of the interdependence of the endocrine system. Its production stimulates the secretion of ACTH by the pituitary gland. And ACTH, as noted above, causes the adrenal cortex to accelerate production of its hormones. Some of these adrenal cortex hormones enable the body to call up the reserves of energy it does not normally need. For example, body proteins are not usually a source of quick energy, but in an emergency situation, the adrenal cortex hormones can convert them to energy-rich sugar compounds.

The Adrenal Glands

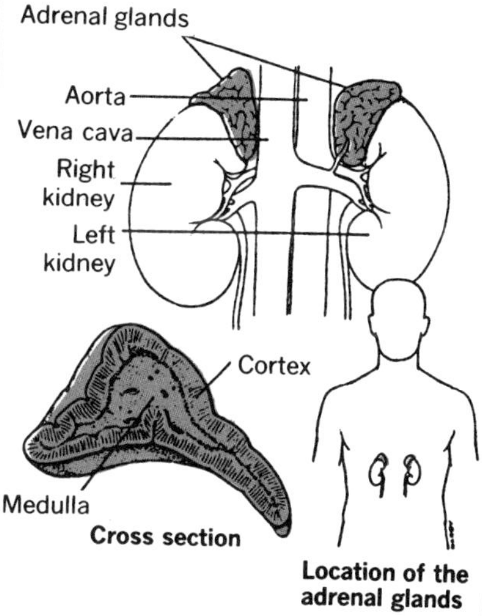

The Corticoids

There are some 30 different hormones, called the *corticoids,* manufactured in the adrenal cortex—the outer layer of the adrenal. A few of these influence male and female sexual characteristics, supplementing the hormones produced in the gonads. The others fall into two general categories: those that affect the body's metabolism (rate of energy use), and those that regulate the composition of blood and internal fluids. Without the latter hormones, for example, the kidneys could not maintain the water–salt balance that provides the most suitable environment for our cells and tissues at any given time.

Corticoids also influence the formation of antibodies against viruses, bacteria, and other disease-causing agents.

Extracts or laboratory preparations of corticoids, such as the well-known cortisone compounds, were found in the 1950s to be almost "miracle" medicines. They work dramatically to reduce pain, especially around joints, and hasten the healing of skin inflammations. Prolonged use, however, can cause serious side effects.

The Islets of Langerhans

Strewn at random throughout the pancreas are hundreds of thousands of tiny clusters of cells. Each of them, when seen under a powerful microscope, forms an "islet" of its own, similar to the other distinct islets, but markedly different from the pancreatic tissue surrounding it. These

The Pancreas and the Islets of Langerhans

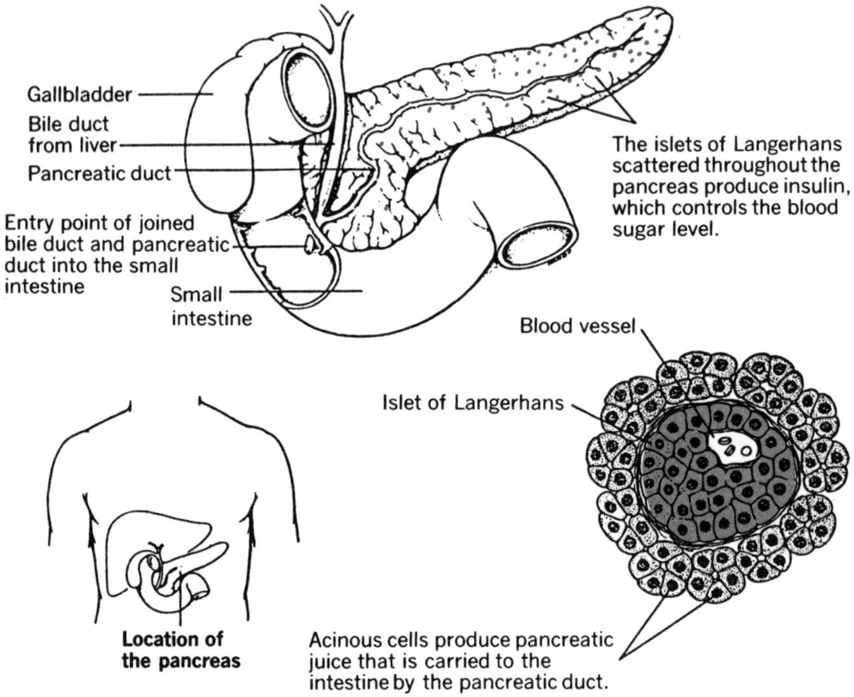

are the *islets of Langerhans,* named after the German scientist who first reported their existence in 1869. Each of these little cell clumps—up to two million or more of them—is a microscopic endocrine gland.

They secrete the hormone *insulin,* and the disease that occurs if they are not functioning properly is *diabetes mellitus.*

Actually, the islets of Langerhans produce not only insulin, but also a

The Pancreas and the Islets of Langerhans

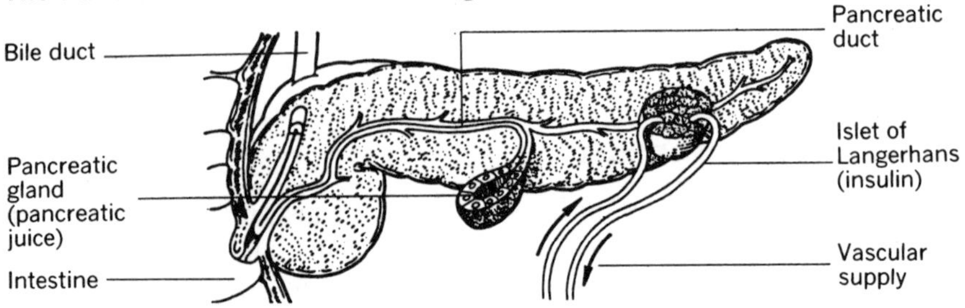

related hormone called *glucagon.* Both regulate the amount of sugar (glucose) that is present in the bloodstream and the rate at which it is used by the body's cells and tissues. Glucose supplies the energy for life and living processes.

When insulin and glucagon are not in sufficient supply, the cells' ability to absorb and use blood sugar is restricted, and much of the sugar passes unutilized out of the body in urine. Because the body's ability to obtain energy from food is one of the very foundations of life, diabetes calls for the most careful treatment.

One of the great advances of twentieth century medicine has been the pharmaceutical manufacture of insulin and its wide availability to diabetics. With regulated doses of insulin, a diabetic can now lead a normal life. See Ch. 15, *Diabetes Mellitus* for a full discussion of this disease.

The Thyroid Gland

The *thyroid gland* folds around the front and either side of the trachea (windpipe), at the base of the neck, just below the larynx. It resembles a somewhat large, stocky butterfly facing downward toward the chest.

Thyroxin

The thyroid hormone, *thyroxin,* is a complex protein-type chemical containing, along with various other elements, a large percentage of iodine. Like a number of other hormones manufactured by the endocrine glands, thyroxin affects various steps in the body's metabolism—in particular, the rate at which our cells and tissues use inhaled oxygen to burn the food we eat.

Hypothyroidism

A thyroid that is not producing enough thyroxin tends to make a person feel drowsy and sluggish, put on weight (even though his appetite is poor), and in general make his everyday activities tiresome and wearying. This condition is called *hypothyroidism.*

Hyperthyroidism

Its opposite—caused by too much secretion of thyroxin—is *hyperthyroidism.* A hyperthyroid person is jumpy, restless, and may eat hugely

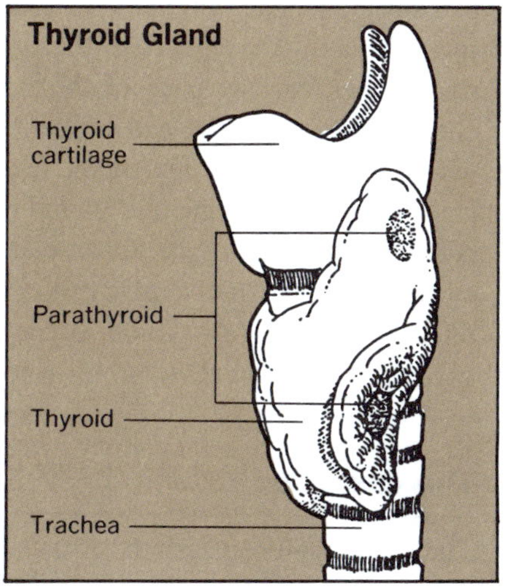

without gaining weight. The difference between the two extremes can be compared to environments regulated by two different thermostats, one set too high and the other set too low.

Although a normally functioning thyroid plays a significant part in making a person feel well, physicians today are less willing than in former years to blame a defective thyroid alone for listlessness or jittery nerves. Thirty or forty years ago it was quite fashionable to prescribe thyroid pills (containing thyroid extract) almost as readily as vitamins or aspirin; but subsequent medical research, revealing the interdependence of many glands and other body systems, made thyroxin's reign as a cure-all a short one.

Of course, where physical discomfort or lethargy can be traced to an underfunctioning thyroid, thyroxin remains an invaluable medicine.

Goiter

One disorder of the thyroid gland—the sometimes massive swelling called *goiter*—is the direct result of a lack of iodine in the diet. The normal thyroid gland, in effect, collects iodine from the bloodstream, which is then synthesized into the chemical makeup of thyroxin. Lacking iodine, the thyroid gland enlarges, creating a goiter. The abnormal growth will stop if iodine is reintroduced into the person's diet. This is the reason why most commercial table salt is iodized—that is, a harmless bit of iodine compound has been added to it.

The Parathyroid Glands

Four small glands, each about the size of a small pea, cling to the base of the thyroid gland, two on each of the thyroid's lobes curving back of the trachea. These are the *parathyroids,* whose main role is to control the level of calcium—as well as other elements needed in carefully regulated amounts by the body—in the bloodstream and tissues. The parathyroids secrete two hormones: *parathormone* when blood calcium is too low; *calcitonin* when the calcium level is too high. These hormones work by controlling the interchange of calcium between bones and blood.

A symptom of defective parathyroids is *tetany*—a chronic or acute case of muscle spasms, which can be controlled by administration of synthetic parathyroidlike chemicals or concentrated vitamin D preparations.

The Gonads

The *gonads* refer to both the two male testicles and the two female ovaries.

There are four hormones secreted by the gonads: the female sex hor-

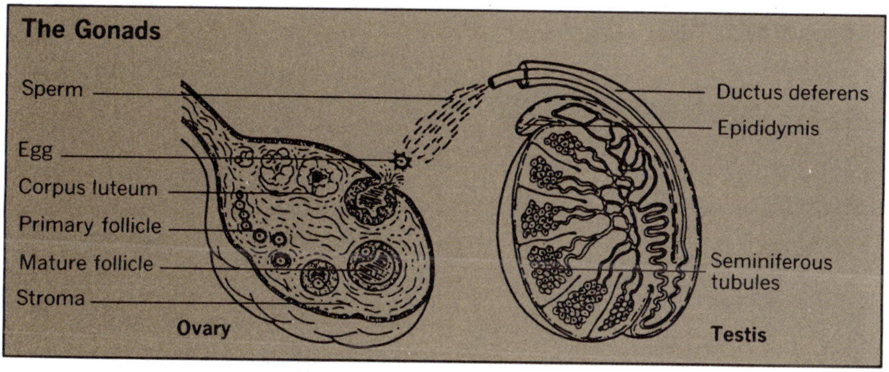

mones, *estrogen* and *progesterone;* and the male hormones, *testosterone* and *androsterone.* Each sex merely has a predominance of one or the other pair of hormones. Men have some of the female hormones, and women some of the male hormones.

In both sexes, puberty is signaled by the release of the gonadotrophic hormones (or *gonadotrophins*) of the pituitary gland. These stimulate the production of sex hormones by the sex glands and the subsequent appearance of secondary sexual characteristics. In men, these include the enlargement of testicles and penis, growth of facial, axillary (armpit) and pubic hair, and enlargement of the larynx, resulting in deepening of the voice. Pubescent women also experience pubic and axillary hair growth, in addition to breast growth and changes in the genital tract that give it child-bearing capability.

Estrogen and progesterone control the cyclic changes within the uterus that involve the development, ripening, and discharge of the egg (ovulation) to be fertilized; the preparation of the lining of the uterus to receive a fertilized egg; and this lining's subsequent dismantling—all the complex biochemical events that occur as part of every woman's menstrual cycle.

The Thymus and Pineal Glands

These are the least known of the endocrine family; in fact, physicians do not know the function of one of them—the *pineal*—and are not even agreed that it is an endocrine gland. Situated near the hypothalamus, at the base of the brain, this tiny, pine-cone-shaped body has follicles that suggest a glandular function and some calcium-containing bits that medical researchers have descriptively dubbed "brain sand."

The *thymus,* only slightly better understood, has the intriguing characteristic of shrinking in size as a person grows up. It is located in the middle of the chest, about midway between the base of the neck and the

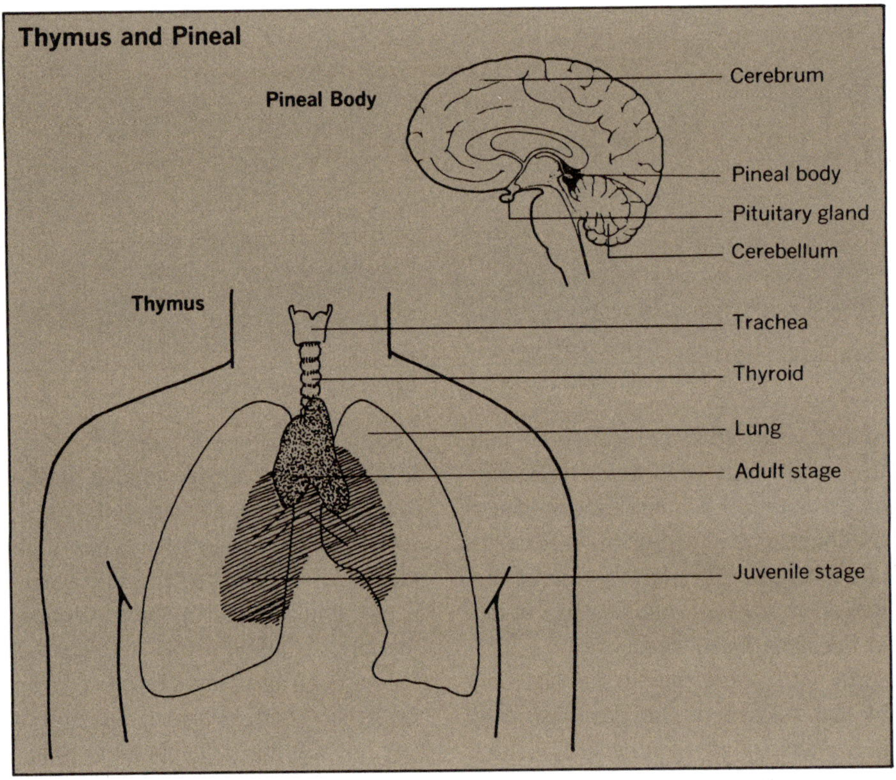

breast line. There is some evidence that the secretions of the thymus play a role in the body's natural immunity defenses. See also Ch. 14, *Diseases of the Endocrine Glands.*

The Sense Organs

Once upon a time, a grade-school teacher would ask, "How many senses do we have?" And his pupils would confidently chorus back, "Five!" People who displayed a knack for predicting future events, or whose quick reactions seemed to give them a jump over most everybody else, were credited with having a "sixth sense."

Scientists now recognize about twice that number—12 or 13 or more. Man, of course, has not grown a number of new senses in addition to the traditional five: sight, hearing, touch, smell, and taste. What has happened is that scientists have discovered many more specific kinds of sense receptor cells. For example, whereas touch was formerly thought of as just one sense, it has now been divided into no less than five different senses, each having its own special kind of receptor cell in the skin.

We can talk with a little more justification of the five sense organs, the five anatomical structures we associate with our senses—the eyes, ears, nose, tongue, and skin. But here, too, it does seem to be oversimplifying things to thus equate the nose—having only a tiny patch of olfactory (sense of smell) receptor cells—with the marvelously complex arrangement of sensing structures that make up the eye. Moreover, the other sense organs are not nearly so specialized as the eye. For example, a good case could be made for the nose being more valuable as an air purifier than as an organ of smell, or for the tongue being more valuable as an aid in digestion than as a source of the taste sensation.

Suppose we accept the proposition that pain is one of the senses of the skin; how then do we explain a pain from inside our bodies—say, a stomachache or a deep muscle pain? The answer, of course, is that there are pain receptors in many other places besides the skin.

What Is a Sense?

A sense is a nerve pathway, one end of which (the receptor end) responds in a certain way to a certain condition affecting our bodies, and whose other end reaches to a part of our brain that informs our conscious mind of what has happened or is happening. A sense is thus distinguished from the body's countless other nerve pathways by the fact that our brain *consciously* registers its impulses, although the impulses themselves are no different from those of the autonomic nervous system.

While remaining aware of the limitations of the traditional list of five sense organs, let us now analyze what they can do and how they operate:

- The eye (vision): Nerve impulses to the brain are stimulated by light waves, from which the brain forms visual images.
- The ears (hearing): Nerve impulses to the brain are stimulated by sound waves, out of which the brain forms meaningful noise, such as speech. Deep within the ear, also, are structures that give us balance.
- The nose (olfaction): Nerve impulses to the brain are stimulated by airborne chemical substances, moistened within the nasal cavity, from which the brain elicits distinctive smells.
- The tongue (taste): Nerve impulses to the brain are stimulated (in presence of water) by chemical substances in food, from which the brain forms sensations of sweet, salty, sour, bitter, savory (umami), or combinations of these tastes.
- Skin (touch): Nerve impulses to the brain are stimulated by the

presence of outside physical forces and changes in the physical environment, including varying temperatures, which the brain registers as feelings of contact, pressure, cold, heat, and pain. (Some medical texts add traction, as when the skin is pulled or pinched, as well as the sensation of tickle.)

The Eye

Rather than take a name-by-name anatomical tour of the eye, let's instead take just three programmed tours of the eye to explore:

- the transformation of light energy into vision;
- focusing, or how the structure of the eye prepares light for transformation into vision; and
- the supporting structures and service units of the eye.

Transforming Light Energy into Vision

If you could look through the opening in the front of your eye (the *pupil*), and see to the very back surface of your eye (as if you could see through the needle valve opening to the inside skin of a basketball), you would see your own *retina.* On your retina are located all the sense receptor cells that enable us to see. There are none anywhere else in the body.

Rods and Cones

A good argument can be made that man's vision is really *two* senses. For on the paper-thin retina are two quite anatomically distinct sense receptors (nerve endings) named, for their appearance under high magnification,

Eye

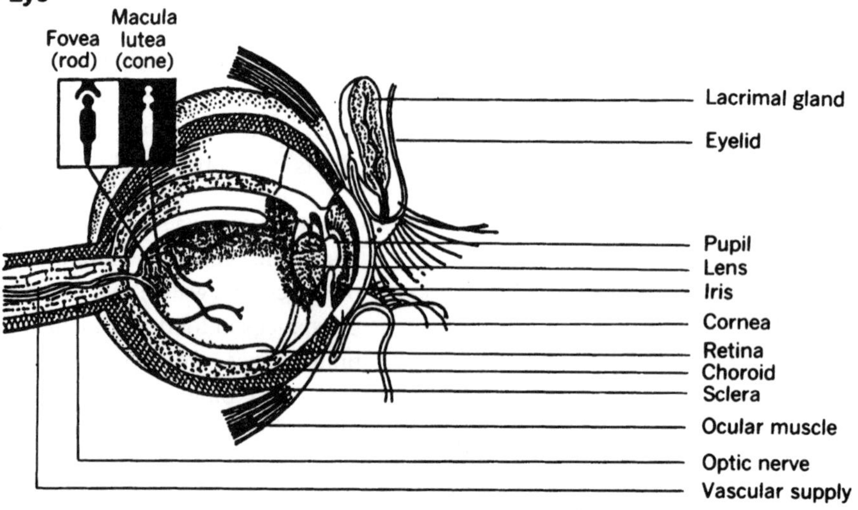

cones and *rods*. The cones are concentrated at a tiny spot on the retina called the *fovea*.

If the focusing machinery of the eye (cornea, lens, etc.) is working just right, light rays from the outside have their sharpest focus on the fovea. Surrounding the fovea is a yellowish area called the *macula lutea* (Latin, "yellow spot"). Together, the fovea and macula lutea make a circle not much bigger than the head of a pin.

All our seeing of colors and fine details is accomplished by the cones of the fovea and the macula lutea. Beyond the yellowish circumference of the macula lutea, there are fewer and fewer cones: rods become the dominant structures on the retina. It has been estimated that there are something less than 10 million cones on the retina of each eye, but more than 10 times as many rods—100 million of them or more.

Although the tight circle of cones in each eye gives man his ability to do close, detailed work (including reading) and to discriminate colors, the cones are virtually useless in detecting objects that are a bit off center from our direct focus, and furthermore operate only in good lighting conditions or in response to bright light sources.

The rods compensate for the specialized limits of the cones. They take over completely in dim light, and also give us the ability to detect peripheral objects and movements—"out of the corner of the eye." Because the rods are not sensitive to colors, our seeing at night is almost completely in black-and-white.

You can give yourself an interesting demonstration of the interacting functions of your own cones and rods if you walk from bright, sunny daylight into a dimly lit theater. In the bright light, your cones have been picking out sharp images and colors. But once in dimness, the cones become inoperative. For a few moments, in fact, you may see almost nothing at all.

Visual Purple

The momentary interval after the cones stop working but before the rods begin to function is explained by a curious pigment present in the eye called *visual purple*. This substance is manufactured constantly by the rods, and must be present for the rods to respond to dim light—but it is destroyed when exposed to bright light. Thus, after entering a darkened room, it takes a few moments for visual purple to build up in the retina. One of the principal constituents of visual purple is vitamin A, which is why this vitamin (present in carrots and other yellow produce) is said to increase our capacity to see in the dark.

The Optic Nerve

Every nerve ending is part of a larger unit, a neuron or nerve cell, and the sense receptors called rods and cones are no exception. Like all nerve cells, each rod and cone sports a long nerve fiber or *axon* leading away from the site of reception. In each eye, fibers serving the hundred-million-plus rods and cones all converge at a certain spot just behind the retina, forming the *optic nerve.* There are no rods and cones at the point where the optic nerve exits from behind the retina at the back of the eyeball: that is why everybody has a "blind spot" at that point. An image passing through that spot completely disappears.

From the retinas, both optic nerves set a course almost directly through the middle of the brain. Right and left optic nerves converge, their individual fibers partially intertwining a short distance behind the eyes. Then this joint optic nerve trunk proceeds toward the rear of the head, where the *occipital lobes,* the brain's "centers for seeing," are located. Just before reaching the occipital lobes, the optic nerve splits again into thousands of smaller nerve bundles (called *visual radiations*) that disappear into the visual cortex or "outer bark" of the occipital lobes. Only at this point are the bits of light energy that have stimulated our rods and cones transformed into images that our brain can "see."

Focusing and Light Control

Lacking the structures of the retina and their connection to the brain via the optic nerve, we could not see. Lacking reasonably normal functioning of the cornea, lens, and iris, we do not see well.

Good vision depends upon the eye being able to bend incoming light rays in such a way that the image being observed falls directly on the retina—in other words, upon proper focusing. The bending or *refraction* of light rays is the joint work of two curves, transparent slivers of specialized tissue through which light passes on its way to the retina. These are the *cornea* and the *lens.* Broadly speaking, the degree of curvature and thickness of these two structures determines whether we see well or poorly, are nearsighted or farsighted.

The Cornea and Lens

The cornea, which does the major light-bending, has a virtually fixed curvature and thickness. The lens puts the finishing touches on the focusing. Its thickness and curvature are adjustable—more or less without our conscious awareness—depending on whether we wish to focus on something nearer or farther away. The lens is made thicker or thinner, a process called *accommodation,* by the relaxing and contracting of tiny, attached *ciliary muscles.* Normally, these muscles do not have to work at all if we are looking at objects more than 20 feet away: but they often are overworked by a great deal of close work.

Focusing

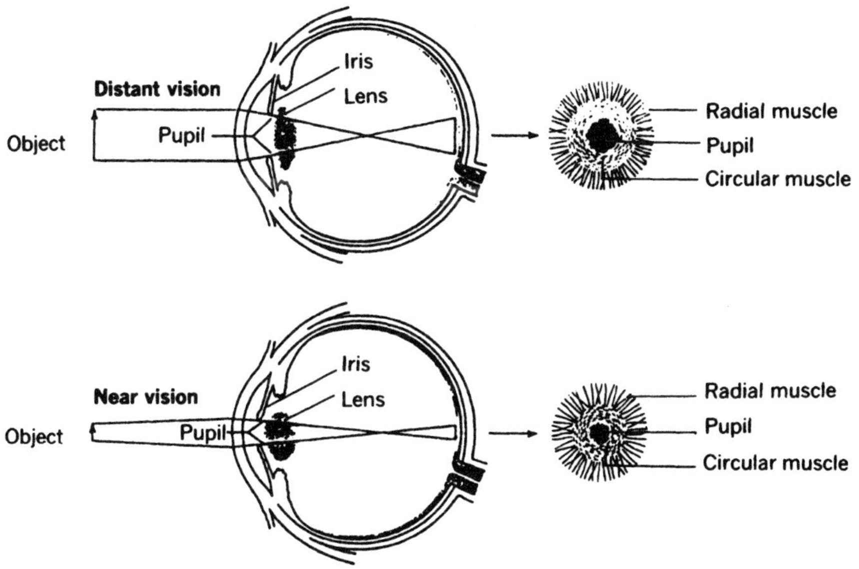

When viewing a distant object (more than 20 feet away), the lens flattens and the pupil dilates, allowing more light to enter the eye. The pupil is dilated by the action of the outer radial muscles of the iris, which contract and thus stretch the previously contracted circular muscles. When viewing a near object, the lens becomes more oval and the pupil contracts as more light enters the eye. This prevents overstimulation of the retina. The pupil is reduced in size by the contraction of the inner circular muscles, which serve to stretch the previously contracted radial muscles.

The Pupil and Iris

Effective focusing in various light conditions also depends upon the diameter of the hole through which light enters the eye. This hole is the *pupil.* Its diameter is controlled automatically—wider in dim light, narrower in bright light—by the muscles of the surrounding *iris.* The iris muscle contains pigment that gives our eyes color (brown, blue, green, etc.). The pupil, opening into the dark interior chamber of the eye, is black. A fully dilated (widened) pupil, as would occur in the dimmest light, illuminates over 15 times more retinal surface than the tiny "pinhole" pupil of an eye exposed to very bright light.

Structural Support and Protection of Eye

Two outer layers protect the eye. The tough outermost layer is the *sclera,* the white of the eye. Underlying the sclera is another layer, the *choroid,* which contains numerous tiny blood vessels that service the sclera and other structures on the eyeball. Both sclera and choroid have concentric openings that allow for the hole of the pupil. The cornea is really

Muscles of the Eye

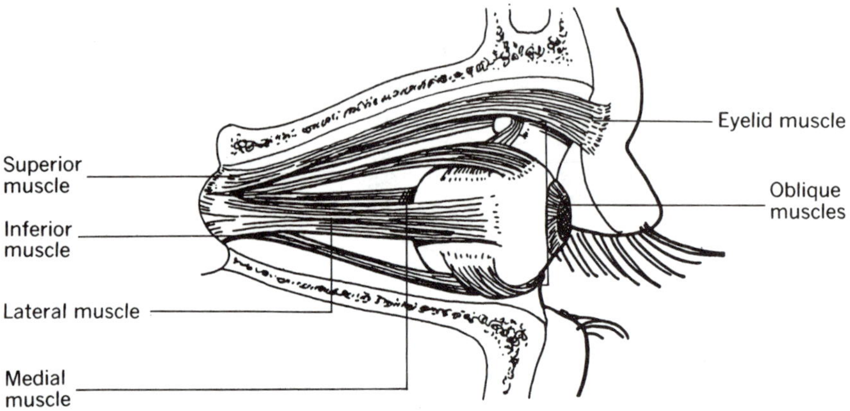

a specialized extension of the sclera, and the iris of the choroid.

Two trapped reservoirs of fluid within the eye are important in maintaining the eye's shape as well as the frictionless operation of its moving parts. These two reservoirs contain fluids called the *aqueous humor* and *vitreous humor.* The tiny space between the cornea and lens, corresponding to the pupil, is called the anterior chamber and is filled with the clear, watery, aqueous humor. The larger interior space behind the lens is called the posterior chamber, and is filled with the vitreous humor.

Muscles for Movement of Eye

In addition to the tiny muscles within the eye that control the opening of the pupil and the shape of the lens, we also have a number of elegant muscles that control the movements of each eyeball, and make both eyeballs move together in unison.

The movements of each eyeball are affected by six muscles attached to its top, bottom, and sides. The teamwork between these muscles—some contracting while others relax—allows the eye to move from side to side, up and down, and at all intermediate angles (obliquely). One of our eyes is always a dominant or leading eye; that is, its movements

Ciliary Muscle Contraction

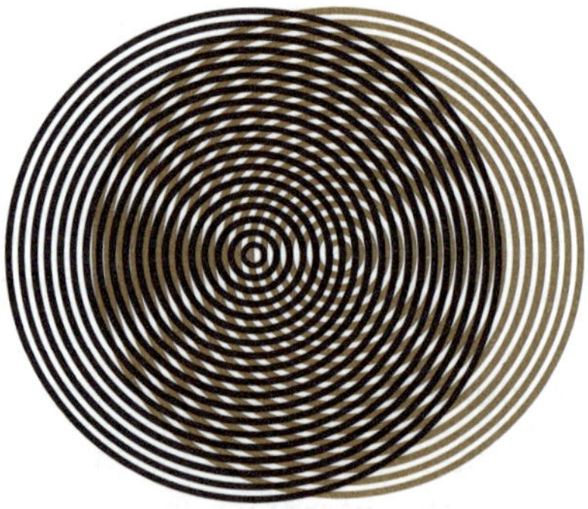

The apparent flickering of the circles is caused by contractions of the ciliary muscles, which control the accommodation (or change in thickness) of the lens for accurate focusing of objects at a variety of distances.

are always followed by the other eye.

Our protective eyelids, of course, are controlled by opening and closing muscles that lie outside the eye proper. These muscles can function both voluntarily and involuntarily.

Lubrication and Hygiene of Eye

Without the moisture provided by tears, our eyeball would scrape excruciatingly on the inside lining (*conjunctiva*) of the eyelid. In addition to lubrication, tears also have a cleansing action, not only because they supply water for washing and rinsing but also because they contain a mild germicide called *lysozyme* that kills bacteria and other potentially harmful microbes.

Tears are produced by the *lacrimal glands* above the eyeball, just under the eyebrow, a bit further toward the temple side than the nose side. They are discharged from several short ducts and spread over the surface of the eyeball by blinking. The *conjunctival sac* at the bottom inner (nose) side of the eye—visible in the mirror as a pinkish flap of tissue—serves as a collecting pool for tears; from there, they drain down a duct into the nasal cavity. This is why somebody who is crying also snuffles and must blow his nose.

There is another tiny drainage network in the eye, located at the interconnection of the cornea and iris, which serves to keep the fluid pressure of the space filled by the aqueous humor within normal limits. Drainage of this area is through microscopic conduits called the *canals of Schlemm.* Improper drainage can cause build-up of pressure, such as occurs in glaucoma, and impairment or loss of vision.

The Ear

Within the tunnels and chambers of the ear lie the two special types of sense receptors that give us, respectively, the sense of hearing and the sense of balance.

The Outer Ear

The *outer ear* includes that rather oddly shaped and folded piece of flesh and cartilage from which earrings are hung, and more important, the external *auditory canal,* a tunnel leading from the ear's opening to the *tympanic membrane,* or *eardrum.*

The Middle Ear

The *middle ear* includes the inner surface of the eardrum and the three tiny, bony *ossicles,* named long ago for their shape (apparently by some blacksmithing anatomist), *the hammer, the anvil,* and *the stirrup;* or in Latin: *the malleus, the incus,* and *the stapes.* These bones respond to the

Ear

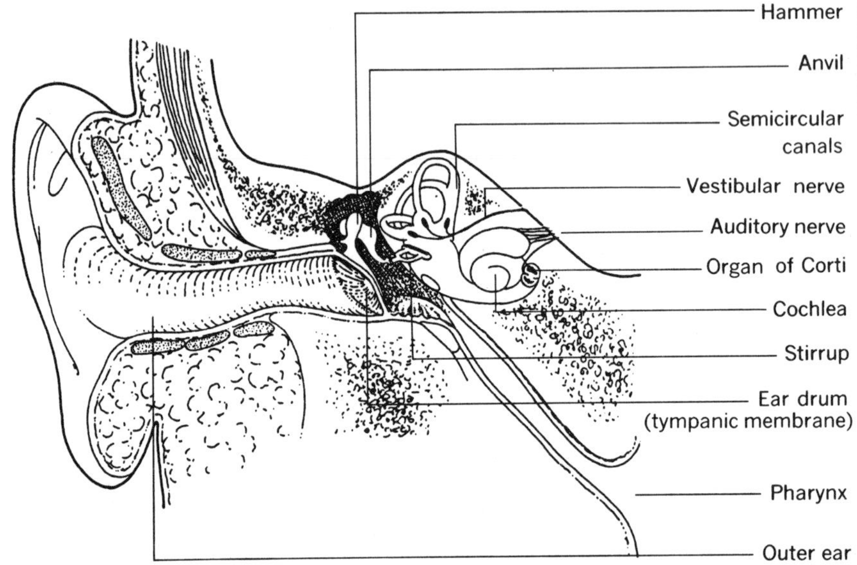

vibrations in the air that are the basis of sound, vibrate themselves, and transmit their vibrations to the inner ear, where the sense receptors for hearing are located, and the *auditory* (or *acoustic*) *nerve* to the brain begins.

The middle ear is connected to the back of the throat (pharynx) by the Eustachian tube. This tunnel between throat and middle ear makes the pressure on the inside of the eardrum, via the mouth, the same as the pressure of the atmosphere on the outside of the eardrum. (Thus yawning helps to equalize pressure.) Without it, or if the Eustachian tube becomes clogged, the taut membrane of the eardrum would always be in imminent danger of bursting.

The Inner Ear

The chambers of the *inner ear* are completely filled with fluid, which is jostled by the ossicles "knocking" on a thin membrane called the oval window, separating the middle from the inner ear. Another flexible membrane, the round window, serves to restrict the motion of the inner ear fluid when the movement is too stormy.

Organ of Hearing

Within the inner ear is a bony structure coiled like a snail shell about the size of a pea. This is the *cochlea,* the actual Latin word for snail or snail shell. Following the internal spiral of the cochlea is the *organ of Corti,* the

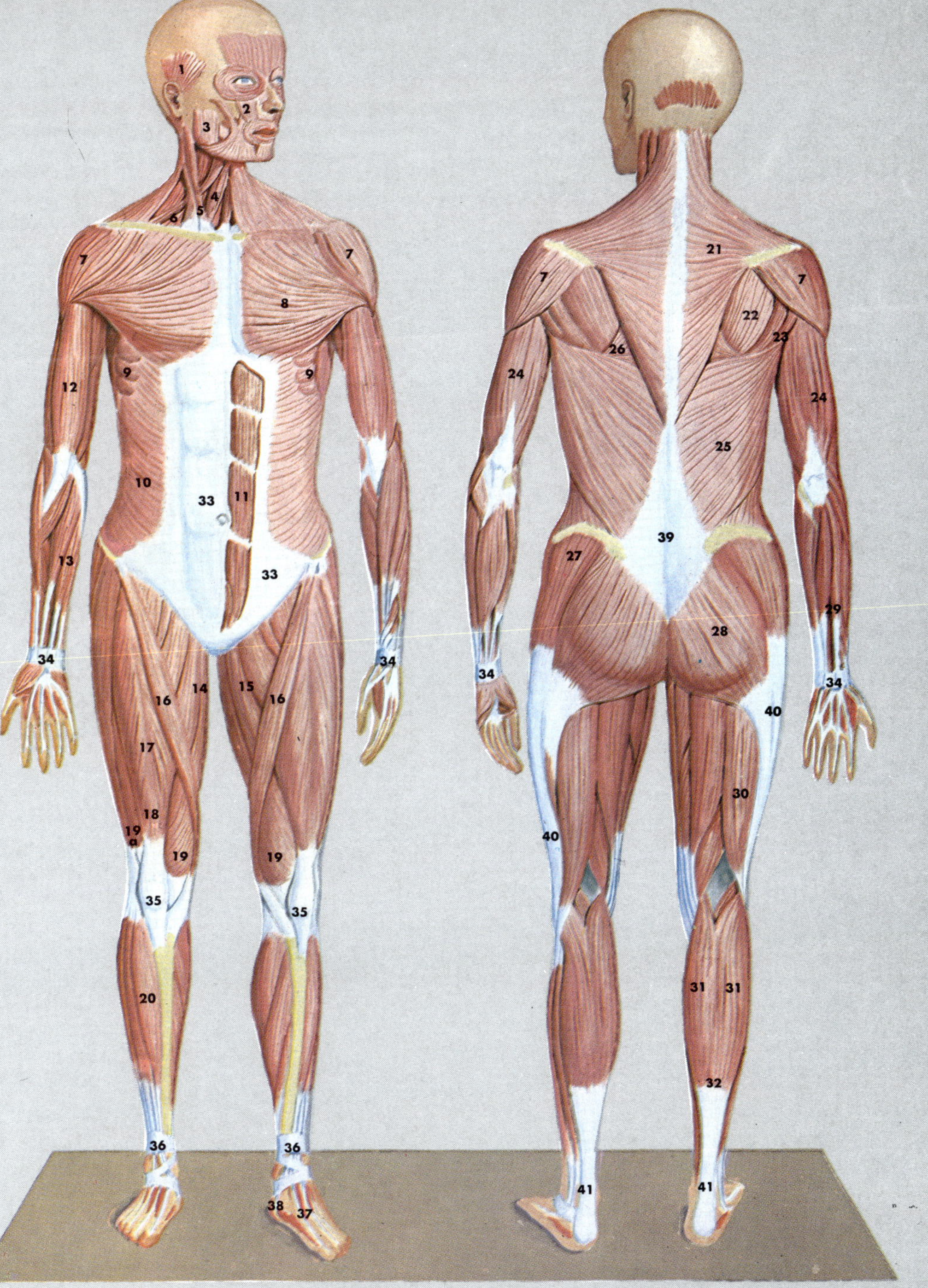

MUSCLES AND TENDONS

MUSCLES

1. Temporal
2. Mimetic muscles
3. Masseter (a muscle of mastication)
4. Infrahyoid muscles
5. Sternomastoid
6. Omohyoid
7. Deltoid
8. Pectoral muscles
9. Serratus anterior
10. External oblique
11. Rectus abdominus
12. Biceps brachii
13. Flexor digitorum superficialis (sublimis)
14. Gracilis
15. Adductor group
16. Sartorius
17. Rectus femoris
18. Quadriceps femoris
19. Vastus medialis

19a. Vastus lateralis

20. Dorsiflexors
21. Trapezius
22. Infraspinatus
23. Teres major
24. Triceps brachii
25. Latissimus dorsi
26. Rhomboideus major
27. Gluteus medius
28. Gluteus maximus
29. Digital extensors
30. Hamstring muscles
31. Gastrocnemius
32. Plantar flexors

TENDONS

33. Rectus sheath
34. Flexor retinaculum of carpal tunnel
35. Patellar tendon
36. Retinaculum of tarsal tunnel
37. Tendons of long digital extensors
38. Tendon of tibialis anterior
39. Lumbodorsal fascia
40. Fascia lata
41. Achilles

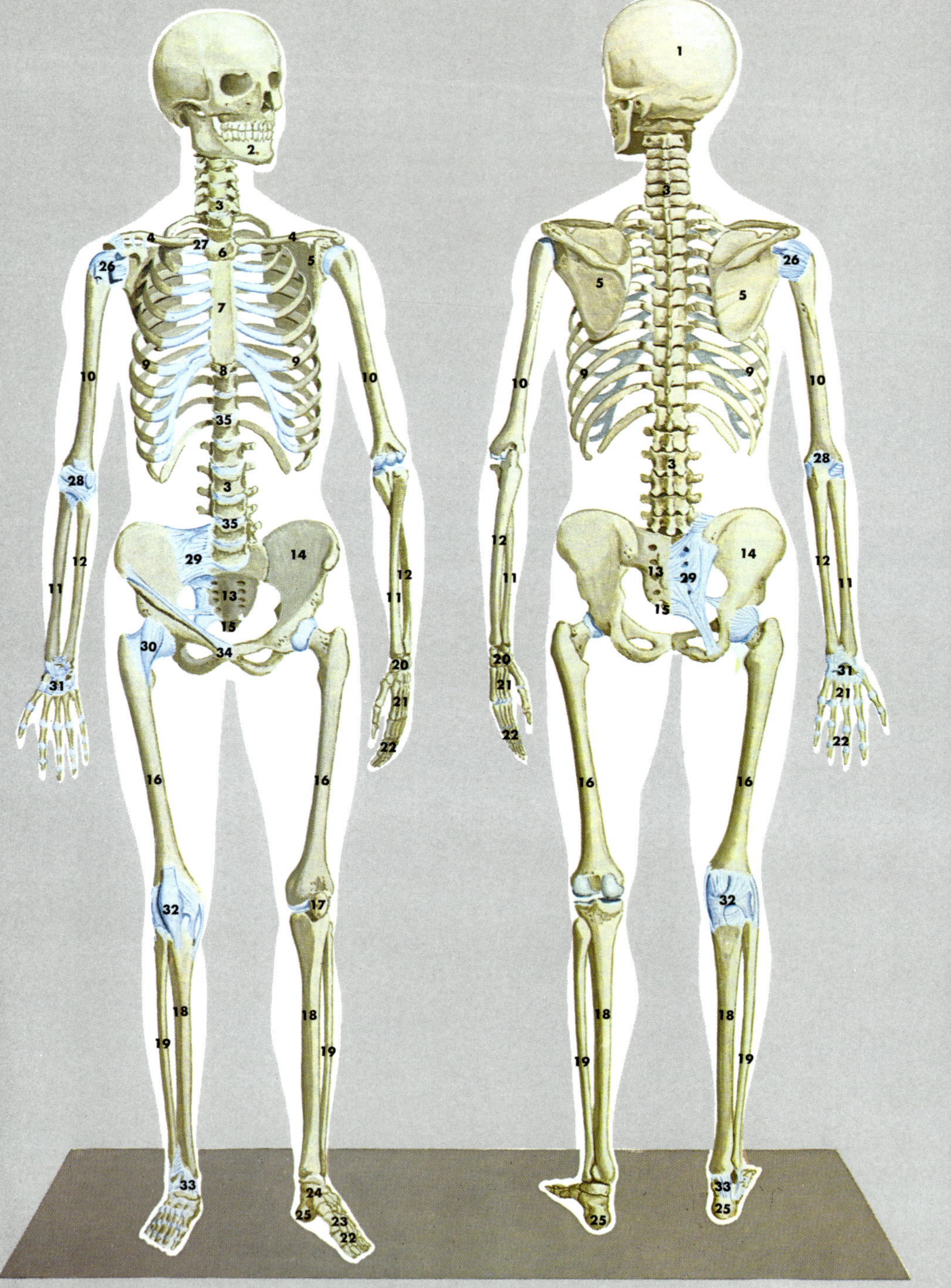

BONES AND LIGAMENTS

BONES
1. Skull
2. Mandible
3. Vertebrae
4. Clavicle
5. Scapula
6. Manubrium
7. Body of sternum
8. Xiphoid process
9. Ribs
10. Humerus
11. Radius
12. Ulna
13. Sacrum
14. Ilium
15. Coccyx
16. Femur
17. Patella
18. Tibia
19. Fibula
20. Carpals
21. Metacarpals
22. Phalanges
23. Metatarsals
24. Tarsals
25. Heel

LIGAMENTS AND JOINTS
26. Capsule of shoulder
27. Sternoclavicular
28. Capsule of elbow
29. Sacroiliac
30. Iliofemoral
31. Wrist
32. Capsule of knee
33. Ankle
34. Pubic symphysis
35. Intervertebral discs

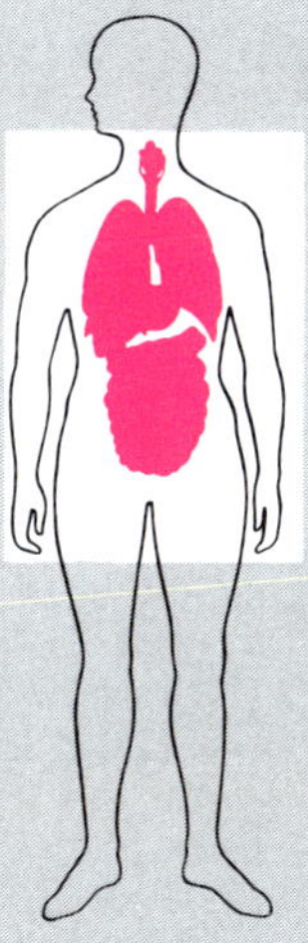

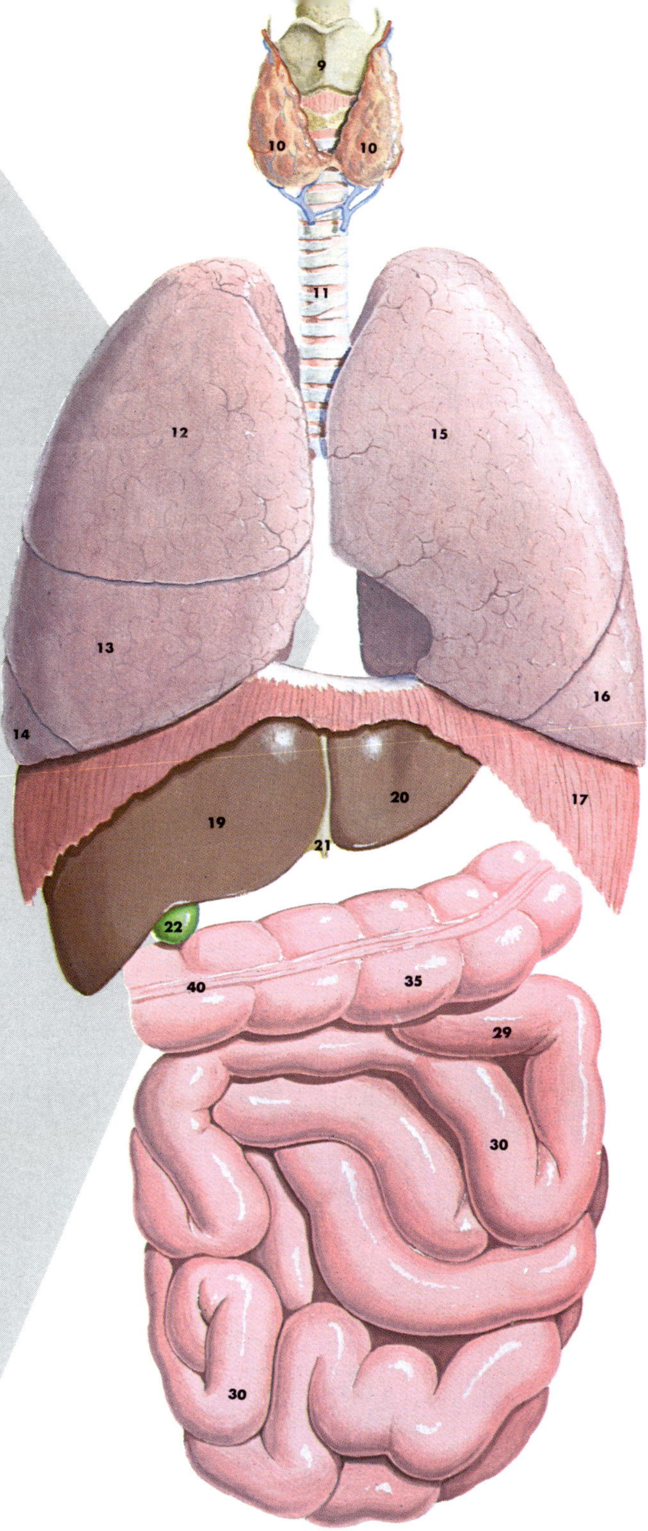

ANTERIOR LUNGS, LIVER, AND SMALL INTESTINE

9. Larynx
10. Thyroid gland
11. Trachea
12. Lung (Right superior lobe)
13. Lung (Right middle lobe)
14. Lung (Right inferior lobe)
15. Lung (Left superior lobe)
16. Lung (Left inferior lobe)
17. Diaphragm
19. Liver (Right lobe)
20. Liver (Left lobe)
21. Falciform ligament
22. Gall bladder
29. Jejunum
30. Small intestine
35. Transverse colon
40. Taenia

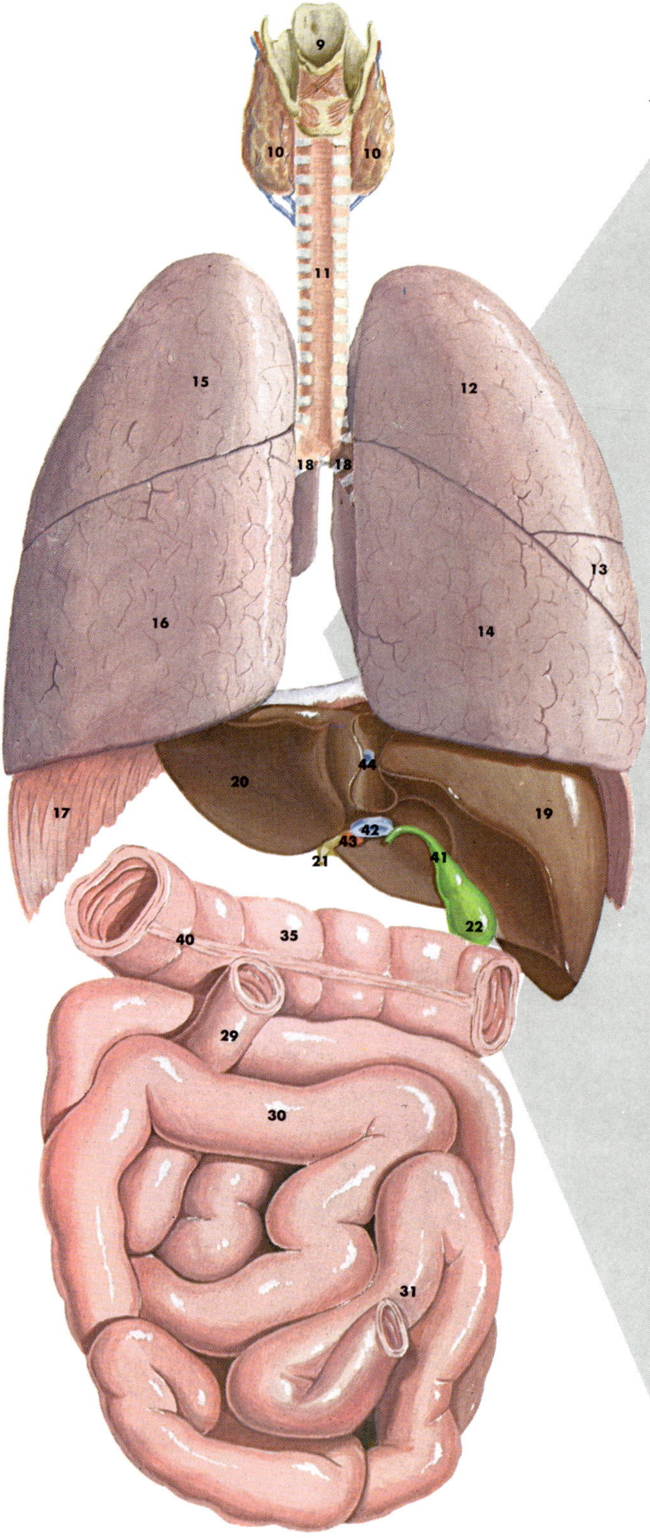

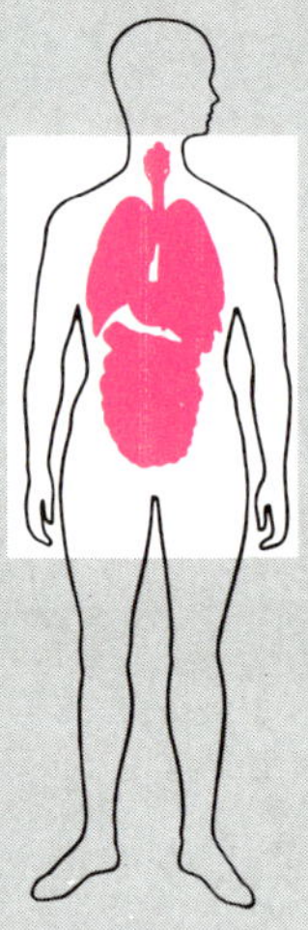

POSTERIOR LUNGS, LIVER, AND SMALL INTESTINE

9. Larynx
10. Thyroid gland
11. Trachea
12. Lung (Right superior lobe)
13. Lung (Right middle lobe)
14. Lung (Right inferior lobe)
15. Lung (Left superior lobe)
16. Lung (Left inferior lobe)
17. Diaphragm
18. Principal bronchi
19. Liver (Right lobe)
20. Liver (Left lobe)
21. Falciform ligament
22. Gall bladder
29. Jejunum
30. Small intestine
31. Ileum
35. Transverse colon
40. Taenia coli
41. Cystic duct
42. Portal vein
43. Hepatic artery
44. Hepatic vein

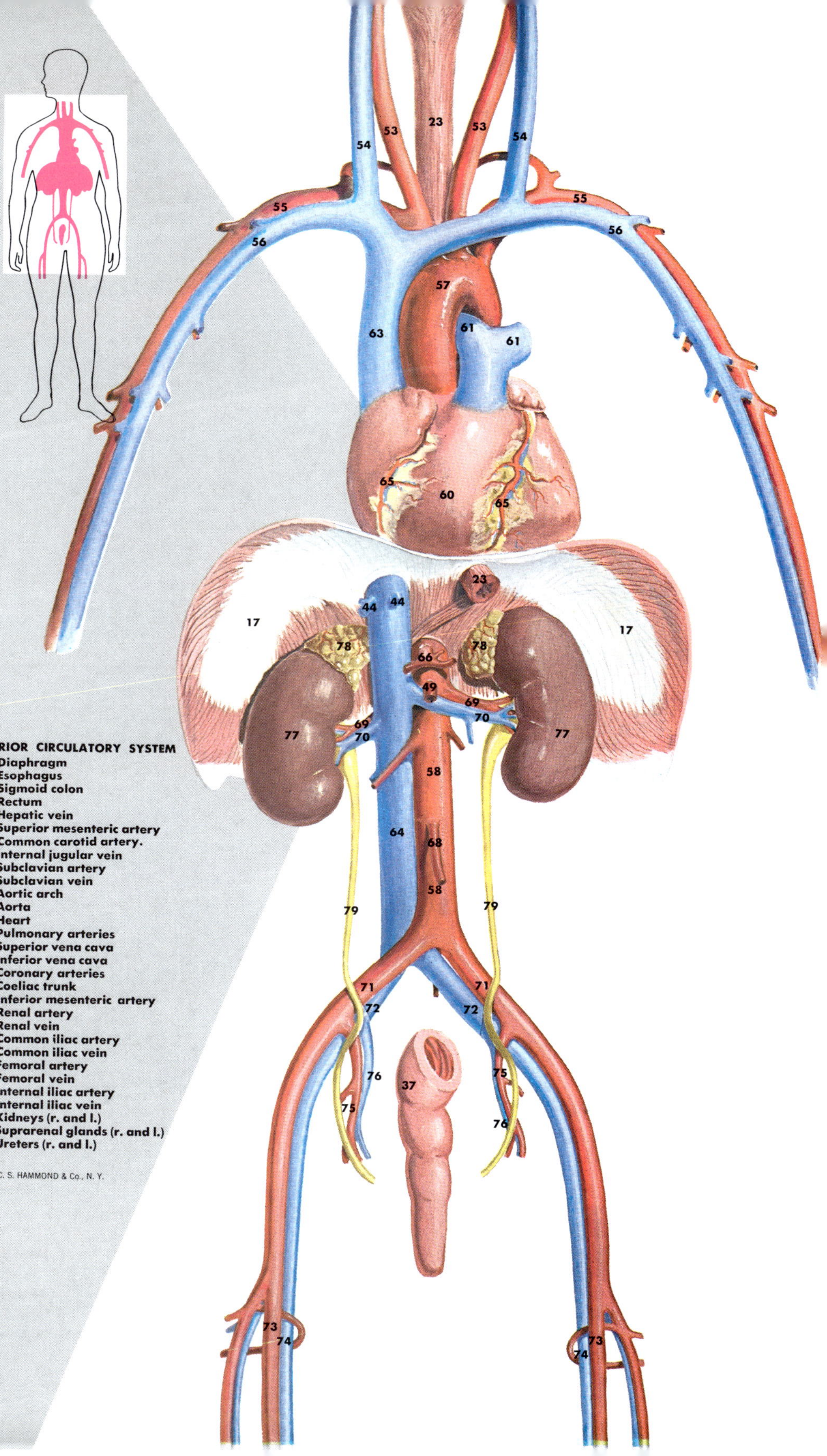

ANTERIOR CIRCULATORY SYSTEM

17. Diaphragm
23. Esophagus
37. Sigmoid colon
38. Rectum
44. Hepatic vein
49. Superior mesenteric artery
53. Common carotid artery.
54. Internal jugular vein
55. Subclavian artery
56. Subclavian vein
57. Aortic arch
58. Aorta
60. Heart
61. Pulmonary arteries
63. Superior vena cava
64. Inferior vena cava
65. Coronary arteries
66. Coeliac trunk
68. Inferior mesenteric artery
69. Renal artery
70. Renal vein
71. Common iliac artery
72. Common iliac vein
73. Femoral artery
74. Femoral vein
75. Internal iliac artery
76. Internal iliac vein
77. Kidneys (r. and l.)
78. Suprarenal glands (r. and l.)
79. Ureters (r. and l.)

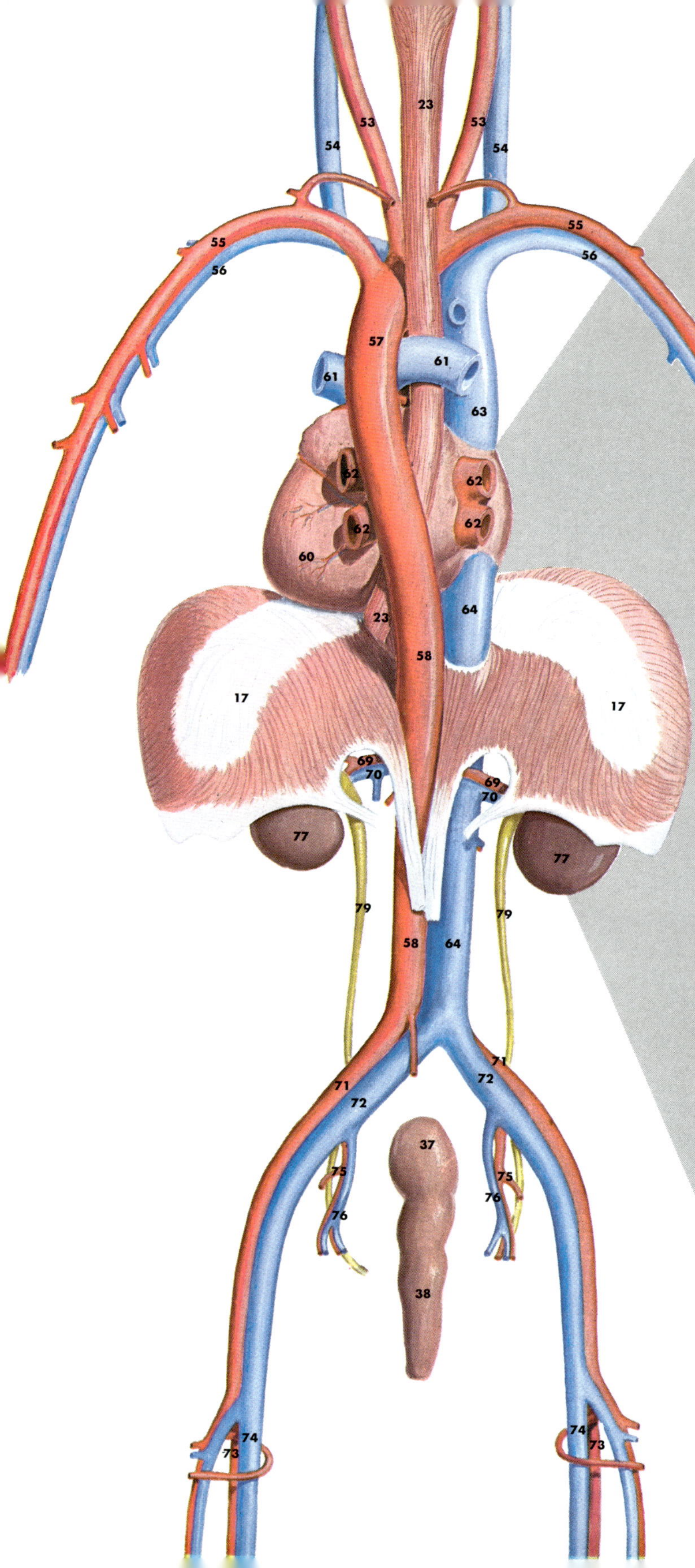

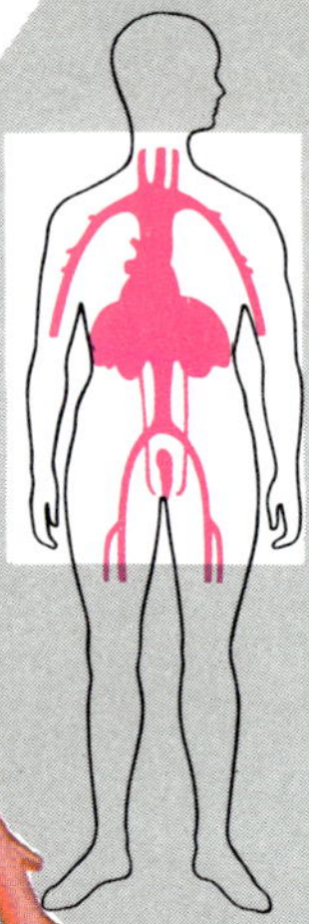

POSTERIOR CIRCULATORY SYSTEM

17. Diaphragm
23. Esophagus
37. Sigmoid colon
38. Rectum
53. Common carotid artery.
54. Internal jugular vein
55. Subclavian artery
56. Subclavian vein
57. Aortic arch
58. Aorta
60. Heart
61. Pulmonary arteries
62. Pulmonary veins
63. Superior vena cava
64. Inferior vena cava
69. Renal artery
70. Renal vein
71. Common iliac artery
72. Common iliac vein
73. Femoral artery
74. Femoral vein
75. Internal iliac artery
76. Internal iliac vein
77. Kidneys (r. and l.)
79. Ureters (r. and l.)

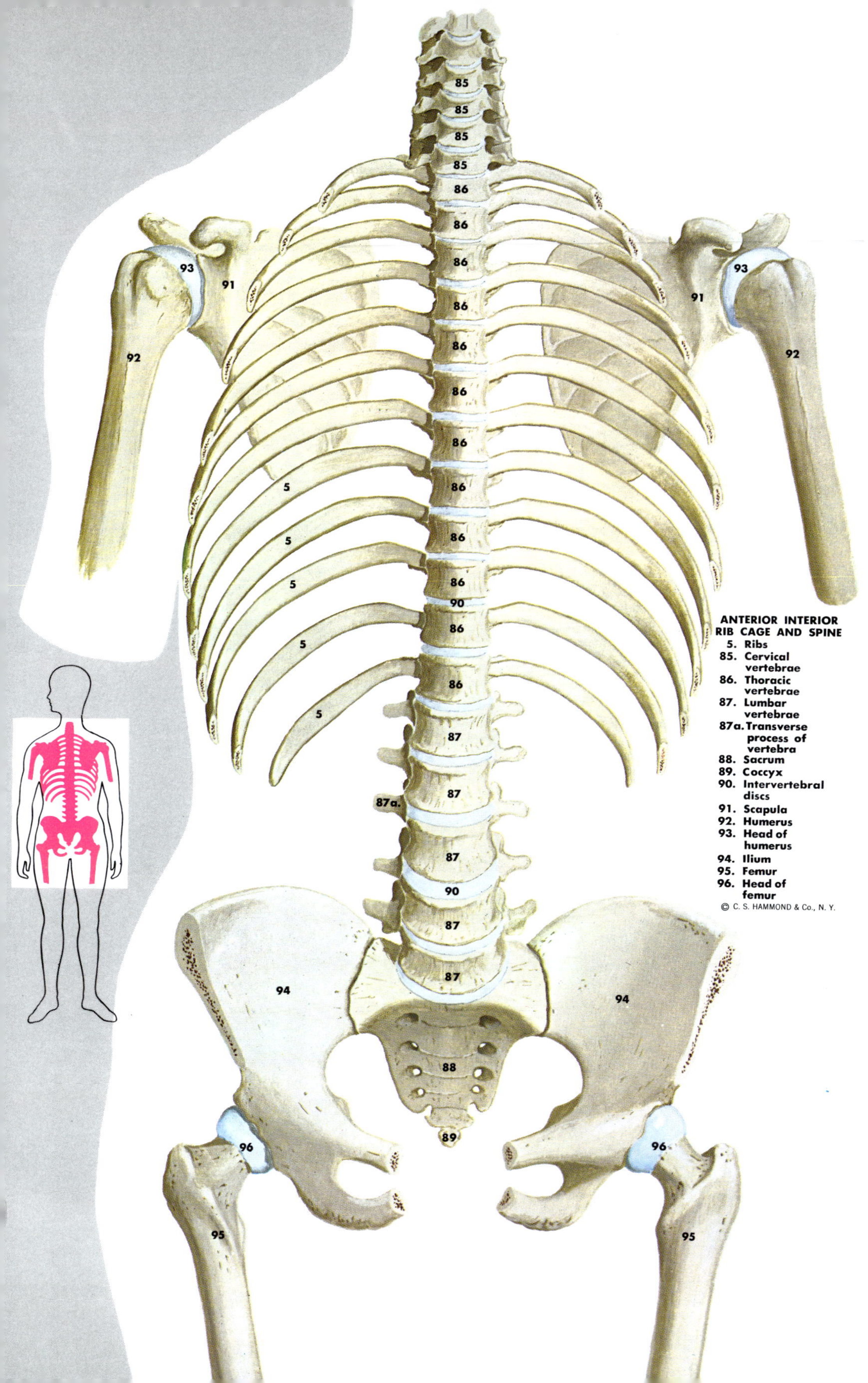

ANTERIOR INTERIOR RIB CAGE AND SPINE

5. Ribs
85. Cervical vertebrae
86. Thoracic vertebrae
87. Lumbar vertebrae
87a. Transverse process of vertebra
88. Sacrum
89. Coccyx
90. Intervertebral discs
91. Scapula
92. Humerus
93. Head of humerus
94. Ilium
95. Femur
96. Head of femur

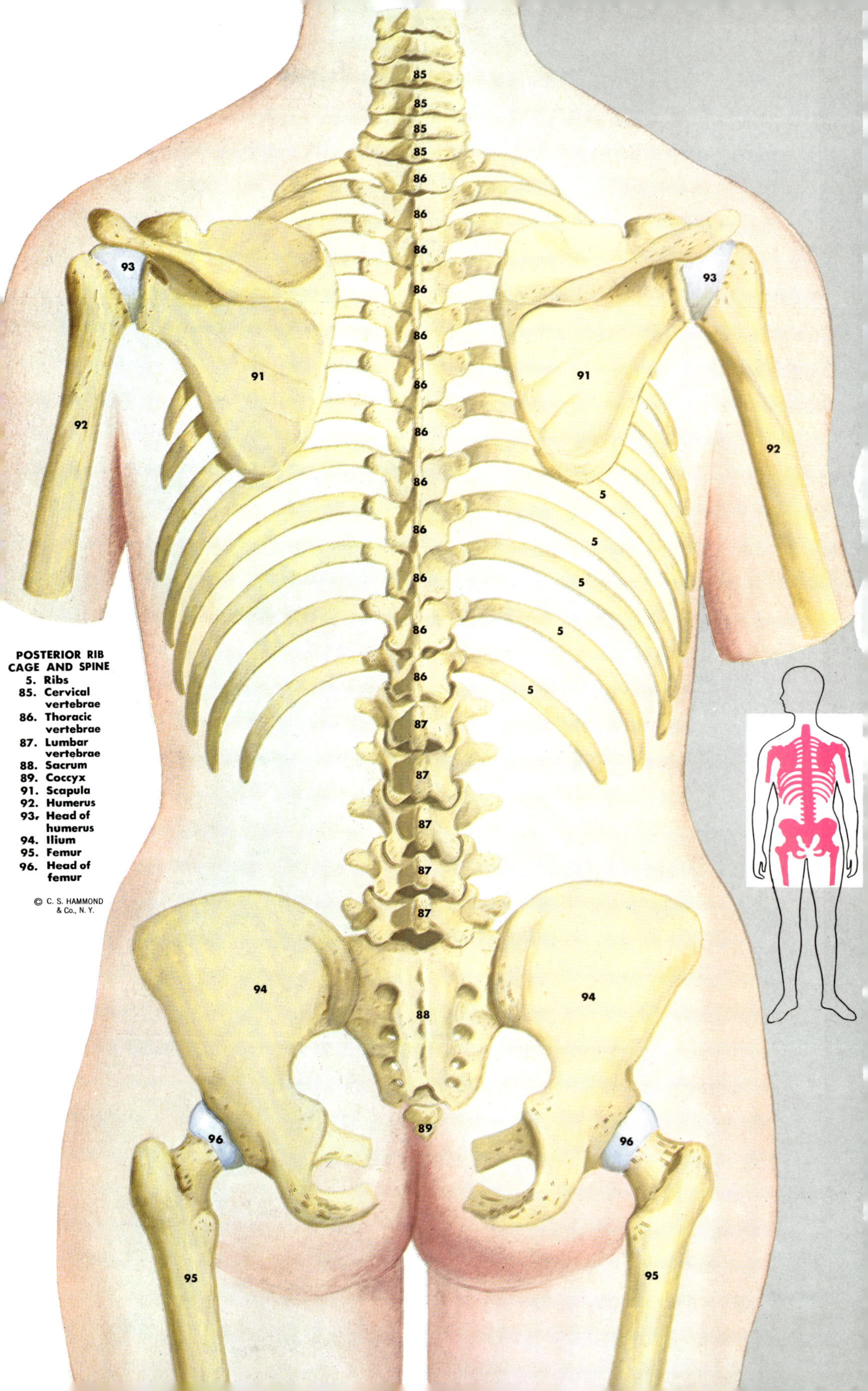

POSTERIOR RIB CAGE AND SPINE

5. Ribs
85. Cervical vertebrae
86. Thoracic vertebrae
87. Lumbar vertebrae
88. Sacrum
89. Coccyx
91. Scapula
92. Humerus
93. Head of humerus
94. Ilium
95. Femur
96. Head of femur

true sense receptors for hearing.

The organ of Corti is made up of thousands of specialized nerve endings that are the individual sense receptors for sound. These are in the form of tiny hairs projecting up from the internal membrane lining the cochlea; they wave like stalks of underwater plants in response to the oscillating currents of the inner ear fluid. There are some 20,000 of these hairs within the cochlea, responsive to almost as many degrees of movement of the fluid. These thousands of nerve endings merge at the core of the cochlea and exit from its floor as the nerve bundle of the *auditory nerve.*

Organ of Balance

The organ of balance, or equilibrium, is also behind the oval window that marks the beginning of the inner ear. The principal structure consists of

The Ear and the Perception of Sound

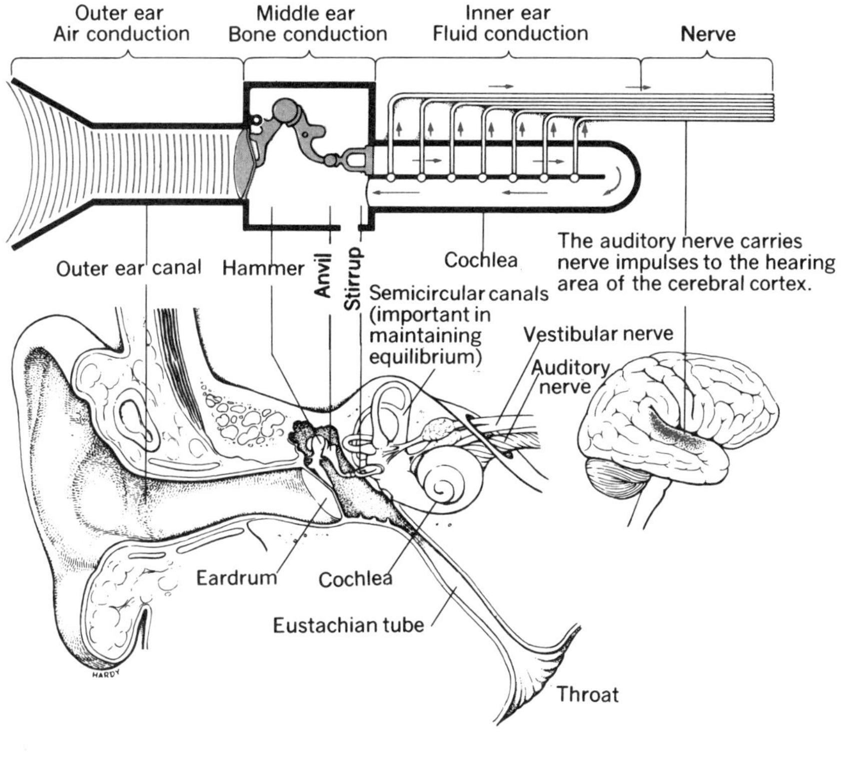

The sound waves are funneled through the outer ear canal to the eardrum. The vibrating eardrum sets into motion the three bones of the middle ear. The bones terminate in an opening in the fluid-filled cochlea. The vibrating bones set the fluid in motion. This stimulates nerve endings, which unite to become the auditory nerve. The nerve impulses are carried to the hearing area in the cerebral cortex.

three fluid-filled *semicircular canals* arranged, like the wheels of a gyroscope spinning on a perfectly flat plane or surface, at right angles to each other. When we are in a normal, upright position, the fluid in the canals is also in its normal resting state. But when we begin to tilt or turn or wobble, the fluid runs one way or another in one or more of the canals. This fluid movement is picked up by crested, hairlike nerve endings lining the inside of the canals and relayed as nerve impulses along the *vestibular nerve* to the brain. Then, the brain sends messages to the muscles that can restore our equilibrium.

The term *labyrinth* is sometimes used to refer collectively to the cochlea, semicircular canals and associated structures of the inner ear. The space or cavity within the labyrinth is called the *vestibule,* which gives its name to the vestibular nerve.

How We Hear

Just as our eye has certain special equipment—its focusing apparatus—to prepare light for the retina, so our ear has special equipment to prepare vibrations for reception by the organ of Corti.

This equipment consists of structures that amplify the vibrations reaching the ear, or, more rarely, damping (decreasing) the vibrations caused by very loud or very close occurrences.

Sound waves are really vibrations in the air that reach the eardrum at the narrow end of the funnel-shaped auditory canal. These vibrations set the membrane of the eardrum vibrating ever so slightly. Behind the eardrum, the first ossicle encountered is the hammer, which is attached to the eardrum by a projection descriptively called the hammer-handle.

From the eardrum, vibrations travel up the handle and set the hammer vibrating. The hammer, in turn, sets the anvil vibrating; and the anvil, the stirrup. The stirrup then knocks like an impatient caller on the oval window of the inner ear, and the then vibrating oval window stirs the fluids within the cochlea. This chain of

The Semicircular Canals

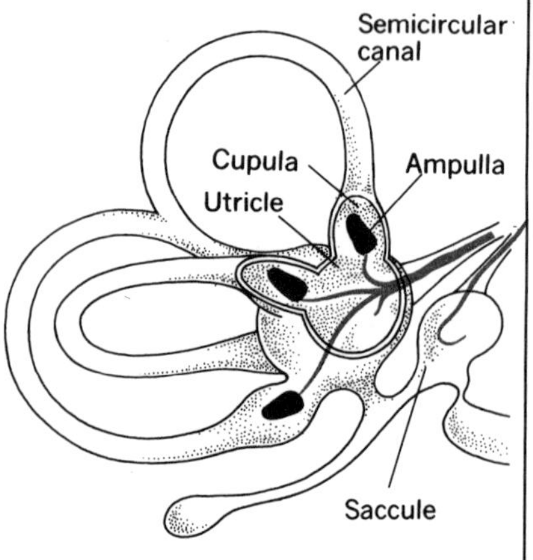

The semicircular canals are swollen at their bases into three ampullae in which receptors are located. When the head moves or accelerates, the fluid within the canals (endolymph), tends to move slower than the head, and the cupula is displaced. This is communicated to the hairlike nerve receptors. Soon the endolymph catches up to the head movement and the cupula returns to its normal position. When movement stops, the endolymph continues to move, the cupula is again displaced, and the nerve receptors are activated until the endolymph ceases to move.

events can account for a tremendous amplification of vibrations—so that we are literally able to "hear a pin drop."

Tiny muscles in the middle ear relax or tighten the eardrum and adjust to changing volumes of sound. For example, a muscle connecting the stirrup and the eardrum relaxes when the stirrup is vibrating violently in the presence of very loud noises. A lax eardrum is less likely to rupture and transmits fewer vibrations to the delicate mechanisms of the middle and inner ear than a taut one. Thus we have to some degree built-in, automatic protection against the assaults of noise pollution—but not nearly enough, according to physicians who are convinced that more and more cases of deafness are caused by the incessant battering of the modern world against our eardrums. Human eardrums are not made to withstand the sound of jet planes taking off, for example.

The Nose and Tongue

The sense receptors on the tongue and within the nasal cavity work very closely together to give us our sense of taste. These five kinds of receptors—the olfactory cell in the nose and the five special cells or taste buds on the tongue for discriminating salty, sweet, sour, bitter, and savory tastes—also have a functional similarity. All are chemical detectors, and all require moisture in order to function. In the nose, airborne substances must first be moistened by mucus (from the olfactory glands) before they can stimulate olfactory cells. In the mouth, the saliva does the wetting.

The general number and distribution of the five types of taste receptors are described earlier in this chapter under "The Digestive System and the Liver." These nerve endings, numbering in the hundreds of thousands, merge into two nerve bundles traveling away from the tongue to the brain's "taste center." The receptors toward the rear of the tongue collect into the *glossopharyngeal nerve;* those at the front and middle are directed along the *lingual nerve.*

Our smell receptors are clustered in an area about a half-inch wide on the ceiling of the nasal cavity. This is called, appropriately enough, the smell patch. The nerve endings pass upward through the sievelike *ethmoid bone,* separating the nasal cavity from the brain, and connect to the olfactory bulb, which is the "nose end" of the *olfactory nerve.* At the other end of the olfactory nerve is the "nose brain" or *rhinencephalon*—a tiny part of the cerebrum in man, but quite large in dogs and other mammals whose sense of smell is keener than man's.

Although man's sense of smell is probably his least used sense, it still has a quite remarkable sensitivity. With it we can detect some chemicals

Taste: The Nose and Tongue

Nose

The *nasal sense receptors,* or *olfactory cells,* which aid in the sense of taste, are chemical detectors stimulated by air-born substances in the nasal passage.

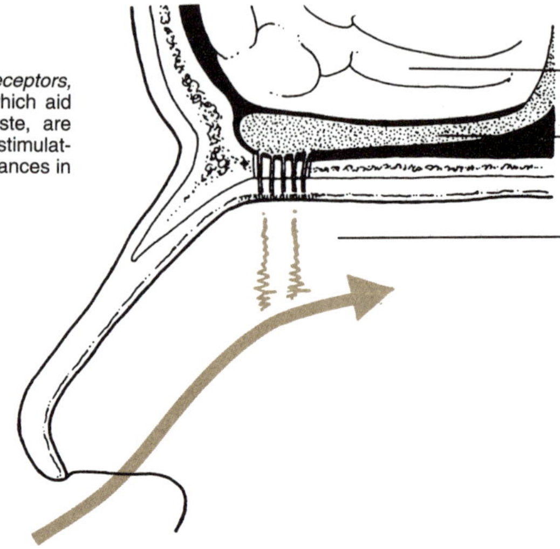

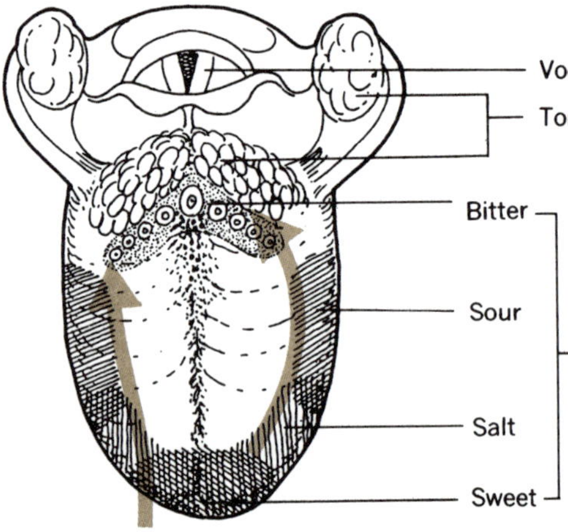

Tongue

The thousands of taste receptors, or "taste buds," are divided into five groups distinguished by the type of taste message each sends to the brain. Receptors from every taste group can be found in all areas of the tongue's surface.

in concentrations as diluted as one part in 30 billion—for example, the active ingredient in skunk spray. Also, man's ability to smell smoke and to detect gas leaks and other warning scents has prevented many a tragedy.

Skin

The sensations stimulated by the various types of sense receptors in the skin are described at the outset of this section. It is worth noting, however, at the end of our tour of the sense organs that the senses associated with the skin are really in a class by themselves. Perhaps the most telling indication of their unique place in the hierarchy of senses is the fact that practically our entire central nervous system is given over to handling the impulses transmitted by these receptors. See also Ch. 16, *Diseases of the Eye and Ear.*

The Urinogenital System and the Kidneys

In large part our good health depends on the quality of the body's internal environment. There is a kind of ecological principle at work within us—if one chain threatens to break, one system becomes polluted, one balance is tilted, then the whole environment is in imminent danger of collapsing. The major responsibility for keeping our internal environment clean and unclogged lies with our two kidneys. They are the filters and purifiers of body fluids: the body's pollution-control stations, its recycling plants, and its waste-disposal units.

The Anatomy of the Kidney

The cortex is the darker, outer part of the kidney. The medulla, the inner part, includes the renal pyramids and the straight tubules associated with them.

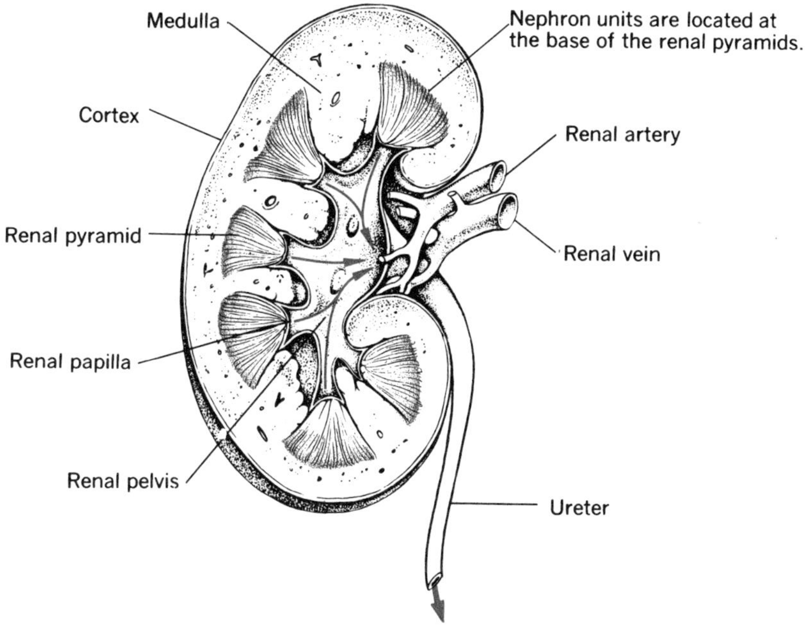

Urine is produced in the nephrons of the pyramids and drains by way of the papillae into the renal pelvis, which empties into the ureter. The ureter carries the urine to the bladder.

The Kidneys

The kidneys are located just behind our abdominal cavity on either side of the spinal cord, their tops usually tucked just under the bottommost rib. Each of our kidneys is four to five inches long and weighs about half a pound. The right kidney is normally placed a bit below the left, to accommodate the bulky liver lying also on the right side above it. Neither kidney is fixed rigidly; both can shift position slightly. Lying outside the muscular sheath of the abdominal cavity, the kidneys are more vulnerable than most internal organs to outside blows, but good protection against all but the severest jolts is afforded by surrounding fatty cushions, the big back muscles, and the bone and musculature associated with the spinal column.

As it has with the lungs, the liver, and most other vital organs, nature has supplied us with a large reserve capacity of kidney tissue—a life-giving overabundance in the event of kidney disease or injury. Indeed, normal function of only one-half of one kidney can sustain a person's life.

The kidney's task of purifying our internal environment—that is, our circulating blood—is really a double task. Each kidney must purify the blood that passes through it, sending back into circulation only "clean blood"; and it must dispose of the impurities it has taken from the blood. The latter is accomplished by the urine draining down a tube, or *ureter,* leading from each of the two kidneys to one common urinary *bladder.* Urine is discharged from the bladder down another tube called the *urethra* to the external opening for urination.

How the Kidneys Process Body Fluids

Blood is brought to the kidney by a renal artery, is treated in the kidney's unique microscopic structures, and exists via the renal vein. (*Renal* means associated with the kidneys.) The sheer volume of blood processed by both our kidneys is prodigious: between 400 and 500 gallons are processed every day.

Internal Structure

Within each kidney are over a million microscopic units called *nephrons.* The nephron is the basic functional unit of the kidney—a little kidney in itself—and is really a superbly engineered and coordinated arrangement of many smaller structures, all working together.

Blood arriving at the kidney from the renal artery is quickly channeled into finer and finer vessels, until finally it flows into a kind of cat's cradle or "ball of wool" structure called a *glomerulus* (composed of intertwining, microscopic vessels called glomerular capillaries). The entire structure of the nephron is built around the microscopic glomerulus (Latin, "tiny

The Nephron

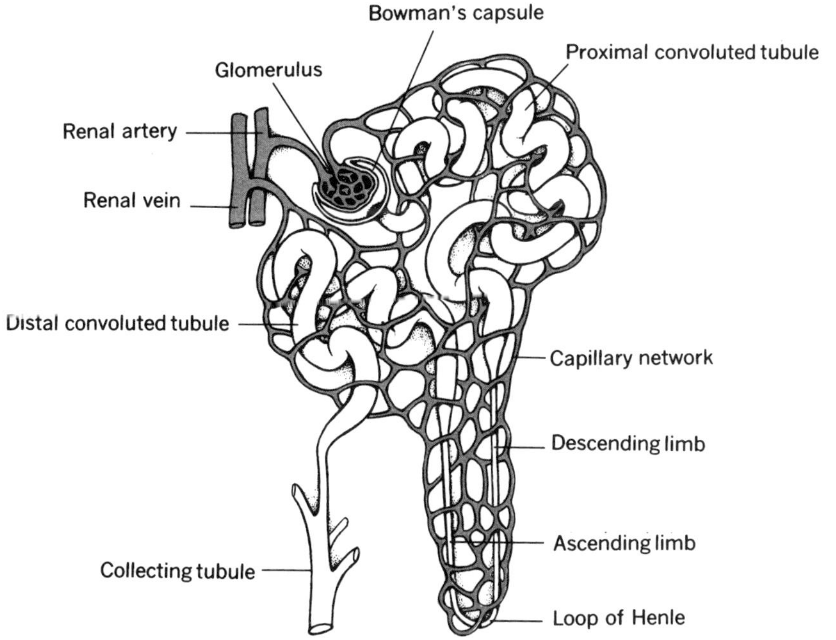

The nephron is a microscopic unit that filters out certain products from the blood. Useful products are reabsorbed by the capillary network. The waste product (urine) is carried to the collecting tubule and emptied into the renal pelvis.

ball"). Surrounding the glomerulus, like a hand lightly cupping a ball of wool, is another structure called *Bowman's capsule.* Fluid and dissolved materials filter out of the blood from the glomerular capillaries through the membranes into Bowman's capsule.

Substances in Bowman's Capsule

The fluids and dissolved materials filtering into Bowman's capsule are by no means all wastes and impurities. In fact, some of the substances must soon be reclaimed. Among the waste substances captured by Bowman's capsule and destined for excretion in urine are various nitrogen salts and other waste products of cellular metabolism, as well as actual or potential poisons that have entered or accumulated in the bloodstream. Nonwaste substances include needed sugars and salts, and water.

Reclaiming Essential Substances

Before we leave the glomerulus altogether behind, it should be noted that like any capillary bed, this small ball of blood vessels has not only an inflow from the renal artery but also outflow vessels leading eventually back to the renal vein.

From the cupped lips of Bowman's capsule, fluid and dissolved substances from the blood trickle into a single tube called a kidney *tubule.* The outflow vessels from the glomerulus wind closely over and around the tubule, forming a capillary network around it. By this means the nonwaste substances are reclaimed and returned to refresh the blood moving away from the nephron.

The tubule itself makes many twists and turns—including one hairpin turn so stunning that it has its own medical name—*Henle's loop.* So much twisting and turning gives the tubule a great deal more surface area than a simple, straight tube would have within the same space, thus increasing the amount of water and dissolved substances that can be recaptured by the encircling capillaries.

If there were no recapturing system in the kidneys, death would probably result from dehydration. Even if that could be avoided, the loss of essential salts and other substances would prove fatal in a short time.

The arithmetic of the situation goes something like this: every day, an estimated 42 gallons of fluid filter out of the glomeruli and into the two kidneys' approximately two and a half million tubules. Dissolved in this 42 gallons—representing about three times the body's weight—are about two-and-a-half pounds of common salt, just one of the many substances in the fluid that our body needs in sufficient amounts. The loss of either water or common salt at a rapid rate would prove fatal in a matter of hours.

But so efficient is the tubule-capillary recapturing system that only an average of less than two quarts of fluid, containing just one-third ounce of salt, pass daily out of the kidneys into the ureter and are excreted as urine. In other words, over 99 percent of both the water and common salt removed from the blood at Bowman's capsules is returned to the blood.

The Kidneys and Blood Pressure

A surprising insight into the critical role played by our kidneys in almost every body function is provided by the relation of blood pressure to kidney function. The blood in the glomerular capillaries must be at higher pressure than the fluid around them, so that the fluid and its dissolved substances can push through the capillary membranes toward Bowman's capsule. If blood pressure in the body falls too low (severe *hypotension*) the formation of urine ceases.

On the other hand, if a portion of the kidney is suffering from anemia due to some disorder, kidney cells secrete *pressor hormones,* which serve to elevate the blood pressure. Thus high blood pressure (*hypertension*) may be a sign of kidney disorder.

The Urinary Tract

From the ends of the million or so tubules in each kidney, urine drains into larger and larger collecting basins (called *calyces,* singular *calyx*) which drain in turn into the kidney's master urine reservoir, the ***kidney pelvis.*** Then, drop by drop, urine slides down each ureter to the urinary bladder.

Urine is held in the bladder by the contraction of two muscle rings, or *sphincters,* one located just inside the bladder before it meets the urethra, and the other encircling the urethra itself. When about a half-pint has accumulated, nerves convey the urge to urinate to the brain, and the person voluntarily causes the sphincters to relax, emptying the bladder. (In exceptional circumstances, the elastic-walled bladder can hold two or three quarts of urine.) Up to the point where the bladder drains, the male and female urinary tracts are very similar, but after the bladder, any similarity stops.

Female Urethra

The female's urethra, normally about one and a half inches long, is not much more than a short channel by which urine is eliminated from the bladder. Its very shortness often gives it an undesired significance, because it

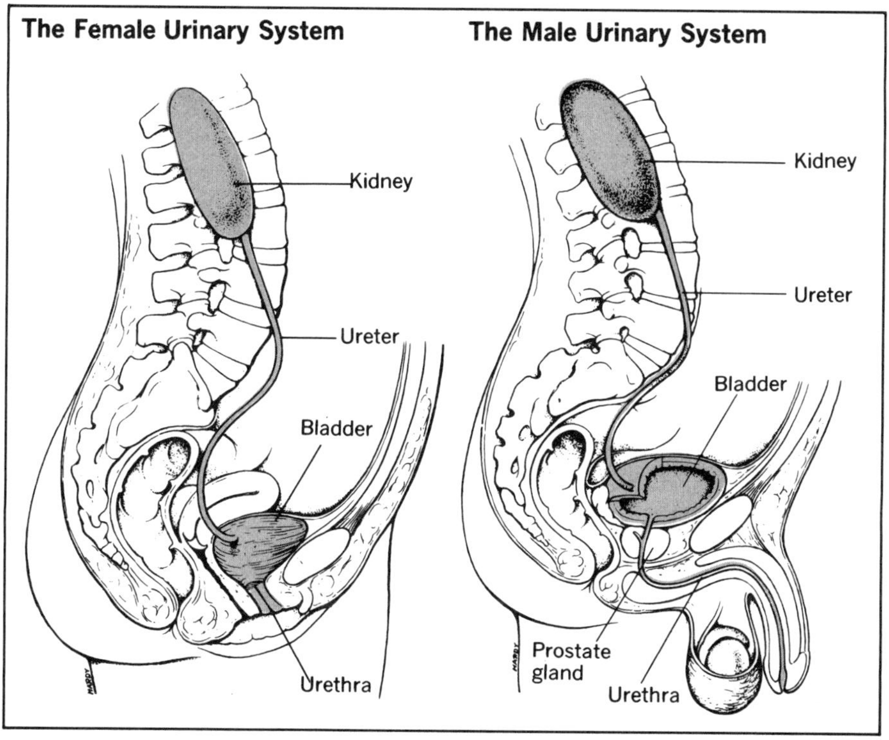

represents an easy upward invasion route for bacteria and other infection-causing microbes from the outside. Acute and painful inflammations of the urethra (*urethritis*) and bladder (*cystitis*) are thus common in women. These lower urinary tract infections, however, can usually be halted before spreading further up the urinary tract by the administration of any of several antimicrobial drugs. See Ch. 25, *Women's Health* for more information on these disorders.

Male Urethra

In contrast to the female, the male's urethra is involved with reproductive functions. So closely connected are the male's lower urinary tract and genital organs that his urethra (from bladder to the outside) is properly called the urinogenital (or genitourinary) tract. This is the reason why the medical specialty known as *urology* deals with both the urinary and genital apparatus of men; but with only the urinary tract of women. The urologist's specialty does not extend to the female genital and childbearing organs, which are the concern of the *gynecologist* and *obstetrician.*

However, all the distinctly male sex glands and organs are linked more or less directly into the eight- or nine-inch length of the male urethra.

The Genitals

The Female Reproductive System

As indicated above, the urinary and genital systems of women are dealt with by two different medical specialties. For this reason, the female genitals are discussed elsewhere. For a description and illustration of the female reproductive system, see Ch. 3, *The Teens.* For a description of infections of the female reproductive tract, see Ch. 25, *Women's Health*

The Male Reproductive System

From its emergence below the bladder, the male urethra serves as a conduit for all the male sexual secretions.

Prostate Gland

Directly below the bladder outlet, the *prostate gland* completely enwraps the urethra. The prostate secretes substances into the urethra through ejaculatory ducts; these substances are essential in keeping alive the spermatozoa that arrive from their manufacturing sites in the *testicles* (or *testes*).

Testicles

The two testicles hang down within a wrinkled bag of skin called the *scrotum.* Although the vulnerable position of the testicles remains something of an evolutionary mystery, one clue is that the optimum production of spermatozoa takes place at a temperature some degrees lower than the normal internal body temperature.

Spermatozoa produced in the testicles travel upward toward the urethra through a seminal duct or tube called the *vas deferens* (one from each testicle). (These are the ducts, incidentally, that are tied and cut in the male sterilization procedure known as a vasectomy.) The sperm cells are then stored, until ejaculation, in little reservoirs called *seminal vesicles* which are situated on either side of the urethra in the area just above the prostate gland.

The portion of the male urethra from the bladder to where it emerges from the encircling prostate, having received the emission of both the prostate and the testicles, is called the prostatic or posterior urethra. The remainder, mainly consisting of the conduit running down the middle of the shaft of the penis, ending in the external opening called the *meatus,* is known as the anterior urethra. See also Ch. 17, *Diseases of the Urinogenital System.*

The Male Reproductive System

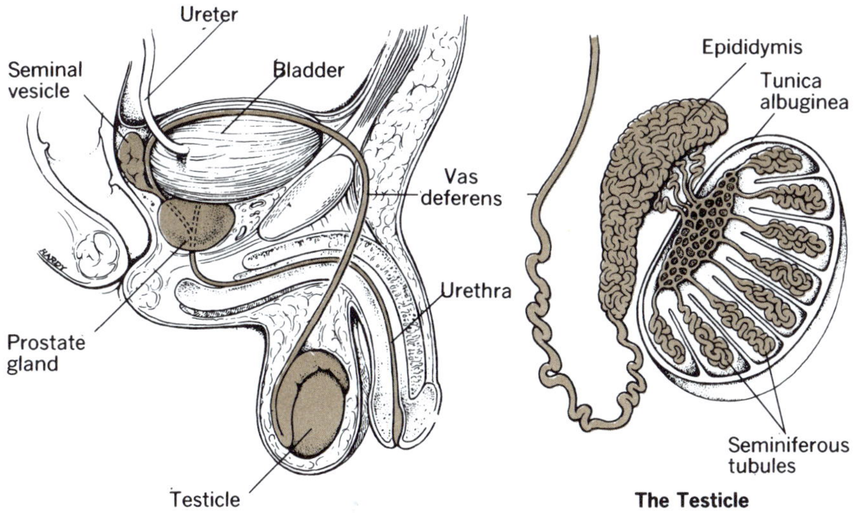

The Testicle

2

The First Dozen Years

Birth, Infancy, and Maturation

Before the Baby Arrives

When a husband and wife decide to have a baby they should both undergo complete physical examinations. This will make it possible to detect and treat abnormalities like diabetes and anemia that might affect the future pregnancy. A pregnant woman should have periodic checkups so that her physician can observe both her progress and that of the growing fetus. Such observation will help to assure a pregnancy and delivery that are free from troublesome complications.

What the Newborn Baby Looks Like

At birth the baby's skin is wrinkled or scaly, and may be covered by a cheesy substance called *vernix caseosa*. During the first two weeks the skin will become quite dry to the touch.

The newborn's head is large in proportion to the rest of its body. The genitals too may seem large, especially in girls. Newborn girls may have swollen genitalia that is a result of *edema* (fluid in the tissues, causing

Newborn Infant

Skull
Because the skull bones are not completely closed at birth, it is possible to see and feel the two most obvious "soft spots" on a baby's head. One is above the brow and the other in back, close to the crown. These *fontanels* close up in the first weeks of life.

Eyes
The eyes appear dark blue and unfocused, with slightly puffy eyelids. Initially, before there is greater muscle control, a baby's eyes may sometimes be turned in a crossed or wall-eyed position.

Skin
The skin is dry and wrinkled especially during the first two weeks of life and some *vernix caseosa* (white prenatal covering) remains. Veins may be visible and downy bodily hair is not uncommon. The bodies of fair skinned babies may temporarily be very ruddy.

Face
The face of the newborn is generally round and pudgy without much definition. Usually it will have a broad, flat nose with very little bridge, a receding chin, and an undersized lower jaw.

Head
The head of a newborn baby normally looks too big for its body. It may appear elongated or lopsided—a temporary condition caused by the physical pressure before birth or during the birth process.

Torso
The torso of a newborn is somewhat startling with its short neck, small sloping shoulders, a round protruding abdomen, and narrow pelvis and hips. The umbilical stump will drop off eventually to form the navel.

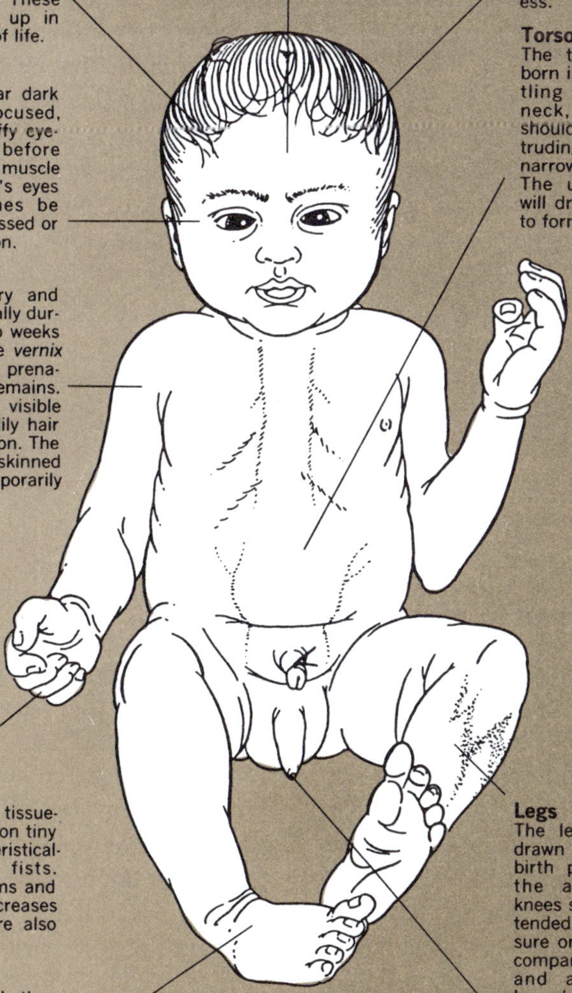

Hand
The hands show tissue-paper thin nails on tiny fingers characteristically curled into fists. Finely lined palms and deep bracelet creases at the wrists are also common.

Feet
The feet, though they look quite complete, contain only one real bone at birth, located at the heel. What will later form into bone is now only cartilage. The skin on a baby's feet may be loose and finely lined.

Size
The average newborn is very tiny, weighing in at only six to eight pounds. Its measure from top to toe is usually anywhere from 18 inches to 21 inches.

Legs
The legs are usually drawn up in the prebirth position against the abdomen with knees slightly bent. Extended, the legs measure on the short side compared to the arms and are somewhat bowed.

Genitals
The genitals of both sexes will seem too large in proportion to other parts of the body, particularly in comparison to scale in the adult.

puffiness), but the swelling is usually present for only a few days after birth.

The eyes can open and react to light, but are unable to focus. Noises produce a *startle response*, a complex involuntary reaction marked by a sudden, jerky, arm and leg movement. The newborn cries a great deal, sucks, and may sneeze.

The infant's stomach may look rather large and protuberant, and, of course, it has the stump of the umbilical cord dangling from it. The umbilical cord has been cut and tied near the navel, and will eventually fall off.

If you feel the front and back of the baby's head, you will notice one or two soft spots, called the *anterior* and *posterior fontanelles*. The posterior fontanelle usually closes at the baby's second month of life, and the anterior at 18 months or earlier.

You also may feel many different ridges in the baby's head. These are the borders of the different skull bones, which fuse as the baby gets older. They are present so that the skull can grow as the baby's brain and head continue to grow.

Soon after birth, you may detect a swelling on the baby's head just under the scalp. This is called *caput succedaneum*. It is nothing to worry about, as it dissolves a day or two after birth. Occasionally, another swelling known as *cephalhematoma* may also be present. This, too, disappears, within a few weeks.

The baby's weight will, of course, vary. Most full-term babies weigh between six and eight pounds. Babies of diabetic mothers are often heavier, and may weigh up to twelve pounds.

Some Advice to New Parents

Now that you are new parents, you may find that anyone—from your mother-in-law to the neighbor down the street to strangers in the grocery store—will be giving you advice on how to be a parent. This is usually because people realize you have entered what can be a most frightening, challenging, exciting, and periodically overwhelming new world, and they only want to help you. Becoming a new parent is a special occasion that can bring with it a rush of conflicting emotions and demands. Even for the parents who are prepared to change their familiar routines, this can be a stressful as well as happy time. Either parent, for example, may feel jealous of the new little person who is receiving so much attention and affection from the other parent. Both new parents are often tired physically and mentally. Relatives and friends may infringe on the new parents' privacy and interfere with their decision making. And, the new mother may find it hard to reconcile her maternal instinct with her desires as a woman and wife.

To adjust to this different phase of life, new parents may want to consider the following:

- The new baby is a shared responsibility. Neither parent should be excluded from the experience of parenthood. New fathers and mothers should learn to feed the baby, change diapers, hold the baby, and get to know him. Parents should take time to assure one another that they are just as important to each other as they were before the child was born.
- Arrange for some kind of assistance at home and don't wait until the baby comes back from the hospital to do it. Plan ahead. New parents are often physically and emotionally tired after the birth experience. During the hospital stay the baby was cared for by a trained staff, but once the family comes home, new parents can feel overwhelmed by old and new responsibilities. A relative, friend, or a housekeeper or other trained person can temporarily stay with you to help out with chores, such as shopping and cooking, to allow you time to adjust to your new life.
- Arrange to have a separate area for the baby even if your home is too small to allow for a nursery. A distinct area or bedroom should be chosen for a crib, a changing table, and a dresser that holds the supplies you will need when changing, dressing, or bathing the baby. Being organized will make life easier for both you and the baby.
- If the baby fidgets and fusses at times, try not to become anxious. If the baby has been fed and is dry and safe, then relax. New parents may be anxious around their baby, and the baby will be sensitive to such emotional responses, especially when being held. Realize that your own occasional feelings of uncertainty are normal, just as it is normal for any baby to periodically fuss.
- It is important for you, as new parents, to be the ones to determine when visitors will be allowed, how long they will stay, and how much the baby may be handled. A new baby should not be subjected to excessive stimulation, and as you get to know your child, you will sense when he is becoming overwhelmed by activity and attention. A baby needs a quiet, organized home, free of upsetting distractions that may come from being startled by loud noises, surrounded by numerous people, and held by many unfamiliar friends or relatives.

Feeding the Baby

One of the first questions a mother-to-be must ask herself is how she will feed her baby.

Breast-feeding is certainly the simplest method, and many women believe that both mother and child get more emotional satisfaction from it than from bottle-feeding. It is also, obviously, less expensive.

Breast-Feeding

Almost any healthy woman who wants to breast-feed her baby can do so. All she needs is the desire and motivation. No special preparation is necessary except, perhaps, some stimulation of the breasts, as prescribed by her physician during pregnancy.

On the other hand, a variety of different factors might necessitate a change from breast to bottle-feeding. Although breast-feeding may be discontinued at any time, some mothers may feel a sense of failure or frustration at being unable to continue having the intimate relationship that so many other mothers enjoy. No harm will come to the baby by being switched to a formula. Once started on a formula, however, it may be difficult to go back to breast-feeding on a regular basis. For a while, at least, the mother will have to stimulate her breasts artificially to increase their milk-producing capacity.

Lactating Breast

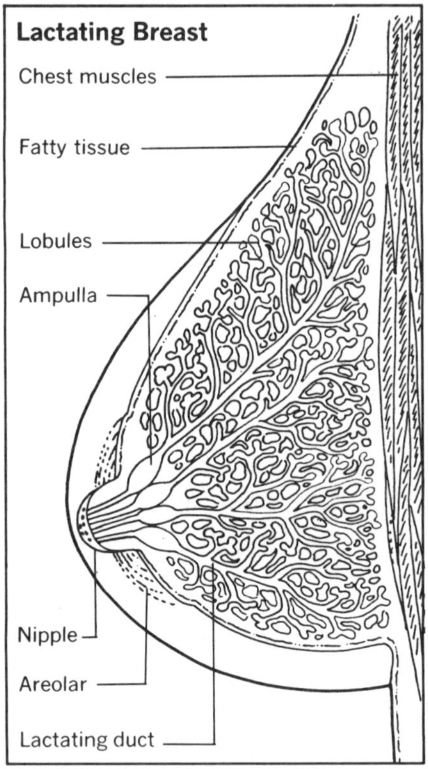

The First Few Days

When a mother first starts to breast-feed, she may be worried that she won't have sufficient milk for the baby. Her breasts are just beginning to fill up with a creamy, yellowish substance called *colostrum*. Transitional and then regular breast milk will not come in for three to five days or longer. Colostrum contains more protein and less fat than breast milk. Secretions of colostrum are small, but during this time the baby does not need very much fluid, and the colostrum will give her adequate nutrition.

Actually, it is important that the milk does not fill the breasts right away because engorgement would be so severe that the baby would not be able to suck well or strongly enough to empty them. During engorgement, the mother's breasts feel extremely tender and full. A good nursing brassiere will lift and support the breasts and alleviate the tender sensation during the one-or-two-day period of the engorgement.

Some Advice to Nursing Mothers

If you do not have enough milk for the first few days, don't worry about it. Let the baby suck on your nipples for three, five, or even ten minutes. Don't keep her on your breasts for twenty or thirty minutes right from the beginning. Start with three minutes the first day, five minutes the second, and so on until you work up to fifteen or twenty minutes. In this way you will toughen your nipples so that your breasts will become accustomed to the baby's sucking. A bland cream may be used to massage the nipple area, particularly if the nipples become sore or cracked.

Be sure to use both breasts. By emptying the breasts, milk production is stimulated; thus an adequate milk supply is dependent upon using both breasts. To avoid any soreness or tenderness, use one breast longer than the other during each nursing period.

Let us assume, for example, that at the first feeding of the day you nurse the baby on the left breast for a long period, then on the right for a short period. During the next feeding the right breast will become the first one on which the baby nurses (for the long period), and the left will be nursed second (for the short period). After a few weeks you should be nursing the baby on the first breast for twenty minutes and on the other for ten minutes.

The Feeding Schedule

Depending on how often the baby wants to feed, you will be wise to adhere to a modified demand schedule. Don't watch the clock and feed the baby every four hours on the dot. You might feed at approximately every fourth hour, which means that you could start a second feeding early—at a three-hour interval—or late—at a five-hour interval. And, needless to say, never wake your baby up at night. She will awaken you.

Bottle-feeding

New parents have a choice between prepackaged formulas and the homemade variety. Either provides the same basic nutritional requirements.

The basic homemade formula for newborns consists of evaporated milk, water, and sugar or one of the sugar derivatives. Twice as much water as evaporated milk is used with one to two tablespoons of sweetening. A similar formula can be made with whole milk in somewhat different proportions. As the baby gets older, the formula will be changed from time to time by your physician.

If one formula does not agree with the baby, it will not help to put her on a similar formula; its ingredients are likely to be virtually the same. You must switch to a radically different formula, such as one containing no milk at all or no carbohydrates. It is up to your physician to advise you which modified formula to try.

As to how much formula should be given at each feeding, let the baby decide. If she is satisfied with two-and-a-half ounces, she is probably getting enough. If she wants up to four-and-a-half ounces, give it to her. The amount is not important as long as your physician feels the baby is in good health.

A final thing to remember about feeding is this: whether you use breast or bottle, you must give your baby the love, warmth, and body contact that she needs. As you feed her, you are not only providing nutritional nourishment for her growing body but giving her emotional and mental food for her developing personality.

The First Six Months

It is extremely important that the baby have regular health supervision. Your baby's physician—whether pediatrician or general practitioner—will check the baby's height and weight on each visit, and make certain she is growing and gaining weight at a satisfactory rate. Often, the first sign of illness in a baby is a change in her height and weight pattern.

Although no two children develop at the same rate, it is possible to make certain generalizations about their development. See the charts in this chapter showing the growth rates for boys and girls.

By two months a baby often holds up her head when she lies on her stomach or when she is being held up. She recognizes large objects, and she knows her bottle or feeding position. She can probably smile.

Sometimes during the second month, your physician should start administering a series of injections against diphtheria, whooping cough, and tetanus (called *DTP*), as well as immunizing agents against polio, influenza, hepatitis B, and pneumonia. See the chart in the "Alphabetic Guide to Child Care" under "Immunization" later in this chapter.

The Three-Month Mark

By three months most babies are eating some solids, which may be specially processed for babies—fruits, cereals, vegetables, meats—in addition to having formula. They may, of course, still be entirely on breast milk. Your physician may also suggest the use of vitamin supplements, which can be added to the baby's milk or solid food. All babies need vitamins A, C, and D. Occasionally, vitamin B is also prescribed. If fluorides are not present in your drinking water, they are often added to the baby's vitamins to retard tooth decay.

At Four Months

By four months the baby will look at moving objects. Do not be surprised if her eyes cross. This is a normal condition during early infancy, and may even persist for a year.

At about this time, the baby may also learn to turn over from front to back—an important milestone. Some babies may have developed bald or flat places on the back of the head from lying more or less in one position. At about this time the condition should begin to disappear.

The Second Six Months

At six months most babies smile when they are brought to the physician's office. At one year of age a visit to the physician is more likely to produce tears and screams. The friendly, sociable attitude of the six-month-old gives way to one in which strangers are shunned or mistrusted, and everyone other than mother may qualify as a stranger.

By the sixth month the baby may roll over when placed on her back. She may learn to crawl, sit, pull herself up, and even stand. By a year she may start to walk, although walking unaided does not often occur so soon.

At this stage the baby is full of life and activity. She won't lie still when you change her diaper, and often needs distraction. She cries if you put her down or leave her alone. Unless you are firm and resist running to her first whimper, you may set the stage for spoiling her as she gets older. Of course, if she continues to cry for any considerable length of time—not more than half an hour—make sure there is nothing wrong with her besides her displeasure at your not appearing like a genie because she screams or fusses.

Other Changes

Other changes occur at this age. Where before she had been a good sleeper, she may now not want to go to sleep or she may awaken at night. Let her know that you are nearby, but don't make a habit of playing with her in the middle of the night—not if you value your sleep.

If you should notice, as many parents do at about this time, that your baby seems to be left-handed, do not try to make her right-handed. Each of us inherits a preference for one hand or the other, and it is harmful to try to change it. In any case, you are not likely to know for sure which hand your child prefers until the second year of her life.

In this second six-month period, the baby will probably take some of her milk from a cup. Don't be surprised if she takes juices out of a cup but insists on taking milk from a bottle. If she tries to hold the bottle or cup herself, let her. Of course, it may be wise to keep a mop handy at first, but after few months her skills will improve. In any case, nonbreakable cups are recommended.

Diet and Teeth

The baby's diet is soon expanded to include pureed baby foods. You might even want to try the somewhat lumpier junior foods; as more of her teeth erupt, the baby will enjoy lumpier food more and more. Teething biscuits can be added to the diet, too. By the time she is one year old she will usually have six teeth (incisors), although, because no two children are alike, she may have none at all. By the end of the first year she will have lost some of her appetite, and her rapid weight gain will cease. This is entirely natural in a period when the outside world is taking more and more interest.

As she starts to move around she wants to investigate everything. Keep dangerous objects—detergents, poisons, and medicines, especially baby aspirin—out of her reach. Tell her "no" to emphasize the seriousness of certain prohibitions. She should understand what "no" means by the time she is one-year-old, and will also probably respond to other simple commands.

It is essential that your baby's health supervision be continued without interruption. During the second six months of life she will complete her protection against diphtheria, whooping cough, tetanus (DTP), and polio (Sabin), and be tested for exposure to tuberculosis (the tuberculin test).

Behavioral Development during Infancy

During a child's first year she needs a warm and loving emotional environment in the home. It is during this time that a child establishes what psychiatrists and psychologists call basic trust. That is, she learns to be a trusting individual who feels that her important needs—those of being cared for, fed, and comforted—will be met by other human beings, initially by her mother.

Emotional Needs

Such activities as holding and cuddling the infant, talking to her, and playing with her in an affectionate, relaxed way are important for her emotional growth. Experiments with animals have shown that if the infant animal does not get sufficient cuddling and physical contact from its mother during its early development, it is unable to perform adequately as an adult later in life. It has also been shown that infants growing up in an environment lacking warm, loving, close physical and emotional contact with a mother or a mother-substitute often fail to thrive and may even die.

Fondling and Sucking

During the first year, most of an infant's satisfactions and gratifications are through the skin's perception of being touched—through physical contact with her mother and other caring adults—and through the mouth, especially sucking. Infants have a great need to suck even when they are not hungry, and this sucking should be both allowed and encouraged.

Parents frequently worry that if they respond to a baby's crying by picking her up they will spoil her, and the baby will cry often in order to get attention. In general, it could be said that during its first year an infant cannot be spoiled. When an infant cries she usually does so because she is uncomfortable, hungry, sick, or needs some physical attention.

Social Responses

As she matures, one of a child's tasks is to begin to see herself as separate from the world around her. During early infancy, the infant does not see herself as an individual who is separate from her mother, from other adults, and from the rest of the world. But, gradually, some time within the first year of life, this feeling of separateness and individuality begins to emerge in the developing infant.

One of the important and gratifying events in the early months of a child's life is the smiling responses. For the first time the infant can respond in a social way to other human beings. It is often at this time that the infant's mother and father begin to think of her as a real person and an individual. Thus the smile could be considered one of the infant's first social communications.

Suspicion of Strangers

Somewhere around the age of eight months, an infant who has in the past without complaint allowed anyone to pick her up begins to distinguish her mother from other individuals. When picked up by another the infant usually cries, acts frightened, and, in general, looks unhappy. This response indicates that she can now tell her mother and other individuals apart—an important and normal step in an infant's development.

Fear of Separation

Some time later, usually around the age of one year, the infant begins to become fearful upon separation from her mother. When her mother walks out of the room or leaves the baby with a sitter, the child may respond with crying, fear, and anger. This again indicates that the infant can now tell her mother from strangers and does not like being separated from her. Although the response is normal and usually subsides within three to four months, parents should learn to leave the child in the hands of a competent sitter, and walk out without guilt or anger. The child must learn that separations are temporary and that parents do return.

The Second Year: The Toddler Stage

It is during the second year of a child's life that he begins to develop independence and separateness from his mother. Beginning with his growing ability to walk, usually some time early in the second year (age 12 to 16 months), an infant starts to explore the world around him more actively. He experiments with greater and greater distances and increasing independence from his mother.

Toward the end of the second year, children frequently become quite independent, trying to do many things for themselves, and resenting their parents or other well-meaning adults doing things for them. Even if the child is not yet capable of performing the tasks he attempts, he should be encouraged in these early moves toward independence. It is also during the second year that speech begins to develop, with the child's first words usually being "ma ma," "da da," "milk," and the ever-present "no."

Developing Relationships with Mother and Father

It is in this phase of the child's life that he develops a real relationship with his mother. In most homes, mother is the loving, warm, secure comforter in his life, the giver of rewards and disciplinarian of his activities, the center of his life. During this period it is imperative that the child's father spend as much time with his son or daughter as possible, so that the child begins to recognize the difference between his relationship to his mother and father.

In some cases the father, because of the demands of business, may find it impossible to spend enough time with his family. This is an unfortunate fact, but one that can be dealt with positively, because it is the quality of the time a father spends with his child rather than the quantity that is most important.

Testing Himself and the World around Him

The toddler is insatiably curious. He wants to explore and investigate everything. Take him outdoors as much as possible. Let him meet children of his own age so that he can play and learn the beginnings of social contact.

Physically, the toddler tries to do many things apart from walking, running, and climbing—including quite a few things that he can't do. He is easily frustrated and may have a short attention span. (Girls are better than boys in this respect.) Don't be impatient with your toddler; don't punish him for his clumsiness. He has a great many experiences ahead of him, and many skills to learn and develop.

You can now expect a negative reaction to your control. Obviously, you must set limits on your child's behavior—on what is acceptable and what is not, while still giving him the freedom to express his emotions and energies in vigorous physical play.

Make the rules easy to understand so that the child will not become confused about what is expected of him. And do not set up impossible standards.

The Third Year

The third year is extremely important. Children are usually toilet trained, show marked growth in their language abilities, and demonstrate a continuing and growing independence.

Negativism

From two to about three and perhaps beyond, a child is extremely negative. When asked to do anything or when asked about anything, he often responds by saying, "No, no, no, no, no." This saying of the word "no" on the slightest provocation indicates a child's wish to become separate and independent from parents, to do what he wants to do when he wants to do it, and to be free from the control of others.

The child's desire for independence can be respected and encouraged by parents within limits, but this does not mean that a parent must give in to a child on every issue. A parent should try to determine what is really important and not make an issue over petty matters that can best be handled with relaxed good humor.

Language Development and Play

A rapid spurt in language development takes place at this time. A child may increase his vocabulary from about 50 words at the beginning of the third year to an almost countless vocabulary at the end of the third year. It is during this year, too, that children first show marked interest in imaginative play activities. Play, including making up stories, using toy trucks and cars, blocks, dolls, and toy furniture, is vital activity for children and should be encouraged by parents. It is through play that children express their feelings, often feelings that cannot be expressed in ordinary ways. The child also experiences what it feels like to be an adult by playing the role of physician, fire fighter, police officer, teacher, mother or father. In addition, during play children discharge tensions and learn to use their muscles and bodies.

Exploring the Body

From very early infancy, all children show a strong interest in their own and in other's bodies. During infancy this takes the form of playing with his own or his mother's body. A baby puts his fingers in his own mouth, in his mother's mouth, ears, eyes, and pats her on the tummy or on the breast. An infant also explores and touches his own body, including the genital region. This interest is normal and need not be discouraged.

Dental Development

The roots of all 20 primary teeth are complete at the child's third year of life. These teeth, which began erupting between 6 and 7 months of age, are called the *central incisors*. The primary teeth, the last of which usually fall out between the eleventh and thirteenth year, are smaller and whiter than the permanent teeth, of which there are 32. The first permanent tooth erupts between 7 and 8 years of age, while the last, the third molars, or *wisdom teeth*, erupt between the seventeenth and twenty-first year.

The Preschooler

This is the age when many children go to school for part of the day and begin learning how to get along with other children in play and in organized activities. They also begin to meet adults other than their parents.

First Separation from Mother

During the ages of three and four, the preschooler develops increasing interest in the world around him, in children his own age, and in himself. One of the key problems that the preschooler has to deal with is his impending separation from his mother when he becomes old enough to go to school. This can often be made less painful by arranging for the child to spend at first short and then increasingly longer periods of time away from his mother. By using baby-sitters both in the evening and during the day, by later having the child spend three or more half-days a week at a preschool, and lastly by enrolling him in kindergarten for either all day or half a day, five days a week, the mother can ease the child's adjustment to the world outside the home.

Although his first nearly full-time separation from mother is difficult for the child, it may be difficult for the mother as well. Mothers often feel that this initial separation from their child will eventually lead to their child's growing up and leaving home. Parents are often nostalgic and somewhat regretful about their children's first going off full time to school. The child's fearful anticipation of a strange situation can be eased by a mother's anticipating school with the child, talking with him about it and reassuring him regarding his fears of abandonment or separation.

Differences between Boys and Girls

A word might be mentioned here concerning differences between boys and girls. At the age of five most girls are ready to attend kindergarten; they can sit in their seats for long periods of time, pay attention to a teacher, and be interested in a task. Boys, because of their somewhat slower rate of maturity, are often less ready than girls for coping with a classroom situation at the age of five.

A child of five grows at a slower rate than in earlier years, but his body is nonetheless changing. The protruding abdomen and knock-knees of the toddler begin to disappear.

Television

Students of the medium suggest that television offers some worthwhile programs for the young child. At the same time, the experts warn that television watching can, over time, become addictive. A basically passive experience, it may also decrease the quality of family life and raise early obstacles to literacy and learning.

The parent's main task, insofar as television watching is concerned, is to find ways to use "the tube" to help the child develop. Parents can, for example, turn on programs that their child enjoys, that do not frighten or overexcite, and that the toddler can learn from. The television should not be used as an "electronic babysitter"; as much as possible, parents should watch when their child does. If a child is 18 months old or older the experts say parents should select the special programs they want their child to see. Television should not, finally, be used as a reward for being good. Such an approach can suggest the TV is more important than interesting games and other worthwhile activities.

Personal Hygiene

Good habits of cleanliness should be established. The child should know that hand-washing before meals is essential even when the hands look clean. He will learn this only if he sees parents do it. As he gets older he should select his own clean clothing and know that dirty clothing should be washed. A daily routine of washing or bathing should be set up, and the child should be encouraged to observe it.

School-Age Children: Parent–Child Relationships

Beginning around the age of four, boys show a decided preference for their mothers. A boy may, for example, tell his mother that when he grows up he would like to marry her and kick father out of the house. At times he may even suggest that he would work to support her and that life would be much nicer if daddy were not around.

This interest in his mother is often expressed in what may be thought of as sexual ways. That is, the child of this age enjoys his mother's affection, including kissing, hugging, and close bodily contact. This wish to have mother all to himself and to have father out of the picture is called the *Oedipal complex* by psychiatrists and psychologists, after the ancient Greek tragedy, *Oedipus Rex*, in which Oedipus kills his father and marries a woman whom he later discovers to be his mother.

At about this same age, similar emotional developments take place in a girl. She will likely be somewhat seductive, coy, and coquettish with her father, and may talk about marrying father (or a man like father) and having mother out of the picture. This phase of emotional attachment between a girl and her father is called the *Electra complex* after the Greek play, *Electra*.

At these times, both the girl and the boy have a strong, although not always conscious, wish to displace the parent of the same sex and have the opposite-sexed parent all to themselves. Strong conflicts disturb children in this phase of development, for they also realize that they love and need the same-sexed parent to instruct them, to guide them, to provide for them, and to love them.

Identification

Both males and females eventually resolve these conflicts by abandoning their so-called sexual attachment to the opposite-sexed parent, forming a closer attachment to the same-sexed parent and trying to be like that parent. This is not a conscious decision, but one that a child makes without realizing it. This process of *identification* with the parent of the same sex starts very early, perhaps as early as the second year, and continues through adolescence, but it is especially noticeable from five to ten.

Much of the energy that had previously been utilized in loving the parent of the opposite sex is now spent in loving the parent of the same sex. The boy follows father around, wants to do whatever he does, and holds as his greatest ambition to be exactly like father when he grows up—even to marrying a woman like the one father did.

The girl during this same period spends the energy that was once expended in love for her father in an attempt to learn to be like mother and perhaps eventually to marry a man resembling in some way her father.

This, however, does not mean that children do not continue to love the opposite-sexed parent; it means only that their primary attachment during these years is to the same-sexed parent. It is this process of identification with the same-sexed parent that facilitates the chief task of the school-age child from 5 or 6 to 11: the task of learning.

Six Years to Adolescence

The years from 6 to 11 have generally been regarded as quiet years as far as emotional development is concerned. Many of the tasks of earlier childhood have been completed, and the relatively stormy years of adolescence have not yet begun. A child's interests begin to turn more and more away from his family and to other children his own age, usually children of the same sex. At this stage, a child's interest in learning is broad and intense.

During this period children begin to be more and more individualistic. Some are solitary, others sociable; some are athletic, others not. One likes only other children, another prefers the company of adults. Some children have imaginary fears that disappear with age or when the fears are discussed with an adult who can explain how or why they originated.

Curiosity about Sex

The child's earlier curiosity about naked people may change to a concern about being clothed and being with people who are clothed. Questions about sex should be answered simply and truthfully.

Adolescence

Adolescence arrives anywhere from 9 to 14 years of age. A girl usually enters adolescence at 10, a boy at about 12.

In female children, there is growth of the breasts and nipples; the pelvis matures, and the external genitalia develop. Axillary (underarm) and pubic hair appear. On the average, girls have their first menstrual period around age thirteen, but it can occur between 10 and 16 years of age. Be sure to explain menstruation to your daughter before the beginning of adolescence.

In male children, the penis and testes develop. Facial, axillary, and pubic hair appear. The voice begins to deepen.

In both boys and girls, there is a rapid growth in height and weight which is related to sexual development. In general the average height of the adolescent is double what is was at age two. See Ch. 3, *The Teens*.

Alphabetic Guide to Child Care

The following Guide is an alphabetically arranged list of articles dealing with many of the problems that confront parents. It includes articles on physical disorders and ailments of childhood; behavioral and emotional problems; and on situations that occur normally in the life of almost every child which may cause tension or distress for parents, child, or both. It is hoped that having information about such normal developmental tensions will help to minimize them.

A note on the cross-references: Where a particular subject is covered elsewhere within this Guide, the reference is printed in small capital letters. (For example: See also TONSILLITIS.) References to sections in other chapters are printed in italic type along with the chapter number. (For example: See "Tonsils and Adenoids" in Ch. 20, *Surgery*.)

Accidents

All children have accidents and injure themselves. Some do more frequently or more seriously than others. Parents should treat the ones that are minor and seek immediate medical attention for ones that are major. The parents' response to an injury can greatly determine the child's response to it. Calm, responsible behavior will keep the child calmer, even in a serious accident.

For minor injuries such as cuts and bruises, treatment can be completed at home. Cuts and scrapes should be washed thoroughly with warm (not hot) water. A skin disinfectant can be applied, only if the cut is not deep. A bandage should be applied during the day to keep dirt out. The cut should be left uncovered when possible, though, to allow it to dry and heal. Once the cut or scrape has scabbed over, a bandage need not be used, unless the scab is damaged or tears off.

Sprains, unless very minor, are difficult to treat at home. It is not likely that a parent can determine the damage to muscle tissue. Sprains can be more painful than breaks and can inflict severe damage to ligaments and tendons. X rays are usually required to determine the damage done to the limb.

Minor sprains that show slight swelling or discoloration of the skin can be treated by applying ice to the injured area as soon as possible after the accident. Keep the limb elevated for ten to twenty minutes with the ice pack on the injured joint. Have the child avoid using the limb for a while. Once movement can be made without serious pain, warm water soaks or baths will help reduce swelling. If pain persists for more than 24 hours, consult a physician.

Bruises are caused by bleeding under the surface of the skin with no cut to the surface of the skin. Black eyes are bruises under the eye tissue. Minor bruises can be treated with cold water or ice packs to the area hurt. (Eyes should receive only water packs, ice against the eye is not recommended.) As the bruise fades a purple or yellow tint to the skin will remain for a few days or so as the body removes the last of the dried blood from the bruised tissue. Bruises can take several days to fade and heal. If it takes longer, a doctor should be consulted.

Head injuries in children are also common. A sharp blow to the head, or a fall, can trigger vomiting in a child. This, in itself, is not a danger signal. Danger signals are:

- Both pupils in eyes not dilated equally.
- Eyes do not move together when following something.
- Child sleeps immediately, or is hard to waken during a nap. Any child should be awakened every three hours to check, for 24 hours after the accident.
- More than one episode of vomiting.
- Any sign of mental disorder—speech or movement difficulties, dazed focus or attention, or any type of non-response.
- Increasing headache.
- Blood or fluid from nose or ears. If any one of these symptoms appear, contact the local hospital emergency facilities immediately.

For more information, see Ch. 35, *Medical Emergencies*, and "The Emergency Room" in Ch. 20, *Surgery*.

Adenoidectomy

See "Tonsils and Adenoids" in Ch. 20, *Surgery*.

Adenoids, Swollen

The adenoids are clusters of lymph tissue located behind the soft palate where the nasal passages join the throat. Along with the tonsils and lymphoid tissues elsewhere in the body, the adenoids are involved in warding off infection. When they themselves become inflamed because of bacterial or viral invasion, they become swollen. Swelling may also occur because of allergy.

Swollen adenoids may block the air passages sufficiently to cause mouth breathing, which in turn will not only give the child an "adenoidal" look, but will lead to more frequent upper respiratory infection, as well as to eventual malformation of the lower jawbone. Chronic swelling may also block the eustachian tube, causing pain in the ear and increasing the possibility of ear infection as well as of intermittent hearing loss. The child's physician can keep track of the severity of such symptoms during periodic checkups and can evaluate the need for surgery. See also TONSILLITIS. For a description of adenoidectomy, see "Tonsils and Adenoids" in Ch. 20, *Surgery*.

Adopted Children

No matter what their individual differences about child rearing, all specialists agree that an adopted child should be told that she was adopted. It doesn't matter that the adoptive parents have come to feel that the child is completely their own. Biologically, she isn't, and it is her human right to find this out not from a neighbor or schoolmate but from the people she loves and trusts as her parents. The fact of her adoption should be talked about naturally in the child's presence even before she can understand what it means. If she is being raised in a loving atmosphere and feels secure in the acceptance of her adoptive parents, the child isn't likely to be upset by the reality of her situation.

When the child becomes curious about the circumstances of her adoption, or if she wants to know about her "real" mother and father, she should be given no more—and no less—information than the adoption agency provided originally.

A widow or divorced woman who remarries when her children are still very young may be faced with the possibility that her second husband wants to legally adopt the offspring of her first marriage. Far-reaching consequences are involved in such a decision, and it should not be undertaken lightly. The problem should be discussed with a lawyer who can present the facts in a detached way so that the decision will cause the least anguish and fewest unpleasant consequences for everyone.

Aggressiveness

In the rough and tumble of play, some puppies are obviously more aggressive than others, and one of them is clearly determined to be top dog. The same is true of children, especially in any society where energy and enterprise are rewarded.

Aggressive tendencies are natural; the form they take is up to the civilizing efforts of the parents. It is they who have the responsibility of helping a child understand that bullying and bossiness are unacceptable. It seems that because of inheritance, body build, or temperament, some youngsters, whether male or female, are more clearly aggressive than others. It is especially for such children that healthy outlets must be provided for aggression—in the form of toys and playground activities when they are little, and in suitable physical and intellectual endeavors when they get older.

Guilt Feelings

Making a child feel guilty about the strength of his aggressive feelings or thwarting them constantly won't wipe out or destroy the feelings; they'll simply be turned inward, or take the form of nail-biting, or express themselves in some sneaky and antisocial way. Parents who are upset by children's play that simulates violence and who disapprove of toy guns should make their feelings clear without making the youngster feel like a monster because he enjoys them. Aggressiveness that expresses itself in violence and bloodshed—as it so often does in movies and in TV programs—should not be the day-in-day-out entertainment to which children are exposed regardless of the parental feelings.

Boy/Girl Differences

As for a boy who doesn't seem aggressive enough to suit a parent's idea of what a boy should be, or a girl who seems too aggressive to conform to family notions about femininity, these stereotypes are being reexamined and discarded by many people because they are too confining and rigid to permit the full development of a child's personality. It's no disgrace for a boy to cry, and it should be a source of pride to have a daughter who is tough and aggressive on the playing field.

Allergies

See NUTRITION, and Ch. 24, *Allergies and Hypersensitivities.*

Anger

Anger is a feeling that everyone is familiar with. There are moments when even the most controlled and civilized adult experiences the kind of anger that might become blind rage. A child whose bike has been stolen has a right to her anger; a child whose baby brother has broken her cherished doll is justifiably angry. Some youngsters seem to be angry all the time because they feel they're always being pushed around by adults. (Many adults are always angry because they feel they're being pushed around by other adults.) Feelings of anger at perceived injustices seem especially common among some children of six, seven, and eight, as well as among some teenagers.

Means of Expressing Anger

When parents know that a child's anger comes from a healthy feeling of outrage or because of confusion, they should allow the anger to be expressed—in words or tears. But it does have to be made clear that smashing things in a fit of rage or having a tantrum is unacceptable. A child at the mercy of powerful feelings of rage can be frightened by them and should be helped to understand and control them. It's also a comfort to children to know that grown-ups can become terribly angry from time to time, but that part of growing up is being able to handle one's feelings and learning how to express them in the right way at the right time. Thus, a father who is in a rage with his boss will find ways of letting him know that he feels an injustice has been done rather than swallow his anger at work and take it out on his wife or children as soon as he comes home.

Animal Bites

See "Animal Bites" in Ch. 35, *Medical Emergencies.*

Anxiety

Children may become chronically anxious when their parents constantly criticize them for failing to measure up to some unrealistic standard of perfection. Likewise, parents become anxious about being parents when they criticize themselves for failing to measure up to some unachievable standard of perfection.

Anxiety is one of the most widespread and most debilitating stresses from which people of all ages suffer in the United States, chiefly because many Americans have been victimized by the notion that everybody can be everything. Thus, a parent will expect a little child to be good, bright, neat, polite, aggressive enough to complete adequately but not so aggressive that the other children don't like him, relaxed and cheerful at the same time that he's supposed to do all his chores and the homework and remember to be nice to his baby-sister. What child burdened with such expectations isn't going to feel anxious about fulfilling them so that he can gain his parents' love and approval?

Parents may waste emotional energy feeling anxious because they think they're inadequate mothers or fathers, perhaps because they lose their tempers from time to time or because they're often too tired to play with their toddler and stick him in the playpen just to keep him out of trouble. A child will also be made chronically anxious if he's always being threatened with punishment, or if he's made to feel that he's bad when he's trying to be good but doesn't know how. The way to keep anxiety at a minimum is to have achievable goals. Is the child healthy, moderately well-behaved, cheerful, and inspiring no complaints from his teachers? Are you as a parent helping him to be healthy, moderately well-behaved, cheerful, and cause no trouble at school? If pressure on the child is small, and he still seems anxious, counseling may be considered.

Asthma

Asthma is a disease of the respiratory system in which there is chronic (long term) inflammation of the lungs and periodic acute episodes called "attacks." During attacks airways contract or go into a spasm, breathing becomes difficult, and a wheezing sound is produced. Lung spasms are also accompanied by secretion of excess mucus into the airways and swelling of the bronchial tubes, causing breathing to be further restricted. Coughing, sweating, and a feeling of tightness in the chest may also accompany an attack.

Both hospitalization for asthma and death from asthma have increased over the past decade. Many physicians and scientists believe this increase is due to such factors as increasing air pollution and improper use of asthma medications. Approximately fourteen million Americans have asthma; of those, about four million are children. Asthma is a leading cause of chronic illness in children.

Triggers and Causes

Asthma may be triggered by a variety of factors, including cold weather, pollen, house dust, cockroaches, mites, animal dander, cigarette smoke, certain cleaning products, and emotional stress. In some cases, asthma may accompany a bacterial or viral infection of the nose or throat.

The Asthma Attack

If an attack occurs, a child may become very frightened, because the attack produces the sensation of suffocating. It can also be frightening to witness a child struggling to breathe. It is important to remain calm, be reassuring to the child, and call the child's pediatrician promptly. Immediate symptoms can be alleviated by prescription medications that are taken as a pill, through an inhaler, or by injection. If the trigger for the attack can be determined, it should be removed from the child's presence as soon as possible.

Treatment and Prevention

Suspected asthma should be assessed by a physician to determine what steps should be taken. Often, desensitization to a certain food or pollen is necessary, or a pet has to be given away. Environmental factors or emotional stress also may play a role. Chronic asthma should never go untreated; frequent attacks can affect overall health. A wide range of medications exist to control asthma. Such medications include corticosteroids, which treat inflammation, and bronchodilators, which may be used when anti-inflammatory drugs are not fully effective. Both of these medicines are available in inhalant form. Allergy injection therapy, which aims to build up immunity, may be recommended for a child whose asthma is triggered by allergens. Other medications come in pill or liquid form. Over-the-counter products may temporarily relieve less severe asthma symptoms.

Aerobic exercise is also recommended for some asthmatics. It raises heart rates and makes the heart pump more blood, thereby improving lung function and overall health.

Autism

See under MENTAL ILLNESS.

Baby-sitters

Whenever anyone other than a parent is responsible for the well-being of children, great care should be taken in selecting the individual. Baby-sitters should get along well with your children, feel comfortable dispensing reasonable disciplinary measures should the children misbehave, and be capable of taking charge in case an emergency situation develops.

Ground Rules

All aspects of the sitter's responsibilities and privileges should be covered in conversations before the first sitting. Parents should explain their expectations of the sitter and details should be ironed out, including pay and whether or not the sitter is allowed to invite company over.

Clear and explicit instructions should always be left with the sitter about what to do and who to call in the event of an emergency, including important telephone numbers, such as where you can be reached.

Beds

Infants should not be left on a full size bed to nap or they could become wedged between the mattress and the solid object and suffocate. Crib mattresses are designed to fit tightly against the frame avoiding the risk of suffocation. To further protect an infant from suffocation, he should not be given a pillow while napping or sleeping. An infant who rolls over and is unable to lift his head may suffocate in the pillow. To help reduce the risk of sudden infant death syndrome, most healthy babies should be put to sleep on their backs on a firm mattress or other firm surface, not on fluffy blankets or comforters. Soft toys or pillows should not be placed in the crib with very young babies.

Bedtime

From babyhood on, the routine of bedtime should be as relaxed as possible for both parent and child. Keeping things peaceful at bedtime doesn't mean giving in to the child's pressures or whims, but involves keeping one's voice calm, pleasant, and firm. Adjustments in the bedtime hour can be made from time to time if you decide that the occasion calls for it.

Bedwetting

Enuresis, the medical term for bedwetting, is the involuntary release of urine, usually during sleep at night. A child who wets his bed recurrently after he has learned to control urination during toilet-training has enuresis. Controlling urination through the night may not occur until after the age of three. About 15 percent of boys and 10 percent of girls are bedwetters at the age of 5; most outgrow it by the time they reach puberty.

Children who are bedwetters should be examined to rule out any physical abnormality in the urinary tract. Obstruction at the neck of the bladder where it joins the urethra or obstruction at the end of the urethra may cause uncontrollable dribbling of urine, but this usually occurs during the day as well as at night. Disease of the nerves controlling the bladder, sometimes hereditary, can cause loss of urine. It can also occur in children who are mentally retarded or mentally ill, or because of an acute or chronic illness. In the latter cases, the problem disappears when the child regains his health.

Emotional problems

If all physical abnormalities for bedwetting have been explored and eliminated as possible causes, the emotional problems of the child and his family should be examined. The condition often develops in conjunction with a stressful change in the child's environment. Typical examples are the birth of a sibling, the absence of a parent, or separation anxiety on the first day of school. An understanding attitude rather than a hostile or punitive one is extremely important in helping a child with enuresis. The bedwetting may be his outlet for emotions he feels he cannot adequately express. Bringing the child's hidden feelings into the open and dealing with them sympathetically usually causes the problem to disappear.

Treatment

Limiting the intake of liquids before bedtime, encouraging the child to urinate before going to bed, or waking the child soon after he's gone to sleep and getting him to go to the bathroom may also help. Behavior modification techniques include the use of positive reinforcement and rewards for dry nights as well as devices with small alarms that awaken the child when he urinates in his sleep. If the condition persists, a doctor may prescribe medication, such as imipramine.

Behavior Problems

See AGGRESSIVENESS, ANGER, DELINQUENCY, DESTRUCTIVENESS, DISHONESTY, DISOBEDIENCE.

Birthmarks

See "Pigment Disorders and Birthmarks" in Ch. 21, *Skin and Hair*.

Biting

Some children learn that their strongest weapon when angry is their teeth. They may bite siblings, friends, and occasionally parents. Because of the enormous risk of infection from the bite, and because it can inflict extreme pain to the person bitten, biting should be strongly discouraged by any child.

Blindness

See HANDICAPPED CHILD.

Booster Shots

See IMMUNIZATION.

Boredom

Babies are usually too hungry or too sleepy—or too cranky—to be bored. Toddlers have so much to investigate around the house that boredom is not likely to be one of their problems. As a child gets older and complains about having nothing to do, you might get him involved in a household chore by saying, "Let's . . ." rather than "Why don't you" or "How would you like to." "Let's tidy the cans on the pantry shelf" or "Let's make some cookies" can make a three-year-old feel useful and interested.

Coping with Boredom Can be Productive

A child who is never allowed to be bored because his parents or older siblings feel that they have to entertain him or play with him is deprived of the possibility of calling on his own resources and learning how to amuse himself. The fact that an only child may have to live through stretches of boredom often contributes to his exploring his own abilities in a creative way. Sometimes just asking a child to "Tell *me* a story" can work wonders. Some parents solve the recurrent problem of boredom by organizing informal play groups of three or four children; others find a nursery school the best solution.

Convalescence

An older child who is recovering from an illness that has kept him out of school and isolated him from his friends may require some special project to work on in addition to catching up on his homework. A period of protracted convalescence is a good time to introduce a new hobby or craft such as model-making or clay sculpture that may solve the boredom problem for years to come.

Brain Damage

Brain damage refers to an organic defect of the brain—that is, tissue destruction—caused by an injury to the nervous system occurring before, during, or after birth. Such injury can be caused by toxic chemicals as well as by physical trauma. It can result in any of a variety of neurological disorders, such as cerebral palsy or other impairment of motor coordination, mental retardation, convulsive seizures, hyperkinesis, or perceptual difficulties.

Minimal Brain Damage

Minimal brain damage (or, more formally, *minimal brain dysfunction*) refers to a condition of some children who suffer from a motor or perceptual impairment that may affect their ability to learn or use language, interfere with memory, or make it difficult for them to control their attention. Some learning disabilities are attributed to minimal brain damage. See also DYSLEXIA.

Brothers and Sisters

Rivalry and jealousy and bickering are inevitable among brothers and sisters; companionship, a helping hand, and good times together are part of the picture too. Parents can keep resentments and quarrels at a minimum by not playing one child off against the other or by refraining from holding up one child as an example of virtue to another. In an atmosphere of equal recognition, brothers and sisters will love and respect each other most of the time and fight only occasionally. Special privileges granted on the basis of such distinctions as "Well, he's the oldest" or "She's the youngest" or exceptions made because "He's a boy" or "She's only a girl" can cause resentments that last a lifetime.

Burns

See "Burns" in Ch. 35, *Medical Emergencies.*

Camps

There seems to be no end to the diversity of camps available for summer enrollment. Most urban and suburban communities have day camps in which children may be accepted for certain minimum periods. They range from expensive groups that offer sightseeing trips, swimming instruction, and other special attractions to groups that cost very little and function more or less like day-care centers. "Sleepaway" camps run by organizations such as the Scouts and the 4-H Clubs are comparatively cheap and will register a child for a week rather than for a month or for the entire summer. Camps subsidized by community funds or private endowment are available for urban children from poor families.

Special Camps

The proliferation of special camps has been a blessing to the parents of disabled children: those with diabetes, muscular dystrophy, learning disabilities, obesity, and other problems need no longer be deprived of a camping experience with their peers. In many cases, particularly for overweight youngsters, the summer experience can be a major health contribution.

In general, an effort should be made to choose a camp that suits the tastes and temperament of the child. A youngster who hates competitive sports is likely to have a miserable time in a camp that emphasizes team spirit. Instead, he may enjoy a place that offers lots of nature study, hiking, and animal care. A child eager to improve his swimming would be better off at a camp with better-than-average water sport facilities rather than one that concentrates on arts and crafts and offers only a nearby pond for all water activities. Information about camps that have official standing can be obtained by writing to The American Camping Association, 5000 State Rd., 67 N, Martinsville, IN 46151-7902; (765) 342-8456.

Cancer

Rare as it may be and affecting only one child in about 7,000 each year, cancer still claims the lives of more children between the ages of one and fourteen than any other single disease. Among the cancers that more commonly affect children in their early years are the following: *acute lymphocytic leukemia,* in which white blood cells proliferate in the bone marrow in such great quantities that they disrupt normal blood production; *neuroblastoma,* which may occur in any part of the body but characteristically involves a tumorous growth in the sympathetic nerve tissues of the adrenal glands; *brain* or *spinal cord tumor; Hodgkin's disease,* or cancer of the lymph nodes; *Wilms' tumor,* a rare kidney cancer that accounts for about one-fifth of all childhood cancers; *retinoblastoma,* an eye tumor that is probably hereditary and is most frequently encountered in children under four; and *bone cancer* that may attack the long bones of the forearm and leg during the growing years. Many of these cancers can now be arrested, and some can be cured if symptoms are detected early enough. See Ch. 18, *Cancer,* for further information about cancer.

Early Symptoms

Early detection is best accomplished by calling to a physician's attention any of the following symptoms that last for more than a few days: continued crying or pain for which there appears to be no explanation; intermittent nausea and vomiting; the development of lumps or swellings in or on any part of the child's body; stumbling or walking unsteadily; a loss of appetite and general lassitude; any marked change in bowel or bladder habits; any unexplained discharge of blood, whether in the stool or urine, or in heavy nosebleeds, or any marked slowness of bleeding to stop after an injury.

Celiac Disease

Celiac disease, officially known as *malabsorption syndrome*, is the designation for a group of congenital enzyme deficiencies in which certain nutrients are not properly absorbed from the intestinal tract. *Celiac* means having to do with the abdomen. Celiac disease is characterized by frothy, bulky, and foul-smelling stools containing undigested fats. Diarrhea may alternate with constipation, the child has severe stomach cramps, and the abdomen becomes conspicuously bloated. If the disease is untreated, anemia results, and the child's growth is impaired. Early symptoms should be brought to a physician's attention so that a correct diagnosis can be made based on laboratory investigation of the stools. Treatment consists of a special, gluten-free diet under a physician's continuing supervision. *Gluten* is a protein component of wheat and rye; special breads, cookies, etc., must therefore be used. If the diet is strictly adhered to, full recovery can be expected although it may take over a year.

Cerebral Palsy

Cerebral palsy is the general term for a group of abnormal conditions commonly associated with a brain disorder that causes the loss or impairment of muscle control. Approximately one child in about 7,000 suffers from some degree of this disability. Damage to the nervous system that results in cerebral palsy may have occurred before birth, during delivery, or in rare cases, as a consequence of accident, injury, or severe illness during infancy or childhood. Because symptoms vary widely, each individual case is assessed for proper treatment by a team of therapists under the supervision of a specialist, usually a pediatrician. One of the most important aspects of treatment involves parental understanding of the fact that it is essential that they help the child to help himself as much as possible. Guiding the youngster towards self-acceptance and independence requires the patience, persistence, and resourcefulness of the entire family, and may require a certain amount of group therapy and counseling. For a discussion of symptoms and treatment, see "Cerebral Palsy" in Ch. 8, *Diseases of the Muscles and Nervous System.*

Cheating

See DISHONESTY.

Checkups

Medical and dental checkups are essential to everyone's health, but they are especially important for the growing child. An infant should be examined by a physician every month for the first six months, and less frequently after that. The pediatrician usually recommends a schedule for immunization and future checkups. If possible, parents should try to maintain continuity with the same physician so that when an illness occurs, the child sees the physician as an old friend rather than a threatening stranger. Continuity also gives the physician a total picture of the child in sickness and in health and enables him to diagnose variations from the normal with more accuracy. Parents who cannot afford the services of a private physician can be assured of good infant and child care at a local child-health station or at the well-baby clinic of a nearby hospital. Between checkups, it's a good idea for parents to keep a running list of questions or problems they would like to discuss with the doctor at the next visit.

Chicken Pox

Chicken pox is caused by a virus. Its incubation period is two to three weeks. Symptoms include those of the common cold, a fever, general malaise, and a rash. It does not usually cause any severe complications in a child, but it can be serious in an adult. It is highly infectious and spreads rapidly.

The rash, which may be either mild or severe, is different from that produced by measles or by rubella. The measles rash is red and blotchy. Chicken pox has bunches of blisters close together. These blisters are filled with fluid, and there is a reddened area around each lesion. As new blisters appear, the older ones become encrusted. The rash may affect the mouth, nose, ears, vagina, penis, or scrotum. In an older child the symptoms may be more severe than in a younger one, and may be accompanied by headache and vomiting. Chicken pox can now be prevented with a vaccine.

Treatment

The only way to treat chicken pox is symptomatically. The rash is very itchy, and an affected child must be prevented from scratching. Otherwise, he may develop a secondary infection and be left pitted and scarred.

Treatment involves the use of lotions, such as Calamine, applied locally to the pox to relieve the itching. If the child is old enough, it's a good idea to let him paint it on himself. Your physician may also prescribe medicine to be taken orally to help the child stop scratching the blisters. In a few days, the rash clears up, the lesions dry, and the crusts fall off.

Child Abuse and Neglect

Child abuse and neglect have been defined in various ways.

In 1962, Dr. C. Henry Kempe, chief pediatrician at the University of Colorado Medical Center, coined the term *battered child syndrome*. According to Dr. Kempe's definition, the victim of battering is "any child who [has] received *nonaccidental* injury or injuries as a result of acts or omissions on the part of his parents or guardians." Under the Child Abuse Prevention and Treatment Act (Public Law 93-247), passed by Congress in 1974 and amended in 1978 and 1996, child abuse and neglect are defined as

> the physical or mental injury, sexual abuse or exploitation, negligent treatment, or maltreatment of a child under the age of 18 by a person who is responsible for the child's welfare under circumstances which indicate that the child's health or welfare is harmed or threatened thereby.

Abuse and neglect clearly take many forms. *Physical abuse* may involve punching, scalding, suffocating, headcracking, and stomping. *Sexual abuse* can mean intercourse, incest, rape, sodomy, or impairing of a minor's morals (see SEXUAL ABUSE). *Physical neglect* occurs when parents or parent surrogates fail to provide the essentials of a normal life. These include food, clothing, shelter, care, and supervision. Under *emotional abuse or neglect* authorities include parental failure to provide love and proper direction, parental rejection, and deprivation of mothering.

Incidence

Figures on the incidence of child abuse and neglect are difficult to confirm. Many such cases are never reported. At least one agency, the National Center on Child Abuse and Neglect, a federal agency, has concluded that just under one million children are maltreated each year. Another estimate indicates that some 3,000 children die annually in New York City alone as a result of physical abuse.

Most of the abuse victims are three years old or younger. Some authorities believe that the cases of neglect are far more numerous than those of actual abuse.

Control

Approaches to control of the problem of child abuse and neglect have been both legislative and social. Laws passed by all 50 states require physicians and other professionals to report suspected cases of child abuse. In increasing numbers the states also require reports from nurses, teachers, counselors, social workers, clergymen, law enforcement officers, attorneys, and coroners. Some states provide for penalties, including fines up to $1,000 or prison sentences of as much as one year, for persons mandated to report but failing to do so.

Control measures have focused in addition on the rehabilitation of abusive parents and protection of abused children. The National Center on Child Abuse and Neglect, established in 1974 as part of the Children's Bureau of the federal Administration for Children and Families, receives funding that makes possible protective services for the short-term care of endangered children outside the home. The Center also provides counseling for parents, foster-care payments, and other services.

On the principle that the abusive parent must be treated if child abuse and neglect are to be controlled, various organizations have instituted parent-oriented programs. Parents Anonymous sponsors therapy sessions in which abusive parents can meet to help themselves and each other. "Helplines" operating in many communities offer aid and counseling to parents who have abused a child but are afraid to contact a social service or other agency. A number of other agencies and groups provide emergency, counseling, outreach, and related services to parents or parent surrogates. Some helplines have workers available to visit homes in life-threatening situations.

Other groups and agencies take a multidisciplinary approach. Alliance, a division of Catholic Charities, brings together existing community agencies that work together in teams to treat child abuse and neglect cases. Hospital-based treatment programs may include a physician, nurse, social worker, and consulting psychiatrist. Lay therapists may visit homes under other programs, and "foster grandparents" over 65 years of age may be recruited to care for battered children who have been hospitalized.

Sources of Help

Persons seeking help or advice on abused and neglected children can look in their communities' yellow pages under the heading "Social Services Organizations." A number of organizations that offer assistance are listed in the SEXUAL ABUSE section. Others include:

- Parents Anonymous, 675 West Foothill Boulevard, Suite 220, Claremont, CA 91711-3475; (909) 621-6184.
- American Humane Association Childrens Division (AHA), 63 Inverness Drive E, Engelwood, CO 80112-5117; (800) 227-4645.
- Parents without Partners Inc., 1650 South Dixie Highway Suite 510, Boca Raton, FL 33432; (561) 391-8833.

Cholesterol

Cholesterol poses two types of problems in children. The first is a lack of cholesterol in children whose parents have kept them from infancy on low-cholesterol diets. Parents should keep in mind that the body requires some cholesterol to function correctly and that the protein derived from meat and eggs is almost essential to growing bodies. Children who are not fed meat, dairy products, or eggs need to have the protein, amino acids, and other nutrients replaced by either pills or a very well balanced diet. Certain vitamins cannot be found in a vegetarian diet, such as one type of vitamin B. Children on restrictive low-fat, low-cholesterol diets can suffer growth failure and malnutrition unless the diet is supervised by a doctor.

The second problem is an extremely elevated cholesterol level. Although general testing of children for high cholesterol is not recommended, one statistic that proved reliable in spotting 9 out of 10 children with raised levels was the amount of television watched. Children who watched two or more hours of television a day were more likely to have cholesterol levels exceeding 200 mg. More importantly, less than half of those children who had raised levels and watched two hours of television came from families who had a history of high cholesterol. This means that these children are not from high-risk families, but they still manage to increase their cholesterol because of their eating patterns and lack of exercise in their daily routine. The flag that points to the problem is excessive TV viewing. Snacking while watching TV, and not exercising, are the suspected culprits.

Circumcision

Circumcision is a surgical procedure in which the foreskin, or *prepuce*, that covers the cone-shaped tip of the male infant's penis is removed. The Book of Genesis speaks of circumcision as a religious rite. Once relatively common in the United States, the procedure has become more rare. The American Academy of Pediatrics has stated that "routine circumcision of the newborn infant lacks medical justification."

Usually performed a few days after birth, the procedure takes only a few minutes and can be done in various ways. A scalpel may be used, for example. Possible complications include excessive bleeding, infection, and urinary obstruction resulting from contraction of the skin at the base of the foreskin. But complications are infrequent.

The parents of the newborn male infant should decide whether to have their son circumcised or not. They may first consult their obstetrician or pediatrician. In most cases, decisions are made on the basis of family, religious, or cultural traditions. However, many family health insurance policies today provide no coverage for the procedure.

Cleft Palate and Cleft Lip

A *cleft palate* is a split in the roof of the mouth sometimes extending to the lip and into the nose. The split is caused by the failure of the two sides of the face to unite properly during prenatal development. The condition occurs in about 1 out of 1,000 births and is sometimes associated with a foot or spine deformity. It is in no way related to mental retardation.

An infant born with a cleft palate cannot suck properly unless a special device, called an *obturator*, is inserted into the split to close it against the flow of air. Where this is undesireable, feeding may be done with a spoon or a dropper.

Because the condition eventually causes speech distortion, it should be corrected at about 18 months of age, before the child begins to talk. The surgery consists of reconstructing the tissue. Sometimes, even at this early age, the child may need some corrective speech therapy following the operation.

If the split occurs only in the lip, commonly called a *harelip*, surgery may be recommended when the infant weighs about 15 pounds, usually at the age of 12 to 15 months. When the operation is performed this early, there is no danger of speech impairment, and the result is only a thin scar.

Clothing

Standards have been set up by the U.S. government for infants' and children's sleepwear to be flame retardant or flame resistent. This does not mean that the material will not burn—even flame retardant material will burn when fire is held against the cloth. The difference is that when the flame is removed, the retardant material ceases to burn. Nontreated material will continue to burn and fuel further flames.

Until recently this meant that sleepwear for small children had to be non-natural fibers. Synthetic material could be coated so that it would not continue to burn after the flame was removed. Cotton does continue to burn and increases the likelihood of serious injuries to a child in case of fire. However, recent improvements in chemical treatment of cotton have provided the clothing industry with flame retardant cotton. Always check clothing labels to see if the cotton is treated. If it is not labeled as flame retardant or flame resistent, it should not be considered for sleepwear.

Labeling should be checked on all clothing that will be used as sleepwear. Often times, manufacturers will produce clothing for infants that looks like sleepwear but is labeled daywear or playwear in order to avoid the need for flame retardant treatment of the cloth. If the clothing is not marked flame retardant, or is not specifically labeled as sleepwear, it should not be used to clothe a sleeping child.

Clubfoot

Clubfoot is a bone deformity characterized by an inturning or outturning of the foot. An orthopedist must put the clubfoot and part of the leg into a cast to correct the condition. If casting does not cure the abnormality, orthopedic surgery may be necessary.

Occasionally, a benign and easily correctable condition involving a child's legs may have been produced by the position the baby was in while still in the uterus.

The mother can help to correct the condition by daily passive exercises of the baby's feet. She does this by turning the feet correctly for a few minutes every day. To maintain the corrected position, the application of plaster is sometimes necessary. Such a procedure requires the attention of an orthopedic surgeon.

Colic

During the first three or four months, many babies have occasional attacks of *colic*, a general term applied to infantile digestive discomfort. After feeding, the baby may cry out in pain and draw up her arms and legs. Her abdomen may feel hard. Apart from making sure the baby is as comfortable as can be, there's not much that can be done for colic. You must try not to let the baby's crying make you a nervous wreck, for your nervousness will be communicated to the baby, which will only create a vicious circle of increasing tension. Usually colic tapers off at about the third month. If the baby's colic attacks are very frequent or persistent, consult your pediatrician.

Color Blindness

Color blindness is a genetic inability to distinguish between certain colors, most commonly between red and green. This defect, which is characteristically male, is inherited through the mother. That is, a woman whose father was color blind can pass the trait to her son without herself suffering the defect. About 8 million people in the United States have the red/green form of color blindness which can neither be cured nor corrected. Many of them are scarcely aware of their deficiency. Parents who suspect that their child may have this minor disability can arrange for simple testing.

Common Cold

By recent count, there are about 150 different viruses that cause common cold symptoms, and because not a single one of them can be treated effectively by medicines, coping with a cold seems to be part of the human condition. Parents who are sniveling, sneezing, and coughing should ask the physician what precautions to take when handling the baby.

Young children with stuffy noses and breathing difficulties should be kept indoors, near a humidifier or steam kettle if the air is especially dry. Nose drops should not be given unless the physician says so. Older children may not want to miss school because of a cold. If they do go, they should be given lots of liquid when they get home and steered in the direction of an afternoon nap. Colds in and of themselves are unavoidable and not serious, but the proper precautions should be taken to prevent complications, such as an ear infection or a sore throat.

Competitiveness

See AGGRESSIVENESS.

Conscience

See GUILT AND CONSCIENCE.

Constipation

Parents who are anxious about the frequency of their own bowel movements or who are excessively refined in their attitudes towards defecation are pretty sure to transmit these feelings to their children unless they make some effort not to. Concerns of this kind are one sure way of constipating a child. Actually, if a child is eating a proper diet, getting enough exercise, and drinking a sufficiency of liquids, constipation is not likely to be a problem.

Frequency of Bowel Movements

Not everyone has a bowel movement every day. On the other hand, some people routinely have more than one movement a day. There is considerable variation among normal patterns of bowel movements. This should be borne in mind before parents conclude that their child is constipated. Children need to be assured that they are not necessarily abnormal if they deviate from the one-a-day pattern.

However, any abrupt change in the normal pattern of bowel movements should be noted, and if it persists contact a physician. Frequent small movements can be a sign of constipation.

A youngster on a light diet because of illness, or one who is dehydrated because of a fever, may suffer from mild constipation that will clear up when he recovers. If constipation becomes chronic, don't resort to enemas or laxatives on your own; discuss the problem with your physician who will want to check on other symptoms that might indicate an intestinal disorder.

Cradle Cap

This condition is marked by yellowish crusts on the baby's scalp. It is usually harmless, and can be taken care of by regular shampooing. Occasionally, a special soap as well as a very fine comb may be helpful.

Crib Death

See SUDDEN INFANT DEATH SYNDROME.

Crossed Eyes (Strabismus)

Do not be alarmed if your baby's eyes do not focus. Crossed eyes are a common condition that usually corrects itself somewhere between the ages of six and twelve months. If crossing of the eyes persists after one year, an ophthalmologist (eye specialist) should evaluate the baby's vision.

If a real problem does develop, one eye—or each eye alternately—may cross, turn outward, or focus below or above the other. Frequently the reason for "turning" is that there is a larger refractive error in one eye than in the other. Eyeglasses will often correct this condition.

Occasionally, eye muscle weakness is the cause of crossed eyes. This is most often true of premature children. The weakness of some muscles causes overaction of other muscles.

Eyeglasses will often prevent the need for eye surgery. Sometimes, however, surgery will be necessary to straighten the eyes. Either before or after surgery the eyes may need further attention in the form of eye drops, a patch to cover one eye, or glasses.

Croup

Croup, a most harassing and terrifying experience for new parents, is a spasm of the windpipe or trachea, especially involving the larynx. When such a spasm occurs, an affected child has great trouble in breathing and produces a cough that sounds like the bark of a dog. In some cases, the child can't breathe at all.

An attack of croup is an emergency. The younger the child, the more dangerous it is. You must get the baby's airway open. The best thing to do is to take the child into the bathroom, shut the door, and turn on the hot water of the shower full force, or of the bathtub and sink if you don't have a shower. The idea is to fill the room with hot steam in order to loosen the mucus plug in the baby's trachea, thus enabling him to cough up the mucus.

Get to your physician as soon as possible so that more effective treatment can begin. If the croup is viral in origin, antibiotics may not help; but when the infection is caused by bacteria, your physician will put the child on one of the antimicrobial agents. If your child is subject to croup, it is a good idea to invest in a hot or cold air vaporizer and use it whenever he has congestion resulting from a cold.

In a really severe emergency, when the windpipe closes completely, a *tracheostomy* must be performed so that the throat can be opened and an airway inserted. A tracheostomy should be performed in a hospital, but if for some reason it is performed elsewhere, the child should be hospitalized as quickly as possible.

Curiosity

If we weren't born curious, we'd never learn a thing. Even before a child can walk and talk, curiosity motivates a good part of her behavior: putting things into her mouth, poking at things, pointing at people, and as the natural urge to speak becomes stronger, holding things up or bringing them to mother or father in order to find out what they're called.

Respecting Curiosity

A parent who respects the child's curiosity will be attentive to it and satisfy it as part of the ongoing learning experience. It doesn't take any extra time when a toddler is sitting in your lap to say the words for the parts of your face (and hers) as she touches them, or the words for her articles of clothing as she tries to help put them on. Dealing with the "why" stage of curiosity is more complicated, especially because in many instances, the child is asking "Why?" for the sheer joy and sense of power of being able to do so.

Many parents who don't know anything about mechanics or astronomy have developed a sense of security by heading for the children's shelves at the local library and reading the simplest books on the subject that interest their preschool children so that they can answer some of their questions. Of course, no one can answer all the questions that a child might ask during an average day. Some should be answered by mother, some by father, and some will have to wait. There's no harm in telling a four-year-old child who wants to know why the wind makes a whistling sound that she'll find out about such things when she goes to school. That's a much better answer than "Don't ask so many questions." Questions should always be listened to even if the answers aren't readily available.

As the child reaches the age of eight and can do a certain amount of reading, it's a good idea to invest in a fairly simple encyclopedia. With such a source of information available, it's possible to respond to some questions with "Let's go find the answer together."

Each family must decide for itself where the line is to be drawn between legitimate curiosity and unacceptable snoopiness or nosiness as children get older and become interested in such matters as how rich the neighbors are, or "What were you and mommy fighting about when I was falling asleep last night?"

Cystic Fibrosis

Cystic fibrosis is an inherited disease in which the child cannot handle the normal secretions of the respiratory tract. There is a lack of ciliary action—the beating movement by the hairs of the cells lining the bronchial tubes of the lungs. Thick mucus collects at the base of the lungs, obstructing the smaller air passages and causing labored breathing and chronic cough.

Respiratory Complications

Bacteria multiply in the accumulated lung secretions, predisposing the patient to chronic bronchitis and other respiratory infections, such as pneumonia. Lung tissue changes can result eventually in severe, permanent damage to the lungs.

Digestive Complications

The abnormally thick, viscous mucus produced by the cystic fibrosis patient tends to obstruct the ducts or openings of the mucus-secreting glands. When such mucus obstructs the pancreas, it interferes with its ability to supply important digestive enzymes to the intestinal tract, thus leading to poor digestion and malabsorption of a number of important nutrients. A child with cystic fibrosis may therefore be poorly nourished in spite of an adequate diet.

Other Complications

Tissue changes in the lungs can restrict blood flow to the heart, leading to increased blood pressure and chronic heart strain. Loss of large amounts of salt through malfunctioning sweat glands can become a very serious problem for youngsters in hot weather, causing dehydration and heat exhaustion. Laboratory tests usually find an abnormally high concentration of salt in the sweat of cystic fibrosis patients. Some tissues may show three times the normal concentration of sodium and twice the normal levels of potassium.

Treatment

There is no known cure for cystic fibrosis. Treatment includes the use of humidifiers and inhalation medication in the form of aerosols to loosen secretions. Another method used is *postural drainage*—lying facedown with the head lower than the feet to let gravity help loosen secretions. Antibiotics are used to control infections; special diets with reduced fat intake and added nutrients are prescribed to compensate for abnormal digestive function. Other medical techniques are utilized in individual cases to maintain normal heart and lung function.

The discovery of the defective gene involved in triggering cystic fibrosis is expected to improve diagnostic testing for the genetic disorder. The subsequent discovery of the cell malfunction that blocks the making of a protein will also enable scientists to improve treatment of the disease with aerosol inhalers and with mucus-thinning medication. Several drugs are being tested with success on patients.

Once considered strictly a disease of early childhood, an increasing number of cases of cystic fibrosis have been detected in recent years among adolescents and adults. Symptoms of the disease, including respiratory difficulty with chronic coughing, may resemble those of an allergic reaction.

How the Disease is Inherited

Cystic fibrosis is transmitted to a child only when both parents are carriers of the trait. When only one parent carries the trait, however, some of the children can become carriers. Through marriage with other carriers, they may then become the parents of a child afflicted with the disorder.

Information on new treatment techniques, the location of treatment centers, and genetic counseling may be obtained from the national headquarters of the Cystic Fibrosis Foundation, 6931 Arlington Rd., Ste. 200, Bethesda, MD 20814.

Daydreaming

See FANTASIES.

Deafness

Major advances have been made in recent years in educating and socializing incurably deaf children who are normal in all other ways. Starting with a proper assessment of the child's degree of deafness at the earliest possible time and the fitting of a hearing aid are two crucial considerations. The child's instruction in lipreading and the use of her own vocal equipment are professionally supervised, and the rest of the family is very much involved in the whole process. Nowadays an important advance in speech therapy is the use of a feedback system that makes it possible for the youngster to be self-corrective. Parents seeking information about special schools and services, summer camps, and other facilities can write to the following agencies: Alexander Graham Bell Association for the Deaf, 3417 Volta Place, N.W., Washington, D.C. 20007; (202) 337-5220; American Speech-Language-Hearing Association, 10801 Rockville Pike, Rockville, MD 20852; (800) 638-8255 [Voice and TTY]. See also HEARING.

Death

Some children's first experience of death is the loss of a grandparent; others may have to confront the fact of death for the first time when a beloved pet dies. A child wants to know where people or animals go when they die. Parents should be as honest as possible in answering such questions and tell their offspring what they themselves truly believe. Those parents who believe that there is life after death should say so; those who do not should say that they do not. Whatever one's beliefs, there are better ways to phrase them than "Grandma is in heaven watching you" or "People who are naughty go to hell when they die."

Death of a Parent

A child who has to cope with the death of a parent may be so disoriented that his behavior will seem odd to the adults around him. He may pretend that the death never happened; others may protect themselves from the shock by burying their feelings and never talking about the dead parent. Still others may feel rage at having been abandoned. Many youngsters are overwhelmed by guilt, feeling that in some magic way they caused the death because from time to time they secretly wished it. In cases where the bereft child cannot cope with the loss, it may be advisable to provide some help in the form of psychiatric therapy.

Delinquency

Juvenile delinquents are minors who are guilty of breaking the law or who are engaged in associations and activities considered harmful to children's morals, such as running errands for gamblers, acting as a lookout during a robbery, or sniffing glue for kicks. Swiping a candy bar or a comic book at the age of ten doesn't define a child as a hardened delinquent, but where such behavior becomes chronic, it's a sign that something is wrong that needs to be corrected. With the guidance of a therapist, it may turn out that the child alone is not entirely responsible for his delinquent tendencies. See also DESTRUCTIVENESS, DISHONESTY, DISOBEDIENCE.

Dental Care

The proper attitude toward dental care is best instilled not by lectures or warnings, but by example. Parents who themselves go regularly to the dentist for checkups, who take care of their teeth by keeping them clean with routine brushing and the use of dental floss, can do more for their child's dental health than those who depend on stern warnings to shape the attitudes of their children. Parents can hardly expect their offspring to be heroic about dental visits when they themselves scarcely ever go unless they have a toothache.

Start Early

Dental care can begin by having the toddler accompany the parent to the dentist so that his baby teeth can be inspected and he can be given a special toothbrush of his own with instructions about how to use it. In communities where the water supply is not fluoridated, the dentist may recommend an ongoing program of fluoride application to the teeth themselves. Some families find that a pediatric dentist who specializes in children's dentistry can deal with a frightened or anxious child more expertly than the family dentist. Other families use the services of the dental clinics that are part of the dental schools of large universities.

No matter who is in charge of the family's dental health, it is important that professional attention is given to the child's dental development at every stage: fillings for decay in the first teeth, routine cleanings and checkups, and preventive orthodontics where advisable. Another aspect of dental care involves keeping the consumption of sweets to a minimum, and making sure that the child's daily diet contains the proper nutrients for building healthy teeth. See also ORTHODONTICS. For full discussion, see Ch. 22, *Teeth and Gums*.

Destructiveness

"It was an accident!" is a common cry when a child destroys a valuable object because of carelessness. And it probably was an accident. Parents who don't want precious bric-a-brac or other delicate possessions broken had better put them out of the reach of curious and clumsy little fingers. Young children should not be punished because their toys always seem to be destroyed; better to give them playthings that are sturdy and comparatively indestructible.

The child who is destructive unwittingly should not be spoken to in the same way as one would speak to a boy who willfully breaks his sister's doll or a girl who spitefully tears her brother's model-making manual. Destructiveness born of anger ("I was so furious, I smashed a dish") may happen rarely, but when it does, it should be commented on as an unsuitable way of dealing with the problem that caused the anger in the first place. When destructiveness gets out of hand or involves group activities amounting to vandalism, parental action should be taken with the guidance of a professional counselor.

Developmental Disability

Any disability that interferes with a child's normal development is a *developmental disability*. The term has been used more specifically, however, to refer to mental retardation, cerebral palsy, epilepsy, and autism.

Diabetes

No one knows why some children develop diabetes. Diabetes is a noncontagious disease that results from the body's inability to produce enough insulin for the normal metabolism of sugar. The diabetic child is thus improperly nourished because the sugar that should be incorporated into the tissues is excreted in the urine. Finding sugar in the urine facilitates early diagnosis. Also, because this disorder causes a disturbance in the metabolism of fat, there is an increase of fat in the blood, detectable in a routine blood count. Juvenile onset diabetes can be more volatile that adult onset diabetes. Control is usually through injectable insulin.

Insulin treatment has undergone some improvements in the past few years. Human insulin is now readily available; beef-pork insulin was common in usage before. There is less likely to be an allergic reaction to human insulin produced through genetic reproduction. Also, doses can be adjusted to the individual through the mix of fast-acting and slow-acting preparations.

Early Signs

Parents who are themselves diabetic will be alert to any symptoms in their offspring. The disease occurs more frequently in children where there is a family history of diabetes. However, because the disorder may occur in children where there is no previous family history of diabetes, alertness to the following signs is advisable: an abnormally frequent need to urinate; an excessive desire for fluids; itching of the genitals; general listlessness; frequent boils and carbuncles; slow healing of cuts and bruises.

If a diagnosis of diabetes is made by the physician, the child may be hospitalized for a few days for a series of definitive tests, and all the members of the family will be educated in the best way to supervise the child's diet and daily routine so that serious complications can be avoided. Professional guidance is also available to ensure that the youngster's emotional adjustment is a healthy one. For a full discussion see Ch. 15, *Diabetes Mellitus*.

Diaper Rash

See RASHES.

Diapers

Some controversy has built up in the past few years over which is more ecologically sound—cloth diapers or paper diapers. Paper diapers in landfills take more than one hundred years to deteriorate. Even if the plastic lining is removed, it is believed that the paper will deteriorate only weeks faster than if the diaper left intact. Effective recycling of paper diapers does not yet exist, and it may be years before the material can be sanitized to the point of recyclability.

Cloth diapers, on the other hand, require strong soaps and chemicals to clean. To insure the sterility and whiteness of the cloth, bleach and harsh detergents are used. These go into the water supply and affect the plant and animal life. The energy used for hot water to wash the diapers also adds to the environmental cost.

Many parents try to use paper diapers only while traveling or in places where having a soiled diaper to carry or clean would be extremely inconvenient. This infrequent use of paper diapers allows for the occasional convenience of the throwaway while reducing paper waste.

Some parents believe that cloth diapers cause more diaper rash; other parents believe that the sealed paper diaper causes more diaper rash. The biggest cause of diaper rash is excessive moisture against the baby's skin, which can be avoided by frequent diaper changes, for whatever diaper used. Excessive use of powders and creams can also increase the problem because of the pasty substance that forms when these encounter moisture.

Diarrhea

Diarrhea, or loose and watery bowel movements, is common in babies because they are more sensitive to certain intestinal germs than older children. They may also be reacting to a change in their formula or to the roughage in a newly introduced fruit or vegetable. In older children, diarrhea may occur not only as a symptom of bacterial or viral infection, or because of food poisoning, but also as an allergic response, or because of overexcitement or anxiety.

Diarrhea in an infant should always be brought to a doctor's attention if it continues for more than 24 hours. The same holds true for an older child, especially when there are also symptoms of cramps, fever, or aches and pains in the joints. Persistent diarrhea from any cause, because it can lead to serious dehydration especially in infants, requires prompt medical attention.

Diphtheria

Diphtheria is a severe and contagious bacterial infection, often fatal if untreated. Once one of the most threatening of all childhood diseases, there are now fewer than 1,000 cases a year in the United States because of widespread and effective immunization.

The first symptoms—fever, headache, nausea, and sore throat—may be confused with the onset of other disorders. However, there is a manifestation of diphtheria that is uniquely its own: patches of grayish yellow membrane form in the throat and grow together into one large membrane that interferes with swallowing and breathing.The diphtheria bacteria also produce a powerful toxin that can eventually cause irreversible damage to the heart and nerves. Diagnosis is usually verified by laboratory identification of the bacteria in a throat culture.

If diphtheria does occur, it is best treated in a hospital. The prompt prescription of antitoxin serum and antibiotics results in recovery in practically all cases. See IMMUNIZATION.

Disabled Child

Whether a handicap is hereditary or acquired, mental or physical, temporary or permanent, it is always a condition that prevents a child from participating fully on an equal footing in the activities of her own age group. But how fully she can participate and her attitude toward her disability are usually a reflection of the attitudes of her parents, teachers, and the community. Of primary importance is an assessment at the earliest possible age of the extent to which the handicap can be decreased or corrected.

Exactly how deaf is the deaf child? Can surgery repair a rheumatic heart? Is a defect of vision operable? Is the child with cerebral palsy mentally retarded or is the seeming mental malfunction a reversible effect of the physical condition? Parents should investigate all the available services offered by voluntary organizations and community groups that might help them and their child. See Ch. 36, *Voluntary Health Agencies*.

One promising development in recent years is the attempt to integrate handicapped children, whenever possible, into the mainstream of education rather than segregate them in special classes. School systems in various parts of the United States are placing deaf, blind, physically disabled, and emotionally disturbed youngsters into classrooms with their nonhandicapped peers and providing them with essential supportive services at various times during the school day. The experience of dealing with nonhandicapped children will provide them with a more realistic preparation for their adult lives.

Discrimination

See PREJUDICE.

Dishonesty

Nobody is honest about everything all the time, and that goes for children as well as adults. It's unrealistic to expect a child never to lie about anything.

Little children like to make things up and can't be held strictly accountable for some of their tall stories when they're still at an age at which fact and fantasy are not clearly distinguished. A colorful exaggeration needn't call for an accusation of lying. It's better to respond with, "That's an interesting story," or "You're just imagining."

Lying and Punishment

As youngsters get older, they should feel secure enough to tell the truth about having been naughty, knowing that although they may be punished, they will get approval for having told the truth. Children shouldn't be so fearful of their parents that dishonesty is their only protection against a beating.

Cheating

Children who are pressured beyond their ability to perform are the ones likeliest to cheat; so are those for whom winning has been held up constantly as a transcendent value. A child who has been caught cheating at school is usually punished by the authorities. If the incident is discussed at home, the parents might reexamine their values before adding to the child's burdens. A youngster who cheats regularly at games will suffer the natural punishment of exclusion by his peers.

Stealing

Young children who embark on group enterprises of stealing "for fun"—whether it's taking candy from the corner market or shoplifting from a department store—needn't be viewed as case-hardened criminals unless the stealing becomes habitual. A nine-year-old who swipes a candy bar once or twice and regrets it belongs in a different category from one who is hired as a lookout for older delinquents. Children usually have respect for other people's property when they have property of their own that they value and don't want anyone else to take.

Disobedience

Father gets a parking ticket because he forgot about alternate sides of the street on Wednesdays; mother has a whipped cream dessert in spite of her physician's orders not to. Are mother and father disobedient? When Junior comes home from the playground at five instead of obeying orders to come home at four, is his disobedience any worse than theirs? Genuine forgetfulness, negligence, or occasional breaking of a rule is only human. Willful chronic disobedience is another matter.

Some children with a strong urge toward independence may test out many parental rules by disobeying them on purpose. A child who has been ordered not to spend any time with another child because the families are feuding, may, by flouting the order, be telling his parents that he has a right to choose his own friends. Where disobedience affects a youngster's health or safety or morals, it's time for parental action, not necessarily in the form of punishment, but in taking stock of the situation to find out why the child won't obey.

Divorced Parents

See "Separation and Divorce" in Ch. 5, *The Middle Years*.

Dreams and Nightmares

Children go through periods of having "bad dreams" or nightmares that wake them up in the middle of the night in a state of terror and bewilderment. It won't do to say, "It's just a dream." To a young child who is just beginning to grasp the difference between what's real and what isn't, nightmare can be extremely threatening. If the child wants to describe the dream after she collects herself, she should be allowed to do so even at 3:00 A.M. She may amplify and exaggerate a little bit, but that's only to let you know that she's been very brave through it all. Parental patience is called for; with a certain amount of reassurance, the child can usually be led back to bed and to sleep.

Youngsters whose sleep is regularly interrupted by nightmares or who are in the grip of the same nightmare may be feeling anxious about a daytime activity or may be feeling guilty about some undiscovered naughtiness. A tactful chat can sometimes reveal what the trouble is so that it can be disposed of during waking hours.

Night Terrors

Some children may have occasional nightmares—often called *night terrors*—in which they scream or tremble in terror. They may sit up in bed while still asleep, or even walk around. Their terror is certainly real, but the parents should remember that the cause of it is purely imaginary. Accordingly, they have no reason to be alarmed; in spite of the child's appearance, she is not in any danger, and no drastic action is called for.

Simply comfort the child, who frequently will be disoriented and confused in a half-awake state, until she can go back to sleep. She will probably have no recollection of the episode the next morning.

If night terrors occur only occasionally, there is no cause for concern, although it might be a good idea to check on the television shows your child is watching before bedtime. If there is a great deal of tension in the household, that could be a contributing cause. If night terrors are persistent or frequent, however, a physician should be consulted. See also SLEEPWALKING.

Dyslexia

Dyslexia is a condition in which an otherwise average or intelligent child suffers from a complex of motor-perceptual disabilities that interfere with the orderly processing and acquisition of language. The disability that results in an inhibition of symbol recognition essential for learning how to read, write, and spell is thought to originate in some form of brain circuitry malfunction that may have been caused by injury or by genetic defect. Recent researchers have established some connection between dyslexia and a faulty pathway between the lower brain—the cerebellum—and the inner ear, causing the dyslexic child to suffer from a mild and permanent form of motion sickness that interferes with learning.

Symptoms

The symptoms of dyslexia vary considerably and may include: garbled or disordered development of speech during the early years; an inability to learn the relationship between sounds and symbols for purposes of reading aloud; an inability to learn how to spell or how to organize written expression; confusion about serial order, as in naming the days of the week or in number concepts; unusual difficulty in doing simple repetitive tasks.

If a parent suspects that a child is suffering from dyslexia, a diagnosis should be made on the basis of tests administered by trained professionals. The child's pediatrician or the school guidance counselor should be consulted about where such tests are best given and assessed. Should the child be diagnosed as dyslexic, an appropriate remedial program or an accredited special school can help surmount some of the learning difficulties.

Earache

Earache is one of the most common complaints of childhood.

As Secondary Infection

Earache is often attributable to bacterial infection of the middle ear and should be treated promptly by a physician. Because the eustachian tube that connects the back of the throat with the middle ear is shorter and wider in a child than in an adult, it affords easier entry to bacteria. Infections of the ear may thus occur as the result of a sore throat or a postnasal drip. Infectious mucus from the nose is often forced into the middle ear by way of the eustachian tube because young children are inclined to sniff it back rather than to blow it out. And when a child is mastering the technique of noseblowing, he should be told that neither one nor both of the nostrils should be pressed closed in the process. Rather, both nostrils should be blown out gently at the same time, and with the mouth open. If gentle blowing doesn't clear the nostrils, the nose should be wiped as necessary.

Recognizing Earache in an Infant

Earache in an infant may be combined with fever and the kind of crying associated with sharp pain. A toddler may indicate the source of discomfort by pulling at the earlobe. Until the pediatrician can prescribe proper medication, discomfort can be relieved by applying a heating pad to the involved ear and giving the child a non-aspirin pain reliever.

Other Causes

Earache may also accompany teething or tooth infection, or it may be the result of pressure caused by water that has been trapped in the ear after swimming or bathing. In small children, an earache may be a sign that the youngster has stuffed a bean or a tiny plastic object so far into his ear that it won't come out as easily as it went in. If you suspect such an occurrence, avoid poking and prodding in an attempt to remove the object. The child should be taken to a physician or to a hospital so that the object can be removed with the proper instruments and the ear examined and treated for possible injury.

Consequences of Neglect of Earache

An earache should always be brought to a physician's attention without delay because untreated middle ear infections can lead to irreversible hearing loss. The leading cause of mild hearing loss in toddlers is believed to be *serous otitis media*, or serous infection of the middle ear. This condition is specifically an inflammation of the middle ear with an accumulation of fluid behind the eardrum. When the condition is chronic or improperly treated during the first three years, it may impair hearing permanently and as a consequence lead to a failure to develop normal language skills. Occasionally the physician may have to make a small opening in the eardrum to drain the fluid, a procedure known as a *myringotomy*. Other treatments may include the insertion of a synthetic tube into the eustachian to expand constricted areas and allow drainage of the inner ear through the auditory tube. The isthmus of the auditory tube is the narrowest point in the canal and may close during swelling or inflammation. To drain the ear properly the tube should be reopened to avoid further infection. See also HEARING.

Eczema

See under RASHES.

Education

See SCHOOL.

Epilepsy

Epilepsy in childhood most commonly takes the form of petit mal or psychomotor episodes.

Petit Mal Seizures

Petit mal episodes are characterized by brief lapses of consciousness, sometimes occurring many times a day. The child does not fall down but simply stops what he is doing and may appear to stare absently.

Psychomotor Seizures

Psychomotor episodes are characterized by the performance of some activity during a brief lapse of consciousness. The child may walk around in circles, or sit down and get up in a purposeless way. During this type of seizure the child may babble nonsensically or chant the same word over and over. Such an attack may last no more than a few minutes, and when the child recovers he is likely to have no memory of its occurrence.

In many instances, parents who expect a certain amount of bizarre behavior from their youngsters may not realize that a form of epilepsy is the cause. Should such incidents occur frequently, they should be called to the attention of the physician who may think it advisable to have the child examined by a neurologist.

A parent witnessing a *grand mal* or convulsive epileptic seizure for the first time may be unduly alarmed and take measures that may harm the child rather than help. For a description of emergency measures during a grand mal seizure, see Ch. 35, *Medical Emergencies.* For a full discussion of epilepsy, see Ch. 8, *Diseases of the Muscles and Nervous System.*

Exercise

Some children seem to sit around a great deal; others are on the move from morning until bedtime. A youngster might be listless or lethargic because there's something the matter that needs to be investigated by a physician. This type of sitting around is quite different from playing with dolls for hours at a time or looking at picture books instead of running around. A young child who really cannot sit still at all may have a problem that needs diagnosing by a physician, too. Practically all children are found between these extremes.

Exercise as a Developmental Need

Toddlers must be allowed to get the exercise necessary for the development of their bodies. They shouldn't be confined in a playpen for most of the day. Three- and four-year-olds who don't go to a nursery school and have no play equipment in their backyard (if they have a backyard), should be taken whenever possible to a local park or playground that has swings, slides, seesaws, jungle gyms, or other devices that are safely designed and installed. Most schools have some kind of supervised gym activity or a free time for yard play, and if they don't, they should. If this scheduled exercise is insufficient for a nine- or ten-year-old, inquiries can be made about athletic facilities at a local YMCA, settlement house, church, or fraternal organization.

Choice of Activities

As children get a little older, they should be permitted to choose the exercise that appeals to them unless there's a good reason for its being forbidden. A girl who wants to join a sandlot baseball team shouldn't be forced to go to a ballet class, and a boy inspired by the dancing he's seen on TV shouldn't be discouraged if the family can afford the lessons. Exercise needn't be synonymous with competition unless the youngster wants it to be. See also "Physical Fitness" in Ch. 3, *The Teens*.

Eyeglasses

Now that infants and youngsters have periodic eye checkups with their physicians, and regular tests are given to all students, more children are wearing glasses than in former years. In addition to *strabismus* (crossed eyes), the three major eye problems encountered in children are *myopia* (nearsightedness), *hyperopia* (farsightedness), and *astigmatism*.

Myopia

The *myopic* or nearsighted child cannot see distant objects well but can see close objects clearly. A very young child so afflicted may stumble and fall easily. An older child attending school may make errors in copying because she has difficulty in making out the words and figures written on the chalkboard. She may be called a behavior problem or may even be said to be mentally retarded. Most cases of myopia can be helped with glasses.

Hyperopia

The *hyperopic* (also called *hypermetropic*) or farsighted eye is shorter from front to rear than the normal eye, and if not corrected will often hinder close work like reading. When a farsighted child reads she often complains of blurring of the printed page, sleepiness, and headache. Farsightedness is often associated with crossed eyes and is usually correctable with glasses.

Astigmatism

In *astigmatism* or distorted vision, there is an uneven curvature of the cornea or lens surface of the eye. This condition causes some light rays to focus further back than others and produces a blurred, distorted image on the retina.

Either a farsighted or nearsighted eye can be *astigmatic;* the abnormality can usually be corrected by properly prescribed eyeglasses.

Fantasies

Every normal child has fantasies, some highly pleasurable, some fearful and frightening. Young children sometimes have a hard time sorting out what they imagine from what's real; this may be especially true when a nightmare interferes with sleep.

Many children quite consciously say, "Let's pretend" or "Let's make believe" when they embark on a dress-up activity; others simply and straightforwardly act out their fantasies by playing games of violence with toy guns. An only child may create a fantasy companion with whom she has conversations; a child who is encouraged to draw may give shape to her fantasies in pictures that mean a lot to her but not much to anyone else.

Daydreaming

Some children infuriate their energetic parents by sitting around and daydreaming (with one sock on and one off) instead of doing their chores. Whatever form fantasies may take, they are an inevitable part of growing up and should be respected, unless they become the equivalent of a narcotic escape from reality rather than a means of enriching it. When a child's fantasy life appears to be turning into a substitute for his real one, the time has come to consult a psychiatric authority.

Fears and Phobias

Babies are fearful about being dropped, and they're frightened by a sudden loud noise. (You *can* make babies cry by saying, "Boo!" When they get older and catch on, they'll think it's fun to be scared.) Toddlers are taught to be afraid of a hot stove, and as children get a little older, they develop night fears that become bad dreams. Many parents transmit, deliberately or unknowingly, some of their fears to their children: fear of dogs, or thunder and lightning, or infection by germs.

Only a thin line separates sensible caution from anxiety. Where a threat of punishment is involved, an anxiety may develop that can last a lifetime. Parents should control the impulse to say such things as, "Don't eat that, it's going to make you sick" or "Don't climb so high, you're going to fall" or "Don't play in the mud; the germs will make you sick." Or, worse yet, "If you do that, the bogey man will get you" or "God will punish you."

Phobias

If fears are often legitimate and usually outgrown through reassuring experiences, phobias are deep-seated unconquerable fears. Many adults suffer from them; two of the most common are *claustrophobia*, the fear of being in an enclosed place, and *acrophobia*, the fear of heights. *Phobia* is a clinical term and shouldn't be used to describe a youngster's aversion to school at a particular time, or his apprehension about elevators and escalators. If parental reassurance can help a child overcome fears of this type, they need not be classed as phobias.

Fever

As every parent knows, babies can run very high fevers. In itself, a rectal temperature of 103° F or 104° F is not necessarily cause for alarm. (Normal rectal temperature is about ½° F to 1° F higher than the oral norm of 98.6° F.) Of course, you should take the immediate step of calling your pediatrician to find out what's causing the fever.

If a baby's fever goes over 104° F, the infant may experience convulsions. To avoid this possibility, he may be bathed with cool water. If convulsions do occur, protect the baby from injuring himself by seeing that his head and body don't strike anything that is hard or that has sharp edges. The convulsion, though frightening, is usually brief and ends of its own accord. Get in touch with your pediatrician without delay.

Although the mechanism that results in fever is not precisely understood, the elevation in temperature is almost always a sign that the child's normal body processes are being disturbed. A child old enough to talk can let you know that his throat is sore or that he has an earache.

Possible Causes

Fever is often the sign of the onset of an infectious disease such as measles or influenza; it usually accompanies severe sunburn; it may be a warning that the infection of a local cut is spreading through the rest of the body. When it comes suddenly and rises quickly, along with cramps or diarrhea, it may indicate a gastrointestinal infection or food poisoning. No matter what a child's age, if temperature by mouth rises above 101° F, a physician should be informed of the fever and accompanying symptoms.

Treatment

Until a diagnosis is made and treatment prescribed, the feverish youngster should be put to bed and kept on a diet of light foods and lots of liquids. If the elevated temperature is combined with stiff neck, aching joints, or headache, nonaspirin medication can be given for relief according to dose instructions indicated.

Fluoridation

Although it has been unequivocally established that fluoridated drinking water is the best safeguard against tooth decay, many parts of the United States continue to resist this public health measure, thus placing a special burden on the parents of preschool children. Families in such communities are strongly urged to consult their dentist or the closest dental clinic connected with a university's college of dentistry for advice on the appropriate measures to be taken to protect their children's teeth. A consultation of this nature is advisable as soon as the baby shows signs of teething, because the fluoride treatments should begin as early as possible.

In many areas where the water supply remains unfluoridated, programs in the public schools supply youngsters with fluoride tablets every day. Although this method of applying the chemical is less effective than its availability in the drinking water, it is a step in the right direction. Concerned parents can make an effort to initiate such programs where none exists by contacting state public health officials.

Foot Care

Unless the child's pediatrician indicates the need for corrective or orthopedic shoes, parents need have little concern for pigeon toes or bowed legs or flat feet. If a shoe salesman suggests remedial footwear, his suggestions should be discussed with a physician before complying with them. A good general rule to follow about the fit of shoes is that they should be about three-quarters of an inch longer than the foot itself. For a child whose feet have a tendency to perspire heavily, sweat socks made of cotton or wool are to be preferred to those made of synthetics. Blisters that form on the instep, heel, or any other part of the foot because of ill-fitting footwear must be treated promptly to avoid serious infection.

Friends

Everyone needs friends. Some children need only one; others seem to enjoy having several. A three-year-old who is just beginning to learn about sharing may be more relaxed playing with just one other child; a ten-year-old may like the hurly-burly of a group of friends to get together with when school is out.

Parents Please Stay Out

Parents should try to steer clear of squabbles between children. One day, Nancy and Harriet are best friends, the next, bitter enemies, because of some real or imagined outrage. Left to their own devices, the children will probably patch things up. If parents get involved, the situation gets magnified out of all proportion. It's not unusual in such situations for the two sets of parents to stop speaking to each other and the two little girls to go back to being best friends again.

Keeping Bad Company

What's to be done about "unsuitable" friends? Some parents may think a particular child is unacceptable because she's too aggressive or too foul-mouthed. If your child seems fond of her nonetheless, voice your opinions, but don't forbid the youngster from coming to the house. Any attempt to break up the friendship is likely to be resisted until your child learns from experience that your judgment was the right one. Children who are discouraged from bringing their friends home because they make a mess or make too much noise are actually deprived of feeling at home in their own house.

Friendships between girls and boys may begin in nursery school and continue for years afterward. Although the tone of the friendship may change, the closeness can be very valuable if it doesn't exclude other relationships.

Frostbite

See Ch. 35, *Medical Emergencies*.

Guilt and Conscience

Children often feel as guilty about bad thoughts as they do about bad deeds. After being angry, a child may feel as badly about having had a fleeting wish to hurt his mother as he would have felt had he actually hurt her. A child should be helped to understand that his thoughts are his own, that his thoughts cannot harm anybody, and that he will not be punished for his thoughts. He should understand that it is only actions of certain kinds that cannot be allowed and that will result in a reprimand or punishment. In other words, a child should not be made to feel guilty for angry or aggressive thoughts toward other members of his family, but only for angry and aggressive acts.

A parent might say to a child, "I understand that you really disliked your brother when you hit him, in fact, even hated him and would have liked to hurt him. It's okay for you to be angry with him, but I am not going to let you hurt him." A clear distinction should be made between hostile feelings and hostile behavior.

Headaches

Children get headaches just as adults do. The difficulty in diagnosing and treating them comes from the different symptoms that children experience. It is believed that up to 10 percent of preadolescents suffer from migraine headaches.

Symptoms of headaches in children include aggression, agitation, vomiting, nausea, visual problems, insomnia, and profuse sweating. Causes are the same as they are in adults: tension, stress, eye strain, migraine, or emotional or physical problems. For a child experiencing frequent or severe headaches, a physician should be consulted to eliminate the possibility of an underlying physical disorder, such as near or farsightedness. Once the doctor has determined that no physical disorder exists, treatment of the psychological cause should be considered. Undue pressure from home or the school can create as much stress on a child as an adult experiences in the workplace.

Medication of children should be taken only under the supervision of a qualified doctor. Children respond to certain medications much differently than adults, and care must be taken in administering the types and quantities of drugs. Also treatment of any child with aspirin should be supervised because of the risk of Reye's Syndrome.

Diagnosis and treatment of children with headaches is difficult. Parents should continue to seek treatment for their children until they are satisfied that the problem has been addressed and is being remedied.

Health Records

It may seem somewhat troublesome to keep orderly health records for every member of the family, but the accumulated information can be extremely helpful if it can be supplied at a moment's notice to a physician or a hospital. Chronologically arranged facts can also provide the material eventually needed by summer camps and school applications and insurance policies.

A notebook containing essential data about past illnesses, accidents, allergies, surgery, and other facts can be extraordinarily helpful and time-saving in supplying a physician with a medical history that simplifies diagnosis and treatment. Such a notebook should have separate sections for immunizations and booster shots and their dates; annual weight and height progress; illnesses with dates and special notations; accidents with dates and any permanent consequences; hospitalization and reason; individual problems relating to allergies, hearing, vision, speech, and the like. Visits to physician and dentist should be recorded, and the blood type entered in a conspicuous place. If possible, parents should also provide a summary at the back of the notebook of their own major illnesses, disabilities, and surgical history.

Hearing

Approximately half of all adult hearing problems are thought to have originated in childhood. About five out of every hundred children reveal some hearing disability when screening tests are given. Total deafness among children is uncommon, and where it does exist, its symptoms become manifest to parents and physicians alike during infancy.

Partial Hearing Loss

Partial hearing disability, on the other hand, is common, and is likely to be overlooked until it may be too late to correct its consequences.

A physician begins to suspect a hearing problem when the mother of a young baby tells him that the child does not react to her voice, to noises, or to other auditory stimuli. As the child gets older, he may not speak properly. Because he has never heard speech, he cannot imitate its sound and may fail to develop normal language skills. Sometimes these children, like visually handicapped children, are mistakenly called mentally retarded or are classified as suffering from hyperkinesis or brain dysfunction. Often the undetected hearing disability stemmed from a middle ear infection that was treated inadequately or not treated at all.

Language Problems

A hearing loss of 15 decibels is considered sufficiently large to produce language problems for a very young child, causing a major handicap in the acquisition of language skills. Specialists therefore recommend that parents ask that their physician test a baby's hearing, especially during and after an ear infection. If a compensatory hearing aid is necessary, the baby should be supplied with one immediately. Speech will not develop normally—that is, the language function of the brain will be impaired—unless the essential sounds of language can be perceived during the first two years of life.

Just as glasses or surgery can help eye problems, simple hearing aids, the surgical removal of excessive lymphoid tissue blocking the eustachian tube, or special instruction in lip reading can often help a hearing problem and open up a new world for the child afflicted with a hearing disability.

Heart Disease

See RHEUMATIC FEVER. See also "Congenital Heart Disease" in Ch. 10, *Heart Disease.*

Hernia

A *hernia* is a condition in which part of an organ protrudes through a weak spot or other abnormal opening in the wall of a body cavity. There are three types of hernias that may occur in children.

Umbilical Hernia

The most common is an *umbilical hernia,* in which there is a protrusion of some of the contents of the abdomen through an opening in the abdominal wall at the navel where the umbilical cord was attached. When the baby cries or strains, the protrusion becomes more obvious, and when the baby is at rest, the bulge recedes. An umbilical hernia usually disappears by the time a child reaches the second year. Because it represents no danger to any of the body functions, the condition need be no cause for concern. It is very common in non-Caucasian children.

Inguinal Hernia

The second most common type of hernia in childhood is known as an *indirect inguinal hernia,* occurring frequently in boys. At birth it may have the appearance of a marble located under the skin at the groin. In time, it may descend into the scrotum that encloses the testicles. This type of hernia is usually corrected by simple surgery that repairs the weakened musculature. The weak muscles are often present on both sides.

Hiatus Hernia

Another congenital hernia is known as a *hiatus hernia* (or *diaphragmatic hernia*) in which part of the stomach protrudes upward through the part of the esophagus that opens into the diaphragm. In some cases, this structural defect is self-healing. Surgical correction is advised only if the hernia interferes with respiration. See also Ch. 11, *Diseases of the Digestive System.*

Hospitalization

Most children at some time in their first 15 years of life require at least one hospitalization, ranging in time from a few days to many months. This can be a frightening experience and may leave permanent emotional scars on a child. Parents can do many things to make the experience less harmful.

Preparing the child for the hospital stay may be the most important task for the parent. There are many books available for different age groups on going to the hospital. Authorities generally agree that parents should:

- Try to answer all the questions the child asks. If you have no answer, try to find one.
- Be as honest as possible. The child will want to know why he or she has to go to the hospital, what will be done there, how long it will take, and whether it will hurt.
- Be reassuring. The child should know that he or she will receive good care and that the hospital visit will be temporary.
- Explain what the hospital is and what it is like—that it has wheeled carts, people in uniform, and so on.
- Using sheets as gowns, role-play to make it clear that the people wearing the gowns will be helpful.
- Let the child know when they will be entering the hospital and how long they will stay.

Most hospitals try to work with parents to make children feel at home and to allay their fears. Many hospitals offer rooms so that parents can "room in"—and stay near the young patient. A playroom may be available. Hospital staff members may hold parent-nurse sessions to introduce mothers and fathers to the hospital's schedule, locations of facilities, and other details. Parents of a child who has to be hospitalized can, by learning as much as possible and cooperating with the staff, help alleviate the child's natural fears of separation, of disablement, and of the strange new situation.

Fear of Separation

Hospitalization for an operation or an illness affects different children at different stages of their development in different ways. Very young children may be particularly worried about separations from their parents. Parents can help with this fear by assuring the child that the separation will not be permanent.

If at all possible, one of the child's parents or another member of the family should stay with the child during much of the hospital stay. During an extended hospitalization, of course, this may become difficult or impossible. Barring accidents, children should always be forewarned of a hospitalization; if they are not, they may feel they were deceived by their parents and could lose trust in them.

Fear of Disablement

Children of about 4 to 10 or 11 may be more worried about possible damage to or disablement of their bodies than about separations from their families. They may have fears that parts of their bodies may be cut out or that in some way they may be permanently harmed. They may feel that when they come back from the hospital they will not be the same as they were when they went in. Matter-of-fact reassurance by the parents can be most helpful in alleviating these fears.

Fear of the Strange

Both younger children and older children aged 10, 11, or 12 may fear the new or strange, such as the anesthetic that goes with an operation. The child should be allowed to talk out fears. Simple explanations usually help. A child can, for example, understand that when you get sick taking medicine can sometimes make you better. At other times an operation, or surgery, is the only thing that will help. In the hospital, physicians or nurses may have to make tests to find out what is wrong. One such test is the X ray, which is simply a "picture" of a part of the child's body.

The parent can prepare the child for the operating room and for the operation. Everything in this special place, for example, must be kept perfectly clean, so nurses and physicians wear long-sleeved gowns. They also wash carefully before the operation begins. They wear sterile gloves so that they can touch patients without passing on germs. They also wear masks, shoe coverings, and caps. They may make a small opening in the patient's skin so that they can take out or get rid of whatever is making the child sick. The physicians and nurses use stitches, or sutures, to pull the skin edges together and allow healing to begin. Some stitches may be under the skin; these simply melt, or dissolve, by themselves.

A dressing may be placed over the part of the child's body that was opened up. These pieces of soft cloth protect the skin opening and keep out germs. When the dressing comes off, a white scar may remain. The scar will not open up and it will not hurt. It will be a sign that the child was sick, got well, and came home.

Hostility

See ANGER.

Hyaline Membrane Disease

Hyaline membrane disease, now technically called the *respiratory distress syndrome*, is a disorder that affects approximately 50,000 newborn babies each year, and until recently was fatal for about half of them. The disorder occurs especially among premature infants, those born by caesarian section, and those with diabetic mothers. In premature infants, the immaturity of the lungs may result in a collapse of the air space within the lungs themselves when the first breath is exhaled. Each new breath then becomes a greater struggle, and with the spread of lung collapse, exhaustion and asphyxiation may occur.

A treatment known as *continuous positive airway pressure* is now being successfully used in many of the special hospital units equipped for newborns with disabilities. The therapy involves a pressure chamber that forces high-oxygen air into the lungs and keeps these air spaces open. The method has already prevented thousands of infant deaths. Newborns who need this assistance acquire the ability to breathe normally in about a week.

Hyperactivity

Hyperactivity, a general term, was formerly used to describe what are now recognized as *attention deficit hyperactivity disorder (ADHD)* and *attention deficit disorder (ADD)*. Recent research indicates that although ADHD and ADD become apparent in childhood, they are not outgrown as previously thought. Neither disorder is a sign of lack of intelligence. There are a number of symptoms of the disorders—such as having difficulty concentrating, being overactive or unusually withdrawn, and not completing tasks—and a child should be evaluated by a professional for an expert diagnosis. ADHD is more common in boys than in girls. Experts estimate that 3 to 5 percent of American children have ADHD or ADD.

ADHD and ADD are believed to be neurological disorders (often inherited) involving the brain mechanisms that regulate attention and impulse control. Treatment usually consists of daily drug therapy with a stimulant, such as Ritalin or Dexedrine, and behavioral therapy. For more information on these disorders contact:

- Attention-Deficit Disorders Association, Southern Region, 12345 Jones Road, Suite 287-7, Houston, TX 77070; (281) 897-0982
- CHADD, Children and Adults with Attention Deficit Disorders, 8181 Professional Place, Suite 150, Landover, MD 20785; (800) 233-4050
- National Attention Deficit Disorder Association, P.O. Box 543, Pottstown, PA 19464, (484) 945-2101

Immunization

Recently developed vaccines against measles, mumps, and rubella (German measles) should eventually wipe out these diseases in the same way that smallpox has been eliminated practically everywhere in the world. Routine immunization follows a schedule of shots administered with minor variations by most pediatricians and child care clinics. Severe reactions are rare, but should they occur, they should be reported to a physician promptly.

Keeping Records

Records should be kept of the child's immunization history so that booster shots can be given at proper intervals. Because families sometimes move from one place to another, changing physicians as they relocate, it saves a great deal of time and trouble if immunization data is written down rather than committed to memory. See HEALTH RECORDS.

DTP or DTaP Injections

DTP stands for diphtheria, tetanus, and pertussis (whooping cough). A newer acellular pertussis vaccine (DTaP) is more commonly used, as it is thought to produce fewer side effects. Children need five doses of DTP or DTaP—at 2, 4, 6, and 15 to 18 months of age, and between 4 to 6 years of age. Injections are usually given in the arm or leg.

Childhood Immunization Schedule*

Age	Vaccine
birth	Hepatitis B†
2 months	DTP or DTaP (diptheria, tetanus, acellular pertussis), Polio, Hib—haemophilus influenza type B, Hepatitis B, Pneumococcal
4 months	DTP or DTaP, Polio, Hib, Hepatitis B, Pneumococcal
6 months	DTP or DTaP, Hib, Pneumococcal
15 months	Chickenpox, DTP or DTap, Polio, MMR (measles, mumps, rubella [German measles]), Hib, Pneumococcal
4 to 6 years‡	DTP or DTaP, Polio, MMR
14 to 16 years**	Tetanus-diptheria booster

*As recommended by the United States Centers for Disease Control and Prevention.

†An additional vaccine (HBIG) should be administered as soon as possible to infants whose mothers test positive for Hepatitis B.

‡Shortly before the child enters school for the first time.

**And every 10 years thereafter.

DTP or DTaP Reactions

DTP or DTaP injections may produce some common, relatively mild, side effects that typically happen one to three days after an injection.

Children may experience pain, swelling, or redness in the area where they were injected. Some doctors recommend applying ice to the area for about 20 minutes. Some children may also develop a fever. For fevers above 120°F, acetaminophen should be given to children younger than seven months of age, while ibuprofen can be used for children older than 6 months. Some additional, relatively common and harmless side effects include fretfulness, mild sleepiness, and poor appetite. It is not unusual for these side effects to last about 24 to 48 hours.

Among the more serious reactions that are relatively uncommon are nonstop crying for more than 3 hours, a high fever (above 105°F), or seizure (staring or jerking about). If any of these reactions occur you should call your doctor or take the child to a doctor immediately.

Some very rare but severe problems can occur after DTP or DTaP vaccinations. These include serious allergic reactions, permanent brain damage, and long-term seizures or coma.

Parents may want to discuss their children's medical histories with their family physicians or pediatricians before taking them in for an inocculaton. In particular, parents should tell their child's doctor if the child has a history of convulsions, allergic reactions to DTP or other vaccines, or if he or she was born prematurely.

Independence

Many parents feel that the most memorable moment in a child's progress toward independence comes when he takes his first steps alone, upright and walking! Most children accomplish this by going independently from the secure arms of one adult to the waiting arms of another. As youngsters move toward greater independence, they will do so with confidence if they can start out from a secure foundation of rules and limits, and return to the security of acceptance and understanding should they come to grief.

The Toddler Stage

The toddler relishes the independence of being able to explore the house or the playground, but he won't go very far before he returns to check in with the person in charge of him so that he can start out all over again. He voices his independence, too: "no" to naps; "no" to outings; "no" to a bath. This is the phase during which parents must be wary of asking "Would you like to" or "Do you want to" instead of just proceeding with the business at hand. Patience is required for the self-assertive fumblings and clumsy efforts at self-feeding and putting on clothes. Assistance should be subtle and tactful, not hurried and bossy: "Baby do, daddy help," is the general idea.

School Age

As the child moves into the larger arena of school and friendships, "I'm not a baby any more" may become a complaint if he wants more freedom than he's permitted to have. At this stage, he begins to learn that responsibility goes hand-in-hand with freedom and independence. Being old enough to ride the bike farther and farther from home means taking on the responsibility of keeping it in good repair and obeying all the traffic rules.

Influenza

See "The Common Cold, Influenza, and Other Viral Infections" in Ch. 12, *Diseases of the Respiratory System*.

Insect Stings and Bites

When a child is bitten or stung by an insect, he often complains about the pain or the itching, but with the application of a lotion or salve to relieve discomfort and a bandage to prevent infection, the incident is soon forgotten. There are times, however, when a sting or a bite may require emergency treatment.

It has been estimated that about four children out of every 1,000 have serious allergic reactions to the sting of a hornet, wasp, bee, yellow jacket, or the fire ant. A child who has sustained multiple stings, or whose body, tongue, or face begins to swell because of a single sting should be taken to the hospital immediately. Tests can clearly distinguish between those children who are highly sensitive to stings and those who are not.

Preventive Measures

A physician should be consulted about the advisability of testing youngsters who are going off to camp for the first time or who are planning long hikes. Rather than curtail the activities of a child who turns out to have an acute sensitivity, it may make sense to plan a series of desensitization treatments against the particular venom. For children who are very allergic to insect stings, an emergency kit containing adrenaline is now available and should always be carried.

Mosquitoes

Every effort should be made to eradicate mosquitoes by eliminating their breeding places. A mosquito bite can be a serious threat to a child's health because these insects transmit several diseases. Where mosquitoes are a problem, infants and children should be protected against them by screens, netting, and the application of repellents.

Ticks

Families that travel and those that have pets should guard against the possibility of infection by disease-bearing ticks. A species of tick known as *Ixodes dammini* can transmit an illness called Lyme disease while another common tick may carry Rocky Mountain spotted fever.

Rashes may appear as symptoms of infection by either tick. The Lyme disease rash may be circular and hot to the touch. It may have a diameter as wide as 28 inches. Untreated in either children or adults, Lyme disease may trigger chills, fever, general feelings of malaise, fatigue, and attacks of arthritis that may last weeks or months to years. Heart and nerve abnormalities may appear. Penicillin is used to bring Lyme disease under control in pregnant women and children.

Less prevalent than Lyme disease, Rocky Mountain spotted fever usually produces a rash on the soles of the feet and the palms of the hands. Prompt medical attention is essential to prevent possible complications. See ROCKY MOUNTAIN SPOTTED FEVER and LYME DISEASE under RASHES.

Intelligence and IQ

Intelligence is a quality, not a quantity. It therefore cannot be measured as precisely as height or weight; nor can it be exemplified as definitely as mechanical skill or athletic ability or musical talent. Although child development authorities and educators may disagree about how to assess intelligence, they generally agree on the following premise: no matter what is inherited and what is instilled by experience, children function best in later life if their earliest years of nurture bring out and develop their inborn capacities.

Encouragement and Enrichment

Beginning with proper prenatal diet and care, a healthy baby is born, and from then on, her intellectual capacities are shaped by experience. Loving and attentive parents give her the self-confidence to explore and learn. She is encouraged to express herself in language. She is exposed to a variety of experiences that will stimulate her curiosity and interest: plants, drawing materials, pets, picture books, outings to the beach. Her efforts to use her intelligence by asking questions are respected and encouraged rather than minimized and ignored.

IQ Tests

Once a child gets to school her capabilities may or may not be measured by a standard IQ test. Such tests, which have been abandoned in some states, assess specific areas of intelligence and are graded according to a statistical norm. Newer techniques for measuring intelligence are designed to compensate for a cultural bias that some authorities believe exists in the standard tests.

Jealousy

See BROTHERS AND SISTERS, NEW BABY.

Kidney Diseases

For a discussion of kidney diseases, see Ch. 17, *Diseases of the Urinogenital System*, and Ch. 18, *Cancer*.

Learning

See CURIOSITY, INTELLIGENCE AND IQ, READING, SCHOOL.

Lead Poisoning

Lead poisoning in children is usually associated with the ingestion of paint and plaster flakes containing high levels of lead. This is a problem in city slums where old buildings are being leveled, or in cases where youngsters manage to gnaw on repainted cribs and other furniture originally covered with lead-base paint. In homes being renovated, the dust from removal of lead paint can cause an increase in lead levels in the blood.

Lead poisoning is a serious danger to the health of approximately half a million children in the United States. Irreversible brain damage and anemia can occur if the condition becomes chronic; convulsions and death may occur in an acute case. To lessen such hazards, legislation now requires new cars to use only lead-free gasoline.

Learning Disability

A child with a learning disability is one who, though otherwise normal, cannot acquire certain skills or assimilate certain kinds of knowledge at the same rate as most other children. Obviously, almost every child lags behind her peers at one time or another in certain subjects; but the difficulties of a learning disabled child are far more severe. A 16-year-old who suffers from a learning disability may, for example, be capable only of third- or fourth-grade math while functioning at her own grade level in other subjects. Some learning disabilities are attributed to minimal brain damage, but in most cases the cause is unknown. See also DYSLEXIA.

Leukemia

See CANCER.

Lying

See DISHONESTY.

Malnutrition

Poor nutrition or undernourishment can occur not only as a result of a faulty diet, but also because a child may have a metabolic defect that prevents her body from making proper use of a particular essential nutrient. Temporary malnutrition may also accompany a long illness in which the child's appetite wanes.

Although malnutrition is usually associated with poverty and child neglect, it can also occur because of ignorance, carelessness, or fanaticism. Children have been found to be malnourished by parents following a macrobiotic diet or a faddish type of vegetarianism. Using vitamins as a substitute for food can also cause certain types of undernourishment.

Older children, especially girls approaching puberty, may embark on starvation diets in an attempt to ward off inevitable body changes and end up seriously malnourished. The general signs of malnutrition are increasing physical weakness, vague and unfocused behavior, as well as the particular symptoms associated with anemia and vitamin deficiencies. See also Ch. 27, *Nutrition and Weight Control*.

Measles

Measles is by far the most dangerous of the common childhood diseases because of its possible complications, such as meningitis, encephalitis, and severe secondary staphylococcus infection. Fortunately, widespread protection is available in the live measles vaccine, which should be given to every child over one year of age.

Symptoms

Measles, a highly contagious disease caused by a virus, has an incubation period of one to two weeks. The most noticeable symptom is the rash that begins on the head and face within a few days after the onset of the disease, and gradually erupts all over the body, blending into big red patches. Other symptoms include fever up to 104° F or higher, a severe cough, sore throat, stuffy nose, inflammation of the *conjunctiva* (the mucous membrane on the inner part of the eyelid and extending over the front of the eyeball), sensitivity of the eyes to light, enlarged lymph nodes, and a generalized sick feeling.

Any child who has contracted measles should be seen by a physician and watched carefully for possible complications. Moreover, if he is of school age, the school should be promptly notified. This, of course, is true for any contagious disease.

Treatment

Measles can be treated only symptomatically. During the incubation period, an injection of gamma globulin will lessen the severity of the disease, or occasionally prevent it. If there are other children at home besides the affected one, they should also receive gamma globulin injections. Antibiotics are of no help unless there is a secondary bacterial infection.

It is now suspected that vaccinations given in the United States and Canada during the 1960s and 1970s were not triggering permanent immunity to measles. Anyone who has been vaccinated during that period should consult his or her physician about reimmunization. The number of cases, including adult cases, of measles has risen dramatically. This is partly because of the need for revaccination in adults; it is also because many parents are not having their children immunized. Measles can be fatal and vaccination can protect against needless deaths from this preventable disease.

All parents should make certain that their children are vaccinated against this potentially serious disease. See IMMUNIZATION.

Medication

New parents can save themselves time and trouble by getting into the habit of writing down a physician's instructions about medication when the child requires it. Although dosages are usually clearly indicated on labels prepared by the pharmacist according to the prescription, the physician may add comments about how or when to change the dosage.

How to Give Medicines to Children

As for administering medication, a calm and assured approach and a minimum of fuss are more effective than wheedling and urging. A very young child may need to be distracted by cheerful conversation as the spoon goes into her mouth; an older child can be given some factual information about the medication and what it will do. No matter what the youngster's age, parents should never trick or fool her about what she's being given, nor should candied medicine be used under any circumstances. Setting up this type of confusion in a young mind can lead to an overdose of "candy" serious enough to require emergency hospitalization.

Overusing Medication

As a child gets older, she will become increasingly conscious of the medication her parents take. Families that are constantly swallowing one or another kind of pill—diet pills, sleeping pills, tranquilizers—might give some thought to their attitude towards drugs and how these attitudes are affecting their children. Generally, it's a good idea to refrain from medicating a child unless the pediatrician recommends it.

Old Medicines

Once the illness for which a particular medication has been prescribed is definitely over, the remains of the bottle or the leftover capsules should be flushed down the toilet. Old, outdated pills can be dangerous. For safety's sake, parents should review the contents of the medicine cabinet on a regular basis and get rid of any medications left over from a previous illness. Basic medications that are essential for occasional emergencies should be reviewed for continuing effectiveness. Some of these might have a limited shelf life and be completely ineffective should they be needed.

Meningitis

Meningitis is an inflammation of the *meninges*, the thin membranes that cover the spinal cord and the brain. The inflammation, which may be caused by a virus or by bacteria, is more common among children than adults, and may occur in epidemics. This is especially true if the infectious agent is meningococcal (*meningococcal meningitis*), because the meningococcal bacteria are also found in the throat and are transmitted by coughing, sneezing, and talking. This type occurs mostly in young adults. Another type of meningitis that commonly occurs among young children during the spring and summer is caused by such organisms as the mumps virus and the coxsackievirus.

Symptoms

Whatever the cause, the symptoms are generally the same: headache, fever, vomiting, and stiff neck. If untreated, the child may go into delirium and convulsions. Drowsiness and blurred vision may also occur, and if the disease develops in an infant, the pressure on the brain caused by the inflamed meninges will create a bulge on the soft spot (fontanelle) of the baby's head. No time should be lost in calling the physician about any of these symptoms.

Meningitis was almost always fatal before the availability of antibiotics, and although it is no longer the threat it once was, it must be treated promptly if irreversible consequences are to be avoided.

Mental Illness

Behind the search for the causes and treatment of mental illness in children is the current research in the relationship between that mysterious entity called the mind and that palpable physical organism called the brain. Parents of children diagnosed as mentally ill are themselves caught up in this distinction, often preferring to call their youngsters "emotionally disturbed." It is now estimated that about one-and-a-half million youngsters under 18 require some kind of treatment for mental illness, and this figure does not include the one million children diagnosed as hyperkinetic. The two most serious forms of childhood mental illness are autism and schizophrenia.

Autism

The term "early infantile autism" was coined in the 1940s to describe babies and young children who show unpredictable deviations in development. Some never learn to speak; others refuse to look anyone directly in the eye. Autistic children may have one or two extraordinary skills and be incapable of remembering their own names. Some authorities used to ascribe autism to a rejecting mother's refusal to love the infant. Most authorities now describe this disorder as an organic condition caused by neurological rather than psychological abnormalities. The same conclusions have been reached about schizophrenia.

The Autism Society of America was organized to initiate schools, offer counseling to parents, and foster research. It can be contacted at 7910 Woodmont Avenue, Suite 300, Bethesda, MD, 20814-3067; (800) 328-8476. See also HYPERKINESIS.

Schizophrenia

In schizophrenia, a child is likely to exhibit any of the following symptoms: confused speech and thinking; lack of emotional responsiveness; withdrawal into fantasy; and, occasionally, hallucinations. There are indications that genetic inheritance plays some role in this disorder, and that environmental influences are also involved.

Studies suggest that symptoms originate in abnormalities of brain chemistry that may be treated with the proper medication. Over the past twenty years, many special schools, including day schools and residential schools, have been established for training autistic and schizophrenic children.

Mental Retardation

An estimated six million people in the United States, are to some degree, mentally retarded—almost three percent of the population. Mental retardation occurs among all nationalities, races, and religions, and among the children of those in the highest social and economic groups as well as those in the lowest.

What Is Mental Retardation?

Mental retardation refers to limitations in an individual's intellectual functioning and in skills, such as the ability to feed oneself, that are needed to live independently. Mental retardation in a child causes the child to develop at a slower pace than a typical child.

Degrees of Mental Retardation

Mentally retarded children (and adults) are often classified into four categories, depending upon the degree of retardation.

Mildly retarded children—those with IQs roughly between 50 and 70—comprise by far the largest category; nearly 90 percent of all retarded people fall into this group. IQ scores by themselves can be misleading, but they are a convenient guide to probable learning and development patterns if understood properly—that is, simply as one of the criteria by which the degree of a child's disability can be estimated. The retardation of mildly retarded children is usually not apparent until they are of school age. With special educational help, such children can achieve satisfying progress in school and, as adults, will be capable with proper training of handling any of a wide variety of regular jobs. They may be indistinguishable from nonretarded people and can be expected to take their places in the life of their community.

Moderately retarded children—those with IQs somewhat below 50—belong to a group that comprises about 6 percent of all retarded people in the United States. The retardation of these children is usually apparent before they begin school, often during the child's first year, in the form of delayed developmental landmarks—for example, late sitting, late standing, late walking, and delayed talking. Many children with Down's syndrome (Mongolism) fall into this group. These children require a more sheltered environment than the mildly retarded, but can be trained as adults to do productive, satisfying work.

Severely and profoundly retarded children often have other handicaps, such as impaired motor coordination or defective vision or hearing. The great majority of these children can be taught to care for their basic needs, and many can do useful work under supervision.

Causes

There are numerous causes of mental retardation. Some cases are specifically caused by congenital factors (conditions existing at or before birth). Among these are the following: deprivation of oxygen to the brain of a baby during the birth process; the mother's contraction of rubella (German measles) during the first three months of pregnancy; complications resulting from Rh factor blood incompatibility between mother and baby; a grossly inadequate prenatal diet of the mother; syphilis; hydrocephalus (accumulation of spinal fluid in the brain); or any other pressure or injury to the brain of the fetus.

Some forms of retardation result from hereditary factors, the genetic makeup of the parents. Down's syndrome and phenylketonuria (PKU) fall in this category.

Mental retardation can also occur as a result of disease. Inflammation of the brain is a possible complication of measles—now wholly preventable by the administration of the measles vaccine. Other causes are brain injuries that result from a severe blow to the head, as from a fall. Some of these injuries are deliberately inflicted, usually by parents. (See CHILD ABUSE AND NEGLECT.) Among environmental hazards, lead and mercury poisoning are of particular importance. Lead-based paint chips have been eaten by unattended children. (See LEAD POISONING.)

If retardation is suspected by parents, medical advice should be sought immediately and a thorough evaluation of the child conducted. Some types of retardation can be greatly benefited by medical and educational treatment. It should be emphasized that all retarded children can learn and that many can be helped to the extent that they can become productive citizens. Parents would like further information about mental retardation or who are in need of counseling should write to the Arc of the United States, 1010 Wayne Avenue, Suite 650, Silver Spring, MD 20910; (301) 565-3842. See also DISABLED CHILD.

Money

Money may not be the root of all evil, but it certainly is the cause of a lot of family quarrels. To communicate to children the value of money and how to use it, spend it, save it, borrow it, lend it, and earn it, parents should try to clarify their own attitudes and settle their own differences.

Young children hear money talked about all the time: "We can't afford it," "That's a bargain," "That's a waste of money." What does it all mean to a preschooler?

The Weekly Allowance

The best way for a child to get first-hand experience in dealing with "I need" and "I want" in terms of cash on hand is to give her a weekly allowance. There isn't any point in doing this until she has mastered addition and subtraction. If the prospect of getting an allowance is motivation for improving her number skills at school, so much the better. The amount of the allowance should be calculated in terms of what it's supposed to cover. These details should be spelled out so that there's no confusion about who is responsible for paying for what. As the child gets older, the amount is adjusted for increasing needs—social occasions such as a ten-year-old might enjoy when she and her friends stop for an ice-cream cone on the way home from school.

Saving

If the family feels that a child should be required to save part of her allowance, a piggy bank and a brief talk about the virtues of saving are essential. Some children get so anxious about money that they turn into misers. When this occurs, it may be advisable to point out that the money is not meant to be hoarded but to be spent on needs and treats. Children who receive birthday or other special presents in the form of money from relatives can open a bank account and learn about interest accrual. Although the money is rightfully theirs, they might be encouraged to consult the family before they spend it all on a passing enthusiasm.

Multiple Births

See Twins and Triplets.

Mumps

Mumps, a mild disorder in most children, is caused by a virus and has an incubation period of from two to three weeks. The most familiar symptom is swollen glands involving the jaw. The glands usually affected are the *parotid glands*—large salivary glands below and slightly in front of the ear—although other glands may be affected, too. Other symptoms include fever and a general sick feeling. No rash is present. Mumps lasts about five days; then the swelling disappears.

In an adolescent boy, the disease sometimes causes an inflammation of the testes (called *orchitis*) and may be very painful. In addition, if it involves both testes, there is a possibility—fortunately only a very slight one—that sterility will result.

In older children mumps occasionally produces the complication called *mumps meningoencephalitis*. The signs of this more serious disease are headache, fever, and extreme debilitation. Finally, there may be an inflammation of the pancreas, which can cause severe abdominal pain and vomiting.

Because mumps is now preventable, every boy and girl should be given the mumps vaccine. Boys should be given the vaccine before puberty.

Muscular Dystrophy

See Ch. 8, *Diseases of the Muscles and Nervous System*.

Nausea and Vomiting

Nausea, the signal that vomiting may occur, is often described as feeling sick to the stomach. The feeling is experienced when irritated nerve endings in the stomach and elsewhere send messages to the vomiting reflex in the brain. When the nerve irritation is acute, vomiting occurs.

Physical Causes

Although nausea and vomiting are usually associated with a child's upset stomach or the sudden onset of a high fever and an acute infection, many youngsters feel nauseated and throw up because of motion sickness in a car or plane, or as the result of severe pain occasioned by a bad fall or other accident. A physician should always be consulted when nausea and vomiting are accompanied by fever, cramps, or diarrhea. For the child who feels sick in a moving vehicle, the physician can prescribe suitable medication. For a youngster who has swallowed a toxic substance, vomiting must often be induced. See Ch. 35, *Medical Emergencies*, for further information on poisoning.

Emotional Stress

Chronic nausea may result from emotional stress. A child who doesn't want to go to school because of some threatening situation, or who is always too anxious before a test because of pressures to do well, or who is fearful about some athletic challenge but ashamed to admit it—children under these pressures are likely to develop symptoms of nausea. However, instead of dismissing the recurrence of nausea and vomiting as typical of an oversensitive child, parents should try to find out the source of the problem and, if necessary, arrange some family therapy sessions with the child.

Nervous Habits

Nervous habits both express and release inner tension, and because growing up isn't an easy process, it's inevitable that most children have one or another way of dealing with their fears, anxieties, and emotional pressures. There's no point in parental scolding or ridicule or punishment, because any of these approaches simply adds yet another pressure to those that exist already. After all, most adults have nervous habits too—whether it's smoking, or picking at a cuticle, or tooth-grinding—and no amount of nagging is likely to put a stop to any of them.

Some nervous habits can be unhealthy, and some can be socially unacceptable but essentially harmless. All are unconscious, and most eventually disappear with age. Among the habits that may need looking into in order to decide that they have no basis in a physical disorder are squinting and throat-clearing. Hair-twirling and foot-shaking can be entirely ignored. Nail-biting may persist for years, or it may yield to vanity or the comments of friends.

Thumb-sucking, abandoned at two, may recur at three because of the arrival of a new baby or because of the stresses of going to nursery school. Many school-age children continue to suck their thumbs when they're going to sleep. There's no need to worry about this habit unless the dentist notices the beginning of an orthodontic problem, in which case, the dentist and not you should discuss it with the child. Nose-picking in public is almost always abandoned when a child enters school. If a big fuss has been made about it, he may continue the habit at home as a gesture of defiance—or because it really is unconscious. When done in private, it's completely harmless.

Masturbation bothers many parents more than it should. In and of itself, there's no harm in it, but as a chronic expression of anxiety, it might be dealt with tactfully and indirectly by trying to get to the source of the tension rather than by punishing or humiliating the child.

New Baby

It's a good idea for parents to talk about the anticipated arrival of a new baby with their child or children before the pregnancy is really obvious. Conversations can be casual, and questions should be answered simply and factually. If any basic changes are to be made—especially if a child is to be shifted to a bed so that the new arrival can have the crib—this transition should be accomplished before the infant appears. Adults should refrain from asking such questions as "Would you like a little brother or a little sister?" or "Isn't it wonderful that there's going to be a new baby in the family?" Preparations made in advance of going to the hospital should, if possible, consider whether the child would prefer to stay at home or with a relative during mother's absence. When the baby is brought home and well-wishers arrive with presents, it's comforting for the first-born to sit in mother's or daddy's lap while visitors coo over the infant in the crib. Thoughtful baby-present givers will always include a little present for the baby's older siblings, too. Parents should do their best to make baby's big brother or sister feel that the new baby is his or hers no less than mother's or father's. See also BROTHERS AND SISTERS.

Nightmares

See DREAMS AND NIGHTMARES.

Night Terrors

See DREAMS AND NIGHTMARES.

Nosebleeds

Children are likely to have nosebleeds more often than adults, and they are usually no cause for alarm. A blood vessel near the nostril may be injured by energetic noseblowing, the presence of a foreign object, or by an accidental blow or an intentional wallop.

Apply Pressure

A minor nosebleed is most effectively stopped by applying pressure over the bleeding area. A child old enough to follow instructions should be told to sit down, hold the head slightly forward, and compress the soft portion of the nose between thumb and forefinger, maintaining the pressure for about five minutes and breathing through the mouth. Application of an ice pack to the outside of the nose is usually helpful. Fingers should be withdrawn very slowly in order not to disturb the clot that should have formed.

Packing the Nostril

If this method doesn't stop the bleeding, a small twist of sterile cotton can be inserted gently into the nostril so that some of it protrudes. Light pressure should be applied once again for five minutes and the cotton allowed to remain in place for a while. Should the bleeding continue in spite of these measures, the child should be taken to a hospital emergency clinic.

Nutrition

Children's nutritional requirements are not the same as adults. Although that may seem like an obvious statement, the fact is many parents do not take it into account when planning meals.

Infants are incapable of digesting many products. Introduction of new food to an infant should be done one item at a time. If the baby has an allergic reaction, the parent then knows what it is in response to. If the baby has eaten two or three new items, it isn't possible to tell without another feeding which one the child is allergic to.

Children can outgrow some intolerances to food. A baby that could not properly digest citrus fruit may be able to handle it well a few months or years later. Some allergies, though, get worse with each exposure. Common food allergies and intolerances include nuts, berries, milk, eggs, and fish.

Children do not require the same quantity of food as an adult. Small children will eat less at a meal, but may need to eat more frequently during the day. Their stomach holds less so they get hungry more frequently.

Children also do not require the same quantity of minerals and vitamins as adults. Childrens' vitamins are available but should not be used to replace a healthy diet. Good eating habits in children establishes a pattern that they are likely to follow for the rest of their lives. Also, children should not become adapted to the idea of taking a pill every day.

Several studies show that children who are obese can diet effectively and that they are more likely to keep the weight off than adults are. Overweight children who diet for a period even as short as 10 weeks are less obese than overweight children who never diet at all. One study demonstrated that dieting in childhood does not completely prevent obesity but it does limit the amount of weight gain to less than half that gained by those who never dieted as children.

Weight is an extremely sensitive subject to children. Adolescents in particular are susceptible to negative self-images based on weight, and to criticism by others. Disorders related to eating are covered in *The Teens* under Anorexia and Bulimia.

Weight gain can commonly be traced to the amount of television a child watches. Obesity and television viewing are related through two habits. The first is that for every hour the child is plopped in front of a television is an hour the child is not playing and exercising. The other is that television watching is usually accompanied by snacking on high-fat, high-salt or sugar pre-processed food.

Orthodontics

Orthodontics is the branch of dentistry that specializes in the correction of *malocclusion* (an improper alignment of the upper and lower teeth at the point where they meet) or to irregularity of tooth positioning. Emphasis is now being placed on the prevention of malocclusion before it can occur. General practitioners of dentistry, *pedodontists* (specialists in children's dentistry), and orthodontists now believe that the need for expensive, time-consuming, and emotionally unsettling orthodontics can sometimes be avoided by beginning treatment as early as the age of four.

The positioning of the permanent teeth is the result not only of inheritance, but of other variables, such as lip-biting and thumb-sucking. Premature loss or partial disintegration of primary teeth also has a strong influence on whether the permanent teeth will be properly positioned.

Preventive Orthodontics

By the time the child is five, an X ray will show exactly how all the permanent teeth are situated in the gums. In some cases, it may be possible to guide these teeth as they erupt. If potential overcrowding and eventual crookedness are indicated, some baby teeth may be pulled to make room for the permanent ones. Normal positioning may also be accomplished by establishing a different balance of muscular forces.

Corrective Appliances

Corrective orthodontics uses many different types of appliances for the repositioning of permanent teeth, all of which operate on the same principle of applying pressure to the bone. Widening the arch of the upper jaw, for example, is accomplished by the use of a screw appliance fixed to the upper teeth so that the two halves of the hard palate are slightly separated along the middle suture, permitting new bone to fill in the space. Specialists point out that a bonus of this orthodontic correction is increased respiratory ease for youngsters who were formerly mouth-breathers.

Parents who have been advised by the family dentist that an orthodontic consultation is advisable for a child, and who are concerned about the eventual economic burden that prolonged treatment might represent, should get a second opinion from the clinical staff of a dental school associated with a university. See also DENTAL CARE.

Pacifiers

Most parents have strong opinions about the use of pacifiers. Whatever the preference, what the baby needs during the early months is satisfaction for the sucking impulse. For most babies, this need seems to taper off at about six months; with those babies in whom the need remains strong, the thumb seems to be a convenient substitute for the pacifier. Whatever decision is arrived at between you and your physician, the important thing to keep in mind is that the pacifier is no substitute for holding and cuddling the baby when she wants comforting, and that sometimes a parent is more dependent on a pacifier than the baby is.

If pacifiers are used regularly, more than one should be available, and they should be inspected periodically to make sure that bits and pieces of rubber haven't been chewed so loose that they may be swallowed and lodge in the windpipe.

Pets

Rural children usually have their own pet animals even if the animals aren't allowed in the house. Suburban families are likely to own a dog that's a pet as well as a discouragement to prowlers. It's the city child who may have to wage a persistent campaign before his parents capitulate to the idea of a pet. Yet even the smallest apartment can accommodate a pet bird or a small fish tank; a cat and a litter box won't cause extra crowding. Of course, dogs offer the greatest companionship but also impose the greatest responsibility; they do have to be housebroken and walked in all weathers at least twice a day. If a child brings a stray animal home, the dog or cat must be checked by a vet before it becomes a household member. Once a youngster can read, the acquisition of a pet hamster or a guinea pig or a pair of gerbils will provide the incentive for trips to the library for books on care and feeding.

Choosing a Dog

When a dog is to be the choice, it's often cheaper and more satisfactory to select one from the litter of a healthy dog you know than to buy one in a pet shop or from a commercial kennel. The Anti-Cruelty Society and other animal shelters can provide families with pets at little or no change. The breed chosen should be suitable in terms of size, temperament, and cost of feeding. Relative advantages and disadvantages should be checked out at the library by the child whose responsibility the pet will be.

For an only child, a pet animal is almost a must, not only for companionship, but so that there's a being in the house who's smaller and more helpless than she is. In families where allergies are a problem, the physician should be consulted about the type of pet that will cause the least discomfort to a vulnerable member of the household.

Pica

Pica is the technical term for an abnormal desire to eat substances that are not fit for food, such as clay, earth, plaster and the like. This tendency is not to be confused with the tendency of babies and toddlers to put unsuitable things into their mouth. Pica is habitual and compulsive, and may result in serious disabilities. Because the phenomenon is especially conspicuous among poor and neglected children, some authorities associate it with nutritional deficiency, others with unsatisfied emotional needs. Signs of pica should be brought to the attention of a physician or a social service agency that can provide guidance on how the child's circumstances should be altered even if the total environment cannot be changed. See also LEAD POISONING.

Pills

See MEDICATION.

Pinworms or Threadworms

See Ch. 11, *Diseases of the Digestive System*.

PKU

PKU stands for *phenylketonuria*, an inherited metabolic defect. Approximately one baby in 10,000 is born with this disease, in which the body is incapable of producing certain enzymes that are essential for the metabolic conversion of the amino acid phenylalanine. The disorder causes the amino acid and some of its byproducts to accumulate in the bloodstream to a dangerous degree. If the condition goes undetected and untreated, irreversible brain damage and mental retardation are the result.

PKU babies are characteristically blond and blue-eyed, with sensitive skin and faulty muscle coordination. In many parts of the United States, state laws require that three days after birth, all babies be given the blood test that detects the presence of PKU so that treatment can begin at once if necessary. Supervised treatment usually continues for several years, and in some communities is available at special therapy centers. Parents or prospective parents who would like to find out whether any member of the family is a carrier of the recessive gene that transmits the PKU disorder can arrange for diagnostic testing and genetic counseling based on the results.

Play

See FANTASIES, TOYS, SAFETY.

Pneumonia

See "Pneumonia" in Ch. 12, *Diseases of the Respiratory System*.

Poison Ivy, Oak, and Sumac Rashes

Poison ivy and poison oak are two plants readily found across the United States. Poison sumac is found in marshes in the southern and eastern states. Children frequently come in contact with the plants while playing, hiking, or camping. The oils from the surface of the plant brush against the skin and usually, within hours, an itchy painful rash appears on the skin.

If contact with poisonous plants is suspected, the first thing one should do is wash the area of skin thoroughly with soap and water as soon after exposure as possible. Removing the poisonous oils can eliminate or reduce the inflammation. Care should be taken not to spread the oils from the infected skin to other skin. Particular care should be given to not touch or rub your eyes after contact with one of these plants. You should also be cautious of rubbing your eyes after scratching infected or exposed skin.

The rash is an itchy red group of small blisters. Cold water dressings can help reduce the itching. Use clean cotton cloth soaked in a solution of one teaspoon of salt per pint of water. Antihistamine medication can help reduce the itching and rash. If the rash persists, becomes infected, is severe, or covers a large part of the child's body, consult a physician immediately.

Poisons and Poisoning

Every year, hundreds of thousands of children swallow some poisonous substance—in too many cases with fatal results—because of parental carelessness, or because the child hasn't been given clear and unequivocal instructions about the difference between "candy" and medicine. Poisoning because of the ingestion of sugar-coated aspirin is a continuing problem; iron-containing multiple vitamins that seem to be a gourmet treat to some children also present a problem because iron in excess doses is a stomach irritant.

Safety Measures

Toddlers can do themselves damage because they're curious about everything, and their sense of taste isn't all that discriminating. Thus it's an absolute necessity to see that all household cleansers and strong chemicals are kept on high shelves rather than on the floor. Many bottles containing medicines come with safety caps that presumably cannot be opened by children—for instance, because pressure must be applied—but can be opened by adults. The experience of many parents, however, is that whereas their children can often open such caps, *they* frequently have a great deal of difficulty. Suffice it to say that the perfect childproof bottle cap has yet to be designed.

Because it's practically impossible for anyone except an expert to know what substances are poisonous to children in what amounts, or which seeds of which plants are harmful if swallowed, many authorities feel strongly that parents should immediately call the closest Poison Control Center for first-aid information rather than try to cope with antidotes or emetics on their own. The Centers are available by phone on a 24-hour-a-day basis. See Ch. 31, *Medical Emergencies*, to find the Poison Control Center nearest you. Make a note of the telephone number and make sure it's available to baby-sitters as well as to all responsible family members.

Poliomyelitis

Until the Salk vaccine was developed in the 1950s, there was no protection against polio (or, as it was then popularly called, *infantile paralysis*). The disease caused paralysis of the extremities and could cause death by paralyzing the muscles used in breathing.

The Salk vaccine utilizes doses of killed virus and is given by injection. Although it is still widely used in many parts of the world, in the United States the Sabin live virus vaccine, which is given orally, has virtually supplanted it. Repeated series of booster shots are unnecessary because the immunity persists for years.

It is advisable that a child receive three doses of the Sabin vaccine, six to eight weeks apart, starting at about the age of two months. One method employs *trivalent* vaccine, in which each dose contains three kinds of vaccine—to give protection against three strains of polio. Three separate doses are necessary, however, to insure full protection. The other method employs *monovalent* vaccines, in which each dose insures protection against a different type of polio.

Posture

"Stand up straight" is an order that many parents issue to their children with the regularity of drill sergeants. Actually, most youngsters tend to slump and have a potbellied look until they're about nine years old. This inelegant posture is not necessarily the sign of any disorder.

Youngsters who are regularly checked by a physician and given a good bill of health are not in any danger of developing a permanent curvature of the spine because they slouch. However, certain kinds of chronically poor posture may be an expression of some disorder that should be checked. Among these are flat feet, nearsightedness or astigmatism, or a hearing loss.

Emotional problems may also be expressed in a child's bearing. Anxiety can lead to carrying one shoulder higher than the other as if warding off a blow. Shyness or insecurity may cause a hangdog stance. For pubescent girls, embarrassment about burgeoning breasts may result in a round-shouldered slump. Some of these causes of poor posture should be discussed with a physician; others may be temporary and shouldn't be turned into major problems by incessant and unproductive nagging. A better corrective is participation in a dancing class or an exercise class. Sports such as ice-skating and bicycle-riding are good posture correctives, too.

Prejudice

The A student (female) who avoids studying mathematics because "girls aren't supposed to be good in math" and the black boy who goes out for the track team even though he'd rather be in the science club "because blacks are better at sports than at brainwork" have unconsciously accepted the prejudiced views of other people about them. What a waste for themselves and society!

Children who are raised in an atmosphere of contempt for and fear and mistrust of Catholics, Jews, Italians, blacks, women, men, are likely to spend the better part of their lives alternating between apprehension and arrogance. It's difficult to believe that adults can have a prejudice such as, "All Orientals are sneaky," which is supposed to describe millions of human beings, or "She's only a girl," which makes a judgment about one-half of the human race.

Being the Object of Discrimination

Parents who have themselves been discriminated against have to prepare their children for the reality of discrimination and how to cope with it. A child raised in an atmosphere of love and respect will have enough self-esteem to refuse to accept anyone else's false notions about him.

Privacy

Every child has a right to a certain amount of privacy even when he's very young. If, for instance, a parent or older child doesn't allow anyone into the bathroom when he's using it, a four- or five-year-old should be given the same option. When children share the same room, or even the same furniture, each one should have a drawer of his own and a shelf of his own for his things. Respecting his private property will lead him to respect other people's. A youngster does like the privacy of playing with his friends without having a parent hovering around all the time, and he certainly doesn't want anyone listening in on his phone conversations by the time he's nine or ten.

Parents have a right to privacy, too! Children should be led to understand—pleasantly but firmly—that some adult conversations are private and not meant for their ears. They should also be taught that when an older member of the family is behind a closed door, it's rude to barge in without knocking.

Puberty

See Ch. 3, *The Teens.*

Punishment

Severe physical punishment should be avoided. Ideally, punishment should be carried out because it has an instructional value for the child rather than because it helps a parent relieve his or her feelings of anger or frustration. Severe physical punishments—for example, the use of sticks, belts, or hard blows to the body—are extremely frightening and may even be permanently injurious to the child. They are also illegal actions, constituting child abuse. Frequently, this kind of discipline can evoke even further anger on the part of the child and lead to further misbehavior.

Duration

Punishments should not be long and drawn out, but should be as immediate as possible and last only a reasonable length of time. For example, withdrawal of television privileges for a month for a seven-year-old's misbehavior would be excessively long, because at the end of the month it would be difficult for her to remember what she had done that was wrong. Excessively long punishments are also difficult to enforce. If possible, a punishment should be related to the misbehavior for which the child is receiving the punishment.

Immediacy

Punishment "when father gets home" or a day later frequently has little meaning for the child and is unlikely to help her stop misbehaving. Rewards for good behavior should also be immediate; affection and approval for most children are often more powerful rewards than candy and money.

Rashes

Rashes of one kind or another are among the most common occurrences of childhood. Whether it's the discomfort of diaper rash soon after birth, the childhood markings of chicken pox, or a case of poison ivy, most skin eruptions aren't too serious and are usually of brief duration.

The First Six Months

Skin rashes are especially common during the first six months. They may result from overheating or overdressing, or to the use of detergents, powders, perfumes, and oils which cause *contact dermatitis*. In addition, certain foods may make the baby break out in facial rashes. Prolonged contact with wet diapers causes *diaper rash*, from the ammonia produced by urine.

Skin rashes can usually be prevented or controlled by:

- Control of temperature
- Proper clothing
- Avoidance of irritating perfumes, powders, and detergents in laundering baby clothes

- Avoidance, in certain circumstances, of milk or other foods, as suggested by your physician
- Avoidance of rubber pants over diapers
- Applications of ointments to rashy areas

If a disturbing skin condition persists or gets worse, your physician will check for special infections like impetigo or fungus, and, should they exist, recommend proper treatment. During the early years, most children develop the characteristic rashes of the contagious childhood diseases, and at these times, a physician's care is usually essential for the prevention of complications.

Eczema

Some children suffer from intermittent eczema that has a tendency to run in families. Eczema can be extremely uncomfortable, because the more it itches, the more it is scratched, and the more it's scratched, the more it itches. This cycle may be triggered by an allergy to a particular food or pollen; it may be a contact dermatitis caused by a particular fabric, or it might flare up because of emotional tension created by family arguments or anxiety about schoolwork. Eczema should be treated by the family physician who may be able to discover its source and prevent further attacks.

Other Allergic Rashes

Other rashes that are essentially allergic in origin are those resulting from contact with poison ivy, oak, or sumac. For information about these and other skin conditions, including hives, see "Disorders of the Skin," in Ch. 21, *Skin and Hair*.

The discomfort of many rashes can be eased by ointments or salves. Plain cornstarch is helpful for prickly heat.

Roseola

Among the more common rashes of early childhood is the one known as *roseola infantum*. It is believed to be caused by a virus. It begins with a high fever that subsides in a few days. There are no other specific signs of illness, and the end of the disorder is signaled by a rash of red spots that disappear overnight. The one aspect of roseola that requires medical attention is the fever. Because high temperature can produce convulsions in infants and babies, efforts should be made to reduce it by sponging and nonaspirin medication.

Pityriasis Rosea

A long-lasting rash thought to be viral in origin is *pityriasis rosea*, easily identifiable because the onset of this infection is preceded by one large raised red scaly eruption known as the herald patch. The rash itself appears symmetrically and in clusters on the trunk, arms, and legs, and in some children on the hands and feet as well as the face. Unfortunately, this rash may last for more than a month.

There is no treatment for it, and, although it leaves without a trace and almost never recurs, it can cause severe itching that should be eased with a salve or ointment. Soap is very irritating and should be avoided.

Rocky Mountain Spotted Fever

Among the diseases caused by organisms known as rickettsiae and transmitted to people by the animal ticks that are infected with them is *Rocky Mountain spotted fever,* also called *tick fever.* In addition to rising temperature, headache, nausea, and malaise, this disease produces a characteristic rash that starts on the ankles, lower legs, and wrists, and then spreads to the rest of the body. Children who wander about in the woods during the summer or whose pets run loose in tick-infested areas should be watched for the presence of a tick on the skin and the ensuing rash. Rocky Mountain spotted fever is a serious disease against which youngsters should be protected by wearing the proper clothing.

Lyme Disease

A rash may be the first visible symptom of Lyme disease, which had been reported in all but a few American states by the late 1990s. Its highest incidence occurs in the northeastern, north-central, and western states. Caused by a tick-carried bacterium, the disease can produce neurological problems, heart disorders, and arthritis. The initial rash can extend over a large area. Antibiotics including tetracycline and penicillin may be used in treatment. The risk of infection may be reduced by frequent inspections of skin areas and prompt removal of the pinhead-sized ticks. If not embedded, a tick can be brushed off; if embedded, it can be pulled out carefully. Care should be taken not to crush the tick's body. The skin should be washed carefully with an antiseptic such as rubbing alcohol.

Lyme disease is treated with antibiotics. If it is caught early, patients can recover completely. For certain groups of people, a vaccine against Lyme disease is recommended.

Reading

Children who see their parents reading or who've heard an older sibling say, "Don't interrupt me when I'm reading" are much more likely to want to learn how to read than those who have never seen an older person absorbed in a book or magazine.

Reading Difficulties

No matter how much the world changes, the child who can't read easily is handicapped. Where a true reading problem exists, parents should confer with the school about a practical solution. If a learning disability appears to be the explanation, tutoring or a special class may be essential. See DYSLEXIA.

Reading for Information

Many youngsters who don't see the point in reading for pleasure when there are many other things they'd prefer to do may go to the library for information about horses or sailing ships or sewing. Families who would like their youngsters to read more than they do have the responsibility of providing a quiet corner, a decent reading light, and an occasional hour of uninterrupted leisure and privacy. Parents who object to a child's habit of "always having her nose in a book" instead of "getting some fresh air and exercise" should withhold their criticism unless the physician recommends a change in the child's activities.

Retardation

See MENTAL RETARDATION.

Reye's Syndrome

Reye's Syndrome is a childhood disease that affects the nervous system and the liver and can result in death. The symptoms normally occur after the child has suffered from the flu or a respiratory illness. The symptoms include vomiting, rash, and disorientation or confusion. If not immediately treated, seizures, respiratory arrest, and coma follow shortly. There is no cure but the dangerous manifestations of the disease can be treated to avoid complications, permanent damage, or death.

The syndrome is believed to be linked to treating the child with aspirin or aspirin-containing medication during the initial illness. Cases of Reye's Syndrome have decreased sharply since 1980, with the increase in public awareness of the link between the disease and the use of aspirin for children.

Given the risk of Reye's Syndrome, it is highly recommended that parents avoid aspirin for children during any illness with fever, flu, diarrhea, or respiratory symptoms. If symptoms persist or if aspirin was given just before the onset of symptoms, please notify a physician. Reye's Syndrome is diagnosed symptomatically.

Rheumatic Fever

Once called growing pains, rheumatic fever is actually a disease of the connective tissues, a secondary manifestation of a primary infection by streptococcus bacteria of the throat or tonsils. Its chief symptoms are pains and tenderness in the joints and sore throat.

Rheumatic fever may be mild enough to escape attention or it may be disabling for a period of months. The insidious aspect of the disease is that it may damage the child's heart in such a way that tissue is permanently scarred and function is impaired in the form of a heart murmur. Acuteness of symptoms varies. Any time from a week to a month after the occurrence of strep throat, the child may complain of feeling tired and achy. Fever usually accompanies the fatigue, and pains in the joints may precede swelling and the development of nodules under the skin in the areas of the wrists, elbows, knees, and vertebrae. The pediatrician can usually detect an abnormal heart finding. The sooner treatment begins, however, the less likely the risk of permanent heart damage.

Close supervision of the affected child may be essential over a long period. Antibiotics, aspirin, hormones (cortisone), and other medicines control the course of the disease and protect the child from its potentially disabling effects. See also "Rheumatic Fever and Rheumatic Heart Disease" in Ch. 10, *Heart Diseases*.

Roseola Infantum

See under RASHES.

Rubella (German Measles)

Rubella was once thought of as a benign disease. Then it was discovered that it could have serious consequences if it were contracted by a woman during the first three months of her pregnancy. The virus that causes rubella is transmitted from the infected woman to her unborn baby, and has been linked to birth defects of the heart, eye, ear, and liver, and to mental retardation.

In addition, a baby who has been exposed to the disease in utero may infect others even though he himself is not affected by it and shows no symptoms. (In fact, most babies are immune to rubella during their first year.) The rubella virus is highly contagious and spreads rapidly.

Rubella has been on the increase in recent years, largely due to the number of young adults who have never been vaccinated. Although it can be a mild illness, it can also cause severe birth defects if contracted by a pregnant woman. Because of the risk of miscarriage and birth defects, pregnant women are advised against getting the immunization during the course of their pregnancy. Anyone who suspects that they or their children were not vaccinated should seek immunization immediately.

The incubation period for rubella is two to three weeks. Symptoms include earache, swollen glands behind the ears, a low-grade fever, and a usually mild, blotchy rash that erupts over the body but lasts only a few days.

Runaways

In growing numbers children and youth ran away from home in the early and middle 1980s. The runaways left home for various reasons. Some were escaping physical or sexual abuse while many others had severe long-term psychological and other problems. A smaller percentage faced temporary or less severe home or school difficulties. Other reasons include "status criminal offense problems"—minor violations of the law that would not be violations at all if committed by an adult—and "poor communication" with parents. Truancy is an example of a status offense. Many children who leave home are not technically "runaways." Professionals call these children *throwaways* because they have in fact been thrown out of the parents' home.

Social service professionals believe many young persons leave home to escape from "dysfunctional families." In such families, parental separation or divorce, poverty, unemployment, and high mobility have, separately or in combination, made the home ineffective as a nurturing environment. The young person may become labeled as a "failure" or "troublemaker"; and a lack of warmth may characterize parent–child relations. In other cases delinquency among a youngster's friends may exert a powerful influence.

The runaways represent diverse age and economic groups. They come from a variety of racial backgrounds. A large proportion are in the 15 to 16 age group. But runaways range in age from 10 or younger to 18.

Parents faced with the fact that a child has run away have to make difficult choices. The child who stays away overnight or for two or more nights has usually not traveled more than 10 miles from home. He or she is usually staying with friends. Only about one in five ventures more than 50 miles from home. The parent or parents of a runaway, considering such facts and not wishing simply to wait, can:

- Look for the youngster themselves. Recommended by many social workers as a logical first step, such a search may involve calls to relatives or the child's friends, checks on favorite haunts, and "driving around" in areas that the young person knows and frequents.

- Report the runaway to police. A "first impulse" alternative, calling the police may not be in the child's best interest. For one thing, the police, especially in large cities, are swamped with such reports. Parental searches actually succeed in finding runaways more frequently than police do. As a second consideration, once reported to police the youngster may be drawn into the juvenile-justice system. In some states, that could result in incarceration with adult offenders or delinquent juveniles. Other states provide that a runaway cannot be held—or cannot be held more than a brief, specified period.

- Contact a local branch of the National Network of Runaway and Youth Services. A private, nonprofit organization with more than 500 community-based shelter programs, the Network serves runaway, homeless, and other "problem" young people. It offers shelter and hotline services 24 hours a day, seven days a week. While not a search operation, the Network also provides crisis and long-term individual and family counseling, outreach, advocacy, referrals for medical, legal, and mental health assistance, and followup services.

- Contact the National Communications System. Supported by the U.S. Department of Health and Human Services, the system operates a nationwide toll-free telephone hotline. Services provided center on referral and crisis intervention aid.

Some national or local services have been established primarily to help runaways obtain clothing, shelter, and food. These organizations also try to mediate between parents and children and to bring families together. Three such groups operate the Runaway Hotline (800/231-6946), the National Runaway Switchboard (800/621-4000), and the National Center for Missing and Exploited Children (800/843-5678).

What happens after a child returns home may determine whether he or she will run away again. Family counselors suggest that parents remain calm. No matter how stressful the runaway incident may have been, parents should try to accept their child as a person. Many runaways, counselors say, are "testing the waters," or experimenting, or seeking a sense of self and identity. If the family can discuss what has happened, the problems that caused the young person to run away may be resolved.

In difficult situations, counseling may be necessary. More and more parents are turning also to inpatient psychiatric services. Usually, these parents have tried other solutions before turning to psychiatry. Contributing to the trend toward hospitalization and professional treatment is the increasing availability of insurance to cover the expected costs.

Safety

See "Accident Prevention" in Ch. 36, *Voluntary Health Agencies*.

Scarlet Fever

Scarlet fever used to be a disease that everyone dreaded. It is highly contagious, and can result in severe aftereffects like rheumatic fever, or the kidney disease known as nephritis.

It is now known that scarlet fever is simply a streptococcal infection—a strain of a specific organism that also causes a diffuse red rash. It can be dealt with quite simply by your physician, the usual treatment being a ten-day course of penicillin, which cures the streptococcal infection and prevents most complications.

Schizophrenia

See under MENTAL ILLNESS.

School

In the United States, an elementary school is a place where children are taught not only how to read, write, handle numbers, and correlate sets of facts, they are also taught how to get along with children different from themselves, how to express themselves creatively, and how to become responsible citizens of a democratic society. If the reality of education falls short of these goals, parents are supposed to exert influence on the proper authorities to see that they are in fact accomplished.

Nursery School

For a child, leaving the protection of the family if only for a half-day in a nearby nursery school is a big step forward. The step is likely to be taken with eagerness if parents present the school as a pleasurable place to be, and not as a dumping ground for a youngster who's in the way of a new baby or a working mother.

Elementary School

The elementary grades represent a major change in many different ways, but most importantly because new authority figures begin to displace parents as the source of all wisdom. Adults and older siblings can help a child make a happy and productive adjustment to school by talking about it with interest and respect. Wherever possible, one or another parent should be present at parent-teacher meetings and participate in the activities of the child's group, such as class trips, visiting days, and the like.

Homework

When youngsters come home with school assignments that they find baffling, parents should feel free to ask the teacher for clearer instructions. If the child is at fault through inattention or ignorance, it might be pointed out to her that whether or not she gets a good education depends on how hard she's ready to work and not how efficiently the teacher can spoon-feed her.

Private Schools

Some families feel that the local public school is not the best place for their children to learn during the lower grades. Alternative private schools, whether denominational, discriminatory, or for gifted children, may have advantages that are less apparent to the child than to the parents, especially if attendance isolates the youngster from her friends in the neighborhood.

Staying Home from School

It's not unusual for a child to avoid going to school once in a while by saying she's sick. She may actually need a rest from the routine every few months. This is quite different from truly getting sick at the thought of facing school. A child who is nauseated in the morning, or who throws up, or who has a stomachache at breakfast, is probably experiencing feelings of anger, resentment, or anxiety beyond her ability to cope with them. Whatever it is in the school situation that's worrying her, she should be given the opportunity to talk about what's going on and the reassurance that efforts will be made to help straighten things out.

For children with disabilities, special facilities are often provided within the structure of the local school so that they can spend at least part of their day with their own age group.

Sex Education

Children need and deserve to have access to correct information about sexual functioning. If there is a natural openness in a family about questions of all types, children first start asking questions about sex when they are three or four; it is then that parents can begin describing sexual functioning to their children.

Questions about Body Parts

The first questions about sex usually have to do with the functioning of body parts. For example, children want to know where urine comes from, what happens to food when they eat it, where feces come from, and where babies come from. Explanations should be given in a straightforward, unembarrassed manner. Children should not be overloaded with information that they do not understand, but parents should be willing to answer questions to the best of their ability.

With older children, particularly 11- and 12-year-olds, it is often helpful for sexual questions to be answered by the parent of the same sex. Reading a book on sexual development with the child can be a good experience for both parent and child. Parents frequently wonder if sex education may not lead children to engage in experimentation. Most of the evidence on this question indicates that children are more likely to experiment sexually when they are ignorant than when their questions about sex are reasonably and accurately answered.

Sexual Abuse and Incest

The sexual abuse of children is much more common than many people realize. It is generally defined as the performance of a sexual act with a child carried out by an adult or an older child. Acts considered sexual include fondling a child's genitals, getting the child to fondle the abuser's genitals, rubbing genitals against a child, oral to genital contact, and anal or vaginal penetration. Sexual abuse is also defined to include showing a child pornographic or sexually explicit materials, making the child perform in pornographic media, and an adult showing his or her genitalia to a child.

Most abusers are known by the abused child and can exert power over him or her. Often the abuser is an authority figure to the child, someone who is loved or trusted. In fact, a large number of abusers are relatives of the abused child. Typically, an abuser convinces, bribes, pressures, or tricks the child into taking part in sexual acts.

Who are the victims of child sexual abuse? They are both males and females, though more girls than boys are the victims of incestuous sexual abuse. Victims range in age from a few months to 16 years or older. The victims represent all socioeconomic groups, all races, and all geographic regions.

Protecting Your Children

Parents have the delicate task of maintaining a loving, touching family relationship while also teaching their child or children to recognize and reject "bad touches." Parents do not want to instill fear, hysteria, or paranoia in their children. But they should teach their child how to escape or avoid abuse within or outside

Safety Tips for Parents

1. Know your children's friends.
2. Never leave your child unattended.
3. Be involved in your child's activities.
4. Listen when your child tells you he or she does not want to be with someone.
5. Pay attention when someone shows greater than normal interest in your child.
6. Have your child fingerprinted and know where to locate dental records.
7. Be sensitive to changes in your child's behavior or attitudes.
8. Take a photograph of your child each year (4 times each year if under age 2).
9. Be prepared to describe your children accurately—including clothing, visible identifying marks, or special characteristics.
10. Develop a set procedure should you and your child become separated while away from home.
11. Do not buy items that visibly display your child's name.
12. Be sure your child's school or day-care center will not release your child to anyone other than you or someone you officially designate.
13. Instruct the school to contact you immediately if your child is absent or if someone other than you arrives to pick up him or her without advance notice from you.

the home. Without dwelling on the details of what *could* happen, show what a bad touch involves—generally, a pinch, hard slap, or a touch in a body area normally covered by a bathing suit. One exception, of course, is a physician's examination. Parental approval makes such an examination acceptable.

Children can and should learn to say "no" to an adult, psychologists tell us. Having said "no," whether the would-be abuser is a friend, relative, or stranger, your child should leave the scene quickly. Then he or she should report the incident to a parent. "Be sure to emphasize that if someone asks them not to tell, they should immediately tell," advises one authority. Parents should make it clear that they will not be angry if they receive such a report.

Parents need to instruct children periodically in the ways to respond appropriately to abusers' approaches. But then they have to listen if the child wants to talk. Children have to be sure both of the parents' love and their willingness to pay attention.

Signs of Sexual Abuse

A child encountering molestation or sexual abuse of any kind is undergoing an emotionally stressful experience. Because the abuser frequently convinces the child not to tell anyone about the abuse, a child's first statements about it might be very vague. The parent should trust the child, be sympathetic, loving, and very supportive. Parents should also try to avoid showing signs of disgust or shock, as this may add to any feelings of guilt the child may be experiencing.

If a parent suspects that their son or daughter has been molested, some authorities suggest asking the child directly if anything has happened to him or her. There are a number of signs that a parent should watch for:

1. Sudden explicit sexual knowledge

2. Precocious sexually related experimentation or speech

3. Toilet training relapses

4. Gagging and unexplained vomiting

5. Regressive behaivor

6. Abrupt changes in behavior, for example, bedwetting

7. Depression and/or self-destructive tendencies

8. Excessive fear of certain individuals and locations

9. Making drawings that show sexual behaviors

10. Irrational fear of a physical exam

11. Unexpected or unusual response when the child is asked if someone touched him or her

12. Unexplained gifts, extra money, or possession of pornography by the child

13. Drug abuse

14. Unexplained bruises or injuries in genital areas

15. Blood spotting or unexplained substances on underwear

16. Vaginal or urinary tract infections

17. Sores or bruising around the lips and the mouth area

18. Infections of the mouth, gums, or throat

Sources of Help

What should a parent do when molestation or sexual abuse is suspected? After you have talked to the child, the next step is to take him or her to a physician to treat any physical injuries and to look for and document physical evidence of the abuse. A physical exam may also be important in reassuring the child that no permanent physical damage has been done to him or her. The police should then be notified, as well as the state or local child protection or social services agency. Depending on need, you may also want to ensure that the child gets counseling. Resource centers that provide diverse kinds of aid include:

- Childhelp USA National Child Abuse Hotline: 800/422-4453
- Child Find hotline: 800/A-WAY-OUT for mediation; 800/I-AM-LOST for abducted children or

people identifying missing or abducted children.

- National Center for Missing and Exploited Children: 800/THE LOST or 703/274-3900
- Runaway Hotline: 800/231-6946
- National Crime Information Center (F.B.I.): 304/625-2000
- National Runaway Switchboard: 800/621-4000

Sibling Rivalry

See BROTHERS AND SISTERS, NEW BABY.

Sickle-cell Anemia

See Ch. 9, *Diseases of the Circulatory System.*

Sisters and Brothers

See BROTHERS AND SISTERS.

Sleep

See BEDTIME, DREAMS AND NIGHTMARES, SLEEPWALKING.

Sleepwalking

Sleepwalking may be distressing to the parent who witnesses it, but it usually does the child no harm. If the child seems to be about to do something dangerous, it's a good idea to wake her up with a few reassuring remarks and guide her back to bed. In most sleepwalking incidents, the child goes back to bed by herself and gets up the next day without the slightest recollection of her nighttime prowl. Parents shouldn't tease or scold or embarrass the child about walking in her sleep. It can be ignored unless it continues over a long period, and then it might be mentioned to your physician.

Smallpox

After smallpox was largely eradicated in 1979, vaccination against the disease was discontinued in the United States.

Smoking

Young children who see older children in the family or other adults smoking cigarettes at home may equate smoking with being grown up, even if their parents don't smoke. A ten-year-old who sneaks off to experiment with a cigarette shouldn't be treated like a criminal, but he should be told that he is harming himself. Parents who smoke and wish they didn't should concentrate on their own efforts to stop and hope that their offspring get the message. In any event, it might help to emphasize to children how hard it is to stop smoking once one has acquired the habit.

Sore Throat

"It hurts when I swallow" is a common complaint of childhood. It may be connected with a cold or tonsillitis, but if there is tenderness at the sides of the neck and a rise in temperature, a physician should be called promptly so that tests can be made to determine whether the child has strep throat. Often a throat culture is necessary. A streptococcus throat infection that is undiagnosed and untreated can have serious consequences. See also STREP THROAT, TONSILLITIS.

Speech Impediments

Among the more common speech defects are *lisping* (the substitution of *th* for *s* and *z* sounds); *lallation* (the inability to pronounce *l* or *r* correctly), and stuttering. Although many children do outgrow their speech disabilities, a considerable number do not.

Therapy

Corrective therapy should be undertaken without too much delay. There have been many advances in the techniques used by speech pathologists, including the audiovisual devices and feed-back systems that promote self-correction. A list of certified speech pathologists can be obtained from the American Speech-Language-Hearing Association, 10801 Rockville Pike, Rockville, MD 20852. See also STUTTERING.

Stealing

See DISHONESTY.

Stepchildren

See Ch. 5, *The Middle Years*. See also ADOPTED CHILDREN.

Stomachache

A wide variety of disorders begins with some kind of abdominal pain, but in most cases, a stomachache is temporary and unaccompanied by any other symptoms. Digestive upsets are frequent in infancy, becoming rarer as the baby approaches the fourth month. See COLIC.

After the baby's first year, a stomachache may signal the onset of a cold or some other infection. The physician should be called if any of the following conditions occurs:

- When the stomach pain is accompanied by fever, vomiting, or diarrhea
- If moderate pain lasts for a considerable time—several hours, for example
- If the pain is obviously acute—the child is doubled over
- If the location off the pain shifts from one place to another

Never give a child a laxative or an enema except on a physician's orders.

A youngster who complains regularly of stomachaches without any other symptoms, and who might also complain of headaches or constipation shouldn't be dismissed as a worrier. The problem should be discussed with your physician so that an investigation can be made of possible causes. In many cases, constipation is the source of stomach pain. When the constipation is cleared up, the stomach pains cease.

Stomach pain may also be of psychosomatic origin, in children as well as in adults. If the pain cannot be explained after a physical examination and tests have been made, parents should consider how they can lighten some of the stresses and tensions in the child's life.

Strabismus

See CROSSED EYES.

Strep Throat

Streptococcal infections, commonly called strep throat, are caused by bacteria that inflame and infect the tissues in the throat. Symptoms include sore throat, swollen glands, redness or blotchy white spots on the throat and tonsils. Severe throat pain may occur for three to four days of the two-week run of the illness. Strep infections should be treated immediately after diagnosis by a physician with antibiotics such as erythromycin or penicillin.

Strep throat poses several risks to the health of both the adult and child sufferer. If left untreated, strep bacteria may produce the toxin that triggers scarlet fever, which also requires treatment with penicillin.

Strep can also lead to rheumatic fever. Rheumatic fever can develop into rheumatic heart disease, leaving the child with a heart murmur. Also treated with penicillin, the disease leaves little damage if caught and treated early.

The last serious problem to arise from a strep infection is relatively new. There a new strep type produces the same symptoms as toxic shock syndrome. The rare form of streptococcus causes low blood pressure, rash, high fever, and rapid organ and blood destruction. It ends in death in 20 percent of the cases. It affects children and adults. Due to the rapid onset of serious and deadly symptoms, it is essential that medical treatment be sought immediately if you or your child suffers any one of the signs of this disease.

Stuttering

Stuttering, or stammering, is a speech dysfunction where the words are spoken with hesitation, repetition, prolongation, or stumbling on one or more syllable of a word. Parents should bear in mind, though, that many children stutter when they are learning to speak. At this stage it is not a permanent problem, and the child will usually outgrow it as ease with language increases.

For a child who continues to show hesitation in speech after the age of four or five, the parents should consider getting professional guidance of a physician, speech therapist, or counselor as recommended by the child's pediatrician. The speech problem may be related to cerebellar disease or a neuromuscular defect or a problem with the voice box. There is also some research being done on hearing problems with stutterers. Some patients respond well to speech therapy when the sound of their voice is played back on a delay through earphones. The slight delay allows them to speak without hesitation. Why this works is not fully understood.

Stuttering can also be related to emotional or psychological problems. Stress from early childhood speech impairment may create a psychological block to speaking. Other problems may enter into the reason for stuttering. It is not uncommon for there to be both emotional and physical reasons for stuttering.

For more information, please call the toll-free hotline for the Stuttering Foundation of America at (800) 992-9392.

Sudden Infant Death Syndrome

Sudden Infant Death Syndrome, sometimes referred to as SIDS and generally known as *crib death*, is the sudden death of an infant prior to one year of age that has no clear cause. Although a number of plausible theories are being investigated—such as the role of swaddling, overheating of nurseries, and colds and other illnesses—the cause of SIDS remains uncertain.

In some cases, autopsies indicate a hidden infection or an unsuspected abnormality, but in most of the deaths, no obvious explanation can be found. One cause appears to be an inherited heart irregularity, and another is respiratory distress, discussed under HYALINE MEMBRANE DISEASE. Improved care of premature babies who are considered to be at higher risk than those born at full term, as well as prenatal tests and ultrasonic alarm systems that monitor breathing are expected to reduce the number of SIDS victims.

Recent findings by the American Academy of Pediatrics suggest a correlation between soft bedding and SIDS. They believe that infants placed facedown to sleep may gradually suffocate as carbon dioxide saturates the bedding material. To reduce this risk, the AAP recommends that parents place their babies on their backs when putting them to sleep.

Parents of infant SIDS victims often suffer intensely—apart from their natural grief—from feelings of guilt, as if they were somehow careless or negligent. They must be reassured that they could not possibly have foreseen the susceptibility of their child to this affliction and that there is therefore no way they could have averted its tragic result.

Swallowed Objects

Babies in a crib or playpen and toddlers playing around the house can certainly be depended on to put all kinds of objects into their mouths. So it's a good idea to make sure that surfaces are cleared of anything that would cause a crisis if swallowed. For example, place cleaning products out of reach, inspect toys for loose or detachable parts, and keep loose buttons and coins in drawers. Some small objects, such as fruit seeds, if swallowed and not choked upon, are unlikely to cause problems when passing through the digestive system. They will be eliminated in regular bowel movements.

Emergencies

Emergencies occur when the object is stuck in the windpipe or when it goes into the bronchial passage. If it is in the windpipe and isn't coughed up right away, use the first aid maneuver for "Obstruction in the Windpipe," Ch. 35, *Medical Emergencies*, without delay. If is doesn't work the first time, do it again—and again. You must clear the windpipe. If all efforts fail, rush the child to a hospital.

Swearing

Sooner or later most children learn swear words, either from hearing their parents use them or from their peers. Young children may use curse words without knowing what they mean or without appreciating how offensive they may be.

Nowadays it is virtually impossible for children to avoid hearing words in everyday use that were strictly taboo when their parents were growing up. However jolting it may be to hear foul words issuing from their angelic-looking children, parents should be neither surprised nor unduly upset if this happens occasionally, especially if they themselves use curse words. They might well point out to the child, however, that many people object strongly to such language, and if they want to be treated courteously by adults, they had better watch their language.

Swimming

Every child should learn to swim, and the earlier the better. Although there's nothing like the ocean for water play, it's not a good place to try to teach a small child how to swim. There are too many extraneous hazards, such as undertow, waves, and unexpected depths. Many communities have outdoor public pools; most large cities have indoor and outdoor pools where professional instruction is available. Even when a child can swim moderately well, she should not be allowed to do so alone, and she shouldn't be allowed to go out in a boat by herself either. Rubber floats, rafts, and the like shouldn't be made available to youngsters until they can swim. A nonswimmer depending on such a device is in trouble if it should drift away from her in deep water.

Talking

The ability to speak is part of the human heritage. How soon and how clearly a child begins to do so depends on several factors. First and foremost is the ability to hear.

Hearing and Speech

Any illness or infection in infancy that has caused even a small hearing loss will interfere with the baby's perception of sounds. This in turn will prevent the normal development of those parts of the brain that govern the imitative aspect of speech.

A Stimulating Environment

How much attention and stimulation the baby gets from his environment and the people around him will have a great effect on how much he tries to say and the age at which he begins to say it. Being listened to and automatically corrected instead of being ignored or teased is the indispensable feedback process that enriches the learning of language. The clarity of the child's speech depends to a large extent on the examples before him; what his ears hear his brain will order his vocal equipment to imitate. Parents who want a child to outgrow baby talk should avoid responding to the baby in kind. Normal adult speech should become the norm toward which the child is constantly striving. See also HEARING, SPEECH IMPEDIMENTS, SWEARING.

Tantrums

See ANGER.

Tay-Sachs Disease

Tay-Sachs disease is an inherited disorder of the nervous system. It causes degeneration of the nerves, starting after six months of age. Infant development through pregnancy and the first six months is normal, but the disease can be detected through genetic testing. The first symptoms to appear are subtle, becoming more obvious with motor deterioration. They include a slowing of development, a loss of vision, and eventually convulsions. A cherry-red spot develops on the retina of the eye. The child will lose the motor coordination that he already had and will deteriorate to the point where he will be unable to lift his head. Normally, the child with Tay-Sachs disease does not survive past the age of four.

Tay-Sachs is found with higher prevalence among the following populations: Ashkenazi Jews, Eastern European Jews, and French Canadians. Testing is recommended for anyone from these populations, and testing is also recommended for all Jews to determine if one is a carrier of the disease.

Tay-Sachs is a form of cerebral sphingolipidosis. It is the infantile onset of the disorder. The others are Jansky-Bielschowsky disease (early juvenile), Spielmeyer-Vogt and Batten-Mayou disease (late juvenile), and Kufs' disease (adult onset). Symptoms are similar and include blindness within two years of the onset of the disorder.

Teething

Babies of four to six months drool a great deal and put their fingers in their mouths. These habits, and the telltale small bumps you may detect on the baby's gums, are the signs of teething. But they don't necessarily mean that the first tooth is about to erupt. That may not happen until he is nearly one year old, although it usually happens earlier.

Teething may or may not be painful. If the baby does fret, medication is available to alleviate the pain. (A little anesthesia, such as Ambesol, rubbed on the gums is a home remedy that often helps.)

Tetanus

Tetanus (also called *lockjaw* because it causes spasms of the jaw) can occur at any age as the result of contamination of a simple wound. The causative organism is usually found in soil, street dust, or feces.

The disease is preventable by immunization. The triple vaccine DTP should be started at about two months of age. See also IMMUNIZATION.

When a child suffers a puncture wound, dog bite, or other wound that may be contaminated, ask your physician about giving the child a booster dose of tetanus toxoid if the child has not had a shot within the past five years.

Tick Fever

See "Rocky Mountain Spotted Fever" under RASHES.

Toilet Training

During the toddler stage, parents begin to teach their child how to control his bowel and urinary functions.

When to Start

A simple question parents frequently ask is, "How do I know when my child is ready to be toilet trained?"

Generally, children do not have muscular control over their bowel movements and urination until about the age of two, so attempting to toilet train a child much before this is usually wasted effort. If it is accomplished, the result is usually a training of the parents rather than of the child. Toilet training should usually take place some time between the ages of two and three and one-half.

A child is emotionally ready when he understands what is meant by toilet training and is willing to perform toilet functions without expressing fear of them. This may occur at any age, but is perhaps most apt to start between the ages of 18 and 24 months. With a first child it usually occurs later than with a second or third child, because the first child has no siblings to emulate. But a first child should usually be trained by the time he is three. Training the child to stay dry through the night may take longer.

Resistance to Toilet Training

Early toilet training—training that is begun during a child's first year—may work, but as a child develops and asserts his personality and independence, he will resent any insistence on manipulating the control of his bodily functions. He may get even by refusing to empty his bowels when put on the potty. Worse yet, if another baby has entered the scene, the early-trained child may revert to wetting and having bowel movements in his training pants.

When you feel the child is ready for training, establish the fact that going to the bathroom is a normal part of daily life. If the child expresses fear, don't struggle with him. Don't fight about it. Take him right off the potty and let him know that you are not concerned or displeased. A genuine complication can arise if the child connects his fear of toilet functions with your displeasure at his failures.

Training can usually be facilitated by praise from the parents for putting the bowel movement and the urine in the proper place, rather than by punishment. Excessive punishment or the threat of it usually results in anger on the child's part and increasing stubbornness and resistance to toilet training. Praise immediately following the proper performance of the act is far more effective in encouraging compliance with the parents' goals.

Tonsillectomy

See "Tonsils and Adenoids" in Ch. 20, *Surgery*.

Tonsillitis

The tonsils are two masses of soft spongy tissue that are partly embedded in the mucous membrane of the back of the throat. Bacterial or viral infection of this tissue is known as tonsillitis. It used to be considered advisable to remove the tonsils if they became enlarged—which they normally do in the process of filtering out mild infections.

Nowadays, an occasional bout of tonsillitis isn't considered sufficient reason for surgical removal of the tonsils, especially because they're likely to be less prone to infection as the child gets older. However, even a mild case of tonsillitis should be called to a physician's attention. Acute symptoms such as swollen tonsils, sudden high fever, swollen neck glands, and severe pain when swallowing must be treated promptly since they might be an indication of a strep throat. The proper antibiotics are always effective in controlling this infection so that it doesn't turn into rheumatic fever or involve the kidneys. Tonsillitis caused by a virus usually responds to a non-aspirin pain reliever, bed rest, and a soft diet. See also ADENOIDS. For a description of tonsillectomy, see "Tonsils and Adenoids" in Ch. 20, *Surgery*.

Toy Safety

Toys come with a recommended age of use. It is important that parents heed the information. Some toys are unsuitable for certain ages, not only because of an inability to use it correctly, but because there may be pieces of the toy that are harmful. These are just a few examples of toys that can be safe at one age and not another; games may have small pieces can be swallowed by little children; electrical toys should only be handled by children old enough to understand the danger. Toys hanging in the crib should not be used by infants old enough to pull themselves up to a standing position because they may strangle on cords and strings of the toy. It should be noted that it is not always the case that only younger children should avoid older children's toys. Toys that are safe for younger children may tip, break, or pinch with the increased size and weight of an older child.

Not all toys come with recommendations or fulfill the safety standards set up by the U.S. government. Cheap imitations may not meet the rigid standards of the more established companies' toys. Several hundred toys are recalled each year, and more may have not yet been tested. It is important that a parent take responsibility for evaluating the safety of any toy to be given to a youngster.

For detailed and important information on age recommendations for toys (*Which Toy for Which Child*) and for a listing of products recommended for their reliability and safety, please write to U.S. Consumer Product Safety Commission, 4330 East-West Highway, Bethesda, MD, or call (800) 638-2772. *The ABC's of Toys and Play* is also a worthwhile publication on how to select toys for children. It is published by Toy Industry Association, Inc., 1115 Broadway, Suite 400, New York, NY 10010.

Tuberculosis

See Ch. 12, *Diseases of the Respiratory System.*

Multiple Births

Multiple births may be *identical*—that is, the result of the splitting of a single egg fertilized by a single sperm—or they may be *fraternal*, which means that they developed from different eggs fertilized by different sperm. Most multiple births are fraternal; except for their birthdays, most twins and triplets are no more alike than other brothers and sisters in the same family.

Although there is no ready explanation for the occurrence of multiple births, the tendency is thought to be genetically determined through the mother. Twins occur about once in every 80 births; triplets and higher order multiples occur much less frequently, although the number of triplets born to American women has quadrupled since the 1970's. Multiple births are much more likely to be premature than are single births. They often require special medical attention after delivery.

Urinary Infections

Urinary infections of either viral or bacterial origin are more common among girls than boys, especially during the preschool years. Such infections are sometimes the explanation for a fever unaccompanied by other symptoms. Any inflammation that creates a burning sensation during urination should be tested and treated promptly because it can spread from the bladder to the kidneys and create a major problem.

Girls can be spared frequent infection if given suggestions at an early age about their toilet routines. Fecal matter is high in bacterial content, so little girls should learn to wipe their bottoms from front to back. This procedure reduces the possibility of contaminating the urethra after a bowel movement.

Vaporizer

A vaporizer is a device similar to a humidifier that moistens the air with steam and thus alleviates some of the discomfort of respiratory congestion. During the winter months when heated interiors are likely to be especially dry and when colds are more common, children and adults can benefit from moist air that keeps the throat, nasal, and bronchial passages from feeling like sandpaper. Medication shouldn't be added to a vaporizer except at the physician's recommendation. If the device is used near a child's bed throughout the night, it should be placed on a surface high enough to prevent it from being bumped into.

Cleaning a vaporizer daily with a weak bleach and water solution will prevent buildup of bacteria.

Vomiting

See NAUSEA AND VOMITING.

Warts

See Ch. 21, *Skin and Hair.*

Water Beds

Because of the softness and the motion of a waterbed, infants up to *at least* twelve months of age should never be left unattended on a waterbed. Infants left even briefly on a waterbed have suffocated. The risks are that the infant will become trapped between the mattress and the frame or wall, or become wedged between a sleeping adult and the mattress, or sink face first into the mattress and be unable to push himself up. Several infant deaths originally attributed to SIDS are now considered suffocation due to a waterbed. At least 24 infants have died while left to nap on the parents' waterbed in the last decade.

Whooping Cough

Whooping cough (also called *pertussis*), like diphtheria a bacterial disease, occurs more frequently than diphtheria because immunity to it wears off, especially in the older child in whom the disease may appear as a severe bronchitis.

Whooping cough can be very serious in young babies because it can cause them to choke and be unable to catch their breath. If your child does contract whooping cough, call your physician immediately. He or she may give a specific drug against the organism that causes the disease as well as a specific antitoxin against the poison that the bacillus releases.

It is advisable to immunize children against whooping cough as early as possible. The effective triple vaccine known as DTP provides immunization not only against whooping cough, but against diphtheria and tetanus as well.

Worms and Parasites

See Ch. 11, *Diseases of the Digestive System.*

3

The Teens

Puberty and Growth

The bridge between childhood and adulthood is a period of growth and change called puberty. There seems to be no standard pattern for the physical changes of puberty. Two boys of the same age who have been nearly identical throughout childhood may appear to set off along entirely different paths of physical development as they enter the teenage years. One may quickly shoot up to a height of five feet eight inches within a couple of years while his companion lags for a while at preteen size, then begins growing into a six-footer. One may develop a heavy beard in his early high-school years while the other boy will have no use for a razor until he is in college. However, both boys are normal youngsters, and each will eventually attain all of the physical attributes of adulthood.

Similarly, one girl may begin menstruating in her 11th year while a classmate will not experience her first menstruation until she is 16. One girl may need a bra while still in grammar school but her friend will fret about a small bustline for many years. But both girls can look forward to normal womanhood. Each has an individual pattern of development, and if there is any rule of thumb about puberty it is that each youngster has his or her own time schedule for the transformation into a mature man or woman.

Puberty: Changes in Girls

The physical changes that occur in the female body during puberty probably are more dramatic than those associated with a boy progressing into manhood. One definite milestone for the girl is her first *menstruation,* commonly regarded as the first sign of puberty. Actually, the first menstruation, known as the *menarche,* is only one of several signs of puberty, along with the slimming of the waist, gradual broadening of the hips, the development of breasts, the appearance of hair about the genitals and in the armpits, and a change in the rate of growth.

The Menarche

The age at which a girl first experiences menstruation generally varies over a period of ten years and depends upon the structural development of the youngster, her physical condition, the environment, and hereditary factors. Menarche can occur as early as the age of 7, and most physicians would not be overly concerned if a girl did not begin to menstruate until she was approaching 17. The age range of 9 to 16 usually is considered normal. The median age for the start of menstruation is around 13½ years, which means that 50 percent of all females are younger than 13 years and 6 months when they reach the menarche, and half are on the older side of that age when they first menstruate. In general, the pubertal experiences of a girl follow a pattern like that of her mother and

Development

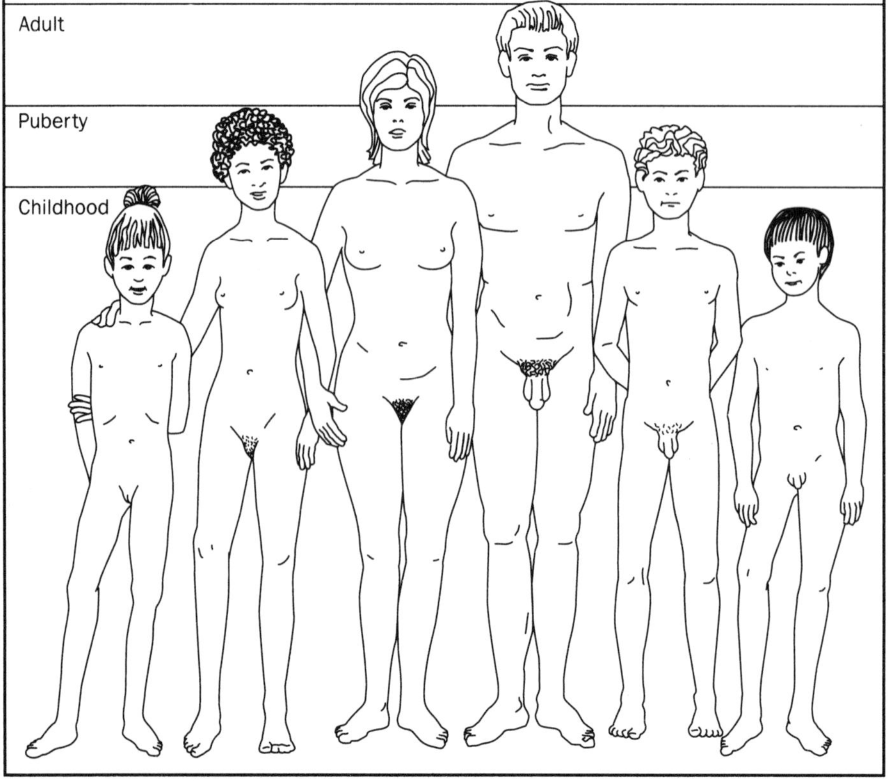

sisters; if the mother began menstruating at an early age, the chances are that her daughters will also.

If the girl has not reached the menarche by the age of 18, she should be examined by a *gynecologist,* a physician who specializes in problems related to the female reproductive system. A medical examination also should be arranged for any girl who experiences menstruation before she reaches the age of eight or nine years.

When menarche occurs on the early side of childhood, the condition is sometimes called *precocious puberty.* The child may suddenly begin menstruating before her mother has told her what to expect, a situation that can prove embarrassing to both child and parents. It may first be detected by a teacher at school; occasionally, a young girl may be aware of bleeding from the vagina but because of fear or false modesty does not report the event to her mother or teacher. For this reason, parents should be alert for changes associated with early puberty and be prepared to explain the facts of life to their children. Also, in the case of precocious puberty, parents should arrange for medical consultation to be certain the bleeding actually is the result of first menstruation and not the effects of an injury or tumor.

Growth Spurt before Menarche

During the year or two preceding the menarche there is a growth spurt of two or three inches. This is because of the hormone changes of puberty. The *hormones* are chemical messengers secreted by glands in various parts of the body and carried rapidly through the bloodstream to organs or other glands where they trigger reactions. The spurt in growth preceding menarche results from the secretion of a growth hormone that is produced by the pituitary gland, and androgen, a hormone secreted by the adrenal glands. They produce rapid growth of the bones and muscles during puberty. The girl who is first among her classmates to menstruate often is larger than those who are of the same age but have not yet reached the menarche.

From numerous research studies of the menarche, it has been learned that poor nutrition and psychological stress sometimes delay the onset of menstruation, that girls reared in cities tend to menstruate earlier, and that climate is a factor, although both tropical and arctic climates seem to be related to early menarche. The first menstrual periods also are likely to occur during the school year, September to June, rather than during the summer vacation.

The First Menstrual Cycles

The first menstrual cycles tend to be very irregular and have been known to be as short as 7 days and as long as 37 weeks. Even when regularity becomes established, the adolescent menstrual cycle usually is longer than the average for adult women. The typical menstrual cycle of a young girl may be about 33 days, compared to an average of 28 days for an adult woman. About three years elapse before the menstrual cycles become regular. In the meantime, irregular menstrual patterns can be considered as normal for girls during puberty.

The first menstrual cycles also are *anovulatory.* In other words, the young girl's ovaries have not matured sufficiently to produce an *ovum,* or egg cell, that can be fertilized by the sperm of a male. There are, of course, the exceptions that make newspaper headlines when a little girl gives birth to a baby. But anovulatory menstruation generally is the rule for the first few months after the menarche.

Delayed Puberty

Delayed puberty probably causes as much anguish as precocious puberty. The last girl in a group of childhood chums to develop breasts and experience the menarche may feel more self-conscious than the first girl in the class to menstruate. If the signs that usually precede menarche have not appeared by the age of 17 or 18, a medical examination should be considered, even though the girl may be a late-late-bloomer at the other end of the spectrum from the 7- or 8-year-old child who has menstruated.

The absence of menstruation after a girl is 18 can be the result of a wide variety of factors. The cause sometimes can be as simple as an *imperforate hymen,* a membrane that blocks the opening of the vagina. It can be the result of a congenital malformation of the reproductive organs, such

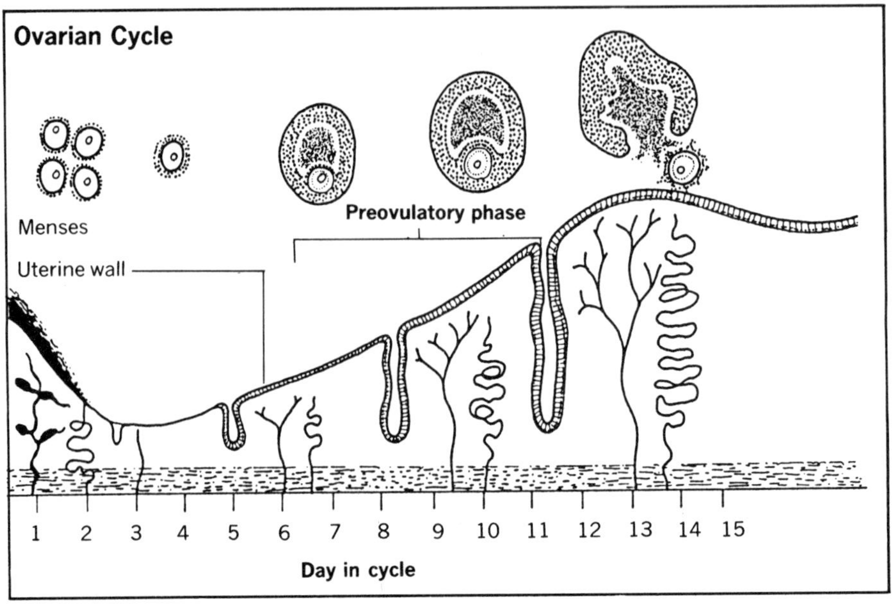

as imperfect development of the ovaries. Accidents, exposure to carbon monoxide gas, or diseases like rheumatic fever or encephalitis in earlier years can result in brain damage that would inhibit the start of menstruation. The relationship between emotional upset and delayed menarche was vividly demonstrated during World War II when some girls who suffered psychological traumas also experienced very late signs of puberty.

Preparing Your Daughter for Menstruation

A mother's main responsibility is to convince her daughter at the beginning of puberty that menstruation is a perfectly normal body function. The mother should explain the proper use of sanitary napkins or tampons and encourage her daughter to keep records of her menstrual periods on a calendar.

The mother also should explain that menstruation usually is not a valid reason to stay in bed or avoid school or work. The girl should be advised that bathing and swimming should not be postponed because of menstruation. There are many old wives' tales about menstruation that are not true. But there may be some truth to stories that loss of menstrual blood can be weakening, particularly if the girl's diet does not replace the body stores of iron which may be lowered during menstrual flow. Iron is a key element of the red blood cell, and if iron-rich foods are not included in the meals of women during their years of menstruation they can eventually suffer a form of iron-deficiency anemia.

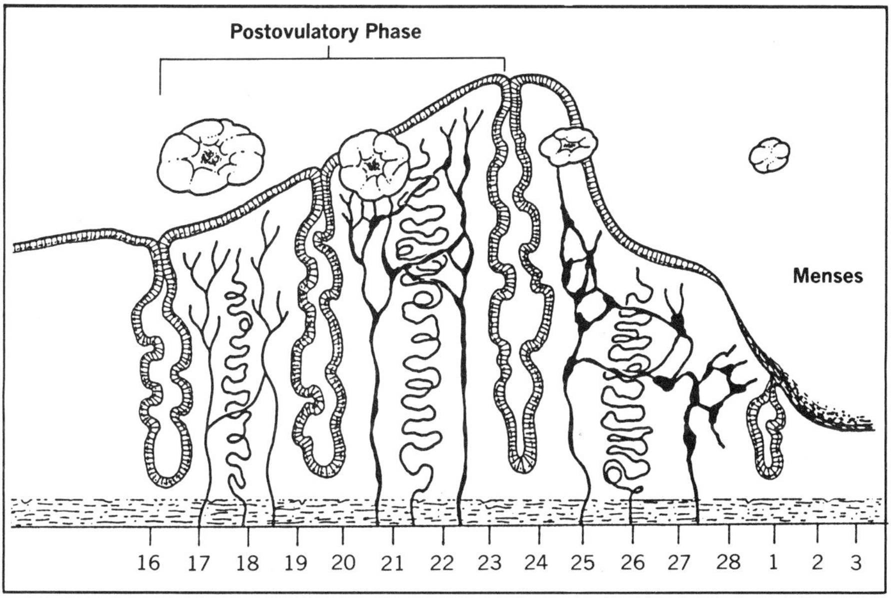

Hormone Activity: Becoming a Woman

Although the sex hormones are the key to what makes girls grow into women and boys into men, both sexes appear to receive secretions of male and female sex hormones in approximately equal amounts for about the first ten years of life. But as puberty approaches, the adrenal glands of girls seem to increase production of a female sex hormone, *estrogen*. Meanwhile, a nerve center in the hypothalamus area of the brain stimulates the pituitary gland, the master gland of the body, to secrete another kind of hormone, *gonadotropin*. Gonadotropin in turn activates a *follicle-stimulating hormone* that causes a maturation of the ovaries, which are part of the original equipment girls are born with but which remain dormant until the start of puberty.

During the second decade of life, the hormone activity stimulates the development of body tissues that not only grow in size but give a girl more womanly contours. However, the fully mature contours of a woman usually do not appear until after the ovaries are functioning and still another female sex hormone, *progesterone*, has been introduced in the system. The ovaries, uterus, Fallopian tubes, and vagina gradually mature as the menarche draws near.

Female Reproductive Organs

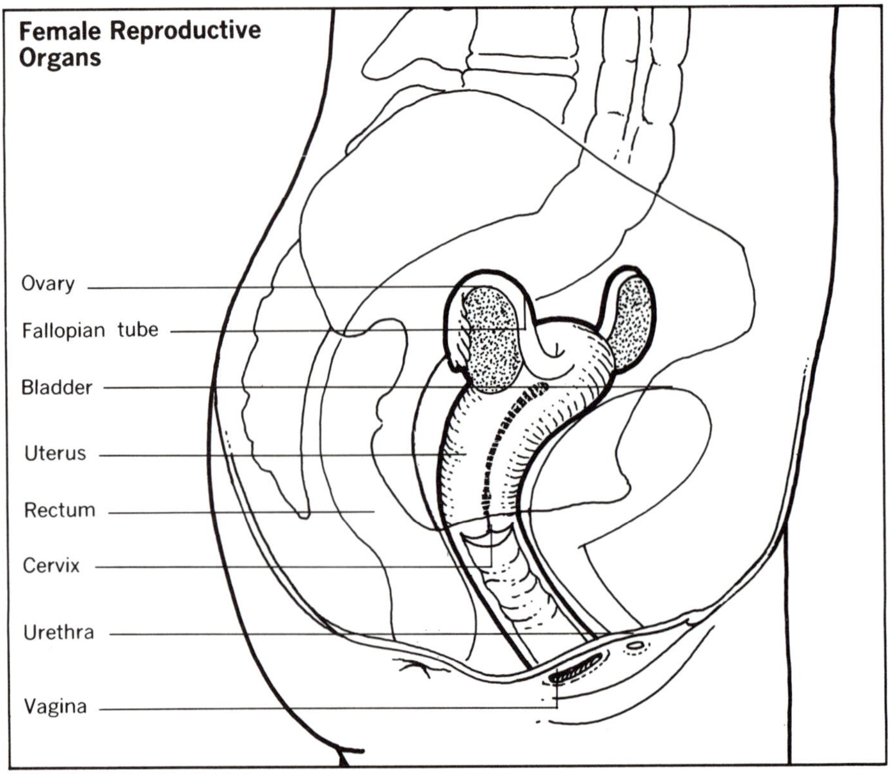

Puberty: Changes in Boys

The appearance of male sexual characteristics during puberty is also influenced by hormonal changes. But the manifestation of male puberty is somewhat more subtle. The pituitary gland in a boy also secretes a gonad otropic hormone that stimulates maturation of *gonads*. In the male, the gonads are the *testicles*, the source of *sperm*. But whereas maturation of the ovaries in females leads to the menarche, there is no obvious sign in the boy that *spermatozoa* are being produced.

However, the secondary sexual characteristics, such as the growth of a beard and pubic hair, the spurt of growth of bones and muscles, the increase in size of the sex organs, and the deepening of the voice, are all indications of puberty. The changes in a boy's characteristics during puberty are usually spread over a period of two years, beginning with an increase in the size of the penis and testicles and reaching completion with the production of spermatozoa in the testicles. During the two-year period there usually is a noticeable increase in the chest size of a boy, with the broad shoulders of manhood appearing during the peak of bone and muscle growth. Generally, the appearance of pubic and facial hair, as well as hair in the armpits, follows the growth of the shoulder and chest area and precedes the change in voice.

The Testicles

The testicles are contained in a walnut-size sac of skin called the *scrotum*. It is held outside the body by a design of nature in order to maintain a temperature for spermatozoa production that is less than internal body temperature. Muscle fibers in the scrotum hold the testicles closer to the body for warmth in cold weather and relax to allow the sperm-producing organ to be farther away from the body when surrounding temperatures are warm.

In some cases, one or both testicles do not descend from the abdomen during the male child's early years. The result is that the undescended testicle or testicles will not produce sperm. An *incompletely descended testicle* always lies somewhere along the normal path to the scrotum. An *ectopic* testicle has deviated from that path and lies somewhere near the inguinal canal, at the junction of the thigh and the lower part of the abdomen. In a third departure from normal development, a *retractile testicle* has stopped short of the scrotum. It can be manipulated into the normal position or may descend to that position at puberty.

The danger of malignant change—of tumor development—usually warrants surgical removal of the incompletely descended and the ectopic testicle. A testicle trapped in the inguinal region may become inflamed because of the pressure of larger body parts in the area. In some cases, physicians are able to assist the de-

The Male Reproductive System

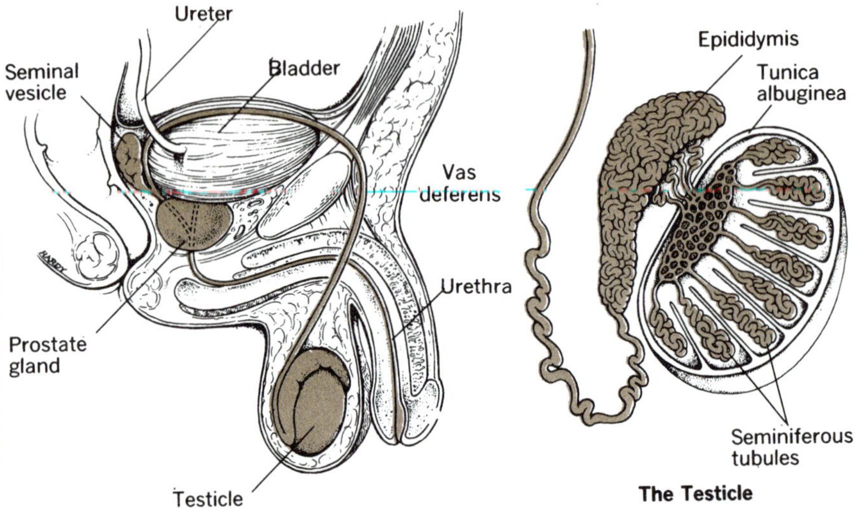

The Testicle

scent into the scrotum through administration of hormones or by surgery. At some point during puberty, a medical examination should include a check on the condition of the testes.

Genital Size

Many boys are as sensitive about the size of their genitals as girls are about breast size. In the case of an empty scrotum because of undescended testicles, it is possible to have the scrotum injected with silicone plastic for cosmetic or psychological reasons so the sac appears less flaccid or larger. The size of the penis may become the subject of discussion in the school shower room. If a boy appears sensitive about the subject, he should be assured that there is a wide variation in normal sizes and that like ears, noses, and other body parts the dimensions have little to do with function.

Nocturnal Emission

Another cause for concern by adolescent boys is the *nocturnal emission.* The nocturnal emission, sometimes called a *wet dream,* is the automatic expulsion of *semen* through the penis while the young man is asleep. The semen is secreted by the *prostate gland,* the *seminal vesicle,* and other glands that open into the *urethra.* The opalescent white fluid carries spermatozoa during intercourse and if the young male does not engage in sexual intercourse or does not masturbate, the semen simply accumulates until it overflows during a nocturnal emission. It is a harmless, normal occurrence.

Bone Growth

As the growth spurt subsides in the late teens, the *cartilage plates,* or *epiphyses,* in the long bones of the body close. Until the growth plates become filled in with calcium deposits, each long bone is in effect three bones—a central shaft separated from the ends by the cartilage growth plates. The growth plates are not completely replaced by bone until a female is about 20 and a male 23 years old. But the rate of growth begins to taper off as sexual maturity is achieved. After that, young women tend to retain fatty tissue and young men gain in muscle mass. Although obesity has been recently linked to genetic mutation, young people can still be diligent in monitoring the quality and amount of food eaten. Proper nutrients and a sensible intake will provide the best fuel for healthy bone growth.

Skin and Hair Problems

Hereditary influences may determine many of the physical and psychological traits that an individual first becomes aware of in the teen years. Because of the various crossovers of the 23 sets of *chromosomes* and the nearly infinite combinations of *genes,* it is not always easy to predict how a child is going to appear as a young adult. But some features, such as hair color and eye color, usually can be identified with one or both parents; other traits may seem to be those of uncles, aunts, or grandparents. Heredity and hormones frequently are involved in the distribution of hair on the body and the oiliness of the skin, both of which can cause concern to teenagers who are plagued by an overabundance or lack of these cosmetic traits. An example of hereditary influences on hair patterns can be seen in early baldness. A receding hairline is not a trait of the parents but rather an influence of the genetic makeup of a grandparent—the trait skips a generation.

Removal of Excess Hair

While not much can be done about baldness that is hereditary, there are ways of handling the problems of excess hair. If a woman has excess hair on her face, arms, and legs, it can be removed by shaving, with wax, by electrolysis, or depilatories. Shaving is the most direct but not always the most satisfactory method of hair removal because it is intended only as a temporary measure. An alternate shortcut is bleaching with diluted hydrogen peroxide; the hair is still there but it is not as noticeable. Another method involves the use of hot wax spread on the skin and allowed to harden. When it is removed quickly, the hair is pulled away.

Depilatories are chemicals that destroy the hair at the skin line. Both hot wax and depilatories have longer-lasting effects than shaving, but they must be repeated at intervals of several weeks.

Depilatories, too, can produce unpleasant allergenic reactions. The only permanent method of removing excess hair is *electrolysis,* which is a time-consuming technique. Each hair root has to be burned out individually with an electric current. Electrolysis is recommended only for small areas and because of the time and expense involved would not be feasible for removing excess hair from regions other than the face.

Acne

There is some evidence that *acne* is partly hereditary. But it is such a common problem among teenagers—it has been estimated that up to 90 percent of all youngsters endure some degree of acne—that it must have been inherited from a mutual ancestor like Adam or Eve. In fact, one of the deterrents to effective control of the skin disorder is that acne is so common that it is neglected by many youngsters. Waiting to outgrow acne can be a serious mistake, because the pimples, blemishes, blackheads, and boils that make life miserable for so many teenagers can be eliminated or considerably reduced. They can also cause scarring. A physician should be consulted in cases of severe or especially persistent acne.

Overactive Oil Glands

Acne can be seriously disfiguring at a time of life when most young people are sensitive about their appearance. It can occur at any time from puberty into early adulthood, and it is caused by poor adjustment of the skin to secretions of sebaceous glands. The imbalance resulting from hormones in the bloodstream will correct itself eventually. But to prevent permanent scarring, a program of simple skin care must be followed faithfully.

Acne is caused by overly active oil glands in the skin. When the oil glands become clogged, blackheads and pimples appear. (Blackheads are caused by a chemical change in the secretions of the oil glands.) To treat acne, a person should wash the skin to clear the pores and oil glands. The skin should be dry enough to peel away soiled layers and remove dirt from the pores. Most topical medications seek to keep the skin sufficiently dry to enhance peeling.

Skin Care

The face should be washed several times a day with warm water and mild soap. It should be dried thoroughly and gently with a clean towel. Careless handling of blemishes, such as squeezing blackheads, and picking at pimples and scabs can result in scarring. Teenagers also should avoid touching their faces. If the condition of the skin is worse than a few mild blemishes, a dermatologist will be able to prescribe topical medication, antibiotics, or hormones to treat the problem. Treatment often takes several months before there is noticeable improvement.

Other Precautions

Young women should not use cold creams or cosmetics unless they have been approved by a physician. Young men who shave must be careful to avoid cutting pimples. A physician also should be consulted about how diet can help control acne. Although the skin disorder is not a dietary disease, there is some evidence that certain foods tend to aggravate it. However, there is a lack of agreement among physicians as to whether chocolate, carbonated beverages, nuts, sweets, and other specific snack items may be the culprits. Because each youngster develops along an individual path, a food item that causes one teenager's face to break out with blemishes will not affect a sibling or classmate in the same way.

Diet

It is no surprise that many American teenagers have poor eating habits. A survey by the Food and Nutrition Board of the National Research Council recently showed that 40 percent of boys between 13 and 19 years of age and 60 percent of the girls in the same age group subsisted on diets that were substandard. Generally, the young people surveyed had abandoned the healthy eating habits of their families. They habitually skipped breakfast and failed to make up the nutritional loss during other meals.

There are several reasons for this phenomenon. Perhaps the most prominent reason is that teens are anxious to break away from their home. They therefore rebel against any form of convention or parental advice. The popularity of fast food institutions and snack shops is a also great contributor to the problem. Such places have become frequent hangouts for teenagers after school and on weekend evenings. With social gatherings in these surroundings, teenagers begin to develop poor eating habits. Frequently, they fill themselves up with non-nutritive foods and have no appetite later for balanced meals. At home, teenagers are great snack-eaters, and much snacking occurs while they are watching television. The combination of inactive television-watching and munching on junk foods leads to an unhealthy physical condition in teenagers.

Calories and Nutrition

A calorie is a unit of energy, and the human body requires a certain amount of energy each day in order to sustain life and continue normal physical activity. The amount of caloric intake varies according to the individual. Much of it depends on physical activity, size, and metabolic rate.

Calories in themselves are not bad. However, excessive intake of calories can lead to severe weight and health problems. Often the problem is not calories but the consumption of "empty calories" from foods high in fat or sugar that are of little or no nutritive value; such as sugary sodas, candy, and potato chips.

To maintain the proper balance between foods consumed and energy used in work and play, a teenager must regulate his or her caloric intake. Much of the regulation occurs naturally. For example, when a person eats a lot, he or she is not hungry for a longer period of time than usual. Often, people crave foods that have been lacking in their diet. Thus, without conscious effort, most people are able to limit their consumption of foods to normal levels.

Nonetheless, teenagers should learn healthy eating habits and be aware of the potential of gaining weight. Regularly checking one's weight on a scale is not a good idea because it may foster unhealthy obsessions that can lead to skewed images of a teenager's physique and perhaps serious eating disorders. It is more important that a teenager monitor weight through the fit of his or her clothing.

Calcium and Phosphorus

Among the important minerals in teenage diets are calcium and phosphorus, which are required for the development of strong bones. Calcium also is required for the effective contraction of muscle tissues and is vital for normal heart function. Milk is the most easily available source of calcium and phosphorus. The recommended daily intake of milk for teenagers is four eight-ounce glasses. It can be served as fluid whole milk, as skim milk, buttermilk, evaporated milk, or as nonfat dry milk. Cheese or ice cream can be substituted for part of the fluid milk allowance. One cup of ice cream is equivalent in calcium to one-half cup of milk. A one-inch cube of cheddar cheese is equal to two-thirds of a cup of milk, which also is equivalent in calcium to one cup of cottage cheese. Two ounces of cream cheese are equal to one ounce of milk.

Iron

Iron is needed for the formation of hemoglobin, the substance that gives red blood cells their red coloration and is responsible for the transport of oxygen and carbon dioxide in the bloodstream. Hemoglobin has such an affinity for oxygen that without it humans would require 60 times as much blood to transport oxygen from the lungs to tissues throughout the body. Girls are five times as likely to need additional supplies of iron in their diets because of blood loss through menstruation. Recommended sources of iron are liver, heart, kidney, liver sausage, meat, shellfish, egg yolk, dark molasses, bread, beans and other legumes. If basic food lists seem dull, the teenager might think of the iron sources in terms of a peanut butter sandwich or two hamburgers; either choice would provide the daily iron needs for a girl. Other minerals that are important to a teenager's diet include the following:

- Sulfur is needed by the body for hair, skin, nails, and cartilage, and is available by eating nearly any protein-rich food.
- Iodine is needed for normal thyroid control of body metabolism and is supplied in the form of iodized table salt.
- Potassium is a tonic for the nervous system and the muscles and is available in adequate amounts in most kinds of meats, as well as bananas, orange juice, and milk.
- Magnesium collaborates chemically with calcium and phosphorus for normal muscle and nerve function, and is found in most forms of protein.

Note: Many of these nutrients are readily available in a normal diet. In most cases, it is not necessary to supplement a teenager's diet with these minerals. Children and teens should not rely on vitamin pills to make up for an unhealthy diet. It is better to eat nutritionally.

Weight Problems

Teens who are seriously overweight or who are contemplating radical weight reduction programs should be examined by a physician. Otherwise, unfair comparisons with other persons of the same age and height may lead to wrong conclusions about the need to gain or lose weight. The weight–height standards are based on averages, and there are many youngsters who are above or below the average but quite healthy and normal.

Another reason for a medical exam is to check the possibility of disease as the cause of the weight problem. The exam will also indicate whether the youngster has some other disorder that could be aggravated by a sudden weight loss.

Achieving optimum weight is only one step toward proper physical conditioning. A youngster who has been able to avoid physical activity could be right on the button as far as weight for his age and height are concerned, but at the same time, his muscular development and heart and lung capacity could be at a very low ebb.

Anorexia Nervosa

One of the most common eating disorders is anorexia nervosa, which occurs most often in teenage girls, but has also been noticed in boys. Anorexics usually have an intense fear of weight gain and a distorted body image. It is believed to be caused by factors including low self-esteem, family conflicts, and societal attitudes toward physical beauty.

The most obvious trait is excessive and unnatural thinness. When anorexics become critically thin, they develop downy hair, called lanugo, all over the body, including the face. Other symptoms include obsession with exercise and eating habits, emphasis on self-control and discipline, high achievement in school, alternating periods of strict fasting and binging, and rituals surrounding food preparation and eating.

Fewer than two-thirds of the children and young adolescents who have anorexia make a sustained recovery from the disorder. Research suggests that about one percent of female adolescents are anorexic. Recovery is crucial; anorexia nervosa may cause dehydration, irregular heartbeat, low blood pressure, poor bone development (increasing the risk for osteoporosis), and, most seriously, permanent brain damage. Anorexics frequently suffer from amenorrhea—cessation or delay of menstruation. Amenorrhea can have serious physical consequences.

Treatment of anorexia nervosa involves psychiatric counseling and, sometimes, hospitalization to ensure weight gain.

Bulimia

When binges become "gorge and purge" sessions—stretches of overeating followed by self-induced vomiting—the condition is called bulimia. Purging can involve vomiting, using laxatives, or taking diuretics. Bulimia may exist in conjunction with anorexia nervosa or it may afflict people who are of average size or are slightly overweight. Like anorexics, most bulimics are female and perceive themselves as larger and fatter than they really are. Studies have shown that 3 percent of the general population and 20 percent of female college students suffer from bulimia.

Factors that may influence the development of bulimia include family problems, social conflicts and insecurities, and cultural emphasis on physical appearance. Physical complications may include a ruptured esophagus, dental caries, and hypoglycemia. Treatment involves counseling and behavior modification. For more information, contact the National Association of Anorexia Nervosa and Associated Disorders, Box 7, Highland Park, IL 60035; 847/831-3438.

Physical Fitness

Good physical conditioning is as important as weight control during the teen years. While not everybody can be a star athlete, almost anyone who has time and determination can improve his or her fitness. Participation in school teams, intramurals, or independent exercise should be encouraged.

Exercise Goals

One of the goals of physical conditioning is to tone and develop muscles. Muscles that are exercised regularly will grow in size and strength. Those that are not will shrink.

Exercise increases the number of individual muscle fibers as well as the number of blood capillaries that supply the muscle tissue with nutritive substances. Consequently, the muscles become more efficient and more toned.

Physical conditioning should also include optimum cardiopulmonary fitness. The increase in heart activity and oxygen consumption is the basis for aerobic workouts. Aerobic means, literally, "with oxygen." Aerobic training involves maintaining a steady rate of physical activity so that the heart, lungs, and muscles work together at a more demanding level than the body's state of rest. Jogging, running, and rapid walking are common examples of aerobic training.

Exercise Precautions

Individual exercise goals should be kept within sensible limits to avoid injury or impaired health. Overexertion can cause dizziness, nausea, and hyperventilation. Teenagers should avoid excessive exercise during severely hot and humid weather. To avoid dehydration, drink plenty of water before and after exercising.

Choosing Proper Equipment

When exercising, it is essential that a teenager use proper athletic gear to avoid injuries. Protective gear such as high-quality athletic shoes, a mouth piece, shin guards, or riding helmets should be used.

The Use of Steroids

In recent years, a number of teenagers have been abusing illegal steroids in the hope of improving physical appearance, self-image, and enhancing athletic performance. Adverse physical effects include acne, stunted growth, vomiting, disturbed hormonal function, heart and kidney disease, liver disorders, and immune system deficiencies. Serious psychological and physiological effects may also occur, including "roid rages," which consist of irritability, violent behavior, mania, psychosis, followed by depression once the drug has left the body. Users risk long-term dependence and addiction. In some cases, suicide has occurred. The National Institute on Drug Abuse (NIDA) offers a confidential information and referral hotline, 800/662-HELP, that directs callers to drug abuse treatment centers in their community.

Care of the teeth

During the teen years, careful supervision by the dentist and cooperation from the teenager are especially necessary. The poor eating habits of many teenagers are reflected in their cavity rate, which is usually higher during adolescence than in later life.

Conscientious oral care can help avoid a high cavity rate and bad breath, problems that are really caused by the same thing—*dental plaque.* For more information on this subject, see Ch. 22, *The Teeth and Gums.*

Need for Frequent Checkups

During adolescence, the dentist will often recommend more frequent checkups. Small cavities are treated before they become deeper and infect the pulp, the inner chamber of the tooth containing nerves and blood vessels. Should the pulp become infected, the tooth may need a root canal or require extraction.

The dentist also treats tooth decay, or *caries,* more popularly known as cavities, to prevent their spread. Cavities begin as a break in the tooth surface, which later enlarges. Food debris can become lodged in the cavity, be attacked by bacteria, and cause a cavity on the next tooth. The only way to avoid such a problem is to have the affected tooth treated immediately.

Front teeth often decay for the first time during this period. They are restored with a silicate or plastic filling close in color to the tooth. Unfortunately, these materials are not permanent and will need to be replaced in time. As a result, neglect of diet and oral cleanliness by an adolescent may mean that he may need many replacement fillings in the same cavity over his lifetime.

Orthodontic Treatment

The development and growth of teeth is completed during the adolescent period. When oral growth is improper, the adolescent needs treatment by an *orthodontist,* a dental specialist who treats abnormalities of the bite and alignment of teeth and jaws. Correction of such conditions as buck teeth, which mar a person's appearance, is a major reason for orthodontic treatment. But there are also major health reasons for orthodontic care. If teeth, for example, come together improperly, efficient chewing of food is impossible. The digestive system is strained because chunks of improperly chewed food pass through it. Orthodontic treatment will, therefore, result in lifelong better health and appearance. For more information, see Ch. 22, *The Teeth and Gums.*

Stimulants and Alcohol

Initial exposure to caffeine, tobacco, drugs, and alcohol usually occurs during adolescence. Teenagers should be fully educated regarding their physical effects and potential danger. They should learn how to use them, if at all, sensibly and in moderation, and to resist peer-group pressures.

Caffeine

Caffeine, which is naturally present in coffee and tea and is used in many carbonated beverages and medications, stimulates the central nervous system to overcome fatigue and drowsiness. It also affects a part of the nervous system that controls respiration so that more oxygen is pumped through the lungs. In large amounts, caffeine can increase the pulse rate, but there are few long-range effects because the substance is broken down by the body tissues within a few hours and excreted. Because of the action of caffeine in stimulating an increased intake of oxygen, it sometimes is used to combat the effects of such nervous system depressants as alcohol.

Nicotine

Nicotine is one of nearly 200 substances in tobacco. It affects the human physiology by stimulating the adrenal glands to increase the flow of adrenaline. The blood vessels become constricted and the skin temperature drops, producing effects not unlike exposure to cold temperatures. When comparatively large amounts of nicotine are absorbed by the body, the pulse becomes rapid and the smoker has symptoms of dizziness, faintness, and sometimes nausea and diarrhea. The release of adrenaline, triggered by nicotine, will produce temporary relief from fatigue by increasing the flow of sugar in the blood. However, the effect is transient, and the feeling of fatigue will return again after the increased blood sugar has been expended.

Other Properties of Tobacco

The nicotine in tobacco can be absorbed simply by contact with the mucous membranes of the mouth; the tobacco does not have to be smoked to get the nicotine effects. Burning tobacco produces a myriad of substances found in the smoke of many plant materials when they are dried and burned. More than 50 different compounds are known to occur in concentrations of one microgram or more in each puff of tobacco smoke. Again, laboratory tests have demonstrated that the substances in burning tobacco do not have to be inhaled; most of the chemical compounds can be absorbed through the mucous membranes while a puff of smoke is held in the mouth for a few seconds. At least ten of the substances in tobacco smoke have been shown to produce cancer in animals. Other chemicals in tobacco tars are known as *cocarcinogens;* although they do not produce cancer themselves, they react with other substances to produce cancers.

Smoking and Disease

The relationship among tobacco smoking and cancer, heart disease, and emphysema-bronchitis is well established, even if some of the cause and effect links are missing. Large-scale studies of the death rates of smokers and nonsmokers have been carried on for more than 20 years. One group, consisting of nearly a quarter-million war veterans, yielded results indicating that smokers are from 10 to 16 times as likely to die of lung cancer as nonsmokers. (The higher ratio is for heavy smokers.) Similar results have been obtained from studies of smokers and nonsmokers with heart disease and lung ailments.

Buerger's Disease

One of the possible, although rare, effects of smoking is the aggravation of symptoms of a particularly insidious circulatory disorder known as *Buerger's disease.* As noted above, one of the effects of nicotine is a drop in skin temperatures. Smoking a single cigarette can cause the temperature of the fingers and toes to drop as much as 15 degrees Fahrenheit; the average is a little more than a 5-degree drop. The temperature change results from constriction of the blood vessels at the extremities. Blood clots may develop in the vessels that have been constricted, cutting off the flow of blood to the tissues of the area. When there is numbness or pain in the extremities, the condition should receive swift medical attention to prevent serious consequences.

Carbon Monoxide Accumulation

Another little publicized effect of smoking is the accumulation of carbon monoxide in the blood. Carbon monoxide is one of the lethal gases emitted in automobile exhaust. It is also produced by burning plant materials such as tobacco. It is a dangerous gas because of its strong affinity for the hemoglobin of red blood cells; locking into the red blood cell chemistry so that the cells are no longer effective for their normal function of transporting oxygen to the body tissues. With the oxygen-carrying capacity of part of the red blood cells wiped out, brain cells and other tissues suffer a mild oxygen starvation and the results are a form of intoxication. Smokers pick up enough carbon monoxide to render up to eight percent of their red blood cells ineffective, increasing the shortness of breath during exercise by approximately 15 percent.

Alcohol

Alcohol usually is not considered a potentially dangerous drug because it is easily available at bars and liquor stores and is served generously at parties. Alcohol has been used by man for thousands of years, at times as a sedative and anesthetic, and when used in moderation has the effect of a mild tranquilizer and appetite stimulant. But when consumed in excess amounts, alcoholic beverages can produce both psychological and physical dependence. It can produce a letdown of inhibitions due to the weakening of some functions of the central nervous system, particularly in the cerebral cortex.

Parents and teachers share an important responsibility to educate young people about the use and misuse of alcohol. Like marijuana, the effects of alcohol on human beings are not thoroughly understood. Some users develop a tissue tolerance for alcohol so that their body tissues require increasing amounts. When alcohol is withdrawn from such users, they develop tremors, convulsions, and even hallucinations. However, there are many varied reactions to the use of alcohol, and an individual may react differently to alcoholic drinks at different times. See Ch. 29, *Substance Abuse.*

Drugs

During the 1960s there was an alarming increase in drug use among teenagers—a problem that deservedly received nationwide attention.

Education concerning the hazards and occasional tragedies accompanying drug use is imperative.

Marijuana

Marijuana affects the central nervous system, including the brain, after it enters the bloodstream. According to some researchers, the substance accumulates in the liver. Some of the effects of marijuana are not unlike those of tobacco. The heart rate increases, body temperature drops, and blood sugar levels are altered. The drug user feels dehydrated, the appetite is stimulated, coordination of movements becomes difficult, there are feelings of drowsiness or unsteadiness, and the eyes may become bloodshot. Taken in higher strengths, marijuana can cause hallucinations or distortions of perception.

Varying Effects

Scientists are uncertain about the pathways of the drug in the central nervous system and its effects on other body systems. The drug's effects seem to vary widely, not only among individual users but also according to the social setting and the amount and strength of the marijuana used. The effects, which usually begin within 15 minutes after the smoke is inhaled and may continue for several hours, vary from depression to excitement and talkativeness. Some users claim to experience time distortions and errors in distance perception. But others sharing the same marijuana cigarette may experience no effects at all.

Although marijuana is not addictive, in the sense that users do not develop a physical dependence upon the substance and that the withdrawal of the drug produces no ill effects, there are dangerous results from the use of marijuana. Marijuana users find it hard to make decisions that require clear thinking, some users develop psychotic reactions or an emotional disorder called "acute marijuana panic," and there is some evidence that the active ingredient is transmitted by expectant mothers to their unborn children.

Hallucinogens

Marijuana sometimes is described as a *hallucinogen* because some users report visual hallucinations, illusions, and delusions after ingesting a large amount of the drug. But marijuana should not be confused with the true hallucinogenic drugs such as *mescaline* and *LSD* (lysergic acid diethylamide), which are known by doctors as *psychomimetic* drugs because they mimic psychoses.

LSD and Mescaline

LSD and mescaline have marked effects on perception and thought processes. Teenagers usually become involved with the use of LSD because they are curious about its effects; they may have heard about its purported "mind-bending" properties and expect to gain great personal insights from its use. Instead of great insight, however, the user finds anxiety, depression, confusion, and frightening hallucinations. The use of LSD is complicated by the reappearance of hallucinations after the individual has quit using the drug; the very possibility of repeated hallucinations causes a sense of terror.

Morphine and Heroin

Besides the hallucinogenic drugs, there are *opium* derivatives, *morphine* and *heroin.* Morphine is one of the most effective pain relievers known and is one of the most valuable drugs available to the physician. Morphine and heroin depress the body systems to produce drowsiness, sleep, and a reduction in physical activity. They are true narcotics, and their appeal is in their ability to produce a sense of euphoria by reducing the individual's sensitivity to both psychological and physical stimuli.

Addictive Properties

A great danger lies in the ability of the body tissues to develop a physical dependence on morphine and its derivative cousin, heroin. The degree to which heroin's "desirable" effects are felt depends in part on how the user takes it. *Sniffing* is the mildest form of abuse, followed by *skin-popping*—subcutaneous injection—and then by *mainlining*—injecting directly into a vein, which is the method used by almost all those dependent on heroin.

The body adjusts to the level of the first doses so that increasingly larger injections of the drug are required to produce the same feelings of euphoria. The ability of the body to adjust to the increasingly larger doses is called *tolerance.* And with tolerance goes *physical dependence,* which means that when heroin or morphine is withdrawn from the user he experiences a violent sickness marked by tremors, sweating and chills, vomiting and diarrhea, and sharp abdominal pains. Another shot of heroin or morphine temporarily ends the withdrawal symptoms. But the user, now dependent upon the drug, must continue regular doses or face another bout of the withdrawal sickness. Heroin has no value as a medicine and is available only through illicit channels at a high price. The heroin addict usually is unable to hold a job because of effects of the drug and often turns to crime in order to finance his daily supply of the narcotic.

Shortened Life Span

The health of narcotics addicts declines so that their life spans are shortened by 15 to 20 years. They are frequently in trouble with the law because of the severe penalties for illegal possession of narcotics. If an addict sells narcotics, as many heroin addicts are driven to do to get enough money to support their habits, the legal consequences may be even more severe.

Amphetamines and Barbiturates

Other commonly abused drugs are *amphetamines,* also known as *uppers* or *pep pills,* and *barbiturates,* sometimes called *downers.*

Amphetamines are central nervous system stimulants. They stimulate the heart rate, increase the blood pressure, cause rapid breathing, dilate the pupils of the eyes, and produce other effects such as dryness of the mouth, sweating, headache, and diarrhea. Ordinarily, amphetamines are swallowed as tablets, but a more extreme form of amphetamine abuse involves injection of the drug, usually methadrine, or methamphetamine, directly into a vein.

Barbituates slow the heart rate and breathing, lower blood pressure, and mildly depress the action of nerves and muscles. Barbituates were commonly prescribed to relieve tension or anxiety and to treat insomnia. They produce physical and psychological dependence. Many doctors now prescribe benzodiazapines instead of barbiturates.

Dangers of Amphetamines and Barbiturates

The danger of using amphetamines is that they can induce people to do things beyond their physical endurance, cause mental disorders that require hospitalization, and, in large doses, can result in death. Although they do not produce the kind of physical dependence observed in the use of narcotics, amphetamine withdrawal for a heavy user can result in a deep and suicidal depression.

Barbiturates are highly dangerous when taken without medical supervision. They distort perception and slow down reaction and response time, contributing to the chances of accidents. Barbituates are a leading cause of accidental poisoning deaths, because they can make the mind foggy and users can forget how many pills they have taken, which may lead to an overdose. They also cause physical dependence, and the withdrawal symptoms range from cramps and nausea to convulsions and death. See also Ch. 29, *Substance Abuse.*

Often Abused Substances

A number of legal substances have increasingly been abused by teenagers in recent years including non-prescription and prescription medications and inhalants. Prescription drugs, such as anti-depressants, antibiotics, and pain-killers, are frequently shared among friends and family members. Borrowed medications can cause severe allergic reactions, particularly if combined with other medications or alcohol. Non-prescription drugs, such as sleep inhibitors and cough syrups, have also been abused, because of their wide availability. When prescription and non-prescription drugs are combined with the abuse of alcohol, the results can be deadly. Inhalants consist of three subgroups: aerosols, solvents, and anesthetics. Abusers sniff or inhale the fumes to achieve a high similar to that of many illegal drugs. Among the aerosol products abused are spray paints, hair sprays, and insecticides. The solvents include paint thinners, airplane cement and glues, and transmission fluid. Anesthetics, not as widely available as inhalants and aerosols, consist of nitrous oxide, ether, and chloroform. The use of inhalants can cause a variety of dangerous side effects including hallucination, mental disorder, nausea, muscular weakness, and fatigue. Long-term abuse may cause kidney, liver, brain, bone marrow, and heart damage, and even death. Some inhalants have also been linked to a variety of cancers.

Adolescent Suicide

Suicides among teenage boys and girls increased greatly in number during the middle 1980s. Health experts termed the phenomenon an "epidemic of self-destruction." In some areas suicides or suicide attempts took place in clusters. Often, groups of close friends were involved. In some cases of cluster suicides or attempts, it appeared that a suicidal attitude was contagious.

By the late 1990s, suicide had become the third leading cause of death among young people 15 to 24 years old; among those 10 to 14, it was the fourth leading cause. These figures represent a tripling of the adolescent suicide rate since the 1950s. A major cause of suicide is untreated depression. It has been estimated that 20 percent of children experience depression before they reach adolescence.

Risk Factors

As educators, social workers, psychiatrists, and others became involved in community efforts to prevent teenage suicides, a number of "risk factors"—signs of an intent to take one's life—were isolated. Changes in a teenager's behavior, whether in peer relationships, school activities, or academic performance, were said to be primary indicators. So were emotional shifts, particularly toward anger or irritability. Depression and withdrawal might accompany the emotional changes. Sadness, changes in eating and sleeping habits, and preoccupation with death were other signs.

Young people considering suicide showed other symptoms. Many reported headaches, stomachaches, and other ailments. Some talked about taking their own lives. A young person who had lost a close friend through suicide was at unusual risk, according to studies. Family histories of suicide and parental depression were cited as indirectly contributing factors.

Parent Involvement

For parents concerned about the possibility of a child's or teen's suicide, such clues are only clues. The parent still has the task of trying to resolve the potential suicide. Authorities make the following suggestions.

Act at Once

Where a preadolescent or adolescent gives clear signals—usually risk factors appearing in combination—that suicide might be contemplated, parents should seek help immediately. Local suicide hotlines or suicide prevention centers should be contacted; counseling may have to be started.

School Help

Many schools cooperate in efforts to prevent suicides. The schools may sponsor group meetings at which students talk out their feelings about suicide, and such meetings may be appropriate as a first or second step. A representative of the community crisis or prevention center normally takes part in such meetings. Many schools have special counselors, psychologists, and others who can serve as direct lines to sources of help.

Out-of-School Contacts

Group meetings provide all teenage participants with the names and locations of out-of-school contact persons who may be able to help them in a crisis. Most crisis agencies operate 24 hours a day, seven days a week, providing aid during the "danger hours" between late afternoon and midnight. Parents may want also to contact clergy, trusted friends or relatives, or others.

Peer Support

Where possible, peer support should be mobilized in the effort to prevent a suicide. Many young people, especially the friends of a depressed or otherwise suicidal teenager, can help—and will do so rather than hear later that a suicide has taken place. But parents should, according to experts, remember that a youngster with high status among his or her peers may influence those peers. In committing suicide, the high-status young person may convince others that "life isn't worth it." Surviving boy- or girlfriends are especially at risk.

Social and Sexual Maturation

The Prospect of Adulthood

As a youngster passes from childhood into adolescence, it is the psychological adjustments rather than the physical changes that are most likely to produce difficulties. The emotional problems, of course, are related to the hormonal activity of the developing body. However, the conflicts that frequently are upsetting to both the adolescent and other members of his family are the result of adjustments that must be made between the young person and the society in which he must live.

In our own culture, the teenager must continually adjust to a complex set of rules and regulations. He frequently may feel that he must accept the responsibilities of adulthood before he is entitled to the privileges of being treated as an adult. Childhood is only a step behind, but he has learned to suppress or ignore childhood relationships. He can easily forget the point of view of children and even resent the ability of his parents to recall the "cute" incidents of his earlier years. At the same time, he may be startled by the suggestion that within a few short years he and his teenage friends will face the selection of a career, marriage, establishment of a home, and a lifetime of responsibilities he may feel ill-prepared to assume.

Future Outlook for Teenagers

While a teenager may feel competent enough to handle adult responsibilities and decisions, he or she may have misgivings about what the future holds. Fear and uncertainty of the unknown can cause anxiety in teenagers, though they may not express it. They are aware that the choices they make—what college or vocational school they select, what profession they choose, who they marry, where they decide to live—can affect their entire lives.

An abundance of educational opportunities and careers choices is available for any teenager. It is the parents' responsibility to expose teenagers to all of the options and to guide them toward attainable goals. Parents should recognize a teen's strengths and weakness and direct him or her to the most appropriate educational institution or profession. Career and college guidance counselors at high school are very helpful.

In the past few decades, the outlook for males and females has become nearly identical, and the career options and lifestyles that teenagers may select are seemingly endless. Traditional social conventions are changing. Many marriages occur after both spouses have established careers, allowing for arrangements that were not possible for many parents of current teenagers. Given the professional opportunities for women, many families are dual-income, or, in some cases, the men choose to stay at home. Much of this depends on the economic needs of a particular family, but the options are there for nearly any kind of work situation and lifestyle.

Need for Independence

Adolescence is a time when a child slowly develops into an adult. With physical changes come psychological changes as well. As such, a teenager wants to be treated like an adult, not a child. These demands are often manifested in rebellious actions and disdainful remarks.

In a desire to act independently, a teenager may exhibit reclusive behavior in order to avoid contact with parents. He or she may be reluctant to divulge information. Sneaking out of the house is a common gesture. These are distinct attempts to dodge unsolicited advice from parents who are only too anxious to give it.

Parents should not be offended by these actions, rather they should allow their child to explore the world independently. Such an education will make them more confident and well-adjusted as adults. Teenagers who are not allowed much freedom are often more difficult to control and can cause more damage out of spite.

Conflicts between Parent and Teenager

Some conflicts between the generations are avoidable. The parents may be protective and slow to cut the apron strings because they love their children and want to prevent them from becoming involved in unhappy situations. The teenager resents the overprotective actions of the parents, regarding them as evidence that they do not trust their own children.

What parents should try to make clear to their children is that they make offering their years of experience as guidelines. Teenagers should value the counsel of more experienced members of the family; they should cooperate by listening to the adult viewpoint. If, after serious consideration of the parents' point of view, the youngster still wants to make his own decision in the matter, it should be understood that he may have to accept the responsibility for the consequences. A keystone in the training for adulthood is the concept that being an adult entails more than just privileges and the authority to make decisions; along with decision-making goes a responsibility to the family and society for the consequences of one's decisions.

Few parents, of course, would refuse to bail out a teenage son or daughter in real trouble. And even when a youngster is rebellious enough to leave home, he should know that the door will always be open to him when he decides to return. Again, limiting the options available to a teenager can lead to a snowballing of bad decisions and resulting complications.

In many cases, the conflicts between parents and teenagers derive from the illusion that a younger child has more freedom of choice. A small child may actually seem to have a freer choice of friends he can bring into his home and the games he can play with them. But there are always limitations to a child's choices, and parents are more understanding of the bad choices by attributing mistakes to the fact that "he's only a child."

Older youngsters become involved in situations in which the decisions are more important. A boy and girl at the age of five can "play house" together in an atmosphere of innocence. However, the same boy and girl could hardly suggest to their parents that they intended to play house at the age of 15. If the boy and girl, although next-door neighbors, are of different social or ethnic backgrounds, they may become aware of parental prejudices in addition to new rules of propriety as they grow into their teenage years.

Decisions of the teen years can involve the use of tobacco, alcohol, owning an automobile, handling of money, overnight trips with friends, association with friends who use drugs illegally, and relationships with members of the opposite sex. The consequences of all alternatives should be outlined for the adolescent.

Search for Identity

Part of the youngster's struggle for independence will involve what sometimes is described as a search for identity. A child accepts without much questioning that he is a member of a certain family and lives in a certain neighborhood. But as he grows older, he becomes aware of his status in the family as well as the status of his family in society. A seven-year-old could not care less about the background of his family or that of his second-grade friends. As he becomes a teenager he learns that such subjects may be matters of concern to parents and their circle of friends. He may imitate the attitudes of his family or disregard them, perhaps inviting criticism that he is rebellious.

More important to the youngster, however, is a growing concern about his position and role in life and where it may lead. He is still in the so-called formative years and is sensitive to countless influences in the world about him. Teenagers become concerned with approaching education and career decisions. It is natural for them to identify with older members in the family, teachers, and celebrities.

Need for Privacy

All teenagers need a good degree of privacy. If a room is shared with a younger sibling, appropriate space should be reserved for their exclusive use. Trunks or other lockable boxes may be required to store personal belongings. Most importantly, parents should respect teenagers privacy by knocking on the bedroom door to get permission to enter. They should resist the urge to search through personal belongings or diaries, or listen-in on phone or other conversations. Proper respect between parents and teenagers concerning privacy is integral to the development of a healthy family-atmosphere.

Contacts with Older Friends

Young teenagers, through part-time jobs as babysitters or errand boys, usually come in contact with young adults outside the family circle for the first time. The young adults may accept the teenagers as peers, which is flattering to the youngsters, who may in turn admire and imitate the young adults. If the teenager has been able to identify closely with his family's sense of propriety, the contacts can be a good social experience. But if the youngster has not been able to identify effectively with his parents and family members, he may be vulnerable to misguiding influences. Because of the urge for adult status, the teenager may find a premature outlet for testing his abilities to live the adult life in the company of young adults. He (or she) can absorb a lot of information—and misinformation—about sex, alcohol, drugs, and other subjects.

Teenagers certainly should not be cautioned against contacts with all young adults, but they should also have a reliable older person aside from their parents with whom they can discuss matters they would not discuss with a mother or father. The alternate adult might be a clergyman, the family physician, a teacher, or even a favorite aunt or uncle. Such an arrangement provides the youngster with a means of learning a bit more about life in an independent manner and from a different point of view than could be obtained within his own immediate family circle.

Relationships with the Opposite Sex

First teenage contacts with the opposite sex tend to be awkward and sometimes embarrassing despite the best efforts and intentions of parents. The meetings may be at school dances or movie dates, perhaps in the presence of a chaperon who is a teacher or parent.

Overcoming Insecurity

Some youngsters will feel more secure than others in social gatherings;

those who feel insecure may not participate at all when such opportunities first arise. As the youngsters grow older, however, they find that more and more of their friends are dating or going to dances or parties to meet members of the opposite sex.

Some boys or girls who feel insecure may find that they are more gregarious or less ill-at-ease if they fortify themselves with a couple of drinks of an alcoholic beverage, or with drugs, before they join their friends. Youngsters who feel the need for stimulants or depressants in order to enjoy parties usually can be helped with psychological counseling to overcome their fears of inadequacy.

Young people should be assured that getting together at parties of mixed sexes is a natural thing to do. It has been going on for generations and although an individual youngster may feel ill-at-ease at his first few dances or parties, he probably will survive. As the boy or girl attends more parties the chances increase that he or she will meet a person of the opposite sex who is particularly attractive. If the feeling is mutual, the acquaintanceship may develop into more or less steady dating.

Going Steady

Steady dating, which leads to a formal engagement and marriage in many cases, should not be encouraged at an early age or before a young person has had an opportunity to date a number of prospective partners. At the same time, it should not be discouraged to the point of producing a rebellious reaction. As was pointed out earlier, some girls admit going steady with a boy for no other reason than to demonstrate their independence of judgment.

Controlling the Sexual Impulse

Teenagers who spend a lot of time together at parties, in their homes, or at recreational meetings such as beach outings are likely to be physically attracted to each other. It may begin with kissing, dancing, holding hands, or simply a natural urge to neck or pet.

Influence of the Mass Media

Complicating sincere efforts of a teenager to make the right decisions in relations with the opposite sex is the constant exposure of youngsters to movies, magazine articles, books, and other media suggesting that sexual relations between unmarried couples are not only acceptable but a common practice. Young males and females need to be made aware of each other's growing sex drives, the consequences of normal sexual attraction, the dangers of unprotected sex, and the influence of the mass media on their perceptions concerning romantic infatuation, intimacy, sex, and adult love.

The Male and Female Sex Drives

Teenagers need to be aware of and responsible for their sexuality, regardless of their gender. While there are no standards or averages for either gender's sex drive, as with adults there is a wide variety of sexual appetite and ability. Because of this variety, creating and establishing relationships appropriate to each individual can be a difficult and complex exchange. It is crucial that both boys and girls openly communicate their true feelings and opinions in order to lessen the possibility of misunderstanding. For example, even when feelings are openly communicated, situations may arise which range from uncomfortable (someone's feelings get hurt) to dangerous (date rape or stalking).

Walking hand-in-hand, or with an arm around the waist, and kissing that is not too passionate, usually are acceptable ways for young teenagers to display affection. And there are activities such as hiking or bicycle riding that afford a boy and girl a chance to be together and apart from the rest of the world. There also are picnics, ball games, movies, and concerts that permit togetherness without setting the stage for hard-to-control sexual impulses.

Masturbation

Another manifestation of the natural sex drives of young persons is masturbation. Discouraged by the rules and standards of society from fulfilling sex urges in the same manner as married couples, teenagers discover they can find sexual satisfaction in masturbation. Despite the stories that warn of physical or mental decay for youngsters who masturbate, the practice is not harmful unless the parents make an issue of it.

If there are dangers in masturbation, they are likely to be the isolation and loneliness associated with the practice and the confusion and anxiety that can result if the young person feels guilty or is punished or criticized for masturbating. Masturbation is such a natural reaction that most youngsters discover it by themselves even if the subject is never discussed by friends or family members. But for many young people, masturbation may violate religious or other beliefs or values. These youngsters may want to discuss the practice with a physician, understanding clergy, or some other trusted person.

Sex Education

Because boys and girls in their teens may be capable of producing children and are known to have strong sexual urges, they should be provided with authoritative information about human reproduction and birth control. It is up to the parents to make decisions regarding the proper sources of such information, how much information should be given, and at what age.

One of the reasons for the popularity of sex education in the schools is that teachers can get the parents off the hook by explaining the facts of life to teens. However, the lessons may be superficial or incomplete, depending upon the teacher and the prescribed curriculum.

Parents should resist the urge to delegate the sex education of their children to a teacher, sex education programs, or even friends and acquaintances. The lessons they receive may be incomplete, superficial, or even incorrect, depending on the teacher, curriculum, or individual experience and viewpoint. Parents need to establish a rapport with their children to be sure that they learn a practical set of facts about adult love, sex, and reproduction, including the possible emotional and physical consequences of premarital or unprotected sexual intercourse.

Although parents may find it difficult or embarrassing to explain the facts of life to their own children, it is one of the most important contributions that can be made to a maturing youngster. At the present time, at least one out of six teenage girls in the United States will have an unwanted pregnancy. Obviously, thousands of parents and teachers are not providing adequate instruction in sex education subjects.

The Male Reproductive System

Any instruction in the facts of life should begin by use of the proper names for the body parts involved. In the male, the external sex organs are the *penis* and the *testicles,* or *testes.* The penis contains a tiny tube, the *urethra,* through which urine is eliminated. Much of the fleshy part of the penis is composed of spongy tissue. When the penis is stimulated sexually, the spongy areas become filled with blood, which makes the penis larger and firm, a condition called an *erection.* The testicles contain male *sperm cells,* also called *spermatozoa.*

The sperm travel up tubules inside the abdomen to a storage organ, or reservoir, the *seminal vesicle.* The sperm storage area also contains a thick white fluid called *semen* that is secreted by glands that open into the urethra. One of the glands, the *prostate,* serves partly as a control valve to prevent urine from mixing with the semen, since both are discharged through the urethra. The semen, containing millions of sperm, empties periodically in a more or less automatic action, being squeezed out of the seminal vesicle by pulsating contractions. The contractions and ejection of semen are called *ejaculation.* During the sex act, or *intercourse,* with a female, the semen is ejaculated into the woman's vagina.

The Female Reproductive System

The *vagina* is the proper name for the tubular female sex organ. At the end of the vagina is an opening, called the *cervix,* which leads into the *uterus.* The uterus, or *womb,* is shaped somewhat like an upside-down pear. When a baby develops within the mother's abdomen, it grows inside the uterus. The uterus also is the source of the bloody discharge that occurs periodically during the fertile years of women. When the blood is discharged it is called *menstruation,* or the menstrual period. The menstrual blood passes out through the vagina, which stretches to become the *birth canal* when a baby is being born. The urethra of a female empties outside the vagina.

The Menstrual Cycle and Conception

Unlike the male reproductive organs, which produce perhaps millions of spermatozoa each day, the female reproductive system ordinarily releases only one germ cell, called an *ovum* or egg, at a time. An ovum is released at an average frequency of once every 28 days. It should always be remembered that the 28-day figure is only an average; the actual time may vary considerably for reasons that are only partly known. The cycles are more likely to be irregular for teenage girls than for mature women. An ovum is released from one of the two *ovaries,* or sex glands, comparable in function to the male testicles, located on either side of the uterus. The ovum, or egg, is transported from the ovary to the uterus through a *Fallopian tube.*

If the ovum encounters male sperm during its passage from the ovary to the uterus, there is a good chance that fertilization, or *conception,* will occur through a union of a spermatozoon and the egg. The fertilized ovum, called a *zygote,* soon divides into a cluster of human tissue cells that become the embryo of a baby. For further information about pregnancy, see under Ch. 4, *The Beginning of a Family.*

During the time that the egg is maturing in the ovary and passing into the uterus after its release, the membrane lining of the uterus becomes thicker because it accumulates blood and nutrients. If the ovum is fertilized, it finds a spot in the membrane where it becomes attached and develops rapidly into an embryo, gaining its nourishment from the blood and nutrient-enriched lining of the uterus. If the ovum is not fertilized, it passes through the uterus, and the blood-rich membrane sloughs off. The blood and some of the cells of the membrane become the discharged material of menstruation. The unfertilized ovum could pass through undetected because it is nearly microscopic.

After menstruation has begun, the female reproductive cycle starts over again. The lining of the uterus once more builds up its supply of blood and nutrients to support a fertilized ovum. Ordinarily, the next ovum will be released about 14 days after a menstrual period begins. If a female does not have intercourse, or avoids intercourse during the time the ovum is released, or in some other manner is able to prevent sperm from reaching an ovum, she will not become pregnant but will experience a menstrual period at intervals that average around 28 days.

When fertilization of an ovum occurs, menstruation ceases and no further egg cells are released until the outcome of the pregnancy has been determined. In other words, the cycles of ovulation and menstruation start anew after the baby is born or the pregnancy has been terminated.

Contraception

The first rule of birth control is that no method is guaranteed to be 100 percent effective. Sexual intercourse nearly always is accompanied by some risk of pregnancy, and the teenagers who try to beat the odds should be willing to take the responsibility for the results. Teenagers should be provided with the basic facts of birth control as soon as they are capable of producing children themselves. But the emphasis should be on the relative unreliability of the techniques which do not require a visit to a physician's office. Many birth control devices and substances can be purchased without a physician's prescription. But if young men and women were aware of their chances of effecting a pregnancy while using such methods, they probably would have second thoughts about taking the risk. See under "Marriage and Parenthood" in Ch. 4, *The Beginning of a Family,* for a full discussion of birth control methods.

Sexually Transmitted Diseases

It is very important to educate teenagers about the hazards of sexually transmitted diseases (STDs). The American Social Health Association and the National Institute of Allergy and Infectious Diseases estimate that at least three million teenagers a year are infected with STDs. In recent years there has been a rise in the occurrence of chlamydia, syphilis, and gonorrhea. This increase is due, in part, to the fact that many with these infections show few or no symptoms and can unknowingly spread the infections to others. Other STDs include genital herpes and warts, trichomoniasis, and chancroid. In addition, hepatitis B and AIDS can be transmitted sexually.

Most STDs, if diagnosed early, can be effectively treated with medications such as antibiotics. However, AIDS and genital herpes are incurable. Medications for these diseases are used to control symptoms but are not effective for everyone. Experts believe that the risk of contracting AIDS is increased in those who have had other STDs.

The rise in many of these diseases is related to the increasing use of oral contraceptives, rather than condoms, during sexual intercourse. Teens are also at high risk because their immature immune systems are less able to combat infection. Drug-resistant bacteria is also a factor in the increase of STDs. Furthermore, many teenagers delay treatment due to social myths and preconceptions, lack of education, embarrassment, or even denial. Other teens may lack health insurance, or do not know how to access free services.

Many parents are frightened to learn that their children are endangering their health with risky behavior. STDs can cause a variety of devastating results if they go undiagnosed and untreated. Untreated syphilis, for example, can result in blindness, heart disease, and insanity. Untreated chlamydia can lead to sterility or ectopic pregnancy. Other STDs may cause brain, nervous system, and bone and joint disease, or destroy the body's immune system. In addition, STDs in women may cause cervical and genital cancer. Risky behavior may be minimized if the teenager can openly communicate with parents or another responsible adult and receive accurate information and advice.

The best way to avoid STDs is not to have sex. If the decision is made to be sexually active, a variety of precautions should be observed. Latex condoms and spermicides, while not 100 percent effective, have been shown to lower the risk of transmission of some STDs and should be used. Teenagers should have frank discussions with their partners regarding their past and present sexual history and STDs. Maintaining a monogamous relationship also lowers the possibility of infections. Additionally, sexually active teens should be taught to identify common symptoms of STDs and conduct self-examinations. If disease is suspected, medical attention should be sought immediately, sexual activity should be stopped, and all past or present sexual partners should be notified. For more information on sexually transmitted diseases, see Ch. 17, *Diseases of the Urinogenital System.*

4

The Beginning of a Family

Family Planning

When and How to Plan

Planning a family basically means figuring out when you want children, how many you want, and how long you choose to wait between pregnancies. It is always recommended that you discuss these things before marriage. It is going to be a major sticking point in a relationship if you want four children and your partner's idea of family is a parakeet.

When to have a family is also important. If you are in your twenties or early thirties and wish to have children, you have several years for doing so. If you are in your late thirties or older, having children may be an immediate priority. This is true for both men and women. Although most men are physically capable of fathering children throughout their lives, they should be young enough to participate actively in the raising of the children. If you father a child when you are 51 years old, you will be 72 when the child graduates from college. This is something to consider when you make the decision to become a parent.

Any plan should leave room for flexibility. Priorities and situations may change during the course of a relationship. Both partners should be aware of this possibility and be flexible to the shifting situations.

Almost no couple expects problems with fertility or conception when they plan a family. Yet approximately 10 percent of all couples have enough difficulty conceiving that they require fertility testing or treatment.

For those whom infertility is not an issue, planning pregnancies involves decisions about birth control and spacing of pregnancies.

Timing Between Pregnancies

The minimum time a couple should leave between pregnancies is set by the period of time the baby is breastfed. Breastfeeding and pregnancy tax the mother's and the fetus's health. It is recommended that any mother who is breastfeeding a child, and is pregnant, wean the child.

For the recovery of the physical health of the mother, two years is the average recommended wait. This puts the children almost three years apart in age.

The length of time between children should take into consideration the age and health of the parents, the number of children the couple wants, and the difficulty they have in conceiving. For a couple that suffers through a miscarriage for every successful pregnancy, a long wait may not be recommended. It should also be noted here, though, that a good gynecologist/obstetrician will be able to recommend what is in the mother's best health interest in spacing of pregnancies. For any couple that experiences difficulties with pregnancies, a doctor's advice on their particular situation should be the primary source of information.

Once physical considerations are understood, it becomes a matter of personal priority for the parents. Some parents prefer to wait until one child is in school, or at least out of diapers, before having another child. Having two toddlers can be quite trying on a parent's energy and patience. For first-time parents, having children close in age may help in arranging the parents' schedule around the children. The problems of arranging for day care may only be extended a year or two if the children are close in age. For children five years apart, working parents have at least one child in day care for ten years. For more discussion on child care and day care, see the end of this chapter.

Conception

Once you decide that you would like to have a child, planning the pregnancy involves two basic schedules. The first is deciding when you want the child to arrive. This includes deciding when pregnancy would be convenient. The second is discovering when fertility occurs each month in the woman's cycle.

When to Get Pregnant

In deciding when the best time of the year to have a baby arrive, several things should be taken into account. If you plan on taking time off from work for the child, you should consider the work you do and when a break in the work load would prove easiest to pull away. If you are a teacher, summer months may provide an ideal time for birth. If you can schedule delivery in

June, the baby will be almost three months old before you start back to school in the fall. For others, a sabbatical or independent project may be timed to coincide with periods at home.

Weather may also help you decide when you wish to get pregnant. Buying winter clothing for the last stage of pregnancy can be costly. Getting a winter coat, and sweaters, and longjohns to fit during the eighth and ninth month of pregnancy may require buying clothes you won't ever wear again. Getting summer dresses and cotton pants for the last trimester of the pregnancy may be cheaper. Some women, however, cannot bear the thought of being eight months pregnant in the August heat.

Holiday schedules are also important. Some children love having birthdays around Christmas and Hanukkah. Other children hate it, feeling that their birthdays are overlooked in the festivities of the season. Preholiday births may allow a family to see distant relatives without taking an added trip across the country. For parents who work, holiday births may allow them to spend vacation time with their newborn.

Each family works on a slightly different schedule than the next. Their needs and what works best for them have to be determined on an individual basis. Even within that family, schedules may shift between the birth of one child and the next. Planning can help ease the burden of time off and child care that may be essential to making a family work.

How to Get Pregnant

Once you have decided on starting or continuing a family, planning the pregnancy involves calculating the fertile period in the menstrual cycle. For some parents, this requires no effort at all. Some women get pregnant immediately after stopping birth control. For others, months of timing ovulation may be required for successful conception.

The best method to figure out an ovulation cycle is to work with your physician. There are some things you can do in advance to help, though. Write down the starting and ending date of your period, for several months. If anything significant happens during the month that may have changed the cycle, such as an illness, note it in your calendar.

Your physician can give your specific information on physical characteristics and signs of ovulation that you should watch for. Basal body temperature fluctuates just before ovulation. If you chart your temperature every day at the same time, usually first thing in the morning, you should notice a slight change in the body temperature approximately two weeks before your period. The rise in temperature of about .4 to .8 degrees Fahrenheit appears normally within 24 hours of ovulation. It should last a few days and then the temperature should return to a normal level.

Some women do not get a sharp increase in temperature. It may be more subtle, more gradual, or even may drop in temperature slightly. It is important that you chart more than a couple months to get a better general view of your own body's rhythm.

Checking the viscosity of mucous production can also give some signs of ovulation. Cervical mucous production becomes more transparent and more elastic as ovulation occurs. There are also physical characteristic changes that can be noted under a microscope.

By establishing and keeping a calendar for these changes, a woman should be able to, with the help of her obstetrician or gynecologist, determine when she is fertile. If, after several months of intercourse during periods of fertility, the couple still has not conceived, the physician will recommend testing for egg and sperm production.

The Menstrual Cycle

The menstrual cycle runs, on average, every 28 days. As many women have cycles longer than 28 days as have cycles shorter than 28 days. Some women's cycles are not always the same length. Cycles may vary each month, with no true regularity. Some may alter between two lengths. For example, a woman may have a cycle that is 28 days, followed by a cycle of 30 days. She may then repeat the pattern. For women who have extremely irregular cycles, birth control pills can help regulate their menstrual flow. When they stop taking the pill, though, they may return to their previous irregularity.

Some women have lower abdominal pain midway through their cycle that accompanies ovulation. Called *mittelschmerz,* the pain can vary from a dull ache lasting hours to a sharp pain that only lasts minutes. The pain is believed to be caused by the release of the ovum from the ovary.

A new cycle is marked from the first day of menstruation. On the first day after menstruation stops, the body's hormonal levels are at their lowest for estrogen and progesterone. The uterine lining is at its thinnest. As the level of estrogen rises the blood-lined wall of the uterus builds. The wall prepares for the embedding of a fertilized egg. For the average cycle (28 days) the wall continues to build for two weeks.

While this is occurring, at least one egg is developing in an ovary. The ovary that develops the egg may alternate from left side to right. How this is controlled by the body's hormonal system is not yet understood. After approximately two weeks, the body releases luteinizing hormone (LH), triggering the release of the ripe egg from the ovary.

The egg travels down the fallopian tube. This may take from one to five days. While the egg is in the fallopian tube, the body continues to prepare the uterine wall for implantation of a fertilized egg.

Male Ejaculation

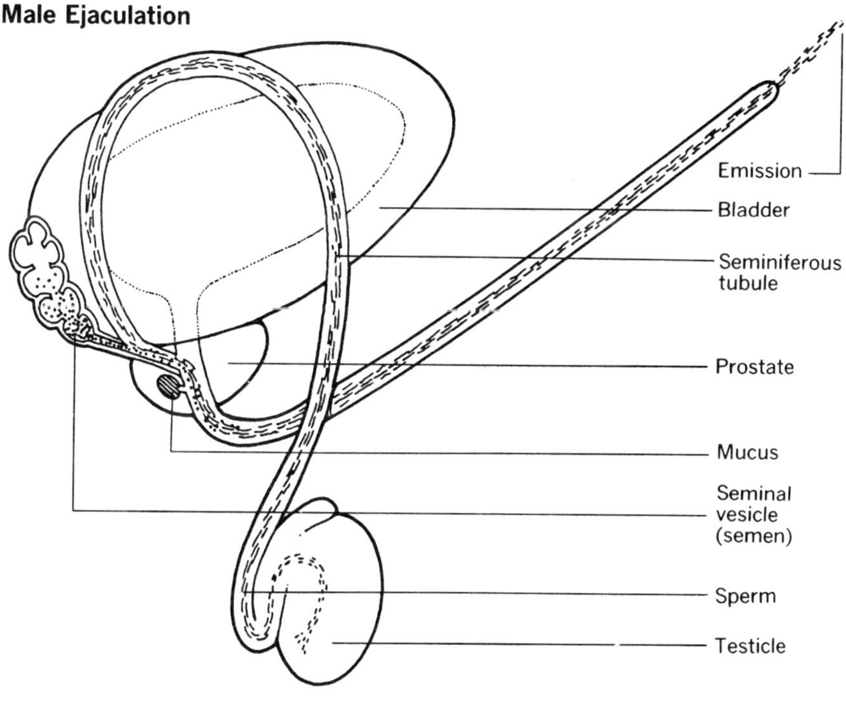

If intercourse takes place during this period of time, the egg and the sperm meet up in the fallopian tube. One sperm will penetrate the egg wall and the egg immediately produces a barrier that prevents a second sperm from penetrating. The fertilized egg, called the blastula during that stage of development, continues to travel down the fallopian tube to the uterus.

If the egg implants on the tube wall, or lodges against something and cannot continue on to the uterus, it will continue growing in the fallopian tube. It will only take a matter of days for the embryo to outgrow the size of the tube. Spots of blood will be the first sign of an *ectopic pregnancy*, or a pregnancy that develops outside the uterus. The accompanying pain will continue to get worse until treatment is sought. After a few days of spotting and pain the fallopian tube will rupture, producing tremendous pain and blood flow. This is an extreme emergency and medical attention should be sought immediately.

If the embryo successfully makes the journey to the uterine lining, it will usually implant against the blood-filled wall. The embryo will develop a cord attachment to the wall, establishing the placental link between the mother and the embryo. Through this cord flows the blood that will keep the embryo alive and nourish its development.

Some eggs will not successfully lodge against the wall. They may pass undetected with the menstrual blood.

The Female Reproductive System

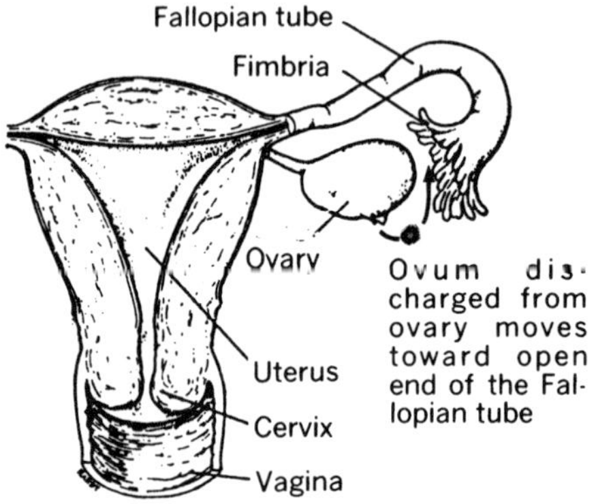

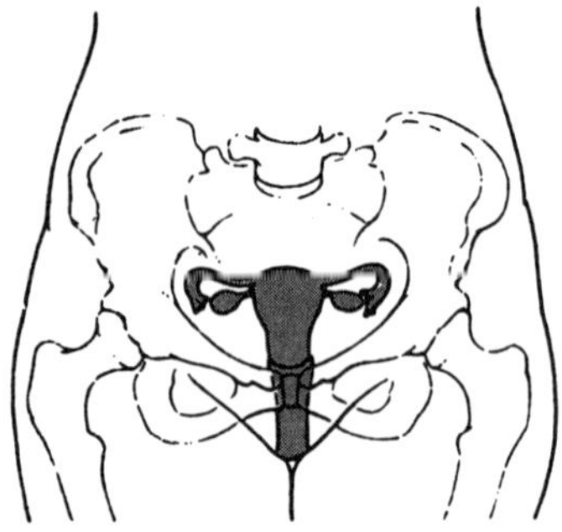
Location of the reproductive organs

They may also temporarily lodge against the wall, delaying menstruation, but then be dispelled by the body. One in ten pregnancies is estimated to end in some form of miscarriage. See the section on Miscarriage, in this chapter, for more information.

If the embryo successfully attaches, it will usually continue to develop normally through to completion of pregnancy. The presence of the embryo triggers hormonal signals that shut off the menstrual cycle. This prevents further development of eggs in the ovaries, keeps the uterine lining intact, and seals the cervix to prevent infection and allow amniotic fluid to fill the uterus.

If the egg is unfertilized during its passage through the fallopian tube, it will either pass into the uterus and then wash out with the menstrual blood or will deteriorate before leaving the body.

Approximately a week past ovulation the ovary will trigger an increase in progesterone production. This, in turn, will cause the deterioration of the uterine wall's blood lining. The deterioration takes about four days before menstruation begins.

Menstruation is the passing of the blood from the uterine wall. The blood is shed, on average, two weeks after the day of ovulation. Menstruation lasts from three to seven days. The flow of blood will vary during the course of menstruation, with the heaviest flow occurring early on after onset.

Extremely heavy periods, called *menorrhagia,* may occasionally occur during one's lifetime. If it is a persistent problem, consult with your gynecologist. *Dysmenorrhea* is the technical term for periods with cramps. As anyone who has had cramps can testify, they can be quite painful. There are several medications that can be taken to ease or relieve the pain of cramping with menstruation. Most require a physician's prescription. Some over-the-counter medications, such as ibuprofen, can also help.

Cramps are the accompanying contractions of the uterus that force the lining to be shed. Many women stop having dysmenorrhea after the birth of their first child. Other women who previously had no problem suffer from cramps after childbirth. Birth control pills can also eliminate or reduce menstrual pain.

Birth Control

Spacing of pregnancies can be controlled by birth control. Several options are available to couples who wish to prevent pregnancy either permanently or temporarily. Temporary measures mean that, once the method of control is stopped, the woman can become pregnant. Permanent birth control is almost always surgically achieved and it involves cutting or removing part or all of the reproductive system. Once a permanent surgical procedure has been done, it is extremely difficult or impossible to reverse. For that reason, it is rarely performed on patients who have never had children.

In the discussion of different types of birth control, a failure rate is given. The failure rate is determined by the number of people who conscientiously use the birth control and still get pregnant. The rate is per year, not per use. So if one person in one hundred has a failure, that means that one woman in hundred gets pregnant during one year of use.

Oral Contraceptives

The birth control pill comes in various types. The main ingredient in all of them is synthetic estrogen. Synthetic estrogen has two common types: mestranol and estradiol. The quantity of estrogen in a pill can vary from .03 milligram to .1 milligram for the average dosage. The pill will also contain synthetic progestogen, of which there are several types. Commonly used progestogens are norgestrel, norethindrone, and ethynodiol diacetate. Levels of progestogen can vary from .15 milligram to 2 milligrams.

The two hormones work in combination to prevent ovulation. Pills with the hormones are taken every day for 21 days. Some pill packages come with seven extra pills containing inactive ingredients. The cycle is 28 days, so the schedule will either be 21 days on pills, 7 days off, or 21 days on hormone pills, and 7 days on placebos (pills with no effect). The reason doctors prescribe the 21/7 set of pills is that the patient is less likely to forget a pill if one is taken every day without exception.

After the 21st pill with hormones is taken, the level of estrogen drops as the placebo (or no pill) is used. After 24 to 48 hours, the menstrual cycle will begin. It will usually be lighter in flow and take fewer days than previous periods. The pill may also eliminate cramping.

The effectiveness rating of the pill is less than one pregnancy for 100 women (a year) for pill doses of .35 milligrams or higher of estrogen. For pill doses of less than .35 milligrams of estrogen, there is a very slightly higher pregnancy rate.

Some women experience side effects with oral contraceptive pills. Side effects may be minor, from headaches to weight gain, or they may be major, from blood clots to strokes. The increase in risk is directly affected by the patient's age and smoking habits. Women over the age of 35 or smokers increase the risk of heart attack, stroke, and blood clots considerably by taking the pill. The pill does not have any linkage to uterine cancer, cervical cancer, or breast cancer. If a woman already has breast cancer, taking the pill is not recommended because it may stimulate tumor growth, but it is not linked to beginning cancerous development.

Oral contraceptives can only be obtained through prescription by a licensed physician. The physician will determine the dosage the woman takes, and will usually start on the lightest effective dosage. Dosage is insufficient if the woman experiences bleeding during the 21 day cycle, heavy menstrual flow, or other unusual symptoms. Consult with your prescribing physician if you experience problems. Occasionally switching from one type of synthetic estrogen to another, without increasing dosage, can remedy a problem.

Once on the pill, women who decide to get pregnant should stop taking the pill. Restarting ovulation may take a few months so it may be a while before the woman becomes pregnant. *It is not dangerous* for a woman to become pregnant immediately after stopping oral contraceptives. It is not a major health concern if pill taking overlaps pregnancy slightly. It may cause some problems if pill-taking continues past the first trimester.

There is no medical reason for stopping the use of oral contraceptives if there are no side effects. It was once believed that a woman should cease pill taking for a period of months, either every year or every ten years. Neither has proved to be of medical benefit.

The Mini-Pill

The mini-pill is the nickname of the progestin-only oral contraceptive. For women who run higher health risks by taking estrogen, the progestin pill may be an alternative. The risk of pregnancy is at least 1 percent higher than for the combination pill, and missing a day increases the likelihood of unwanted pregnancy (a higher risk than missing a combination pill). The risk of ectopic pregnancy (the fetus develops outside the uterus, usually in the fallopian tube) is also greater. Ectopic pregnancy can be an extremely painful, serious complication with the risk of sterility to at least one fallopian tube. Any woman on the mini-pill who suffers from lower stomach pain should be tested immediately for a possible ectopic pregnancy.

IUDs

Intrauterine devices (IUDs) are small metal pieces inserted semi-permanently into the woman's uterus. Barring complications they remain in place for one to two years. One type sold in the United States is a form called the Copper T. It is made of copper and is t-shaped, measuring less than 1 inch in length. The other is a double s-shape. Two small threads descend from the tail of the device, through the cervix into the vagina. These threads are used to check position of the IUD and to withdraw the IUD after the prescribed period of time.

IUDs are recommended only for women who have already had one successful delivery, are active in a mutually monogamous relationship, and who do not plan on getting pregnant for a few years. The device is inserted at the doctor's office after verification that the woman is not pregnant, has no current pelvic infection or disease, and has never had an ectopic pregnancy.

Because of the problematic history of the IUD, most of the devices were taken off the market. The Dalkon Shield was associated with a number of serious problems and triggered numerous lawsuits against the company. Since then, research and testing of IUDs has improved. However, there are still serious potential complications from using an IUD, so a woman who gets one is required by the IUD manufacturer to sign a Patient Consent, after the side effects have been explained by her doctor. The side effects are too numerous to list here, but the major ones are septic or spontaneous abortion, perforation of the uterus or cervix, ectopic pregnancy, or fetal damage during pregnancy. Common minor complaints are cramping, heavy menstrual flow, anemia, or amenorrhea (no period).

Pregnancy rates for IUDs vary from less than 1 pregnancy for 100 women using the device, to 8 pregnancies per 100. Individual devices have varying rates and their effectiveness is also determined by the size of the woman's uterus. The larger the uterine cavity, the less likely she will conceive while using the IUD. Some women accidently expel the IUD; this occurs less frequently with the large size IUDs inserted into larger width uteruses.

Condoms

Condoms are rubber or natural material sheaths that fit over the glans and shaft of the penis. Natural material condoms are usually made from sheep intestinal tissue and will protect against unwanted pregnancy but may allow the AIDS virus to pass through. For this reason, rubber condoms are preferred for both protection against pregnancy and disease.

Several types of condoms are available to the general public. They are purchased without a prescription at a drug store, pharmacy, or other general merchandise shop. They come with or without lubrication on the rubber, and with or without a reservoir tip. The reservoir tip is intended to hold the semen after ejaculation.

Similar to the male-worn condom is the female-worn condom—a rubber sheath inserted into the vagina. The physical appearance of the female-condom is a tube, with a sealed ring at the top. The plastic ring, similar to a diaphragm ring, fits against the cervix at the top of the vagina. Attached to the diaphragm-like ring is the long, round sheath of rubber. The sheath covers the entire vaginal wall and the end of the sheath (another, larger ring) remains outside the body around the vaginal opening.

Condoms, even without the use of a spermicide, have a low failure rate. When used correctly, the rate is 2 pregnancies for every 100 users. In actuality, the pregnancy rate is closer to 10 percent, since the condom is frequently used incorrectly. One of the more common errors is placing the tip of the condom too close to the glans of the penis, leaving no room for the semen after ejaculation. Other reasons are tearing or mispositioning of the condom during intercourse, although this is extremely rare. Another, more common problem is the use of petroleum jelly for lubrication. Petroleum products deteriorate rubber material. Only water-based lubricants should be used. Also, the penis should be withdrawn while still erect, to insure that the condom remains in place throughout intercourse. Correct storage of the condom, away from heating sources, helps keep the condom in good condition.

Condoms, when used with spermicides, have an even lower failure rate. The spermicides kill sperm that may pass beyond the condom barrier. Condoms, and condoms with spermicides, offer the best protection against contracting sexually transmitted diseases during intercourse.

Spermicides

Spermicides are sold as creams, foams, jellies, tablets, or suppositories. They can be inserted into the vagina with a plastic applicator or in tablet or suppository form. Directions, which vary from type to type, must be followed carefully. Usually the spermicide must be applied less than 30 minutes before intercourse. It must be reapplied for each episode of intercourse and remain in place for about 8 hours afterward. Spermicides are most commonly used with diaphragms, condoms, and cervical caps. On their own, spermicides have an estimated failure rate of 20 percent. Some people may have allergic reactions to spermicides.

Diaphragms and Other Barriers

Barrier methods of birth control work by placing a physical barrier, usually of rubber, over the cervical opening to the uterus. The barrier remains in place for at least several hours after intercourse to prevent sperm from entering into the uterus. Barriers are used in conjunction with spermicidal creams, foams, or jellies to enhance protection against sperm passage.

The single-most common form of barrier is the diaphragm. The diaphragm is prescribed by a health professional after sizing a women for the dimensions of the diaphragm. If a woman loses or gains more than ten pounds, or becomes pregnant, she should be checked to see if the diaphragm size has to be changed.

The diaphragm is coated with a spermicide and inserted before intercourse. The device will protect for up to 6 hours, but reapplication of spermicide is required for each episode of intercourse. After the last intercourse the diaphragm should be left in place for at least 6 hours but no longer than 24. The diaphragm should then be washed thoroughly before reuse.

Although the diaphragm used with spermicide can be an effective method of birth control, it is difficult to use this method correctly. The success rate depends on a number of factors, including the proper positioning of the diaphragm, use of a diaphragm of the correct size, and the timing of its use. The failure rate with this method can be as high as 20 percent.

Cervical caps are smaller types of rubber barriers designed to fit around the cervix. They must be prescribed and sized by a health professional. They are also used with spermicides and can remain in place for up to 48 hours. Again, due to such variables as correct positioning and size, the failure rate is high and can be as much as 40 percent.

The vaginal sponge is a doughnut-shaped device with spermicide that covers the cervix. The failure rate for this method can be as high as 25 percent.

Injection or Implantation Devices

In 1992 the FDA approved Depo-Provera, a contraceptive for women that contains the hormone progestin. It is available only through prescription. A health professional must administer an injection of Depo-Provera to the woman once every three months. The failure rate is extremely low, approximately 1 percent.

Norplant is an implantation device that was first approved for use in 1990. Norplant 2 was approved in 1996. Both devices contain progestin that is held in small rubber tubes about the size of matchsticks. A health professional surgically places these tubes under the skin of a woman's upper arm. Norplant provides protection for up to five years. Norplant 2 protects for up to three years. Also, either device may be surgically removed to stop its contraceptive properties. The failure rate is about 1 percent. Possible side effects include inflammation at the surgical site and irregular menstrual bleeding. In addition, it is sometimes difficult to remove these devices.

Natural Birth Control Methods

Natural birth control is called that when it requires no outside prevention method for pregnancy. Natural methods include rhythm method, withdrawal, and abstinence.

The rhythm method involves determining the characteristics of the woman's ovulation cycle and avoiding intercourse during the days before and after ovulation. Ovulation occurs *on average* 14 days before the next period. This is only reliable for a woman who has an exact 28-day cycle with the normal ovulation timing. (Many women do not have such a cycle.) To determine ovulation patterns, it is first necessary to chart changes in vaginal body temperature and monitor vaginal secretions for several months. Anyone using the rhythm method should consult with a doctor for specific details of monitoring temperature and secretion patterns. This is a complex birth control method and requires a great deal of commitment by both partners to make it effective. When used correctly the rhythm method has a failure rate as high as 20 percent. The failure rate is much higher when it is used by couples inexperienced in monitoring ovulation.

Withdrawal method refers to the withdrawal of the penis prior to ejaculation, during intercourse. The risk in this method is that preejaculative liquids can contain enough sperm to impregnate a woman. Also, semen on the exterior of the vagina, or the labia, can also travel back into the uterine cavity and fertilize an egg. Timing on withdrawal is essential and should be done prior to any ejaculation. Because of this, withdrawal is often considered an inadequate form of birth control. It can be emotionally and physically dissatisfying. It also has an exceedingly high failure rate, estimated between 20 and 40 percent. This is only slightly better than no birth control at all.

Abstinence is the decision to not engage in intercourse. It is the only method of birth control that is 100 percent effective. For individuals who are not involved in mutually monogamous relationships, it is the most effective method of preventing AIDS and other sexually transmitted diseases.

Permanent Birth Control

Permanent birth control is obtained surgically. It is usually nonreversible. Surgical sterilization is available to both women and men.

Tubal Ligation

Tubal ligation is the surgical blocking of the fallopian tubes. The fallopian tubes transport the egg from the ovary to the uterus. By blocking the path that the egg travels, the egg is no longer capable of making contact with the sperm. Tubal ligation is done by cutting, tying, banding, cauterizing, or removing a section of each tube so the path is no longer contin-ous. Depending on the surgical method used to block the tube, the ability to reverse the procedure (should you decide later to have children) may be nearly impossible. Also depending on the method used to tie off the tubes, the number of women who become pregnant after a tubal ligation is, at the highest, 2 in 1000.

Tubal ligation can be done immediately following childbirth, if the doctor is briefed on the decision well in advance of the delivery. It can also be done by scheduled surgery at any time. Fifteen percent of all women over the age of 45 have elected to have a tubal ligation.

Tubal Ligation

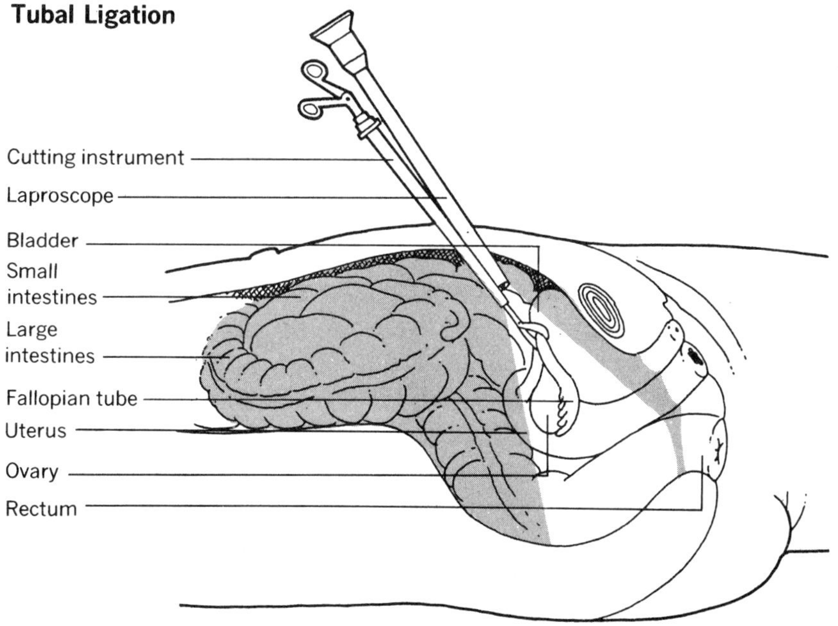

Hysterectomy

Hysterectomy is the removal of the uterus and, perhaps, the cervix. This procedure is completely irreversible. Chances of pregnancy following the procedure are none.

A *subtotal hysterectomy* is the removal of the uterus, leaving the cervix, fallopian tubes, and ovaries in place. A *total hysterectomy* is the removal of the cervix as well as the uterus. *Oophorectomy* and *ovariectomy* are both used to describe the surgical removal of one or both of the ovaries. *Ovariohysterectomy* is the removal of the ovaries, fallopian tubes, and uterus. The quantity of tissue removed will be determined by the patient and the doctor, based on the reasons for the operation. For removal of cancerous tissue, all the organs may need to be removed. For sterilization, only a subtotal hysterectomy may be necessary.

Hysterectomies have become increasingly used to correct problems that may be remedied by medication, or which may be temporary in nature and not warrant surgery. To recommend a hysterectomy solely for birth control is unusual. It should only be done in cases where tubal ligation is not sufficient in correcting problems, or where some underlying physical problems require surgery. Although hysterectomies are common, they are still considered major surgery and should be approached as such, by both the doctor and the patient. Recoveries can take six weeks or longer.

Vasectomy

Vasectomy is sterilization of the male by cutting the vas deferens, the tubes that transport the sperm. The surgery is normally performed in the doctor's office with local anesthesia. Incisions are made either on each side of the scrotum or on the center midline of the scrotum. The tubes are then cut, and tied or cauterized on each end. Pain following the procedure is usually responsive to nonaspirin painkillers. Heavy lifting or strenuous exercise should be avoided for a week.

Vasectomy

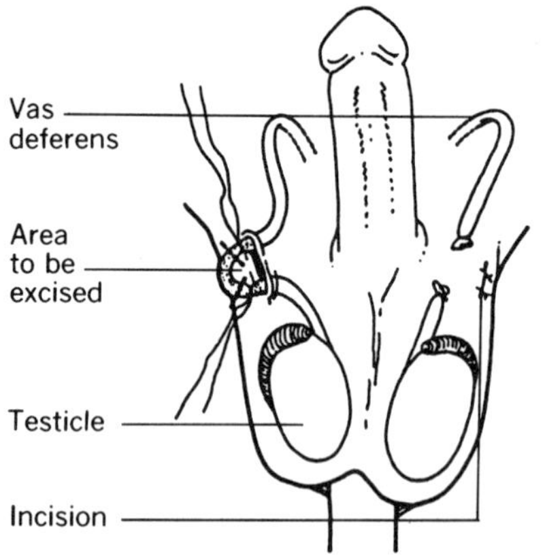

Vasovasotomy is the surgical procedure that attempts to reconnect the vas deferens after a vasectomy. This operation is done for men wishing to reverse the surgical sterilization. Success at this procedure can vary from 30 to 75 percent, depending on the type of initial sterilization procedures, and on the skill of the surgeon in reconnection of the tubes.

Infertility

Infertility can stem from numerous problems. It is estimated that as high as one in ten couples cannot conceive a child. There are an estimated 1.8 million women in the United States who are classified as infertile, which is about 5 percent of the female adult population of reproductive years.

Infertility can stem from the male

reproductive system about 40 percent of the time, the female system about 40 percent of the time. But it also is a combination of problems shared by both partners a majority of the time.

A couple is considered for fertility testing after a prolonged period of time in which they have actively been trying to conceive and have been unable. A prolonged period of time should be considered at least several months, and probably one year. After that, you should consult with your doctor about the need to test for fertility problems.

Blockage of the Fallopian Tubes

Thirty percent of the women who are infertile suffer from blockage of both of the fallopian tubes. Blockage can stem from scar tissue that develops from surgery, injury, diseases such as pelvic inflammatory disease (PID), or birth defects. Abnormal tissue growth from ailments such as endometriosis can block the passageway with excess tissue growth. Some of these blockages can be treated surgically; others are irreparable and the women will not be able to conceive naturally.

Hysterosalpingography

This is a long name for the X-ray technique that is used to check for defects and blockage in the fallopian tubes and uterus. (Hystero refers to the uterus, salpingo for the fallopian tube, and graphy for the X-ray technique.) A radiopaque dye is injected into the uterus and fallopian tubes. Then an X ray is made to check for unusual formations and blockages that may be obstructing the path of the egg to the uterus. Two X rays will be taken; one on the day of the dye insertion, and one 24 hours later.

Transcervical Balloon Tuboplasty (TBT)

One of the surgical techniques used to unblock damaged fallopian tubes is called transcervical balloon tuboplasty (TBT). A deflated balloon at the end of a flexible guiding tube is inserted into the fallopian tube and inflated. As angioplasty works on blocked arteries, the tuboplasty works by inflating in the area that is restricted, forcing the tube open. The inflation is done several times to force the scar tissue open and clear the passageway. The surgery is done through outpatient care, which means that it can be performed without a costly overnight stay at a hospital. It is shown to be effective for more than half of the women deemed treatable for fallopian tube blockage.

Treatment of Uterine Disorders

Several problems can arise from uterine dysfunction or disease. Tumors, polyps, and endometrial growth can prevent implantation of fertilized eggs in the uterine lining. There are several surgical procedures, mostly done in the doctor's office, that can correct the problems. *Dilation and curettage (D and C), endometrial biopsy,* and *endometrial curettage* are procedures that allow the physician to remove unusual growths from the cervix and uterine walls.

Hormonal Deficiencies

Hormones regulate the development and release of the ovum from the ovary and prepare the uterine wall for reception of the fertilized egg. Low levels of certain hormones can disrupt any one of the numerous stages of the menstrual cycle. Hormonal problems affect one third of all infertile women.

Anovulatory cycles are menstrual cycles in which no egg is released. *Amenorrhea* is when there is no menstruation, with or without ovulation. *Inadequate endometrium* is when the lining of the uterus is not sufficient for the fertilized egg to lodge on. All of these conditions can be treated with synthetic hormones. Many couples are able to conceive after hormonal treatment. The physician determines the hormone levels through a series of exams. Urine testing, mucous testing, and biopsies will give the different hormone levels for the various hormones required for successful fertilization.

Sperm Count and Formation

The single largest contributing factor to male infertility is sperm count or formation. Testing of sperm involves three studies: count, motility, and morphology.

Sperm Count

The number of sperm present in a single ejaculation should be at least 20 million in one milliliter. For a full determination of sperm count before a male is diagnosed as infertile, testing should be performed more than once. *Oligospermia* is the reduced count of sperm; *azoospermia* is the complete absence of sperm.

Several factors influence sperm production. Alcohol consumption, drug use, and restrictive clothing all reduce sperm count. Blocked ducts in the epididymis or in the vas deferens can also reduce the number of sperm present during ejaculation. Low hormone levels may reduce sperm count. Methods for reversing or correcting low sperm count problem can range from the simple—elimination of affecting factors such as alcohol—to the difficult—surgical reparation of the vas deferens to remove blockage.

Sperm Motility

Motility is the ability of the sperm to travel through the fluid present. A normal score for sperm motility is that two hours after ejaculation, 50 percent of the sperm are still actively swimming. If the sperm die unusually quickly, it is less likely that one will make the passage through the female cervix and uterus and meet up with the egg in the fallopian tube.

Sperm Morphology

The structure of the sperm (morphology) is a small oval body with a whiplike tail that is used to propel the sperm through the uterus. The tip of the sperm body has a cap with enzymes that deteriorate the protective coating on the ovum when the two press together. Sperm that is misshapen, or missing a tail or the enzyme cap, will not be able to successfully penetrate an ovum. In a morphology test, at least 60 percent of the sperm should be normally structured.

Motility and morphology problems present barriers to natural fertilization. Some men are able to successfully impregnate their spouses without surgical intervention, despite deficient sperm; others may require extensive intervention.

Immunological Problems

In some partners, the female will develop an immunological response to the male's semen. This means that her immune system attacks the sperm, responding the same way it would to an invasion by a virus. The immune system destroys the sperm before it can reach the ovum. Why this occurs is unknown, but the response fades if exposure to the sperm is eliminated. The treatment for immunological attacks is eliminating intercourse or using condoms for several months until the female's immune system shuts off the mechanism that responds to the sperm.

Alternative Forms of Conception

There have been a number of breakthroughs for couples experiencing difficulty in conceiving. There are methods for overcoming problems in sperm production, egg production, and fertilization.

Drug Therapy

In certain cases of infertility, drug therapy may be used to correct the problem. For example, Metrodin, a drug containing a natural hormone, is used to stimulate egg development. Pergonal, another hormonal drug, may be used to promote egg or sperm development. Pills containing clomiphene citrate, a nonsteroidal drug, are used to stimulate ovulation. Drug therapy can also be used with the following methods.

Artificial Insemination

Artificial insemination is the nonsurgical insertion of sperm into the vagina or uterus. This technique can be done to provide a more concentrated sperm count from the father or provide sperm from a donor if the man is infertile. It is mainly successful on women who are not experiencing infertility problems themselves.

IVF

IVF is the procedure in which an egg is fertilized by a sperm in a laboratory glass dish. Typically in this process a woman is treated with drug therapy to stimulate egg production. Eggs are then drawn from the ovaries and placed in the dish with the man's sperm in order to be fertilized. After approximately two days, several fertilized eggs are implanted in the woman's uterus. More than one egg is implanted because it is likely that not all will develop. The success rate for a pregnancy is about 20 percent.

GIFT

GIFT (gamete intrafallopian transfer) is a procedure in which a doctor inserts both the eggs and the sperm into a woman's fallopian tube for fertilization inside the woman's body. The resulting fertilized egg then travels to her uterus, as in the natural process of conception. The success rate for this method is about 25 percent.

ZIFT

ZIFT (zygote intrafallopian transfer) is a procedure in which the eggs and sperm are combined in the laboratory. Then the fertilized eggs are inserted in the fallopian tube so that they may travel to the uterus as they would in natural conception. The success rate is about 25 percent.

ICSI

ICSI (intracytoplasmic sperm injection) is a laboratory procedure in which a doctor injects a single sperm into a single egg for fertilization. The fertilized egg is then implanted in the woman's uterus. This procedure is especially useful for men with low sperm counts, low sperm motility, or sperm that cannot penetrate the egg on their own. The success rate with this method is about 25 percent.

Donor or Frozen Eggs and Sperm

Donor eggs, donor sperm, or both may be used in fertilization techniques. Donor eggs and sperm are donated by healthy women or men whom the parents may or may not know. Technological advances have also made it possible to freeze sperm or eggs for later attempts at pregnancy.

Surrogacy

If a woman is unable to carry a fetus to term in a pregnancy, an alternative is to have another woman carry the fetus. Depending on the type of fertility problem, the surrogate mother may carry the egg of the infertile mother or a donor egg. The egg may be fertilized by the father or by donor sperm. In some cases the surrogate provides the egg and undergoes one of the above fertilization techniques with the father's sperm. A surrogate may be a relative, friend, or hired woman. The legal involvement is complicated and the necessary arrangements require serious discussions.

Pregnancy

Once you have conceived, the baby has nine months of growth and change to prepare itself for the outside world. There are numerous physiological changes to the mother as the baby grows inside her, and many emotional changes and discoveries for both parents.

As soon as a women realizes she may be pregnant, she should schedule an appointment with a gynecologist/obstetrician. The doctor will perform a blood test that can confirm the mother's pregnancy status. Once a women finds that she is pregnant and decides to proceed with the pregnancy, her doctor will schedule her for monthly exams, through the 28th week of pregnancy. Then she may see her doctor every other week from the 30th week to the 36th. After the 36th week of pregnancy, she should be seen every week until delivery. Delivery should occur before the 42nd week.

First Trimester

The first three months of pregnancy take the embryo from a single free-floating cell to a formed two-inch recognizable fetus. The mother's breasts enlarge to prepare for the production of milk. The uterus increases in size to make room for the growing fetus and the surrounding liquid, called *the amnion*. The placenta forms to process the mother's blood and carry nutrients and water to the fetus. The umbilical cord is the connection between the mother and her child. Nutrients travel through it to the baby and waste material travels back to be processed out by the mother's system.

Because of the direct link between the mother's blood and the baby's blood, the mother must be diligent about the foods and drugs she ingests. Many chemicals can pass through the placenta; some will do irreparable harm to the forming baby. Alcohol, caffeine, chemicals from cigarette smoke, and some medications will pass through the placenta and have been shown to harm the developing fetus. In large quantities, they can cause brain damage, deformity, or death. Any medication should be approved by the pregnant woman's obstetrician before use.

The first examination should be to confirm your pregnancy and run an initial screening for health problems and general health history. A complete physical will either be done then or at a following appointment.

At your first visit with your obstetrician, after you know you are pregnant, your doctor should give you information on what to expect.

During Pregnancy

A pregnant woman needs special foods to maintain her own health as well as to safeguard the health of her baby. She should have additional vitamin D, folic acid, and iron, usually recommended as dietary supplements. More important for most women is the provision of adequate protein in the diet to prevent toxemia of pregnancy or underweight babies. Between 70 and 85 grams of protein a day should be eaten during pregnancy, even if this results in a weight gain of as much as 25 pounds. Adequate nutrition is more important than restricting weight gain to 20 pounds or less.

Morning Sickness

During the second and third months of pregnancy, usually, morning sickness may plague the expectant mother. With the raised hormone levels, and the increased pressure on the internal organs from the growing uterus, the stomach can become easily upset. Morning sickness usually occurs during the first hours after awakening, and can start immediately upon rising.

Although the mechanism of morning sickness is not understood, it is believed that the combination of having gone all night without food and the pressure on the stomach from lying down create the nausea. Munching on crackers and dry toast before arising and continuing to snack through the day will help. Some women experience morning sickness throughout the day; others never experience it. Morning sickness can range from slight nausea to regular vomiting and increased inability to hold down food and tolerate ordinary odors.

Frequent Urination

As the uterus grows it puts pressure on the surrounding organs. This pressure will shift during the pregnancy from the bladder to the intestines, then to the lungs, as the size of the uterus expands. During the first trimester the main pressure occurs on the bladder, creating the need for the pregnant woman to urinate more frequently. It may cause her to awaken at night to use the bathroom.

Fatigue

Many women experience fatigue during the first trimester of pregnancy. Some women will also continue to experience fatigue throughout the preg-

The Fetal Environment in the Uterus

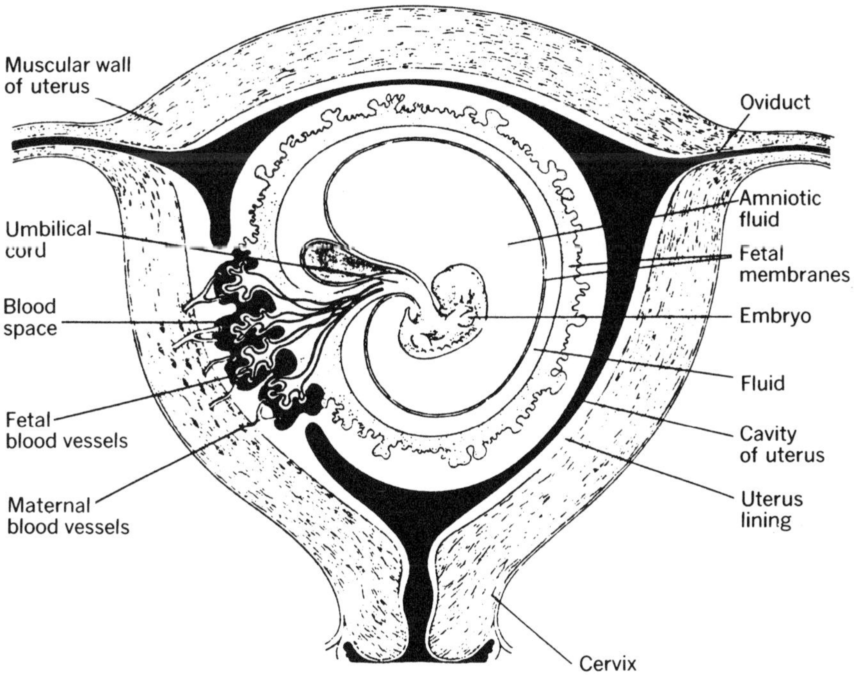

nancy. Others experience a respite from being tired during the second trimester. Some of the fatigue may come from restless sleep or interrupted sleep caused by changes in the mother's body. It also stems from the shift of energy to the developing fetus, taxing the mother's body. This new draw of energy requires an increased intake of food by the mother to compensate for the increased need. Despite the fact that the mother may not look pregnant, her nutritional needs increase immediately upon becoming pregnant and vitamin supplements are sometimes prescribed.

Second Trimester

It is usually sometime during the fourth month that a woman starts "showing." This means that the stomach becomes slightly, but visibly, distended with the growth of the fetus. This may not be noticeable when the woman is fully clothed.

By the end of the second trimester, the pregnant woman will probably have felt the baby move. The baby will begin by rolling and moving about in the amnion surrounding it. It eventually fills the space to keep from moving extensively, but arm and leg jabs will become more apparent and more vigorous as the baby grows. The baby will double in size during the second trimester, getting to an average length of 13 inches by the end of the sixth month. All of the organs and all of the features are in place and developing.

Constipation

The pressure of the growing uterus will shift slowly from the bladder to the intestines. This will relieve the need to urinate as frequently as before, but there will be increased difficulty with bowel movements because of the added pressure. This will result in constipation for some pregnant women.

Varicose Veins

With increased body weight concentrated in the pelvic area, some women experience problems with varicose veins. Leg veins are under increased pressure and may bulge into visible bubbles on the surface of the skin. This may be caused by weakened venal (vein) walls, expanded blood volume, and decreased tension in the muscles. By using aids such as support panty hose and avoiding prolonged standing, the pregnant woman can alleviate some of the problems. Her physician can guide her to other methods of avoiding or exacerbating the problem.

Breathlessness

Breathlessness can start in the second trimester, triggered by hormonal changes that affect the capillaries in the lungs. It will continue into the last trimester because the uterus will push up on the diaphragm, the muscle that controls lung expansion.

Third Trimester

The baby continues to grow, adding fat cells and filling out. The eyes, ears, and mouth are all functioning. The lungs are beginning to expand and contract, taking in amniotic fluid in preparation for breathing air. During the eighth or early ninth month, the baby will rotate into a head down position to prepare for descent through the birth canal. By the ninth month the baby is too big in the womb to make large movements. The sensations the mother feels are the baby jabbing and poking with arms and legs.

Depending on the status of lung development and on the emergency care available, a baby born during the third trimester can survive. The lungs are ill-equipped to deal with the intake of oxygen, but new treatments are available to help the child survive.

Contractions

Some women experience mild uterine contractions throughout the second and third trimester of pregnancy; others only experience contractions toward the end of the third trimester. These contractions can be thirty seconds to several minutes in duration. They usually start at the top of the uterus and the woman experiences a tightening sensation that moves down the uterus to the pelvic floor. The contractions should not be extremely painful, and if they become uncomfortable, changing position or lying down may relieve them. The contractions, known as *Braxton Hicks contractions*, are preparing the uterine muscles for delivery. The contractions may be difficult to distinguish from true labor toward the end of the pregnancy. False alarms, where the expectant mother thinks labor has begun, are caused by this. Lying down should alleviate Braxton Hicks contractions, but not true labor.

Fatigue

As in the first trimester, fatigue can become a daily obstacle. The pregnant woman's body is carrying a large weight and large drain on her energy system. As the baby gets closer to delivery, the amount of energy required increases, increasing the likelihood that the mother will tire easier.

Awkwardness

Falling, tripping, dropping things; and general inability to get into and out of chairs and cars is a normal part of pregnancy. The shift in a woman's center of gravity can occur rapidly during the last trimester, giving her little time to adjust. Moving and stepping over things becomes more difficult as the woman's line of vision with her feet and the ground becomes blocked. Her added weight can make some movements more difficult. And the swelling that comes from general edema can make handling small objects more cumbersome. All of these problems disappear after delivery.

Edema

General swelling of the extremities, the hands and feet particularly, is a normal aspect of pregnancy. About 75 percent of pregnant women experience some swelling from retention of fluids. It is usually helpful to *increase* water intake to alleviate some of the swelling. Increased fluids help the body flush out excess liquids. Talk to your doctor if swelling becomes a problem. *Pre-eclampsia* and *toxemia* occur in a small percentage of women, where swelling is extreme and life threatening if not treated. Your doctor will monitor for pre-eclampsia by checking your blood pressure, weight gain, and degree of swelling.

Breathing Difficulties

As the size of the baby grows, the baby and the uterus will push on the diaphragm muscle that controls breathing. This added pressure keeps the woman from deep breathing and can be painful. Also the baby may temporarily lodge a foot against her ribs or diaphragm, causing sharp pains. During the last two weeks or so, the baby will drop into the pelvic girdle and the pressure will be relieved on the diaphragm. This is called *lightening.* (Note: Shortness of breath, rapid and shallow breathing and/or rapid pulse should be reported immediately to a doctor.)

Prenatal Diagnosis and Tests

During your pregnancy, you will undergo a few or many of the following examinations. Depending on your health and potential health risks, these tests may be performed more than once; some may be done each month. Other tests may be added. Each provides you and the physician with information about your health and the health of the developing baby. Prenatal care increases the chances of having a healthy baby tremendously. Less than 2 percent of the women who see their obstetrician regularly after the second month of pregnancy have an underweight baby.

Home Pregnancy Tests

Home pregnancy tests can now be purchased in almost any pharmacy or drugstore. The prices range from $5.00 to more than $20.00. All the tests work on the same principle—they test for the presence of the hormone Human Chorionic Gonadotropin (HCG), which is present at high levels during pregnancy. A chemical in the home testing kit will change colors when HCG is present. The tests are 99 percent accurate in labs, but probably around 95 percent accurate in home use, where circumstances are not as controlled. A false-negative test will register if the HCG levels are not high enough yet. A false-positive reading may occur if you have unusually high HCG readings or another chemical which mimics HCG in the test. If you have not had your period and you suspect that you may be pregnant, it is advisable to have a doctor's test regardless of the results of the home kit. You should seek medical advice as soon as possible.

Blood tests

Blood is tested during your first examination to determine if you are pregnant. Either during the same examination or at a follow-up examination, blood is tested for the following: anemia; infectious diseases, including sexually transmitted diseases and AIDS; immunities to childhood diseases, especially German measles; and diabetes. Sometime before delivery blood will be checked again for diabetes, sexually transmitted diseases, and hepatitis.

Rh Compatibility Test

Rh is the part of the blood type that labels the blood positive or negative. The only time this poses a problem is when the mother is Rh negative and the father is Rh positive and the offspring develops Rh positive blood. This used to pose serious threat to the pregnancy, but can now be treated adequately with drugs.

Urine tests

The physician will check your urine, probably at each visit, for sugar (diabetes), protein (toxemia), bacteria (infection), and perhaps drug use.

Pelvic Exams

Pelvic exams are done throughout pregnancy to check the position of the fetus and the status of the vaginal walls and the cervix. As you approach delivery, the cervix muscle will *efface* and *dilate*, meaning that the walls will thin and the cervical opening will increase. During your early visits to the doctor, a pap smear will be performed to check for infections and unusual growths on the cervix. Other smear tests will be done for diseases such as chlamydia. These tests may be repeated late in pregnancy.

Ultrasound

By using sound waves to reflect off the fetus in the uterus, the doctor is able to determine the size, position, and occasionally the sex of the forming baby. Ultrasound can be performed anytime after about the fifth week of pregnancy. Your physician will let you know what scheduling is used in his or her office. Some obstetricians perform ultrasound to get an accurate date on the pregnancy by the size of the fetus; others may wait to do one reading later to determine general position and health.

Ultrasonography is performed *transabdominally* (across the stomach) or *transvaginally* (through the vagina). If the ultrasound is done transabdominally, then the woman must drink plenty of fluids beforehand to fill the bladder. This allows the bladder to push the uterus up for better positioning as well as provide an obvious sighting for the bladder so it is not misidentified.

Amniocentesis

To determine the genetic makeup of the developing baby, a small portion of the amniotic fluid can be drawn out of the womb to pick up floating cells, which contain the baby's genetic information. This allows the doctor and the pregnant woman the opportunity to screen for different inheritable diseases. Amniocentesis is usually performed on higher risk patients during the fourth or fifth month of pregnancy. Armed with the information provided, the parents can choose to carry the baby to term, abort the fetus, or have intrauterine surgery performed to remedy problems with the fetus.

The fluid is drawn out by a syringe that is inserted into the woman's naval to the level of the uterus. Using ultrasound to avoid the placenta and the fetus, the needle draws up fluid. This procedure runs about a one in one hundred risk of causing amniotic leaking, and a one in two hundred risk of infection. The risk of triggering spontaneous abortion is even lower.

Chorionic Villus Sampling (CVS)

A newer procedure than the amniocentesis, the CVS samples the tissue that forms between the interior uterine wall and the beginning placenta. The needle-like tube is inserted either through the vagina or the stomach and guided by ultrasound to the chorionic villus. This testing procedure is usually performed during the third month of pregnancy.

The benefits of the test are that it can be performed earlier in the pregnancy, and a determination to discontinue the pregnancy poses less risk to the woman when decided during the first trimester. Amniocentesis can only be done after the start of the second trimester. The risk is that, because it is a newer procedure, the spontaneous abortion rate following CVS is higher than the rate for amniocentesis. As doctors become more practiced with the procedure it is believed the rate will even out.

Fetal Monitoring

External and internal monitoring of the fetus are done to check on the heart rate and stress of the fetus. External monitoring involves registering the heartbeat via ultrasound readings and, if needed, a pressure gauge to measure contractions.

Internal monitoring is done only during delivery and if some level of distress is suspected or likely in the fetus. The monitoring electrode is placed on the baby's scalp through the opening in the cervix. This can only be done after dilation has started. A catheter that measures pressure can also be inserted into the uterus to measure contraction pressure. Both of these units can be connected to the monitor reader by cord or by radio wave.

Monitoring is now a regular procedure during delivery. It allows the doctors to check on the health of the baby and provides an early warning if the baby is in distress. It should be set up so that it does not interfere at all with the birthing process.

Apgar Test Score

When the baby is born, you will probably be given an Apgar score that refers to the general health of the baby. The scores range from 0 to 10 and are based on five criteria: skin color and appearance, heart rate, respiratory effort, muscle tone, and reflex responses. Stillborns rate a zero with no pulse, blue skin, and no response system; extremely healthy babies can score a 10 with good coloration, good crying, and strong pulse and muscular activity.

Birthing

There are three basic stages to birthing: labor, delivery, and placental delivery. The average length of birthing is 14 hours for the first birth and 8 hours for births after that. This is only an average though. Some women will experience mild true contractions for 24 hours before significant dilation begins. Some women have labors that last an hour or less. Although it may seem ideal for women who have experienced extremely long labors to have a 20 minute birthing process, there are risks with short labors. The most likely thing with short labors is that you won't get to the hospital on time. Since no one knows when labor will begin or how long it will last, it is extremely important for every woman who is pregnant to have a good understanding of what happens during birthing and what to do as soon as labor begins.

Labor

Labor is marked with the beginning of regular contractions of the uterus. In some women this will be similar to the Braxton Hicks contractions they have been experiencing during the days preceding labor. For others the true labor contractions will be much harder and much more severe in pressure and duration than the Braxton Hicks contractions.

Latent Phase

During the initiation of labor the contractions will be some distance in time apart—up to a half hour. Contractions may be regularly spaced or may come irregularly. Because of the possible differences in pressure and duration, some women do not recognize the early stages of labor.

Contractions should come more rapidly, eventually getting to a pace of every five minutes. The contractions are slowly opening the cervix (dilatation) and thinning the cervical muscle (effacement) to allow for the passage

Birth Sequence

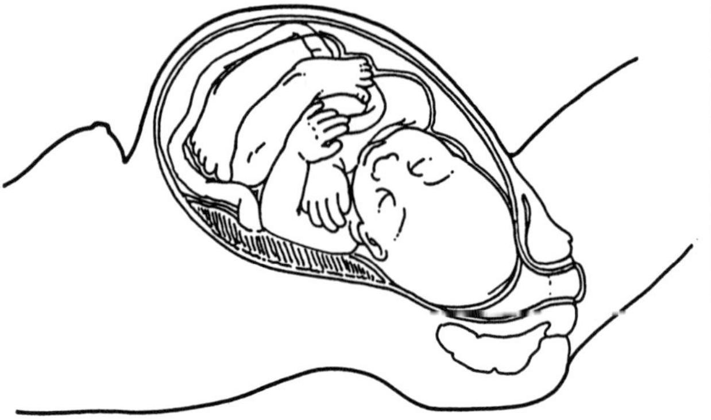

Dilated cervix
During the first stage of labor the cervix dilates to form a passageway into the vagina, the birth canal. Contractions of the uterus may occur at intervals of approximately 5 to 15 minutes, with brief periods of rest in between, which permit oxygen to flow to the fetus.

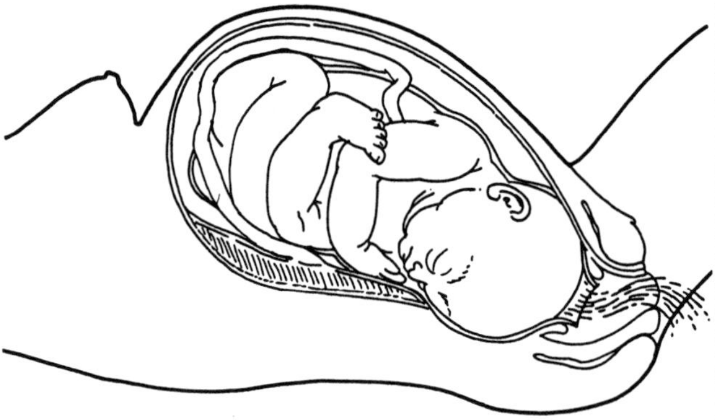

Ruptured amniotic sac
Ruptured amniotic sac ordinarily signals the onset of the second and generally shorter stage of labor. Contractions during this stage occur in more frequent succession and are more intense. The so-called *bag of waters,* which contains the amniotic fluid, is ordinarily discharged during a strong contraction but may even rupture before labor begins.

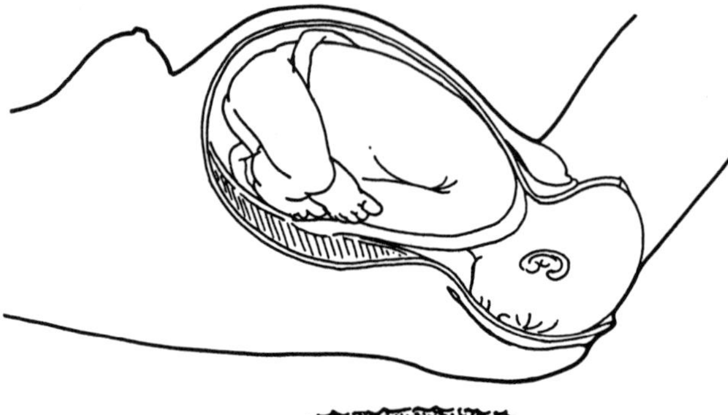

Delivery
As the fetus moves into the lower pelvic region the mother naturally experiences a conscious impulse to bear down and help its entry into the world. She may feel a few moments of increased pressure or pain as the infant's head gradually appears and is followed by the rest of its body.

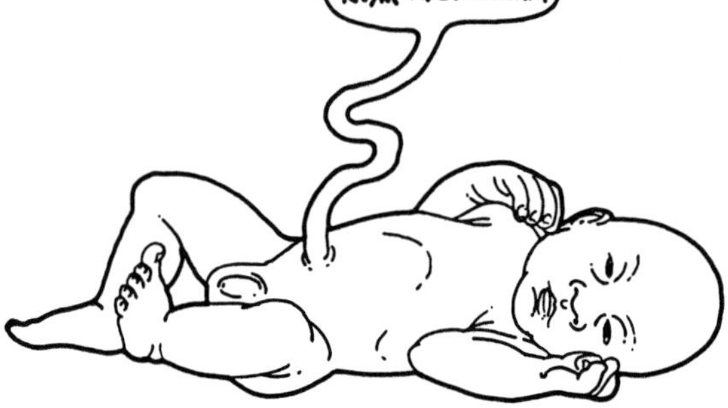

Placental stage
Placental stage is the third stage of labor and is characterized by the expulsion from the womb of the placenta, or *afterbirth,* to which the baby is connected by the umbilical cord. This cord is not cut until all the placental blood has pulsed into the baby's body.

of the baby into the vaginal canal. The muscle will eventually thin and open to 10 centimeters during the last part of labor.

Call your doctor when you know labor has begun. Most doctors recommend that women wait out this period at home. Talk to your doctor about what activities are recommended and what should be avoided during this phase. Since the latent phase of labor can last up to one full day, resting is important.

Active Phase

The contractions come more rapidly, last longer, and are stronger in pressure. The contractions force the cervical muscle to dilatation of 7 centimeters. If the amniotic sac did not break during the latent phase, it will break now. The attending physician may choose to break the sac to help the baby's head to *crown*. Crowning occurs when the baby's head moves into the pelvic bone region and becomes visible through the vaginal canal. The act of crowning will normally break the amniotic sac if it has not already ruptured.

By the active phase you should be attended by your health care person. Contractions will reduce to every two or three minutes and may last one full minute. If the attending physician decides that the vaginal canal is not wide enough to accommodate the size of the baby's head, he or she may decide to perform an *episiotomy*. This procedure involves a small incision in the tissue between the vagina and the anus or off to the side of the vagina. The majority of first births have this procedure; about half the women who have given birth before have an episiotomy again.

Transitional Phase

This can be the most difficult part of the birthing process because it comes at the end of the hard work of labor. The extremely strong contractions are still two to three minutes apart but are now lasting over a minute. The contractions have peaks in pressure that are much stronger than previous contractions. The cervix dilates to a full 10 centimeters, usually in less than an hour. This is the point where breathing exercises learned in birthing classes will come in handy. You may be too anxious, annoyed, or fatigued to consider them though. The coach is there to help with this. At the end of the transition the baby's head forces through the canal and the largest width of the head passes the cervical opening.

Delivery

At this point you can start to push. The point from the end of transition to the actual delivery of the baby should be less than one hour and in some women can take less than fifteen minutes. The baby will usually descend head first with the head facing the back of the mother's body. Other possible positions include the baby facing front, the baby descending feet or butt first (breech delivery) or an arm or leg descending first. All fetal positions except head first, face back, may require medical intervention.

Placental Delivery

The last part of the birthing process is the delivery of the placenta. The delivery of the placenta usually follows the birth of the baby by less than one hour. It can occur within five minutes or it may take some time. Nursing the baby during this period helps because the stimulation of the nipples causes uterine contractions that help separate the placenta from the uterine wall, arrest bleeding, and shrink the size of the uterus. The placenta should be delivered in one solid piece.

It is during this time that any tears or surgical cuts will be repaired by the doctor. The episiotomy will be stitched.

Caesarian Sections

In some cases the mother is not able to deliver a baby through the vaginal canal. This can be due to several possible circumstances. If the baby is in one of several breech positions, such as arm or leg descended, the doctor may elect to perform a caesarian instead of attempting to shift the baby for vaginal delivery. If the baby's head is too large to pass through the pelvic girdle bones, or if the pelvic opening is too small to accommodate even a normal size infant, caesarian section will be performed. Also, if the mother does not dilate entirely or if the contractions are not adequate to push the baby into the birth canal, a caesarian will be performed.

In all these circumstances, caesarians are performed to avoid undue stress on the fetus and the mother during the birthing process. The uterus will only be able to provide life support to the infant for a few days after labor has begun. As the physical status of the placenta deteriorates, the loss of oxygen-rich blood will harm the fetus. The pressure from continued contractions will also eventually stress the fetus. Vaginal walls and the cervical muscle will swell from the extended pressure of contractions. It becomes essential to the health of both the mother and the child that labor not continue for too long.

A caesarian section begins with a local anesthesia to the mother that numbs the belly region. An incision is made after anesthesia that opens a small section of the stomach (usually right above the pubic hair). A second incision is made into the uterine wall. If amniotic fluid remains in the uterus, it will be suctioned away with the same type of tube the dentist uses. The baby is then lifted from the uterus either by hand or by forceps. The umbilical cord is clipped. The placenta may be delivered through the surgical opening. Then both layers of the incision are stitched closed (frequently with metal or plastic clips).

Birthing Places

There are several alternatives for where you can have your baby delivered. Check with your community and your attending physician to see what is available and review what you are comfortable with.

Hospitals

Some hospitals offer a variety of options to the traditional sterile delivery rooms that were common for women over the past forty years. They may have private patient rooms where the mother can decide who attends the birth. All the equipment that will be needed is in the room. The baby may still sleep in the nursery, but will be brought to the mother for feeding.

Birthing Room

Birthing rooms are a step away from private patient rooms. The room is equipped for most emergencies, except caesarians. The father and others can be present throughout the delivery. The atmosphere in the room is designed to be homey and comfortable. For most of the labor the woman will remain on a traditional bed. The bed can then be broken down into a birthing bed for the final stage of labor and delivery. The baby will most probably remain in the room with the mother during her recovery.

Home Delivery

Not usually recommended for first-time pregnancies, the home delivery is just that—delivering the baby in your home. Your attending medical personnel will be there for assistance, but except in emergencies, the full labor and delivery will take place in the home. Screening for this is intensive, because there is little that can be done in emergencies except to take the woman to the hospital in an ambulance.

Birthing Assistants

Along with the choices one can make on where to give birth, one also has choices for who will assist.

Problems during Delivery

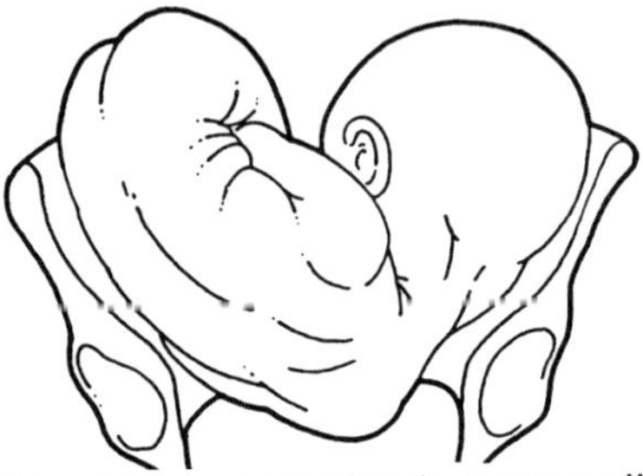

Shoulder presentation (transverse lie): delivered through Caesarian

Complete breech: Caesarian delivery recommended

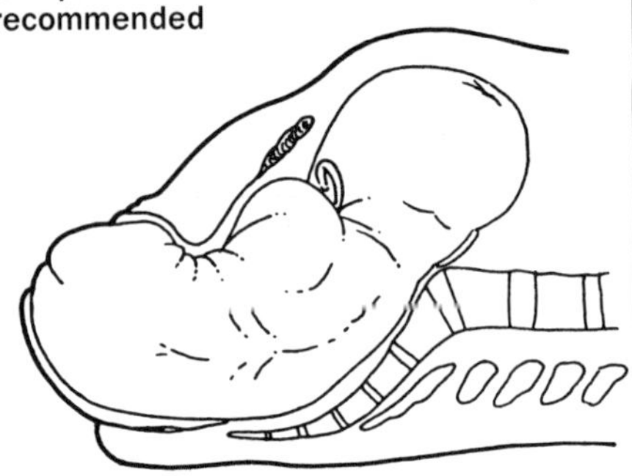

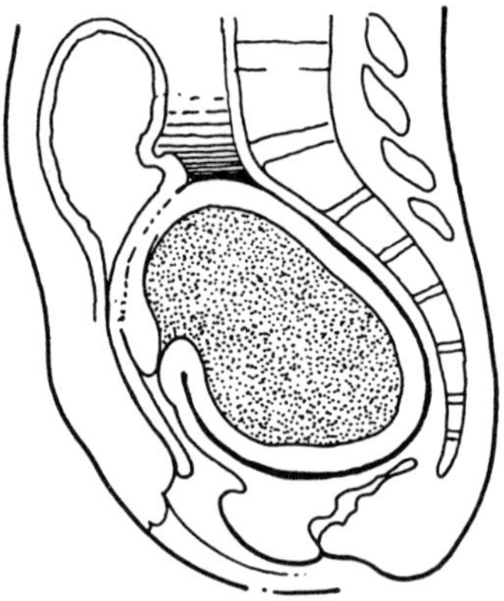

Uterine Disorder from Pregnancy

Hydatidiform mole: a growth that forms from cells from the pregnancy. It simulates the early stages of pregnancy, with morning sickness, expansion of the uterus, and lack of menstrual cycle. It usually grows faster than a normal pregnancy, though, and can be diagnosed through ultrasound and tissue examination.

Obstetricians

Traditional medical practitioners, obstetricians, are fully trained medical doctors who specialize in pregnancy and birth. They usually assist in deliveries in the hospital, either in delivery rooms or birthing rooms. There may be some in your community, though, who will perform home births.

Nurse Practitioners

Nurse practitioners have several years of medical training although there are procedures that a doctor can perform that a nurse practitioner cannot. The nurse practitioner specializing in birthing will be able to assist in all deliveries, with an attending physician for caesarian sections.

Although arrangements vary from clinic to clinic, there is usually one obstetrician on staff with several nurse practitioners. It is likely that you would only see the doctor once or twice during the course of your pregnancy. The nurse practitioner would be able to handle most of your concerns.

Midwives

Certified midwives may also hold nursing degrees, although this is not a requirement in all states. They will assist in all deliveries, but, like the nurse practitioner, cannot perform caesarian sections. They are trained for all aspects of pregnancy and delivery.

Complications of Pregnancy

Occasionally something goes wrong during pregnancy or childbirth. This may be some problem that can be treated either with medication or surgically. There are some problems, though, that cannot be remedied. In some cases, the mother may lose the fetus.

Miscarriage

When the body rejects the embryo or developing fetus for whatever reason, this is considered a miscarriage or *spontaneous abortion.* There are numerous reasons why a miscarriage may take place. A shift in hormone level, a defect in the embryo, or another factor that interferes with the normal development of the fetus.

Early Miscarriage

Occurring in the first trimester of pregnancy, early miscarriage may be as frequent as one in ten pregnancies. Many miscarriages go undetected because the woman may not realize she has conceived and the body sheds the developing egg before any signs of pregnancy occur. In most of these miscarriages, it is believed that the egg would not have survived to delivery because of physiological defects. Other reasons may include inadequate hormonal development of the uterine lining and a faulty immune reaction to the embryo.

Symptoms

Symptoms of early miscarriage include cramps from the uterine area, not unlike menstrual cramps. This is caused by the uterine contractions that force the lining to be shed. Heavy bleeding accompanies or follows the

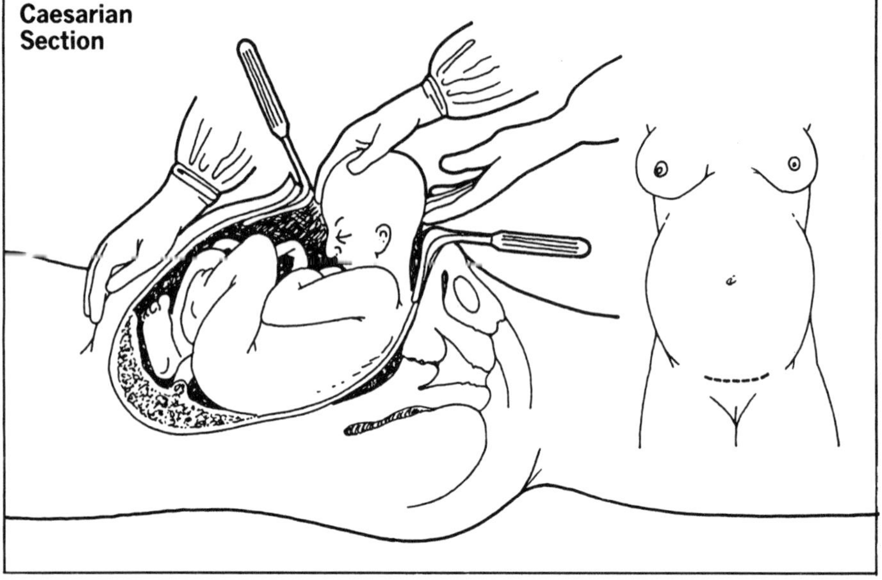

Caesarian Section

cramping when the lining is expelled. The bleeding may also be present without accompanying pain. Light bleeding that persists for a few days or more can also signal an impending spontaneous abortion. With any of these symptoms, the attending physician should be contacted immediately. Upon examination the doctor will determine if the cervix has become dilated—a sign of miscarriage. The physician will guide you through treatment that follows a miscarriage, or will help to arrest the symptoms if a miscarriage has not yet taken place.

Late Miscarriage

Occurring during the second or early third trimester, late miscarriages are physically more difficult to endure. (Psychologically both early and late miscarriages can be difficult if the woman has prepared for the upcoming baby.) Late miscarriages can be caused by trauma, insufficient uterine or cervical capability, or exposure to chemical or drug substances that trigger a miscarriage.

Symptoms

Bleeding, a pink discharge, a brown discharge, or cramping may precede a late term miscarriage. Some women will experience uterine contractions and spotting without it signaling difficulty with the pregnancy. However, any changes in the mother's condition or any experience of the symptoms above should be discussed with the attending physician immediately.

The mother will be examined by the attending medical person to see if the cervix has begun to dilate. If a miscarriage has begun, several steps may be used to prevent it continuing. Continual bed rest, hospitalization, and surgery are just a few of the possible remedies, depending on the reasons for the threat of miscarriage. If the miscarriage does occur, the doctor will try to determine the reasons for it to prevent a reoccurrence in subsequent pregnancies.

Late miscarriages will follow the stages of labor in some women, once miscarriage has become inevitable. The woman will have to expel the fetus and the uterine lining, along with the placenta. A dilatation and curettage (D & C) may be required to clean the uterus after a miscarriage to ensure that no infection sets in. Once the doctor determines that the uterus is sound, and that the reason for miscarriage has been remedied (if possible) then a new pregnancy may begin.

Stillbirths

A baby delivered after about the 20th week of pregnancy will be diagnosed as a stillbirth instead of a miscarriage.

Symptoms

Following the pattern of the late miscarriage, stillbirths can be late miscarriages or they can be full deliveries. The fetus may have already died *in utero* or may die during the labor and delivery. Many of the reasons that apply to late miscarriage also apply here. Other reasons for stillbirths can include deterioration of the uterus, umbilical strangulation, infection of the amnion or uterine lining, or other physiological defects.

Abortions

Different than a spontaneous abortion, an *induced abortion* is when the doctor ends the pregnancy medically. This can occur for several reasons. The woman may elect to have the pregnancy terminated. This is legal through the first trimester in all states, and through the second trimester in some states. If the fetus threatens the life of the mother or has died *in utero*, the pregnancy can be terminated at any point.

There are several methods of inducing an abortion. All involve opening the cervical muscle to remove the fetus. This requires local anesthesia in a first trimester abortion, and can require general anesthesia after the first trimester. Performed in a doctor's office or in the hospital, the medical procedure is considered less risky than birthing. If performed by unqualified personnel or in unsanitary conditions, the risks increase greatly. When the tissue from the pregnancy remains after an abortion, infection can set in. It is therefore extremely important that competent medical personnel be sought to perform abortions.

During the first trimester a D & C can be used to remove the embryo. The uterus can also be aspirated by vacuum. This is a method that removes all the embryonic tissue at once. Second trimester abortions usually involve a chemical injected into the uterus that triggers the body to expel the fetus and induce labor. A pill, RU 486, has been introduced in Europe that triggers spontaneous abortion. It is still being tested for use in the United States.

Genetic Disorders

There are 4,300 genetic defects that can be passed on to offspring. Of those 4,300 there are about 600 that are common enough to be tested for in couples where the risk is considered high. It is estimated that three percent of all births are to parents carrying a genetic defect. These can range from mild disorders such as night blindness to serious and life threatening disorders such as Tay-Sachs and sickle cell anemia. If one grandparent or immediate family member carries a known genetic disorder, the attending physician may recommend genetic testing and counseling. Even if abortion is not considered by the parents, genetic testing will allow the parents to prepare for any eventuality.

Child Care

Bringing the Baby Home

Once the child is born, the mother will spend a couple days to a couple weeks in the hospital, depending on her condition after delivery. Caesarian deliveries can keep a woman in the hospital for several days to assist in recovery from the surgery.

Preparation for the baby should be made before delivery, if at all possible. This includes preparing the baby's sleeping area, buying clothes, diapers, and other essentials for the baby. Some parents worry about how they would handle coming home to a nursery if the baby did not survive or was required to remain at the hospital for some time.

Many parents find that, if they did lose the child, disassembling the nursery helped in the mourning process. It may be more difficult for parents to come home to a house where there are no signs of the infant, than to return to a nursery where they have to confront their loss.

In most circumstances, though, the

parents return home from the birthing process with baby in hand. It is more than likely that the new mother will be tired from the hard work of delivery. The father will also have been functioning with little sleep if he assisted in delivery and is helping with the feeding and care of the newborn. So having the nursery set up with essentials is one way of assuring that the new family is not adding to the increased demand in their time with this new member.

Essentials in the nursery should include: diapers (cloth, disposable, or both) t-shirts in more than one size, a washtub, a car seat, a crib with a mattress that fits snugly against the sides, blankets, a bunting suit and clothing appropriate to the season, soft terry towels and washcloths, flame resistant pajamas, and a chair for the parent to sit in during feedings. Other items to consider are: a baby monitor that lets you hear the baby when you are in another room, a nightlight, a little music box or recorder that plays lullabies, bottles for feeding, a bottle warmer, pacifiers, clips to hold the pacifier to the baby's clothes, a mobile that hangs over the crib, a stroller, a baby carrier (sling or backpack), a diaper bag, baby oil, powder, shampoo, hypoallergenic soap, and other assorted toiletries. Some of these you may receive as gifts; others you will no doubt want to supply yourselves.

It is important when purchasing items such as carriers, cribs, car seats, and other equipment where safety plays a major role, that you consult with consumer guides, professional recommendations, and that you contact the U.S. Consumer Product Safety Commission, 4330 East West Highway, Bethesda, MD, (800) 638-2772 to find out if any complaints are registered on the products you are considering. It is worth your baby's safety to take the time to research the things that your baby will spend so much time using. You cannot determine quality by price and, remember, the manufacturer isn't going to put warnings about defects on products they sell.

When buying clothes for the baby, keep in mind that many babies are born bigger than the newborn size of clothing. There is no guarantee for your baby's size, so you should be equipped with several sizes of clothing in case you come home with a big baby. You don't want a nine pound baby and a roomful of six-pound size t-shirts.

Post-Partum Depression

It is estimated that 50 percent of all women suffer from some form of the blues when returning home with their baby. This can be caused by several things. There is a let-down that comes from having an event that you have prepared months for be over. This can be accompanied by the fact that the pregnant woman is the center of attention until the baby comes. Then the baby is the center of attention.

The physical fatigue that comes with birthing, nursing, and caring for a child that has to be fed night and day can also lead to exhaustion and depression.

Some parents take several weeks to bond with their babies. The baby may feel like a stranger when the parent (not just the mother) holds him. The baby, for all practical purposes, *is* a stranger. You are just getting to know his wants, needs, and desires. Each baby is unique in the way he wants to be held, in what the different types of crying mean, and how he responds in general to life around him. Even experienced parents must get used to this new being and his new personality. This takes time. So the sensation that you are not madly in love with or attuned to the child is neither unusual nor incomprehensible. The feelings will develop as you become more comfortable with your baby.

The feelings of inadequacy that arise from all of these potential sources of depression may increase the depression. You may feel like an inadequate or deficient parent because you are not as good a parent as you expected. The ability to be a parent takes time and learning. You should allow adequate time to develop the skills that make you comfortable with your new baby.

If, after several weeks, you still have feelings of depression and inadequacy, talk to your doctor about counseling. It may be a passing problem or it may be tied to other aspects of your life. A good counselor should be able to help you sort everything out and get to the root of your insecurity with your baby. But, again, allow yourself a normal amount of time to adjust without brow-beating yourself about it.

Both fathers and mothers can suffer from post-partum depression. It is important that the new parents communicate with each other about their feelings and their needs. Chances are that the other parent will not only understand what you are feeling, but will be experiencing some of the same feelings as well.

Other methods of handling this period can include talking with other parents about the new stresses that accompany parenthood. Support groups, new parent groups, and other such gatherings may already exist in your community. If not, try to start one, provided it doesn't add a major burden on your time.

If you miss some aspect of your life before baby, such as going out, then make some effort to treat yourself to such an occasion. Talk with friends and keep from isolating yourself if you feel a need to share company. If, however, the problem is too much company and no private time, then feel free to establish visiting hours, as you would have in a hospital when someone else is watching out for your health and well-being.

Serious post-partum depression

Severe post-partum depression that requires immediate counseling has the same symptoms that require immediate counseling even without a baby. The symptoms include: suicidal thoughts, violent urges (particularly directed inward or toward the baby), chronic insomnia, extreme lethargy, loss of appetite, complete inability to function, and general sense of despair. Any of these symptoms should be discussed thoroughly with your physician and/or a counselor as soon as possible.

Diet for Nursing Mothers

A nursing mother has special dietary needs in addition to those satisfied by the normal adult diet. She should drink an extra quart of milk and eat two more servings of citrus fruit or tomatoes, one more serving of lean meat, fish, poultry, eggs, beans, or cheese, and one more serving of leafy green or yellow vegetables.

After the Birth: Physical Changes

The mother's body will take several weeks to get back to something resembling the pre-pregnancy state. Weight gain, uterine expansion, and breastfeeding all change the body and take some time to undo.

Weight gain

Depending on how much weight the mother has gained during the course of the pregnancy, it can take several weeks to several months to get back down to her pre-pregnancy size. If you have gained the recommended 20 to 25 pounds during pregnancy, it will take about two months to lose the extra weight if you don't diet. If you are breastfeeding, dieting should only be done under strict supervision of your doctor.

The uterus will remain distended for several weeks following delivery. Breastfeeding helps reduce the size of the uterus because a hormone (oxytocin) that increases uterine contractions is released during breastfeeding.

Extra water is maintained in the mother's body during the pregnancy, and this water takes some time to eliminate. The extra fluids will be eliminated from the mother through frequent urination and heavy sweating. It is important that the new mother continue to replenish her fluids despite this apparent flood of liquids leaving her body. Increased intake may help increase the speed with which the body eliminates the unneeded fluids.

The body will also pick up extra weight in the breasts if the mother continues to breastfeed. For mothers who are bottlefeeding, it will take several days for the breasts to reduce in size.

Exercising to help tone and shape the pelvic, stomach, and thigh muscles is a good method of speeding your return to your usual size. Talk with your physician for post-partum exercises that will not tax your muscles but will help build them up and firm them.

Lochia

Following a delivery, whether vaginal or caesarian, the body will excrete through the vagina a discharge that will shift from bright red to reddish-brown to yellowish-white. This discharge, called *lochia,* is normal and is the result of the body shedding the last particles of blood and fluids from the uterus. Lochia may last from three to eight weeks after delivery.

Warning signs that the lochia is abnormal include: bright red blood after about the fourth day, heavy bleeding that requires pad changes of more than one an hour (at any time following delivery), foul-smelling discharge, heavily clotted blood, or an absence of discharge during the first two weeks after delivery. Other symptoms to watch for include: lower abdominal pain after the second day and/or lower abdominal swelling. *All of these symptoms require immediate consultation of your doctor.*

Perineal pain

With or without an episiotomy, the perineal area is normally sore following vaginal deliveries. The head of the baby has pushed against the muscles and the muscles are likely to be bruised. Talk to your physician about methods of alleviating soreness if it becomes severe. For relief of mild pain, try soaking baths, sitting on inner tubes or cushions, lying on your side instead of sitting up, and continuing with Kegel exercises.

Fever

Puerperal fever is a sign of infection of the placental site following delivery. Although it is extremely uncommon now (it was once a major killer of post-partum women), any fever that lasts for more than a few hours or becomes higher than 100 degrees should be reported immediately to your doctor. It may be just a virus or from the changes taking place for breastfeeding, but your doctor should be notified of any fever during the first month you are home.

General fears and concerns

Most parents have some fears and concerns surrounding the birth of their baby and the general routine that is required once the baby is home. Other concerns are around the various changes and symptoms that both the mother and the baby go through following birth. Some may involve simple things like dry skin; some may be more disconcerting, like rashes and red patches. If you cannot find any answers in your stock of books on pregnancy and babies, or if you are really concerned, you should not hesitate to call your doctor. If he or she feels that you need guidance and are panicky, then request some good books to help you understand what to expect. In any case, no concerned and caring doctor will object to a new parent needing reassurance about the mother's and the baby's health. It is better to ask questions and find out that there is nothing to worry about than to not ask questions and leave a potentially serious problem ignored.

Child Care and Day Care

Once you have a child, you make a choice about how that child is to be cared for during the years before school. The majority of families in the United States can no longer afford to have one parent stay home to raise a child. This means that, for at least part of the week, the child will be cared for by someone other than a parent.

Most parents have caretakers either come to their home or they drop the child off at the caretaker's place. The child will be there three to eight hours a day. Some children are in child care for up to twelve hours, depending on the parents' schedule.

For children with only one primary caretaker, and this counts for more than one quarter of American children, time in day care is essentially the same amount of time as the average adult full-time employee. The quality of the care is as influential on the child's upbringing as the quality of the parental care received during nonwork hours. Because of this, child care selection is extremely important to the safety and well-being of any child entrusted to someone else.

Child Care in the Home

Nannies, au pairs, child care workers, and babysitters are the names for people who come to, or live in, the homes of the child for whom they care. The arrangements can range from one caretaker to one child, to one caretaker for two or three families' small children. The ability of the parents to pay for child care determines the type of care selected.

Few families can afford the salary and the living space required of the live-in nanny. For those who can, the nanny provides a registered, reliable, trained caretaker who will supervise the child for as many years as the parents deem necessary. Au pairs are much the same type of worker, except they usually do not have educational training for child care. They tend to be younger workers, less likely to stay for more than a year or two in the same position. Many au pairs are foreign students seeking a chance to live abroad for a while.

Child care workers and babysitters may come to take care of the child during assigned hours. They may live somewhere else and their work hours are scheduled for regular work patterns. They may work for one family, or a few families may pool together resources and use one caretaker for several children. One child care worker should care for no more than four or five children at a time, to provide the best safety and education for the children.

When hiring someone to come watch your children in your home, several things should be considered. The most important is to check the personal history of whomever is being considered. This now means going beyond personal recommendations. Check for police records, work papers, history of employment, and any other documentation that the person can provide to show stability, reliability, honesty, and integrity *while working with children.* In most situations, the caretaker will be unsupervised while working with your small children. Children's versions of events may not fully explain events you should know about, or may exaggerate problems with the caretaker that are not important. You have to have complete faith that this person is delivering the service you expect in a manner that meets with your full approval. If you have the opportunity to observe at least one full day of activity under the care of the worker, you should take it. This gives you a sample of how your child will spend important hours of his development. It also allows you to watch how a worker deals with the frustrations and problems that come up every day when dealing with youngsters.

Child Care Centers and Programs

Many states are now requiring registration of child care centers. Even for individuals who run informal-style child care in their own home, licensing may be required. The state will set up rules of how much space is needed per child, how many staff employees per child, what kind and variety of food is to be served, what activities are allowed, and what type of insurance is needed to cover for accidents while at the center. Check to see if your state has a licensing program, and what the licensing requirements are. If your state does have such a program, you should only use licensed facilities for your child. If there is no mandatory licensing, find out if there is a voluntary licensing program for day care. You should check references thoroughly for programs that have no governmental inspection. Even with licensing, you want to ask the same types of questions that the licensor asks:

- How many staff per student?
- With whom is a sick staff member replaced?
- What food is provided for the children?
- What activities are provided for?
- What instruction and education is the child given?
- What are the age ranges of the children enrolled?
- How many children does the facility accommodate?
- How many children per classroom or room?
- Are any activities off the center grounds? Is permission obtained in advance to take the child off the grounds?
- What is the policy for sick children? Are they allowed in the classroom? If a child is brought to the center, obviously sick, what procedures are followed by the day care staff?
- If a child gets sick or injured while at day care, what procedures are followed?
- What is the policy of allowing children to leave with someone other than a parent? Is advance notice required? Is the parent the only acceptable guardian to be picking up a child? (Although it may seem initially that you would only want a parent picking a child up, you may wish to carpool, or have a babysitter or a relative pick up a child. You want to make absolutely sure, though, that the child cannot leave with anyone who walks in and asks to take the child home.)
- What are their hours? What are their pickup times? If you are late, what do they do with the child?
- What is the discipline policy of the center? (This is of fundamental importance that the policies be explained in advance of enrollment.)
- Do they expel children? For what reasons?

Look around the facilities. Are they clean, well kept, and brightly lit? Are there appropriate ranges and types of toys for your child's age? Are there any safety violations or potentially dangerous aspects to the room's design (such as an open staircase without guardgates).

Attend the facilities while day care is in session. Observe the interaction of the children to see if they are well cared for, occupied in a manner you find suitable, and playing or interacting positively. Get references from parents whose children are the same age as yours and are currently using the day care program.

Once you have enrolled in the program, continue to monitor the classroom atmosphere. Occasionally drop by early before picking a child up to watch the activities. Continue to talk to other parents who have children in the same program. And, above all, continue to talk to and listen to your child about how he has spent his day.

Day care can be one of the most influential and rewarding experiences for a child. Your child will learn to interact with other adults, and perhaps other children, depending on the type of care you select. It will provide him or her with early educational experience that will be the foundation of the entire learning experience. If it is a positive experience from the start, it is likely that your child will continue to enjoy learning throughout his or her lifetime.

5

The Middle Years

Maintaining good health over the years is far simpler, less expensive, and more comfortable than restoring health that has become poor. Because some diseases cannot be cured after they are contracted, it is only logical to try to prevent all possible health problems. The techniques of modern preventive medicine are available to Americans of every age.

All people are not beautiful or handsome, but nearly everyone can have the kind of attractiveness and vitality that comes from good health. The health of an individual depends upon the kind of body he inherits and the care he gives it. Good health can be thought of as a state of social, physical, and mental well-being, a goal virtually everybody can attain—if the responsibility for maintaining one's own health, with occasional help from the health experts, is accepted.

Keeping Fit

Physical Changes

Physically, middle age should be a pleasant plateau—a time to look back on a vigorous youth, enjoy an active present, and prepare for a ripe old age.

Middle age should not be measured by chronological age but by biological age, the condition of various parts of the body. You might say that the middle-aged body is like a car that has been driven a certain number of miles. It should be well broken in and running smoothly, but with plenty of reserve power for emergencies, and lots of mileage left.

Biological age should be measured by the state of the heart, arteries, and other essential organs, the length of life and comparative health of parents and grandparents, temperament and outlook on life, and outward appearance. The way you have fed or treated yourself is important. Eating the wrong kinds of food, being overweight, smoking too much, or worrying too much can add years to biological age.

However, no one should be surprised if he is not in quite the shape he was when he was 25 or 30 years old. At age 40 to 50 it is perfectly normal to have only 80 percent of the maximum breathing capacity, 85 percent of the resting cardiac output, 95 percent of the total body water, and 96 percent of the basal metabolic rate. These factors, however, should not slow anyone down very much.

There is one difference, though, that can be anticipated in middle age. Reaction time and decision-making processes may be a bit slower. This is because the nervous system is one of the most vulnerable to aging. The cells of the central nervous system begin to die early in life and are not replaced, while other organs are still growing and producing new cells. Specific response to input is delayed because it takes a greater length of time for an impulse to travel across the connections linking nerve fibers.

Thus, though you may function as usual under normal conditions, you may find it a little harder to respond to physical or emotional stress. However, if you have followed a sound health maintenance program, including good nutrition, enough mental and physical exercise and rest, and moderate living habits, you should respond to unusual physiological or emotional stress quite adequately.

The Importance of Checkups

Physical disabilities associated with chronic disease increase sharply with age, starting with the middle years. While more than half (54 percent) of the 86 million persons who have one or more chronic conditions are under age 45, the prevalence of disability from illness is greatest in the 45 and older age group. Of those under 45 who have chronic conditions, only 14 percent are limited in activity as compared with almost 30 percent of the 45 to 64 age group. And only 1 percent of those under 45 with chronic illness are completely disabled, as compared with 4 percent in the 45 to 64 age group.

These figures suggest that it is wise to have an annual checkup so that any disease process or condition can be nipped in the bud. Further evidence of the value of medical checkups comes from the Aetna Life Insurance Company, which compared two groups of policyholders over a five-year period. Those who did not have checkups and health counseling had a death rate 44 percent higher than the group who did. Regular checkups will not only help prolong life, they will also help you to live it more comfortably.

Here are some other good reasons for having a physical checkup:

- If an organ has been attacked by serious disease in youth, it may deteriorate at an early adult age.
- Heredity may play an important role in determining the speed at which various organs age. If your parents and grandparents had arteriosclerosis, there is a chance you might develop this condition in your middle years.
- Your environment (smog, poor climate, etc.) might affect the rate at which your body ages, particularly the skin.
- Individual stresses and strains or abuses or overuse (of alcohol, for example) may create a health problem in middle age.
- The endocrine glands (pituitary, thyroid, parathyroids, adrenals, ovaries, testicles) play important roles in aging. Serious disease of one or more of these glands may lead to premature aging of an organ dependent upon its secretions.
- At middle age you are more likely to be beset by emotional strains at work or at home that could make you an early candidate for heart disease, arteriosclerosis, and other degenerative disorders.
- The earlier a chronic disease is detected, the better the chance that it can be arrested before permanent damage is done. This is especially true in the case of glaucoma, diabetes, heart disease, cancer of the lung or breast or other cancers—all of which could have their onset in middle age.

To help detect disease and other debilitating conditions, many physicians utilize automated medical screening, which combines medical history with selected physiological measurements and laboratory tests to give the physician a complete health profile of the patient. This profile should indicate the probability of any chronic condition, which the physician could then pinpoint with more thorough tests.

Also, annual checkups enable the physician to observe changes taking place over a period of time. For example, he is able to observe gradually changing blood chemistry levels or a progressive increase in eye pressure that could signal the onset of disease.

Don't Try To Be Your Own Physician

A panel of medical specialists from the University of California at Los Angeles recently found that many men of 40 years and older were dosing themselves with unnecessary pills and "conserving" their energy by increasing bed rest to the point that it actually became enervating.

These physicians point out that increasing dependence on pills can be harmful as well as expensive. Laxatives are a good example of a popular commercial medicine taken unnecessarily by large numbers of people. Perhaps only one person in 100,000 may have an actual motor disability of the bowels, and most constipation can be easily corrected through proper foods and exercise, without resorting to laxatives. Also, taking vitamin pills or avoiding all high-cholesterol foods is unnecessary—unless recommended by a physician.

But, most important, "conserving" energy through prolonged bed rest or avoiding exercise can be fatal. The panel members pointed out that before age 40, a person exercises to improve his performance, but that after age 40 he exercises to improve his chances of survival.

Physical Fitness and Exercise

In middle age most of us stop performing most forms of exercise other than those that we enjoy doing. In other words, we find it easier to bend an elbow than lift weights. This is unfortunate, because in middle age most of us need regular exercise to maintain both mental and physical fitness and to increase endurance, strength, and agility.

As noted earlier, in middle age there is some decrease in breathing capacity, cardiac output, and metabolic rate; yet exercise can improve these functions. The more often the normal heart and circulatory system are required to move blood to active regions of the body through exercise or movement, the more efficient they become. Protracted exercise also improves the work of the lungs by increasing their ability to expand more fully, take in more air, and utilize a greater proportion of the oxygen in the inhaled air.

While exercise alone cannot eliminate obesity, it can help prevent it by improving digestion and bowel movements and by burning up excess calories. Exercise can also make you feel, look, and think better. Some traditional formal exercises, however, like touching the toes while keeping your knees stiff, or doing deep knee bends, are potentially harmful in middle age; they put too much stress on weak parts of the back and legs.

Despite protests about not having enough time, everyone has time to exercise, particularly if it is worked into the daily routine—for example, walking instead of riding to the train, office, store, or bus stop. You might find you'll get there faster, especially in traffic-clogged metropolitan areas, and you'll save money as well. More important, those minutes of "stolen" exercise accrue over the years in the form of improved health.

healthy for the foot was the formerly fashionable spike heel and pointed toe.

Any heel two inches or higher will force the full weight of the body onto the smaller bones in the front of the foot and squeeze the toes into the forepart of the shoes. This hurts the arch, causes calluses on the sole of the foot, and can lead to various bone deformities.

The major solution to this problem is to buy good shoes that really fit. The shoes should be moderately broad across the instep, have a straight inner border, and a moderately low heel. To fit properly, shoes should extend one-half inch to three-fourths inch beyond the longest toe.

Avoid wearing shoes that have no support; also, avoid wearing high heels for long periods of time. Extremely high heels worn constantly force the foot forward and upset body balance. Changing heel height several times a day will rest the feet and give the muscles in the back of the legs a chance to return to their normal position. It's highly desirable to wear different shoes each day, or at least alternate two pairs. This gives the shoes a chance to dry out completely. Dust shoes with a mild powder when removed.

Shoes should not be bought in the morning. They should be tried on near the end of the day, when the feet have broadened from standing and walking, and tightness or rubbing can be more easily detected.

As to hosiery, socks and stockings should extend a half-inch beyond the longest toe. Stretch socks are fine in many cases, but plain wool or cotton socks help if your feet perspire a lot.

Foot Exercises

Exercise your feet by trying these simple steps recommended by leading podiatrists:

- Extend the toes and flex rapidly for a minute or two. Rotate the feet in circles at the ankles. Try picking up a marble or pencil with your toes; this will give them agility and strength.
- Stand on a book with your toes extended over the edge. Then curl your toes down as far as possible, grasping the cover.
- After an unusually active day, refresh the feet with an alcohol rub. Follow this with a foot massage, squeezing the feet between your hands. When you are tired, rest with your feet up. Try lying down for about a half-hour with your feet higher than your head, using pillows to prop up your legs.
- Walk barefoot on uneven sandy beaches and thick grass. This limbers up the feet and makes the toes work. Walking anywhere is one of the best exercises for the feet if you learn to walk properly and cultivate good posture. Keep toes pointed ahead, and lift rather than push the foot, letting it come

down flat on the ground, placing little weight on the heel. Your toes will come alive, and your feet will become more active.

Foot Ailments

Doing foot exercises is particularly important in middle age, because the foot is especially vulnerable to the following problems.

Bunions

A bunion is a thickening and swelling of the big joint of the big toe, forcing it toward the other toes. There is also a protuberance on the inner side of the foot. Unless treated, this condition usually gets progressively worse. Surgery is not always necessary or successful. Often, special shoes to fit the deformed foot must be worn.

Stiff Toe

People suffering from this problem find that the big joint of the big toe becomes painful and stiff, possibly due to a major accident or repeated minor trauma. This condition usually corrects itself if the joint is protected for a few weeks, usually by a small steel plate within the sole of the shoe.

Hammer Toe

This clawlike deformity is usually caused by cramping the toes with too small shoes. The pressure can be eased with padding and, in some cases, the deformity can be corrected by surgery.

Ingrown Toenail

Cutting the nail short and wearing shoes that are too tight are major causes of ingrown toenails; the edge of the nail of the toe—usually the big toe—is forced into the soft outer tissues. In some cases the tissues can be peeled back after soaking the foot in hot water, and the offending part of the nail can be removed. To prevent ingrown toenails, the nails should be kept carefully trimmed and cut straight across the nail rather than trimmed into curves at the corners. For severe or chronic cases of ingrown toenails it is best to seek professional treatment.

Morton's Toe

This is the common name for a form of *metatarsalgia,* a painful inflammation of a sheath of small nerves that pass between the toes near the ball of the foot. The ailment is most likely to occur in an area between the third and fourth toe, counting from the large toe, and usually is due to irritation produced by pressure that makes the toes rub against each other. In most instances, the pressure results from wearing improperly fitted shoes, shoes with pointed toes, or high heel shoes, which restrict normal flexing of the metatarsals (the bones at the base of the toes) while walking.

Temporary relief usually is possible through removal of the shoes and massaging of the toes, or by application of moist, warm heat to the afflicted area. In cases of very severe pain, a doctor may inject a local anesthetic into the foot. Additional relief sometimes can be obtained by wearing metatarsal arch supports in the shoes. However, continued irritation of the nerves can result in the growth of a tumor that may require surgical removal.

Care of the Teeth

An attractive smile is often the first thing that one notices about others. In addition to creating an attractive appearance, healthy teeth and gums are a basic requirement for good overall health. The dentist should be visited at whatever intervals he recommends, usually every six months.

Neglect of oral hygiene and the forgoing of dental checkups are commonplace in the middle years. An often-heard excuse is that the eventual loss of teeth is inevitable. Years ago, loss of teeth really was unavoidable. Today, however, thanks to modern dental practices, it is possible for nearly everyone to enjoy the benefits of natural teeth for a lifetime.

Problems of Aging

When the human body reaches middle age, a number conditions that are the result of advancing years begin to make themselves felt. These include wrinkling of the skin, baldness, varicose veins, and the body's decreased ability to deal with nicotine, caffeine, alcohol, and excess calories.

Skin

The skin usually starts to show its age in the mid to late 30s. At that time it starts to lose its elasticity and flexibility, and becomes somewhat thinner. Little lines—not yet wrinkles—start to show up, usually crow's feet around the eyes.

Wrinkling takes place at different times with different people, and sometimes in different areas of the skin. Heredity may play a part.

Treatment for Wrinkles

While wrinkles do not hurt, many people want to do something about them. Experienced physicians and dermatologists have a number of techniques for removing or minimizing wrinkles. One accepted method is dermabrasion, or planing of the skin with a sanding instrument. Laser resurfacing is another surgical procedure to smooth out wrinkles by removing the top layers of the skin. Chemical peels have a similar effect.

Dermal fillers such as collagen may be injected to fill out deeper wrinkles and creases. Another injectable treatment is the botulinum toxin, or botox, which temporarily paralyzes the muscles that create creases in the skin. The facial lines then gradually lessen with disuse.

The use of retinoic acid, or tretinoin (available as the topical prescription medications Retin A™ and Renova™), for the treatment of fine wrinkles has become popular. Retinoic acid was originally used for the treatment of acne and has not yet been studied for long-term use for wrinkles. Side effects may include heightened sensitivity to sunlight and skin irritation or rash. Alpha and beta hydroxy acids, available in many over-the-counter cosmetics, peel off the top layers of skin to speed rejuvenation.

Skin Texture Change

Besides wrinkling, the skin has a tendency in some people to become thinner, leathery, and darkened as they move towards the 40s and 50s. This effect can be minimized if the skin is toned up with cold cream and other emollients that provide the moisture and oil the skin needs. Also, overexposure to the sun—one of the prime agers of the skin—should be avoided.

In fact, most physicians feel that the sun is a lethal agent. Its aging effects on the skin are well documented, as is the role of excessive sun exposure in causing skin cancers.

Cosmetic Surgery

Cosmetic surgery for both men and women is becoming increasingly popular and sophisticated. Cosmetic surgery procedures include *rhinoplasty* (nose); *facial plasty* or *rhytidoplasty* (face lift); *blepharoplasty* (upper eyelids and bags under the eyes); breast augmentation and reduction; as well as the dermabrasion and other methods mentioned earlier. See "Plastic and Cosmetic Surgery" in Ch. 20, *Surgery*.

Baldness

The occurrence of baldness (medically known as *alopecia*) and attempts at concealing or reversing it can be traced back thousands of years. For example, in ancient Egypt bald men used a mixture of fats to cover their heads. Today there are several options for treating baldness, though baldness is typically caused by factors that cannot be altered, such as aging and heredity.

Other causes of male baldness include infections, systemic diseases, drugs that have a toxic effect, mechanical stress, friction, and radiation. Diet does not usually affect baldness, but chronic starvation or vitamin deficiencies can contribute to dryness, lack of luster, and hair loss. Also, excessive intake of vitamin A can cause hair loss.

In women, loss of hair is quite common toward the end of pregnancy, after delivery, and during menopause. A hysterectomy, crash dieting, severe emotional stress, high fever, a major illness such as thyroid disease or diabetes, certain allergies, and the use of systemic drugs such as steroids and amphetamines—all can produce hair loss.

The most common form of baldness is *androgenetic alopecia*. It is commonly known as either male pattern baldness or female pattern baldness (depending, of course, on whether the affected person is male or female). With this type of baldness, hair follicles shut down, becoming unproductive. Experts believe that hormones play some role in this process. *Alopecia areata* is an autoimmune disease in which hair may suddenly fall out in patches. Other body hair, such as eyebrows and eyelashes, may also be lost. In many cases, the hair will grow back, although it may be thinner than before.

Male Pattern Baldness

Male pattern baldness may begin as early as the late teens, the 20s, or 30s. With this type of baldness the hairline at the forehead recedes and hair begins to fall out at the crown of the head. Eventually only a fringe of hair remains at the sides and along the back of the head.

Female Pattern Baldness

Female pattern baldness may begin in the 30s or 40s and become more noticeable after a woman experiences menopause. This type of baldness is characterized by an overall thinning out of the hair.

Treatments

Although many people are perfectly comfortable with their baldness, others find it a distressing condition they wish to change. Today there are several methods of treatment for these people.

Two surgical methods are *hair transplantation* and *scalp reduction*. For hair transplantation a doctor removes, usually from the back of the patient's head, small sections of follicle-bearing tissue and hair called *grafts*. These grafts are placed in recipient incisions in the bald areas of the head. This can be an expensive, time consuming, and painful process.

Scalp reduction is the process in which sections of bald scalp are surgically removed and the remaining hair-covered areas are pulled more closely together. Sometimes elastic expanding devices are first placed under hair-covered areas of the scalp, stretching the hair-covered skin so that it will cover a larger area. This can be a costly and painful process.

Drug therapy is used for the nonsurgical treatment of baldness. The most commonly used drug is minoxidil, a topical drug (a drug placed directly on the scalp) that has been approved by the FDA for promoting hair growth. Minoxidil is now available over-the-counter in such products as Rogaine. It must be used twice daily and works best for younger patients whose hair loss is fairly recent. Minoxidil, however, does not work effectively for many people. If hair regrowth does occur, the patient must continue to use minoxidil or the new hair will fall out. It can take from four months to a year to see results. The FDA has also approved Propecia, a prescription medicine in pill form, for hair growth. Propecia, however, can only be used to treat male pattern baldness. As with minoxidil, if hair regrowth occurs, a patient must continue to take the pill or the new hair will fall out.

Hair weaves and hairpieces are also options for those wishing to change their appearance. A hair weave is a wig that is attached by sewing it to existing hair. Hairpieces, or toupees, are wigs that are attached to the scalp with such methods as glues or tapes.

Excess Hair

For some middle-aged women, the problem is too much hair in the wrong place, instead of too little. Excess hair can grow on the face, chest, arms, and legs. In some instances, unwanted hair may be a sign of an endocrine disorder that can be detected by a physician. In other cases, it can be caused by chronic irritation, such as prolonged use of a cast, bandage, or hot-water bottle; it can also be due to excess exposure to the sun, iodine or mercury irritation, or localized rubbing.

Excess hair can be bleached, shaved, tweezed, waxed, or removed by chemical depilatories and electrolysis. Only electrolysis is permanent. See “Hair Removal” in Ch. 21, *Skin and Hair.*

Varicose Veins

Another complaint of middle-aged men and women is *varicose veins.* About half the women over 50 years of age have these enlarged veins with damaged valves in their thighs and calves.

Varicose veins can occur in various parts of the body. They are, however, most common in the legs.

Varicose veins are usually caused by years of downward pressure on the veins, causing the valves to break down. This often happens to people who must stand for many hours at a time. The large, bluish irregularities are plainly visible beneath the skin of the thighs and calves, and they cause a heavy dragging sensation in the legs and a general feeling of tiredness and lack of energy.

Treatment

Discomfort from varicose veins may be relieved by wearing support hose, by elevating the legs when possible, and by not standing or sitting in the same position for long periods of time. Severe cases of varicose veins may require further treatment, such as *sclerotherapy,* injecting the vein with a solution that scars and closes the vein; *ligation,* the removal of the vein; or *vein stripping,* tying off the main veins and removing superficial veins. Laser surgery may be used in some cases to close smaller veins.

Complications from vericose veins include *varicose ulcers,* skin ulcers near the ankle; and *phlebitis,* inflammation and clotting in a vein.

Menopause

The permanent end of a woman's menstrual cycle is called *menopause.* It is defined as the time after which 12 months have passed since a women's last period. The duration of time it takes for the body to change over to a non-menstruating hormonal structure varies. It may be as short as a year; some women may experience menopausal signs and occasional periods for up to ten years.

The average age that a woman experiences menopause is 51. However, menopause can normally occur in women at any time between the ages of 40 and 55.

The *premenopausal stage* is the length of time before frequently irregular menstruation or the cessation of menstruation. The body begins to undergo changes that may go unnoticed. Ovulation may be irregular and may not occur with every menstrual cycle. The estrogen and progesterone levels in the body may decline.

Signs that accompany the premenopausal stage include increasing or lessening menstrual flow, skipped or shortened periods, and occasional irregularly occurring menstruation.

The *perimenopausal stage* is the onset of noticeable changes. The menstrual cycle may abruptly cease, or become unpredictable and irregular. Hormone levels of estrogen and progesterone continue to decline. Egg production becomes increasingly irregular or ceases entirely. Egg production may or may not correspond to menstrual flow. A woman can continue ovulating without having a period, or may have periods without ovulating.

The most familiar signs of menopause occur during the perimenopausal period. These occurrences should be considered "signs" and not "symptoms," since they do not represent anything going wrong. They are not a sign of illness.

The one sign that everyone is aware of is the "hot flash." Referred to as flashes or flushes, this is a rapid increase in blood vessel dilation at the surface of the skin. The skin temperature can rise between four and eight degrees. The internal body temperature may drop with the increase of the surface temperature. A common hot flash pattern is a sudden feeling of extreme warmth, occasionally accompanied by heavy sweating, and chills following, as the internal body temperature cools. For some women, flashes occur daily; for others they may only occur once every several weeks. Some menopausal women never experience them. Many women experience flashes but are not disturbed by them.

Hot flashes at night, which produce heavy sweating and chills, are sometimes referred to as "night sweats." They may just be nighttime flashes. They can, though, lead to loss of sleep and thereby trigger fatigue, irritability, and insomnia. Problems with sleep should be discussed with your physician.

Dressing for fluctuations in body temperature may help reduce some undesirable side effects. Wear layers of clothing so when you are warm you can take off the top layer. The top layers are available, then, if you get cold later. It is commonly feared by some women that others can tell when one is experiencing a hot flash. This is rarely true; the usual physical response is a slight blush that goes unnoticed by others. Reassurance by friends can help relieve anxiety.

Other signs of menopause that may be problematic or startling when they occur include flooding. This is the sudden onset of a very heavy menstrual flow. It can occur without warning and normal amounts of menstrual protection may not be adequate. As with the hot flashes, this may never happen, or it may happen extremely infrequently, or it may be a recurrent problem. It is, however, usually only a problem in terms of hygiene and embarrassment. Flooding alone is not normally a symptom of an underlying problem. If there is no underlying disease, no surgery or treatment is required for this. If you are distressed by flooding and need reassurance, or *if it is accompanied by pain* please see a physician.

Vaginal changes that occur during menopause can include a thinning of the vaginal wall. This is normally associated with the reduction of estrogen production. The vagina will produce less lubrication and hold less moisture. The signs of this may include perceived dryness, itching, irritation from walking, and pain or discomfort during intercourse. Because the loss of lubrication may be the underlying cause, using douches and feminine hygiene sprays are not recommended. A water-based lubricant, such as K-Y Jelly™, or moisturizer such as Replens™, is recommended for discomfort, particularly with intercourse. You should avoid oil-based lubricants, such as Vaseline™, as they are more difficult for the body to absorb and may create problems with infection.

Mood swings are also commonly cited as a sign of menopause. They may accompany the hormonal swings of the early stages of menopause or they may occur later. Many women do not have noticeable mood change at all.

The change of mood may be sudden or it may be gradual. Depression has been noted by some women, and will most likely pass as the body adapts to the new hormonal levels. Knowing that it is caused by hormonal changes may help some women adjust to temporary shifts in mood. Debilitating or distressing changes should always be discussed with your doctor.

The *post-menopausal stage* is the rest of one's life after menopause. The menstrual cycle has ceased entirely. The production of eggs has stopped. The body's production of estrogen and progesterone is very low. The body has returned to a stable, predictable physical pattern.

A physician may prescribe estrogen or combined estrogen and progesterone supplements to reduce or eliminate some of the adverse reactions to menopause. Hormonal treatment may reduce or eliminate hot flashes, as well as vaginal wall thinning and drying, and it can reduce heavy menstrual bleeding. Hormone therapy may also protect against osteoporosis, but it may also increase a woman's risk of breast or uterine cancer. Research continues on new types of synthetic estrogen that may be risk-free. The risks and benefits of any hormone therapy should be discussed with a physician before treatment is begun.

Hysterectomies

When problems arise with the reproductive organs or with the body's response to the fluctuation in hormone production, surgery may be a solution.

Hysterectomy, the surgical removal of the uterus, and oophorectomy, the surgical removal of the ovaries, are medical procedures that alleviate major medical problems or remove cancerous tissue. Cancers of the uterus, ovaries, or cervix are frequently treated with removal of the cancerous and surrounding tissue. Hemorrhaging that has not responded to hormonal or other less invasive surgery may be corrected with a hysterectomy.

Other problems that can be alleviated surgically are noncancerous fibroid growths, endometriosis (in which the uterine tissue invades other tissues), and physical impairment or deterioration of the uterus or ovaries, as often occurs when the uterus collapses through the cervix.

There are several types of hysterectomies, differing in how much of the reproductive system is removed.

A *subtotal hysterectomy* is the removal of the uterus, leaving the cervix, fallopian tubes, and ovaries in place. A *total hysterectomy* is the removal of the cervix as well as the uterus. *Oophorectemy* and *ovariectomy* are both used to describe the surgical removal of one or both of the ovaries. *Ovariohysterectomy* is the removal of the ovaries, fallopian tubes, and uterus. The quantity of tissue removed will be determined by the patient and the doctor, based on the reasons for the operation. For removal of cancerous tissue, all organs may need to be removed. For sterilization, only a subtotal hysterectomy may be necessary.

If a woman has not already been through menopause, removal of the ovaries will initiate it.

Although hysterectomies are common, they are still considered major surgery and should be approached as such, by both the doctor and the patient. Recovery can take six weeks or longer.

It has been estimated that four out of five hysterectomies may be unnecessary. Women with abnormal uterine bleeding, fibroid tumors, and other gynecologic conditions should investigate alternatives to hysterectomy, always following the best available medical advice.

Male Sexuality and Aging

Most men are capable of having intercourse, and fathering children, throughout their lives. Aging can reduce some physical capacity in sexual performance, but the vast majority of men remain sexually capable through old age.

Physical problems that can be encountered, however, involve testicular failure and testicular cancer.

Testicular cancer is relatively rare, affecting less than 2 percent of the adult male population with cancer. Symptoms include include a lump in the the testicle, swelling, and some alteration in the consistency of the affected testicle. The symptoms may also include dull aching from the lower abdomen, groin, or scrotum. Men should do a monthly physical check for lumps, because testicular cancer, when caught early, has a very high survival rate. If left unchecked until the yearly physical, the cancer has a chance to spread.

Testicular failure is when the body shuts off the functions of the testes. This may be caused by hormonal deficiency and can be cured through hormonal replacement therapy. Since hormonal therapy can lead to prostate problems, it is recommended that a physician closely monitor any medication for testicular failure.

Vasectomy

Vasectomy is the sterilization of the male by cutting the vas deferens, which are the tubes that transport the sperm. The surgery is normally performed in the doctor's office with local anesthesia. Incisions are made either on each side of the scrotum or on the center of the scrotum. The tubes are then cut, and tied or cauterized on each end.

Vasovasotomy is the surgical procedure that attempts to reconnect the vas deferens after a vasectomy. This operation is done for men wishing to reverse the surgical sterilization. Success at this procedure can vary from 30 to 75 percent, depending on the skill of the surgeon and the type of initial sterilization procedures.

Drugs, Chemicals, and Alcohol

Most substances consumed in excess cause temporary problems at the least, and permanent damage to your health at the worst. As you age your body is less and less able to tolerate excesses. An additional problem is that the effects of over-indulgence accumulate during your lifetime. This accumulation can increase your chances for such health problems as cancer, cirrhosis (a liver disease), and heart disease. Use of tobacco products, alcohol, caffeine, and other chemicals can have both short-term and long-term effects.

- Cigarettes and other tobacco products contain a substance called nicotine that experts now recognize to be an addictive drug. Cigarette and cigar smoke also contain at least 40 known carcinogens (cancer-causing agents). Continued use of a tobacco product has a cumulative effect on your body. For example, your body becomes less able to remove carcinogens. The delicate tissues of the kidneys, liver, lungs, or other vital organs can become damaged. You increase your chances of developing lung cancer or cardiovascular disease. Some damage may be reversed if you break your habit. Other effects, however, may be permanent. By using a tobacco product, you risk scarring tissue, developing cancer, and premature death.
- Binge drinking or drug taking puts you at risk for an overdose, which causes major trauma to the body and can result in death. Binging on cigarettes, food, or caffeine may not result in such an immediate response, but the short-term damage to your body can be substantial.

Nicotine

Nicotine is both psychologically and physically addictive. When you smoke, nicotine enters your body through the membranes of your mouth, throat, lungs, and related areas. When you chew tobacco, nicotine enters your body through the membranes of your mouth. When the nicotine reaches your brain, it produces feelings of pleasure, satisfaction, calm, or alertness. As you repeatedly expose your body to nicotine, you become used to having a certain amount every day.

Although the nicotine habit is hard to break, there are many benefits to doing so. Lung cancer, which is primarily caused by smoking, kills about 160,000 Americans a year. People with lung cancer have only a 14 percent survival rate for living five years after diagnosis, even with treatment. In addition, cigarette smoking is believed to be a major cause of *emphysema* (a disease that decreases efficiency of the lungs), which kills more than 15,000 people a year. Approximately 100,000 smokers die from heart attacks each year. According to the American Cancer Society, however, breathing becomes easier and coughing decreases one to nine months after you quit smoking. Five years after you quit, your chance of developing lung cancer decreases by 50 percent. After 15 years of not smoking, your chance of developing cardiovascular disease, which can cause a heart attack, is not much greater than that of someone who has not smoked.

It is therefore important to stop smoking. Today there are several methods to help you quit.

The *nicotine patch* is a bandage-shaped patch that is placed on the skin each day. Nicotine on the patch is absorbed through the skin. The patches are used in a series that contains less and less nicotine, allowing you to wean yourself from the drug. Patches are available over-the-counter or through prescription.

Nicotine gum is a gum that, when chewed, releases nicotine into the body through the mouth. A chewing pattern must be followed when using nicotine gum. It is chewed slowly until a peppery taste comes out. It is then placed between the cheek and gums until this taste disappears. Then the gum is discarded. Most people chew about 10 pieces a day. The gum is available over-the-counter.

Nicotine nasal spray is a spray containing nicotine that you inhale through your nose. The nicotine is absorbed into your body through your nasal lining. This product is available only through prescription.

The *nicotine inhaler* is composed of a mouthpiece and a plastic cartridge containing nicotine. When you use the inhaler, you release nicotine into your mouth and throat. This product is available only through prescription.

Pills containing bupropion hydrochloride (marketed under the name Zyban) are also available. Zyban contains no nicotine. Medication in the pill is absorbed into the body through the digestive system. Experts believe the medicine works by raising levels of certain chemicals in the brain. This increase causes a person to feel good and experience decreased nicotine cravings. These pills are available only through prescription.

When using any of the medical products described here, it is important not to smoke or chew tobacco. This is necessary to avoid having an overdose of nicotine. Also, if you have such medical problems as high blood pressure, you should consult with your doctor before using any type of stop-smoking aid. Women who are pregnant or breast-feeding should also consult with their physicians before using any of the stop-smoking aids, even those available over the counter.

Caffeine

Experts believe that caffeine works on the central nervous system: fatigue and drowsiness fade while mental activities quicken. Too much caffeine, however, can produce headaches, irritability, and confusion. Some experts also believe that postmenopausal women who get little calcium and consume a large amount of caffeine may increase their risk of bone loss.

Caffeine is found both in foods and beverages. Tea leaves have almost twice as much caffeine as an equal weight of coffee. However, the amount of caffeine in a cup of tea is less than that in a cup of coffee because the amount of tea leaves used is relatively small. Coffee, colas, and chocolate are other popular items containing caffeine. Consult with your physician if caffeine consumption is a problem for you. If you find that you need a caffeine beverage to keep going, you might be better off taking a rest instead.

Alcohol

Studies in recent years have shown that the moderate use of alcohol can have some surprising benefits. Experts still agree, however, that there are no health benefits to heavy drinking, binge drinking, or alcoholism. (For a discussion of alcoholism, see the section "Alcohol Abuse" in Ch. 29, *Substance Abuse*.) Moderate drinking in middle age means no more than one drink per day for a woman, two per day for a man. By the time people reach their mid-60's, their daily intake of alcohol should decrease from these levels. A drink is defined as 12 ounces of beer or 5 ounces of wine or 1½ ounces of 80-proof liquor.

Studies indicate that the potential benefits of moderate drinking are a lowered risk of developing heart disease, a lowered risk of developing diabetes, a higher level of HDL cholesterol (the "good" cholesterol), and a lower risk of developing dangerous blood clots. Not everyone, however, may benefit from moderate drinking. For example, there are indications that such drinking may increase a woman's risk of developing breast cancer. There is also the possibility that drinking may increase the chance for cancers of the mouth, throat, or liver for both men and women.

Other factors, such as your medical history and medications that you take, may also influence the amount of benefit you receive from moderate drinking. It is important, therefore, to discuss the health benefits of drinking with your doctor who will know your individualized needs. It is not generally recommended that someone *start* drinking for health reasons.

Alcohol and Responsibility

Alcohol in any amount will affect your body, decreasing your ability to concentrate, your coordination, and your ability to react quickly. Remember, it is *never* safe to drink and drive. If you are at a party, meeting, luncheon, or other gathering where alcohol is offered but you do not wish to drink, there are a number of ways to politely pass up alcohol. Say "no thanks" if you do not want an alcoholic beverage. There should be plenty of other beverage options, such as juices, soda pops, or mineral waters. There is nothing socially improper about not drinking alcohol. You may also consider volunteering to be the designated driver. Designated drivers agree before a party or other gathering not to have any alcoholic drinks so that they then are able to safely drive others home. Alcohol is high in calories, and dieters may wish to avoid it. Whatever your reason, however, never allow yourself to be pressured into drinking when you do not want to.

Hangovers

Alcohol is toxic and is deadly in large quantities. It is not unheard of for people to die of alcohol poisoning after they have ingested too much. Blacking out, passing out, vomiting, and headache are all signs of having overindulged in alcohol. A hangover is the unpleasant feeling you may experience after you have had too much alcohol. Hangovers are characterized by such symptoms as headache, dry mouth, and upset stomach. Although there are numerous suggestions to speed recovery from a hangover—such as drinking warm broths, eating sugary foods, or having cup after cup of coffee—these quick fixes are not effective. Medicines, such as antacids and pain relievers, and vitamins, such as C and B-complex, may relieve symptoms, but there is no cure for a hangover. Your body needs time to recover.

Proper diet

Proper diet is an important contribution an individual can make to his good health, because foods build body tissues and provide energy for the body to work. Adequate diet planning is not difficult. The basic rules of good nutrition must be learned. See Ch. 27, *Nutrition and Weight Control,* for a full treatment of diet and nutrition. Applying these rules to a daily diet will take only a few minutes of planning when the menu is decided upon, and will reap enormous rewards in good health and appearance. The hardest part of planning a balanced diet is to avoid selecting food solely on the basis of taste or convenience and ignoring nutritional value.

Vitamins

Optimal vitamin intake is essential for good health. Besides protecting against vitamin deficiency disorders such as scurvy and pellagra, research indicates that adequate vitamin intake can also protect against such chronic illnesses as osteoporosis, cancer, and heart disease. Eating a proper, balanced diet should fulfill vitamin and other nutritional requirements. Unfortunately, most people do not eat enough of the nutritious foods they need to satisfy these requirements. For that reason, it is recommended that all adults take a multivitamin pill daily.

Breakfast

Many Americans do not eat breakfast, an important contribution to good diet. Studies prove that men, women, and children need an adequate breakfast. A good breakfast can provide a start in meeting the day's vitamin and mineral requirements. Studies show that people who eat a good breakfast are more alert and productive than those who skip breakfast. Eating breakfast also boosts the body's metabolism, thus helping the body to burn calories more efficiently throughout the day.

Weight and Health

Overweight is one of the biggest deterrents to successful middle age and is one of the greatest threats to health and longevity. As one physician said, "Consider how few really obese persons you see over 60 years of age." Unfortunately, in middle age most of us maintain the eating habits of our youth while we cut down on our exercise. The result: added weight that acts as a deterrent to our physical well-being.

The overweight person is more likely to develop arthritis, diabetes, heart disease, high blood pressure, kidney trouble, and many other disabling or fatal disorders.

As reported in *Nation's Business,* "If you are overweight by 10 percent, your chances of surviving the next 20 years are 15 percent less than if you had ideal weight; if you are 20 percent overweight, your chances are 25 percent less; if you are 30 percent overweight, 45 percent less." In other words, the odds are against the overweight person.

If you do not know what your ideal weight should be, a physician can tell you. To check yourself, try the "pinch" test. Take a pinch of skin on your upper arm just below the shoulder. If more than a half-inch separates your fingers, you might be overweight. Try the same test on your stomach when you're standing erect. Your mirror can also reveal the telltale signs of middle-age fat—the double chin, sagging belly, flabby arms and legs.

Good Eating Habits

Is there any magic way to reduce? The only sure way is to *eat less,* and to continue this practice all the time. It will not help if you go on a crash diet and then resume your normal eating habits. And while exercise will help control weight and burn up excess calories, probably the best exercise is to push yourself away from the table before you've overeaten.

Calories do count, and usually the caloric intake of a person in the 40- to 55-year age bracket should be about one-third less than that of a person between ages 25 and 40. Again, your physician or a good calorie-counter can help you determine what to eat and how much.

Here are some additional tips from nutritionists to help you lose weight:

- *Cut down on quantity.* Eat just enough to satisfy your appetite—not as much as you can. Even low-calorie foods will add weight if you eat enough of them.

- *Eat less more often.* Spread your food intake over several meals or snacks. Some hospitals have been experimenting with five meals a day, spreading the recommended total food intake over two full meals a day (brunch and dinner) and three snacks (continental breakfast, afternoon snack, and before-bedtime). They find that the stomach handles small amounts of food better, that metabolism keeps working at a good pace all day, and that blood sugar levels (your energy reserve) do not drop between meals. Also, the process of digestion burns up calories.

- *Avoid high-calorie foods.* Cut out breads, rolls, jellies, jams, sauces, gravies, dressings, creams, and rich desserts. These are the villains that add calories and are not as rich in nutrients.

- *Look for natural flavors.* Cultivate an interest in the natural flavor of what you eat. Try vegetables without butter, coffee and tea without cream and sugar. You might want to substitute a pinch of salt or a squeeze of lemon on your vegetables or noncaloric sweeteners in your beverages, but chances are you will find the natural flavors new and interesting.

- *Serve only just enough.* Keep portions small and put serving dishes with leftovers out of sight. Taking seconds is often just a habit. Cultivate the idea of just one serving, and you will find it satisfies the appetite. Another idea: serve meals on smaller plates. the portion will look big if only in relationship to the size of the plate.

In order to maintain a healthy body and a youthful appearance while dieting, you must make sure you eat the necessary proteins and nutrients. This can be done by selecting a healthful variety of foods. See Ch. 27, *Nutrition and Weight Control.*

As a panel of experts on middle age has said: "Two factors are vital to successful middle age: physical activity and a variety of interests. Move around but don't rush around. Keep an open mind and a closed refrigerator. Remember that variety is more than the spice of life—it's the wellspring of life. The person who pursues a variety of activities will usually stay fit long after middle age."

Living Life to the Fullest

No wise man ever wished to be younger. —Jonathan Swift

Staying young is looked on by most of the rest of the world as a peculiarly American obsession. This obsession is certainly fostered and exploited by the advertising industry, but its causes have to be looked for elsewhere.

In many countries, it is the old who are venerated for their wisdom and authority. This point of view is likely to prevail in societies that stay the same or that enjoyed their greatest glories in the past.

The United States is another matter. It is a yound country with a relatively short history. It is also a nation built on the idea of progress and hope in the future. And to whom does the future belong if not to youth?

Keeping up with change is unfortunately identified by too many people with how they look rather than how they think or feel. To be young in heart and spirit has very little to do with wearing the latest style in clothes—no matter how unbecoming—or learning the latest dances. Maintaining an open mind receptive to new ideas, keeping the capacity for pleasure in the details of daily living, refusing to be overwhelmed by essentially unimportant irritations can make the middle years more joyful for any family.

A Critical Time

Nowadays, the average American can expect to reach the age of 70. Thus, for most people, the middle years begin during the late 30s. Ideally, these are the years of personal fulfillment accompanied by a feeling of pride in accomplishment, a deeper knowledge of one's strengths and limitations, and a growing understanding and tolerance of other people's ideas and behavior.

Emotional Pressures

In many families, however, the pleasures of maturity often go hand in hand with increased pressures. It's no simple matter for the typical husband and wife in their 40s to maintain emotional health while handling worries about money, aging parents, anxiety about willful teenagers, tensions caused by marital friction, and feelings of depression about getting older. To some people, the problems of the middle years are so burdensome that instead of dealing with them realistically—by eliminating some, by compromising in the solution of others—they escape into excessive drinking or into sexual infidelity. It doesn't take much thought to realize that those escapes do nothing except introduce new problems.

Physical Symptoms of Emotional Problems

For others, deep-seated conflicts that come to a head during the middle years may be expressed in chronic physical symptoms. Many physicians in the past intuitively understood the relationship between emotional and physical health, but it is only in recent years that medical science has proved that feelings of tension, anxiety, suppressed anger, and frustration are often the direct cause of ulcers, sexual impotence, high blood pressure, and heart attacks, not to mention sleeplessness and headaches.

Of course, there are no magic formulas that guarantee the achievement of emotional well-being at any time of life. Nor does any sensible person expect to find a perfect solution to any human problem. However, it is possible to come to grips with specific difficulties and deal with them in ways that can reduce stress and safeguard emotional health.

Sexuality during the Middle Years

In spite of the so-called sexual revolution and all its accompanying publicity, it is still very difficult for most people to sort out their attitudes towards sexual activity. It is a subject that continues to be clouded by feelings of guilt and anxiety, surrounded by taboos, and saddled with misinformation. For each individual, the subject is additionally complicated by personal concepts of love and morality.

Many people were shocked when the Kinsey reports on male and female sexual behavior appeared. More recently, militant efforts have been made in various communities to prevent the schools from including sex education in their courses of study. Yet marriage counselors, family physicians, ministers, and all other specialists in human relations can attest to the amount of human misery caused by ignorance about sex—all the way from the ignorance that results in a 15-year-old's unwanted pregnancy to the ignorance of a 50-year-old man about his wife's sexual needs.

Sexuality After Menopause

Sexual relations between partners can continue throughout the life of the marriage. There is no reason that a person cannot remain sexually active, barring medical complications, for one's entire life.

Sexual function will change with aging. It takes longer for a man to obtain an erection and it takes longer to achieve orgasm for both partners. Women may suffer from thinning and drying of the vaginal walls following menopause, but the difficulties that this may cause are easily remedied. Lubricants that are water-based (unlike petroleum jelly, which is oil-based) can be used to replace natural lubricants. If it takes longer to arouse one partner, then set aside a little more time for romance.

It may be easier for the couple to enjoy lovemaking in the morning, after a good night's rest, rather than the end of the evening when they both may be tired. Since it is likely that there will be no children in the house to interrupt, couples may find that there is a renewed interest in sex, because of a new-found freedom that comes with having grown children and having no fear of an unplanned pregnancy.

There are circumstances, though, that may arrive that hinder or block sexual relations. These are discussed in brief here.

Problems with Sexual Activity

Occasional problems with sexual drive or capabilities are normal. Most people will experience some fluctuation during their lifetime. If a problem persists beyond a few weeks, or if any pain is associated with sexual intercourse, you should consult with your doctor. Although the causes may be psychological, it is best that you do not draw this conclusion without speaking with a medical expert first. Some of the problems that may be experienced follow.

Impotence

Impotence, or *erectile dysfunction,* is defined as a lack of an adequate erection necessary to complete intercourse. Physical factors, rather than psychological factors, are the origin of most cases of impotence.

Physical causes of impotence include diseases such as diabetes, kidney disease, hypertension, alcoholism, and multiple sclerosis. These diseases can cause physical damage to the body, leading to impotence. Surgeries for prostate, bladder or rectal cancer may sometimes cause impotence. Spinal cord injuries and injuries to the pelvic area can also cause impotence. Impotence is also an unfortunate side effect of many medications, such as antidepressants, tranquilizers, antihistamines, and high blood pressure medicine.

Psychological causes include guilt, stress, and anxiety in any area of a man's life; fatigue; diminished self-esteem; depression; and fear of sexual inadequacy.

Although physical factors cause most cases of impotence, psychological factors are often present. This is usually due to the man's reaction to the physical cause of his impotence.

Diagnosis

Your doctor will ask about your medical history and when the impotence began. The first step will likely be a physical exam followed by blood tests.

To distinguish between psychological causes and physical causes, your doctor may have you take one of the following three tests, which operate on the accepted medical principle that most men have approximately 3 to 5 erections during every sleep period. In what is called the *stamp test,* a strip of stamps is wrapped around the penis before the subject retires for the night. The strip tears along one of the perforated edges if the subject experiences an erection while sleeping.

Two other tests are more reliable. In one, a *snap gauge band* is wrapped around the penis; the band has snaps designed to open at various stages of penile rigidity. A third test utilizes an electronic monitor to tell exactly when erections occur, with what rigidity, and for how long. Two circular elastic silicone bands are attached to the penis; sensor wires connect the bands to an apparatus similar to an electrocardiograph machine.

Treatment

Counseling is often used to treat impotence stemming from psychological reasons. Common interventions include talking with the therapist and your partner regarding sexual expectations, and learning techniques that help decrease any apprehension associated with sexual intercourse.

Drugs to combat impotence can be taken orally or injected into the body. Alprostadil can be injected into the penis or inserted into the urethra in the form of a tiny pellet. Alprostadil usually produces an erection within 20 minutes that may last for an hour.

Perhaps the most well-known anti-impotence drug is sildenafil, or Viagra. It is taken orally up to one hour before sexual activity and works by enhancing response to sexual stimulation. Unlike drugs administered by injection, which trigger an uncontrolled erection, Viagra provides the man an opportunity to achieve an erection in response to sexual stimulation.

Testosterone replacement therapy may help to reduce impotence in men whose levels of natural testosterone are low.

Vacuum devices are another treatment option. These devices create a vacuum aroung the penis, which causes blood to be drawn into the penis, producing an erection.

Surgery to repair damage to the penis is done in instances where the blood flow to the penis has been blocked. The long-term effectiveness of this procedure is unclear.

When other treatment options fail, surgically implanted prostheses (penile implants) may be considered. One implant, made of flexible, plastic-covered metal wire, maintains the penis in a constantly erect state but can be bent into an erect or downward position. A second type works hydraulically to pump the penis into a naturally erect state. Two expandable metal tubes implanted in the penis function with an attached tiny pump in the scrotum and a water reservoir placed behind the muscles of the lower abdomen. Pressure on the pump causes the penis to become erect; valves make possible penile relaxation.

Self-Image Problems

If you do not believe yourself to be physically appealing, it is possible that you may regard a partner with suspicion and hostility if he or she finds you physically appealing. You may be willing to perceive insult and ill-intent where none is meant if you do not believe yourself to be a desirable partner.

Self-image is one of the most important aspects of sexuality. Believing that one is too old, too fat, too thin, or too wrinkly can be a huge obstacle to a satisfying sex life. Self-image is estimated to be a problem for half of the male population and the majority of the female population. One cannot change the view others have of beauty, but one can improve a self-image. This may require counseling, but it is worth the effort, because the ability to be happy rests with the ability to be happy with oneself.

Sexual Activity and Disability

Disabilities, whether the result of genetics, disease, accident, or aging, need not be a complete barrier to sexual satisfaction. Most disabilities allow some form of sexual gratification, and with an understanding partner, this can be worked out. Counseling and training may be needed to develop the emotional support and understanding necessary to achieve a fulfilling relationship with your partner, but if both are willing participants in the learning process, this can be achieved. Talk with your physician or a therapist specializing in disabilities about your situation. If they cannot provide guidance, they can direct you to someone who can.

Coping With Retirement

As the average age of men and women extend into the seventies, the number of years spent in retirement increases. These years can be fulfilling and exciting, or they can pass slowly, with little to look forward to. It is important that people consider their retirement before they get to it. If they have not done so and find themselves at retirement age, it is important that they set goals and prioritize regarding how they will spend their days.

Preparation for Retirement

The single biggest concern to most retirees is their financial condition. With Social Security under constant scrutiny by the government, it is important that everyone consider sources of money they can count on other than the Social Security program.

Start planning for your retirement by figuring out *exactly* what money you will have coming in, and when, for your retirement. Questions you will need to investigate include:

- What are you and your spouse's pension benefits from work?
- How are these benefits affected by the death of the spouse, before and after retirement age?
- What are you scheduled to receive from Social Security?
- What are your savings and other benefits worth?
- What other sources of income will be available to you after retirement?

You should fill in the *Request for Earnings and Benefit Statement* form SSA-7004 every three years to insure that the government records of your earnings are accurate. They are only obliged to correct your records for the previous three years. This also keeps you informed of what you are entitled to for your income credits. The form is available through all Social Security offices.

You should also be aware that the age of retirement for Social Security is no longer strictly held at 65 years of age. For people born between 1954 and 1960, the age is 66. For those born in 1960 and after, the age is 67. There is a reduction of payments related to your age, if you retire early.

Once you have figured out what money you have coming in, you need to do a budget for what you will be spending after retirement. This is tricky since inflation and property-cost fluctuations can be hard to predict. However, it is better to guess than to just ignore this step.

You need to figure out basic expenses, and then extra expenses and perks. If you would love to sail around the world, don't just assume you can't do it. Calculate it into your retirement needs and see if you can save enough now with investments to allow for your dreams.

Basic expenses should include as a minimum:

- Property and income taxes
- House repairs, rent, and other living quarter expenses
- Medical insurance and expenses
- Food, clothing, and day-to-day purchases
- Expenses remaining for children (college, etc.)
- Emergency income for nursing homes, catastrophic illness or other incapacitating problems
- General entertainment and activity costs

Once these are down on paper, discuss what your goals and ambitions are for the years ahead. Budget in those expenses. Some possibilities include, but certainly are not limited to:

- returning to school
- traveling
- pursuing a hobby
- moving to another climate
- starting another career or business

Assume that you will live to at least 95. This way you likely to have enough for the majority of your retirement. You are better off overpredicting, rather than underpredicting, your age at death.

Calculate your expenses for the total of the thirty years. You can set inflation at 5 or higher, or use a guide to retirement earnings. Then figure out what you will have as income when you retire. If you have enough saved, and enough pension to provide for all your needs, then you are set for retirement. If not, you need to calculate what you have still to save.

There are several guides available for a more exact method of predicting costs and savings. AARP is an organization that can guide you to sources. Their address is: 601 E Street, NW, Washington, DC 20049; (888) 687-2277.

When to Retire

Once you have figured out your financial needs and earnings for retirement, you can estimate how many years you have saved for, and how many years you still need to work to gain enough income to provide for retirement. If you can afford early retirement, and you have activities that would fulfill you, it should be considered as an option. If you find that you have to continue working beyond the time you had assumed for retirement, you may be able to manage with fewer hours or a job with less pressure without influencing your pension.

Beyond Retirement

Once you have the finances figured out for your retirement (or if you have retired), you need to figure out how you are going to spend your time. These years can be the most rewarding and exciting of your life. There are literally hundreds of ways for you to spend your time. If you are thoughtful about your retirement planning, you may find that you still don't have enough time in the day to do everything that you want.

Volunteer Work

Volunteer work can be one of the most rewarding ways to spend your time. Depending on your community, there will be a variety of places that are happy to train and utilize volunteers in different positions. Depending on your personal needs, volunteer positions can range from basic tasks—such as greeting visitors, assisting patients in reading, or escorting people—to jobs that resemble working positions, such as accounting, staff management, and teaching. You can select what you want to do with the level of effort you are interested in putting in. You can do more than one volunteer position to fill different needs. You may want to work one or two days with children, and then take on a more pressured, or less pressured, position elsewhere for another day of activity. You should research and ask around about the organizations that take volunteers.

Most arts organizations, museums, zoos, hospitals, schools, day care centers, and nonprofit organizations rely on their volunteers for many jobs.

Community Activism

You may be interested in pursuing your volunteer work in another arena entirely. Political and social activism is based on volunteer support. That support is both financial- and assistance-based. You are in a position, once you retire, to take your expertise to an organization that fights for the positions you support and believe in. If no organization exists in the area you want to dedicate your time, then start one. Chances are good that if you are interested in something, others in the community are also interested. This resolves two potential problems in retirement: lack of activity and social contact. You will meet people with similar interests by participating in community organizations.

Home Management

Once you have retired, you will probably be spending a few more hours, at least, in your home. This is when the dripping faucet, the faded carpet, and the stained walls will become more annoying. Do not take on more repair work than you can manage physically or financially. Plan repairs and redecorating to accommodate your time and your budget. Overhauling your home may be a goal, but it should be planned as such and not decided on impulsively. The stress of remodeling and renovating should be taken into account with your physical health.

Children Leaving Home

One of the major turning points in many adults' lives is when their children grow up and leave the house. Children usually move out of their parents' house, for at least part of the year, between the ages of 18 and 21. The majority of children leave their parents' house sometime in their twenties.

For many families, this shift from full-time caregiver for a child to parent of independent adults is a difficult one. Regardless of the continued contact through visits and calls, the fact that their child no longer lives with them may be difficult for the parent to adjust to. It may also be difficult for the child to adjust to this change; transition to adulthood can be rocky.

Once the children are off on their own, parents may find themselves with a sense of loss, lack of purpose, or anxiety. All of this may be attributed to the last child moving out, or it may be to a combination of events, such as a child leaving and a sixtieth birthday. If you or your spouse experience any prolonged or severe bouts of depression, it is important to consult with a therapist, even if you are sure you recognize the source of the depression. Recovering from the depression is what you should be working toward.

Many parents, however, find the empty home an enjoyable change. After adapting to the new patterns of living without children, they find that the respite from caring for others can be exhilarating. For some parents, this may be the first time in two decades when their days are completely their own to decide. They find they have the opportunity to put themselves first. Although there may be some residual guilt about self-indulgence, it generally passes quickly. This is the opportunity to nurture and care for yourself and your spouse as you have cared for your children. And, as any parent will attest, your children will continue to provide you with parenting concerns for the rest of your life.

Your biggest consideration during this transition should be your emotional and mental state. As with any major life change, this period of transition may create stress, mood changes, and susceptibility to depression. If you experience any of the warning signs of depression (lethargy, prolonged sadness, changes in appetite, or insomnia or excessive sleeping are some of the signs), please contact your physician or therapist.

Separation and Divorce

Marriage in this country is based on the highly personal concept of love rather than on such historical foundations as a property merger between two families or an arrangement determined by the friendship of the young people's parents. It is often assumed, therefore, that if mutual love is the basis for embarking on a marriage, its absence is a valid reason for dissolving it, either by legal separation or divorce.

The idea of divorce is not particularly modern; in practically every time and place where a form of marriage has existed, so has some form of divorce, with reasons for it that range from physical abuse to failure to deliver a piece of land mentioned in the marriage contract.

Facts About Divorce

Statistics indicate that in the United States as a whole, almost half of all marriages end in divorce. However, these figures by no means indicate that the family as an institution is on the way out, because most people who get divorced will marry again.

There are many reasons for the high rate of separation and divorce:

- Over the last 50 years, a large percentage of the population has been getting married.
- Although the trend toward earlier marriages has leveled off in recent years, a significant number of people still marry at earlier ages than was common in the past. (The divorce rate is highest among poorly educated groups who married before the age of 21.)
- The legal requirements for separation and divorce are less rigid than before. No-fault divorces are now allowed in most states.
- With increased independence and earning capacity, women are less frightened of the prospect of heading a family than they may have been in the past.

Other facts about divorce:

- Most first marriages that end in divorce last an average of 7 to 8 years.
- College graduates are more likely to marry and less likely to divorce than high school graduates and people with less than a high school education.

Telling Children the Truth

Many parents who are contemplating a breakup of their marriage generally make every effort to seek professional guidance that might help them iron out their differences. When these efforts fail and steps are taken to arrange for a separation or divorce, it is far healthier for parents to be honest with each other and with their children than to construct elaborate explanations based on lies.

A teenager who is given the real reason for a divorce is less likely to brood about it than one who is told lies that he can see through. If the real reason for a divorce is that the parents have tried their best to get along with each other but find it impossible, the child who is in his teens or older will most likely understand this. If the marriage is ending because the husband or wife wants to marry someone else, the explanation given to the child should avoid assigning blame. When the rejected parent tries to enlist the child's sympathy by blackening the character of the parent who is supposedly the cause of the divorce, the results are almost always unpleasant. Under no circumstances and no matter what the child's age should he be called on to take the side of either parent or to act as a judge.

In addition, children should not be told any more about the circumstances of the breakup of their parents' marriage than they really want to know. Young people have a healthy way of protecting themselves from information they would find hurtful, and if they ask few questions, they need be told only the facts they are prepared to cope with. Of course, as they grow older and live through their own problems, they will form their own view of what really happened between their parents.

After the Separation

Traditionally, in separation and divorce proceedings, the children have remained in the custody of the mother, with financial support arrangements and visiting rights spelled out for the father. Although an increasing number of fathers have been awarded custody of their children in recent years, it is still commonly the mother who must face the problems of single parenthood after divorce. Although teenage children may need some extra attention for a while, there is no need for a mother to make a martyr of herself, nor should she feel guilty when she begins to consider remarrying.

The father should be completely reliable in his visiting arrangements, and if he has remarried, should try to establish good relationships between the offspring of his former marriage and his new family.

Losing a Spouse

As you and your spouse get older, you should begin to prepare for the fact that one of you will probably survive the other. This can be the most difficult challenge you face. Having a spouse or a child die can be the most strenuous and difficult parts of life. It can occur at any time during adulthood. Widows and widowers are not just people in their 70s and 80s. One can lose a spouse at 21 or 41 and experience the same sense of loss and confusion.

Depending on the preparations made before the spouse dies, the concerns of the surviving spouse may range from mourning and adjusting to single life to attempting to arrange financial support, dividing inheritance, and struggling to sort through all the legal and financial matters that may be left by the deceased.

Preparing a will is one of the things you can do in preparation for your own and your spouse's death. You cannot assume that everything will be easily handled if you die and your spouse is surviving. Wills provide some legal assistance to the surviving spouse to sort through finances during the difficult times that follow the spouse's death.

It is important for anyone, of any age, to maintain a strong support group of friends and family. Without this, any change in one's life will be confronted alone. With a strong group of supporters, almost any tragedy can be weathered. Meeting people and making friends can be a difficult thing to do. By joining clubs, support groups, and organizations, you are reaching out to people with similar backgrounds or interests. It is likely that you will be able to establish some contacts through such activities. You and your spouse may wish to pursue this together, or you may each seek out friends of your own interest. If you have relocated or do not, for whatever reason, have a circle of friends you can turn to, it is important to establish one. It makes the transition to widowhood easier if your support group is in place.

If you have already lost a spouse and have not prepared for it, you can still seek out a support group in your community. This may be found in churches and synagogues, community centers, and in local organizations. As explained before, it is important to watch for any warning signs of serious depression and seek professional counseling immediately if any are experienced.

Loss of a Parent

The loss of a parent may affect your family when you or your partner lose a parent, or when you lose a spouse and your children have lost a parent.

It is important to work through the mourning period. Some people respond to death by attempting to plow through the time, as if unscathed by the event. Others shut down entirely and refuse consolation or assistance in coping. Neither response may be in the best interest of the mourner.

Coping with death is a personal experience. Each individual will respond uniquely to a loss of a family member. And each individual may respond differently to different losses. Mourning one's parent will be different than mourning one's spouse. It is important for everyone to remember this when adjusting to a death in the family.

The mourning period can range from several days to several months. There is no correct period of time to spend in mourning. If you are not comfortable with the amount of time you are taking to get over the loss, then feel free to speak to someone about it. But there is no rule for how long you should spend mourning.

Any inability to function through day-to-day activities, such as eating, sleeping, bathing, grocery shopping, or other mundane events, should be taken as a sign of serious depression and not part of general mourning. You may not feel like socializing, but you should still have the energy to take good hygienic care of yourself. As always, any behavior that is threatening to life and health should be referred to professional counseling immediately. You should watch for such signs in yourself, your parents and your children after experiencing any family member's death.

6

The Later Years

Aging and What To Do About It

Growing older could mean growing healthier. In many ways you are as old as you think and feel. Consider these points:

- No disease results just from the passage of years.
- We age piecemeal—each organ separately rather than uniformly.
- In retirement you have less daily stress and strain, and you have more time to take care of yourself.

What, then, makes a person think and feel old?

The Aging Process

Physically, we mature at about 25 to 30, when the body reaches maximum size and strength. Then, body tissues and cells are constantly being rebuilt and renewed. Nutrition, rest, exercise, and stress influence the length of time that the body can maintain a balance between the wearing down and rebuilding of body tissues. When more cells die than can be reproduced, they are replaced by a fibrous, inert substance called *collagen*. The living process slows down to compensate, and we begin aging; strength and ability start to decline.

But this happens at various intervals. For instance, vision is sharpest at age 25; the eye loses its ability to make rapid adjustments in focus after age 40. Hearing is sharpest at about age 10, then diminishes as you grow older. Sensitivity to taste and smell lessens after age 60.

The decline in strength and muscle ability is long and gradual; there are even gratifying plateaus. At age 50, a man still has about four-fifths of the muscle strength he had when he was 25.

Although physical abilities may decline, mental abilities may actually improve during the middle years, and memory and the ability to learn can remain keen. Dr. Alfred Schwartz, dean of education at Drake University, was asked: "Can a 70-year-old man in reasonably good health learn as rapidly as a 17- year-old boy?" Dr. Schwartz answered:

> Indeed he can—provided he's in the habit of learning. The fact that some older people today are not active intellectually is no reflection on their ability to learn. There is ample proof that learning ability does not automatically decline with age.

Regardless of what you may have heard, organic brain damage affects less than one percent of those over age 65.

But in thinking about physical change, remember that this is just one aspect of aging. Age is determined by emotional and intellectual maturity as well as by chronological years.

Can a person do anything to retard aging?

Most *gerontologists* feel that the reason more people don't live longer is that they are not willing to follow a regimen of diet, exercise, rest, recreation—coupled with the exclusion of various excesses. And while there isn't anything you can do to set back the clock, you can keep in good health by making sure to have regular physical examinations, sufficient exercise, adequate rest, nutritious food, and a positive mental attitude.

A Positive Mental Attitude

Mark Twain once said: "Whatever a man's age he can reduce it several years by putting a bright-colored flower in his buttonhole." A lively, fresh outlook is essential for enjoyable living at any age. Most physicians believe there is a direct connection between one's state of mind and physical health. This is especially true when you are faced with the challenges of retirement. Plato said: "He who is of a calm and happy nature will hardly feel the pressure of age, but to him who is of an opposite disposition, youth and age are equally a burden."

Experts in the field of aging have found that most older people can relieve transitory depression by a deliberate shift of thought or by physical activity. If you look upon retirement as an opportunity to take better care of yourself and to pursue old and new interests, you'll go a long way toward better health.

The Annual Checkup

For peace of mind and to maintain and improve your health, make it a habit to see your physician at least once a year. To remind themselves, many people make an appointment on their birthday. An annual checkup is especially important in later years and should not be put off or neglected.

During a routine checkup, the physician pays special attention to enlarged lymph nodes of the neck, armpits, and groin, and the front of the neck. He or she also checks the condition of veins and arteries and looks at your knees and arches—which are of particular importance to older people.

The physician makes tests for arteriosclerosis, high blood pressure, diabetes, brain tumors, and other diseases. He can feel and tap your body to check your lungs, liver, and spleen, and he can take electrocardiographs to detect changes in your heart. Simple tests can note bladder and kidney conditions.

In addition, physicians usually ask about personal habits—smoking, drinking, eating. They also want to know about any unusual symptoms you might have. Be completely frank with your physician, answer his questions as directly as possible, and give all information that might be helpful.

When explaining the nature of your ailment or symptom, explain what part of the body is involved, what changes are associated with the symptoms, and whether symptoms occurred after a change of diet or medicine. Mention any previous experiences with this condition and what treatments you might have had.

It is extremely important to tell your physician about any pills you are taking—including aspirin, tranquilizers, and sleeping tablets. Even the most common drug can affect the potency of medication he might prescribe.

After your physician has taken your case history and has all the reports from your tests, he or she will want to talk with you, explain any findings, and perhaps make some recommendations.

If you have questions, don't be afraid to ask them. Ask about the nature of your ailment, how long it may take for relief or cure, how the therapy or medication is expected to work, and the possible impact on your everyday activities.

Hopefully, by following your physician's advice you'll stay healthy and well.However, if you are at home and feel ill, call your physician if:

- Your symptoms are so severe you can't endure them.
- Apparent minor symptoms persist without explainable cause.
- You are in doubt.

For more information, see "The Physical Examination" in Ch. 26, *Physicians and Diagnostic Procedures*.

Oral Health

It is especially important in later years to have regular dental checkups. After age 50, over half of the American people have some form of *periodontal disease*, and at age 65 nearly all persons have this disease.

Brushing teeth at least twice a day is a defense against periodontal disease. Use dental floss to remove all food particles and plaque from areas between the teeth, especially after each meal. See "Periodontal Disease" in Ch. 22, *The Teeth and Gums*, for more information on this subject.

Dentures

If you do lose some teeth, they should be replaced with bridges or partial or full dentures, because the cheeks and lips will otherwise sag and wrinkle and make you look older than you really are. Chewing ability and the clarity of speech are also impaired if missing teeth are not replaced. See "Dentures" in Ch. 22, *The Teeth and Gums.*

Diet and Health

Just what are your food requirements as you grow older? Basically you need the same essential nutrients that you have always needed, except that you face special problems. You need to:

- Select food more carefully to eat adequate proteins, vitamins, and minerals—while cutting down on calories.
- Get the most nutritious food for the least money and make the most of what you buy.
- Avoid bad eating habits—make mealtime a pleasure rather than a chore.
- Learn new techniques to stretch meals, use leftovers, and substitute lower-priced items with the same nutritional value for higher-priced foods. In other words, learn how to shop well.

Basic Requirements

How can you get the essential nutrients every day? A good rule is first to eat recommended servings from the Food Guide Pyramid (see below) established by the U.S. Department of Agriculture. Then, eat other foods that you like, as long as they do not go over the recommended daily caloric intake. Some older and sedentary adults require only 1,600 calories a day. For more active older adults, an intake of 2,200 calories is recommended, which is less than the 2,800 calories needed by teenage boys and active young adults. As you grow older, your physical activity decreases and your metabolism slows, causing body fats to build up and making you more prone to hardening of the arteries and certain heart conditions. Make sure you balance your eating with sufficient exercise. Use vitamin supplements as recommended by your physician.

Here is an explanation of the Food Guide Pyramid:

Bread, Cereal, Rice, and Pasta Group

Six to 11 servings from this group are recommended. Typical servings are a slice of bread, 1 ounce of dry cereal, and ½ cup of cooked cereal, rice, or pasta. These foods provide complex carbohydrates, a source of energy. These foods also supply vitamins, minerals, and fiber. Try to choose whole-wheat and whole-grain products, which have more fiber. Watch out for fat and sugar in the foods you buy, and limit high-calorie and high-fat spreads and condiments in serving them.

Vegetable Group

Three to five servings of vegetables daily are recommended. A serving is a cup of raw leafy vegetables, ½ cup of other vegetables, or ¾ cup of juice. Vegetables provide vitamins (such as A and C) and minerals (such as iron and magnesium). They are low in fat and provide fiber. Eat different types of vegetables—dark green and leafy (spinach, broccoli, dark lettuce), deep yellow (carrots, sweet potatoes), and starchy (potatoes, corn, peas). Also include legumes, such as chickpeas and beans. Legumes, high in protein, are also a good substitute for meat. Go easy on fats, such as butter, mayonnaise, and salad dressings.

Fruit Group

Two to four servings of fruit per day are suggested. A serving is a medium banana, apple, or orange; ½ cup of chopped fruit; or ¾ cup of juice. Fruits provide vitamins A and C and potassium and are low in fat and sodium. Choose whole fruits, which have more fiber, more often than juices. Choose fresh fruits and juices, and frozen, canned, or dried fruits. Limit or eliminate fruits packed or frozen in heavy syrup and juices that have added sugar. Include citrus fruits, melons, and berries, which have vitamin C. Be sure that your juice is 100 percent fruit juice, not stretched with sugary water. Fruit-flavored sodas, such as grape and orange, do not count.

Meat, Poultry, Fish, Dry Beans, Eggs, and Nuts Group

Two to three servings from this group are needed daily. These foods supply protein and nutrients such as B vitamins, iron, and zinc. You should have the equivalent of five to seven ounces of cooked lean meat, fish, or poultry. For example, two to three ounces of cooked lean meat or fish (about one medium chicken breast half or an average hamburger) is a serving. For the other foods in this group, count ½ cup of cooked dry beans, one egg, two tablespoons of peanut butter, or ⅓ cup of nuts as equivalent to an ounce of lean meat. Choose lean or skinless meat, dry beans and peas, and fish often. Trim away all visible fat on meat, and broil, roast, or boil instead of frying. Limit egg yolks; try substituting extra whites. Go easy on nuts and seeds, which are high in fat.

Milk, Yogurt, and Cheese Group

Two to three servings a day are recommended. Milk products provide protein, vitamins, and minerals, including important calcium. A serving is a cup of milk or yogurt (a cup of cottage chesse is only ½ a serving because of its lower calcium content), 1½ ounces of natural cheese, or 2 ounces of processed cheese. Choose low- and non-fat products often.

Eating Habits

If you find that mealtime is a chore rather than a pleasure, try these tips to enhance your meals:

- Drink a glass of water as soon as you wake up to promote good digestion, weight control, and bowel movements.
- Try a walk or light exercise to stimulate appetite and to regulate body processes. Moderate exercise also will help regulate weight.
- You might sip glass of wine before dinner. This can improve appetite and digestion. Port, a light sherry, and vermouth with a dash of soda are good appetite stimulators.
- Make meals interesting by including some food of distinctive flavor to contrast with a mild-flavored food; something crisp for contrast with softer foods, even if it is only a pickle or a lettuce leaf; some brightly colored food for eye appeal.
- Pep up your food with a judicious use of herbs and spices or flavor-enhancers like wine, bottled sauces, fruit juices, and peels.
- If some food causes you distress, eliminate it and substitute something else of equal nutritive value. Green salad may include too much roughage for the intestinal tract; ham or bacon may be supplying your body with too much salt, which increases water retention. Or you may be drinking too much coffee, tea, or soft drinks.
- Be realistic about your chewing ability. Food swallowed whole may be causing digestive problems. If your teeth are not as good as they were or if you are wearing dentures, try cubing, chopping, or grinding foods that are difficult to chew. Let your knife or meat grinder do part of the work.
- Try a different atmosphere or different setting for your meals. Use candlelight, music, and your best linen on occasion. Move outdoors when the weather is good; eat your lunch in the park and dinner on the patio.
- Occasionally invite a friend or relative to dine with you. It's surprising what stimulating conversation and an exchange of ideas can do to boost your mood and appetite.
- Try a new recipe or a new food. Thanks to modern transportation, foods are available in larger cities from many areas and other countries. Eat eggplant or okra, avocado or artichoke, gooseberry jam, or garbanzo beans in a salad. And why not have a papaya with lemon juice for breakfast?

Cooking Hints

Try these ideas for preparing food more easily; they are especially useful if you have only a single gas or electric burner:

- Combine your vegetables and meat—or some other protein food—in a single pot or pan. You can cook many hot, nourishing meals of this kind: Irish stew, braised liver or pot roast with vegetables, ham-and-vegetable chowder or fish chowder, a New England boiled dinner.
- Combine leftovers to make a one-dish meal. Leftover meat combines beautifully with vegetables, macaroni, or rice. Add a cheese or tomato sauce or a simple white sauce and heat in a baking dish. Chopped tomatoes or green onions or chives will give extra flavor and color to the dish.
- Round out one-dish meals with a crisp salad topped with cut strips of leftover cooked meat or poultry or another raw food, bread, a beverage, and perhaps a dessert.
- Mix leftover cooked vegetables with raw fresh ones, such as chopped celery, cucumber slices, tomatoes, green pepper, shredded cabbage, to make an interesting salad.
- Cream vegetables, meat, fish, or chicken. Or serve them with a tasty sauce. Use canned tomato or mushroom soup for a quick and easy sauce. If the dish is a bit skimpy, a hard-boiled egg may stretch it to serving size.
- Add a bit of relish, snappy cheese, or diced cucumber to a cooked dressing for meat or vegetable salad.
- If you cook a potato, an ear of corn, or some other vegetable in the bottom of a double boiler, you can use the top to warm rolls, heat leftover meat in gravy, or heat such foods as creamed eggs or fish.

The Value of Exercise

As you grow older, exercise can help you look, feel, and work better. Various organs and systems of the body, particularly the digestive process, are stimulated through activity, and, as a result, work more effectively.

You can improve your posture through exercise that tones supporting muscles. This not only improves appearance but can decrease the frequency of lower-back pain and disability.

Here are some other benefits of exercise: it can increase your ability to relax and tolerate fatigue; it improves muscle tone; reduces fat deposits; increases working capacity of the lungs; improves kidney and liver functions; increases volume of blood, hemoglobin, and red blood cells, leading to improved utilization of oxygen and iron.

Also, physically active people are less likely to experience a heart attack or other forms of cardiovascular disease than sedentary people. Moreover, an active person who does suffer a coronary attack will probably have a less severe form. The Public Health Service studied 5,000 adults in Framingham, Mass., for more than a decade. When any member of the group suffered a heart attack, his physical activity was reviewed. It was found that more inactive people suffered more fatal heart attacks than active members.

Walking for Exercise

Exercise need not be something you *must* do but rather something you *enjoy* doing. One of the most practical and enjoyable exercises is walking. Charles Dickens said:

> Walk and be happy, walk and be healthy. The best of all ways to lengthen our days is to walk, steadily and with a purpose. The wandering man knows of certain ancients, far gone in years, who have staved off infirmities and dissolution by earnest walking—hale fellows close upon eighty and ninety, but brisk as boys.

The benefits of walking were revealed in a recent Health Insurance Plan study of 110,000 people in New York City. Those who had heart attacks were divided into two groups—walkers and nonwalkers. The first four weeks of illness were reviewed for both groups. At the end of the time 41 percent of the nonwalkers were dead, while only 23 percent of the walkers were. When all physical activity was considered, 57 percent of the inactive had died compared to only 16 percent of those who had some form of exercise.

Walking is as natural to the human body as breathing. It is a muscular symphony; all the foot, leg, and hip muscles and much of the back musculature are involved. The abdominal muscles tend to contract and support their share of the weight, and the diaphragm and rib muscles increase their action. There is automatic action of the arm and shoulder muscles; the shoulder and neck muscles get play as the head is held erect; the eye muscles are exercised as you look about you.

Other Types of Exercise

Swimming and bicycling exercise most of the muscles, and gardening is highly recommended. The fresh air is beneficial, the bending, squatting, and countless other movements exercise most parts of the body.

Surprisingly, most games do not provide good exercise. According to a physical fitness research laboratory at the University of Illinois, the trouble with most games is that the action is intermittent—starting and stopping—a burst of energy and then a wait. The bowler swings a ball for two and one-half seconds and gets about one minute of actual muscular work per game. Golf is a succession of pause, swing, walk—or, more often, a ride to the next pause, swing, and so on. Also, you spend a lot of time standing and waiting for the party ahead and for your partners. Tennis gives one more exercise but it too involves a great deal of starting and stopping, as does handball. No game has the essential, tension-releasing pattern of continuous, vigorous, rhythmic motion found in such activities as walking, running, or jogging.

For formal exercises, you could join a gym, but you might find your enthusiasm waning after a few weeks. You could also exercise at home; there are many excellent books on exercise that provide programs for you to follow at home on a daily basis.

But everyone's exercise capacity varies. It is best to discuss any new exercise program with your physician, especially if you have some illness or are out of practice. Then select an exercise which is pleasant for you and suitable to your condition.

It is most important always to warm up before any strenuous exercise. The U.S. Administration on Aging's booklet, *The Fitness Challenge in the Later Years*, states:

> The enthusiast who tackles a keep fit program too fast and too strenuously soon gives up in discomfort, if not in injury. A warm-up period should be performed by starting lightly with a continuous rhythmical activity such as walking and gradually increasing the intensity until your pulse rate, breathing, and body temperature are elevated. It's also desirable to do some easy stretching, pulling, and rotating exercises during the warm-up period.

The booklet outlines an excellent program—*red* (easiest), *white* (next), and *blue* (the most sustained and difficult). Each program is "designed to give a balanced workout utilizing all major muscle groups."

A Word of Caution

You may be exercising too strenuously if the following happens:

- Your heart does not stop pounding within 10 minutes after the exercise.
- You cannot catch your breath 10 minutes after the exercise.
- You are shaky for more than 30 minutes afterwards.
- You can't sleep well afterwards.
- Your fatigue (not muscle soreness) continues into the next day.

Sensible, moderate exercise geared to your own physical capacity can help to give you a sense of all-around well-being. As Dr. Ernest Simonson, associate professor of physiological hygiene at the University of Minnesota Medical School, has said:

> Those who exercise regularly never fail to mention that it makes them feel better in every way. It's common logic if one feels better, his attitude towards others will be more congenial. When one is in a cordial, happy frame of mind, he will likely make wiser decisions, and his world in general will look better.

Weight Control

Importantly, both diet and exercise affect the individual's ability to control his weight (see Ch. 27, *Nutrition and Weight Control*; "Weight Problems" in Ch. 23, *Aches, Pains, Nuisances, Worries*; and Ch. 37, *Physical Fitness*). Healthy habits in both areas provide a complete answer for many older persons. For others, some additional effort is required.

The same diet rules that help the older person feel well and function adequately will make weight control simpler. But persons beyond middle age who have weight problems should make extra efforts to bring their weight down. Extra pounds of fat only make it harder for the vital organs to function; excess poundage also forces the heart to work harder. A variety of diets may be used to bring your weight back to where it should be. But the calorie-counter program may suffice for most persons.

Exercise provides the second key to weight control. Many physicians feel that older persons of both sexes should walk at least a mile daily. Other exercises acclaimed by physicians include golf, gardening, working on or around the house, and similar activities. Some other basic rules regarding exercise and diet should be noted:

- Avoid junk, or high carbohydrate, food where possible.
- Make certain you are eating foods that provide enough protein.
- Eat to assuage hunger, not to drive away boredom.
- Remember that appetite usually decreases with age, and act accordingly.
- Avoid vitamins unless they are prescribed by your physician, and use them accordingly.
- Try every day to eat foods in the four basic groups.
- Keep moving; walk daily—to the store, post office, church, around the block.
- If you exercise already, do it regularly; a little exercise daily is better than a lot on weekends.
- If you don't exercise but are thinking of starting a program of workouts of some kind, start slowly and build up—following your physician's recommendations.
- If stress gives you problems, find ways to relax without eating or drinking; consider light exercises, yoga, meditation, breathing exercises, or some other method.

Skin Problems

As a person grows older, his skin begins to wrinkle; oil and sweat glands slow down, causing the skin to become dry. Also, the skin may lack the elasticity and tone of normal skin, and this might cause changes in facial contours.

However, the skin, like other parts of the body, tends to age according to various factors. Among prime agers of the skin are exposure to sunlight and weather; the sailor and chronic sunbather may have older-looking skin than their years. Also, hereditary and racial factors influence skin age.

Itching

The skin often itches as one grows older. Itching usually stems from external irritations or internal diseases. External irritations may be more severe in winter because of lack of humidity and because the skin oil does not spread properly. Too many baths or wearing wool garments could also cause itching. You can correct this by cutting down on bathing, maintaining correct temperature and humidity, and applying skin creams.

If itching does not clear up in about two weeks, the trouble may be due to any of a number of internal diseases, some of them serious. Thus, it is wise to see your physician if itching persists.

Skin Cancer

Skin cancer can be easily diagnosed and treated. The two most common types are *basal cell* and *squamous cell.*

The basal cell type begins with a small fleshy *nodule*, usually on the face. It may take several months to reach one-half to one inch in diameter. In about a year it begins to ulcerate and bleed. Then it forms a crust, which it sheds at intervals, leaving another ulcer. A physician can usually remove the ulcer by a local operation.

Smoking and exposure to the sun aid squamous cell cancer. Lesions or horny growths may appear on the lips, mouth, and genitalia, and they tend to spread and increase in size. Again, your physician can treat or operate effectively. See also Ch. 18, *Cancer*.

Vitiligo

Vitiligo is an autoimmune disease that causes loss of pigment in skin. No cure exists for vitiligo, which affects about 1 percent of the U.S. population, but treatments include drugs and exposure to ultraviolet A radiation. The condition, itself, is not physically painful, but it is emotionally damaging.

Senile Purpura

Sometimes the skin develops *senile purpura* as one grows older. The characteristic hemorrhages of this condition usually appear on the extremities, and the purple color gradually fades and leaves mottled areas of yellow-brown. Generally, the skin is thin, fragile, and transparent in appearance.

Statis Dermatitis

Sometimes in association with such conditions as varicose veins, the skin may develop *stasis dermatitis*, an acute, chronic condition of the leg, associated with swelling, scaling of the skin, and in some cases, ulcer formation. It may exist for years with or without ulceration.

If any of the above conditions develop, it is wise to consult your physician rather than try to treat yourself.

Other Skin Conditions

Other skin conditions that may develop in the later years may include an increase in coarse hairs on exposed places such as the upper lip or chin. The downy hairs in the ears and nose become thicker and more apparent, and the eyebrows may become bushy. Graying hair is popularly associated with aging, but its onset often depends upon genetic factors and varies so much that it cannot be used as a reliable measure of age.

The earlobes may elongate as you grow older and the nails may become coarse and thickened or thinner and brittle.

Relieving Skin Conditions

As mentioned earlier, you can use some creams to relieve dryness and scaliness in older skin. The best of such creams are the water-in-oil emulsions (cold creams) such as Petrolatum Rose Water Ointment USP XVI, or oil-in-water emulsions such as Hydrophilic Ointment USP XVI. Wrinkle creams will not help much, but some conditions may be masked by regular cosmetic items such as powder, rouge, mascara, hair dyes, etc.

Sunscreens may aid in preventing acute and chronic overexposure to the sun's rays.

Various types of surgery may be performed to correct older skin conditions, but they won't work for everyone. Among some of the more common types of surgery are plastic surgery, dermabrasion (skin planning), chemosurgery (chemical cautery), cryosurgery (freezing of the skin), and electrosurgery (employing electricity). See "Plastic and Cosmetic Surgery" in Ch. 20, *Surgery*.

Hearing Loss

About three out of ten persons over age 65 have some hearing loss; at age 70 to 80 this percentage increases greatly.

Causes

While some hearing loss can be blamed on bad listening habits (tuning out people and conversation a person does not want to hear), the two major causes are conduction loss and nerve defects. A person with conduction loss hears high-pitched sounds best; a person with nerve impairment hears low sounds best. A combination of the two is called mixed hearing loss.

Conduction loss can be caused by excessive ear wax, diseases of the ear, disturbances of the eardrum, or abnormalities inside the ear. It can also be caused by *otosclerosis,* a bony growth over the window to the inner ear. Most of these conditions can be treated by an ear doctor (*otologist*). He can remove wax from the ear, repair or replace eardrums, remove bony growths, and loosen or remove fixed ear bones.

Nerve defects (sensorineural hearing loss) may be another story. They are caused by wear and tear on the ear, disease, certain drugs, and blows and skull fractures, and usually cause permanent damage that cannot be helped by surgery or medical treatment.

Some persons complain about ringing in the ears (*tinnitus*) that may start without warning and vary in intensity and quality. What causes tinnitus in one person may not cause it in another, but often it is caused by wax in the ear, middle ear infection, arteriosclerosis, tension in the jaw muscle, or certain drugs.

Hearing Aids

In most cases a hearing loss can be helped with a hearing aid or surgery. But if you think you have a hearing problem your first task is to see your physician. If your physician believes a hearing aid will help you, you should see a dispensing audiologist. The American Speech-Language-Hearing Association, 10801 Rockville Pike, Rockville, MD 20852, will supply a directory of certified practitioners on request. If you have trouble finding an audiologist, an experienced hearing-aid dealer may be able to advise you on the device best suited to your needs. The National Hearing Aid Help Line (800/521-5247), a service of the National Hearing Aid Society, provides lists of dealers certified as dispensing audiologists.

A hearing test at a hearing aid clinic may be your next stop. Here trained audiologists will scientifically measure your hearing and assist you in trying on different kinds of aids. The audiologists do not sell hearing aids, but can tell you what kind is best for you. There are four basic kinds of aids:

- Body Aids operate with a cord running to the receiver mold in the ear from the aid, carried in a pocket or worn in a special carrier.
- Behind-the-Ear hearing aids fit behind the ear. A plastic tube leads from the microphone, amplifier, and receiver to the earmold that fits in the ear.
- Canal Aids fit inside the ear canal.This model is hardly visible.
- In-the-Ear hearing aids fit in the outer ear.

When hearing aids are not effective, other options include *cochlear implants* and *middle ear hearing devices*. Both devices are surgically implanted. Cochlear implants, which are placed in the inner ear, are generally used in cases of very severe or profound hearing loss. Middle ear hearing devices, which are attached to a bone in the middle ear, are generally used for people with hearing loss no longer helped by hearing aids, but not severe enough to warrant a cochlear implant.

Buying a Hearing Aid

No single hearing aid is ideal for every hard-of-hearing person. Thus testing is essential if you are to find the right aid (which is why you should not buy one through the mail). You may want to bring a friend or relative when you are being fitted. A familiar voice serves as a yardstick to help you judge which aid is best. Some things to consider are the quality of the sound, the aid's ability to help you understand speech in both noisy and quiet places, comfort, ease of use, and price—including the earmold and the expected costs of upkeep.

It takes time to get used to a hearing aid. An aid amplifies all sounds—wanted and unwanted. It also changes most sounds, giving them an "electronic" character. Voices may sound unnatural and tinny. Normal noises may be harsh and grating. But special circuiting in many of today's aids limits the sound level reaching the eardrum. These *automatic gain controls* prevent discomfort but may distort speech. A still newer approach is to use filters to screen out background noises.

In addition to greatly reducing the sizes of many hearing aids, technological advances are expanding the usefulness of hearing aids continually. Noise blockers filter out sounds that do not fit with speech patterns. Tiny microphones reduce the buzzing noises picked up by some older hearing aid models. Treble and bass dials give the wearer a way to adjust sound quality to background noises. With the dials the wearer can also make adjustments to the hearing fluctuations resulting from bodily changes.

If you do not want to wear a hearing aid, or cannot adjust to one, you can try lip reading or speech reading. Each involves watching the lips and vocal chords to determine what another person is saying.

Talking to the Hard-of-Hearing

If you are talking to someone who has some hearing difficulty, he'll understand you better if you speak slowly and distinctly and use the lower range of your voice. Face him when you speak; let him see the movements of your lips. It also helps to point to visible objects.

Above all, don't shout. In fact, raising your voice sometimes pitches it into a higher frequency which a hard-of-hearing person may find difficult to understand.

Other Health Problems

The following health problems might also confront an older person. (Many of these conditions are discussed at greater length elsewhere in the book; in such cases, cross-references are supplied for your convenience at the end of the section.)

Heart Disease

The heart is the strongest, toughest muscle in the body. It is like an engine that could run 70 years or more without an overhaul. The heart has a complete maintenance and repair system, enabling many heart disease victims to continue long and useful lives.

While heart disease is not necessarily a product of aging, some heart and blood vessel problems become more acute as one grows older.

The following symptoms do not necessarily indicate heart disease, but it is wise to see a physician if you notice any of them:

- Shortness of breath
- A feeling of tightness in the chest or pain directly related to exertion or excitement
- Swelling of the feet and ankles
- Unusual fatigue

There is much that physicians can do to prevent heart conditions or to relieve them once present. But there is much that you can do to help yourself.

Weight

Extra pounds of fat mean more work for the heart.

Diet

The rules of sound nutrition apply to proper heart care.

Smoking

Heavy cigarette smokers suffer three times as many heart attacks as do pipe or cigar smokers. Nonsmokers are safest.

Exercise

Exercise improves the pumping action of the heart as well as circulation, digestion, and general health.

Worry

Worry increases tension and elevates blood pressure. Try to cultivate a philosophical approach to the daily ups and downs. See Ch.10, *Heart Disease*.

Strokes

Strokes are not hopeless; even severely paralyzed patients may make remarkable progress. A *stroke* occurs when the blood supply to a part of the brain tissue is cut off and, as a result, the nerve cells in that part of the brain can't function. When this happens, the part of the body controlled by these nerve cells can't function either.

Whenever the blood supply is cut off from an area, small neighboring arteries get larger and take over part of the work of the damaged artery. In this way nerve cells that have been temporarily put out of order may recover, and that part of the body affected by the stroke may eventually improve or even return to normal. See Ch. 9, *Diseases of the Circulatory System.*

Once a stroke has occurred, treatment and rehabilitation program options—which may include surgery, medication, and physical and occupational therapy—can help the patient resume as many normal activities as possible. A plan can be worked out with the physician, patient, family, and local organizations.

Arthritis

There are two main types of arthritis: *rheumatoid arthritis* and *osteoarthritis.*

Rheumatoid arthritis—which can cause pain and swelling in joints, nerves, muscles, tendons, blood vessels, and connective tissue in the whole body—can strike at any age, but it occurs mainly in the 25-to-40-year age group. The exact cause of rheumatoid arthritis is unknown.

Osteoarthritis is a degenerative joint disease that affects almost everyone who lives long enough; it is a product of normal wear and tear on the joints over the years. Poor posture and obesity are contributing causes, as are heredity and trauma.

Osteoarthritis is usually mild, and it seldom cripples. Pain is generally moderate. Unlike rheumatoid arthritis, which is inflammatory, spreads from joint to joint, and affects the whole body, osteoarthritis confines its attack locally to individual joints. Rarely is inflammation a problem.

Osteoarthritis is likely to develop in any joint that has been required to take a lot of punishment or abuse: the knee or hip joints of someone who is overweight; joints injured in an accident; joints injured or overused in sports; joints subjected to unusual stresses and strains in work or play; joints with hidden defects that were present at birth.

There is no specific cure for arthritis, but the pain and swelling can be controlled. In other than acute cases, common aspirin has proved the safest and most popular medication.

Adequate rest for both the body and the affected joint is a fundamental treatment. Heat, controlled exercise, hydrotherapy, and massage are all effective if done under a physician's supervision. See "Arthritis and Other Joint Diseases" in Ch. 7, *Diseases of the Skeletal System.*

Cancer

Cancer can strike at any age, but it does strike more frequently in the later years. Many factors are believed to contribute to cancer; these include frictional and chemical irritations like cigarette smoking; irritation of the skin and mouth (such as poor dentures); and exposure to the sun, X rays, or radioactive elements. Common sites are the lips, mouth, stomach, intestines, rectum, liver, pancreas, lungs, breast, kidney, bladder, skin, uterus, and prostate.

Early detection and prompt treatment are the best protection against cancer. If any of the following seven danger signals lasts longer than two weeks, be sure to get a checkup.

1. Unusual bleeding or discharge

2. A lump or thickening in the breast or elsewhere

3. A sore that does not heal

4. Change in bowel or bladder habits

5. Hoarseness or cough

6. Indigestion or difficulty in swallowing

7. Change in a wart or a mole

Great strides have been made in treating cancer with surgery, radiotherapy, and chemotherapy. See Ch. 18, *Cancer.* For cancers affecting women only, see "Cancers of the Reproductive System" and "Cancer of the Breast" in Ch. 25, *Women's Health.*

The Eyes

The eyes do age. After age 40, failing vision is usually caused by natural hardening of the lens, making it difficult to see close objects. However, failing vision may also be the first symptom of a serious bodily disorder, of glaucoma, or of a cataract, all of which require a physician's immediate attention.

Both glaucoma and cataracts can be treated effectively. About 90 percent of glaucoma cases can be checked with eye drops, and about 95 percent of cataracts can be removed by a painless operation.

Other diseases that may develop in later years affect the blood vessels of the eye. A common disease is *macular degeneration,* which causes impaired central vision. See Ch. 16, *Diseases of the Eye and Ear.*

Diabetes

The most likely candidates for diabetes are overweight persons over age 40, particularly those who have a hereditary history of diabetes, and especially older women.

The exact cause of diabetes is not known, but it is a disorder in which the body cannot easily process certain foods—mainly sugars and starches. Symptoms include increased thirst, constant hunger, frequent urination, loss of weight, itching, easy tiring, changes in vision, and slow healing of cuts and scratches.

Treatment and control consist of planned diet, exercise, and, in many cases, insulin shots or oral medication. Well-controlled diabetics can lead active lives. See Ch. 15, *Diabetes Mellitus*.

Constipation

There is no truth in the notion that a daily bowel movement is necessary for good health. A movement every day or twice a day may be all right for one person; for another every three or four days may be enough.

The two most common causes of chronic constipation are physical inactivity and poor food and water habits. Ironically, constipation may be caused by swallowing a cathartic nightly to induce a bowel movement. The habit eventually leads to chronic constipation because normal bowel movement ceases and bowel evacuation depends on using a cathartic.

To maintain proper bowel movement, try the following:

- Drink eight to ten glasses of water a day. Take two glasses of water on an empty stomach as soon as you get up.
- Drink more fruit juices and eat more dried and fresh fruits.
- Get at least one-half hour of moderate exercise daily. Walking, for example, is excellent, particularly if you relax while you walk.
- Give yourself enough time for normal bowel movement and set up a regular time for evacuation.
- If you are constipated, consult your physician to make sure it is simple and functional. See under Ch. 23, *Aches, Pains, Nuisances, Worries*.

Back Problems

As we grow older, the back muscles—weakened by inactivity, poor posture, and almost unavoidable wear and tear—start to complain.

Other causes of back problems are muscle and joint strain, changes in the spine, psychological tension, and internal diseases. Here are some tips to help avoid backache:

- Learn to lift correctly. Use your leg muscles, which are stronger than back muscles, by placing your feet closer to the base of the object, bending your knees outward, and pushing up with your legs.
- Avoid subjecting your back to any sudden, erratic motion.
- Try to improve your posture when sitting and walking.
- Sleep on a firm bed; a bed board may be helpful.
- Get regular exercise of a type that stimulates all your muscles rather

than just a few.

- If you sit for a long period, get up and stretch occasionally.
- Beware of excess weight. Extra weight on the abdomen pulls on the vertebrae at the small of the back, increasing the spine's normal curve and causing pain.
- Try never to become overfatigued or exhausted, either physically or mentally. Emotional pressure, from work or personal problems, causes muscle tension. See "Backaches" in Ch. 23, *Aches, Pains, Nuisances, Worries.*

Because the feet are farthest away from the heart's blood supply, they are often the first areas affected by circulatory diseases. Also, arthritis and diabetes might first show up in the feet.

Warning signs include continued cramping of the calf muscles, pain in the arch and toes, and unusually cold feet—especially if accompanied by a bluish skin. Brittle or thickened toenails or burning, tingling, and numbness may also signal a circulatory disease.

Foot ulcers may be one of the first signs of diabetes. Some***bunions***—swollen, tender, red joints—are caused by arthritis. Swelling around the feet and ankles suggests a possible kidney disorder.

If you have these symptoms, go to a *podiatrist* (a foot doctor) or to your own physician. They are trained to recognize these symptoms.

Most older people, however, suffer from minor aches and pains in the feet that are caused by poor foot care or abuse. See "The Vulnerable Extremities" in Ch. 23, *Aches,Pains, Nuisances, Worries.*

Care of the Feet

To prevent these problems, treat yourself to daily foot care. Dry your feet thoroughly and gently after bathing and inspect the skin for abrasion, rough spots, or cracks. Dry carefully between the toes. If the skin is dry or scaly, lubricate it with lanolin or olive oil. If recommended by your physician, apply a medicated foot powder as a preventative measure against athlete's foot.

When you cut your nails, do it with a strong light and be careful to cut straight across the nail to prevent ingrown toenails. Avoid the use of strong medications containing salicylate and strong antiseptics like iodine, carbolic acid, lysol, or bleach. Harsh chemicals that attack toughened skin can irritate normal tissue and cause infection. Avoid using hot water bottles, electric pads, or any form of extreme heat or cold. Diabetics should visit a podiatrist regularly.

The Prostate

Men over 50 may have an enlarged *prostate,* a condition known as benign prostate enlargement. (This is not caused by sexual excesses or venereal disease.) The exact cause is not known, but it's estimated that some type of enlarged prostate afflicts 10 percent of 40-year-olds and up to one half of all men over 60.

The prostate is a rubbery mass of glands and muscle tissue about the size and shape of a horse chestnut. It is wrapped around the urethra and base of the bladder at the point where they join. The prostate functions as part of a man's sexual apparatus, providing a fluid that transports and nourishes the spermatozoa.

Symptoms of an enlarged prostate include difficulty in urination. There might be an initial blocking of the urine, or the stream may lack force. You may feel that you can't empty the bladder, and you may have urgent needs to urinate. You may have pain or blood in the urine from straining.

If you have any of these symptoms, your physician can easily check for enlarged prostate by a simple rectal examination. If he discovers an enlargement, he can usually treat it in early stages with simple massage. But if it has progressed too far, he may have to operate, although other options exist, including drug therapy, electrovaporization, laser therapy, balloon dilation, and stents.

If surgery is chosen an operation is usually performed through the urethra or by an incision in the lower abdomen. The choice depends upon the individual problems of the patient and the judgment of the surgeon. In either case, the patient usually recovers completely in a short time.

A rectal examination can also discover early stages of cancer of the prostate, the second most common form of cancer among men after skin cancer, and the second leading cause of cancer death among men after lung cancer. Some 20 percent of men over 60 have this condition, and it is most common in men over 70.

Unfortunately, this disease does not manifest itself early, so it is important that men over 40 have the diagnostic rectal examination.If the disease is detected early and treated—usually by surgery, hormonal therapy, and possibly radiation—the cure rate is very high. If found late, the cure rate is low.

When treatment is by surgery, the entire prostate and upper urethra may be removed. In some cases, the disease may be retarded or relieved by treatment with female hormones.

In both enlargement and cancer of the prostate, early detection is vital to a successful cure. That is why it is important to have a rectal examination. See also "Cancer of the Prostate" in Ch. 18, *Cancer*.

Alzheimer's Disease

Alzheimer's disease is a group of brain disorders marked by progressive deterioration and affects both memory and reasoning abilities. Victims of Alzheimer's, which is a form of dementia, or mental deterioration (see "Dementia" in Ch. 8, *Diseases of the Muscles and Nervous System*), undergo various behavioral changes. These include an inability to concentrate, anxiety, irritability, agitation, withdrawal, and petulance. Persons suffering from Alzheimer's may wander about and lose their way. They may have temper tantrums and engage in obsessional behavior, such as repeatedly washing dishes. Time and place disorientation may be accompanied by delusions and depression. In the later stages of the disease, bladder and bowel control may be lost.

Diagnosing Alzheimer's in its early stages is difficult despite its numerous symptoms. Laboratory tests that could identify the disorder do not exist. Adding to the problems of diagnosis, various other disorders have similar symptoms. The best medical alternative, a complete physical examination, generally includes a review of any drugs or medications the patient has been taking as well as standard laboratory tests. The latter help to rule out other diseases or disorders that may be treatable. A clinical evaluation can include a CT (computed tomography) scan, an EEG (electroencephalogram), and assessment of evidence from family members and the patient regarding the latter's (or patient's) mental state.

Even when diagnosed with relative certainty, Alzheimer's disease cannot be cured. But some symptoms, including depression and delusions, can be treated. The effect is to slow the progress of the disorder. Where Parkinson's disease or heart problems accompany Alzheimer's, treatment can focus on alleviation of those conditions.

A small proportion of Alzheimer's cases have been linked to the possession of a flawed gene that causes cells to produce too much of a protein called beta amyloid. It is not known, however, whether excess beta amyloid protein is the cause, or the result, of brain devastation. Scientists have also linked the possession of another gene, apolipoprotein E4, to an increased susceptibility to the most common form of Alzheimer's.

According to the American Academy of Neurology, there is building evidence that physical and mental exercise, adequate vitamin intake, good cardiovascular health, and anti-inflammatory drugs may be protective against Alzheimer's. They also found that 1,000 I.U. of vitamin E twice a day may slow the progression of the disease.

Meeting the Challenge of Leisure

Leisure Activities

In ten years of retirement, you will have the leisure time equivalent of working 40 hours a week for 21 years. You cannot fish this time away and you cannot rest it away. Anything you do for a long time must have meaning; it must satisfy some basic need and want. Certain needs remain constant throughout life:

- Security—good health, income, and a recognized role in society
- Recognition—as an individual with your own abilities and personality
- Belonging—as a member of a family, social group, and community
- Self-expression—by developing abilities and talents in new areas and at new levels
- Adventure—new experiences, new sights, and new knowledge

There are many activities that can satisfy these basic needs and wants and keep you in top shape.

Travel

Travel can satisfy your need for adventure in many ways. If you travel offseason at bargain rates, you may be able to cut costs significantly. Most travel problems stem from rushing to meet a schedule. Making every minute count on a fast-paced European tour can be expensive and exhausting. A simple or leisurely trip can be more relaxing and cheaper.

Wherever you travel, you might try to center your trip around an interest or a hobby. You can take art or music tours—tours that stress education, night life, culture, or special interests. You can travel on your own or with a group. But whatever you do, participate; don't just observe.

Doing things instead of just observing adds new dimensions to the pleasure of going places. For people who participate, travel means the adventure of enjoying exciting new places, people, and experiences. To help plan your trip, contact the government tourist offices of foreign countries (ask your library for mail and Internet addresses), the National Park Service, and the state or local chambers of commerce.

Gardening

Gardening can satisfy one's need for self-expression in many ways. Being outside in the fresh air and planting living things can bring satisfaction and peace of mind.

Gardening is a multifaceted hobby that offers many challenges. You can go into plant breeding, growing for resale, introducing new plants, collecting rare and unusual plants, selecting plants, or simply cultivating what you find personally appealing and satisfying.

Your local library or bookstore has many books on the subject. There are local and national garden clubs you can join to learn about your hobby and to meet other people who are interested in gardening. One such organization is the American Community Gardening Association, 1916 Sussex Road, Blacksburg, VA 24060, (540) 552-5550. In addition, state extension directors at state colleges and universities, county agricultural agents, and local plant nurseries can give expert advice and information.

Reading

Reading offers excitement, adventure, pursuit of knowledge, and an introduction to new people and places. Your local library is the best place to launch a reading program—and you may be surprised to find that it offers more than books. Most libraries have art and music departments, audiovisual services (films and microfilm copies), foreign language departments, periodical rooms (newspapers and magazines), writing classes, genealogy workshops, and special courses of general interest.

Hobbies

A hobby can be any physical or mental activity that gives you happiness, relaxation, and satisfaction. It should not be just a time killer—it should offer some tangible reward. Also, it should have continuity, not be too expensive, and not make undue demands on time and energy. Perhaps you would prefer a series of hobbies, some serious and some just for fun. They can be related to your work or completely unrelated. In any event, a hobby should be something you've always wanted to do.

Before selecting a hobby, consider these points:

- Do you like to do things alone? Consider arts, crafts, reading, sewing, fishing—activities that are not dependent on others, although you can enjoy them with others.
- Do you like groups? Seek hobbies that include other people—organizational, sport, game, or craft activities.
- Do you like to play to win? Try your luck in competitive or team games that stress winning.
- Do you have to be an expert? Too many of us are afraid to try new activities because we hate to fail or look clumsy. But be fair; judge your efforts in light of your past experience and present progress.
- Do you put a price tag on everything? Many people will not engage in an activity if it costs too much. Yet, many hobbies fail because they're tried on a shoestring without adequate equipment. Also, some people do not want to do anything unless it brings in money. If so, perhaps you should look for something that's an offshoot of the work or business you know best.

Creative Crafts

Creative crafts are difficult for most of us because we are conservative, afraid to make mistakes, sensitive because of buried and almost forgotten blunders. Yet creativity is essential to life. Without it we don't live fully; through creative skills we refurbish old interests and develop new ones.

Most of us are happiest with creative crafts that do not require intricate work or fine detail and that are not too demanding physically. Some crafts best suited to retirement years include weaving, rug making, sewing, ceramic work, knitting, plastic molding, woodwork, leather craft, and lapidary.

You can learn these and other crafts and also market your products through senior centers, adult education classes, and senior craft centers.

Volunteer Work

Through community service and volunteer work, thousands are not only helping others but are serving themselves. Such activities keep time from hanging heavy, give purpose to retirement, and in some cases may lead to paying jobs and a second career.

Participating in community activities is not difficult. In some communities a call to the city clerk is enough to get started. In others, a letter to the mayor will bring faster results. In larger cities, call the Volunteer Bureau in your area; this is a United Fund agency that acts as a clearing house for volunteer jobs.

If you wish to have the type of volunteer job that leads to a second career, you might consider doing work for one of the government programs utilizing the skills of older people. There are several such programs administered by the Corporation for National and Community Service. These include the Foster Grandparent Program, the Retired Senior Volunteer Program, AmeriCorps, and the National Senior Service Corps. For additional information about any of these organizations, write the Service at 1201 New York Ave. NW, Washington, DC, 20525.

The Peace Corps also needs the skills of retirees. However, you must be skilled in some trade or profession, pass a tough physical examination, and complete a rigorous orientation and training program. For more information, contact the Peace Corps at (800) 424-8580 and ask for a copy of the brochure Older Volunteers in the Peace Corps. It lists specific skills needed in the Peace Corps.

The Service Corps of Retired Executives also needs senior volunteers. It is a federally funded non-profit organization that advises aspiring entrepreneurs. It has hundreds of offices around the country and can be reached at (800) 634-0245.

There are other volunteer jobs that may not pay a salary, but do fill a basic need by allowing you to pass along your skills and ideals to younger people. You can do this through the Boy Scouts, Girl Scouts, Boys Clubs of America, YMCAs and YWCAs, hospitals, organizations which serve people with mental and physical disabilities, and many other organizations.

Continuing Social and Intellectual Activities

The one organ we can depend upon in old age is the brain. At 80, a person can learn at approximately the same speed he could when he was 12 years old. But like any organ, the brain must be kept active and alert by constant use.

One of the best ways to exercise the brain is through some process of continuing education. This does not have to mean going back to school or taking formal classes. Continuing education can take the form of participating in discussions in senior centers, "Y's," town meetings, or study courses. You can find out about educational opportunities and possibilities by contacting local, state, or national offices of education; state employment offices; the Adult Education section of the U.S. Department of Education, Office of Vocational and Adult Education, 4090 MES, 400 Maryland Avenue, SW, Washington, D.C. 20202; the State Commission on Aging (write to your state capital).

Your local library may have some suggestions (and perhaps offers some classes), and your local "Y" is probably offering some programs.

The federal government continues to be a prime source of educational literature. Each year the government prints about 50 million books, pamphlets, brochures, reports, and guidebooks on everything from astrology to zoology. For a free price list of specified subjects, write to the Superintendent of Documents, U.S. Government Printing Office, Mailstop: SDE, 732 N. Capital Street NW, Washington, DC 20401.

Formal and informal learning situations can help you keep pace with change and the future. Continuing education prepares you to live contentedly with a free, independent spirit and mind—while providing you with the means for improved social integration, participation, and satisfaction.

Sexual Attitude and Activity in the Aged

We have come far since the Victorian era when talk about sex was taboo. Now science is taking a candid look at sex in the later years and is exploding old myths as well as exploring new truths. Such enlightenment can help reduce any remaining guilt in this area.

After Age 60

In one study to determine the pattern of sexual behavior after 60, researchers at Duke University quizzed 250 people aged 60 to 93 about their sexual activities. Of the 149 who were married, 81 reported they were still sexually active; even in the single group, 7 of the 101 questioned reported "some sexual activity."

Dr. Gustave Newman, who conducted the study, reported 10 percent of the couples over 60 as having sexual relations more than once a week, though couples over 75 unanimously reported less activity.

"No age is an automatic cut-off point for sex," claims the late Dr. Isadore Rubin in his study, *Sexual Life After Sixty*. "But," he continues,

> sexuality cannot flourish in a climate where rejection of aging as a worthwhile stage of life leads inevitably to self-rejection by many older persons . . . the men and women who "act old" in their sexual activity before their bodies have really called a halt become sexually old long before their time.

Physiological and Psychological Changes and Sex

Postmenopausal women may experience painful intercourse due to a decrease in vaginal lubrication. This problem is easily remedied with the use of nonpetroleum-based vaginal creams or jellies.

Many women take a renewed interest in sex after menopause. Dr. William H. Masters and Mrs. Virginia E. Johnson in their study *Human Sexual Response* credit the tendency of many women to experience a second honeymoon in the early 50s to the fact that they no longer have to worry about pregnancy and usually have resolved most of the problems of raising a family.

On the other hand, they tell us:

> Deprived of normal sexual outlets, women exhaust themselves physically in conscious or unconscious efforts to dissipate their accumulated and frequently unrecognized sexual tensions. Many demonstrate their basic insecurities by casting themselves unreservedly into their religion, the business world, volunteer social work, or overzealous mothering of their mature children or grandchildren.

While some women become more responsive as they grow older, Masters and Johnson point out, "There is no question that the human male's responsiveness wanes as he ages."

Men may experience less sexual urgency, delayed or partial erection, and less defined ejaculations because the body's secretion of the male hormone testosterone decreases with age and the conduction of nerve impulses is less rapid. Also, arteries in the penis are less able to maintain the blood pressure necessary for a full erection.

Another common concern for older men is impotence, that is, diminished or no sexual response. Nearly everyone experiences impotence from time to time, often from such routine problems as fatigue, stress, or illness. The incidence of impotence, however, definitely increases with age. (By age 65, 30 percent of men report chronic impotence; by age 75, 55 percent do.)

Impotence has been linked to such problems as diabetes, Parkinson's disease, liver or kidney disease, and lower back problems. Other causes are certain medications, excessive alcohol consumption, drug abuse, and smoking. Most cases of impotence, however, can be traced to psychological problems such as anxiety, depression, or marital problems. About 80 percent of these cases can still be overcome with psychotherapy.

Sexual dysfunction in women is often called *frigidity* and implies a *cold* woman who cannot become excited sexually. As with men, there are both organic and psychological causes which can often be treated.

Although sex for most healthy men and women over 60 may not be quite the same as it was for them in their 20s, that does not mean it cannot be good, or even better. A change in attitudes and expectations about sex may have surprising results. Couples may find new enjoyment in reducing the pace of lovemaking and exploring different ways of giving each other pleasure besides intercourse.

Health Concerns

For those not so healthy older men and women, especially most of those who have suffered heart attacks, there is no reason for them not to have sex. After a heart attack most are able to resume sexual activity within a few months, although patients with angina pectoris may be advised to proceed cautiously.

According to Dr. Philip Reichert, former executive secretary of the American College of Cardiology:

> We must get rid of the notion that every heart patient lives under an overhanging sword and that he faces the constant threat of sudden death. The congenial married couple, accustomed to each other and whose technique is habituated through many years of companionship, can achieve sexual satisfaction without too great an expenditure of body energy or too severe a strain upon the heart. . . .

Hypertension sufferers may sometimes indulge in a restricted form of sexual activity with medical supervision. And modern therapy and surgical methods can often prevent or delay impotence caused by prostate disease or diabetes.

Where any health problem is involved, it is best to analyze your sex needs and those of your partner; consult with your physician and partner as to how you can both attain satisfaction without harm to your health; see your physician regularly and report accurately distress symptoms.

Recent research has dispelled other long-held ideas about sex, too—among them the myth that masturbation is childish and harmful to health. Moreover, Rubin points out: "All studies of older persons have shown that autoerotic activity, while not as common as in the younger years, is far more prevalent in later years than most of us have imagined."

Dr. Lester W. Dearborn, marriage consultant, in pointing out the role masturbation plays in the lives of the single or widowed, comments:

> It is to be hoped that those interested in the field of geriatrics will . . . encourage the aging to accept masturbation as a perfectly valid outlet when there is a need and other means of gratification are not available.

Cellular Therapy and Hormone Treatment

To keep older people vigorous and active, some researchers have experimented with *cellular therapy* as a means of retarding aging. Dr. Paul Niehans, a Swiss physician, introduced the idea of cellular therapy in the 1930s with his theory that organs begin to deteriorate in old age when the body fails to replace the cells that compose it. He prescribed a treatment whereby a person is injected with cells from healthy embryonic animal organs. (He used sheep, pigs, and calves.) He believed that the animal cells from a particular organ would migrate to the same organ in the aging body and reactivate it. Thus, kidney troubles could be cured with cells from an embryonic animal kidney. Although such notables as Sir Winston Churchill, Pope Pius XII, Somerset Maugham, and Dr. Konrad Adenauer submitted to it, cellular therapy is not widely accepted in the United States today as an effective agent against aging.

More to the point, most researchers feel, are the current experiments with hormones. Hormones help women through the tension of menopause and are used to treat impotence and loss of sexual desire. However, some studies have linked estrogen hormone therapy statistically with uterine cancer. For this reason and because of side effects, hormones face many years of testing before they will be used extensively to retard aging.

Mental Outlook

Good health plus a romantic outlook promote sex appeal at any age. Showing affection, whether sexually or not, keep you sparkling and lively no matter what your age.

A good wholesome attitude toward life, a hearty sense of humor, a sympathetic interest in other people—all help make up the indefinable something that makes us appealing to the opposite sex. Cleanliness, neat suitable apparel, and good posture all add to the image we create of ourselves in other people's minds. So do the manners we reflect in the courtesies we show the people around us—the thoughtful little things we do for them, our reactions to the things they do for us.

If you're a woman over 65 who is

looking for companionship, you'll probably find a good personality uplift will get you farther than a face or bust lift. If you're a man who is hoping to find feminine companionship, you will probably find a good spiritual overhaul more image-enhancing than dyeing your hair. Also, a good night's sleep is the best aphrodisiac.

The Right Housing

Selecting retirement housing is like selecting a spouse; there are many possibilities, but few that are right.

Ideally, the right housing should take care of you rather than requiring you to take care of it. It should give you shelter, security, and privacy; allow you freedom; and keep you near friends, relatives, and a grocer who delivers.

To Move or Not to Move

What is the right housing for you—the one that you are in or some other place? The answer to this question depends upon the state of your pocketbook and the state of your health.

Advantages of Moving

Right now you might be in good health, but this could change. Would stairs become a problem? Could you keep up the house and garden? Would you want more adequate heat? Older people are more comfortable when the temperature is over 75° F. You might also need better lighting in several rooms.

If you are retired, you might find that you cannot keep up expenses on the old house. You might find that your larger, older house does not suit the reduced size of your family or your need for work or recreation. You could probably save money by living in a smaller place that requires less upkeep. You could also arrange to move nearer children and grandchildren, or into an area where you could find new opportunities for work and recreational activities.

Advantages of Staying Put

But by staying in your home you would remain in familiar surroundings and near old friends. You could maintain your comfortable routine and remain independent as long as possible. If you have unused space, you could move into the first floor and shut off the second floor to save on heat and maintenance. Or you could convert part of the house into apartments.

Where to Live?

Many older persons fulfill ambitions of long standing by moving to warmer climates after retirement. The question whether such a move should be undertaken should be considered with other questions relating to housing.

Moving to a different climate makes sense for many reasons. Many elderly persons feel threatened or restricted by cold winters and their usual accompaniments—snow, sleet, and high winds. Having more leisure time, older persons feel that warmer temperatures will make it possible to take part in more activities for more hours of the day than if they "stay put." Some persons move so that they can live closer to friends who have already moved—or to children or other relatives. Some move to play golf or tennis outdoors the year around.

An individual or couple considering a move to a warmer climate should look at a number of basic considerations. A key one relates to the cost of living in the new area or state. Living on incomes that may have been substantially reduced by retirement, older persons without special preferences may select that state that offers the cheapest living.

"Retirement to the sun" entails many other decisions. States like New Mexico offer a wide range of sites, from urban to desert, from high mountains to empty plains. Some of the states with favorable tax laws and cheap living costs have little to offer in the way of cultural attractions. Other states may lack recreational activities.

Psychological Trauma

Moving 100 or 1,000 or 2,000 miles to live in a warmer climate obviously involves some pain of separation and loss. The psychological trauma occasioned by a departure from old friends and familiar surroundings has caused major problems for some older persons. For that reason, the psychological challenge should be given deep consideration *before* any move is made.

How to alleviate the trauma of leaving the familiar for the unfamiliar? Some persons spend a year in the new locale, return home, and *then* make up their minds to move or not to move. Others, including those who cannot afford such trial living, at least visit the target region to "get a feel" for it and its way of life.

Requirements of Retirement Housing

Whatever you plan to do, your retirement housing should be located near or be easily accessible to shops and recreation centers by public transportation. To make living arrangements more pleasant, individual housing units should contain at least 400 square feet, and there should be two or more rooms.

The new dwelling unit should be equal to or better than the housing you have been used to in the past. It should be suitable for comfortable living in both health and sickness—easily adaptable to convalescent needs with either two bedrooms or a bedroom and sleeping alcove.

In addition, retirement housing

should incorporate the following:

- All rooms on one floor, and that floor reached by few, if any, steps
- No thresholds or tripping hazards
- Non slip surfaces in hallways, bedrooms, and kitchens
- Handrails by all steps and inclines
- Adequate illumination in halls, near steps, and in other potentially hazardous areas
- Fully automatic central heating
- Doors and halls wide enough to accommodate a wheelchair

Public Housing

If you decide to move and to rent instead of buying, consider public housing projects. These projects are available to single men and women 62 or older, as well as to families whose head is 62 or older or has a spouse at least 62. Local housing authorities build, purchase, or lease the units and set entrance requirements and maximum income limits. Rents are comparatively low.

The Department of Housing and Urban Development also makes loans for nonprofit (and profit) sponsors that will build housing for senior citizens with moderate or higher incomes.

Retirement Hotels and Communities

You might also consider retirement hotels, which are especially numerous in Florida, California, and Texas. These hotels are usually refurbished former resorts that provide room and board at a fixed monthly rent.

Retirement communities offer housing of various types, usually apartments, cooperatives, and individual units. Costs at such facilities vary widely depending on location, amenities, availability, and demand.

Would you like retirement community living? It's usually the life for people who like people and who enjoy being active. For those who don't, it can be a bit tiring. Some people do not like the closeness and activity found in a retirement community and prefer living in a less social environment.

Assisted Living Facilities

Assisted living facilities allow seniors who need medical attention to live in an environment that offers more independence and privacy than traditional nursing homes. They are the fastest growing type of senior housing in the United States. Typical facilities offer 24-hour supervision, assistance with medication, meals, and private or semi-private rooms. These facilities are generally not well-suited for seniors who require 24-hour skilled nursing care. The AARP has reported that the average monthly fees for assisted living facilities are approximately $2,000.

Cooperatives and Condominiums

In addition to lifetime care facilities, many church, fraternal, and union groups offer other types of housing. In the case of church-sponsored housing, residence usually is not restricted to members of the sponsoring faith.

Some of these units are operated as *cooperatives;* others as *condominiums.* The major difference in the two is that condominium owners have titles to their units, while cooperative residents are stockholders in the cooperative association with occupancy rights to specific units. Condominium owners pay their own taxes; cooperative residents pay taxes in their monthly charges.

Mobile Homes

You might also want to consider a mobile home. A suitable one must be at least 10 feet wide and 50 feet long.

What is it like to live in a mobile-home park? Certainly, there is a closeness in these parks that you would not have in a normal neighborhood. Typically, the mobile home is placed on a lot 25 to 30 feet wide and 75 feet deep. This means that you could have 12 families within a radius of 100 feet.

Residents visit back and forth and hold frequent picnics, barbecues, and other social activities. This would not be the way of life for someone who did not enjoy group activities.

Be Realistic

To find out what type of housing is best for you, look around the area to see where you want to live. Each community is different, shaped by the people who live there. Talk to the residents and do some serious thinking before you move, not forgetting to carefully consider your financial position in regard to the new locale. Try to be realistic; don't expect to find the perfect climate for health and happiness. The nearest thing to it would be a place that encourages outdoor life, is neither too hot nor too cold, has a relative humidity of around 55 percent, and enough variety in weather, with frequent but moderate weather changes, to be interesting and not too monotonous.

If you have any doubts about the location as far as health is concerned, check with your physician.

When Faced with Ill Health

How can you help yourself or others when faced with a serious or terminal illness?

Alvin I. Goldfarb, M.D., former consultant on Services for the Aged, New York State Department of Mental Hygiene, notes the importance of self-esteem, self-confidence, sense of purpose, and well-being to a person who is seriously ill or dying. Supported by the idea, "I've led a good and full life," older people can face a serious or terminal illness with dignity. Sometimes this acceptance may be almost an unspoken and tacit understanding between the aging and society to help the separation process along.

When a person is terminally ill, the chances are that he is not in severe pain. With the increasing supply of pain-relieving drugs and the possibility of sedation, very few elderly patients suffer greatly with pain. While a fear of death probably exists in most people, when death is actually encountered the fear is seldom overwhelming, even though it may deeply affect others directly involved with the dying patient.

Most patients are at least aware of the possibility of dying soon; those with lingering conditions are particularly adept at self-diagnosis. But more often, they notice a change in social relationships with friends, family, and medical personnel.

Patient–physician relationships can be vital in helping the seriously ill patient retain peace of mind. It is the physician's responsibility to give compassion and recognize fear, even when it is hidden. Likewise, he should respond to a patient's hidden wish to discuss his illness. Of course, there is no set formula for communicating with seriously ill patients. Each individual needs a different approach, and most physicians are sensitive to this.

Many physicians report that death, except in unusual cases, is not accompanied by physical pain. Rather, there is often a sense of well-being and spiritual exaltation. Physicians think this feeling is caused by the anesthetic action of carbon dioxide on the central nervous system and by the effect of toxic substances. Ernest Hemingway wrote, "The pang of death, a famous doctor once told me, is often less than that of a toothache."

Stages of Death

According to physicians, people die in stages—rapidly or slowly, depending on circumstances. First comes *clinical death,* when respiration and heartbeat cease. The brain dies as it is deprived of oxygen and circulating blood, and *biological death* occurs.

Life can be restored in the moments between clinical death and brain death if circulation and respiration are continued through the use of medical devices that stimulate the heart and lungs.

After the brain ceases to function, cellular death begins. Life is not considered to be completely lost until the brain stops functioning. It is possible for surgeons to remove viable organs after biological death for transplant or other use.

Many clergymen and physicians insist that we need more honest communication about death, as such communication is probably the single most useful measure to avoid unnecessary suffering. Sound knowledge never made anyone afraid. And although death will probably always remain essentially a mystery, scientists will continue to search for a better understanding of its nature. By such means they may learn a great deal more about life.

When Death Comes . . . a Medical Perspective

Family members adjusting to the death of a loved one may face the question of whether or not an autopsy should be performed. More and more, medical experts are underscoring the need for an autopsy as a means of confirming the cause of death. The postmortem examination may also "provide a reasonable context for accepting death," according to Daniel W. McKeel, director of autopsy pathology at Washington University School of Medicine. From a family and genetic point of view, the autopsy may reveal information about specific conditions or medical problems in the deceased that survivors can use to guide their own health practices and concerns.

Contrary to some reports, the autopsy need not delay funeral arrangements or disfigure the body so as to require a closed casket. Autopsies are generally mandatory in homicide, suicide, burn deaths, deaths resulting from on-the-job injuries, operating room deaths, and questionable or unwitnessed deaths.

The Complete Reference Guide to

MEDICINE AND HEALTH

The Complete Reference Guide to MEDICINE AND HEALTH

EDITED BY
Richard J. Wagman, M.D., F.A.C.P.
Assistant Clinical Professor of Medicine
Downstate Medical Center
New York, New York

Volume Two

FACTS ON FILE/NEW YORK

ISBN 0-8160-6144-0 (hardcover)

Printed in the United States of America

Editor
Richard J. Wagman, M.D., F.A.C.P.
Assistant Clinical Professor of Medicine
Downstate Medical Center
New York, New York

Contributors to The New Complete Medical and Health Encyclopedia

Consultant in Surgery

N. Henry Moss, M.D., F.A.C.S.
Associate Clinical Professor of Surgery
Temple University Health Sciences Center and Albert Einstein Medical Center;
Past President, American Medical Writers Association;
Past President, New York Academy of Sciences

Consultant in Gynecology

Douglass S. Thompson, M.D.
Clinical Professor of Obstetrics and Gynecology and Clinical Associate Professor of Community Medicine
University of Pittsburgh School of Medicine

Consultant in Pediatrics

Charles H. Bauer, M.D.
Clinical Associate Professor of Pediatrics and Chief of Pediatric Gastroenterology
The New York Hospital-Cornell Medical Center
New York, New York

Consultants in Psychiatry

Julian J. Clark, M.D.
Assistant Professor of Psychiatry
and
Rita W. Clark, M.D.
Clinical Assistant Professor of Psychiatry
Downstate Medical Center

Consulting Editor

Kenneth N. Anderson
Formerly Editor
Today's Health

Bruce O. Berg, M.D.
Associate Professor
Departments of Neurology and Pediatrics
Director, Child Neurology
University of California
San Francisco, California

D. Jeanne Collins
Assistant Professor
College of Allied Health Professions
University of Kentucky
Lexington, Kentucky

Anthony A. Davis
Vice President and Education Consultant
Metropolitan X-Ray and Medical Sales, Inc.
Olney, Maryland

Peter A. Dickinson
Editor Emeritus
Harvest Years/Retirement Living

Gordon K. Farley, M.D.
Associate Professor of Child Psychiatry
Director, Day Care Center
University of Colorado Medical Center

Arthur Fisher
Group Editor
Science and Engineering
Popular Science

Edmund H. Harvey, Jr.
Editor
Science World

Helene MacLean
Medical writer

Ben Patrusky
Science writer

Stanley E. Weiss, M.D.
Assistant Attending Physician, Renal Service
Beth Israel Hospital and Medical Center, New York

Jeffrey S. Willner, M.D.
Attending Radiologist
Southampton Hospital
Southampton, New York

Contents

Volume II

7

Diseases of the Skeletal System

The bones and joints of the human body, although designed to withstand a great deal of stress, are subject to a variety of disorders that can affect people of all ages. Some skeletal deformities are the result of congenital defects, and can be treated by physical therapy or surgery with varying degrees of success. Arthritis and related joint diseases, caused by wear and tear over the years, probably affect more people than any other skeletal disorder.

Man's erect posture makes the spine especially vulnerable to problems of alignment, often causing considerable pain. Bone tissue can also be invaded by tumors and by infections of the bone marrow. Also, stress to bones and joints can cause fractures or dislocations, which require prompt medical treatment to prevent deformity or loss of mobility.

Congenital Defects

As the fetus develops in the womb, its bony skeleton first appears as soft cartilage, which hardens into bone before birth. The calcium content of the mother's diet aids the fetus in bone formation and in the development of the normal human skeleton. Thus the basic skeletal structure of an individual is formed before his birth. In some instances, the bones of the fetus develop abnormally, and such defects are usually noticeable soon after delivery.

The causes of skeletal birth defects are not always known. Some may result from hereditary factors; others have been traced to the mother's exposure to X rays, radiation, chemicals, drugs, or to disease during pregnancy. Among the more common birth defects are extra fingers, toes, or ribs, or missing fingers, hands, toes, feet, or limbs. Sections of the spine may be fused together, often without causing serious problems later in life, although some fused joints can hinder the motion of limbs. The sections of the skull may unite prematurely, retarding the growth of the brain.

Defects of the Skull, Face, and Jaw

Various malformations of the skull, face, and jaw can appear at birth or soon after. They include *macrocephaly* (enlarged head) and *microcephaly* (very small head). Microcephaly is caused by the premature fusion of the cranial sutures in early childhood. If brain growth increases very rapidly during the first six months of life in infants whose skulls have fused prematurely, the brain cannot expand sufficiently within the rigid skull, and mental retardation results. Surgery is used to widen the sutures to permit normal brain development.

Cleft lip and *cleft palate* are common facial deformities and are visible at birth. These are longitudinal openings in the upper lip and palate. They result from failure of the area to unite in the normal manner during embryonic stages of pregnancy. They should be corrected at an early age. If surgery is performed in infancy there is a good chance that the child will mature with little or no physical evidence of the affliction and with no psychological damage as a result of it. See "Cleft Palate and Cleft Lip" in Ch. 2, *The First Dozen Years*, for further information.

Defects of the Rib Cage

Every normal human being has 12 pairs of ribs attached to the spine, but some people are born with extra ribs on one or both sides.

Although such extra ribs are usually harmless, one that projects into the neck can damage nerves and the artery located in that area. In adults extra neck ribs may cause shooting pains down the arms, general periodic numbness in the arms and hands, weak wrist pulse, and possible diminished blood supply to the forearm. Surgery may be required to remove the rib and thereby relieve the pressure on the nerves or artery. Minor symptoms are treated by physiotherapy.

Congenital absence of one or more ribs is not uncommon. An individual may be born with some ribs fused together. Neither condition creates any serious threat to health.

Congenital Dislocation of the Hip

Dislocation of the hip is the most common congenital problem of the pelvic area. It is found more often in girls than in boys in a five to one ratio.

Babies born from a breech presentation, buttocks first, are more likely to develop this abnormality than those delivered head first. The condition may be the result of inherited characteristics.

Clinical examination of infants, especially breech-born girls, may reveal early signs of congenital hip dislocation, with the affected hip appearing shorter than the normal side. If the condition is not diagnosed before the infant is ready to walk, the child may begin walking later than is normal. The child may develop a limp and an unsteady gait, with one leg shorter

The Human Skeleton

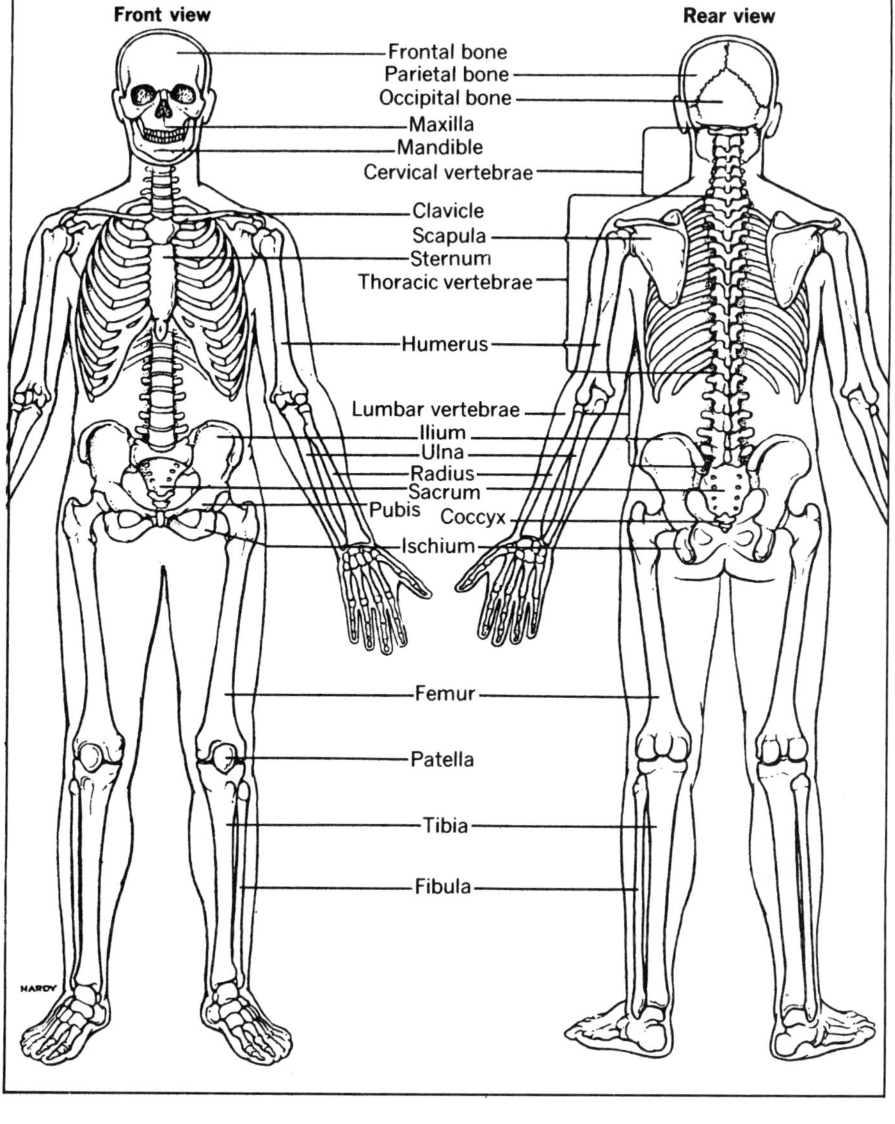

than the other.

Early diagnosis of this condition is important, followed by immediate reduction and immobilization by means of a plaster cast or by applying traction. Permanent deformity, dislocation, uneven pelvis, retarded walking, limping, and unsteady gait are possible complications if this condition remains untreated. Surgery is sometimes required.

Arthritis and Other Joint Diseases

Arthritis is probably the most common of all disabling diseases, at least in the temperate areas of the world. It has been estimated that almost 20 percent of the population suffers from one of the many forms of arthritis. In the United States alone, more than 13 million persons each year seek professional medical care for arthritis. Of this number, some seven million must restrict their daily activities, and about 750,000 are so disabled by arthritis that they are unable to attend school, work, or even handle common household tasks.

Arthritis apparently is not associated with any stage of civilization; it has been diagnosed in the skeletons of prehistoric humans. There is even evidence that arthritic diseases afflict a variety of animals, including the dinosaurs that inhabited the earth more than 100 million years ago. Arthritis caused pain and suffering to such famous people as Goethe, Henry VI, Charlemagne, and Alexander the Great.

Arthritis and *rheumatism* are terms sometimes used interchangeably by the layman to describe any abnormal condition of the joints, muscles, or related tissues. Many rheumatic or arthritic diseases have popular names, such as "housemaid's knee," "baseball finger," or "weaver's bottom." Physicians usually prefer to apply the term *arthritis* to disorders of the joints, especially joint disorders accompanied by inflammation. More than 75 different diseases of the joints have been identified; they are classi-

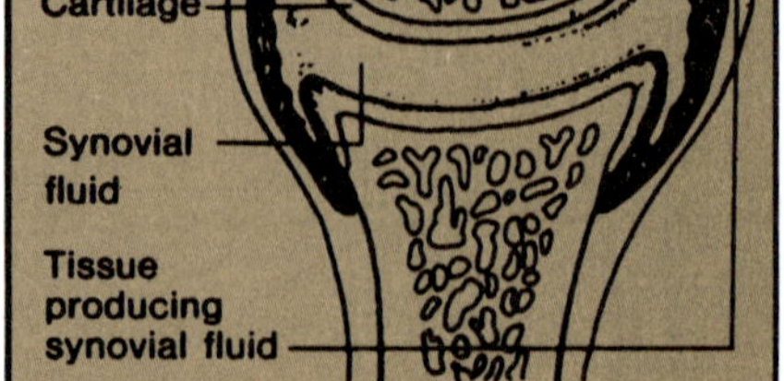

All of the body's joints allow movement of the bones through this combination of ball and socket contours. Cartilage allows the bones to move without scraping or catching. Synovial fluid helps reduce friction in the movement.

fied according to their specific signs, symptoms, and probable causes. The list includes bursitis, gout, and tendinitis in addition to the major disorders, rheumatoid arthritis and osteoarthritis.

Rheumatoid arthritis and osteoarthritis are examples of two types of arthritic ailment that are quite different diseases. Rheumatoid arthritis usually develops from unknown causes before the age of 45 and is marked by a nonspecific inflammation of the joints and in body organs; the inflammation is accompanied by changes in substances found in the blood. A victim of rheumatoid arthritis may develop limb deformities within a short period of time. Osteoarthritis, on the other hand, is most likely to produce symptoms after the age of 45. Here the cause is simply wear and tear on the cartilage cushions of the joints, mainly weight-bearing ones such as the hips and knees. Both kinds of joint disorders afflict millions of persons with painful and disabling symptoms.

Osteoarthritis

The most common form of arthritis is *osteoarthritis*, which is also known by the terms *hypertrophic arthritis* and *degenerative joint disease*. It can be said quite accurately that if you live long enough you will experience osteoarthritis. In fact, osteoarthritis is most common in areas of the world where people have the greatest longevity. The first signs of osteoarthritis may appear on X-ray pictures of persons in their 30s and 40s, even though they have not yet felt pain in the weight-bearing joints, the hips and knees, where discomfort usually appears first. Studies show that nearly everybody has at least the beginning signs or symptoms of osteoarthritis after they reach their 50s. It affects both men and women, although women may not experience symptoms until after they have reached menopause.

Causes

A somewhat simplified explanation of the cause of osteoarthritis is this: the joints between the bones of a young person are cushioned and lubricated by cartilage pads and smooth lining membranes; normal wear and tear on the joints during a lifetime of activity gradually erodes the protective layers between the bones. In addition, the bones may develop small growths at the joints, a factor that aggravates the situation. There is evidence that heredity plays a role in the development of these bone growths, which are ten times more likely to occur in women than in men.

While hips and knees are among the most likely targets of osteoarthritis, the disease also can involve the hands, the shoulders, or back. Weight-bearing joints are commonly involved when the patient is overweight and spends a great deal of time standing or walking.

Symptoms

Except for the descriptions of aches and pains by victims of osteoarthritis and X-ray examination of the joints, a physician frequently has little information to go on in making a diagnosis of this disease. In some cases, there may be enlargement of the joint and some tenderness. But few cases are marked by the excessive warmth, for example, associated with rheumatoid arthritis. There are no laboratory tests that can distinguish the disorder from other rheumatic or arthritic diseases.

Osteoarthritis seldom causes the degree of discomfort experienced by patients afflicted by rheumatoid arthritis; the disease is not as disabling for most patients, and even the stiffness associated with osteoarthritis is milder, usually lasting only a few minutes when activity is attempted, while the stiffness of rheumatoid arthritis may continue for hours.

Arthritis of the Hip

Although most cases of osteoarthritis are not seriously disabling, arthritis of the hip is a prominent cause of disability in older persons. It produces pain in the hips, the inner thigh, the groin, and very often in the knee. Walking, climbing steps, sitting, and bending become very painful, because the joint is destroyed by degeneration of bone and cartilage. Stress and strain on the hip joint further aggravate the condition, which becomes worse with advancing age.

Surgery to replace the head of the femur or the entire hip joint with metal or plastic parts has brought relief from pain and restored mobility to some patients suffering from severe arthritis of the hip.

Small children sometimes suffer from transient arthritis of the hip, of unknown cause, manifested by pain, limitation of hip movement, and impeded walking. Because the condition usually disappears within six weeks, the only treatment is bed rest. Transient arthritis must not be mistaken for the more serious pyrogenic hip arthritis of children and adults, marked by high fever.

Spinal Arthritis

The aging process is the prinicipal cause of spinal arthritis. Other contributing factors are disk lesions and injury. Spinal arthritis causes pronounced bone degeneration and disability. The sufferer experiences severe back pain radiating to the thighs as a result of interference of the nerve roots from *osteophytes*, or spurs, formed in the joints. In mild cases, physical therapy may be the only treatment required.

Treatment of Osteoarthritis

For most patients, osteoarthritis is not likely to be crippling or disabling. The effects generally are not more serious than stiffness of the involved joints, with occasional discomfort and some pain. When weight-bearing joints are involved, the basic remedies are weight control and adequate rest for the areas affected. In some instances, the patient may have to learn new postural adjustments; symptoms often appear in another joint after the first has been affected because the patient tends to favor the joint that first caused pain and shifts weight or muscle stress to the second joint.

Physical therapy and corrective exercises are helpful. A physician may recommend the use of aspirin or another analgesic for the pain. Steroid drugs may be injected into an injured joint, but usually only for temporary relief. Surgery is sometimes recommended for removal of troublesome bone spurs or to correct a serious problem in a weight-bearing joint, where a metal cup or other device may be inserted as part of an artificial joint.

Hip Disorders

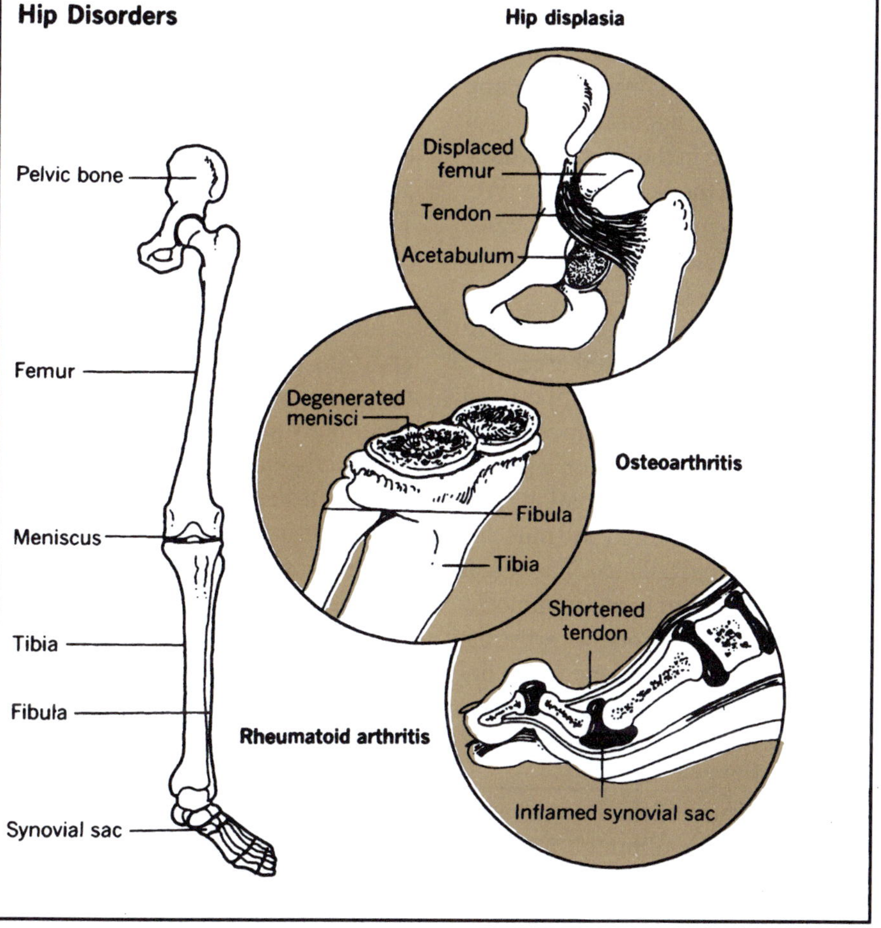

Rheumatoid Arthritis

Rheumatoid arthritis occurs at a much earlier age than osteoarthritis, appearing at any time from infancy to old age, but most commonly afflicting persons between the ages of 20 and 45. Women are three times as likely to be victims of rheumatoid arthritis as are men, although men seem to lose that advantage after the age of 50. All races seem to be equally vulnerable. Recent studies suggest a tendency to develop the disease may be inherited in some people. It is also thought that allergies, infections, or homonal disturbances play a role in initiating the disease.

Symptoms

Rheumatoid arthritis can begin as part of an acute illness, with high fever and intense inflammation of the joints, or it can develop insidiously with little or no discomfort except for fatigue, loss of appetite, weight loss, and perhaps a mild fever. Sometime later the victim becomes aware of aches and pains in the joints and muscles and seeks medical attention. Frequently, deformities develop before the patient realizes that rheumatoid arthritis may be the cause of swollen joints, pain, redness, or excessive warmth about the affected area.

The inflammation of a joint caused by rheumatoid arthritis may continue for weeks or it may last for a period of years. During inflammation, tendons become shortened and muscles lose their normal balance. The result is the deformity of joints commonly associated with rheumatoid arthritis, such as a swan-neck shape in the fingers. Muscular weakness develops and there is a loss of grip strength in the hands when that area is affected. Patients may be unable to make a tight fist.

A common symptom of rheumatoid arthritis is a stiffness that develops during periods of rest but gradually disappears when activity resumes. After a night's sleep, the stiffness may persist for a half hour or much longer. The stiffness may result, at least in part, from the muscular weakness that accompanies the disease.

Although the effects of rheumatoid arthritis are most commonly observed in the hands or feet of patients, other body joints such as the elbows, shoulders, knees, hips, ankles, spine, and even the jawbones may be involved. It is possible for all of a patient's joints to be involved, and the involvement often is symmetrical; that is, both hands will develop the symptoms at the same time and in the same pattern.

Probable Causes

The exact cause of rheumatoid arthritis is unknown, although a variety of factors have been associated with the onset of the disease. Emotional upsets, tuberculosis, venereal disease, psoriasis, and rheumatic fever are among conditions associated with the beginnings of the disease. Various viruses and other microorganisms have been isolated from the inflamed tissues of patients, but medical researchers have been unable to prove that any of the infectious agents is the cause. Efforts have also been made to transmit rheumatoid arthritis from a known victim to a normal volunteer by transfusions and injections of substances found in the victim's tissues, but without success in tracing the causative factor.

Treatment

The symptoms of rheumatoid arthritis intensify or abate spontaneously and unpredictably. Available methods of treatment do not cure the disease but relieve the symptoms so that the pain is reduced and some normal movement is facilitated. Proper nutrition, heat, rest, and exercise are also helpful. A number of drugs can reduce the inflammation of the joints, but they may have undesirable toxic side effects. Accordingly, before any drug therapy is embarked upon, the patient should seek the advice of a physician specializing in arthritic disorders.

Aspirin

The most common drug used to treat all kinds of arthritis is aspirin, an analgesic; it is also the most economical. Occasional side effects, such as irritation of ulcers or other gastrointestinal upsets, as well as buzzing in the ears, can result from aspirin use, especially in massive doses; such complications can sometimes be avoided by the use of specially coated aspirin tablets. The size of the dose usually is started at a minimum level and gradually increased until the physician finds a level that is most helpful to the patient but does not result in serious side effects. Celebrex, a new type of analgesic that is less irritating to the stomach, was approved for use in 1999.

There are several other drugs used in the treatment of rheumatoid arthritis. Non-steroidal antiinflammatory drugs (NSAIDs) such as ibuprofen, fenoprofen, naproxen, and indomethacin work about as well as aspirin but with less severe side effects. NSAIDs do however have side effects such as abdominal pain, nausea, and constipation. Most NSAIDs are generally taken twice a day. In 1993 the FDA approved oxaprozin (sold as Daypro), which needs to be taken only once a day.

In 1998 the first of a new class of drugs was approved for the treatment of rheumatoid athritis. Etanercept, an intravenous medication marketed as Enbrel, blocks the activity of tumor necrosis factor, believed to play a part in the inflammation process. This new class of drugs represented a major breakthrough in treatment; patients using it reported significantly less pain and swelling. Side effects include rashes at the site of injection and upper respiratory tract reactions.

Another new class of drugs, called disease modifying anti-rheumatic drugs, were also approved in the late 1990's. Leflunomide, sold as Arava, was the first of this new class to be marketed. It affects the function of immune cells known as T lymphocytes. Arava too can cause side effects, some of which can be very serious. It can cause intestinal distress, hair loss, or reversible liver damage. It has also been shown to cause birth defects; therefore, premenopausal women who take it also have to use birth control. Women taking the drug who decide to have a baby must discontinue using it and undergo a drug elimination process under doctor supervision.

Many other drugs promising relief for victims of arthritis have made their appearance in recent years. For example, penicillamine (trade name: Cuprimine) was found to help patients with rheumatoid arthritis. Experiments with many other drugs—including aclofenac, flurbiprofen, and proquazone—are under way.

Steroids

The cortisone-type (steroid) drugs have proven effective in controlling severe cases of rheumatoid arthritis. They can be given orally or injected directly into the affected joints. However, these drugs generate a number of undesirable side effects, and withdrawal often results in a severe recurrence of the original symptoms. Thus, steroid drug therapy is a long-term process that can make the patient totally dependent on the medication. Some physicians are reluctant to inject steroid drugs into the joints because the effect is temporary and there is a danger of introducing infection by repeated use of the needle. In addition, some patients do not seem to respond to the steroid drugs and X-ray studies of the joints may show progressive destruction of the tissues despite the medications.

Rest

Bed rest is recommended for acute cases and up to 10 hours of sleep per day is advised for mild cases of rheumatoid arthritis. The patient also should take rest periods during the day whenever possible, reducing fatigue and stress on the affected joints. As in severe cases of osteoarthritis, the patient should try to adjust his daily work habits to avoid strain on weight-bearing joints.

Exercise

Patients tend to avoid moving arthritic joints because of pain and stiffness. Exercise of an arthritic joint, however, helps prevent the adjoining muscles from shrinking and weakening. A program of physiotherapy—including hot packs and exercise—can be extremely helpful.

The exercise program should carry the joints through their normal range of movement. Exercises should be performed every day but not carried to the point of fatigue. In addition to exercises intended to prevent limitation of normal joint movement, isometric-type exercises should be used to maintain or increase muscle power in other parts of the body that might otherwise be neglected because of limited activity by the patient.

Posture

The patient should be encouraged to maintain proper posture as much as possible, through correct positioning of the body when standing, sitting, or reclining in bed. A sheet of thick plywood may be used under a mattress to prevent it from sagging. Chairs should be firm with straight backs. Pillows should be avoided whenever possible.

Crutches, canes, leg braces, and other devices may be needed by the patient in advanced stages of rheumatoid arthritis. In some cases, orthopedic surgery is recommended to help reconstruct the limbs and joints as a part of rehabilitation.

Heat

Massages or vibrating equipment are not recommended as part of the therapy for rheumatoid arthritis patients. Heat in the form of hot baths, hot compresses, or heating pads, however, may be helpful. Paraffin baths are particularly helpful in treating hands or wrists.

Diet

While osteoarthritis patients are advised to lose as much weight as possible, rheumatoid arthritis patients tend to suffer from weight loss and nutritional deficiencies. Part of the cause may be a loss of appetite that is a characteristic of the disease and part may be the gastrointestinal problems that frequently accompany the disorder and that may be aggravated by the medications prescribed. Some physicians advise that rheumatoid arthritis patients include adequate amounts of protein and calcium in their diets as a preventive measure against a loss of bone tissue.

Juvenile Rheumatoid Arthritis

A form of arthritis quite similar to adult rheumatoid arthritis afflicts some children before the age of 16. Called *juvenile rheumatoid arthritis* or *Still's disease*, it includes a set of symptoms that nevertheless differentiate it from adult rheumatoid arthritis. In addition to the rheumatoid joint symptoms, the patient may have a high fever, rash, pleurisy, and enlargement of the spleen. The onset of the disease may appear in the form of an unexplained childhood rash and fever, with arthritic symptoms developing as much as several weeks later. A possible complication is an eye inflammation that can lead to blindness if untreated.

Treatment

Juvenile rheumatoid arthritis is treated with aspirin or steroid drugs, or both, along with other kinds of therapy used for the adult version of rheumatoid arthritis. Steroid therapy is often more effective against rheumatoid arthritis in children than in adults. There may be a complete remission of the disease or the patient may experience rheumatoid symptoms into adult life.

Ankylosing Spondylitis

A kind of arthritis that affects the spine, causing a fusion of the joints, is known as *ankylosing spondylitis*. About 90 percent of the patients are young adult males. There is some evidence that it may be a hereditary disease.

Like other forms of arthritis, ankylosing spondylitis is insidious in its start. The patient may complain of a backache, usually in the lumbar area of the back. Some victims of the disease have claimed they were without pain but felt muscle spasms and perhaps tenderness along the lower part of the spine. Then stiffness and loss of motion spread rapidly over the back.

Along with fusion of the spine, the ligament along the spine calcifies like a bone. X-ray photographs of the spinal column may show the backbone to resemble a length of bamboo. A complication is that the spine is bent and chest expansion is limited by the fusion so that normal breathing is impaired.

Treatment of the disease consists of physical therapy and exercises to prevent or limit deformity and the use of aspirin or other drugs to reduce pain.

Gout

Gout is an arthritic disease associated with an abnormality of body chemistry. There is an excessive accumulation of uric acid in the blood resulting from the chemical abnormality, and the uric acid, in the form of sharp urate crystals, may accumulate in the joints, where they cause an inflammation with symptoms like those of arthritis. A frequent target of the urate crystals is the great toe, which is why gout patients occasionally are pictured as sitting in a chair with one foot propped upon a pillow.

Primary Gout

There are two forms of gout, primary gout and secondary gout. Primary gout is presumed to be linked to a hereditary defect in metabolism and afflicts mostly men, although women may experience the disease after menopause. The painful inflammation may develop overnight following an injury or illness or after a change in eating habits. The patient may suddenly feel feverish and unable to move because of the tenderness of the affected joint, which becomes painfully swollen and red.

Although the great toe is a common site for the appearance of gout, it also may develop in the ankle, knee, wrist, hand, elbow, or another joint. Only one joint may be affected, or several joints might be involved at the same time or in sequence. The painful attack usually subsides within a week or so but it may return to the same joint or another joint after an absence of a few years. The inflammation subsides even if it is not treated, but untreated gout may eventually result in deformity or loss of use of the affected joint. During periods between attacks the patient may show no signs of the disease except for high blood serum levels of uric acid and the appearance of *tophi*, or *urate* (a salt of uric acid) deposits, visible in X-ray photographs of the joints.

Secondary Gout

Secondary gout is related to a failure of the kidneys to excrete uric acid products or a variety of diseases that are characterized by overproduction of certain types of body cells. Failure of the kidneys to filter out urates can, in turn, be caused by various drugs, including aspirin and diuretics. Gout symptoms can also be caused by efforts to lose weight rapidly through a starvation diet, because this speeds up the breakdown of stored body fats. Among diseases that may precipitate an attack of secondary gout are Hodgkin's disease, psoriasis, and some forms of leukemia.

Chronic Gouty Arthritis

A form of arthritis called *chronic gouty arthritis* is associated with patients who have abnormal levels of uric acid in their blood. While they may or may not be plagued by attacks of acute joint pain, the urate deposits apparently cause a certain amount of stiffness and soreness in various joints, especially during periods of stormy weather or falling barometric pressure. The tophi or urate crystals may spread to soft tissues of the body, such as bursae, the cartilage of the ear, and tendon sheaths. More than ten percent of gout patients eventually develop kidney stones formed from urate deposits in the kidney.

Treatment of Gout

Because gout was traditionally associated with certain meats that are rich in chemicals called *purines*, special diets were once a routine part of the treatment. In recent years, there has been less emphasis placed on maintaining a low-purine diet for gout patients. This change in therapy is mainly the result of the relatively good success in maintaining proper uric-acid levels in gout patients with medications. However, adequate fluid intake is still recommended to prevent development of urate kidney stones.

Infectious Arthritic Agents

There are at least 12 types of arthritis and rheumatism that are associated with infections involving bacteria, viruses, fungi, or other organisms. One of these diseases is known as *pyrogenic arthritis*. The arthritis-causing organisms infect a joint and induce pain and fever and limitation of joint movement by muscle spasm and swelling. Treatment includes bed rest and antibiotics. If untreated, destruction of the joints is possible.

Gonococcal Arthritis

This disease is transmitted by the gonococcal bacteria associated with venereal disease. As in the venereal disease itself, the arthritic effects are more likely to be treated at an early stage in men than in women because men are more likely to develop obvious infections of the urethra and thus seek medication from a physician. In females, the initial infection is likely to go unrecognized and untreated by antibiotics. The infection, meanwhile, may spread to body joints and produce acute attacks of arthritis. The symptoms tend to appear first in the wrists and finger joints; there may also be skin lesions that occur temporarily in areas near the joints.

Tuberculous Arthritis

As the name suggests, this disease is associated with tuberculosis and can be serious, leading to the destruction of involved joints. The infection spreads to the joints from other areas of the body. The early symptoms include pain, tenderness, or muscle spasm. In children and young adults the infection tends to settle in the spinal joints. If there is an absence of pain, the disease may go unnoticed until changes in posture or gait are observed. If untreated, the disease may progress toward spinal deformity. When detected early in the course of the disease, treatment with antituberculosis drugs and physical therapy may control the disorder. In some cases, surgery may be required.

Rubella Arthritis

This form of arthritis derives from an infection involving the rubella virus. The arthritis symptoms may appear shortly after a rash appears, or they may be delayed until after the rash has faded. The onset of the arthritis effects may be accompanied by fever and a general feeling of illness; pain and swelling are most likely to occur in the small joints of the wrists, knees, or ankles. The physician usually advises aspirin for the pain while it lasts, usually about a week. Eventually all signs and symptoms may subside without joint destruction.

Bacteria That Cause Arthritis

A type of bacteria that causes spinal meningitis also may cause symptoms of arthritis. The pain usually is not severe and may be limited to a few body joints. Antibiotics are administered to control the infection, although this form of the disease does not respond as rapidly to the medication as some of the other versions of arthritis caused by infection.

Several other kinds of bacteria may invade the joints and precipitate or aggravate arthritic symptoms. They include the increasingly common strains of bacteria that have become resistant to control by antibiotics. Patients who are being treated with steroid drugs or those whose resistance to infection has been lowered by disease are among the most vulnerable victims.

Fungal Arthritis

While fungal infections are relatively rare causes of arthritis, there are at least four kinds of fungus that have been identified as the responsible organisms in joint inflammations. The fungus seems to be carried by the bloodstream to the area of the joint where it causes an inflammation in the tissues surrounding the bony structures. The infection usually can be treated with special antibiotic remedies that destroy fungal organisms, but surgery is occasionally necessary to ensure eradication of the source of the inflammation.

Psoriatic Arthropathy

Arthritis also may be associated with psoriasis (a chronic skin condition marked by bright red patches and scaling) in a disease known as *psoriatic arthropathy.* This variation of the disease is marked by a deep pitting of the nails along with a chronic arthritic condition. The disease may be mild or very destructive and the sacroiliac region of the spine may be involved. The uric acid levels associated with gout frequently are elevated in patients with psoriasis, so gout symptoms also can appear. Unfortunately, one of the medications commonly used in the treatment of rheumatoid arthritis and gout, chloroquine, cannot be used as therapy for psoriatic arthropathy symptoms because the drug aggravates the psoriasis. Otherwise, the treatment is quite similar to that used for rheumatoid arthritis—analgesics such as aspirin and steroid drugs. In severe cases, methotrexate may be administered to control both the joint and skin symptoms.

Other Arthritic Diseases

Two kinds of arthritis once associated with venereal diseases are no longer considered a hazard of intimate contact. One is syphilis-caused arthritis, which is a possible problem but actually quite rare because of improved control of syphilis. The second is *Reiter's syndrome,* a form of arthritis in which there is also involvement of urethritis, or inflammation of the urethra, and conjunctivitis, an inflammation of the eye. The disease also may be accompanied by skin lesions and a fever, pain in the heels, and a urethral discharge. Perhaps because Reiter's syndrome seems to affect young men and symptoms may be similar to those of gonococcal arthritis, it was once assumed that this form of arthritis was a kind of venereal disease. However, there is a lack of evidence that the disease is transmitted by sexual contact.

Rheumatic Fever

This generalized inflammatory disease, which affects the entire body with pain and swelling of the joints, sometimes is classified as a form of arthritis. Rheumatic fever usually follows a sore throat or tonsillitis caused by streptococcus bacteria; however, the disease is not regarded as a streptococcal infection by itself. A common effect of rheumatic fever is a scarring of the heart valves due to inflammation of that tissue. The heart valve damage is permanent. The streptococcal infection itself can be controlled by antibiotic medications. For further information, see "Rheumatic Fever and Rheumatic Heart Disease" in Ch. 10, *Heart Disease.*

Bursitis

The *bursa* is a fluid-filled sac located in the muscle near most joints. The fluid lubricates the joint, thereby providing smooth joint movement. Infection or injury may cause inflammation of the bursa. This condition is known as *bursitis* and can be very painful. The most commonly affected joints are the shoulder, knee, and hip.

Calcium deposits in the shoulder tendon or calcification of the bursa (*calcific bursitis*) leads to more painful shoulder problems. This may be similar to *interstitial calcinosis,* a condition in which calcium deposits are found in the skin and subcutaneous tissues of children. Recovery from calcific bursitis is achieved by medical care, minor surgery, and resting the inflamed joint. Radiation treatments can sometimes speed the recovery process.

Living with Joint Diseases

The control of arthritis requires skilled medical supervision over extended periods of time. The causes of the major forms of arthritis are still

Bursitis

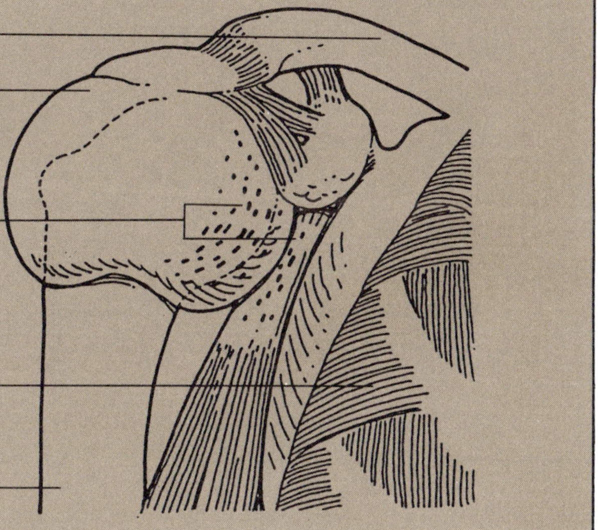

unknown, although various theories have been formulated to explain it based on metabolic, biochemical, and microscopic tissue studies. Despite years of intensive research, it has not been possible to isolate a microorganism that is generally agreed to be a cause of rheumatoid arthritis. Viruses have been implicated in a number of arthritic diseases and may be a cause of rheumatoid arthritis; the evidence remains elusive, however, and the virus theory will remain a theory until the specific causative organism has been isolated and tested.

Whatever the mystery surrounding the causes of osteoarthritis and rheumatoid arthritis, severe crippling can be prevented in 70 percent of the cases if the patient seeks medical care early in the disease and receives proper medical treatment. The course of the disease varies from patient to patient and in many cases is confined to a few joints, causing little or no impairment of function. Commonly, however, there is a tendency toward relapse or continued inflammation.

The arthritis patient needs to develop a sense of coexistence with the disease, a tolerant attitude toward the problems of possible pain or disability without surrendering to arthritis. Millions of people have learned to live with arthritis and have found that it is possible to work, travel, raise families, and enjoy many of the recreational activities pursued by people not afflicted by the disease.

Joint Replacement

Over the years, various methods of replacing joints have evolved. Like artificial hips, artificial knee, elbow, ankle, shoulder, toe, and finger joints

Joint Replacement (Hip)

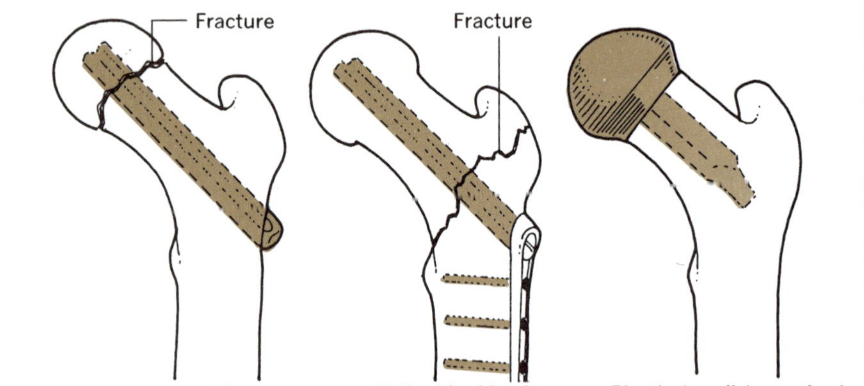

are becoming more and more common. Technically known as arthroplasty, joint replacement both relieves pain, including the pain of arthritis, and improves function.

Materials used in joint replacement operations include metal, plastic, and ceramic components. Because of the tasks they perform in bodily movement, hip, knee, and ankle arthroplasties are undertaken much more often than those involving other parts. Developments in knee replacement surgery include a "cementless knee" that has a porous surface of chrome cobalt beads; aided by the beads, the patient's bone cells grow right into the knee replacement.

In each type of operation, the surgeon faces special problems. The elbow, for example, is not a simple hinge or joint but has three sections. Each involves one of the three arm bones that meet at that point: the humerus, the radius, and the ulna.

Surgical joint replacement techniques are continually evolving. In all cases, the patient faces some risks. Patients are also told usually that joint replacements do not really cure arthritis or osteoarthritis even though they normally relieve pain.

Defects and Diseases of the Spine

Spinal Curve Deformities

When looked at from the side, the normal human spine follows a shallow S-shaped curve. If there is an exaggerated forward curvature of the spine, that condition is described as a *lordosis*. This type of spinal curvature is uncommon except in late pregnancy, and is caused by hip deformity or a defect in posture.

Kyphosis

Kyphosis is an exaggerated backward spinal curvature characterized by a humpback appearance. A person with this disorder develops an abnormal-looking thorax (or chest) due to the hump in the back and may sometimes find it difficult to lie on his back. The condition is brought on by untreated fractures of a vertebral body, a spinal tumor, osteoporosis, or spinal tuberculosis. If the principal cause is diagnosed and treated, recovery is possible.

Scoliosis

Scoliosis is a lateral curvature of the central part of the spine and appears mostly in children from birth and young adults up to age 15. Early diagnosis and proper orthopedic care are important. If scoliosis appears in early adulthood, the prognosis is better than if the disease starts in infancy. Growth of the curvature ends when the individual's skeletal development ceases.

Scoliosis creates an ugly spinal deformity, and this is usually the only symptom. Sometimes there may be an acute attack of sciatica. Treatment of scoliotic children requires hospital-

Vertebral Column

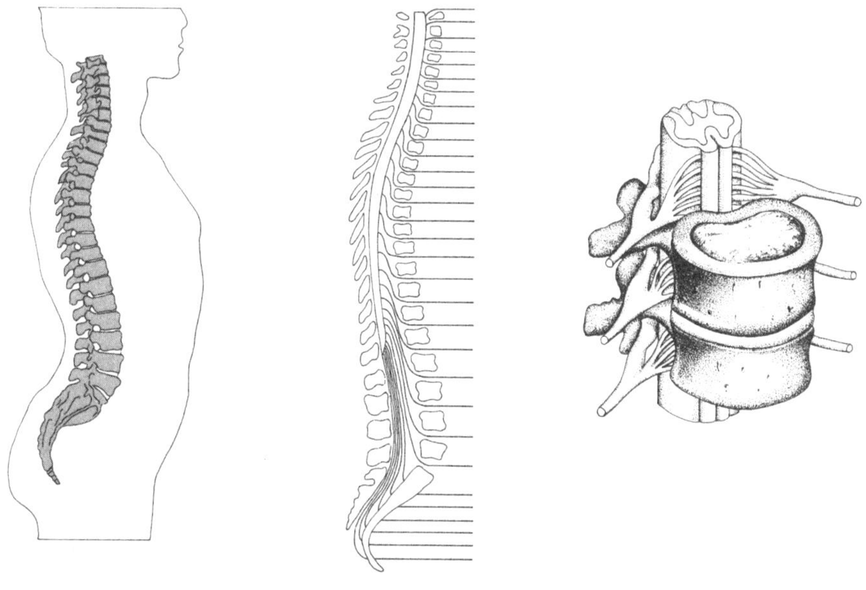

Scoliosis

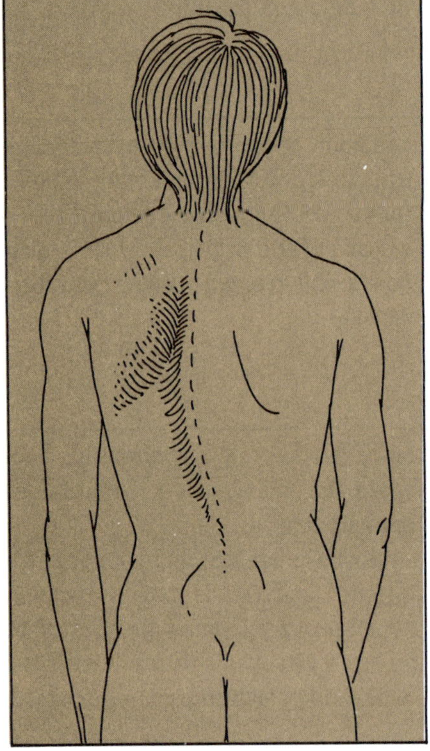

ization. In simple cases, a cast is applied from the chest to the waist to reduce the curvature. Fusion of the vertebral bodies with bone grafting to maintain the fusion may be necessary.

Spinal Tuberculosis

Chronic pulmonary tuberculosis can spread to the skeletal system, including the vertebral column. Spinal tuberculosis, also known as *Pott's disease*, affects one or more vertebrae in children and young adults. It is currently a relatively rare disease.

The diseased vertebrae may collapse because of the pressure from the vertebrae above, resulting in a humpback deformity and possible paralysis of the lower limbs. The usual symptoms are back pain, stiffness, and limited movement. Antibiotics are administered to combat and cure the infection.

Spinal Infections

Fever-inducing microorganisms may reach the spine via the blood and lymph channels, resulting in spinal osteomyelitis or a general inflammation of the vertebrae. This results in bone destruction, pressure on the spinal cord, and paralysis of the legs. Successful treatment includes bed rest, drug therapy, and sometimes a body jacket (for immobilization) made from plaster of Paris.

Tumors

The spinal column is affected by both malignant and benign tumors. They can either destroy the bony makeup of the affected vertebra, apply pressure to the spinal cord with resultant paralysis, or interfere with the nerve roots.

Spinal tumors are generally destructive. Some, like *meningiomas* and *neurofibromas*, result in lack of control over bowel and bladder function in addition to the loss of functioning of the lower extremities. Malignant tumors of the spinal column may originate from cancer of the prostate, uterus, bladder, lungs, or breast.

The symptoms of spinal tumors are pain, deformity, weakness, and lower limb paralysis. Diagnosis requires careful study of the subjective symptoms, as well as special tests and radiological examinations. Treatment may involve radiation therapy and chemotherapy; some tumors can be surgically removed. In many instances, the patient may be given analgesics to relieve the pain.

Back Pain and Its Causes

Most adults have experienced some form of back pain. Back pain is a serious physical impairment in persons of all ages, but it occurs more frequently in older persons.

Lumbago and Sciatica

Lumbago refers to general pain in the lower back. Technically, it is not a disease but a symptom that is accentuated by bending, lifting, turning, coughing, or stooping. Pain from neuritis of the sciatic nerve adds to one's misery, with pain shooting down the legs. This form of back pain is commonly known as *sciatica*, and, like lumbago, can be considered a symptom of some other condition. Treatment depends on the underlying cause of both.

Slipped and Herniating Disks

Between each two vertebrae is a fibro-cartilaginous disk that acts as a cushion. These disks are subjected to strain with every movement of the body, especially in the erect position. Increased pressure may cause a disk to protrude or herniate into the vertebral canal, causing what is referred to as a *slipped disk*. This condition can also be brought on by injury, degeneration caused by aging, unaccus-

Sciatica

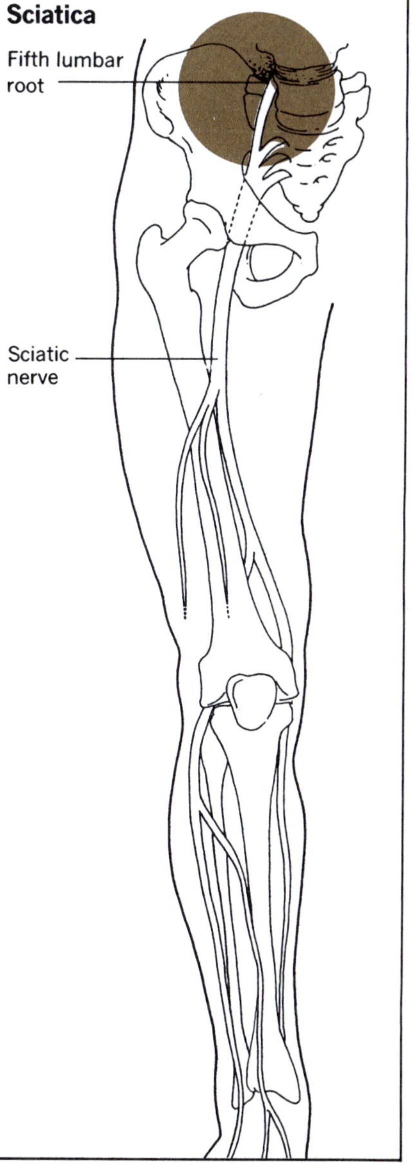

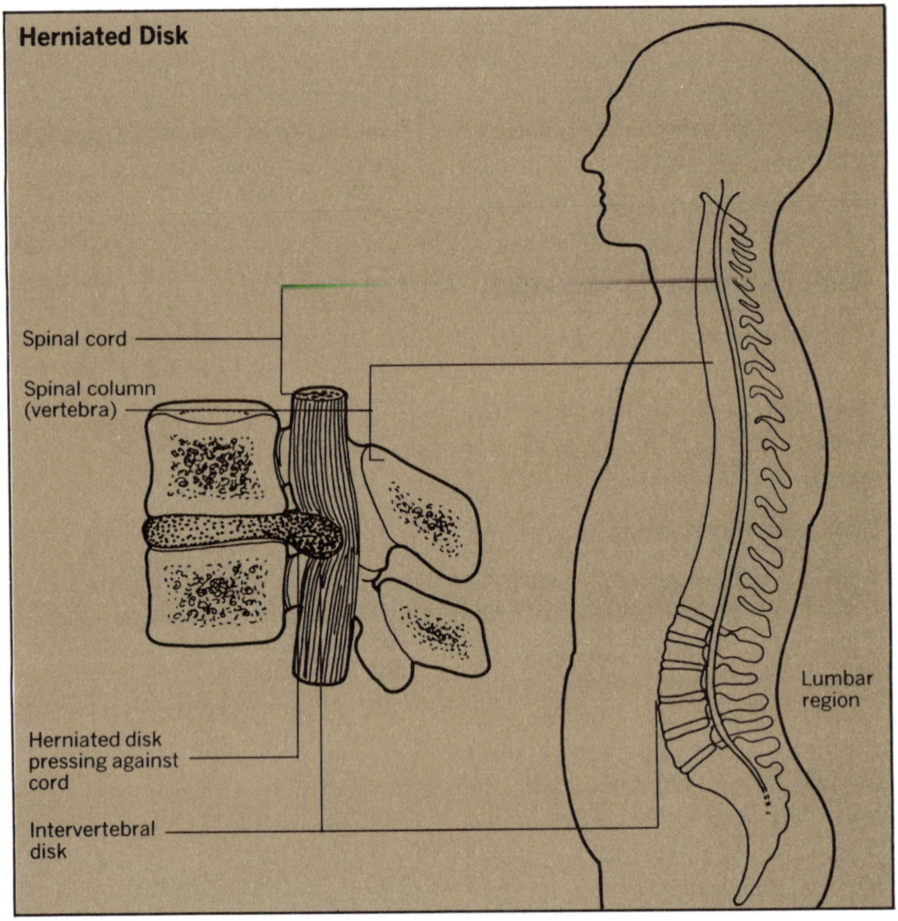

tomed physical activity, or heavy lifting.

The herniating disk presses against nerves in the area, resulting in low back pain, sciatica, and in some instances, disabling muscle spasm. Back rest and a surgical corset may help milder forms of slipped disk by allowing natural healing to take place. Treatment may also include bed rest with intermittent traction to the legs for several weeks. Spinal fusion may be required in severe cases.

A severely herniated disk can be surgically removed to relieve pain and other symptoms. Disk removal is followed by fusion of the vertebral bodies on both sides of the removed disk. Fusion is accomplished by bridging the vertebral space with a bone graft. For a fuller description of surgical repair of a slipped disk, see under "Orthopedic Surgery" in Ch. 20, *Surgery*.

Spondylolisthesis

A forward displacement of one vertebral body over another results in a painful condition known as *spondylolisthesis*. In mild cases there may be no symptoms at all. But in more advanced forms, there is severe low back pain when in the erect position and on bending, with the pain radiating to the legs. The displaced vertebra interferes with nerve roots in that area.

Mild cases require no treatment. Severe cases may require fusion of the vertebral segments with bone grafting; less severe symptoms can be relieved by a specially fitted corset.

Muscle Spasms and Strained Ligaments

Lack of physical exercise and unaccustomed bending can cause acute backache from undue muscle strain. Backache from strain on the ligaments is not uncommon in women following childbirth. The symptoms are similar to general low back pain. Physiotherapy with moist heat and massage helps restore muscular tone and relieve the pain. Muscle-relaxing drugs are sometimes prescribed.

Sacroiliac Pain

The *sacroiliac* joints in the lower back, where the *iliac* (hipbone) joins the sacrum, are a common location for osteoarthritic changes, rheumatoid arthritis, tuberculosis, and ankylosing spondylitis. The most common site of pain is in the lower lumbar region, radiating to the thighs and legs. X-ray diagnosis helps to pinpoint the cause of this particular form of back pain.

Other Disorders of the Skeletal System

Because bone consists of living cells, it is constantly changing as old cells die and new cells take their places. Any systemic disease during the growing period may temporarily halt the growth of long bones. As the aging process continues, dead bone cells are not replaced as consistently as in earlier life. The bony skeleton thus loses some of its calcium content, a process known as *decalcification* or *bone atrophy*, and the bones become fragile.

Pelvis and Hip Disorders

The hip joint presents most of the problems in the pelvic area. Symptoms may appear in early infancy in the form of congenital hip dislocation, in older children as tuberculous and transient arthritis, as slipped epiphysis in young adults (discussed below), and as osteoarthritis in adults and the aged. Early diagnosis of these conditions is very important in reducing the possibility of permanent deformity.

Diagnosis is achieved by physical examinations for signs of abnormal joint stability and mobility, postural changes, unstable and painful hip movement, fixed joint deformity, and pain in the lower back. Measurement of both lower limbs may indicate the presence of abnormal hip structure. X-ray examination of the pelvic area and both hips aids in diagnosis, as does blood analysis, which may yield evidence of early signs of gouty or arthritic conditions.

Slipped Epiphysis

This condition occurs in late childhood, between the ages of 9 and 18. The head of the *femur*, or thighbone, slips from its normal position, affecting one or both hips. The individual feels pain in the hip and knee, has limitation in joint movement, and walks with a limp. Usually there is evidence of endocrine disturbances.

Legg-Perthes' Disease

This is an inflammatory condition of unknown origin involving the bone and cartilage of the femoral head. It is found mostly in children between 4 and 12 years old and usually affects one hip. The symptoms are thigh and groin pain, joint movement limitation, and a walking impediment.

Successful treatment requires extended hospitalization with weight traction applied to the diseased hip and limitation of body weight on the affected side. Untreated Legg-Perthes' disease leads to permanent hip joint deformity and possible osteoarthritis around middle age.

Coxa Vara

This hip deformity is caused by a misshapen femur and causes shortening of the leg on the affected side; as a result, the person walks with a limp. The condition may be related to bone softening brought on by rickets, poorly joined fractures of the hip, or congenital malformation of the hip joint. Some cases may require surgical correction.

Any attack of persistent unexplained hip pains, limitation of movement, and walking impediments should be referred to the family physician for further investigation. Early diagnosis is crucial in controlling and eradicating many of the crippling diseases of the pelvic area.

Other Bone Disorders

Osteoporosis

This metabolic disorder is marked by porousness and fragility of the bones. When the condition is associated with old age, it is called *senile osteoporosis.* While the exact cause of the disorder is unknown, most physicians believe that calcium deficiencies—or inadequate calcium intake—may be a primary cause. Other contributing causes may be protein deficiency and a lack of the sex hormones androgen and estrogen. Postmenopausal women experience a dramatic decrease in the production of estrogen, which maintains bone strength. Because of its link with estrogen, osteoporosis is quite common among postmenopausal women.

Researchers stress the need for both good diet and exercise as means of arresting or preventing osteoporosis. Calcium and vitamin D supplements may help. A calcium-rich diet includes foods such as low-fat cheeses and milk; yogurt; red kidney, lima, and soybeans; fish; and green, leafy vegetables. Several types of drugs to treat osteoporosis are also available; they include estrogen, bisphosphonates, calcitonins, and estrogen receptor modulators (SERMs), such as raloxifene.

New methods of diagnosis have made earlier detection possible. Noninvasive methods include *absorptiometry,* a measure of bone loss in the wrist and foot; *dualphoton absorptiometry,* a measure of bone loss in the spine and hip; and the use of a CT scan to measure loss of spinal bone. Blood tests, today the subject of research, may provide a means of very early detection. Once bone loss has been found to be too rapid, physicians can suggest ways to slow the rate of loss before fractures occur.

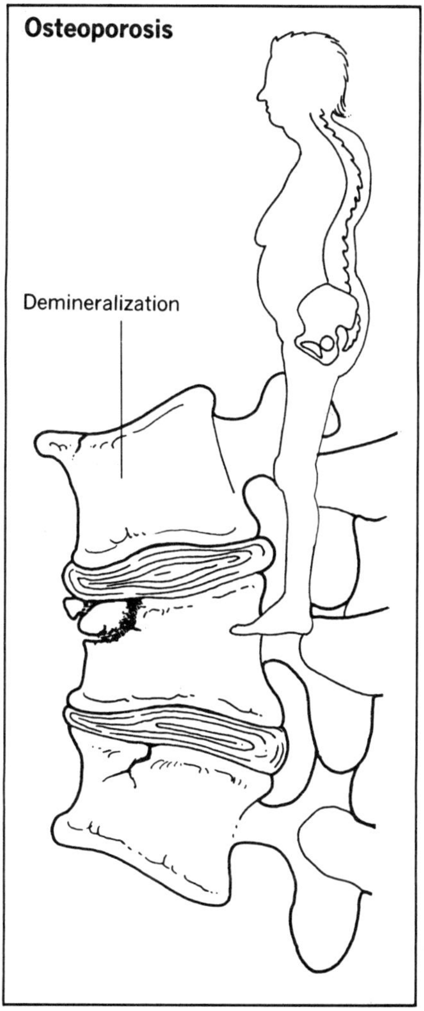

Osteogenesis Imperfecta

During the formation and development of bones, a process called *osteogenesis,* the bones may grow long and thin but not to the required width, becoming brittle so that they fracture easily. This condition is known as *osteogenesis imperfecta.* The individual may grow out of the condition in the middle twenties after suffering numerous fractures while growing up. A child thus afflicted cannot participate in games or other strenuous activities.

Paget's Disease

Paget's disease is characterized by a softening of the bones followed by an abnormal thickening of the bones. Its cause is unknown, and it manifests itself after the age of 30. It may cause pain in the thighs, knees, or legs, as well as backache, headache, and general fatigue. Symptoms include deafness, deformity of the pelvis, spine, and skull, and bowed legs. Although there is no known cure, Paget's disease is not usually fatal, but is eventually disabling.

Osteomyelitis

Osteomyelitis is an inflammation of the bone caused by fever-inducing bacteria or mold organisms. The invading microorganisms usually reach the bone through the bloodstream after entering the body through a wound or ulcer; the infection also can begin through a compound fracture or during surgery. The staphylococcus germ is most frequently the causative agent, and the most frequent site is the shaft of a long bone of a child. In adults, osteomyelitis usually occurs in the pelvis or spinal column.

Symptoms

Symptoms are fever, chills, and pain, with nausea and vomiting, especially in younger patients. There also may be muscle spasms around the affected bone. The infected bone usually is sensitive to the touch but X rays may reveal no abnormality during the early stages. Redness and swelling sometimes appear in tissues above the inflamed bone, and as the disease progresses the patient may find that simply moving the affected limb is painful. The infection can involve a joint, producing misleading symptoms of arthritis.

Causes

Examination by a physician usually reveals signs of a recent wound, ulceration, or similar lesion that may have been accompanied by pus from the invading bacteria. Laboratory tests of the blood usually will show an abnormal number of white cells and the presence of the infectious microorganism. Signs of anemia also may be found.

Treatment

Treatment may include the use of antibiotics for a period of several weeks. In difficult cases, surgery may be required to drain abscesses or to remove dead bone tissue. Before the advent of antibiotic drugs, osteomyelitis could be a fatal disease; early and proper treatment with modern medications has virtually eliminated that risk.

Diet and Bone Disorders

A proper diet is necessary to maintain the health of the skeletal system. The body's retention of the bone-building minerals, phosphorus and calcium, depends on vitamin D, which is manufactured in the human skin through the action of the sun's ultraviolet radiation.

Rickets

An insufficient supply of vitamin D and a lack of exposure to sunlight leads to a vitamin deficiency disease known as *rickets*. It can occur in infants and small children who live in northern latitudes and thus are not exposed to sufficient sunlight to permit their body to manufacture vitamin D. Rickets slows growth and causes bent and distorted bones and bandy legs. Symptoms first appear between the age of six months and the end of the first year. If rickets is recognized in time, it can be cured by a diet containing adequate vitamin D and by exposure to sunlight. If the disease is unchecked, the bones may develop permanent curves.

Bone Tumors

Benign and malignant tumors can occur in bone and bone marrow, although these growths are far less common than tumors of the body's soft tissues. Children and adolescents are more susceptible to bone tumors than adults. Since X rays cannot show whether a bone tumor is benign or malignant, surgical biopsy of the affected tissue is necessary in all cases.

Benign Tumors

These tumors usually take the form of an overgrowth of bone tissue, often near a joint, with many cysts or hollow spaces in the affected tissue. These growths often cause pathological fractures, in which a bone breaks for no apparent reason. Swelling, pain, and limited mobility in the joint nearest the tumor are the most common symptoms. Treatment consists of surgical removal of the tumor, after which the surrounding bone gradually repairs itself as it does after a fracture.

Malignant Tumors

Bone cancers may be primary (originating in the bone tissue itself) or caused by metastasis of cancer cells from a site elsewhere in the body. The most common types of primary bone cancer are *osteogenic sarcoma,* a rapidly growing form of cancer that often spreads into nearby muscles; *chondrosarcoma,* which begins in cartilage at the end of a bone; and *Ewing's sarcoma,* a highly malignant cancer of the shafts of the long bones in children.

Bone cancer of the extremities is treated by amputation of the affected limb, followed by radiation therapy. If treatment is begun early enough and all the cancerous tissue is removed, the prognosis for survival is favorable.

Injury to Bones and Joints: Fractures and Dislocations

Bones can be broken or displaced when the body is subjected to a violent impact or when a limb is suddenly wrenched out of its normal position. Auto and bicycle accidents and accidents in and around the home account for many such injuries. See Ch. 31, *Medical Emergencies,* for information on accidents and how to provide treatment.

A *fracture* is a break in a bone as a result of injury or pathological weakness. Tumors, for example, can destroy bones to such an extent that a spontaneous fracture occurs due to pathological weakness. Osteoporosis can also cause such fractures.

A *dislocation* is a displacement of any part, especially a bone. During this process the joint-capsule ligaments and muscle may be torn. The displaced bones must be reset by a bone specialist in their original position and immobilized until healing is complete. If this is not done, there is every possibility that the unhealed muscles will not provide the necessary support, thereby causing chronic spontaneous dislocation.

Injury (*trauma*) to bones and joints should not be dismissed lightly, especially if pain persists. If untreated, fractures and dislocations may heal with the bones out of alignment. Permanent deformity and joint degeneration are two possible complications.

Crush injuries, such as those occurring in some industrial and automobile accidents, may result in the clogging or blockage of blood vessels that supply blood to an extremity. When this happens, tissues below the blockage may die, and wounds do not heal because of lack of oxygenated blood and nutrition. If the fractures and wounds are not properly treated, *gangrene*, or the death of soft tissues, can sometimes result, requiring amputation just above the site of blockage and at a location that will make the healing process possible.

Kinds of Fractures

Incomplete fractures are those that do not destroy the continuity of the bone. In a *complete fracture*, the bone is completely broken across. A *simple* or *closed fracture* is one in which the fragments are held together under the surface of the skin by the muscles and soft tissues. In a *compound* or *open fracture* one or both fragments pierce the skin, resulting in an open wound. In some cases the bony fragments can be seen protruding through the skin.

Comminuted fractures are the result of crushed bones. Several fragments appear at the trauma site. *Greenstick fractures* occur when one side of the bone is broken and the other bent. This type of fracture is more common in long bones, especially the forearms, clavicle, and legs of young children. *Stress fractures*, tiny cracks in the bone, can occur in the bones of the foot or leg of athletes who put these bones under repeated stress, such as ballet dancers and long-distance runners.

Types of Bone Fractures

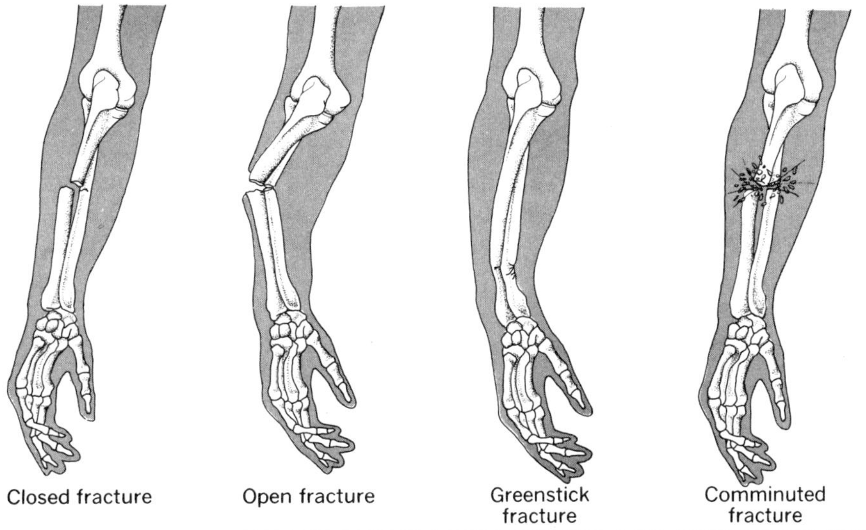

Healing of Fractures

When a bone breaks, new bone cells called *callus* are laid down at the ends of the fracture to unite the fragments. This is the beginning of the healing process, the speed of which is dependent on the nature of the fracture.

Simple, incomplete, and greenstick fractures heal readily. Rest is usually sufficient to heal stress fractures. However, compound fractures have wounds and fragments to complicate the healing process. Cleaning and suturing the wound and administering antibiotics reduce the chance of infection and promote healing.

Comminuted fractures may have to be disimpacted and all fragments reset, usually by an orthopedic or general surgeon. Some very serious fractures of the extremities may require surgical insertion of metallic pins, nails, plates, wires, or screws to hold the fragments in proper position, thereby promoting rapid healing with minimal deformity. Such devices must be made from corrosion-free and rustproof metals because they may remain in the body for a few months or throughout the person's lifetime.

Age and the Healing Process

The age of the fracture victim determines the speed of healing. In healthy, normal children, broken bones mend quickly because a rapid bone-cell manufacturing process is constantly in progress during the growth of the child. This is further advanced by proper diet, including daily intake of milk and milk products to provide the calcium required to build healthy bones.

In young adults, new bone cells do not develop as rapidly as in the growing child, but under normal circumstances, this will not present problems with the healing of fractures. Fractures in the aged heal slowly or not at all, depending on the age and health of the individual.

Treatment of Fractures

Correction of a fracture or dislocation is called *reduction* and is usually performed by an orthopedic surgeon. Bones that are merely cracked do not require reduction; they heal with the aid of immobilization. More serious fractures require manipulation, pressure, and sometimes, as mentioned above, wires, pins, nails, and screws, to bring the fragments together so that they can unite.

Healing of fractures and dislocations following reduction requires proper immobilization, which also reduces pain by preventing movement of the fragments. Immobilization is usually accomplished by the use of splints or plaster casts or by applying *traction*. Traction subjects the fractured member to a pulling force by means of a special apparatus, such as a system of weights and pulleys.

After a fracture or dislocation is reduced and immobilized in a cast, the injury is X-rayed to ensure that the immobilized reduction will heal without deformity. If the reduction is not satisfactory, the cast is removed, the fragments are remanipulated to provide better reduction, and a new cast or bandage is applied. Periodic X-ray rechecks help the physician ascertain the degree of new bone formation as the healing continues. Casts are also checked to make sure there is not excess swelling of tissues and compression of blood vessels in the area.

How long a cast must remain depends on the extent of the injury and the rapidity of healing. A broken wrist may heal in four to six weeks while a fractured tibia may require four months of immobilization in a plaster cast.

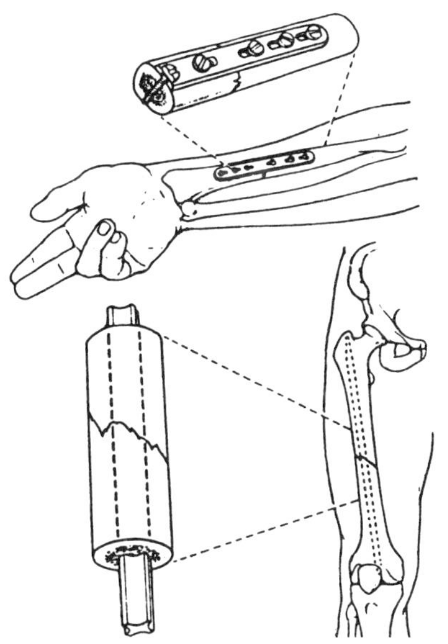

(Top) A metal plate is fastened with screws to secure a fractured bone in the arm (the radius). The enlarged portion shown in cross section is also shown as it appears in the patient's arm. *(Bottom)* A steel rod has been driven through the center of the femur of the leg to hold the jagged ends of the fractured bone in proper alignment. Such appliances are sometimes left in place indefinitely when there are no adverse reactions.

Fracture of the Pelvis

Pelvic injuries are most often caused by falls in the home or on slippery streets and by industrial or automobile accidents.

The pelvis bears the entire weight of the body from the waist up and must bear the stress of general body motion during daily activity. The bony architecture of the pelvis does not readily permit the use of a plaster cast to immobilize a fracture. Consequently, fractures of the pelvis require bed rest for at least three weeks, depending on the nature of the injury and the age of the patient.

Simple fractures in children and young adults heal readily with complete bed rest and proper home care. Among the aged, the creation of new bone cells occurs more slowly, and this complicates the management of serious pelvic fractures in people over 65. Prolonged inactivity from extensive bed rest presents other health hazards for the aged, such as sluggish digestion and respiratory or vascular complications.

Fracture of the Hip

Falls are a major cause of hip fractures—the most common type of pelvic injury. Intense pain with limitation of hip movement and external rotation of the lower leg are indications of a hip fracture. When this occurs, a physician should be contacted immediately. The patient should be placed flat in bed until medical advice has been obtained. Proper diagnosis requires X-ray examinations.

Patients with hip fractures must be hospitalized. Although a hip fracture may be treated with traction, this method requires months of bed rest and is rarely used. The best method for treating such fractures is to nail the hip together with a metallic pin. The operation is performed by a surgeon, usually an orthopedist, who uses X-ray examinations during surgery to ascertain that the pin is in the correct position. Some hip fractures may also require a metallic plate screwed to the bone to help immobilize the fracture.

After plates and pins have been inserted, the patient can be out of bed within a day. This speeds recovery and prevents the complications of prolonged bed rest. Hip nails are usually left in the patient, depending on the nature of the fracture and the patient's age. Recuperation includes periodic medical checkups and X-ray examinations.

Hip Replacement

In recent years the technique of total hip replacement has become well advanced. The technique can be used where the hip joint has been injured or severely weakened by disease.

Called *total prosthetic replacement of the hip*, the operation involves removal of the upper portion of the large leg bone, the femur, and of the ball-like joint that holds it in the hip socket. A substitute piece shaped like the removed section of bone is attached to the femur. Care has to be taken during the operation to make certain the new part is firmly attached—by embedding the replacement part in the shaft of the bone. In addition, the surgeon tries not to destroy or damage the muscles and other tissues surrounding the hip. The replacement part is usually made of metal; a commonly used material is a durable cobalt-chromium alloy that produces no painful reactions in surrounding bones and tissues.

With modern techniques, hip replacement surgery can restore most patients to virtually normal levels of functioning. The implanted parts can carry weight and stand the strains of everyday use. Metal screws and a grouting agent (mortar of plastic cement or other material) help to join the metal implant to the leg bone. Patients may begin to walk one to three days after surgery. While they can later play golf or other nonstrenuous games, they are usually told to avoid more demanding activities, such as tennis or handball, because of the danger that they might fall and injure the replacement hip.

Some patients have had successful hip replacement surgery on both their right and left sides. Later they were able to function with good mobility and without pain.

Pubic Fracture

Pubic fractures can cause ruptures of the bladder with urine leaking into the pelvic cavity. Routine urinalysis for the presence of blood cells is always necessary in cases of pelvic fractures. Surgical repair of the bladder may be required.

Skull Injury

Although the skull is very thick, it is not invulnerable. Head injuries can result from sports or playground accidents, falls, automobile or industrial accidents, or sharp blows to the head. Head injuries can cause linear or hairline skull fractures, depressed skull fractures (dents), brain injury due to fracture fragments or foreign bodies piercing the brain (as in the case of a bullet wound), or *concussion* with or without bone damage. The effects of concussion can show up as dizziness, nausea, irritability, the tendency to sleep deeply or lose consciousness, a weak pulse, and slowed respiration.

Any of these injuries can cause blood vessels to rupture and bleed. The resulting blood clots form what is known as a *subdural hematoma,* which may cause increased pressure on the brain. Patients with a subdural hematoma feel dizzy, slip slowly into unconsciousness, and may die unless immediate hospital care is available. Usually half of the body on the opposite side of the clot becomes paralyzed.

A depressed fracture can also apply pressure on the brain at the area of the depression. Surgery is required to relieve the pressure.

No skull injury should be treated lightly. A child may hit his head in a playground or in the backyard and conceal this from his parents, or a baby-sitter may be afraid of losing her job if she reports such a fall. An alcoholic may slip on the street and strike his head on the sidewalk. Anyone who suffers a blow to the head or who falls on his head should be observed carefully for possible later complications. If such incidents are followed by vomiting, drowsiness, and headaches, immediate medical attention should be sought.

Facial Injury

A blow to the eye may fracture the upper or lower borders of the eye socket. It can also cause what is commonly known as a black eye, the blue-black appearance of which results from bleeding under the skin. The swelling can be reduced by applying an ice pack to the area.

Fractures of the facial bones, jaw, and nose result from a direct blow to these areas. The impact may rupture blood vessels and cause facial deformity. Dislocation of the jaw is a common problem caused by trauma. It may also occur spontaneously in certain individuals by an unusually wide-mouthed yawn or laugh. It is an uncomfortable rather than painful experience.

Serious facial injury requires hospitalization and surgical restoration. Skin lacerations may have to be sutured and the scars removed by plastic surgery; fractures of the jaw and mouth may require surgical wiring for stabilization and immobilization before healing can take place. In some instances both jaws may be wired together until healing takes place.

Injury to the Rib Cage

Accidents, athletic injuries, and fights account for most injuries to the rib cage. Any blow to the chest can cause rib fractures, which hurt when one coughs or inhales. Hairline and incomplete fractures are less serious than complete fractures, where the fragments are usually sharp and pointed. Such fractured ribs can tear the lungs, causing air to leak into the pleural space, with possibly serious results. The lung can collapse as a result of being punctured. Punctured blood vessels can hemorrhage into the pleural space. The accumulated blood may have to be withdrawn before it reduces the capacity of the lungs to carry out their normal function.

Severe chest injuries—crush injuries with multiple fractures—require hospitalization. The patient must be confined to bed and kept under constant medical observation and treatment. If the lung has collapsed, it has to be reinflated. In simple rib fractures the chest may be strapped to immobilize the fragments and promote rapid healing. Generally, analgesics alone are enough to relieve pain.

Fractures of the sternum are caused by direct blows to the sternal area, as is usually the case with automobile accidents when the steering wheel hits the driver's chest. This injury can be avoided if the driver wears a shoulder-restraining belt, and if his car is equipped with a collapsible steering column.

Chest pains following a blow to the area of the sternum should be medically investigated by means of X-ray diagnosis for possible fracture. The fracture fragments may have to be wired together and remain in place until the injury has healed. For simple fractures, rest may be the only treatment required. The serious complication of a fractured sternum in a steering-wheel accident is contusion of the heart; it should be evaluated by means of an electrocardiogram.

Spinal Injury

Most spinal injuries originate from automobile accidents, industrial mishaps, falls, athletics, or from fights and beatings. Spinal injuries can create fractures that compress or sever the spinal cord, with resultant paralysis. A diving accident or headlong fall may cause a concussion and possible fractures of the cervical spine. Head-on collisions in the sports arena and automobile accidents are the chief causes of cervical spine fractures.

An individual who jumps from a considerable height and lands on his feet, especially on his heels, may easily fracture his spine. Sudden pain in the thoracic spine following a jump should receive immediate medical attention and investigation.

Whiplash

These injuries, the most common form of injury to the spine, occur most often during head-on and rear-end automobile accidents that suddenly jerk the neck and injure the cervical vertebrae. Accident victims thus injured may undergo months of agonizing headaches and pain in the neck. Immobilization of the neck by a surgical collar will reduce some of the pain and aid the healing process.

First Aid for Spinal Injuries

Victims of spinal injuries should be moved as little as possible. While waiting for professional help, the patient should be placed on his back and made as comfortable as possible. If an accident or explosion victim is wedged between debris, attempts should be made to free him, but his body should be kept flat with as little movement as possible. No attempt should be made to have the person sit up or stand before he has been examined by a physician. Unnecessary movement of victims of spinal injury can damage the spinal cord and cause permanent paralysis.

Decompression of Fractures

Anyone with a spinal injury should be taken to the emergency ward of the nearest hospital for X-ray examinations that will reveal possible fractures. If the fracture compresses against the spinal cord, the extremities may be paralyzed. In such cases, a neurosurgeon or an orthopedist may perform a delicate operation, lifting the fracture fragments away from the spinal cord, thereby relieving the pressure and reestablishing control and movement of the paralyzed extremities.

Fractures of the cervical spine can be decompressed by applying traction to the neck. Frequent X-ray rechecks are required to assess the degree of healing and new bone formation. Patients with fractured vertebrae undergo a lengthy rehabilitation with frequent medical rechecks and physical therapy. In some severe cases of spinal fractures that result in paralysis, the individual is never able to walk again.

8

Diseases of the Muscles and Nervous System

If any part of the brain has developed abnormally, the usual function of that structure would be expected to be altered. Abnormalities present at birth are called *congenital* defects. If the nervous system does not receive a normal blood supply because of the obstruction of a blood vessel, or if there is a tear in the vessel with subsequent hemorrhage, the cells are deprived of blood and will die. These lesions are *vascular* or *cerebrovascular* accidents. Cerebral injury, or *trauma,* can destroy brain tissue, with consequent loss of normal function; infections of the nervous system may also permanently injure tissue. Finally, brain function can be altered by *metabolic, toxic,* or *degenerative* changes in normal body chemistry. It is not surprising, then, that such a beautifully organized nervous system is vulnerable to the hazards of living.

Diagnostic Tests

A patient who has been referred to a *neurologist,* a physician who specializes in diseases of the nervous system, will be asked to tell the history of the problem in great detail, for that history will describe

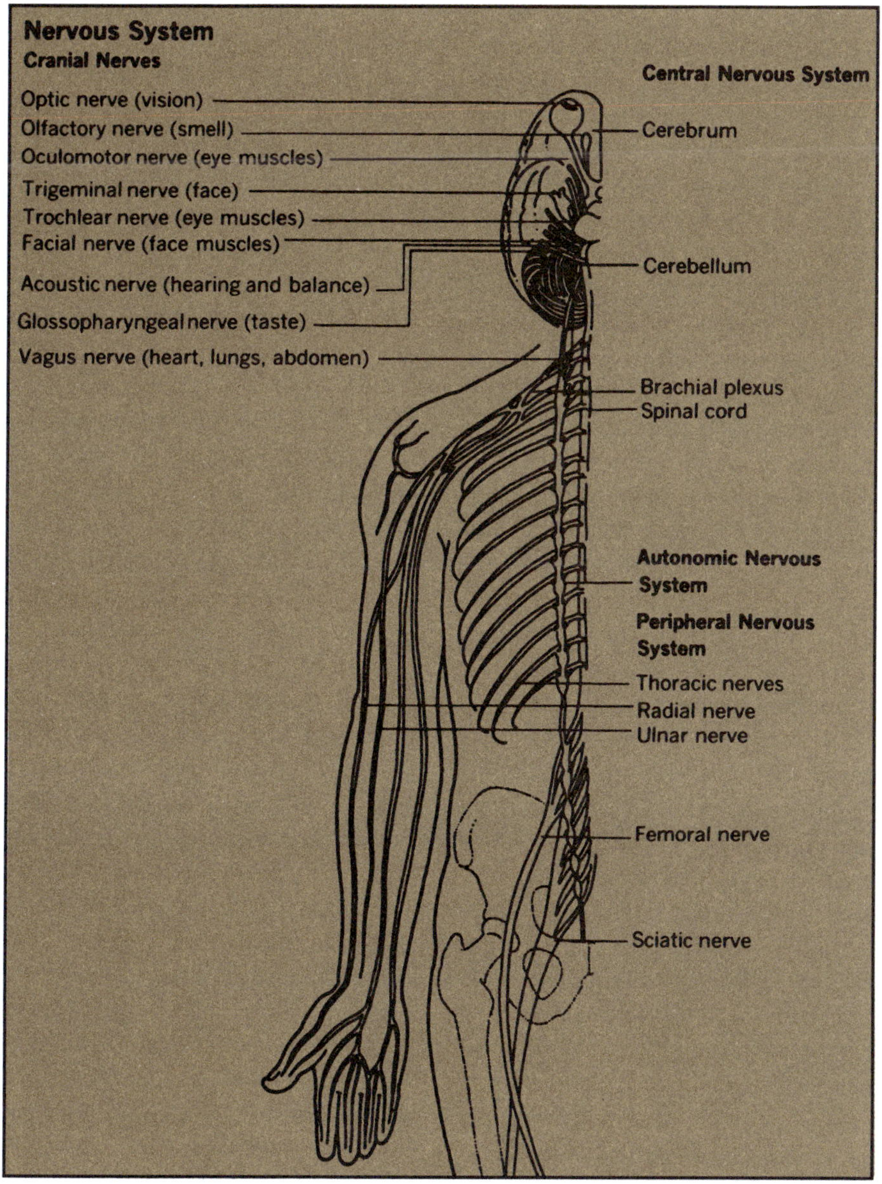

the nature of the disorder; the neurological examination will help locate the site of the problem. After the neurological examination has been completed, the physician may order radiographs (X-ray pictures) of the skull and spinal column and an electroencephalogram. The *electroencephalogram* (EEG), or brain wave recording, assists the physician in locating such brain abnormalities as tumors and in determining the characteristics of convulsive disorders.

It may also be necessary to perform

a *lumbar puncture (spinal tap)* in order to obtain a specimen of the *cerebrospinal fluid* (CSF), the fluid that bathes the brain and spinal cord. For this test a needle is inserted through the patient's lower back into the spinal canal. A sample of CSF is then withdrawn for analysis.

Occasionally, other specialized tests are used to provide the physician with an image of the brain, spinal cord, or veins. For example, *ultrasonography,* a test using high-frequency sound waves to produce images, can be used to examine major veins in the neck for damage or blockages. Ultrasound tests are noninvasive and can also be used to examine other areas of the body, such as the liver, heart, or kidneys.

Another specialized test is the *cerebral arteriography,* also known as an angiography. In this test a material that is opaque to X rays is injected into the blood vessels that supply the brain. The vessels can then be seen plainly on X-ray film, and abnormalities in the vessels can be diagnosed. In some cases this test has been replaced by noninvasive tests, such as computed tomographic scanning and magnetic resonance imaging.

Myelography is another invasive test using radiopaque liquid dye similar to that used in angiography. The dye is injected with a spinal needle into the sac-enclosed space around the spinal cord. X rays are then taken that can show problems with the spine, such as compression or disc injuries, or tumors in the lower brain.

Computed tomographic scanning, also known as *CT scanning,* is a noninvasive procedure in which X-ray beams from many angles are directed at a patient lying on a special table. As the X rays pass through the body, different tissues absorb different amounts of the X rays. The strength of the beams emerging from the patient's body is measured by an X-ray detector. The measurements are processed by a computer that then makes an image of the interior of the patient's body. One function of this test is to generate pictures that look like slices of the brain. CT scans can be used to locate such problems as tumors and fluid accumulation in the brain. CT scans can also be used to diagnose problems in other parts of the body.

Magnetic resonance imaging, also known as *MRI* and *nuclear magnetic resonance (NMR) imaging,* is a noninvasive process using a magnetic field instead of X rays to create images of the inside of a patient's body. For this test a patient lies on a special table that passes into a tube-like structure that contains a large magnet. Atoms in the body react to the magnetic field and this reaction is recorded by a scanner that sends the information to a computer. The computer then creates images of the interior of the patient's body. This test can be used in diagnosing problems in the structure of the brain or other parts of the body. The *functional MRI* shows brain function as well as its structure.

Another test that can show brain function is *positron emission tomography,* also known as *PET.* In this test very small amounts of radioactive substances are injected into a patient's body. When these substances decay they emit particles called positrons. A scanner records this process and sends information about the emission of positrons to a computer. The computer then creates an image from the information. Besides showing brain function, PET scans can be used on other parts of the body to show such problems as muscle damage.

Cerebral Palsy

The term *cerebral palsy* is not a diagnosis but a label for a problem in locomotion exhibited by some children. Definitions of cerebral palsy are many and varied, but in general refer to nonprogressive abnormalities of the brain that have occurred early in life from many causes. The label implies that there is no active disease process but rather a static or nonprogressive lesion that may affect the growth and development of the child.

Included in the category of cerebral palsy are such problems as limpness (flaccidity), *spasticity* of one or all limbs, incoordination, or some other disorder of movement. In some patients, quick jerks affect different parts of the body at different times (*chorea*); in others, slow, writhing, incoordinated movements (*athetosis*) are most pronounced in the hands and arms. Incoordination of movement may also occur in muscles used for speaking and eating, so that speech becomes slurred, interrupted, or jerky; the patient may drool because incoordinated muscle action prevents efficient swallowing of saliva. This does little to improve the physical appearance of the child and, unfortunately, he may look mentally subnormal.

The fact that a patient has an abnormality that is responsible for difficulty in locomotion or speech does not mean that the child is mentally retarded. There is some likelihood that he will be mentally slow, but patients in this group of disease states range from slow to superior in intelligence, a fact that emphasizes that each child must be assessed individually.

A complete examination must be completed, and to determine the patient's functional status complete psychological testing should be performed by a skilled psychologist.

Treatment

Treatment for cerebral palsy is a continuing process involving a careful surveillance of the patient's physical and psychological status. A physical therapist, under the physician's guidance, will help to mobilize and maintain the function of the neuromuscular system. Occasionally, an orthopedic surgeon may surgically lengthen a tendon or in some way make a limb more functional. A speech therapist can provide additional speech training, and a vocational therapist can help the patient to find appropriate work. The key professional is the primary physician, usually the pediatrician, who with care and understanding guides the patient through the years.

Bell's Palsy

Bell's palsy is a paralysis of the facial nerve that was first described by Sir Charles Bell, a Scottish surgeon of the early nineteenth century. It may affect men and women at any age, though it occurs most commonly between the ages of 30 and 50. The onset of the facial paralysis may be abrupt: the patient may awaken one morning unable to move one side of his face. He can't wrinkle one side of his forehead or raise the eyebrow; the eye will not close on the affected side, and when attempting to smile, the face is pulled to the opposite side. Occasionally the patient may experience discomfort about the ear on the involved side. There is no difficulty in swallowing, but because the muscles about the corner of the mouth are weak, drooling is not uncommon, and food may accumulate in the gutter between gum and lip.

Bell's palsy may affect the branch of the facial nerve that supplies taste sensation to the anterior part of the tongue and the branch that supplies a small muscle in the middle ear (the *stapedius*) whose function it is to dampen loud sounds. Depending on the extent to which the facial nerve is affected, the patient may be unable to perceive taste on the side of the paralysis and may be unusually sensitive to sounds, a condition known as *hyperacusis*.

The most probable causes of Bell's palsy are inflammation of the facial nerve as it passes through a bony canal within the skull or inflammation of that bony canal with subsequent swelling and compression of the nerve. It is not uncommon that the patient has a history of exposure to a cold breeze, such as sleeping in a draft or riding in an open car. Any patient who has a facial weakness should be carefully evaluated by a physician, preferably a neurologist, to be quite certain that there is no other neurologic abnormality. When the diagnosis of Bell's palsy is certain, some therapeutic measures can be taken.

Treatment

There is no specific treatment for Bell's palsy, but many physicians recommend massage, application of heat, and exercise of the weak muscles, either passive (by external manipulation) or active (by use). These therapeutic measures do not specifically influence the course of the facial nerve paralysis, but they are thought to be useful in maintaining tone of the facial muscles and preventing permanent deformity. Occasionally a V-shaped adhesive tape splint can be applied to the affected side of the face, from the corner of the mouth to the temple. Some physicians treat the condition with steroids such as cortisone, which may hasten recovery if begun at the onset of the illness.

In treating Bell's palsy, it is important to remember that when the eyelid does not close normally, the conjunctiva and cornea are not fully lubricated, and corneal lesions may develop from excessive dryness or exposure to the air. For this reason, some ophthalmic lubrication may be recommended by the physician.

About 80 percent of the patients with Bell's palsy recover completely in a few days or weeks, and about 10 to 15 percent recover more slowly, over a period of three to six months. The remaining 5 to 10 percent will have some residual facial deformity.

Parkinson's Disease

Parkinson's disease is a potentially devastating neurological disease that results in a progressive loss of muscle control. Patients with *parkinsonism* are easily recognized because of the characteristic symptoms of gradually worsening tremors, rigidity, decreased ability to make voluntary movements and, in many cases, loss of cognitive functions.

Scientifically described nearly a century and a half ago, the disease is associated with the death, or degeneration, of the brain cells that supply dopamine, a chemical that transmits signals between nerve cells. These brain cells are called the *substantia nigra*. Such degeneration is normal in the human brain, but in patients suffering from Parkinson's disease the loss of the substantia nigra, or the dopamine-producing neurons, occurs at an accelerated rate.

The onset of parkinsonism may follow encephalitis, a brain injury, or exposure to toxic substances, but the symptoms usually occur in patients who are middle-aged or older and, in these instances, there is no known cause for the degeneration of the nerve cells.

The tremors or shaking usually involve the fingers and the wrist, but sometimes the arms, legs, or head are involved to the extent that the entire body shakes. Characteristically, the tremors occur when the patient is at rest. The tremors stop or are much less marked during a voluntary muscle movement. Tremors do not occur when the patient is asleep.

Early in the disease, the patient notices what appear to be the normal signs of aging—a little shakiness, stiffness, jerky motions, and difficulty with movements such as rising out of a low, deep chair. Very gradually the signs increase. The shaking begins to interfere with daily activities and other signs develop, including what most patients with parkinsonism perceive as the most distressing symptom, *bradykinesia,* the gradual loss of spontaneous movement. In advanced stages of the disease, such bradykinesia results in periods when the patient's body is completely unable to move itself. These "frozen" periods are known as *akinesia*. And, while the emotional balance of the parkinsonian patient is generally unaffected by the disease, he may lose the ability to control the facial and vocal muscles which allow him to convey a range of different emotions. Although the patient may continue to have natural emotional responses, he cannot indicate them in the normal manner, by smiling or frowning or by raising or lowering his voice. Instead, his face appears expressionless, his voice flat. The patient frequently experiences periods of depression and tremendous frustration.

While most patients with Parkinson's disease continue to retain their cognitive abilities, in severe or advanced cases, the patient may suffer some degree of mental deterioration or dementia.

Treatment

Once it was determined nerve pathways in the brains of patients with parkinsonism were depleted of dopamine, modern treatment of the disease began to focus on providing the remaining healthy nerve cells with the means to make the crucial chemical. First introduced in the 1960s, levodopa, a natural brain chemical also used by the nerve cells to make dopamine, is the traditional treatment for sufferers of Parkinson's disease. Levodopa (or L-dopa), and levodopa-containing compounds, force the dying nerve cells in the brain to produce more dopamine. L-dopa also reduces all of the main symptoms of the disease. However, because the dopamine-producing cells continue to die, levodopa is usually rendered useless within ten years. For this reason, physicians sometimes delay treatment until a patient shows more severe symptoms. The drug, selegiline, also known as deprenyl, works to increase and extend the effects of Levodopa.

Side effects associated with L-dopa include nausea, involuntary movements, some mental changes, cardiac irregularities, and urinary retention. The undesirable side effects of nausea and confusion have been somewhat countered by the use of drugs like carbidopa, an *extracerebral decarboxylase inhibitor,* that prevent the levadopa from changing into dopamine before it enters the brain. "End-of-dose" akinesia, the return of symptoms a few hours after taking medication, can be relieved in some cases by taking the patient off drug treatments entirely for several days. Patients are usually hospitalized during this "drug holiday" and some take part in speech and physical therapy programs.

Other drugs include those in the anticholinergic and dopamine agonist categories. Anticholinergic drugs are used to treat the early stages of the disease and include: trihexyphenidyl hydrochloride, benztropine mesylate, diphenhydramine hydrochloride, biperiden, and procyclidine hydrochloride. All of these drugs reduce tremors and rigidity to a modest degree, but none affects bradykinesia. Patients using the drugs may experience such side effects as gingivitis or inflammation of the gums, constipation, mild dizziness, nausea, nervousness, and slightly blurred vision. More serious side effects could include urinary retention, confusion, and psychosis. The two drugs in the dopamine agonist category, bromocriptine and pergolide, stimulate the brain's dopamine receptors, "convincing" the receptors they are dopamine. Bromocriptine and pergolide are used alone and in conjunction with levodopa.

While drug therapy remains the primary course of treatment, research advances have been made in other areas, such as studies of possible environmental causes and experimental surgeries. One procedure, *deep-brain stimulation,* is now approved by the FDA. A small electrode is implanted in the brain, which is connected to a device under the skin of the chest, which produces electrical impulses that eliminate the tremors.

Epilepsy

Epilepsy is a common disorder of the human nervous system. In the United States, alone, more than four million people suffer from epilepsy.

Epilepsy affects all kinds of people, regardless of sex, intelligence, or standard of living.

Causes and Precipitating Factors

A single epileptic seizure usually occurs spontaneously. In some cases, seizures are triggered by visual stimuli, such as a flickering image on a television screen, a sudden change from dark to very bright illumination, or vice versa. Other patients may react to auditory stimuli such as a loud noise, a monotonous sound, or even to certain musical notes. A seizure is accompanied by a discharge of nerve impulses, which can be detected by electroencephalography. The effect is something like that of a telephone switchboard in which a defect in the circuits accidentally causes wrong number calls. The forms that seizures take depend upon the location of the nervous system disturbances within the brain and the spread of the nerve impulses. Physicians have found that certain kinds of epilepsy cases can be traced to specific areas of the brain where the lesion has occurred.

Epilepsy can develop at any age, although nearly 85 percent of all cases appear before the age of 20 years. Hence, it is commonly seen as an affliction of children. There is no indication that epilepsy itself can be inherited, but some evidence exists that certain individuals inherit a greater tendency to develop the condition from precipitating causes than is true for the general population. According to the Epilepsy Foundation, studies show that if neither parent has epilepsy, the chances are one in 100 that they will have an epileptic child, but the chances rise to one in 40 if one parent is epileptic.

About 70 percent of epilepsy cases are *idiopathic*—that is, they are not attributable to any known cause. In the remaining 30 percent, the recurrent seizures are *symptomatic*—they are symptoms of some definite brain lesion, either congenital or resulting from subsequent injury. Because it can reasonably be assumed that some of the idiopathic cases are a result of lesions that have not been identified, epilepsy is perhaps best regarded not as a specific disease but as a symptom of a brain abnormality due to any of various causes.

Aura Preceding a Seizure

Unusual sensory experiences have been reported to occur before a seizure by about half the victims of epilepsy. The sensation, which is called an *aura,* may appear in the form of an unpleasant odor, a tingling numbness, a sinking or gripping feeling, strangulation, palpitations, or a gastrointestinal sensation. Some patients say the sensation cannot be described. Others report feeling strange or confused for hours or even days before a seizure. Such an early warning is known as a *prodrome.*

The various types of epilepsy can be broadly grouped under four general categories: grand mal, petit mal, focal, and psychomotor. Only one feature is common to all types of epilepsy—the sudden, disorderly discharge of nerve impulses within the brain.

Grand Mal Seizure

The *grand mal* is a generalized convulsion during which the patient may initially look strange or bewildered, suddenly groan or scream, lose consciousness and become stiff (*tonic phase*), hold the breath, fall to the ground unless supported, and then begin to jerk the arms and legs (*clonic phase*). There may be loss of bowel and bladder control. The tongue may be bitten by coming between clenched jaws. The duration of the entire seizure, both the tonic and clonic phases, is less than two minutes—frequently less than one minute—followed by postconvulsive confusion or deep sleep that may last for minutes or hours.

Variations in the Pattern

The sequence of events in grand mal seizures is not invariable. The tongue-biting and urinary and fecal incontinence do not occur as frequently in children as in adult patients. Children may also demonstrate a type of grand mal seizure in which the patient suddenly becomes limp and falls to the floor unconscious; there is no apparent tonic or clonic phase and the muscles do not become stiff. Other cases may manifest only the tonic phase, with unconsciousness and the muscles remaining in a stiffened, tonic state throughout the seizure. There also is a clonic type of seizure, which begins with rapid jerking movements that continue during the entire attack. In one very serious form of convulsive seizure known as *status epilepticus,* repeated grand mal seizures occur without the victim's becoming conscious between them.

Petit Mal Seizure

Petit mal seizures are characterized by momentary staring spells, as if the patient were suspended in the middle of his activity. He may have a blank stare or undergo rapid blinking, sometimes accompanied by small twitching movements in one part of the body or another—hands, legs, or facial muscles. He does not fall down. These spells, called *absence* or *lapse attacks,* usually begin in childhood before puberty. The attacks are typically very brief, lasting half a minute or less, and occur many times throughout the day. They may go unnoticed for weeks or months because the patient appears to be daydreaming.

Focal Seizure

Focal seizures proceed from neural discharges in one part of the brain, resulting in twitching movements in a corresponding part of the body. Usually, one side of the face, the thumb and fingers of one hand, or one entire side of the body is involved. The patient does not lose consciousness and may in fact remain aware of his surroundings and the circumstances during the entire focal convulsion. Focal convulsions in adults commonly indicate some focal abnormality, but this is less true in a child who may have a focal seizure without evidence of a related brain lesion.

With their knowledge of the nerve links between brain centers and body muscles, physicians are able to determine quite accurately the site of a brain lesion that is involved with a focal seizure.

Jacksonian Epilepsy

One type of focal seizure has a distinctive pattern and is sometimes called a *Jacksonian seizure,* and the condition itself *Jacksonian epilepsy.* The attack begins with rhythmic twitching of muscles in one hand or one foot or one side of the face. The spasmodic movement or twitching then spreads from the body area first affected to other muscles on the same side of the body. The course of the twitching may, for example, begin on the left side of the face, then spread to the neck, down the arm, then along the trunk to the foot. Or the onset of the attack may begin at the foot and gradually spread upward along the trunk to the facial muscles. There may be a tingling or burning sensation and perspiration, and the hair may stand up on the skin of the areas affected.

Psychomotor Seizures

Psychomotor seizures, or *temporal lobe seizures,* often take the form of movements that appear purposeful but are irrelevant to the situation. Instead of losing control of his thoughts and actions, the patient behaves as if he is in a trancelike state. He may smack his lips and make chewing motions. He may suddenly rise from a chair and walk about while removing his clothes. He may attempt to speak or speak incoherently, repeating certain words or phrases, or he may go through the motions of some mechanical procedure, like driving a car, for example.

The patient in a psychomotor seizure usually does not respond to questions or commands. If physically restrained during a psychomotor episode, the patient may appear belligerent and obstreperous, or he may resist with great energy and violence. Usually, the entire episode lasts only a few minutes. When the seizure ends, the patient is confused and unable to recall clearly what has happened.

The aura experienced by victims of psychomotor seizures may differ from that of other forms of the disorder. The psychomotor epileptic may have sensations of taste or smell, but more likely will experience a complex illusion or hallucination that may have the quality of a vivid dream. The hallucination may be based on actual experiences or things the patient has seen, or it may deal with objects or experiences that only seem familiar though they are in fact unfamiliar. This distortion of memory, in which a strange experience seems to be a part of one's past life, is known as *déjà vu,* which in French means literally "already seen."

Other visual associations involved in various forms of epilepsy include those in which the patient experiences sensations of color, moving lights, or darkness. Red is the most common color observed in visual seizures, although blue, yellow, and green also are reported. The darkness illusion may occur as a temporary blindness, lasting only a few minutes. Stars or moving lights may appear as if visible to only one eye, indicating that the source of the disturbance is a lesion in the brain area on the opposite side of the head. Visual illusions before an epileptic attack may have a distorted quality, or consist of objects arranged in an unnatural pattern or of an unnatural size.

Auditory illusions, on the other hand, are comparatively rare. Occasionally a patient will report hearing buzzing or roaring noises as part of a seizure, or human voices repeating certain recognizable words.

Treatment of the Epileptic Patient

Usually the physician does not see the patient during a seizure and must rely on the description of others to make a proper diagnosis. Because the patient has no clear recollection of what happens during any of the epileptic convulsions, it is wise to have someone who has seen an attack accompany him to a physician. First, the physician begins the detective work to find the cause of the seizure. He will examine the patient thoroughly, obtain blood tests, an electroencephalogram, and a lumbar puncture, if indicated. Even after all these studies, however, the physician often can find no specific cause that can be eradicated. Efforts are then made to control the symptoms.

The treatment of epilepsy consists primarily of medication for the prevention of seizures. It is usually highly effective. About half of all patients are completely controlled and another quarter have a significant reduction in the frequency and severity of attacks. The medication, usually in tablet or capsule form, must be taken regularly according to the instructions of the physician. It may be necessary to try several drugs over a period of time to determine which drug or combination of drugs best controls the seizures. Phenobarbital and diphenylhydantoin (Dilantin) may be prescribed for the control of grand mal seizures and focal epilepsy, and the physician may find that a combination of these drugs or others offers the best anticonvulsant control. Trimethadione frequently is administered to petit mal patients; primidone or phenobarbital may be prescribed for psychomotor attacks.

Antispasmodic drugs such as diazepam have been shown to be useful in controlling prolonged, repeated, generalized seizures. A new diazepam gel reduces the numbers of seizures that occur in clusters.

Surgery is an option for those who do not respond to drug treatment, but is not always effective.

However, medicine and surgery are not the only treatments for epilepsy. Emotional factors are known to influence convulsive disorders. Lessening a patient's anger, anxiety, and fear can help to control the condition. An understanding family and friends are important, as are adequate rest, good nutrition, and proper exercise. The exercise program should not include vigorous contact sports, and some activities such as swimming should not be performed by the patient unless he is accompanied by another person who understands the condition and is capable of helping the epileptic during a seizure.

There is nothing permanent about epilepsy, although some patients may endure the symptoms for much of their lives. It is a disorder that changes appreciably and constantly in form and manifestations. Some experts claim that petit mal and psychomotor cases if untreated may progress to more serious cases of grand mal seizures. On the other hand, epilepsy that is given proper medical attention may eventually subside in frequency and severity of attacks. In many cases, seizures disappear or subside within a short time and treatment can be discontinued gradually.

While some effort has been made by medical scientists to determine if there is an "epileptic personality," evidence indicates there is no typical personality pattern involved. Whatever behavior patterns and emotional reactions are observed are the result of individual personality makeup rather than being directly related to epilepsy. Most epilepsy patients are capable of performing satisfactory work at various jobs; one study showed that only nine percent were partially dependent and four percent were incapable of holding a job. In some areas there may be restrictions on issuing driver's licenses to epileptics or other legal regulations that limit normal activities for epilepsy patients. As a result, some epileptics may conceal their condition or avoid medical treatment that might be reported to government agencies.

Because of ignorance and misinformation, some people regard epilepsy as frightening or mysterious, and patients may suffer unnecessarily and unjustly. In fact, behavioral abnormalities in patients with seizures are commonly the reflection of how they are viewed by others.

When epilepsy has been diagnosed in a child, the parents must be instructed about the condition and the need for continuous careful medical supervision. If the child is old enough to understand, he also should learn more about the nature of the condition. Misbeliefs should be corrected. Both parents and child should understand that seizures are not likely to be fatal and that a brain lesion does not lead to mental deterioration. Parents and child should learn what actions should be taken in the event of a seizure, such as loosening clothing and taking steps to prevent injury. Natural concern should be balanced with an understanding that overprotection may itself become a handicap. The child should be encouraged to participate in social and physical activities at school and in the neighborhood as long as they do not strain his capabilities. Finally, parents should not feel guilty about the child's condition and think that some action of theirs contributed to the child's condition. See "Epileptic Seizures" in Ch. 31, *Medical Emergencies,* for a description of what to do when a seizure occurs.

Further information about epilepsy, including causes, effects, treatment, rehabilitation, and laws regulating employment and driver permits, can be obtained from the Epilepsy Foundation of America, 4351 Garden City Dr., Landover, MD 20785; U.S. Department of Health and Human Services, 200 Independence Avenue, S.W., Washington, D.C. 20201; and National Institutes of Health (NIH), 9000 Rockville Pike, Bethesda, MD 20892.

Amyotrophic Lateral Sclerosis

Amyotrophic lateral sclerosis, ALS, is a degenerative neurological disease in which the nerve cells that control muscles die, resulting in loss of muscle movement and the wasting away of muscles from lack of use.

The first signs of ALS, commonly known as Lou Gehrig's Disease (named for the New York Yankees player who died of it at 38), are the inability to do simple tasks, such as turn a door knob or button a shirt. The condition starts on one side of the body, then moves to the other side. As muscles begin to degenerate, the person loses weight. Eventually, ALS sufferers lose control of their ability to speak, to move, to swallow, or sometimes even to breathe. Mentally, they remain alert, trapped in a withering body.

Treatment

Since there is no cure for ALS, treatment focuses on controlling symptoms. One drug, riluzole, has been shown conclusively to prolong survival of ALS patients. Scientists have also discovered a defective gene believed to be the cause of the inherited form of the disease (about ten percent of the cases). Antispasmodic drugs, such as diazepam, are available as are drugs to help patients with impaired ability to swallow.

Multiple Sclerosis

Multiple sclerosis is a disease in which the myelin sheath that insulates nerves is progressively destroyed through attacks by white blood cells of the immune system. The disease affects mainly the brain and spinal cord. It is termed *multiple* because there are distinct and separate areas of the nervous system involved, seemingly distributed in a random pattern.

Multiple sclerosis rarely appears before the age of 15 or after 55. A person aged 30 years is statistically at peak risk of developing the disease. The typical patient, statistically speaking, is a woman of 45 who was born and raised in a temperate climate. Women are more susceptible to the disease than men by a ratio of 1.7 to 1, and women are more likely than men to experience the onset of symptoms before the age of 30.

There are no laboratory tests that are specific for multiple sclerosis, although there are certain tests that may suggest the presence of the disease. Diagnosing the disorder depends to a large extent upon tests that rule out other diseases with similar signs and symptoms. The first symptom may be a transitory blurring of vision or a disturbance in one or more of the limbs, such as numbness, a tingling sensation, clumsiness, or weakness. There may be a partial or total loss of vision in one eye for a period of several days, or the patient may experience double vision, dizziness or pain when moving the eye. In some cases, the patient may develop either a lack of sensation over an area of the face or, paradoxically, a severe twitching pain of the face muscles. In more advanced cases, because of involvement of the spinal cord, the patient may have symptoms of bladder or bowel dysfunction and male patients may experience impotence.

When brain tissues become invaded by multiple sclerosis, the patient may suffer loss of memory and show signs of personality changes, displaying euphoria, cheerfulness, irritability, or depression for no apparent reason.

Multiple sclerosis is marked by periods of remission and recurrence of symptoms. Complete recovery can occur. About 20 percent of the patients may have to spend time confined to bed or wheelchair. In severe cases, there can be complications such as infections of the urinary tract and respiratory system.

Treatment

There is no known cure for multiple sclerosis and, until recently, treatment techniques generally were aimed at relieving symptoms, shortening the periods of exacerbation, and preventing complications that could be crippling or life-threatening. Most patients experience recurrences of symptoms that last for limited periods of days or weeks, followed in cycles by periods of remission that may last for months or years, making it difficult to determine whether the therapy applied is actually effective or if the disease is merely following its natural fluctuating course.

Among the medications now used are anti-inflammatory drugs such as adrenocorticotrophin (ACTH), a hormone that seems to reduce the severity and duration of recurrences. Cortisone and prednisone, two steroid hormones, also can be used and have an advantage over ACTH in that they can be taken by mouth rather than by intramuscular injection. Not all patients react favorably to steroid drugs and serious side effects may be experienced.

Beta interferon, the first drug to be approved by the FDA for any form of multiple sclerosis, significantly reduces the number of acute episodes of the disease and lessens the severity of the episodes that occur. Recent studies show that it can also significantly delay progression of the disease and reduce the frequency of attacks in people with secondary progressive MS. Brain scans reveal that nerve damage is reduced in patients taking beta interferon.

Physical therapy and antispasmodic medications may be employed for patients suffering weakness or paralysis of the limbs. Bed rest during periods of exacerbation is important; continued activity seems to worsen the severity and duration of symptoms during those periods. Muscle relaxants and tranquilizers may be prescribed in some serious cases and braces could be required for patients who lose some limb functions.

Causes

The cause of multiple sclerosis has not been established.

A theory that researchers consider promising suggests that a virus similar but not identical to HTLV-I (human T-cell leukemia virus-I) may cause multiple sclerosis. HTLV-I causes an unusual form of leukemia. Some T-cells, a type of white blood cell, have been found to contain genetic material from this virus. These T-cells were taken from the cerebrospinal fluid of MS victims, establishing a possible link between the cells and the virus.

Infections of the Nervous System

Like any other organ system, the brain and its associated structures may be host to infection. These infections are usually serious because of the significantly high death rate and incidence of residual defects. If the brain is involved in the inflammation, it is known as *encephalitis;* inflammation of the brain coverings, or *meninges,* is called *meningitis.*

Encephalitis

Encephalitis is usually caused by a virus and, because the symptoms are not specific, the diagnosis is usually made by special viral immunologic tests. Both sexes and all age groups can be afflicted. Most patients complain of fever, headache, nausea or vomiting, and a general feeling of malaise. The mental state varies from one of mild irritability to lethargy or coma, and some patients may have convulsions. The physician may suspect encephalitis after completing the history and the physical examination, but the diagnosis is usually established by laboratory tests that include examination of the cerebrospinal fluid (CSF), the EEG, and viral studies of the blood, CSF, and stool. Because there is no specific treatment for viral encephalitis at the present time, particular attention is paid to general supportive care.

Meningitis

Meningitis can occur in either sex at any time of life. The patient often has a preceding mild respiratory infection and later complains of headache, nausea, and vomiting. Fever and neck stiffness are usually present early in the course of the disease, at which time the patient is commonly brought to the physician for examination. If there is any question of meningitis, a lumbar puncture is performed and the CSF examined. It is not possible to make a specific diagnosis of meningitis without examination of the cerebrospinal fluid.

Meningitis is usually caused by bacteria or a virus. It is important to learn what the infectious agent is in order to begin appropriate therapy. Bacterial infections can be treated by antibiotics, but there is no known specific treatment for viral (*aseptic*) meningitis. Meningitis is a life-threatening disease and, despite modern antibiotic therapy, the mortality rate varies from 10 to 20 percent.

Poliomyelitis

Poliomyelitis is an acute viral illness affecting anyone at any time of life, though most commonly before the age of ten. It is also called *polio* or *infantile paralysis.*

Polio is caused by a virus that probably moves from the gastrointestinal tract via nerve trunks to the central nervous system, where it may affect any part of the nervous system. The disease, however, most often involves the larger motor neurons (*anterior horn cells*) in the brain stem and spinal cord, with subsequent loss of nerve supply to the muscle.

There are two categories of polio patients: *asymptomatic,* those who have had no observed symptoms of the disease, but test positive for antibodies to polio; and *symptomatic*, those who have the clinical disease, either with residual paralysis (paralytic polio) or without paralysis (nonparalytic polio).

The symptoms of poliomyelitis are similar to those of other acute infectious processes. The patient may complain of headache, fever, head cold, runny nose, or he may have loose stools and malaise. One-fourth to one-third of patients improve for several days only to have a recurrence of fever with neck stiffness. Most patients have a progression of their symptoms, marked by neck stiffness and aching muscles. They are often irritable and apprehensive, and some are rather lethargic.

Whether or not the patient will have muscle paralysis should be evident in the first few weeks. Some have muscle paralysis with the onset of symptoms or by the 5th day of the disease; others become aware of loss of muscle function several weeks after the onset. Patients experience a muscle spasm or stiffness, and may complain of muscle pain, particularly if the muscle is stretched.

The extent of the muscle paralysis is variable, ranging from mild localized weakness to inability to move most of the skeletal muscles. Proximal muscles (those close to the trunk, like the shoulder-arm or hip-thigh) are involved more often than distal muscles (of the extremeties), and the legs are affected more often than the arms. When the neurons of the lower brain stem and the spinal cord at the thoracic level and above are affected, the patient may have a paralysis of the muscles used in swallowing and breathing. This circumstance is life-threatening, and particular attention must be paid to the patient's ability to handle saliva and to breathe. If independent, spontaneous respiration is not possible, patients must be given respiratory assistance with mechanical respirators.

Treatment

There is no cure for polio. The patient should be given general supportive care, assuring adequate nutrition and fluid intake. Muscle spasm can be treated with hot compresses and pain medication. Physical therapy will aid with rehabilitation.

In 1953, Dr. Jonas Salk developed the first successful polio vaccine. Today, vaccination is accomplished with either the Salk vaccine (killed virus), which is given intramuscularly, or the Sabin (live attenuated virus), given orally. Immunization with poliomyelitis vaccine has proven to be highly effective in eradicating the disease, and it is now a part of routine immunization for all children.

West Nile Virus

West Nile virus is a virus that generally infects animals and is spread by mosquitoes. Humans can become infected after being bitten by a mosquito that has previously fed on an infected animal.

About one-fifth of the persons bitten by an infected mosquito will develop *West Nile fever*. Symptoms usually appear within 3-14 days. In mild cases, symptoms include fever, headache, body aches, nausea, vomiting, and swollen lymph glands.` A skin rash on the back, chest, and stomach may sometimes develop. Symptoms in more serious cases include high fever, headache, neck stiffness, stupor, tremors, coma, conclusions, vision loss, numbness, and paralysis.

There are no vaccines or treatment available for West Nile virus. Symptoms in mild cases generally disappear on their own within a few days. Symptoms in severe cases require hospitalization.

The virus was first identified in Africa in 1937, and is commonly found in the Middle East, West Asia, Europe, and Africa. It appeared in the United States in 1999 for the first time, and spread quickly through the country during the next few years.

Dementia

Dementia is a term for mental deterioration, with particular regard to memory and thought processes. Such deterioration can be brought about in various ways: infection, brain injury, such toxic states as alcoholism, brain tumors, cerebral arteriosclerosis, and so forth.

The presenile dementias (*Alzheimer's disease*) represent a group of degenerative diseases of the brain in which mental deterioration first becomes apparent in middle age. Commonly, the first clue may be demonstrations of unusual unreasonableness and impairment of judgment. The patient can no longer grasp the content of a situation at hand and reacts inappropriately. Memory gradually fades and recent events are no longer remembered, but events that occurred early in life can be recalled. The patient may wander aimlessly or get lost in his own house. There is progressive deterioration of physical appearance and personal hygiene, and, finally, the command of language deteriorates. Unfortunately, there is a relentless progression of the process, and the patient becomes confined to bed and quite helpless.

Whether the mental deterioration seen in some aged patients, senile dementia, is a specific brain degeneration or is secondary to cerebral arteriosclerosis is not yet settled. It does appear, however, that senile dementia is probably secondary to a degenerative process similar to that of Alzheimer's disease but occurring late in life.

Whether or not dementia can be halted depends upon its cause. If, for example, the dementia is secondary to brain infection or exposure to toxic material, eradication of the infectious agent or removal of the toxin may be of distinct benefit in arresting the dementing process. Unfortunately, there is no specific treatment for the brain degenerative processes.

Muscle Diseases

When one hears the words "muscle disease," one may think of only muscular dystrophy and picture a small child confined to a wheelchair. But there are many diseases other than muscular dystrophy in which muscle is either primarily or secondarily involved, and many of these diseases do not have a particularly bad prognosis. Muscle diseases may make their presence known at any time, from early infancy to old age; no age group or sex is exempt.

Any disease of muscle is called a *myopathy*. The hallmark of muscle disease is weakness, or loss of muscle power. This may be recognized in the infant who seems unusually limp or *hypotonic*. Often the first clue to the presence of muscle weakness is a child's failure to achieve the developmental milestones within a normal range of time. He may be unusually clumsy or have difficulty in running, climbing stairs, or even walking. Occasionally a teacher is the first one to be aware that the child cannot keep up with classmates and reports this fact to the parents. The onset of the muscle weakness can be so insidious that it may go unnoticed or be misinterpreted as laziness until there is an obvious and striking loss of muscle power.

Muscles of the Abdomen and Thorax

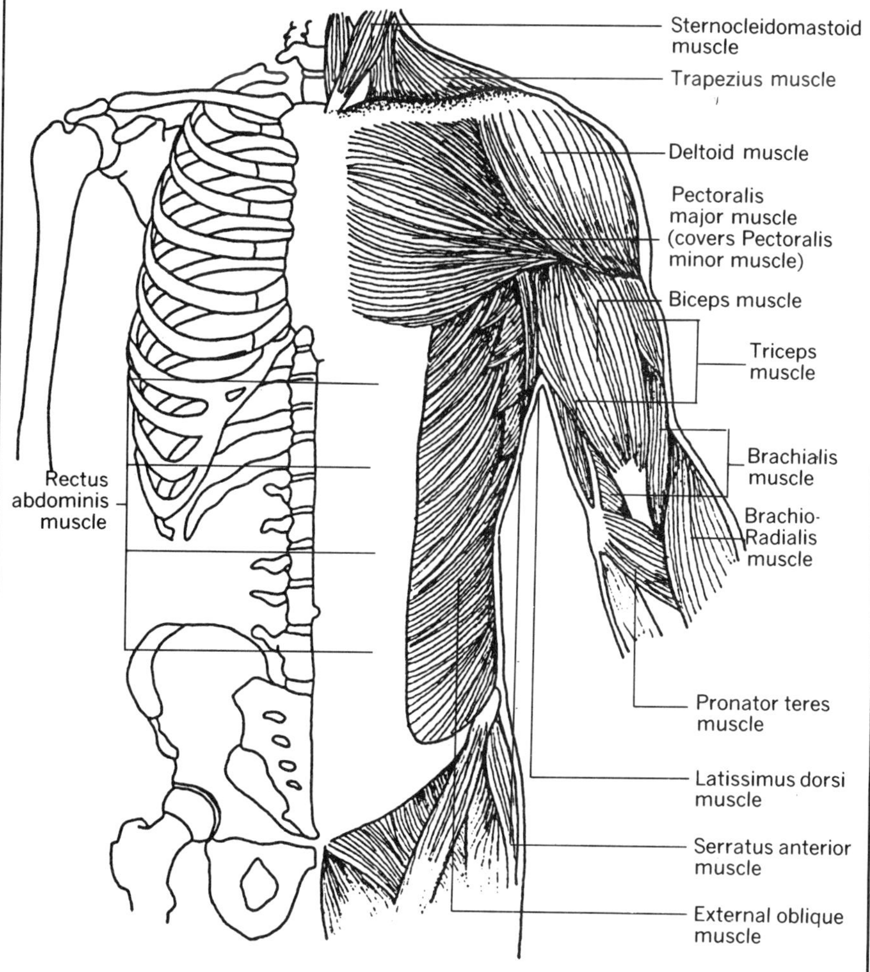

This is true in the adult as well who at first may feel tired or worn out and then realize that he cannot keep up his previous pace. Often his feet and legs are involved in the beginning. He may wear out the toes of his shoes and may then recognize that he must flex his ankles more to avoid tripping or dragging the toes. Or he finds that he must make a conscious effort to raise the legs in climbing stairs; he may even have to climb one step at a time. Getting out of bed in the morning may be a chore, and rising from a

Muscles of the Back

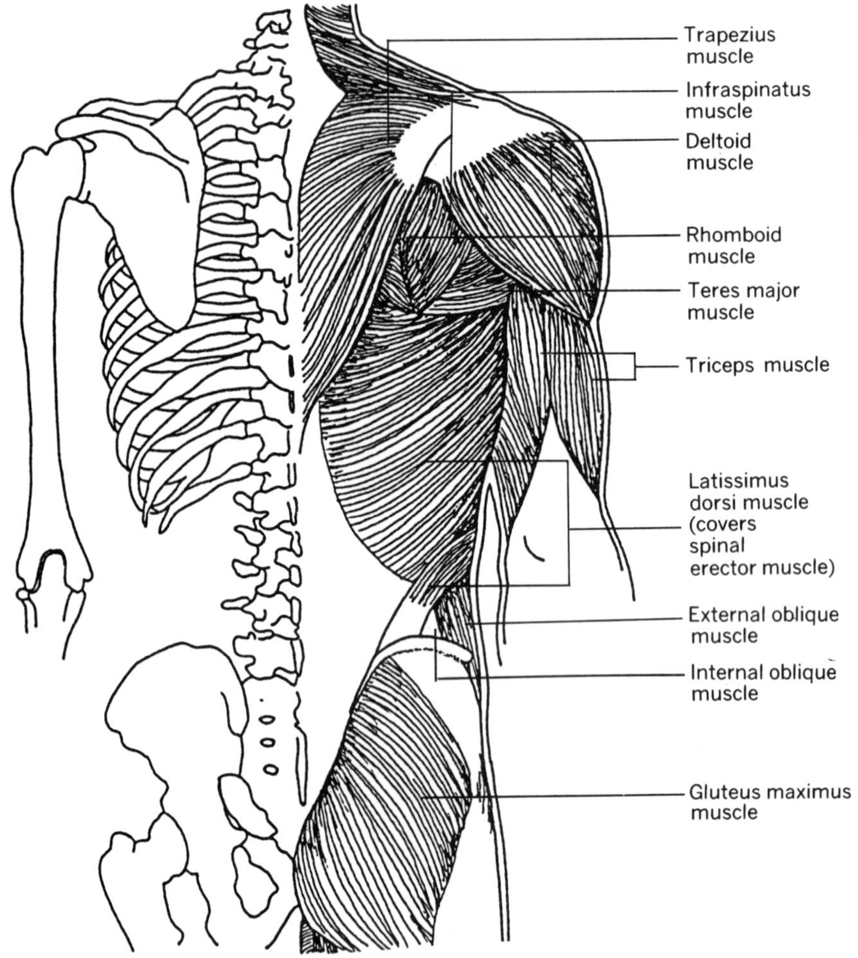

seated position in a low chair or from the floor may be difficult or impossible. Those with arm involvement may recognize that the hands are weak; if the shoulder muscles are involved, there is often difficulty in raising the arms over the head. The patient may take a long time in recognizing the loss of muscle power because the human body can so well compensate or use other muscles to perform the same motor tasks. If the weakness is present for a considerable length of time, there may be a wasting, or a loss of muscle bulk.

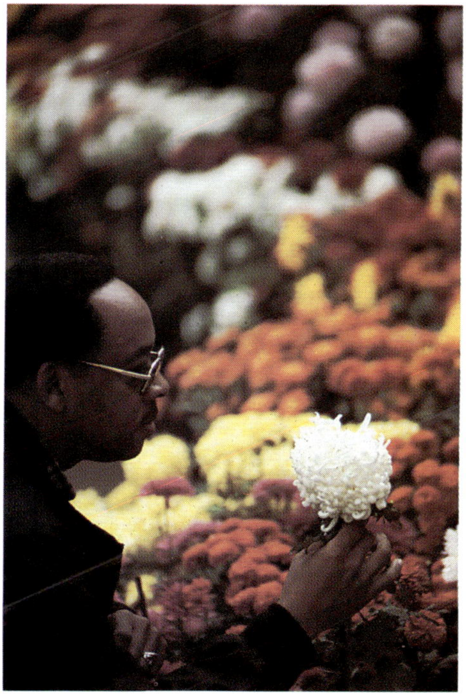
Myopia

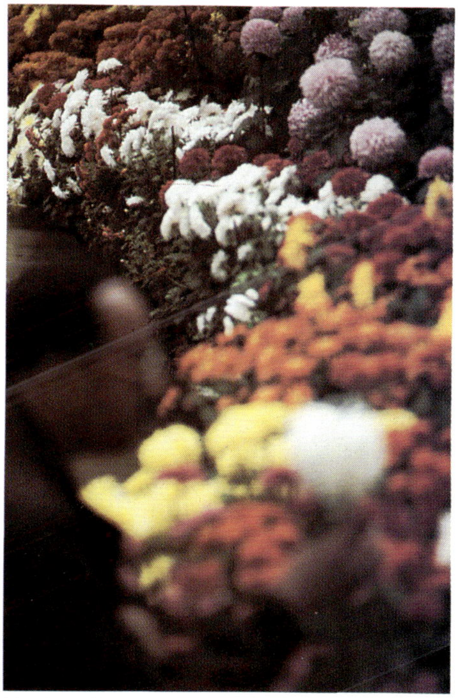
Hyperopia

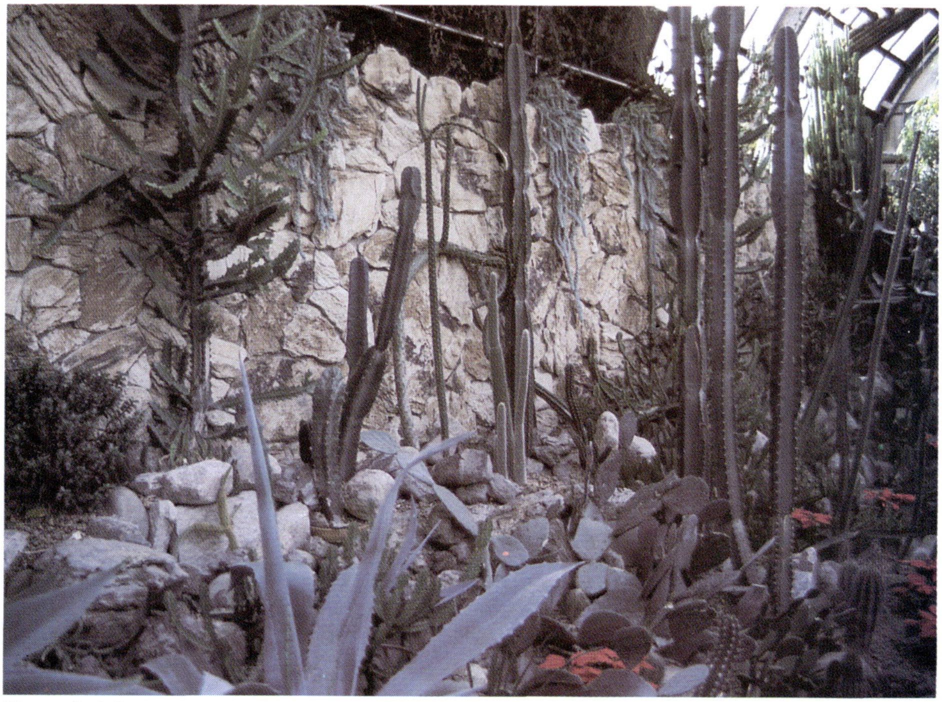
Normal vision

(All photographs © R. Flanagan–Image Finders)

(Photos on the following four pages demonstrate normal and abnormal eyesight.)

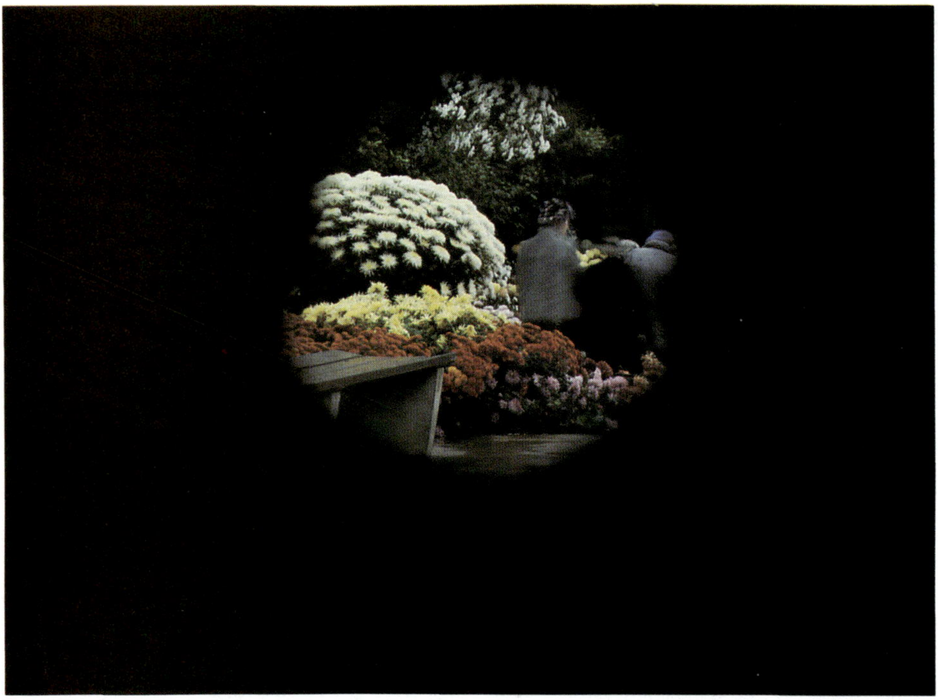

Glaucoma

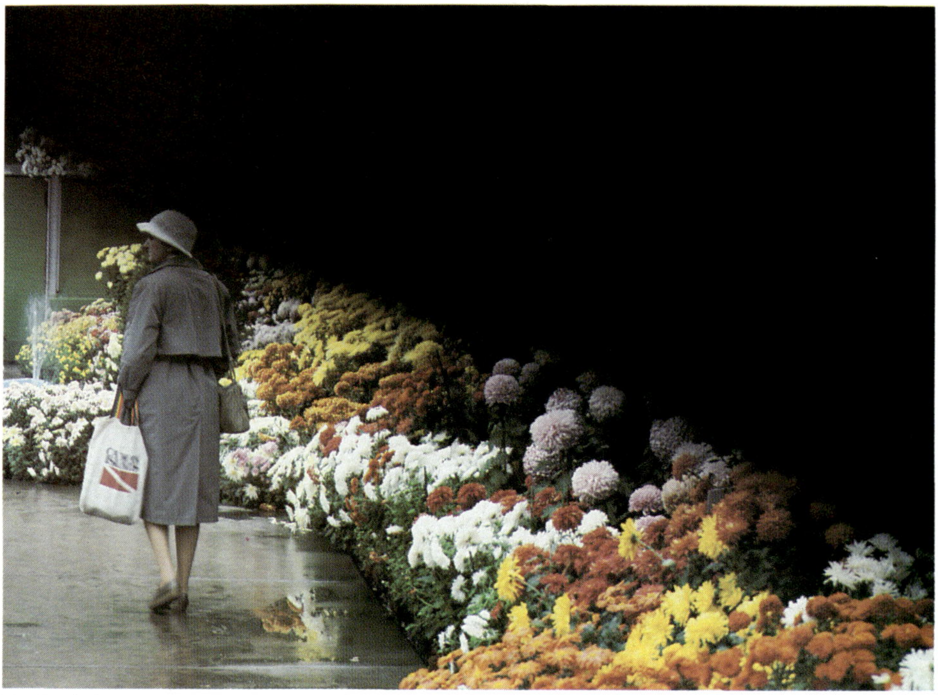

Retinal detachment

(All photographs © R. Flanagan—Image Finders)

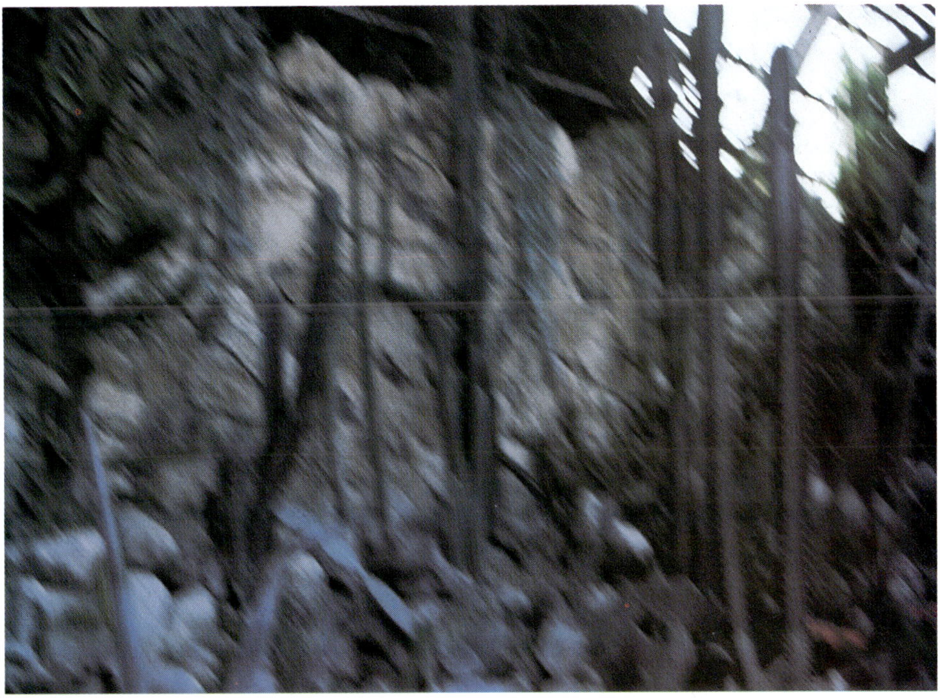

Astigmatism

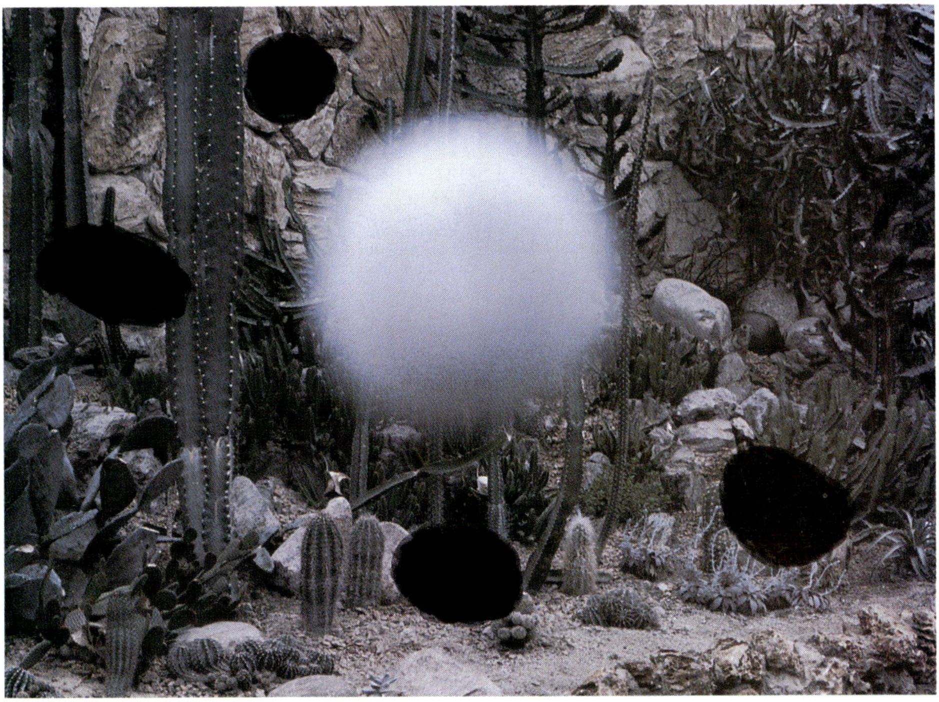

Diabetic retinopathy

(All photographs © R. Flanagan—Image Finders)

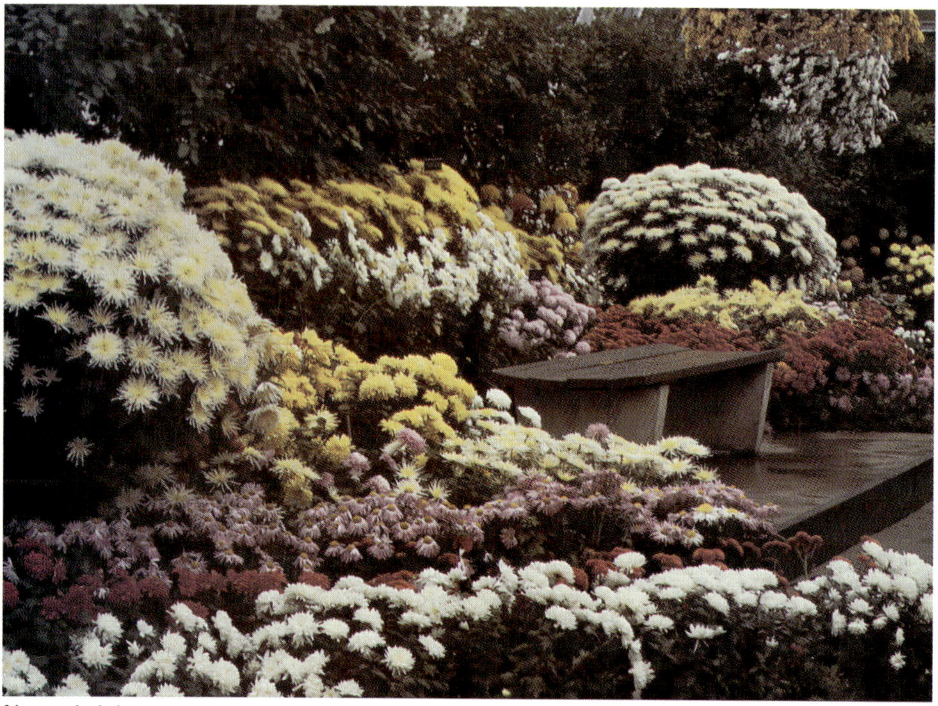
Normal vision

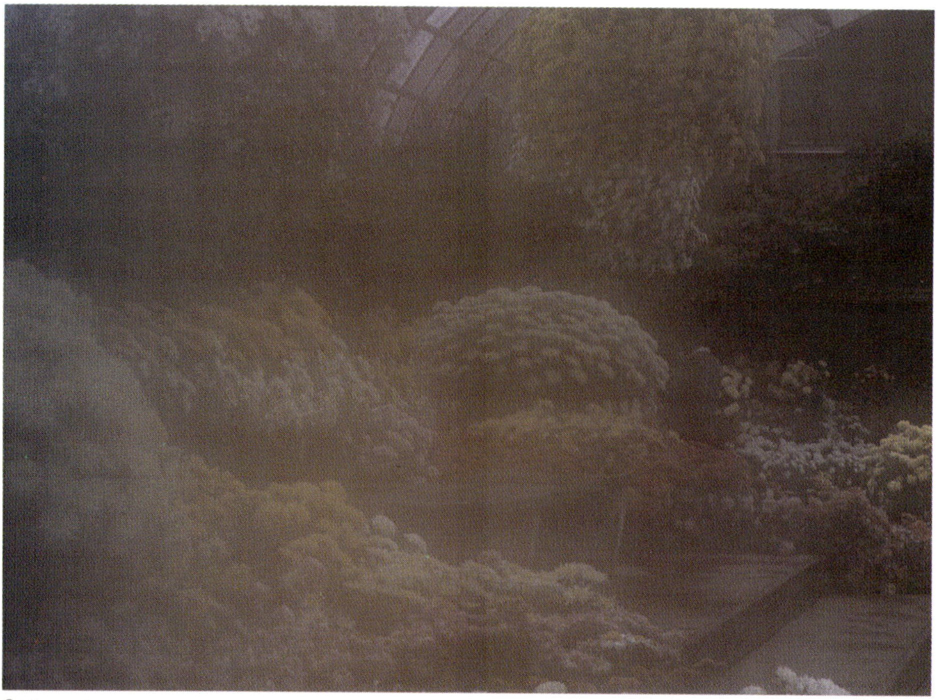
Cataract

James P. Rowan

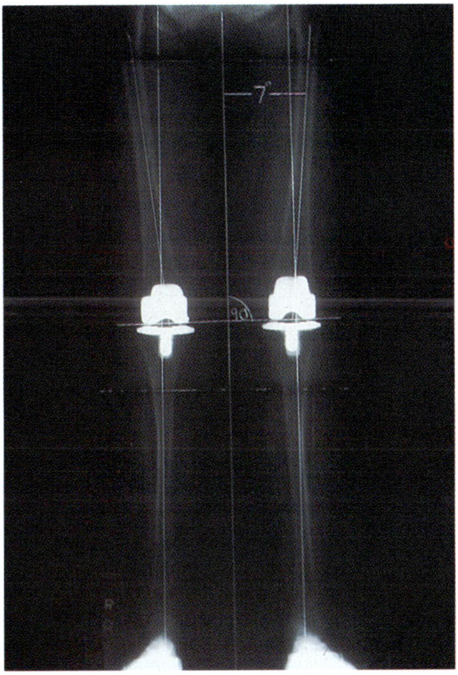

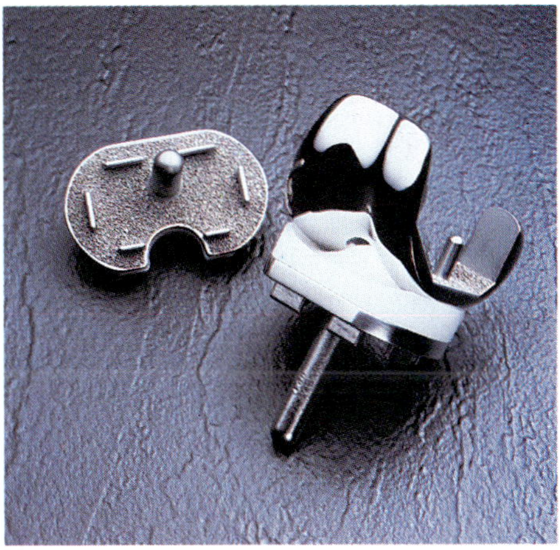

Total knee system
(Courtesy Dow Corning Wright)

Total knee system implanted
(Courtesy Dow Corning Wright)

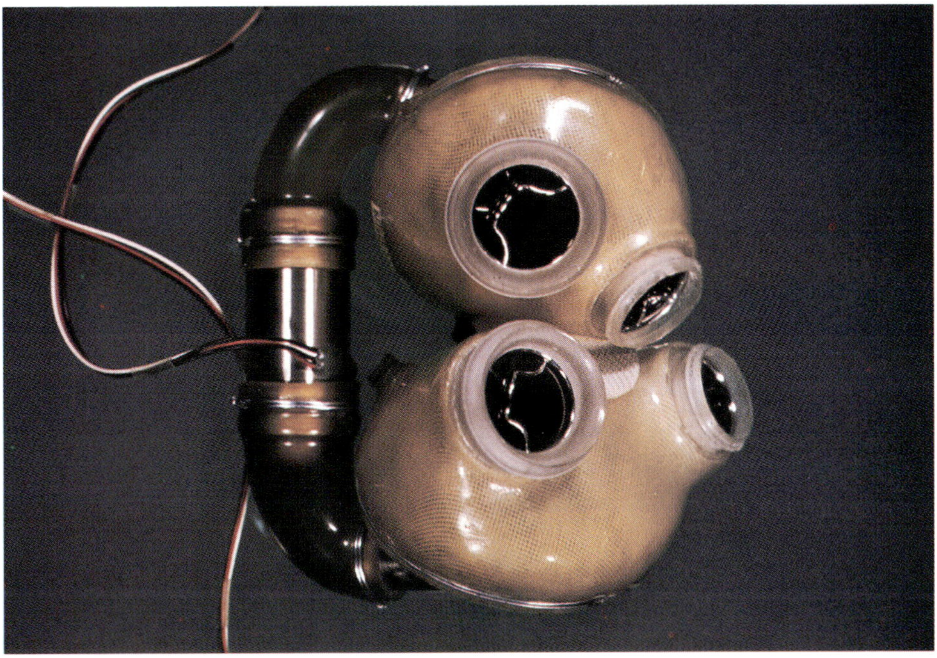

Jarvik-7 artificial heart
(© Hank Morgan, Photo Researchers, Inc.)

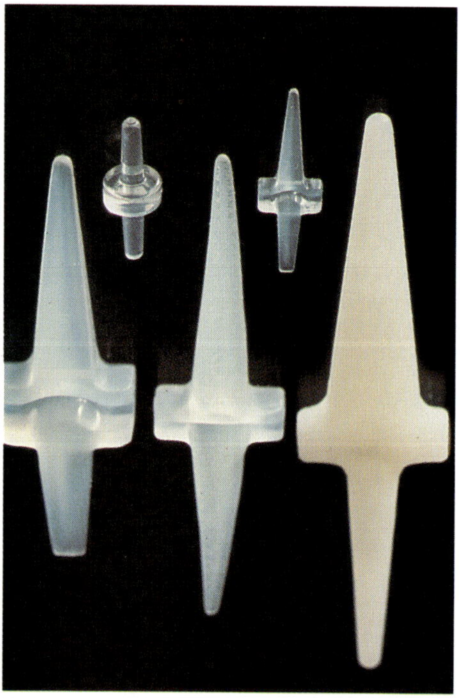

Various hand implants

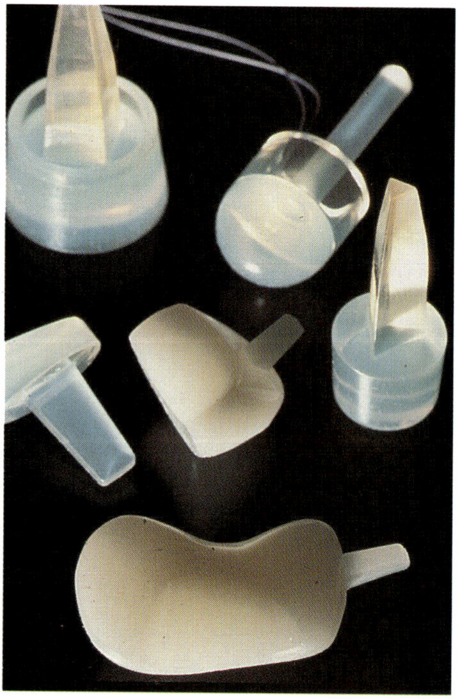

Toe, finger, wrist implants

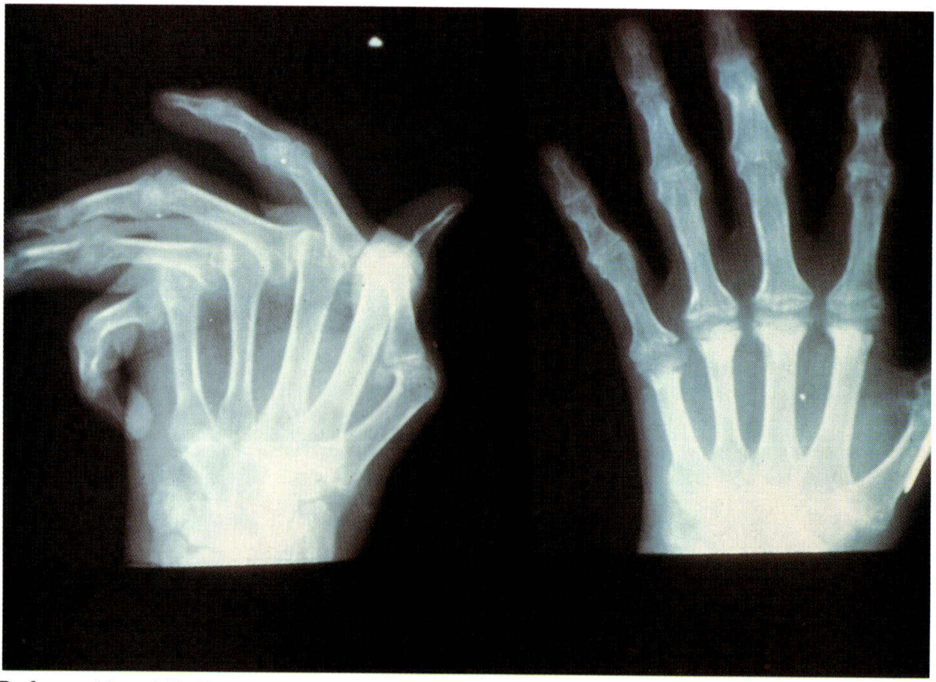

Deformed hand (left) and same hand after flexible implant resection arthroplasty

(All photographs courtesy Dow Corning Wright)

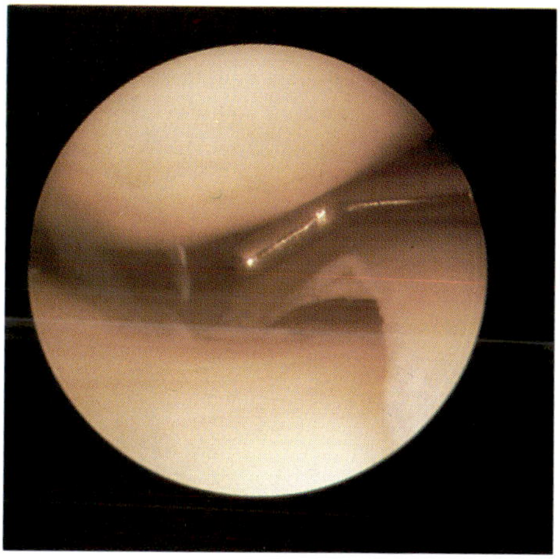

Arthroscopic knee surgery on torn ligaments

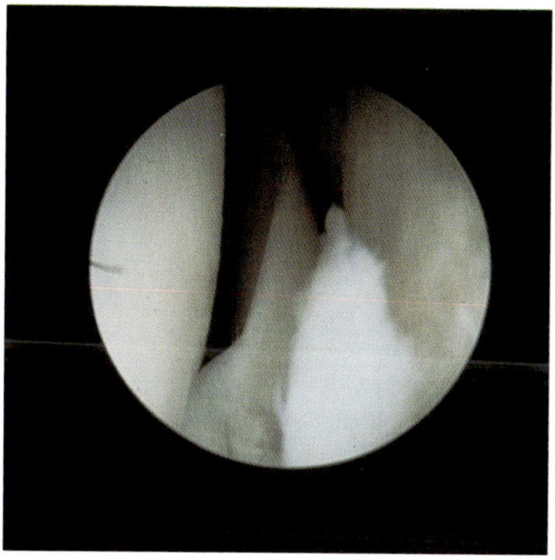

Arthroscopic photograph of knee joint

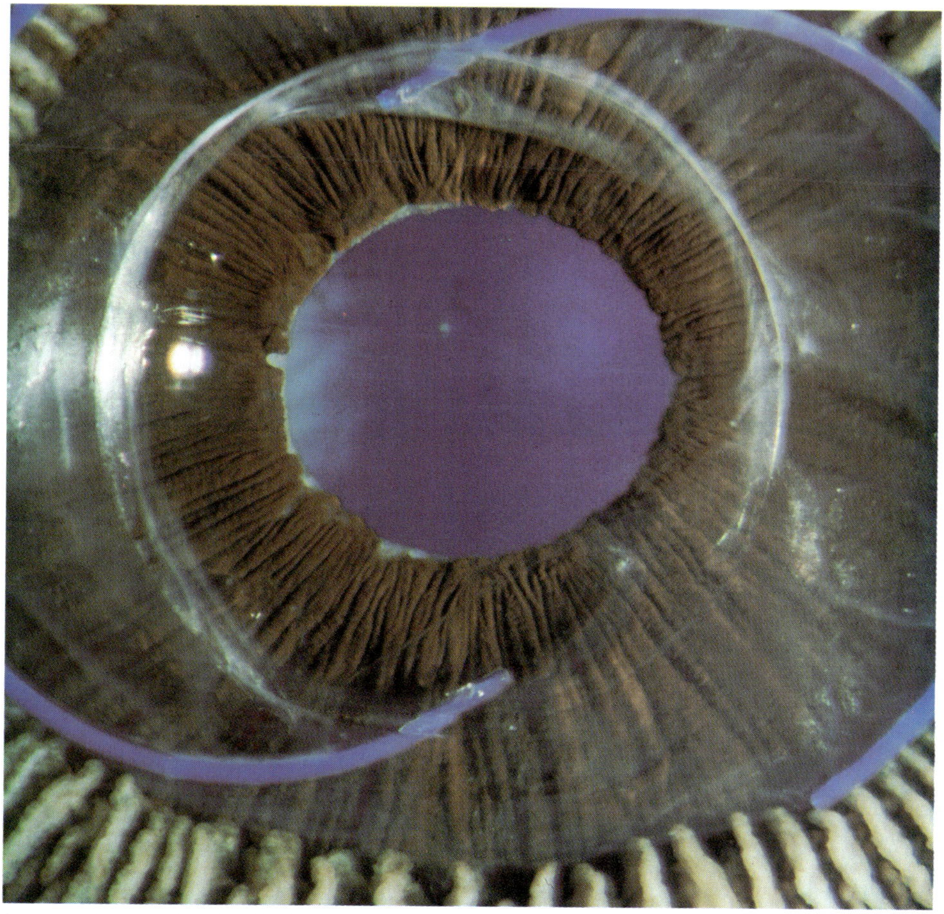

Intraocular lens implant in human eye

(All photographs © Photo Researchers, Inc.)

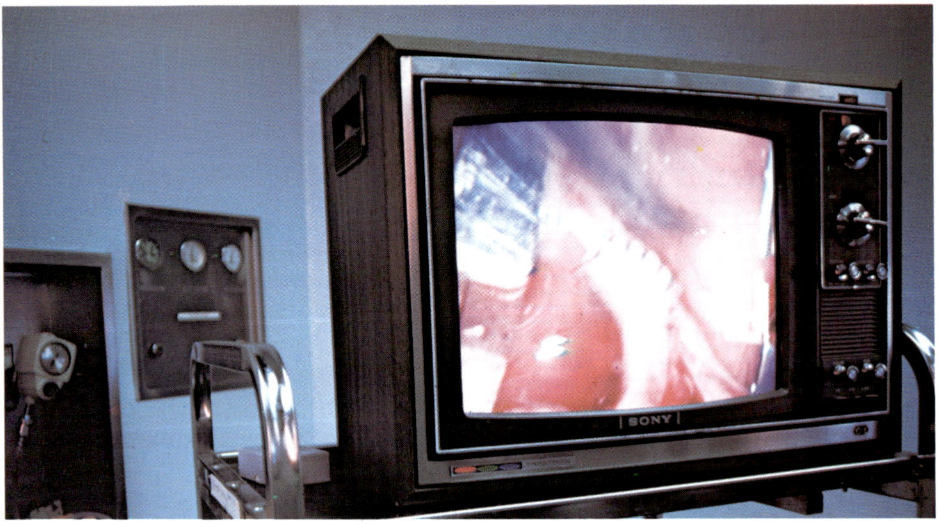

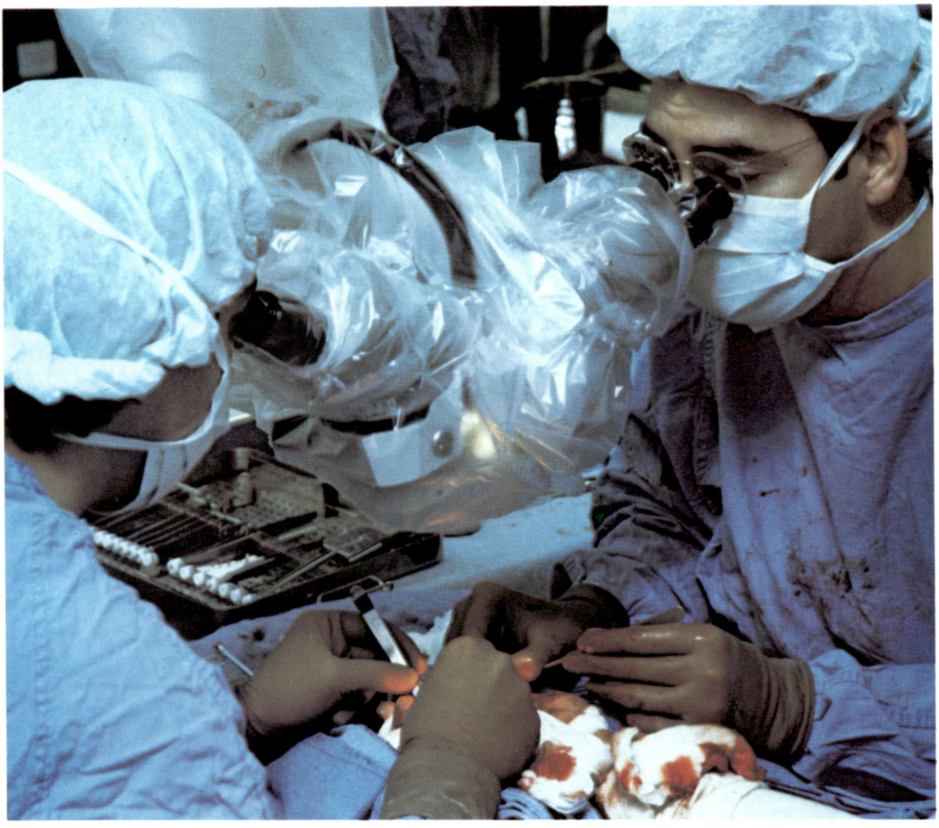

Monitoring device (above) used to assist vascular reconstruction surgery (below)

(© Dan McCoy—Rainbow)

Diagnostic Evaluation of Muscle Disease

In evaluating patients with motor weakness, the physician must have a complete history of the present complaints, past history of the patient, and details of the family history. A general physical and neurological examination is required, with particular reference to the motor, or musculoskeletal system. In most cases, the physician will be able to make a clinical diagnosis of the disease process, but occasionally the examination does not reveal whether the nerve, the muscle, or both are involved. In order to clarify the diagnosis, some additional examinations may be required, mainly determination of serum enzymes (a good indicator of loss of muscle substance), a muscle biopsy, and an electromyogram.

Serum Enzymes

Enzymes are essential for the maintenance of normal body chemistry. Because the normal concentration in the blood serum of some enzymes specifically related to muscle chemistry is known, the determination of concentrations of these enzymes can provide additional evidence that muscle chemistry is either normal or abnormal.

Muscle Biopsy

The first step is the surgical removal of a small segment of muscle, which is then prepared for examination under the microscope. The examination enables the physician to see any abnormality in the muscle fibers, supporting tissue, small nerve twigs, and blood vessels. The muscle biopsy can be of great value in making a correct diagnosis, but occasionally, even in good hands, there is not sufficient visible change from the normal state to identify the disease process.

Electromyograph (EMG)

This is a technique for studying electrical activity of muscle. Fine needles attached to electronic equipment are inserted into the muscle to measure the electrical activity, which is displayed on an *oscilloscope,* a device something like a television screen. It is not a particularly painful process when performed by a skilled physician, and the information gained may be important in establishing a diagnosis.

Muscular Dystrophy

Muscular dystrophy (MD) is defined as an inborn degenerative disease of the muscles. Several varieties of MD have been described and classified according to the muscles involved and the pattern of inheritance. There is no specific treatment for any form of MD, but the patient's life can be made more pleasant and probably prolonged if careful attention is paid to good nutrition, activity without overfatigue, and avoidance of infection. Physical therapists can be helpful in instructing the patient or the parents in an exercise program that relieves joint and muscle stiffness. Sound, prudent psychological support and guidance cannot be overemphasized.

Duchenne's Muscular Dystrophy

In 1886, Dr. Guillaume Duchenne described a muscle disease characterized by weakness and an increase in the size of the muscles and the supporting connective tissue of those muscles. He named the disease *pseudohypertrophic* (false enlargement) *muscular paralysis,* but it is now known as *Duchenne's muscular dystrophy.*

Duchenne's MD is observed almost entirely in males. It is inherited, however, like many other sex-linked anomalies, through the maternal side of the family. The mother can pass the clinical disease to her son; her daughters will not demonstrate the disease but are potential carriers to their sons. More than one-quarter of the cases of Duchenne's MD are sporadic, that is, without any known family history of the disease. There are rare cases of Duchenne's MD in females who have *ovarian dysgenesis,* a condition in which normal female chromosomal makeup is lacking.

The disease process in Duchenne's MD may be apparent during the first few years of life when the child has difficulty in walking or appears clumsy. The muscles of the pelvis and legs are usually affected first, but the shoulders and the arms soon become involved. About 90 percent of the patients have some enlargement of a muscle or group of muscles and appear to be rather muscular and strong; however, as the disease progresses, the muscular enlargement disappears. Most patients progressively deteriorate and at the age of about 10 to 15 are unable to walk. Once the child is confined to a wheelchair or bed, there is a progressive deformity with muscle contracture, with death usually occurring toward the end of the second decade. A small percentage of patients appear to have a remission of the disease process and survive until the fourth or fifth decade. Despite herculean attempts to unravel the riddle of muscular dystrophy, the problem is yet unsolved.

A benign variety of MD, *Becker type,* begins at 5 to 25 years of age and progresses slowly. Most of the reported patients with Becker type are still able to walk 20 to 30 years after the onset of the disease.

Facio-Scapulo-Humeral Muscular Dystrophy

This type of muscular dystrophy affects males and females equally and is thought to be inherited as a dominant trait. The onset may be at any age from childhood to adult life, but is commonly first seen in adolescence.

There is not false enlargement of the muscles. The muscles affected, as indicated by the name of the disease, are those of the face and shoulders, usually with abnormal winging of the *scapula* (either of the large, flat bones at the backs of the shoulders). There is also a characteristic appearance of lip prominence, as if the patient were pouting. Occasionally there is an involvement of the anterior leg muscles and weakness in raising the foot. The disease progresses more slowly than Duchenne's type, and some patients can remain active for a normal life span.

Limb-Girdle Muscular Dystrophy

This type of muscular dystrophy is less clearly delineated than the others. Males and females are equally affected and the onset is usually in the second or third decade, but the process may start later. It is probably inherited as a recessive trait, but many-cases are sporadic. It may first affect the muscles of the pelvis or the shoulder, but in 10 to 15 years both pelvis and shoulder girdles are usually involved. The disease varies considerably from patient to patient; sometimes the disease process appears to be arrested after involvement of either the pelvis or the shoulder, and the course thereafter may be a benign one. Most, however, have significant difficulty in walking by middle age.

Other Varieties of Muscular Dystrophy

These include ocular, oculopharyngeal, and a distal form (involving the muscles of the hands or feet).

Ocular MD

This type involves the muscles that move the eye as well as the eyelids; occasionally, the small muscles of the face and the shoulder girdle are affected.

Oculopharyngeal MD

This type involves not only the muscles that move the eye and the eyelids but may also affect the throat muscles, so that patients have difficulty in swallowing food (*dysphagia*).

Distal MD

This type is rare in the United States but has been reported in Scandinavia. Both sexes can be affected. Usually after the fifth decade, the patient recognizes weakness of the small muscles of the hands and anterior leg muscles that assist in raising the toes. The disease is relatively benign and progresses slowly.

The Myotonias

This is a group of muscle diseases characterized by *myotonia,* a continuation of muscle contraction after the patient has voluntarily tried to relax that contraction. It is best observed in the patient who holds an object firmly in his hand and then tries to release his grasp suddenly, only to realize that he cannot let go quickly. There are two major members of this group of diseases and several other less common variants.

Treatment

As in the case of muscular dystrophy, there is no specific treatment for myotonia. Some drugs, such as quinine, have limited value in decreasing the abnormally prolonged muscular contractions, but as yet no treatment has been completely effective.

Myotonia Congenita

This condition is usually present at birth, but is recognized later in the first or second decade of life when the child complains of stiffness or when clumsiness is noted. A child with this condition appears very muscular and has been called the "infant Hercules." The unusual muscular development persists throughout life, but the myotonia tends to improve with age.

Myotonic Dystrophy

The other major variety of myotonia, *myotonic dystrophy,* is a disease in which many organ systems in addition to muscle are involved. Both males and females are affected equally, and the onset may occur at any time from birth to the fifth decade. It is not unusual for a patient to recognize some clumsiness, but he may not be aware that he has a muscle disease. The myotonia may range from mild to severe. There is a striking similarity in the physical appearance of patients with myotonic dystrophy, the features of which include frontal baldness in the male, wasting and weakness of the temporal muscles (that control closing the jaws), muscles of the forearm, hands, and anterior leg muscles. Other physical abnormalities include cataracts in about 90 percent of the patients, small testicles, and abnormality of the heart muscle. Thickening and other bony abnormalities have been seen in the skull radiogram and, with time, many patients become demented.

Polymyositis

Polymyositis is a disorder of muscular and connective tissues affecting both sexes, males more commonly than females. It can occur at any age, although usually after the fourth decade. It is characterized by muscle weakness with associated muscle wasting; about half of the patients complain of muscle pain or tenderness. The disease may begin suddenly, but often follows an earlier mild, febrile illness. Changes in the skin are common, including a faint red-violet discoloration, particularly about the eyelids, and these changes are often associated with mild swelling. There may be a scaly rash. Some patients have ulcerations over the bony prominences. About one-quarter of the patients with polymyositis complain of joint stiffness and tenderness and an unusual phenomenon in which the nail beds become blue (*cyanotic*) after minor exposure to cold.

Treatment

The treatment involves the administration of cortisone preparations, which may be required for many years. General supportive care, including appropriate physical therapy, is recommended.

Myasthenia Gravis

Myasthenia gravis is characterized by muscle weakness and an abnormal muscle fatigability (pathologic fatigue); patients are abnormally weak after exercise or at the end of the day. The disease affects males and females at any period, from infancy to old age, but it is most common during the second to the fourth decades. There is no complete explanation for myasthenia gravis, but it is believed that there is some defect in the transmission of a nerve impulse to the muscle (*myoneural junction defect*). The disease may occur spontaneously, during pregnancy, or following an acute infection, and there appears to be a curious association with diseases in which there is an immunologic abnormality, such as tumors of the thymus gland, increased or decreased activity of the thyroid gland, and rheumatoid arthritis.

Usually there is an insidious onset of generalized weakness or weakness confined to small groups of muscles. Normal muscle power may be present early in the day, but as the hours pass the patient notices that one or both eyelids droop (*ptosis*) or he may see double images (*diplopia*). If he rests and closes his eyes for a short time, the ptosis and the diplopia clear up, only to return after further muscle activity. The weakness can also be seen in the trunk or the limbs, and some patients have involvement of the muscles used in speaking, chewing, or swallowing (*bulbar* muscles). Some are weak all the time and have an increase in that weakness the longer they use their muscles. The muscles used in breathing may be affected in patients with severe myasthenia, and these patients must be maintained on a respirator for varying periods of time.

Treatment

Myasthenia gravis is treated with drugs that assist in the transmission of the nerve impulse to the muscle. Medication is very effective, but the patient should be carefully observed by the physician to determine that the drug dose and the time of administration are adjusted so that the patient may have the benefit of maximal muscle power. Surgical removal of the thymus gland, *thymectomy,* may prove of benefit to some patients in lessening the symptoms of muscle weakness; however, not all patients have clinical improvement of the disease after thymectomy, and patients must be selected very carefully by the physician. Myasthenia gravis is another chronic disease in which long-term careful observation by the physician is most important in obtaining an optimal medical and psychological outcome.

9

Diseases of the Circulatory System

It's called the river of life, the five or six quarts of blood that stream through the 60,000 tortuous miles of arteries, veins, and capillaries.

Blood contains many elements with specific functions—red cells to transport oxygen from the lungs to body tissues, white cells to fight off disease, and tiny elements called *platelets* to help form clots and repair tears in the blood vessel wall. All float freely in an intricate complex of liquid proteins and metals known as *plasma.*

Because of the blood's extreme importance to life, any injury to it—or to the grand network of channels through which it flows—may have the most serious consequences. The troubles that beset the circulation may be grouped conveniently into two categories: diseases of the blood and diseases of the blood vessels.

Diseases of the Blood

Diseases of the blood include disorders that affect the blood elements directly (as in the case of *hemophilia,* where a deficiency in clotting proteins is at fault) as well as abnormalities in the various organs involved in maintaining proper blood balance (i.e., spleen, liver and bone marrow). The various ills designated and described below are arranged according to the blood component most affected (i.e., clotting proteins, red blood cells, and white blood cells).

Hemorrhagic or Clotting-Deficiency Diseases

The blood has the ability to change from a fluid to a solid and back to a fluid again. The change to a solid is called *clotting*. There are mechanisms

The Circulatory System

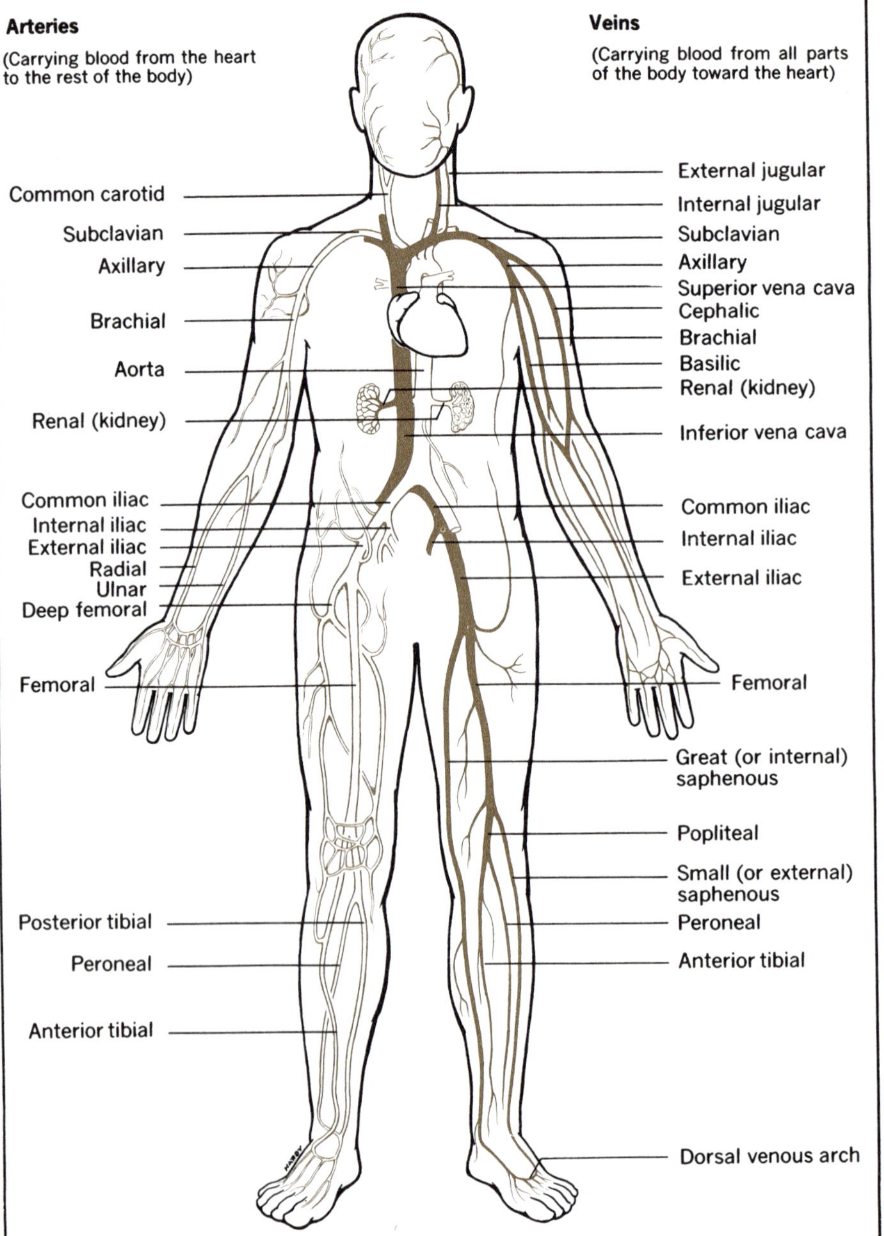

not only for sealing off breaks in the circulatory system when serious blood loss is threatened, but also for breaking down the seals, or clots, once the damage has been repaired and the danger of blood loss is eliminated. Both mechanisms are in continuous, dynamic equilibrium, a delicate balance between tissue repair and clot dissolution to keep us from bleeding or literally clogging to death.

Clotting involves a very complex chain of chemical events. The key is the conversion of an inactive blood protein, *fibrinogen,* into a threadlike sealant known as *fibrin.* Stimulus for this conversion is an enzyme called *thrombin,* which normally also circulates in an inactive state as *prothrombin* (formed from vitamin K in the daily diet).

For a clot to form, however, inactive prothrombin must undergo a chemical transformation into thrombin, a step requiring still another chemical—*thromboplastin.* This agent comes into play only when a tissue or vessel has been injured so as to require clot protection. There are two ways for thromboplastin to enter the bloodstream to spark the chain of events. One involves the release by the injured tissue of a substance that reacts with plasma proteins to produce thromboplastin. The other requires the presence of blood platelets (small particles that travel in the blood) and several plasma proteins, including the so-called antihemophilic factor. Platelets tend to clump at the site of vessel injury, where they disintegrate and ultimately release thromboplastin, which, in the presence of blood calcium, triggers the prothrombin-thrombin conversion.

The clot-destroying sequence is very similar to that involved in clot formation, with the key enzyme, *fibrinolysin,* existing normally in an inactive state (*profibrinolysin*). There are also other agents (e.g., *heparin*) in the blood ready to retard or prevent the clotting sequence, so that it does not spread to other parts of the body.

Naturally, grave dangers arise should these complex mechanisms fail. For the moment, we shall concern ourselves with hemorrhagic disorders arising from a failure of the blood to clot properly. Disorders stemming from excessive clotting are discussed below under "Diseases of the Blood Vessels" because they are likely to happen as a consequence of preexisting problems in the vessel walls.

Hemophilia

Hemophilia is probably the best known (although relatively rare) of the hemorrhagic disorders, because of its prevalence among the royal families of Europe. In hemophilia the blood does not clot properly and bleeding persists. Those who have this condition are called *hemophiliacs* or bleeders. The disease is inherited, and is transmitted by the mother, but except in very rare cases only the male offspring are affected. Hemophilia stems from a lack of one of the plasma proteins associated with clotting, *antihemophilic factor* (*AHF*).

The presence of hemophilia is generally discovered during early childhood. It is readily recognized by the fact that even small wounds bleed profusely and can trigger an emergency. Laboratory tests for clotting speed are used to confirm the diagnosis. Further investigation may occasionally turn up the condition in other members of the family.

In advanced stages, hemophilia may lead to anemia as a result of excessive and continuous blood loss. Bleeding in the joints causes painful swelling, which over a long period of time can lead to permanent deformity and hemophilic arthritis. Hemophiliacs must be under constant medical care in order to receive quick treatment in case of emergencies.

Treating bleeding episodes may involve the administration of AHF alone so as to speed up the clotting sequence. If too much blood is lost a complete transfusion may be necessary. Thanks to modern blood bank techniques, large quantities of whole blood can be made readily available. Bed rest and hospitalization may also be required. For bleeding in the joints, an ice pack is usually applied.

Proper dental hygiene is a must for all hemophiliacs. Every effort should be made to prevent tooth decay. Parents of children with the disease should inform the dentist so that all necessary precautions can be taken. Even the most common procedures, such as an extraction, can pose a serious hazard. Only absolutely essential surgery should be performed on hemophiliacs, with the assurance that large amounts of plasma are on hand.

Purpura

Purpura refers to spontaneous hemorrhaging over large areas of the skin and in mucous membranes. It results from a deficiency in blood platelets, elements essential to clotting. Purpura is usually triggered by other conditions: certain anemias, leukemia, sensitivity to drugs, or exposure to ionizing radiation. In newborns it may be linked to the prenatal transfer from the maternal circulation of substances that depress platelet levels. Symptoms of purpura include the presence of blood in the urine, bleeding from the mucous membranes of the mouth, nose, intestines, and uterus. Some forms of the disease cause arthritic changes in joints, abdominal pains, diarrhea and vomiting—and even gangrene of the skin, when certain infectious organisms become involved.

To treat purpura in newborns, physicians may exchange the infant's blood with platelet-packed blood. Sometimes drug therapy with *steroids* (i.e., cortisone) is prescribed. In adults with chronic purpura it may be necessary to remove the spleen, which plays an important role in eliminating worn-out blood components, including platelets, from the circulation. Most physicians prescribe large doses of steroids coupled with blood transfusions. Purpura associated with infection and gangrene also requires appropriate antibiotic therapy.

Red Cell Diseases

Half the blood is plasma; the other half is made up of many tiny blood cells. The biggest group in number is the red blood cells. These cells contain a complicated chemical called *hemoglobin,* which brings oxygen from the lungs to body cells and picks up waste carbon dioxide for expiration. Hemoglobin is rich in iron, which is what imparts the characteristic red color to blood.

Red blood cells are manufactured by bones all over the body—in the sternum, ribs, skull, arms, spine and pelvis. The actual factory is the red bone marrow, located at bone ends. As red cells mature and are ready to enter the bloodstream, they lose their nuclei to become what are called *red corpuscles* or *erythrocytes.* With no nucleus, a red corpuscle is relatively short-lived (120 days). Thus, the red cell supply must be constantly replenished by bone marrow. And a busy factory it is because 20 to 25 trillion red corpuscles normally travel in the circulation. The spleen is responsible for ridding the body of the aged corpuscles, but it is not an indiscriminate sanitizer; it salvages the hemoglobin for reuse by the body.

To measure levels of red cells, physicians make a blood count by taking a smidgen of blood from a patient's fingertip. The average number of red cells in healthy blood is about five million per cubic millimeter for men, and four and one-half million for women.

Anemia

Anemia exists when the red cell count stays persistently below four million. Abnormalities in the size, shape, or hemoglobin content of the erythrocytes may also account for anemic states. Any such irregularity interferes with the red cell's ability to carry its full share of oxygen to body tissues. It also tends to weaken the red cells so that they are more likely to be destroyed under the stresses of the circulation.

Anemia may result from:

- nutritional deficiencies that deprive the body of elements vital to the production of healthy cells
- diseases or injuries to organs associated with either blood cell formation (bone marrow) or blood cell destruction (spleen and liver)
- excessive loss of blood, the consequences of surgery, hemorrhage, or a bleeding ulcer and
- heredity, as in the case of *sickle cell anemia* (where the red cells are misshapen)

Hemolytic Anemia

There are also several kinds of disorders known as ***hemolytic anemias*** that are linked to the direct destruction of red cells. Poisons such as snake venom, arsenic, and lead can cause hemolytic anemia. So can toxins produced by certain bacteria as well as by other organisms, such as the parasites that cause malaria, hookworm, and tapeworm. Destruction of red cells may also stem from allergic reactions to certain drugs or transfusions with incompatible blood.

The various anemias range from ailments mild enough to go undetected to disorders that prove inevitably fatal. Many are rare; following are the more common.

Pernicious Anemia

Pernicious anemia, or *Addison's anemia,* is associated with a lack of hydrochloric acid in the gastric juices, a defect which interferes with the body's ability to absorb vitamin B_{12} from the intestine. Because the vitamin acts as an essential stimulus to the production of mature red blood cells by the bone marrow, its lack leads to a reduced output. Moreover, the cells tend to be larger than normal, with only half the lifespan of the normal erythrocyte.

The symptoms are characteristic of most anemias: pale complexion, numbness or a feeling of "pins and needles" in the arms and legs, shortness of breath (from a lack of oxygen), loss of appetite, nausea, and diarrhea (often accompanied by significant weight loss). One specific feature is a sore mouth with a smooth, glazed tongue. Advanced stages of the disease may be marked by an unsteady gait and other nervous disorders, owing to degeneration of the spinal cord. Red cell count may drop to as low as 1,000,000. Several kinds of tests may be necessary to differentiate pernicious anemia from other blood diseases—a test for hydrochloric acid levels, for example.

Pernicious anemia, however, is no longer so pernicious, or deadly, as it once was—not since its cause was identified. Large, injected doses of vitamin B_{12} usually restore normal blood cell production.

Sickle Cell Anemia

Sickle cell anemia, an inherited abnormality, occurs almost exclusively among black people. Widespread in tropical Africa and Asia, sickle cell anemia is also found in this country, affecting perhaps 1 in 500 American blacks. The red blood cells are sickle-shaped rather than round, a structural aberration arising from a defect in the manufacture of hemoglobin, the oxygen-carrying component. Such mis-shapen cells tend to clog small blood vessels, depriving organs and tissues of oxygen. Sickle cells live

Sickle Cell Anemia

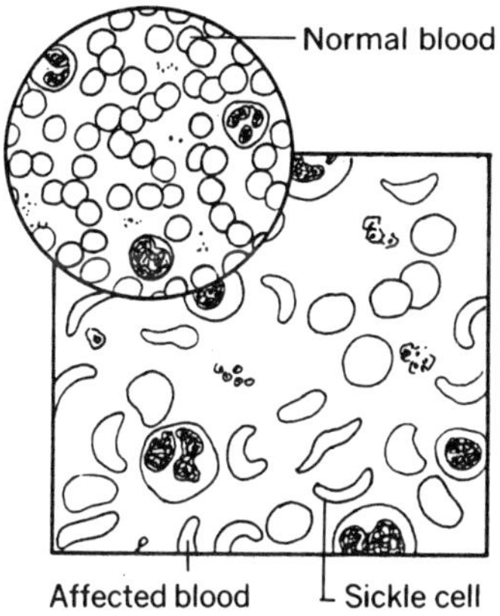

only 10 to 20 days, as compared to 120 for normal red blood cells. They cannot be replaced fast enough, causing anemia.

A differentiation should be made between sickle cell anemia, the full-blown disease, and sickle cell trait. Anemia occurs when the offspring inherits the sickle cell gene from both parents. In some patients the symptoms are mild; in others, they are severe. The disease can cause pain and swelling in the feet and hands, along with fever; fatigue, paleness, and shortness of breath; severe pain that can last from hours to weeks, sometimes requiring hospitalization; retinal damage that can be serious enough to cause blindness; jaundice; delayed growth and puberty in children and slightness of build in adults; infections; susceptibility to strokes in children; and acute chest syndrome, a life-threatening condition caused by infection or trapped sickle cells in the lung. Sickle cell anemia is a very serious disease for which there is no cure, but there are treatments that can help, including painkilling drugs, penicillin, and blood transfusions. The anticancer drug hydroxyurea reduces the frequency of painful episodes and of acute chest syndrome and lessens the need for transfusions.

Sickle cell anemia was once fatal to most of its victims by the age of 30. Today, with good medical care, many people with sickle cell anemia can live into their 40s and even beyond.

Those with only one gene for the disease have *sickle cell trait.* They are not likely to have too much trouble except in circumstances where they are exposed to low oxygen levels (the result, say, of poor oxygenation in a high-altitude plane). Administration of anesthesia or too much physical activity may also bring on some feverish attacks. Those with the trait can pass it on to the next generation. One in 12 black Americans carries the trait.

Iron-Deficiency Anemia

Iron-deficiency anemia is a common complication of pregnancy, during which time the fetus may rob the maternal blood of much of its iron content. Iron is essential to the formation of hemoglobin. The deficiency can be further aggravated by digestive disturbances (e.g., a lack of hydrochloric acid) that may hinder the absorption of dietary iron from the intestines. Some women may not observe proper dietary habits, thereby aggravating the anemic state. Successful treatment involves increasing iron intake, with iron supplements and an emphasis on iron-rich foods, including eggs, cereals, green vegetables, and meat, especially liver.

Polycythemia

Polycythemia is the opposite of anemia; the blood has too many red corpuscles. The most common form of the disease is *polycythemia vera* (or *erythremia*). In addition to the rise in corpuscle count, there is a corresponding rise—as much as threefold—in blood volume to accommodate the high cell count, and increased blood viscosity. Symptoms include an enlarged spleen, bloodshot eyes, red mouth, and red mucous membranes—all resulting from excess red cells. Other common characteristics are weakness, fatigue, irritability, dizziness, swelling in the ankles, choking sensations, vise-like chest pains (angina pectoris), rapid heartbeat, and sometimes severe headaches. There is also an increased tendency toward both clotting and hemorrhaging.

The disease occurs primarily in the middle and late years and is twice as prevalent in males as in females. The cause is unknown, but polycythemia is characterized by stepped-up bone marrow production activity.

Radioactive phosphorus therapy is one method for controlling this hyperactivity. Low iron diets and several forms of drug therapy have been tried with varying degrees of effectiveness. A one-time panacea, bloodletting—to drain off excess blood—appears to be of considerable value. Many patients survive for years with the disease. Premature death is usually the result of vascular thrombosis (clotting), massive hemorrhage, or leukemia.

The Rh Factor

Rh disease might also be considered a form of anemia—in newborns. The disorder involves destruction of the red blood cells of an as-yet unborn or newborn infant. It is brought about by an incompatibility between the maternal blood and fetal blood of one specific factor—the so-called Rh factor. (Rh stands for rhesus monkey, the species in which it was first identified.) Most of us are Rh positive, which is to say that we have the Rh protein substance on the surface of our red cells. The Rh factor is, in fact, present in 83 percent of the white population and 93 percent of the black. Those lacking it are classified as Rh negative.

A potentially dangerous situation exists when an Rh negative mother is carrying an Rh positive baby in her uterus. Although the mother and unborn baby have separate circulatory systems, some leakage does occur. When Rh positive cells from the fetus leak across the placenta into the mother's blood, her system recognizes them as foreign and makes antibodies against them. If these antibodies then slip across into the fetal circulation, damage is inevitable.

The first baby, however, is rarely

affected because it takes time for the mother's body to become sensitized to the Rh positive cells. But should she become pregnant with another child, the now-sensitized mother's blood produces a large quantity of destructive antibodies that could result in stillbirth, death of the infant shortly after birth or, if the child survives, jaundice and anemia.

Modern medicine has reduced the fatality rate and considerably improved the prognosis. Severely affected newborns are being treated by complete blood transfusion—even while still in the womb—to draw off all the Rh positive cells. After birth and as it grows older, the child will once again produce Rh positive cells in its bone marrow—but by that time the danger from the mother's antibodies is past. Recently an Rh vaccine to prevent the problem from ever occurring was developed. After Rh negative women give birth to their first Rh positive baby, they are immunized with the anti-Rh serum to prevent them from manufacturing these dangerous antibodies.

White Blood Cell Diseases

For every 600 to 700 or more red corpuscles, there is one white blood cell, or *leukocyte.* White cells, unlike red corpuscles, have nuclei; they are also larger and rounder. About 70 percent of the white cell population have irregularly-shaped centers, and these are called *polymorphonuclear leukocytes* or *neutrophils.* The other 30 percent are made up of a variety of cells with round nuclei called *lymphocytes.* A cubic millimeter of blood normally contains anywhere from 5,000 to 9,000 white cells (as compared with the four to five million red cells).

White cells defend against disease, which explains why their number increases in the bloodstream when the body is under infectious assault. There are some diseases of the blood and blood-forming organs themselves that can increase the white count. Disorders of the spleen, for example, can produce white cell abnormalities, because this organ is a major source of lymphocytes (cells responsible for making protective antibodies). Diseases of the bone marrow are likely to affect neutrophil production.

Leukemia

Leukemia, characterized by an abnormal increase in the number of white cells, is one of the most dangerous of blood disorders. The cancerlike disease results from a severe disturbance in the functioning of the bone marrow. Chronic leukemia, which strikes mainly in middle age, produces an enormous increase in neutrophils, which tend to rush into the bloodstream at every stage of their development, whether mature or not. Patients with the chronic disease may survive for several years, with appropriate treatment.

In acute leukemia, more common among children than adults, the marrow produces monster-sized, cancerous-looking white cells. These cells not only crowd out other blood components from the circulation, they also leave little space for the marrow to produce the other elements, especially the red cells and platelets. Acute leukemias run their fatal course in a matter of weeks or months—although there have been dramatic instances of sudden remission. The cause is unknown, but recent evidence strongly suggests that a virus may be responsible for at least some forms of the disease.

Modern treatment—radiation and drugs—is aimed at wiping out all of the malignant cells. A critical stage follows treatment, however. For with the disappearance of these abnormal cells and the temporary disruption of marrow function, the patient is left with his defenses against infection down. He also runs a great risk of hemorrhage. Therefore, he is usually kept in isolation to ward off infections. In addition he may be given white cell and platelet transfusions along with antibiotic therapy. Eventually—and hopefully—the marrow will revert to normal function, freed of leukemic cell production. For additional information on leukemia, see Ch. 18, *Cancer.*

Other White Cell Diseases

Agranulocytosis

Agranulocytosis is a disease brought on by the direct destruction of neutrophils (also called *granulocytes*). Taken over a long period of time, certain types of drugs may bring about large-scale destruction of the neutrophil supply. Symptoms include general debilitation, fatigue, sleeplessness, restlessness, headache, chills, high fever (often up to 105° F.), sore mouth and throat, along with psychologically aberrant behavior and mental confusion. White cell count may fall as low as 500 to 2,000. Sometimes agranulocytosis is confused with leukemia.

Treatment involves antibiotic therapy to ward off bacterial invasion, a likelihood that is increased owing to the lowered body resistance. In advanced cases, hospitalization and transfusions with fresh blood are necessary. Injections of fresh bone marrow may also be prescribed.

Leukopenia

Leukopenia is less severe than agranulocytosis. It too involves a reduction of circulating white cells to counts of less than 5,000. It is usually the result of allergic reactions to some chemical or drug.

Infectious Mononucleosis

Infectious mononucleosis, also known as *glandular fever* or *kissing disease,* is characterized by the presence in the bloodstream of a large number of lymphocytes, many of which are abnormally formed. The disease is mildly contagious—kissing is thought to be one popular source of transmission—and occurs chiefly among children and adolescents. The transmitting agent, however, has yet to be discovered, though some as yet unidentified organism is strongly suspected.

The disease is not always easy to diagnose. It can incubate anywhere from four days to four weeks, at which point the patient may experience fever, headache, sore throat, swollen lymph nodes, loss of appetite, and a general feeling of weakness.

The disease runs its course in a matter of a week or two, although complete recovery may take a while longer. Bed rest and conservative medical management is often enough for complete patient recovery. A few severe cases may require hospitalization because of occasional complications, such as rupture of the spleen, skin lesions, some minor liver malfunctions, and occasionally hemolytic anemia or purpura.

Diseases of the Blood Vessels

Diseases of the blood vessels are the result primarily of adverse changes in the vessel walls, such as hardening of the arteries, stroke, and varicose veins.

A healthy circulation depends to a large extent not only on the condition of the blood-forming organs but on the pipelines through which this life-sustaining fluid flows. The arteries, which carry blood away from the heart, and the veins, which bring it back, are subject to a wide range of maladies. They may become inflamed, as in the case of arteritis, phlebitis, and varicose veins; or they may become clogged—especially the arteries—as a result of atherosclerosis (hardening of the arteries) or blood clots (thrombosis and embolism), which can prevent the blood from reaching a vital organ.

The Inflammatory Disorders

Arteritis

Arteritis, or inflammation of the arterial wall, usually results from infections (e.g., syphilis) or allergic reactions in which the body's protective agents against invading organisms, the antibodies, attack the vessel walls themselves. In these instances, the prime source of inflammation must be treated before the arterial condition can heal.

Phlebitis

Phlebitis is an inflammation of the veins, a condition that may stem from an injury or may be associated with such conditions as varicose veins, malignancies, and infection. The extremities, especially the legs, are vulnerable to the disorder. The symptoms are stiffness and hot and painful swelling of the involved region. Phlebitis brings with it the tendency of blood to form blood clots (*thrombophlebitis*) at the site of inflammation. The danger is that one of these clots may break away and enter the bloodstream. Such a clot, on the move, called an *embolus,* may catch and become lodged in a smaller vessel serving a vital organ, causing a serious blockage in the blood supply.

Phlebitis

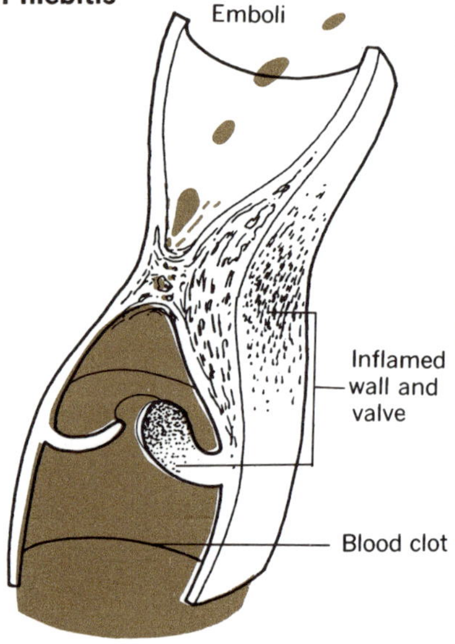

Physicians are likely to prescribe various drugs for phlebitis—agents to deal with the suspected cause of the disorder as well as *anticoagulants* (anticlotting compounds) to ward off possible thromboembolic complications.

Varicose Veins

Varicose veins, which are veins that are enlarged and distorted, primarily affect the leg vessels, and are often troublesome to people who are on their feet for hours at a time. Varicose veins develop because either the walls or the valves of veins are weakened. Some people may be born with weakened veins or valves. In others, the damage may develop from injury or disease, such as phlebitis. More women than men seem to have this condition, but it is common among both sexes. In women, the enlarged veins sometimes occur during pregnancy, but these may well diminish and disappear after delivery. Some elderly people are prone to this condition because the blood vessels lose their elasticity with aging, with the muscles that support the vein growing less sturdy.

In most instances, the surface veins lying just beneath the skin are involved. If there are no other complications, these cases are seldom serious, although they may be disturbing because of unsightliness. Physicians have remedies, including surgery, for making varicose veins less prominent.

When varicose veins become severe, it is usually because the vessels deeper in the leg are weak. Unchecked, this situation can lead to serious complications, including swelling *(edema)* around the ankles and lower legs. Occasionally, very painful skin ulcers may form near the ankle. A brownish discoloration of the skin often precedes the development of such ulcers.

Most of the complications can be averted with early care and treatment. For mild cases of varicose veins, self-care measures can provide relief and keep the condition from worsening. Physicians often recommend wearing compression stockings as a first approach before trying other treatments. The stockings work by steadily squeezing the legs, which helps the veins and muscles move blood more efficiently. Other effective self-help measures include elevating the legs, losing weight, exercising, and avoiding wearing tight clothing. It is also important to avoid long periods of either sitting or standing. Changing position frequently helps to encourage blood flow.

Severe cases of varicose veins may require treatment, such as *sclerotherapy,* injecting the vein with a solution that scars and closes the vein; *ligation,* the removal of the vein; or *vein stripping,* tying off the main veins and removing superficial veins. Laser surgery may be used in some cases to close smaller veins. See "Vascular Surgery" in Ch. 20, *Surgery,* for more information about surgical treatment of varicose veins.

Varicose Veins

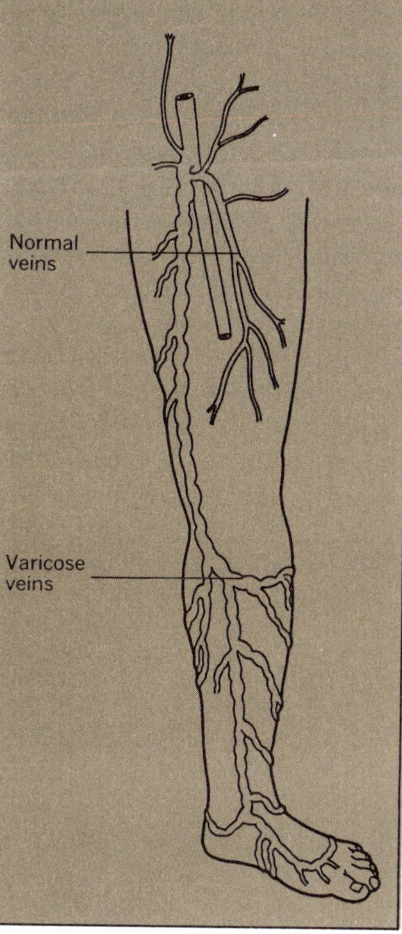

The Vessel-Clogging Disorders

Atherosclerosis

Atherosclerosis (hardening of the arteries) is the nation's most serious health problem, the underlying cause of a million or more deaths each year from heart attack and stroke. It is the process whereby fats carried in the bloodstream gradually pile up on the walls of arteries, like rust in a pipe. The vessels become brittle and roughened; the channel through which blood flows grows narrower. Eventually the organs and tissues supplied by the diseased arteries may be sufficiently deprived of their normal oxygen delivery so as to interfere with proper function. Such a cutback in the pipeline supply is called *ischemia*. This fat deposit poses its greatest hazard when it occurs in the vessels serving the heart, brain and, sometimes, the lower extremities.

A reduced supply of blood to the lower extremities may cause irreversible damage and ultimately lead to death of the leg tissues unless proper circulation is restored. Bacterial invasion may follow; the area may swell, blacken, and emit the distinctly offensive smell of the deadly infection. Such a condition is known as *gangrene,* a severe disorder that may require amputation above the site of blockage if other measures, including antibiotic therapy, fail. Diabetics more commonly than others may develop atherosclerotic obstructions in

Atherosclerosis and Its Influence in Thrombosis, Stroke, and Embolus

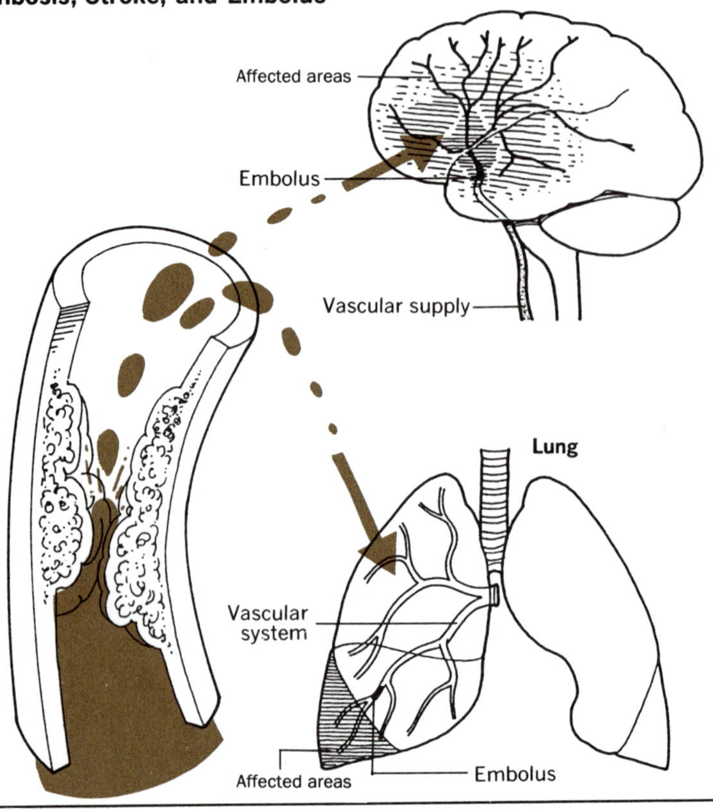

leg arteries. Such persons must take care to avoid leg injuries, because even minimal damage in an already poorly served tissue area can bring on what is termed *diabetic gangrene.*

When the coronary arteries nourishing the heart are involved, even a moderate reduction in blood delivery to the heart muscle may be enough to cause angina pectoris, with its intense, suffocating chest pains.

Thrombosis

Thrombosis, a blood clot that forms within the vessels, is a great ever-present threat that accompanies atherosclerosis. The narrowed arteries seem to make it easier for normal blood substances to adhere to the roughened wall surfaces, forming clots. If the clot blocks the coronary arteries, it may produce a heart attack—damage to that part of the heart deprived by vessel obstruction. For a detailed account of atherosclerosis and heart attack, see under Ch. 10, *Heart Disease.*

Stroke

Stroke, like heart attack, is a disorder usually resulting from blockage brought on by the atherosclerotic process in vessels supplying the brain. This sets the stage for a *thrombus,* or blood clot fixed within a vessel, which would not be likely to occur in arteries clear of these fatty deposits. A stroke may be a result of an interruption of blood flow through arteries in the brain or in the neck vessels leading to the brain.

Sometimes the shutoff of blood flow, or *embolism,* may be triggered by a wandering blood clot that has become wedged in cerebral vessels. This kind of clot, known as an *embolus,* is a thrombus that has broken free into the circulation.

A stroke may also stem from hemorrhaging, where a diseased artery in the brain bursts. A cerebral hemorrhage is most likely to occur when a patient has atherosclerosis in combination with hypertension (high blood pressure). (For a discussion of hypertension, see "Hypertensive Heart Disease" in Ch. 10, *Heart Disease.*) Hemorrhage is also a danger when an aneurysm forms in a blood vessel. An *aneurysm* is a blood-filled pouch that balloons out from a weak spot in the artery wall. Sometimes, too, pres-

Brain Hemorrhage

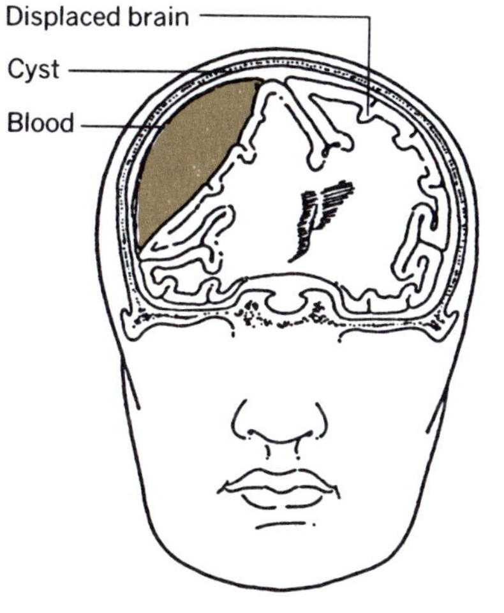

sure from a mass of tissue—a tumor, for example—can produce a stroke by squeezing a nearby brain vessel shut.

When the blood supply is cut off, injury to certain brain cells follows. Cells thus damaged cannot function; neither, then, can the parts of the body controlled by these nerve centers. The damage to the brain cells may produce paralysis of a leg or arm; it may interfere with the ability to speak or with a person's memory. The affected function and the extent of disability depend on which brain region has been struck, how widespread the damage is, how effectively the body can repair its supply system to this damaged area, and how rapidly other areas of brain tissue can take over the work of the out-of-commission nerve cells.

Symptoms

Frequently there are symptoms of impending stroke: headaches, numbness in the limbs, faintness, momentary lapses in memory, slurring of speech, or sudden clumsiness. The presence of these symptoms does not always mean a stroke is imminent; sometimes they are quite harmless. But should they be stroke warning signals, the physician can take some preventive action. He may recommend anticoagulant therapy as well as drugs to bring down elevated blood pressure. In some cases, he might decide to call for surgical replacement of diseased or weakened sections of arteries leading to the brain.

Treatment

After a stroke, medical personnel may use *single photon emission computed tomography* (SPECT) to assess quickly the effects of a stroke. A refinement of nuclear scanning (See Chapter 26, Physicians and Diagnostic Procedures), SPECT shows the nature and extent of brain damage. The next critical steps are careful control of blood pressure and intensive rehabilitation. Not everyone needs a rehabilitation regimen; some strokes have little effect. Some persons recover quickly from what appears to be a severe stroke. Others may suffer serious damage and may take a long time to recover even partially. A great deal can usually be done to help—especially those who are partially paralyzed and those with *aphasia,* the inability to speak properly because of damage to the brain's speech center.

Preventing Future Strokes

Determining the reason that a stroke occurred is a crucial step toward the prevention of future strokes. In addition, various medical options can help prevent future strokes. One important option involves medication. To decrease the risk of a stroke resulting from atherosclerosis, the first drugs of choice are cholesterol-lowering statin drugs, such as lovastatin, pravastatin, and simvastatin. The statin drugs not only effectively lower blood cholesterol levels, they also have few short-term side effects. Other drugs used to prevent future strokes are the anticoagulants aspirin, clopidogrel, ticlopidine, warfarin, and heparin. These drugs improve blood flow by keeping blood platelets from sticking together as they pass through narrowed arteries.

Surgery may also be used as a preventive measure. *Carotid endarterectomy* clears vessel-blocking plaque deposits from moderately or severely narrowed carotid arteries. An alternative to carotid endarterectomy is *angioplasty,* in which a small wire tube is placed down a narrowed artery. In the tube is a balloon that inflates to widen the artery. In some cases, a *stent* (a short, narrow tube of plastic or metal) may be inserted in the widened artery to keep it from narrowing again.

Embolism

An embolus, or thrombus that has broken away into the bloodstream, is, as we have seen, sometimes the direct cause of a stroke. A heart attack may also cause a stroke. Bacterial action may soften a thrombus so that it separates into fragments and breaks free from its wall anchorage. Thrombi are not the only source of emboli; any free-floating mass in the bloodstream, whether an air bubble, clumps of fat, knots of cancer cells, or bacteria, can prove dangerous.

Usually, however, emboli originate as thrombi in the veins, especially the leg veins. Breaking free, the clump of clot material wanders into the bloodstream to be carried toward the right chamber of the heart and then onward into the lungs, unless dissolved before that. Once in the pulmonary arteries, there is a growing threat that the moving mass will catch in one of the smaller branches of the lung circulation. This life-threatening blockage is called a *pulmonary embolism.*

This disorder takes at least 50,000 lives a year; most occur during or following prolonged periods of hospitalization and bed rest. The lack of activity slows the blood flow and increases the danger of thrombi—and ultimately emboli. Prevention requires getting the patient out of bed as soon and as often as possible to stimulate leg circulation. The nonambulatory patient, meanwhile, is encouraged to move his legs by raising them, or changing positions so as to step up blood flow.

The detection of a large embolus—symptoms include shortness of breath and chest pains—may require emergency surgery for removal. In most instances, however, treatment involves administering anticoagulants to prevent new clots from emerging while allowing the body to rid itself of the embolus.

10

Heart Disease

Heart disease is the commonly used, catch-all phrase for a number of disorders affecting both the heart and blood vessels. A more apt term is cardiovascular disease, which represents America's worst health scourge. More than 68 million Americans of all ages have some kind of cardiovascular disease. When considered together heart and circulatory system diseases, including stroke, account for more than one-half of all deaths each year in the United States. Men's risk of a heart attack is greater than women's, and men tend to have heart attacks earlier in life than women do. Cardiovascular disease comprises several symptoms and disorders: coronary artery disease, hypertensive heart disease, rheumatic heart disease, and congenital heart disease.

Coronary Artery Disease

To keep itself going, the heart relies on two pencil-thick main arteries. Branching from the aorta, these vessels deliver freshly oxygenated blood to the right and left sides of the heart. The left artery is usually somewhat larger and divides into two sizable vessels, the circumflex and anterior branches. A clot near its mouth is common and can lead to a serious and often fatal heart attack. These arteries wind around the heart and send out still smaller branches into the heart muscle to supply the needs of all cells. The network of vessels arches down over the heart like a crown—in Latin, *corona*—hence the word coronary.

Coronary artery disease is a form of

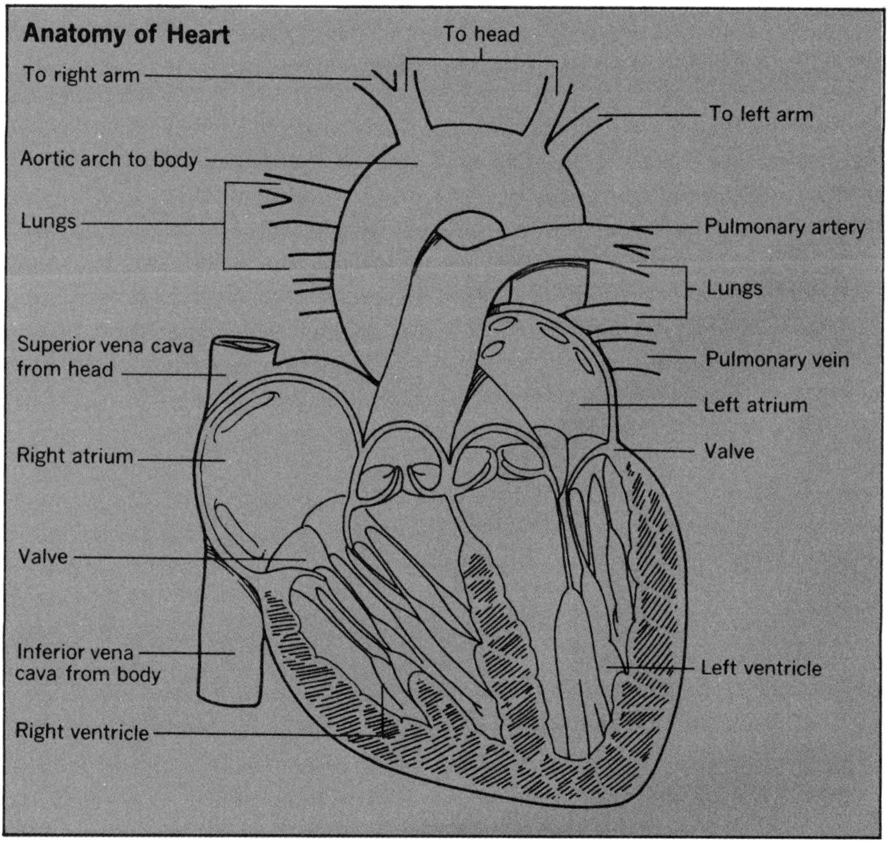

Anatomy of Heart

cardiovascular disease. It refers to the narrowing or blockage of the coronary arteries that is usually the consequence of *arteriosclerosis*—the buildup of fatty deposits within the arteries. Two conditions are a common result of coronary artery disease. One is *angina pectoris,* pain in the chest (and sometimes left arm) caused by insufficient delivery of oxygen to the heart. The other is *myocardial infarction,* or heart attack. Heart attack is the country's leading cause of death among adults.

Heart attacks strike about 1.6 million Americans annually and kill about 600,000. Overall, more than six million adults either have or are suspected of having some degree of coronary artery disease.

Risk Factors of Coronary Artery Disease

1. Sedentary lifestyle.
2. High cholesterol.
3. High blood pressure.
4. Obesity.
5. Cigarette smoking.
6. Diabetes.
7. Family history of coronary disease.

Controlling the Risk Factors of Coronary Artery Disease

- Exercise regularly. Consult your physician for the best program for your age and physical condition.
- Eat less saturated fat and cholesterol. Substitute polyunsaturated vegetable fats or monounsaturated fats. Eat more poultry, fish, fruits, vegetables, and complex carbohydrates.
- Undergo periodic tests of your total cholesterol level. A total cholesterol reading under 200 is desirable; a reading from 200-239 ranks as "borderline high" and indicates the need for dietary adjustments; levels above 240 are considered "abnormal" and indicate a need to consult a physician and possibly undergo drug therapy.
- Monitor your blood pressure and control it if it is high. Adults should have their blood pressure checked at least every two years. Those whose blood pressure is consistently 140/90 or higher are considered to have high blood pressure.
- Don't smoke. The risk of heart attack in smokers is more than twice that of nonsmokers. The sudden death rate from heart attack is two to four times higher among smokers than for nonsmokers. Giving up the habit can decrease the coronary risk to that of nonsmokers within two years.
- Get down to your proper weight and stay there. Excess weight taxes the heart, making it work harder.
- An aspirin every other day or daily has been shown to lessen the chance of heart attack for persons at risk. Because aspirin inhibits blood clotting, it should not be taken by those with high blood pressure, a family history of stroke, bleeding disorders, ulcers, or impaired liver or kidney function. Consult your physician before taking aspirin regularly.

Arteriosclerosis

Coronary artery disease exists when flow of blood is impaired because of narrowed and obstructed coronary arteries. In virtually all cases, this blockage is the result of atherosclerosis. Atherosclerosis is a form of *arteriosclerosis,* a thickening and hardening of the arteries. Arteriosclerosis refers to the process by which a buildup of fatty deposits called *plaque* piles up on the inner wall of the arteries. As more plaque accumulates, the once-smooth wall becomes thicker, rougher, and harder, and the blood passageway becomes narrower.

This process goes on slowly and imperceptibly and begins early in life. If the plaque buildup becomes severe, it can greatly reduce the flow of blood through an artery. Plaques can rupture; when they do, they can form clots that can either block blood flow or break off and travel to another part of the body. If a blood clot blocks a vessel that feeds the heart, it causes a heart attack. To some extent, the body protects itself by developing, over a long period of time, alternative arterial connections, a process termed *collateral circulation,* through which the blood flow bypasses the diseased arteries. Eventually, however, blood flow may become significantly obstructed, prompting the brief, episodic chest pains of angina pectoris.

The preventive measures for arteriosclerosis are the same as those for coronary artery disease: exercise regularly, cut down on cholesterol and fat, don't smoke, control your blood pressure, and keep your weight down. Adopting these measures greatly decreases the chance of developing arteriosclerosis.

Angina Pectoris

Angina pectoris is a symptom of inadequate blood flow through the coronary arteries to the heart. It means chest pain (from the Latin *angere* meaning choke and *pectoralis* meaning chest). Angina pectoris occurs when some part of the heart muscle is not getting enough blood, usually during times of exertion or stress. At such times, the heart must work harder and faster. If one or more of the heart's arteries is narrowed by disease, the extra blood and oxygen required to nourish the heart cannot reach a region of the heart muscle. *Anginal* pain is a signal that muscle cells are being strained by an insufficiency of oxygen; they are, in effect, gasping for air.

The attacks are usually brief, lasting only a matter of minutes, and they normally stop when the person rests. Angina pectoris seldom causes permanent damage to the heart muscle.

Symptoms

Angina attacks are likely to appear when sudden strenuous demands are placed on the heart. They may come from various kinds of physical exertion, or from watching an exciting movie or sporting event. An attack can occur even when an individual is lying still or asleep—perhaps the result of tension or dreams. Extreme temperatures, heavy meals, alcohol, and cigarette smoking can also trigger an angina attack. The most obvious characteristic of an angina attack is pain.

Usually the pain is distinctive and feels like a pressing or squeezing sensation in the chest. Sometimes it eludes easy identification. As a rule, however, the discomfort is felt behind the breastbone, occasionally spreading to the arms, shoulders, neck, and jaw. Not all chest pain is angina; in some cases it may simply be gas in the stomach.

Angina Pectoralis

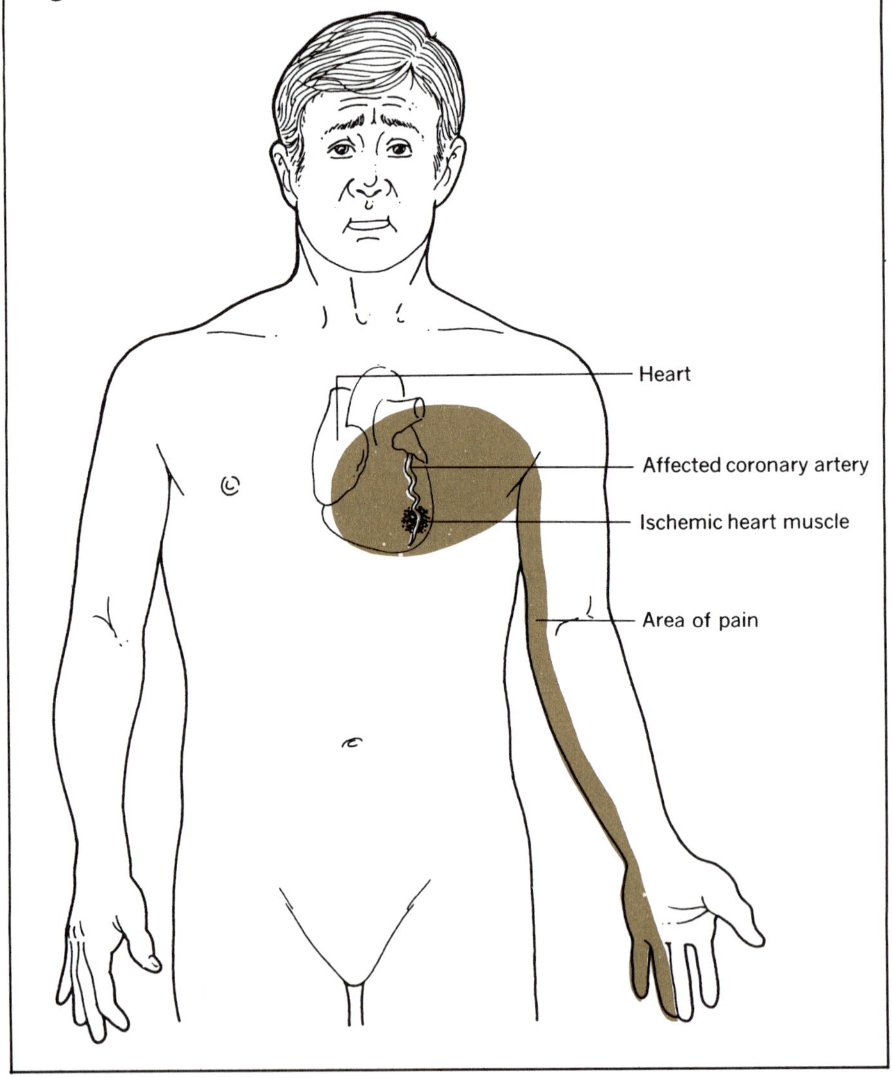

Treatment

It is important to note that angina pectoris is not a heart attack. It is a symptom, not a disorder. In most cases it is the result of arteriosclerosis, and thus recommendations for reducing the risk of arteriosclerosis also apply to angina. In addition, treatment may involve avoiding overly taxing physical labors or emotional situations likely to induce discomfort. The medication most often prescribed for angina is *nitroglycerin*. It dilates small coronary blood vessels, allowing more blood to get through within minutes. Nitroglycerine pellets are not swallowed but are placed between the cheek and gum, where they are quickly absorbed by blood vessels there and sped to the heart, reducing pain within minutes. Nitroglycerin is also available in a sprayable form. Often anginal attacks can be headed off by taking the medication before activities that are likely to trigger an attack. Some people experience temporary, mild headaches as a side effect of taking nitroglycerin.

Drugs that have been found to relieve chronic angina include beta-blockers. Beta-blockers block the release of stressful hormones and decrease the heart's need for blood and oxygen by reducing its workload. They may cause shortness of breath. For that reason, physicians usually prescribe other medications for persons with asthma.

The first of the beta-blockers to come into use was *propranolol.* But more than ten other chemically related drugs may be prescribed; among them, atenolol, timolol, carteolol, carvedilol, metoprolol, nadolol, and pindolol. Physicians generally try to fit one of these drugs to the problems of the individual patient. There is some evidence that propranolol and nitroglycerin taken together may increase the effectiveness of the therapy.

Other drugs for chronic angina are the calcium channel blockers. They prevent coronary spasms, one cause of angina chest pains, by blocking the flow of calcium ions into the cells of the heart and blood vessels, thus dilating the arteries and increasing blood flow to the heart. The heart's demand for oxygen is lessened, and blood pressure is lowered. Some chemically different calcium channel blockers in use are verapamil, nifedipine, and diltiazem.

Angina does not mean a heart attack is inevitable. Many angina patients never have one. If angina begins to worsen, however, coronary bypass surgery or the insertion of a *coronary stent,* a device that helps keep the artery unblocked, may be necessary.

Heart Attack

Heart attack is the common term for *myocardial infarction,* or death of heart muscle, which is also described as *coronary occlusion* (total closure of the coronary artery).

A heart attack is not a stationary, one-time episode. It is a process that usually evolves over four to six hours. As time elapses, more of the heart tissue is deprived of blood and deteriorates or dies.

Although heart attacks can occur at any age, the frequency of heart attacks builds rapidly between the ages of 30 and 55. In this age group, men experience heart attacks about 4 times as often as do women. However, nearly half of all deaths among women age 50 and older are due to some form of cardiovascular disease. The decline of estrogen levels after menopause is thought to increase women's risk of heart attacks. By the age of 65, women are about as likely as men to experience heart attacks.

Symptoms

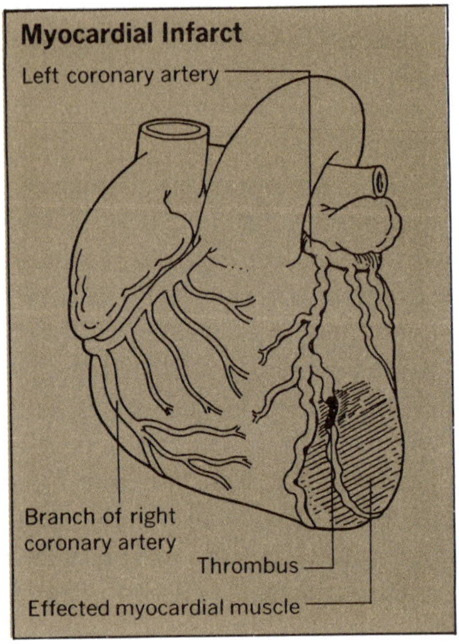

Sometimes the symptoms are so vague or indistinct that the victim may not know he has had a heart attack. Often a routine electrocardiogram turns up an abnormality indicative of an *infarct,* or injured area; thus the importance of periodic checkups. Special blood tests can also detect an elevation in the number of white blood cells or a rise in the enzyme content, resulting from leakage when heart cells are injured.

Most heart attacks, however, have well-recognized signs and symptoms. The most common are:

- A squeezing pain or feeling of pressure or fullness in the center of the chest that lasts for more than a few minutes
- An intense pain that extends beyond the chest to the shoulder, back, or either arm, or that radiates up the neck into the teeth and jaw
- Abnormal perspiring
- Sudden, intense shortness of breath
- Nausea or vomiting (because of these symptoms, an attack is sometimes mistaken for indigestion; usually, coronary pains are more severe)
- Occasionally, lightheadedness or fainting.

Treatment

Knowing the warning signals and taking the proper steps may make the difference between life and death. Call a physician or get to a hospital as soon as possible. Time is crucial. Most deaths occur in the initial hours after attack. About 50 percent, for example, die within 3 or 4 hours after onset of a major heart attack.

Often, death is not due to any widespread damage to the heart muscle, but rather to an irregularity in the heart's electrical system that causes a disruption in the signals that initiate heart muscle contraction. The results of these out-of-kilter rhythms, or *arrhythmias,* include complete heart stoppage or cardiac arrest, and are often reversible with prompt treatment.

For a patient whose heart attack is

the result of a blood clot (thrombus), the administration of clot-dissolving drugs limits the extent of damage to the heart and increases the survival rate. Other drugs used to treat the heart include antiarrhythmics, which restore a regular beat to an irregularly beating heart, and vasopressors or inotropic agents that stimulate the heart and enhance heart function. Among the many cardiostimulants, or inotropic drugs, is a large group called partial beta 1 agonists that accelerate the rehabilitation process and increase exercise tolerance.

Of two other classes of therapeutic drugs, calcium and beta channel blockers are used to slow the heart rate, while angiotensin converting enzyme (ACE) inhibitors increase blood flow to the kidneys. The ACE inhibitors also block an enzyme that raises blood pressure. Among the diuretics are Dyazide and furosemide, marketed as Lasix. Both help to prevent fluid accumulation in the lungs.

Because most heart attacks are the result of reduced blood flow due to clots or buildup of deposits on arterial walls, following a heart attack the problem arteries must be identified. This is done in a procedure called *coronary arteriography* (cardiac catheterization), where blocked arteries are identified by X-ray "movies" taken of an injected opaque dye. Another technique, magnetic resonance imaging (MRI), uses magnetic forces to identify problems in specific areas of the heart and its arteries.

Once clogged arteries are identified, they must be cleared. The procedures that clear arterial blockages begin with the pushing of a catheter through an artery in the leg or arm and into a coronary artery that has been narrowed by the buildup of plaque, which cuts off the flow of blood.

In one common procedure, *balloon angioplasty,* a balloon attached to a catheter is maneuvered to the site of arterial blockage and then inflated. The inflation forces open the artery by crushing the plaque against the arterial walls. The balloon and catheter are then removed.

Another procedure, atherectomy, removes the blockage. After one catheter is guided through the artery to the obstruction, a second catheter —equipped with a cutting tool—is guided through the first. The tool is then used to remove the blockage.

In about a third of the cases treated using these techniques, the plaque returns within six months. One solution to this problem, called re-stenosis, is the use of a stent—a small, tubular structure. After an angioplasty or atherectomy, a catheter is used to guide the stent into place at the site of the blockage. Lattice-like in structure, the stent can be expanded to press against the artererial wall once it is in place. It remains there permanently, keeping the artery open. Some stents are coated with drugs and are more effective, but they are also much more expensive. For this reason, both types of stents are in use.

In cases where the blocked section of the artery is too long or difficult to reach, coronary artery bypass surgery must be performed.

Coronary Care Units

Special hospital centers called coronary care units (CCUs) have been created to provide for heart attack victims. Headed by a cardiologist and staffed by highly trained nurses, the CCU provides around-the-clock electronic devices that keep watch over each patient's vital functions, particularly the heart's electrical activity. The critical period is the first 72 hours, when up to 90 percent of heart attack patients experience some type of electrical disturbance or *arrhythmia* (irregular heartbeat).

Patient rooms in the CCU are designed to ensure privacy and a tranquil, cheerful environment. Rooms may be separated from one another by curtains or partial or full walls.

Each patient is connected via electrodes attached to the skin to a heart monitor, which records the rhythm and rate of the heartbeat and the blood pressure. An alarm system notifies the nurse when a major change is taking place in the patient's condition.

Other CCU equipment includes defibrillators for treatment of the condition called ventricular fibrillation (see section on arrhythmias), electroshock equipment, intravenous pacemakers, and a crash cart stocked with such items as the drugs needed for emergency cardiac care (ECC) and endotracheal tubes.

The advent of coronary care has produced striking results. Where in use, these units have reduced heart attack deaths among hospitalized patients up to 30 percent. If all heart victims surviving at least a few hours received such care, more than 50,000 lives could be saved annually.

Emergency Care

Many heart attack victims never reach the hospital. About one-third die before they receive medical care. Evidence suggests that many of these sudden deaths result from ventricular fibrillation or cardiac arrest—reversible disturbances when treated immediately. If the patient is alive two hours after an attack the prognosis for recovery generally is good.

These considerations led to the concept of mobile coronary care units that bring the advanced techniques of heart resuscitation to the victims. Originated in 1966 in Belfast, Northern Ireland, mobile coronary care units, or emergency medical services (EMS), are specially equipped ambulances, with medical emergency personnel onboard, that are ready to race with on-the-spot aid to heart attack patients. Their use has significantly reduced mortality among heart attack patients. Typically, medical emergency personnel carry oxygen; heart medication, such as nitroglycerin; drugs, such as morphine for pain relief; and defibrillators to restart the heart if it stops beating.

An emergency technique called *cardiopulmonary resuscitation* (CPR), has also reduced out-of-hospital heart attack mortality figures. Used in conjunction with mouth-to-mouth resuscitation, CPR is an emergency procedure for treating cardiac arrest. The lower part of the breastbone is compressed rhythmically to keep oxygenated blood flowing to the brain until appropriate medical treatment can be applied to restore normal heart action. Often, CPR alone is enough to restart the heart. Training for the technique is widely available at hospitals or local branches of the Red Cross. Regular refresher courses are important, however, because improper use of the technique could fracture a rib or rupture a weakened heart muscle if too much pressure is applied.

Coronary Artery Bypass Surgery

In situations in which coronary artery blockage is severe, or when a patient's heart disease does not respond to medications, coronary artery bypass surgery may be appropriate. If the patient has had a heart attack, the heart should be given time to recover before bypass surgery is performed. Coronary artery bypass surgery involves removing a short length of vein from the leg and using it to create a route for blood to go around (bypass) severely blocked coronary arteries.

It is often preferable to use either of the two (or both) internal mammary arteries for the bypass instead of a leg vein. One problem with using a leg vein is that the vein tends to develop blockages similar to those in the arteries it was intended to bypass. The mammary arteries are more resistant to the buildup of atherosclerosis.

Although coronary artery bypass surgery relieves debilitating angina or reduces the risk from severely blocked arteries by restoring adequate blood flow to the heart, it does not cure the underlying disease—atherosclerosis. The patient must take care to follow the recommended dietary and lifestyle changes for reducing atherosclerosis.

Heart Surgery

Heart surgery can correct congenital defects, repair heart valves damaged by infection, bypass diseased arteries by means of a coronary bypass, correct arrhythmias with the implantation of a pacemaker, and even replace the heart (heart transplantation).

In some heart surgeries, such as coronary bypass, a heart-lung machine is used to keep blood and oxygen flowing to the body while the heart and lungs are stopped. Other, less invasive, types of heart procedures, such as angioplasty, do not require the use of a heart-lung machine.

In *stenosis,* in which one of the major valves of the heart is obstructed or in *regurgitation,* in which the valve does not close properly, surgical valve repair or replacement may be performed. *Valvoplasty,* a nonsurgical procedure, may also be used to widen a constricted valve opening.

A heart transplant may be required when such diseases of the heart as *cardiomyopathy* (heart muscle disease), *myocarditis* (inflammation of the myocardium), and *pericarditis* (inflammation of the sac surrounding the heart) do not respond to lifestyle changes or medication.

Heart transplantation has been performed with increasing success for more than 20 years. The best candidates for transplantation are psychologically stable, otherwise healthy individuals under age 60. About 80 percent of transplant patients survive for at least a year. Some have lived for more than a decade.

Two problems associated with heart transplantation are the acquisition and storing of donor hearts and overcoming the body's rejection response to transplants. The former means a long waiting list for potential transplant patients. Immunosuppressive drugs help control the latter. For more information, see "Heart Surgery" in Ch. 20, *Surgery*. See also "Organ Transplants" in Ch. 20., *Surgery*.

Recuperation

Cardiac rehabilitation is crucial not only for heart-attack patients, but also for those who have had coronary artery bypass surgery, angioplasty, insertion of a stent, valve replacements, and congestive heart failure, among others. In this section, the recuperation of heart-attack patients will be discussed.

In the first phase of recovery, most heart-attack patients may, within the first day or two after an attack, gradually participate in daily activity. For example, by the second day, patients may bathe their upper body and are encouraged to move from the bed to a chair for one to two hours per day. By the fourth day, most may shower and dress themselves and take supervised walks of 100 to 600 feet several times a day. By the third to seventh day, patients may walk up to 600 feet three times a day and can begin supervised stair climbing. Most heart-attack patients who do not have other complications are commonly discharged from the hospital 5 or 6 days after admission.

The second phase of recovery generally covers a 2- to 12-week period and begins after the patient goes home from the hospital. During this period, patients continue rehabilitation under supervision, usually at a medical center. Because the needs of a person who has had a mild heart attack are different from one who has had an extensive bypass operation, a rehabilitation program must be tailored to the individual. Strategies for rehabilitation combining elements of lifestyle modification that include diet, exercise, and other factors are usually required. By the third phase of recovery (6 to 12 weeks after discharge), patients have usually developed their own exercise routines and are making progress controlling risk factors such as smoking, obesity, or high blood pressure. Sometimes medication is prescribed for the first few weeks or months after a heart attack. Such medications might include warfarin, which is a blood-thinner, amiodarone, to treat arrhythmias, diuretics, and beta-blockers.

After rehabilitation, most heart-attack patients are able to regain their independence and can return to their jobs. The level of activity that the patient ultimately can resume is something that the patient and physician must determine together.

Before or after a heart attack victim returns to work and more normal life habits, physicians may want to know how he or she will react to stresses, medicines, and other factors and conditions. This is done by using ambulatory electrocardiographic monitoring, or *Holter monitoring,* which delivers electrocardiographic readings for 24 to 48 hours or longer while the patient goes about his or her normal activities. Electrodes are placed on the chest and taped to the body. The electrodes connect with a tape recorder that makes electrocardiograms. Completely portable because of its light weight, the monitor is carried in a pocket or a strap hung over the patient's shoulder.

The monitor's recordings are especially useful in diagnosing arrhythmias, which may occur at unpredictable times. Patients using the ambulatory monitor are generally asked to supplement the cardiographic record by keeping notes on their activities. These notes show the physician the activities in which the patient was engaged from hour to hour during the day. The notes may be matched up with the EKG to show what stresses accompanied particular activities. Some monitors have a special band on which the patient can record oral reports of his or her activities. The monitor's tape record and the patient's written or dictated notes help the physician give more specific instructions to the patient regarding the activities that will facilitate recovery.

Arrhythmias

A disturbance in the rhythm of the heart is termed *arrhythmia* and can range from a mild "skipped beat" to a life-threatening failure to pump. The latter is called *ventricular fibrillation,* and it is the most common cause of *cardiac arrest,*, in which the heart suddenly stops beating. Death can follow in minutes unless medical help is provided immediately. People who have had a heart attack or who are elderly are at a much higher risk of developing a life-threatening arrhythmia.

In ventricular fibrillation, the heart's electrical activity becomes disordered. As a result, the heart's lower (pumping) chambers rapidly contract in an unsynchronized way. In effect, the ventricles flutter rather than beat, and the heart pumps little or no blood. Symptoms may include palpitations, lightheadedness, chest discomfort, shortness of breath, or loss of consciousness. If a more normal rhythm is not restored within three to five minutes, the patient will suffer brain and heart damage and will die.

Treatment involves the use of an instrument called a *defibrillator.* The most common type of defibrillator is a portable, external device with electric plates that are applied to the chest.

The device sends a massive jolt of electricity into the heart muscle to get the heart back on the right tempo.

Another kind of defibrillator can be implanted in the chest. The implantable cardioverter-defibrillator (ICD) is inserted surgically, just as a pacemaker is. It constantly monitors heart rhythm, and when it senses that the rhythm is abnormal, it gives the heart a small shock to return the rhythm to normal.

There are many different types of arrhythmias. Many of them are harmless and occur in people who do not have underlying heart disease. Such arrhythmias, called "premature beats," can be caused by stress, caffeine, tobacco, alcohol, or cold medicines. Other arrhythmias are caused by heart disease. In most such cases, the heart disease, not the arrhythmia, poses the greater risk to the patient.

In a small number of people with serious symptoms, however, the arrhythmias themselves can be dangerous. These arrhythmias require medical treatment to keep the heartbeat regular. For example, some people have a very slow heartbeat (bradycardia), which causes them to feel lightheaded or faint. If not treated, the heart may stop beating and the person could die.

Less serious arrhythmias than ventricular fibrillation include *atrial flutter* (where the atria contract too often), *atrial fibrillation* (where they contract in an ineffective and uncoordinated manner), and *paroxysmal atrial tachycardia* (where the heart rate may race at between 140 and 240 beats per minute for minutes or even days). Other arrhythmias are caused by a malfunctioning mitral valve of the heart or the sinus node (the area of the heart that sends electrical signals to the chambers, controlling the beat; i.e., the heart's pacemaker).

Arrhythmias that are associated with heart disease or heart attacks can be controlled with lifestyle changes and medications designed to pace the heart.

Hypertension

Hypertension is the most common cardiovascular disease, affecting more than 45 million Americans, with more than half having some degree of heart involvement. A little more than 60,000 deaths are directly attributable to hypertension and hypertensive heart disease.

Hypertension, or elevated blood pressure, results from a persistent tightening of the body's very small arterial branches, the *arterioles*. This clenching increases the resistance to blood flow and sends the blood pressure up, just as screwing down the nozzle on a hose builds up pressure in the line. The heart must now work harder to force blood through. Over a period of time, the stepped-up pumping effort may cause the heart muscle to thicken and enlarge. Eventually, the overworked circulatory system may break down, with resultant failure of the heart or kidneys, or the onset of stroke. The constant hammering of blood under high pressure on the walls of the arteries causes them to thicken, making them less flexible (a condition called arteriosclerosis) and also accelerates the development of atherosclerosis and heart attacks.

How Blood Pressure is Measured

Blood pressure is measured in millimeters of mercury with an instrument called *sphygmomanometer.* The device consists of an inflatable cuff attached to a mercury meter. The physician wraps the cuff around the arm and inflates it with air from a squeeze-bulb. This drives the mercury column up toward the top of the gauge while shutting off blood flow through the brachial artery in the arm. With a stethoscope placed just below the cuff, the physician releases the air and listens for the first thudding sounds that signal the return of blood flow as the blood pressure on the wall of the artery equals the air pressure in the cuff. He records this mercury meter reading. This number represents the *systolic* pressure, the force developed by the heart when it contracts.

By continuing to let air out, the physician reaches a point where he can no longer hear the pulsing sounds of flowing blood. He marks the gauge reading as the *diastolic* pressure, the pressure on the artery when the heart is relaxing between beats. Thus, two numbers are used to record blood pressure: the systolic followed by the diastolic.

Normal systolic pressure for most adults is between 100 and 120, and diastolic between 60 and 80. Many factors, such as age and sex, account for the wide variations in normal readings from individual to individual. Systolic blood pressure, for example, tends to increase with age.

Normally, blood pressure goes up during periods of excitement and physical labor. Hypertension is the diagnosis when repeated measurements show a persistent elevated pressure of 140 or higher for systolic and 90 or more for diastolic.

In addition to the sphygmomanometer reading in the examination for high blood pressure, the physician shines a bright light in the patient's eyes so that he can look at the blood vessels in the retina, the only blood vessels that are readily observable. Any damage there resulting from hypertension is usually a good index of the severity of the disease and its effects elsewhere in the body.

The physician may also perform some tests of kidney function to ascertain whether the hypertension is of the essential or secondary kind, and whether there has been any damage to the kidneys.

Causes

The vast majority of all hypertension cases are classified as *essential.* This simply means that no single cause can be defined. Rather, blood pressure may be elevated for a number of reasons—none of which has yet been firmly implicated—operating in some complex interplay.

In fact, less than one person in 20 with hypertension has a specific disease causing their high blood pressure. If a cause can be determined, the high blood pressure is classified as *secondary.* Some of the causes of secondary hypertension include certain medications, such as birth control pills or decongestants; kidney disease; adrenal disease; thyroid disease, abnormal blood vessels; and use of illegal drugs, such as cocaine or amphetamines.

In addition, certain risk factors are related to hypertension. Although not in themselves causes of the condition, they can be contributing factors. Risk factors over which the patient has no control are age, race, gender, and family history. Risk factors that can be controlled or managed include obesity; inactivity; cigarette smoking; a high-salt diet; too little potassium; excessive alcohol consumption; and high levels of stress.

In addition, some chronic conditions, such as diabetes and high blood cholesterol levels, can increase the risk of developing hypertension.

Symptoms

Essential hypertension usually first occurs when a person is in his or her thirties. In the early stages, one may pass through a transitional or prehypertensive phase lasting a few years in which blood pressure rises above normal only occasionally, and then more and more often until finally it remains at these elevated levels.

Symptoms, if they exist at all, are likely to be something as nonspecific as headaches, dizziness, or nausea. As a result, without a physical examination to reveal its presence, a person may have the disease for years without being aware of it. That can be dangerous, because the longer hypertension is left untreated, the greater the likelihood that the heart will be affected.

About 10 percent of causes fall under the *secondary hypertension* classification because they arise as a consequence of another known disorder. Curing the underlying disorder also cures the hypertension. Usually it is brought on by an obstruction of normal blood flow to the kidney because of atherosclerotic deposits in one or both of its major supply lines, the renal arteries. Adrenal gland problems such as Cushing's Syndrome or a tumor of the adrenal gland can also cause hypertension. Many patients can be cured or substantially improved through surgery.

Treatment

Essential hypertension cannot be cured, but it can be treated. The best initial treatment strategy for controlling or reducing it is modification of lifestyle. Lifestyle modifications should include eating a nutritionally balanced diet; reducing sodium intake (if the patient is sodium-sensitive); limiting alcohol and caffeine; not smoking; controlling weight; getting regular exercise; and managing stress. Such self-care measures may make drug therapy unnecessary. But if they do not significantly improve blood pressure within three to six months, medication may be required. A wide variety of antihypertensive drugs are available, and almost anyone with hypertension can control it with an individually tailored drug regimen.

Diuretics are often the first drugs prescribed. They work by helping the kidneys eliminate salt and water, which decreases the amount of fluid throughout the body, thereby decreasing blood pressure. Adrenergic blockers, the most common of which are beta-blockers, are another type of antihypertensive. These drugs lower blood pressure by blocking the effects of the sympathetic nervous system. Other drugs include angiotensin converting enzyme inhibitors, calcium antagonists, and direct vasodilators. Direct vasodilators are usually added as a second medication when another drug alone is not effective. For malignant hypertension, which requires rapid lowering, drugs such as diazoxide and nitroprusside are usually administered intravenously.

Rheumatic Fever and Rheumatic Heart Disease

Rheumatic heart disease involves permanent damage to the heart muscle and heart valves caused by rheumatic fever. Rheumatic fever generally strikes children between the ages of 5 and 15. It is less common in the United States than it used to be, but a few outbreaks have occurred since the 1980's. Triggered by streptococcal attacks in childhood and adolescence, rheumatic fever may leave permanent heart scars. The heart valves are most often affected. Damage to the valves may not appear for 10 to 30 years after rheumatic fever.

Causes

The exact cause of rheumatic fever is still not entirely understood. Rheumatic fever is preceded by an invasion of bacteria belonging to the group A beta hemolytic streptococcus family. Many people develop a strep infection, such as strep throat, at some point in their lives. Most recover without any complications. But in about 3 percent of individuals, the strep infection produces rheumatic fever within a few weeks.

The invasion of strep sparks the production of protective agents called antibodies. For some reason, the antibodies attack not only the strep but also the body's own tissues—the very tissues they are called upon to protect. Researchers have suggested the possible reason, although all the evidence is not yet in. According to a widely held theory, the strep germ possesses constituents (*antigens*) that are similar in structure to components of normal, healthy cartilage and connective tissues—found abundantly in joints, tendons, and heart valves—in susceptible individuals. Failing to distinguish between them, the antibodies attack both. The result is rheumatic fever involving joint and valve inflammation and, perhaps, permanent scarring.

Symptoms

Rheumatic fever is not always easy to diagnose. No laboratory test can confirm rheumatic fever. Diagnosis is based on the presence of several criteria and symptoms, both major and minor.

Major:

- Fever
- Arthritis, which involves swelling or pain in one or more joints; usually, several joints are involved one after the other in migratory fashion
- Carditis or heart inflammation
- A raised, nonitching skin rash, which often disappears in 24 to 48 hours
- Chorea, which involves uncoordinated, jerky and involuntary motions of the arms, legs, or face, which result from rheumatic inflammation of brain tissue. These symptoms usually disappear within a few weeks or months
- Abdominal pain
- Hard lumps, under the skin and over the inflamed joints, usually indicating severe heart inflammation

Minor:

- Joint aches without inflammation
- Previous rheumatic fever or evidence of rheumatic heart disease
- Abnormal heartbeat on EKG
- Blood test indicating inflammation

Rheumatic fever does not always involve the heart; even when it does, permanent damage is not inevitable. Nor does the severity of the attack have any relationship to the development of rheumatic heart disease.

The real damage arises when heart valve tissue becomes inflamed, affecting the valve's ability to close properly. When the acute attack has passed and the inflammation finally subsides, the valves begin to heal, and scar tissue forms.

Scar tissue may cause portions of the affected valve leaflets to fuse together. (*Leaflets* are the flaps of the heart valves.) This restricts leaflet motion, impeding the full swing action and thereby blood flow through the valve. This condition is called valvular *stenosis*. The leaflets may become shrunken or deformed by healing tissue, causing *regurgitation* or backspill because the valve fails to close completely.

Both stenosis and regurgitation are often present. Most susceptible are the *mitral valve*, which regulates flow from the upper to the lower left chambers of the heart, and the *aortic valve*, the gateway between the left ventricle and the general circulation. Rarely attacked are the two valves in the right chambers.

Treatment

During the acute stages of rheumatic fever, the patient is given heavy doses of antibiotics to rid the body of all strep traces and aspirin to control swelling and fever. For severe heart inflammation, a corticosteroid, such as prednisone, can reduce inflammation. A strong risk of recurrence is associated with rheumatic fever; therefore, antibiotics may have to be taken for several years as a preventive measure.

The patient with valve damage can in many cases be treated medically, without the need for surgical intervention. He may, of course, have to desist from certain strenuous activities, but in all other ways he can lead a relatively normal life. Surgical relief or cure is available, however, for patients with severe damage or those who may, with age, develop progressive narrowing or leakage of the valves.

Surgery

Stenotic valves can be scraped clear of excess scar tissues, thereby returning the leaflets to more normal operation. In some cases individually scarred leaflets are replaced with synthetic substitutes. The correction of severe valvular regurgitation requires replacement of the entire valve with an artificial substitute, or, as some surgeons prefer, with a healthy valve taken from a human donor dying of other causes.

Diagnosis and Prevention

The development of antibiotics has made rheumatic fever preventable. These drugs can knock out the strep before the germs can set off the inflammatory defense network sequences, but early detection is necessary. Among the symptoms of strep are sudden onset of a sore throat with redness and swelling; high fever; swollen lymph nodes in the neck; and sometimes nausea and vomiting. Diagnosis is often made with a rapid test kit, which can check throat secretions for bacterial infections within minutes in the doctor's office. Alternatively, a throat culture may be done. A positive identification using a throat culture, which can take up to two days in a laboratory, calls for prompt treatment (usually an antibiotic) to kill the germs before the complications of rheumatic fever have a chance to set in.

Unfortunately, many strep infections may be mild enough to escape detection. The child may recover so quickly that the parents neglect to take the necessary precautions, but the insidious processes may still be going on in the apparently healthy child. This is a major reason why rheumatic fever is still with us, though in severe decline.

Heart Murmurs and Damaged Heart Valves

The prime sign that rheumatic heart disease has developed is a heart murmur—although a heart murmur does not always mean heart disease. The murmur may be only temporary, ceasing once the rheumatic fever attack subsides and the stretched and swollen valves return to normal. To complicate matters more, many heart murmurs are harmless. Such functional murmurs may appear in 30 to 50 percent of normal children at one time or another.

As many as three in five patients with rheumatic fever may develop murmurs characteristic of scarred valves—sounds of blood flowing through damaged valves that fail to open and close normally.

There is some encouraging evidence that rheumatic fever patients who escape heart damage the first time around will do so again should a repeat attack occur. On the other hand, those with damaged valves will probably sustain more damage with subsequent strep-initiated attacks.

Endocarditis

One of the additional bonuses of antibiotic therapy is that it has all but eliminated an invariably fatal complication to which rheumatic patients were especially vulnerable—an infection of the heart's lining, or *endocardium,* called *subacute bacterial endocarditis.* The scar tissue provides an excellent nesting site for bacteria to grow.

The germs are found in most everyone's mouth and usually invade the bloodstream after dental surgery. Fortunately, it is easy to prevent or cure because the germs offer little resistance to antibiotics. As a precaution, dentists usually give rheumatic fever patients larger doses of penicillin (or other antibiotics to those allergic to penicillin) before, during, and after dental work to prevent endocarditis from occurring.

Congenital Heart Disease

Congenital heart disease includes heart and major blood vessel deformities that exist at birth. In the United States, about 30,000 children are born with a heart defect each year.

Research is ongoing, but at least 35 types of congenital heart malformations have been identified. Most—including all of the 15 most common types—can be either corrected or alleviated by surgery. The defects result from a failure of the infant's heart to mature normally during development in the womb in the early part of pregnancy.

The term *blue baby* refers to an infant born with a heart impairment that prevents blood from getting enough oxygen, a condition known as *cyanosis.* Because blood low in oxygen is

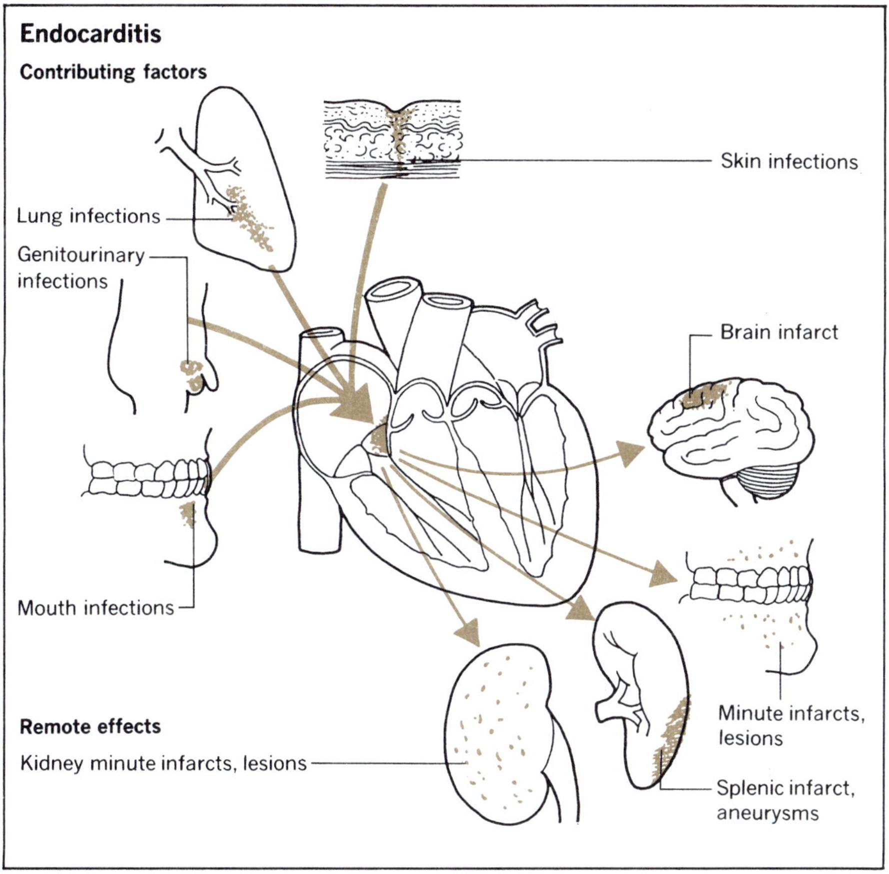

dark bluish red, it imparts a blue tinge to the skin and lips.

The cause of inborn heart abnormalities is not known in most cases. Some defects can be traced to maternal viral infection, such as German measles (rubella), during the first three months of pregnancy when the fetus' heart is growing rapidly. Certain drugs or, possibly, genetic mutations, are among other factors that are known or thought to be associated with such defects.

Heart abnormalities may come singly or in combination. There may, for example, be a hole in the walls separating the right and left heart chambers, or a narrowing of a valve or blood vessel that obstructs blood flow, or a transposition in major blood vessel connections—or there may be a combination of all of these.

Diagnosis

A reasonably complete diagnosis can often be made on the basis of a conventional physical examination, including visual inspection of the infant's general condition, blood pressure reading, chest X-ray, blood tests, Doppler echocardiogram, and electrocardiogram. A more complex diagnosis may require *cardiac catheterization.* In cardiac catheterization, a thin, flexible tube or catheter is inserted into an arm or leg vein. A dye or contrast material may be injected through the catheter into a blood vessel or chamber of the heart, enabling an X-ray motion picture to be recorded. While the physician watches with special X-ray equipment, the tube is advanced carefully through the vein until it reaches the heart chambers. Once there, it can provide information about the nature of the defect.

Advanced techniques known as computed axial tomography (CAT) scan, positron emission tomography (PET), and magnetic resonance imaging (MRI) may also be used. Both the CAT and the PET scanners require injection of a contrast fluid so that a "picture" can be taken. The CAT scanner takes X-ray images of "slices" of the patient's body with the aid of a computer. The PET scanner works on an electronic principle, with detectors located in a circle around the subject. Also computerized, MRI diagnoses by employing magnetic forces to "see" through bones, revealing such details as the differences between healthy and diseased tissues.

Treatment

From these tests, the cardiologist and a surgeon can decide for or against surgery. Depending on the severity of the disease, some conditions may require an immediate operation, even on days-old infants. Until recently, specialists often recommended waiting until the infant was older before surgery was undertaken. In a number of instances, however, the defect may not require surgery at all.

Open-heart surgery in infants with inborn heart defects carries a higher risk than does the same surgery in older children. Risks must be taken often, however, because about one-third will die in the first month if untreated, and more than half within the first year.

Refinements in surgical techniques and postoperative care have given surgeons the confidence to operate with remarkable success on infants who are merely hours old. Specially adapted miniature heart-lung machines may also chill the blood to produce *hypothermia,* or body cooling. This slows metabolism and reduced tissue oxygen needs so that the heart and brain can withstand short periods of interrupted blood flow. A good deal has been learned, too, about the delicate medical management required by infants during the surgical recovery period. All of these advances account for the dramatic increases in survival for infants who would have been given up for lost only a couple of decades ago.

Congestive Heart Failure

Heart failure usually occurs as a result of underlying heart diseases that have damaged or weakened the heart, causing it to work harder. Contributing cardiac conditions may include coronary artery disease or hypertension. The heart, however, has not stopped beating. It continues to contract, but it lacks the strength to keep blood circulating normally throughout the body. Physicians sometimes refer to the condition as cardiac insufficiency.

When the heart fails to pump efficiently, the flow slows down, causing blood returning to the heart through the veins to back up. Some of the fluid in the blood is forced out through the thin walls of small blood vessels into surrounding tissues. Here the fluid pools, or congests.

The result may be swelling, or *edema,* which can occur in many parts of the body but most commonly occurs in the legs and ankles. Fluids sometimes collect in the lungs, interfering with breathing and making the person short of breath. Heart failure also causes the kidneys to retain excess sodium and water, adding to the edema.

Congestive Heart Failure

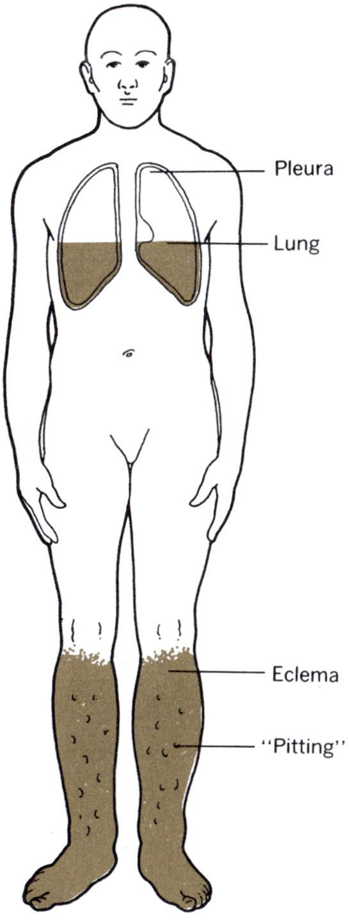

Treatment

Treatment usually includes a combination of rest, drugs, diet, and restricted daily activity. The main drugs used are the angiotensin-converting enzyme (ACE) inhibitors, which lower blood pressure and decrease the heart's workload. *Digitalis,* in one of its many forms, is often prescribed to strengthen the action of the heart muscle. It also slows a rapid heartbeat, and promotes excretion of excess fluids. Dosage varies from person to person. When edema is present, diuretics are prescribed to speed the elimina-

Pacemaker Implantation

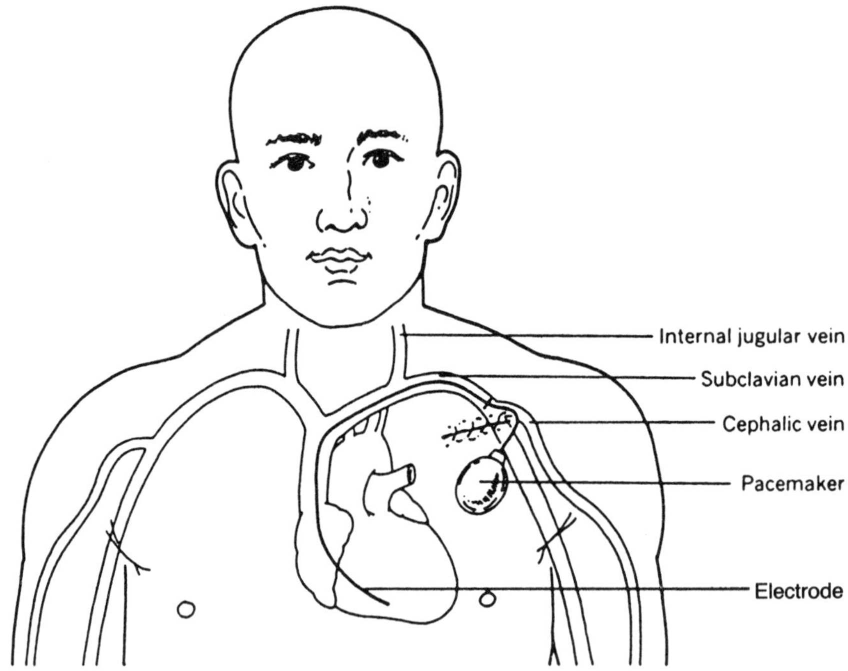

tion of excess salt and water. A sodium-restricted diet is generally necessary to reduce or prevent edema. Patients may also need bed rest for awhile, with a gradual return to slower-paced activity.

Most important, however, is adequate treatment of the underlying disease that led to heart failure in the first place.

Heart Block

Sometimes the scars resulting from rheumatic fever, heart attack, or surgical repair of the heart may damage the electrical network in a way that blocks normal transmission of the signal between the upper and lower chambers. The disruption, called *atrioventricular block,* manifests in three degrees of intensity. First degree heart block is detectable only with an EKG and is merely a short delay in the normal transmission. Second degree heart block shows up as an irregular pulse—some of the beats are blocked. In third degree heart block, none of the beats reach the lower chambers; they begin beating on their own, but at a much slower rate, meaning that blood flow, especially to the brain, is seriously affected. Blackouts and convulsions may ensue.

For first degree heart block and many forms of second degree, nervous system stimulants may be used to keep the heart from lagging. For third degree heart block and some forms of second degree, however, drugs are not enough. An artificial electronic pacemaker, implanted in the body and connected to the heart by wires, has been successful for many people with this condition. The pacemaker fires electrical shocks into the ventricle wall to make it beat at the proper rate. Most devices are powered by tiny lithium batteries that last 7 to 8 years, on average.

11

Diseases of the Digestive System

Digestive Functions and Organs

The function of the digestive system is to accept food and water through the mouth, to break down the food's chemical structure so that its nutrients can be absorbed into the body, a process called *digestion,* and to expel undigested particles. This process takes place as the food passes through the entire *alimentary tract.* This tract, also called the *gastrointestinal tract,* is a long, hollow passageway that begins at the mouth and continues on through the esophagus, the stomach, the small intestine, the large intestine, the rectum, and the anus. The salivary glands, the stomach glands, the liver, the gallbladder, and the pancreas release substances into the gastrointestinal tract that help the digestion of various food substances.

Digestion

Digestion begins in the mouth where food is shredded by chewing and mixed with saliva, which helps break down starch into sugars and lubricates the food so that it can be swallowed easily. The food then enters the *esophagus,* a muscular tube that forcibly squeezes the food down toward the stomach, past the *cardiac sphincter,* a ring of muscle at the entrance of the stomach that opens to allow food into the stomach.

The stomach acts as a reservoir for food, churns the food, mixes it with gastric juices, and gradually releases the food into the small intestine. Some water, alcohol, and glucose are absorbed directly through the stomach into the bloodstream. Enzymes secreted by the stomach help break down proteins and fats into simpler substances. Hydrochloric acid secreted by the stomach kills bacteria and prepares some minerals for absorption in the small intestine. Some food may leave the stomach one minute after it enters, while other parts of a meal may remain in the stomach for as long as five hours.

The food passes from the stomach to the first section of the small intestine, the *duodenum,* where it is acted on by pancreatic enzymes that help break down fats, starches, proteins,

The Digestive System

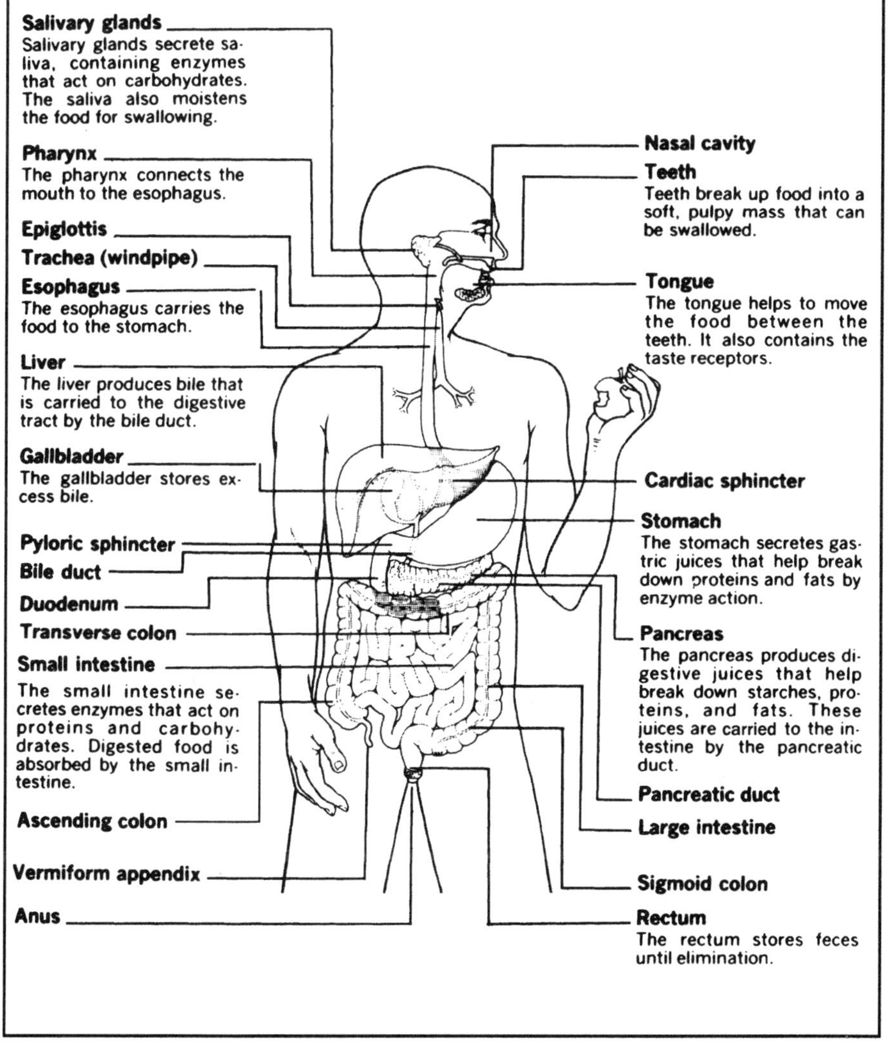

and other substances. While the food is in the duodenum it is also digested by *bile,* which is produced by the liver and stored in the gallbladder. During a meal, the gallbladder discharges its bile into the duodenum. The bile promotes the absorption of fats and vitamins.

The semidigested food is squeezed down the entire length of the intestines by a wavelike motion of the intestinal muscles called *peristalsis.* Digestion is largely completed as the food passes through 20 feet of small intestine, which absorbs the digested food substances and water and passes them into the bloodstream. The food nutrients are distributed by the bloodstream throughout the body and used by the body cells.

Those parts of the food that are indigestible, such as the skins of fruits, pass into the large intestine, or *colon,* along with bacteria, bile, some minerals, various cells, and mucus. This combination of substances makes up the *feces,* which are stored in the colon until *defecation.* Some water and salts in the feces are absorbed through the walls of the colon into the bloodstream. This conserves the body's fluids and dries the feces. The formation of a semisolid fecal mass helps precipitate defecation.

The Passage of Food through the Alimentary Canal

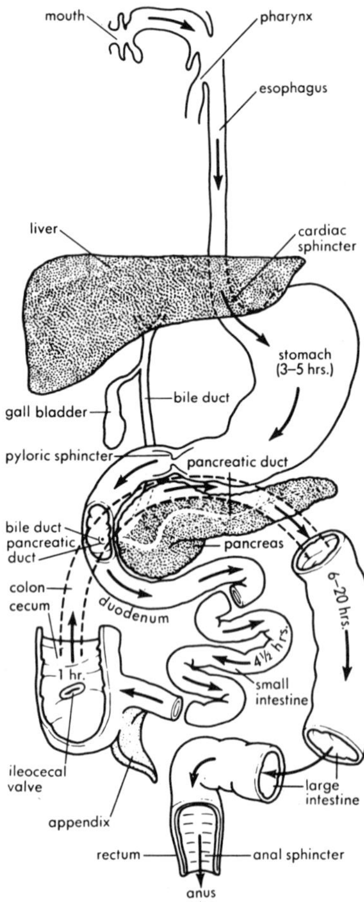

This drawing indicates the duration of each digestive process. Food enters the mouth and is passed through the pharynx and esophagus into the stomach, where it is partly digested. The small intestine completes digestion and absorbs digested food. The large intestine absorbs excess water. Indigestible residue collects in the rectum for later disposal.

The Oral Cavity

The Salivary Glands

The smell of food triggers the salivary glands to pour saliva into the mouth; that is what is meant by "mouth-watering" odors. During a meal, saliva is released into the mouth to soften the food as it is chewed.

Stones

Stones will sometimes form in the salivary glands or ducts, blocking the ducts and preventing the free flow of saliva into the mouth. After a meal, the swollen saliva-filled glands and ducts slowly empty. The swelling may sometimes be complicated by infection. Surgical removal of the stones is the usual treatment; sometimes the entire gland is removed.

Tumors

Tumors sometimes invade the salivary gland. An enlarged gland may press on the auditory canal and cause deafness, or it may result in stiffness of the jaw and mild facial palsy. The tumors can grow large enough to be felt by the fingers, and surgery is required to remove them.

Inflammation of the Parotid Glands

Inflammation of the upper (*parotid*) salivary glands may be caused by an infection in the oral cavity, by liver disease, or by malnutrition.

Mumps

One of the commonest inflammations of the salivary glands, called *mumps,* occurs especially in children. It is a highly contagious viral disease characterized by inflammation and swelling of one or both parotid salivary glands, and can have serious complications in adults. See "Alphabetic Guide to Child Care" in Ch. 2, *The First Dozen Years,* for a fuller discussion of mumps.

Bad Breath (Halitosis)

Poor oral hygiene is the principal cause of offensive mouth odor, or *halitosis.* It can result from oral tumors, abscesses from decaying teeth, and gum disease or infection. The foul smell is primarily a result of cell decay, and the odors are characteristic of the growth of some microorganisms.

When halitosis results from poor oral sanitation, the treatment is obvious—regular daily tooth brushing and the use of an antiseptic mouthwash. If the halitosis is because of disease of the oral cavity, alimentary tract, or respiratory system, the cure will depend on eradicating the primary cause.

Nonmalignant Lesions

The oral cavity is prone to invasion by several types of microorganisms that cause nonmalignant lesions. The most prominent follow.

Canker Sores

These are of unknown origin and show up as single or multiple small sores near the molar teeth, inside the lips, or in the lining of the mouth. They can be painful but usually heal in a few days.

Fungus Infections

Thrush is the most common oral fungus infection and appears as white round patches inside the cheeks of infants, small children, and sometimes adults. The lesions may involve the entire mouth, tongue, and pharynx. In advanced stages the lesions turn yellow. Malnutrition, especially lack of adequate vitamin B, is the principal cause. Thrush is also one of the opportunistic infections commonly found in persons with AIDS. See also "AIDS" in Ch. 19, *Other Diseases of Major Importance.* Fungus growth may be aided by the use of antibiotics, which kill normal oral bacteria and permit fungi to flourish.

Tooth Decay and Vitamin Deficiencies

Lack of adequate vitamins in the daily diet is responsible for some types of lesions in the oral cavity. Insufficient vitamin A in children under five may be the cause of malformation in the crown, dentin, and enamel of the teeth. Lack of adequate vitamin C results in bleeding gums. Vitamin D insufficiency may lead to slow tooth development.

An inadequate and improper diet supports tooth decay, which in turn may be complicated by ulcers in the gums and abscesses in the roots of the decaying teeth. A diet with an adequate supply of the deficient vitamins will cause the symptoms to disappear. Infections, abscesses, cysts, or tumors in the mouth require the attention of a physician, dentist, or dental surgeon. See Ch. 22, *The Teeth and Gums.*

Chancres

These are primary syphilis lesions, which commonly develop at the lips and tongue. They appear as small, eroding red ulcers that exude yellow matter. They can invade the mouth, tonsils, and pharynx. Penicillin therapy is usually required.

The Esophagus

Varices

Varices (singular: *varix*) are enlarged and congested veins that appear in the esophagus because of increased blood pressure to the liver in patients with liver cirrhosis. This disease is most common in chronic alcoholics. Esophageal varices can be complicated by erosion of the mucous lining of the esophagus as a result of inflammation or vomiting. This causes hemorrhaging of the thin-walled veins, which can be fatal.

Bleeding esophageal varices may require hospitalization, immediate blood transfusions, and surgery.

Hiatus Hernia

The lower end of the esophagus or part of the stomach can sometimes protrude through the diaphragm. This *hiatus hernia,* sometimes referred to as a *diaphragmatic hernia,* can be a result of congenital malformation; in adults, the principal cause is weakness of the muscles around the opening of the esophagus leading into the stomach.

In individuals who are obese and who have large stomachs, the stomach contents may be forced back into the lower esophagus, causing this area to herniate. Other causes include stooping, bending, or kneeling, which increases pressure in the stomach. Pregnancy may increase abdominal pressure in the same manner as obesity.

Typical symptoms are vomiting when the stomach is full, heartburn with pain spreading to the ears, neck, and arms, swallowing difficulty with the food sometimes sticking in the esophagus, and a swollen abdomen. The vomiting may occur at night, with relief obtained by getting up and walking about for a few minutes. Belching will relieve the distension, and *antacids* (acid neutralizers) may be prescribed to counter gastric hyperacidity.

Conservative treatment involves

Hernia

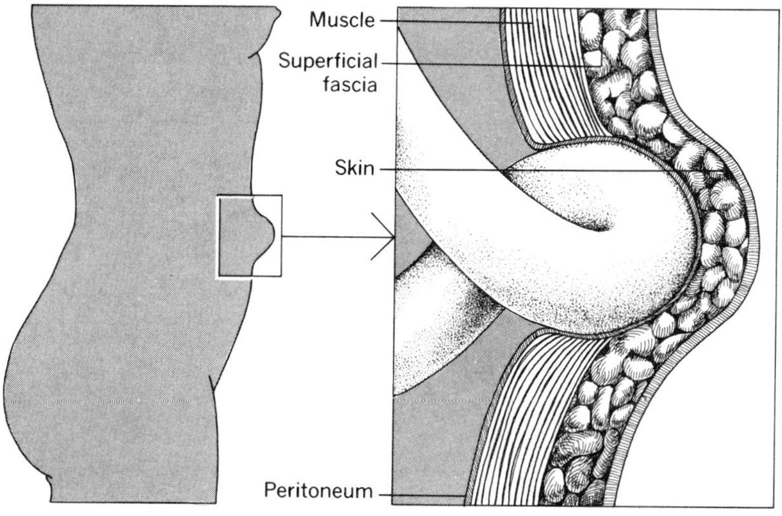

Hernias result when a part of the intestine pushes through layers of muscle against the body's layers of skin.

eating small portions at frequent intervals. Dieting and a reduction in weight cause the symptoms to disappear. When the symptoms are due to pregnancy, they disappear after delivery. When medical management is not successful, surgical repair of the hernia is necessary. See also "Hernias" later in this chapter.

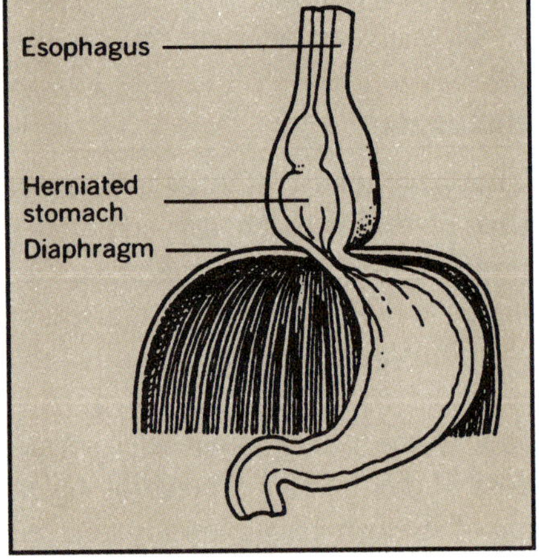

Achalasia

Achalasia is abnormal dilation of the lower esophagus caused by failure of the cardiac sphincter to relax and allow food to enter the stomach. Food collects in the esophagus and does not flow into the stomach. The patient feels as though the food is sticking in the middle of his chest wall. Small amounts of food may eventually pass into the stomach, and the mild pain or discomfort disappears.

If the condition persists, the pain may increase to become a continuous burning sensation at each meal, due to inflammation of the esophagus by accumulated food. If the patient lies down, some of this esophageal content will regurgitate and enter the pharynx. If the vomitus gets into the lungs, the end result may be *aspiration pneumonia,* a form of pneumonia caused by inhaling particles of foreign matter.

The disease is difficult to control, and the condition tends to return, so that surgery is often used to create a permanent opening between the esophagus and stomach.

Swallowing Difficulty

Difficulty in swallowing is called *dysphagia,* which should not be confused with *dysphasia,* a speech impairment. Dysphagia may be caused by lesions in the mouth and tongue, acute inflammatory conditions in the oral cavity and pharynx (mumps, tonsillitis, laryngitis, pharyngitis), lesions, cancers, or foreign bodies in the esophagus. Strictures in the esophagus—from esophageal ulcers or from swallowing corrosive liquids—will also impair swallowing.

Stomach and Intestines

Indigestion (Dyspepsia)

There are times when the gastrointestinal tract fails to carry out its normal digestive function. The resulting indigestion, or *dyspepsia,* generates a variety of symptoms, such as heartburn, nausea, pain in the upper abdomen, gases in the stomach (*flatulence*), belching, and a feeling of fullness after eating.

Indigestion can be caused by ulcers of the stomach or duodenum and by excessive or too rapid eating or drinking. It may also be caused by emotional disturbance.

Constipation

Constipation is the difficult or infrequent evacuation of feces. The urge to defecate is normally triggered by the pressure of feces on the rectum and by the intake of food into the stomach. On the toilet, the anal sphincter is relaxed voluntarily, and the fecal material is expelled. The need to defecate should be attended to as soon as possible. Habitual disregard of the desire to empty the bowels reduces intestinal motion and leads to constipation.

Daily or regular bowel movements are not necessary for good health. Normal bowel movements may occur at irregular intervals due to variations in diet, mental stress, and physical activity. For some individuals, normal defecation may take place as infrequently as once every four days.

Simple Constipation

In simple constipation, the patient may have to practice good bowel movement habits, which include a trip to the toilet once daily, preferably after breakfast. Adequate fluid intake and proper diet, including fresh fruits and green vegetables, can help restore regular bowel movement. Laxatives can provide temporary relief, but they inhibit normal bowel function and lead to dependence. When toilet-training young children, parents should encourage but never force them to have regular bowel movements, preferably after breakfast.

Chronic Constipation

Chronic constipation can cause feces to accumulate in the rectum and *sigmoid*, the terminal section of the colon. The colonic fluid is absorbed and a mass of hard fecal material remains. Such impacted feces often prevent further passage of bowel contents. The individual suffers from abdominal pain with distension and sometimes vomiting. A cleansing enema will relieve the fecal impaction and related symptoms.

In the overall treatment of constipation, the principal cause must be identified and corrected so that normal evacuation can return.

Intestinal Obstructions

Obstruction to the free flow of digestive products may exist either in the stomach or in the small and large intestines. The typical symptoms of in-

Intestinal Obstructions

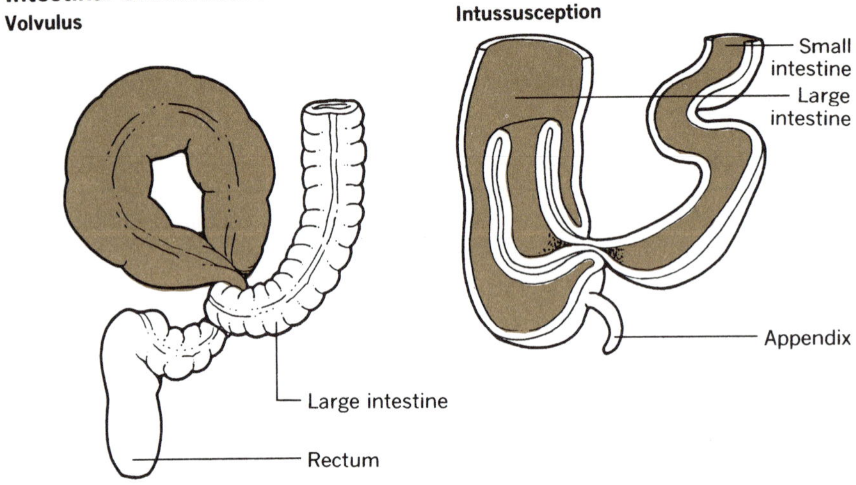

testinal obstruction are constipation, painful abdominal distension, and vomiting. Intestinal obstruction can be caused by the bowel's looping or twisting around itself, forming what is known as a *volvulus*. Malignant tumors can either block the intestine or press it closed.

In infants, especially boys, a common form of intestinal obstruction occurs when a segment of the intestine folds into the section below it. This condition is known as *intussusception,* and can significantly reduce the blood supply to the lower bowel segment. The cause may be traced to viral infection, injury to the abdomen, hard food, or a foreign body in the gastrointestinal tract.

The presence of intestinal obstructions is generally determined by consideration of the clinical symptoms, as well as X-ray examinations of the abdomen. Hospitalization is required, since intestinal obstruction has a high fatality rate if proper medical care is not administered. Surgery may be needed to remove the obstruction.

Diarrhea

Diarrhea is the frequent and repeated passage of liquid stools. It is usually accompanied by intestinal inflammation, and sometimes by the passing of mucus or blood.

The principal cause of diarrhea is infection in the intestinal tract by microorganisms. Chemical and food poisoning also brings on spasms of diarrhea. Long-standing episodes of diarrhea have been traced to inflammation of the intestinal mucosa, tumors, ulcers, allergies, vitamin deficiency, and in some cases emotional stress. Diarrhea, in conjunction with other symptoms, can also indicate infection with human immunodeficiency virus (HIV), the suspected cause of

AIDS. See "AIDS" in Ch. 19, *Other Diseases of Major Importance.*

Patients with diarrhea commonly suffer abdominal cramps, lose weight from chronic attacks, or have vomiting spells. A physician must always be consulted for proper diagnosis and treatment; this is especially important if the attacks continue for more than two or three days. Untreated diarrhea can lead to dehydration and malnutrition; it may be fatal, especially in infants.

Dysentery

Dysentery is caused by microorganisms that thrive in the intestines of infected individuals. Most common are *amoebic dysentery,* caused by amoebae, and *bacillary dysentery,* caused by bacteria. The symptoms are diarrhea with blood and pus in the stools, cramps, and fever. The infection is spread from person to person through infected excrement that contaminates food or water. The bacteria and amoebae responsible can also be spread by houseflies which feed on feces as well as on human foods. It is a common tropical disease and can occur wherever human excrement is not disposed of in a sanitary manner.

Dysentery must be treated early to avoid erosion of the intestinal wall. In bacillary dysentery, bed rest and hospitalization are recommended, especially for infants and the aged. Antibiotic drugs may be administered.

In most cases the disease can be spread by healthy human carriers who must be treated to check further spread.

Typhoid

Enteric fever or *typhoid* is an acute, highly communicable disease caused by the organism *Salmonella typhosa.* It is sometimes regarded as a tropical disease because epidemic outbreaks are common in tropical areas where careless disposal of feces and urine contaminates food, milk, and water supplies. In any location, tropical or temperate, where unsanitary living predominates, there is always the possibility that the disease can occur. Flies can transmit the disease, as can shellfish that live in typhoid-infested waters.

The typhoid bacilli do their damage to the mucosa of the small intestines. They enter via the oral cavity and stomach and finally reach the lymph nodes and blood vessels in the small bowel.

Symptoms

Following an incubation period of about ten days, general bodily discomfort, fever, headache, nausea, and vomiting are experienced. Other clinical manifestations include abdominal pain with tenderness, greenish diarrhea (or constipation), bloody stools, and mental confusion. It is not unusual for red spots to appear on the body.

If untreated, typhoid victims die within 21 days of the onset of the disease. The cause of death may be perforation of the small bowel, abdominal hemorrhage, toxemia, or other complications such as intestinal inflammation and pneumonia.

Treatment and Prevention

A person can best recover from typhoid if he receives diligent medical and nursing care. He should be isolated in a hospital on complete bed rest. Diet should be restricted to highly nutritious liquids or preferably intravenous feeding. Destruction of the bacilli is achieved by antibiotic therapy, usually with Chloromycetin.

The best way to prevent the spread of typhoid is to disinfect all body refuse, clothing, and utensils of the person infected. Isolation techniques practiced in hospitals prevent local spread. Milk and milk products should always be pasteurized; drinking water should be chlorinated.

Human beings can carry the disease and infect others without themselves becoming ill; they are usually not aware that they are carriers. Within recent years, a vaccination effective for a year has been developed. People traveling to areas where sanitation practices may be conducive to typhoid should receive this vaccination. In such areas, it is usually a good practice to boil drinking water as well.

Foreign Bodies in the Alimentary Tract

Anyone who accidentally swallows a foreign body should seek immediate medical aid, preferably in a hospital. Foreign bodies that enter the gastrointestinal tract may cause obstruction anywhere along the tract, including the esophagus. For emergency procedures, see "Obstruction of the Windpipe" in Ch. 31. *Medical Emergencies*.

Dental plates and large chunks of meat have been known to cause fatal choking. A foreign body in the esophagus may set off a reflex mechanism that causes the trachea to close. The windpipe may have to be opened by means of a *tracheostomy* (incision in the windpipe) to restore breathing. If the object swallowed is long and sharp-pointed, it may perforate the tract.

Foreign bodies in the esophagus are usually the most troublesome. Small fish bones may stick to the walls of the esophagus; large pieces of meat may block the tract. X-ray studies aid the physician in locating the swallowed object and in determining how best to deal with it.

Small objects like coins and paper clips may pass through the digestive tract without causing serious problems. Their progress may be checked by X rays of the abdomen. Examination of stools will indicate whether or not the entire object has been expelled. With larger objects, the problem of blockage must be considered.

It is sometimes necessary for a surgeon to open the stomach in a hospital operating room and remove the foreign object.

Ulcers

A *peptic ulcer* is an eroded area of the mucous membrane of the digestive tract. The most common gastrointestinal ulcers are found in the lower end of the esophagus, stomach, or duodenum and are caused by the excessive secretion of gastric acid which erodes the lining membrane in these areas.

Scientists have discovered a bacteria, Helicobacter pylori, that causes 80 percent of gastric ulcers and 95 percent of duodenal ulcers, and that also figures in a small amount of peptic ulcers. The bacteria dwells in the mucous lining of either the stomach or duodenum. It is unclear why ulcers appear in only a portion of those testing positive for the bacteria. The cause of non-Helicobacter pylori ulcers is also uncertain, but any factor that increases gastric acidity may contribute to the condition.

Symptoms

Early ulcer symptoms are gastric hyperacidity and burning abdominal pain that is relieved by eating, vomiting, or the use of antacids. The pain may occur as a dull ache, especially when one's stomach is empty, or it may be sharp and knifelike.

Other manifestations of a peptic ulcer are the following: nausea, associated with heartburn and regurgitation of gastric juice into the esophagus and mouth; excessive gas; poor appetite with undernourishment and weakness in older victims; and black stools resulting from a bleeding ulcer.

The immediate goal of ulcer therapy is to heal the ulcer; the long-term goal is to prevent its recurrence. An ulcer normally heals through the formation of scar tissue in the ulcer crater. The healing process, under proper medical care, may take several weeks. The disappearance of pain does not necessarily indicate that the ulcer has healed completely, or even partially. The pain and the ulcerative process may recur at regular intervals over periods of weeks or months.

Although treatment can result in complete healing and recovery, some victims of chronic peptic ulcers have a 20-to-30-year history of periodic recurrences. For such patients, ulcer therapy may have to be extended indefinitely to avoid serious complications. If a recurrent ulcer perforates the stomach or intestine, or if it bleeds excessively, it can be quickly fatal. Emergency surgery is always required when perforation and persistent bleeding occur.

Detection and Treatment

Conventional treatment options include a combination of ulcer diets, which consist of bland foods such as milk, eggs, and jellos; rest and the reduction of stress; and antacids and antispasmodic medication to reduce stomach contraction and acidity and slow digestion. In severe cases, hospitalization and surgery may be necessary. Although these treatments remain common today, the emergence of H. pylori as a factor has brought about new treatment options that may eventually replace the vast majority of previous therapies.

Ulcer sufferers should consider a variety of treatments based on cost, severity, and the presence of H. pylori. Patients with mild-to-moderate ulcer symptoms are urged to undertake a one-to-two month treatment of an H2 blocker, which reduces secretions of gastric acid, and Prilosec, an acid-suppressing drug. H2 treatment is successful in a third of ulcer cases, with the ulcers reappearing on the average of one year after treatment. Side effects of H2 therapy include mental confusion, fever, and a slowed pulse. Other gastric and limiting drugs have been found to attack the leukocytes, or white cells, of the blood.

Endoscopy, a costly and sometimes uncomfortable test, is the preferred procedure for patients whose ulcers do not respond to H2 therapy or other treatments, or when the presence of the H. pylori bacteria is suspected. This ten-to-fifteen-minute test, usually done on an outpatient basis, consists of inserting a lighted tube down the throat into the duodenum and stomach in order to procure a tiny portion of the gastric or duodenal lining for testing. If H. pylori is detected along with an ulcer, the patient undertakes a two-week combination of two antibiotics—Flagyl and either tetracycline or amoxicillin, as well as bismuth subsalicate (Pepto Bismol). Some physicians may add an H2 blocker such as Tagamet or Pepcid to relieve symptoms and hasten healing. Those with a confirmed history of ulcers can skip endoscopy and be tested for infection alone with blood tests that specifically check for the presence of antibodies to H. pylori.

Hospitalization may be an option if the ulcer does not respond to H2, antibiotic, or other treatments; if pain persists; or if an active gastric ulcer is present. A patient may be hospitalized for three weeks to ensure proper diet and the reduction of emotional stress from work and personal relationships. During this time, the healing process is monitored by X-rays and other tests.

If there is no improvement after three or four weeks, surgery may be advised. Such surgery is elective, as opposed to the emergency surgery required by large, bleeding, or perforated ulcers. After the removal of the acid-producing section of the stomach, some patients may experience weakness and nausea as their digestive system adjusts to the reduced size of the stomach. A proper diet of special foods and fluids, plus sedatives, can alleviate this condition. The chances for complete recovery from surgery are good. For a full description of surgical treatment of peptic ulcers, see “Peptic Ulcers” in Chapter 20, *Surgery*.

Diverticula

A *diverticulum* is an abnormal pouch caused by herniation of the mucous membrane of the digestive tract. The pouch has a narrow neck and a bulging round end. Diverticula are found in the esophagus, stomach, duodenum, colon, and other parts of the digestive tract.

The presence of diverticula in any segment of the digestive tract is referred to as *diverticulosis*. When diverticula become inflamed the condition is known as *diverticulitis*. The latter is a common form of disease of the sigmoid colon and is found in persons past the age of 45.

In mild cases, there may be no symptoms. On the other hand, a diverticulum may sometimes rupture and produce the same symptoms as an acute attack of appendicitis—vomiting and pain with tenderness in the right lower portion of the abdomen. Other symptoms are intermittent constipation and diarrhea, and abdominal pain.

Diverticulosis is treated by bed rest, restriction of solid food and increase of fluid intake, and administration of antibiotics. Surgery is recommended when diverticulosis causes obstruction of the colon or creates an opening between the colon and the bladder, or when one or more diverticula rupture and perforate the colon. The outlook for recovery following surgery is good.

Diverticulosis

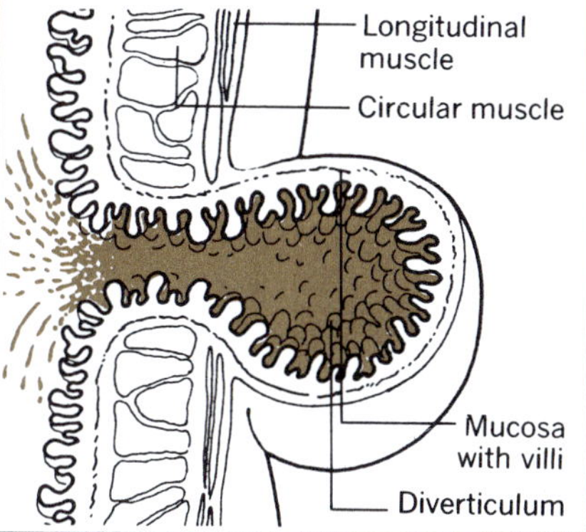

Hemorrhoids (Piles)

Hemorrhoids, or *piles,* are round, purplish protuberances at the anus. They are the results of rectal veins that become dilated and rupture. Hemorrhoids are very common and are often caused by straining because of constipation, pregnancy, or diarrhea.

Hemorrhoids may appear on the external side of the anus or on the internal side; they may or may not be painful. Rectal bleeding and tenderness are common. It is important to emphasize, however, that not all rectal bleeding results from hemorrhoids. Small hemorrhoids are best left untreated; large painful ones may

Hemorrhoids

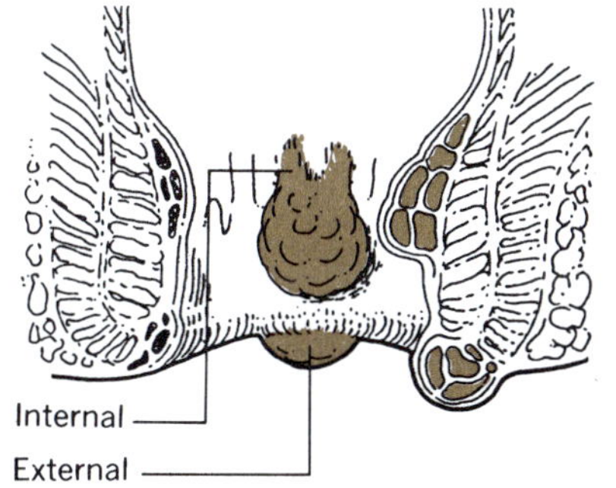

be surgically reduced or removed. *Prolapsed* piles—those that have slipped forward—are treated by gentle pressure to return the hemorrhoidal mass into the rectum. The rectal and anal opening must be lubricated to keep the area soft. Other conditions in the large bowel can simulate hemorrhoids and need to be adequately investigated.

Hernias

Hernias in the digestive tract occur when there is muscular weakness in surrounding body structures. Pressure from the gastrointestinal tract may cause a protrusion or *herniation* of the gut through the weakened wall. Such hernias exist in the diaphragmatic area (*hiatus hernias,* discussed above), in the anterior abdomen (*ventral hernias*), or in the region of the groin (*inguinal hernias*). Apart from hiatus hernias, inguinal hernias are by far the most common.

One of the causes of intestinal obstruction is a *strangulated hernia.* A loop of herniated bowel becomes tightly constricted, blood supply is cut off, and the loop becomes gangrenous. Immediate surgery is required since life is threatened from further complications.

Except for hiatus hernias, diagnosis is usually made simple by the plainly visible herniated part. In men, an enlarged scrotum may be present in untreated inguinal hernias. The herniating bowel can be reduced, that is, manipulated back into position, and a truss worn to support the reduced hernia and provide temporary relief. In all hernias, however, surgical repair is the usual treatment.

Hernias

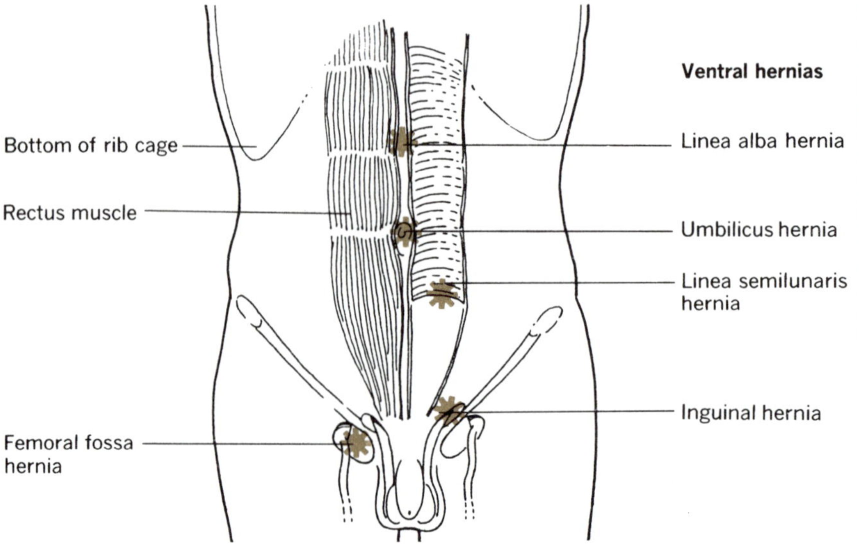

Gastritis

Gastritis is inflammation of the mucosa of the stomach. The patient complains of *epigastric* pain—in the middle of the upper abdomen—with distension of the stomach, loss of appetite, nausea, and vomiting.

Attacks of acute gastritis can be traced to bacterial action, food poisoning, peptic ulcer, the presence of alcohol in the stomach, the ingestion of highly spiced foods, or overeating and drinking. Occasional gastritis, though painful, may disappear spontaneously. Gastritis may also cause serious bleeding. The general treatment for gastritis is similar to the treatment of a gastric ulcer.

Enteritis

Enteritis, sometimes referred to as *regional enteritis,* is a chronic inflammatory condition of unknown origin that affects the small intestine. It is called regional because the disease most often involves the terminal ileum, even though any segment of the digestive tract can be involved. The diseased bowel becomes involved with multiple ulcer craters and ultimately stiffens because of fibrous healing of the ulcers.

Regional enteritis occurs most often in males from adolescence to middle age. The symptoms may exist for a long period before the disease is recognized. Intermittent bloody diarrhea, general weakness, and lassitude are the early manifestations. Later stages of the disease are marked by fever, increased bouts of diarrhea with resultant weight loss, and sharp lower abdominal pain on the right side. This last symptom sometimes causes the disease to be confused with appendicitis, because in both conditions there is nausea and vomiting. Occasionally in women there may be episodes of painful menstruation.

Treatment involves either surgical removal of the diseased bowel or conservative medical management and drug therapy. In acute attacks of enteritis, bed rest and intravenous fluids are two important aspects of treatment. Medical management in less severe occurrences includes a daily diet rich in proteins and vitamins, excluding harder foods such as fresh fruits and vegetables. Antibiotics are prescribed to combat bacterial invasion.

Colitis

Colitis is an inflammatory condition of the large intestine, of uncertain origin, and often chronic. It may result from a nervous predisposition which leads to bacterial or viral infection. The inflammation can cause spasms that damage the colon, or can lead to bleeding ulcers that may be fatal.

In milder forms, colitis first appears with diarrhea in which red bloody streaks can be observed. The symptoms may come and go for weeks before the effects become very significant. As the disease process advances, the diarrhea episodes become more frequent; more blood and mucus are present in the feces. These are combined with abdominal pain, nausea, and vomiting. Because of the loss of blood, the patient often becomes anemic and thin. If there are ulcer craters in the mucosa, the disease is called *ulcerative colitis.*

Ulcerative Colitis may be treated with medication, surgery, and hospitalization is sometimes necessary. Surgery may be needed if an acute attack has been complicated by perforation of the intestines or if chronic colitis fails to respond to medical management.

Nonoperative treatment includes control of diarrhea and vomiting by drug therapy. Antibiotics are given to control infection and reduce fever, which always accompanies infection. A high protein and vitamin diet is necessary. But if the diarrhea and vomiting persist, intravenous feeding becomes a must. Blood transfusions may be required for individuals who have had severe rectal bleeding. Because there is no absolute cure, the disease may recur.

Appendicitis

The *vermiform appendix* is a narrow tubular attachment to the colon. It can become obstructed by the presence of undigested food such as small seeds from fruits or by hard bits of feces. This irritates the appendix and causes inflammation to set in. If it is obstructed, pressure builds within the appendix because of increasing secretions, a situation that can result in rupture of the appendix. A ruptured appendix can be rapidly fatal if *peritonitis,* inflammation of the peritoneal cavity, sets in.

In most cases the onset of appendicitis is heralded by an acute attack of pain in the center of the abdomen. The pain intensity increases, shifts to the right lower abdomen with nausea, vomiting, and fever as added symptoms. Some individuals, however, suffer from recurrent attacks of dull pain without other signs of gastrointestinal disease, and these may not be significant enough to warrant immediate hospitalization.

Diagnosis of appendicitis is usually dependent on the above symptoms, along with tenderness in the appendix area, increased pulse rate, and decreasing blood pressure. The last two are very significant if the appendix ruptures and peritonitis sets in. Whenever these symptoms are observed, the patient should be rushed to the nearest hospital.

Immediate surgical removal of the diseased appendix by means of a small incision is necessary in all nonperforated acute cases. This type of operation (*appendectomy*) is no longer considered major surgery. If the appendix ruptures and peritonitis is evident, emergency major surgery is necessary to drain the infection and remove the appendix. In the absence of postoperative complications, the patient recovers completely. One of the major problems of appendicitis is early diagnosis to prevent dangerous complications.

Intestinal Parasites

Not all the diseases of man are caused by microscopic organisms. Some are caused by parasitic worms, *helminths,* which invade the digestive tract, most often via food and water. In recent years government health agencies have largely eliminated the prime sources of worm infection: unwholesome meat or untreated sewage that finds its way into drinking water. Nevertheless, helminths still exist. Drugs used to expel worms are called *vermifuges* or *anthelmintics.*

The following are among the major intestinal parasites.

Tapeworms (Cestodes)

These ribbon-shaped flatworms are found primarily in beef, fish, and pork that have not been thoroughly cooked. There are several species ranging from inch-long worms to tapeworms that grow to about 30 feet and live for as long as 16 years.

Tapeworms attach themselves to intestinal mucosa and periodically expel their eggs in excreta. If such feces are carelessly disposed of, the eggs can reach drinking water and be taken in by fish or ingested by grazing cattle. The eggs hatch in the animal's large bowel and find their way into the bloodstream by boring through the intestinal wall. Once in the blood they eventually adhere to muscles and live a dormant life in a capsule.

People who eat raw or partially cooked meat and fish that are infested with tapeworms become infected. The worms enter the bowel, where they feed, grow, and produce eggs. When the egg-filled segments are excreted, the cycle begins anew. Tapeworm infection is usually asymptomatic. It is discovered when egg-laden segments in feces are recognized as such.

Medication must be given on an empty stomach, followed later by a laxative. This will dislodge the worms and enable the body to purge itself of them. A weekly check of stools for segments of the worms may be necessary to confirm that the host is free of the parasites.

Hookworms

There are many species of these tiny, threadlike worms which are usually less than one centimeter long. They are found principally in tropical and subtropical areas of China, North Africa, Europe, Central America, and the West Indies, but they are by no means extinct in the United States.

The eggs are excreted in the feces of infected individuals, and if fecal materials are not well disposed of, the eggs may be found on the ground of unsanitary areas. In warm, moist conditions they hatch into larvae that penetrate the skin, especially the feet of people who walk around barefooted. The larvae can also be swallowed in impure water.

Hookworm-infected individuals, most often children, may experience an inflammatory itch in the area where the larvae entered. The host becomes anemic from blood loss, due to parasitic feeding of the worms, develops a cough, and experiences abdominal pain with diarrhea. Sometimes there is nausea or a distended abdomen. Diagnosis is confirmed by laboratory analysis of feces for the presence of eggs.

Successful treatment requires administration of anthelmintic drugs, preferably before breakfast, to destroy the worms. Weekly laboratory examination of the feces for evidence of hookworm eggs is a necessary precaution in ascertaining that the disease has been eradicated. Untreated hookworm infestation often leads to small bowel obstruction.

Trichinosis

This sometimes fatal disease is caused by a tiny worm, *Trichinella spiralis,* which is spread to man by eating improperly cooked pork containing the tiny worms in a capsulated form. After they are ingested the worms are set free to attach themselves to the mucosa of the small intestines. Here they mature in a few days and mate; the male dies and the female lays eggs that reach the muscles via the vascular system.

Trichinella organisms cause irritation of the intestinal mucosa. The infected individual suffers from abdominal pains with diarrhea, nausea, and vomiting. Later stages of the disease are marked by stiffness, pain, and swelling in the muscles, fever with sweating, respiratory distress, insomnia, and swelling of the face and eyelids. Death may result from complications such as pneumonia, heart damage, or respiratory failure. Despite government inspection of meats, all pork should be well-cooked before eating.

Threadworms (Nematodes)

These worms, also called pinworms, infect children more often than adults. Infection occurs by way of the mouth. The worms live in the bowel and sometimes journey through the anus, where they cause intense itching. The eggs are laid at the anal opening, and can be blown about in the air and spread in that manner. The entire family must be medically treated to kill the egg-laying females, and soothing ointment should be applied at the rectal area to relieve the itching. Good personal hygiene, especially hand washing after toilet use, is an essential part of the treatment.

Roundworms (Ascaris)

These intestinal parasites closely resemble earthworms. The eggs enter

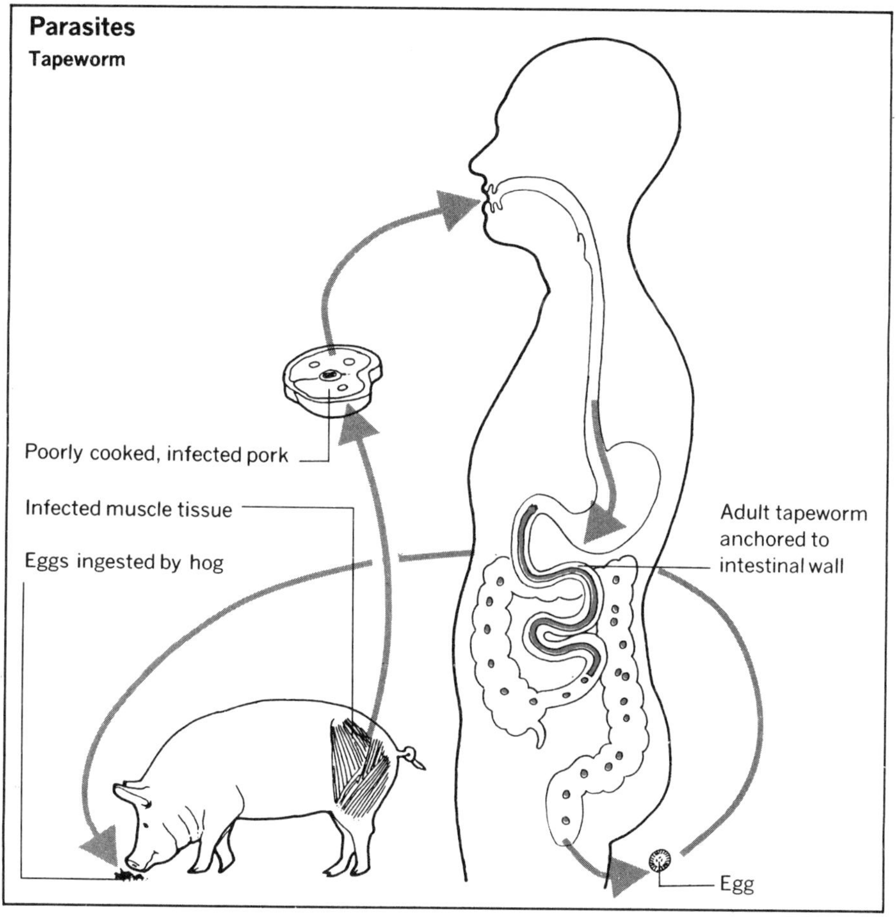

the digestive tract and hatch in the small bowel. The young parasites then penetrate the walls of the bowel, enter the bloodstream, and find their way to the liver, heart, and lungs.

Untreated roundworm infestation leads to intestinal obstruction or blockage of pancreatic and bile ducts caused by the masses of roundworms, which usually exist in the hundreds. Ingestion of vermifuge drugs is the required treatment.

Food Poisoning

Acute gastrointestinal illnesses may result from eating food that is itself poisonous, from ingesting chemical poisons, or from bacterial sources. The bacteria can either manufacture *toxins* (poisonous substances) or cause infection. Improperly canned fish, meats, and vegetables may encourage the growth of certain toxin-manufacturing organisms that resist the action of gastric juice when ingested. A person who eats such foods may contract *botulism,* a type of food poisoning. Symptoms include nausea, abdominal pain, vomiting, blurred vision, dryness in the mouth and throat, and poor muscular coordination. If the toxins become fixed in the central nervous system, they may cause death. Emergency hospitalization is required, where antitoxins are administered intravenously and other measures are taken to combat the effects of botulism.

Food poisoning caused by the *Salmonella* bacteria is spread by eating contaminated meat, or by eating fish, egg, and milk products that have not been properly cooked or stored. The organisms are also transmitted by individuals who handle food with dirty hands. Victims suffer from vomiting, diarrhea, abdominal pain, and fever. This type of food poisoning can be fatal in children and the aged, especially if they are ailing. Medical treatment with hospitalization, administration of broad-spectrum antibiotics, and intravenous fluids (to replace water loss due to vomiting) is required.

Escherichia coli, or *E.coli,* is a bacteria that can also cause food poisoning. The most commonly found harmful strain in the United States is E.coli O157:H7. It produces toxins that damage the intestinal lining in victims, causing them to suffer from nausea, fatigue, abdominal cramps, and watery or bloody diarrhea. E.coli may be spread by swimming in water contaminated by human feces; or consuming foods or beverages that are contaminated with the bacteria—most commonly, raw or undercooked ground beef. Most people do not require treatment and recover in 5 to 10 days. Antidiarrheal medications are not recommended and may cause complications.

Liver Disease

Cirrhosis

Chronic disease of the liver with the destruction of liver cells is known as *cirrhosis.* A common cause is excessive intake of alcoholic beverages along with malnutrition. However, there are other predisposing factors, such as inflammation of the liver (*hepatitis*), syphilis, intestinal worms, jaundice or biliary tract inflammation, and disorders in blood circulation to the liver.

Victims of cirrhosis are usually anemic and have an elevated temperature, around 100° F. Alcoholics very often lose weight, suffer from indigestion, and have distended abdomens.

Accurate diagnosis of cirrhosis depends on complex laboratory tests of liver function, urine, and blood. If liver damage is not too far advanced, treatment of the complications and underlying causes can aid the liver cells in the process of regeneration. In long-standing chronic disease, liver damage may be irreversible. Alcoholics who forgo alcohol may be restored to health, depending on the extent of liver damage, with a proper diet rich in proteins and vitamins.

Successful treatment of liver cirrhosis may require long hospitalization with drug therapy and blood transfusions. During alcoholic withdrawal, the patient may require close medical observation and psychiatric help. If the patient's jaundice improves and his appetite returns, recovery in milder cirrhosis cases is possible.

Jaundice

In diseases of the liver and biliary tract, excessive bile pigment (*bilirubin*) is recirculated into the bloodstream. It enters the mucous membranes and skin, giving them the characteristic yellow pigmentation of the disease.

Gallstones or tumors that obstruct the free flow of bile are one cause of jaundice. Other causes include hepatitis, overproduction of bile pigments with resultant accumulation of bile within the liver, cirrhosis, and congenital closure of the bile ducts, the last a common cause of jaundice in infancy.

Apart from the typical yellow appearance of the skin, jaundice generates such symptoms as body itching, vomiting with bile (indicated by the green appearance and bitter taste), diarrhea with undigested fats present in the stools, and enlargement of the liver with pain and tenderness in the right upper abdomen.

Treatment of jaundice requires continued medical care with hospitalization. Surgery may be necessary to remove stones in the biliary tract or other obstructions. If there is bacterial infection, antibiotic therapy is necessary.

Hepatitis

Infectious hepatitis or hepatitis A virus (HAV) is spread in food and water contaminated by the feces of infected individuals. HAV often infects day care workers and travelers in Third World countries. The incubation period of HAV lasts from one to six weeks. Symptoms include fever, nausea, vomiting, aching muscles, fatigue, loss of appetite, and sometimes jaundice. HAV can usually be cured by a few weeks of bed rest. Treatment with immune globulin will halt the virus if given early enough to those exposed. It is important to note that those infected with HAV will not become carriers upon full recovery. Vaccines against HAV are available. Good sanitary practices can halt the spread of HAV. Vigorous handwashing after restroom use or changing diapers and before preparing and eating food is strongly recommended.

The hepatitis B virus (HBV) is more serious than HAV because it often causes long-term infection and chronic liver disease, such as cancer and cirrhosis. Most HBV is transmitted through exposure to blood and other bodily fluids via sexual contact, the sharing of needles in illicit drug use, being stuck with an infected needle in a hospital setting, and the use of unsterilized instruments in body piercing or tattooing. A newborn can also be infected if the mother is a carrier. The incubation period of HBV is from forty days to six months. Symptoms, while similar to those of HAV, are usually more severe, and often lead to chronic infection. A small percentage of adults and a high percentage of babies who contract HBV will become chronic carriers of the virus, placing them at risk for serious health problems later in life. Vaccines for hepatitis B exist, and vaccination is recommended for children and adolescents and for high-risk groups such as health care workers, intravenous drug users, and those with multiple sex partners. Treatment with alpha interferon or lamivudine also reduces the severity of infection.

The hepatitis C virus (HCV) is transmitted through blood transfusions or blood to blood contact. HCV is spread through sexual contact in about 10 percent of cases. Many people infected with the HCV remain healthy for years and even decades before symptoms appear. Those with asymptomatic infection eventually develop serious liver ailments. About 75 percent develop cirrhosis of the liver and 20 percent develop liver cancer; necessitating liver transplants. Symptoms include darkening of the urine, abdominal discomfort, loss of appetite, nausea and vomiting, severe fatigue, muscle pain and tenderness, accumulation of fluid in the abdomen and sometimes the legs, and sometimes jaundice. No vaccine exists for HCV. Treatment can be interferon injections alone or interferon and the oral drug ribavirin. The methods have different success rates in clearing the virus from the blood. If liver damage becomes too great, a transplant will be necessary. End-stage hepatitis C patients account for half of all liver transplants.

The hepatitis D virus (HDV) appears only in those infected with HBV. HDV is transmitted through contaminated blood and sexual contact. Those infected with both HBV and HDV are at greater risk of severe infection and death than those infected with HBV alone. Prevention methods used for HBV, such as vaccination and immune globulin, will prevent the contraction of HDV.

The hepatitis E virus (HEV) is transmitted in the same manner as HAV. The incubation period for HEV averages forty days. Symptoms of HEV are similar to other forms of the virus, but severe infection and increased mortality are common, especially in pregnant women. There is no treatment for HEV. Cases of HEV have not been documented in western Europe or the United States.

Hepatitis G (HGV) is transmitted through the blood and possibly through sexual contact. It is sometimes found in association with HCV. The initial acute infection apparently does not become chronic, although the virus does persist in the blood. Hepatitis G is the most recently identified type, and more research is needed on transmission, treatment, and other aspects.

Gallbladder Disease

The biliary tract is very often plagued by the presence of stones, in the gallbladder or one of the bile ducts. Gallstones are mostly a mixture of calcium carbonate, cholesterol, and bile salts, and can occur either as one large stone or a few smaller ones.

When fats from the daily diet enter the small intestines, the concentrated bile from the gallbladder is poured into the duodenum via the bile ducts. Bile is necessary if fats are to be digested and absorbed. If stones are present in the biliary tract, the gallbladder will contract, but little or no bile will reach the fats in the small bowel.

Untreated gallbladder disease leads to several possible complications. The obstructed bile pigments may be recirculated in the bloodstream, causing jaundice. Obstruction of the ducts causes increased pressure and may also result in perforation of the gallbladder or ducts. Acute inflammation of the biliary tract is always a possibility due to the irritation caused by the concentrated bile.

A gallbladder that is full of stones or badly diseased must be surgically removed for the patient's health to improve. In milder cases, other treatment and special diet can prevent attacks.

Treatment and Diagnosis of Gastrointestinal Disorders

Some medications used in treating gastrointestinal disorders, such as antacids and laxatives, can be purchased without prescription, but should be taken only upon a physician's advice.

Treatment of gastrointestinal diseases may require low-residue diets—that is, a diet of foods that pass through the digestive tract very readily without a large amount of solid fecal residue. Included are low-fat meals, liquids, and finely crushed foods. Diagnostic tests may require overnight fasting, fat-free meals, or eating specific foods. Raw fruits and vegetables, salads, alcohol, and coffee do not belong in a bland diet. See under Ch. 27, *Nutrition and Weight Control,* for further information on special diets.

GI Series

By filling the digestive tract with *barium sulfate,* a substance opaque to X rays, a radiologist can locate areas of abnormality. Barium sulfate can be mixed as a thin liquid or paste and be swallowed by the patient during studies of the esophagus, stomach, and small intestines. The type of radiological examination that utilizes such a barium meal is known as a *GI* (gastrointestinal) *series.* The large bowel is examined with the barium mixture administered through the rectum like a standard enema, known as a *barium enema.* This procedure makes it possible to visualize the inner walls of the colon. For further information on diagnostic procedures, see Ch. 26, *Physicians and Diagnostic Procedures.*

12

Diseases of the Respiratory System

The human body cannot survive for more than a very few minutes in an environment that lacks oxygen. Oxygen is required for the normal functioning of all living body cells. This vital gas reaches the body cells via the bloodstream; each red blood cell transports oxygen molecules to the body tissues. The oxygen comes from the atmosphere one breathes, and it enters the bloodstream through the very thin membrane walls of the lung tissue, a fresh supply of oxygen entering the bloodstream each time a person inhales. As the red blood cells circulating through the walls of the lung tissue pick up their fresh supply of oxygen, they release molecules of carbon dioxide given off by the body cells as a waste product of metabolism. When a person exhales, the lungs are squeezed somewhat like a bellows, and the carbon dioxide is expelled from the lungs.

The automatic action of breathing in and out is caused by the alternate contraction and relaxation of several muscle groups. The main muscle of breathing is the *diaphragm,* a layer of muscle fibers that separates the organs of the chest from the organs of the abdomen. Other muscles of respiration are located between the ribs, in the neck, and in the abdomen. As the diaphragm contracts to let the lungs expand, the other muscles increase the capacity of the *thorax,* or chest cavity, when one inhales. The muscles literally squeeze the lungs and chest when an individual exhales.

Any disease of the muscles and bones of the chest wall or of the passages leading from the nose to the lung tissue—containing the small air sacs where the gases are actually exchanged—will interfere to some extent with normal function. As with any organ of the body, there is a great

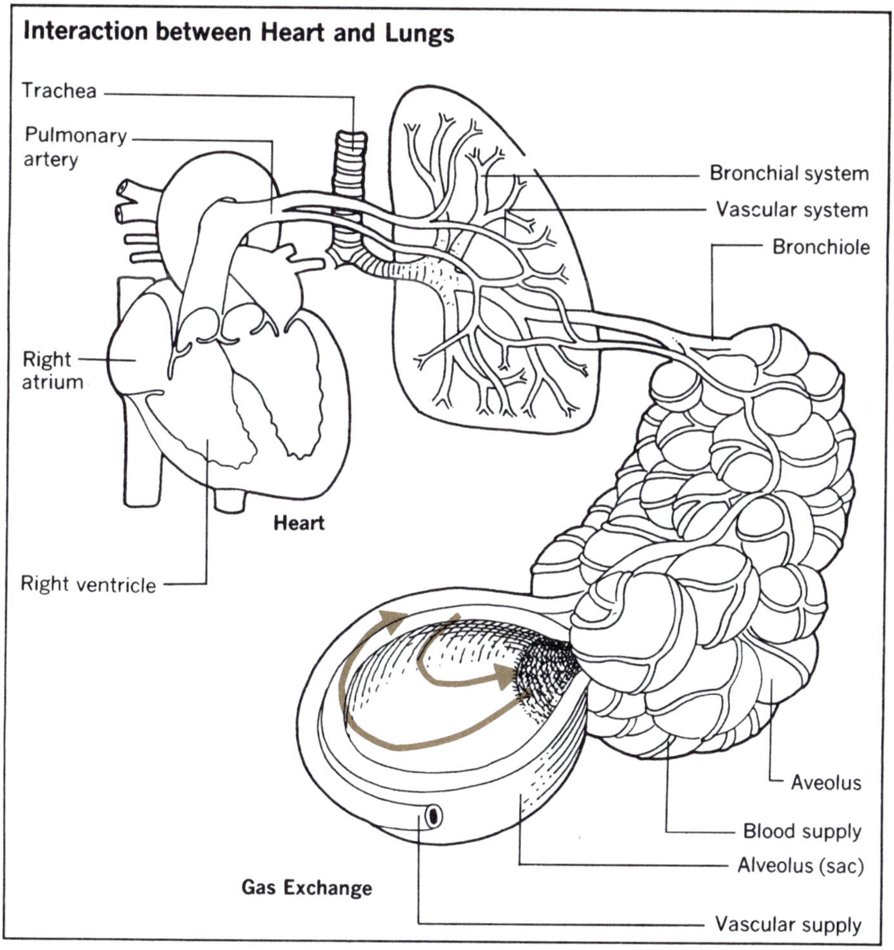

reserve built into the lungs that assures that small to even moderate amounts of diseased tissue can exist without compromising their ability to sustain life. However, when disease of the lungs, air passages, thoracic (rib) cage, or any combination of these parts decreases the capacity of the reserve areas, then the oxygen supply to all the organs and tissues of the body becomes deficient, and they become incapable of performing their vital functions.

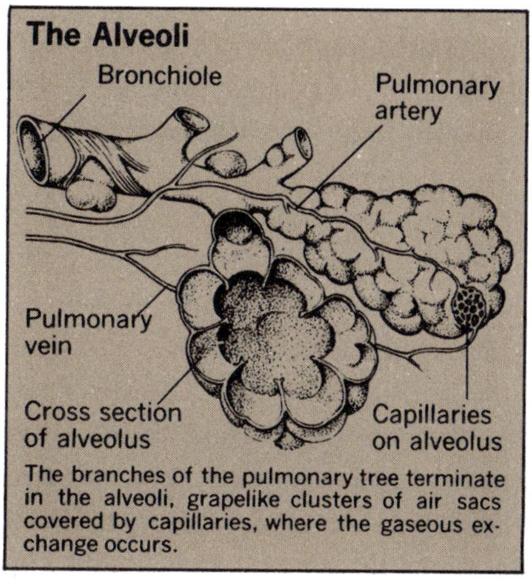

The branches of the pulmonary tree terminate in the alveoli, grapelike clusters of air sacs covered by capillaries, where the gaseous exchange occurs.

Diseases of the thoracic cage are relatively uncommon. Certain forms of arthritis cause fixation of the bony cage and limit expansion when breathing. Various muscle and nervous system diseases weaken the muscles used to expand the chest for breathing.

Diseases of the *bronchi* or air passages tend to narrow those tubes and thereby limit the amount of air that can pass through to the tiny *alveoli,* or air sacs. Other conditions affect the alveoli themselves, and, if widespread enough, allow no place for the oxygen and carbon dioxide to be exchanged.

The most common forms of lung disease are infections caused by viruses, bacteria, or fungi. Infection is always a potential threat to the lung because this organ is in constant contact with the outside air and therefore constantly exposed to infectious agents. It is only through elaborate defenses that the body is able to maintain normal functions without interference by these agents.

The major defenses are simply mechanical and consist mainly of the hairs in the nose and a mucous blanket coating the inside of the bronchi. The very small hairs (called *cilia*) in the breathing passage act as a filtering system; mucous membranes of the bronchi help to intercept small particles as they are swept along by the action of the cilia. Whenever these structures are diseased, as in chronic bronchitis, there is a much greater likelihood of acquiring infection.

The Common Cold, Influenza, and Other Viral Infections

The Common Cold

The common cold is the most prevalent illness known to mankind. It accounts for more time lost from work than any other single condition. The infection rate varies from one individual to another.

Surveys indicate that about 25 percent of the population experience four or more infections a year, 50 percent experience two or three a year, and the remaining 25 percent have one or no infections in a year. There is also some variation from year to year for each person, explained often by the amount of exposure to young children, frequent extreme changes in weather, fatigue, and other factors.

For years it has been felt that chilling plays a role in causing the common cold, and, although difficult to prove, there is almost certainly some truth to the idea. By some as yet unclear process, chilling probably causes certain changes in our respiratory passages that make them susceptible to viruses that otherwise would be harmless.

The common cold affects only the upper respiratory passages: the nose, sinuses, and throat. It sometimes is associated with fever. Several viruses have been implicated as the cause for the common cold. But in the study centers that investigate this illness, isolation of a cold virus is only achieved in about one half of the cases. These viruses are not known to produce any other significant illnesses. Most likely they inhabit the nose and throat, often without producing any illness at all.

Symptoms

The major part of the illness consists of about three days of nasal congestion, possibly a mild sore throat, some sneezing and irritation of the eyes (though not as severe as in hay fever), and a general feeling of ill health often associated with some muscle fatigue and aching. After three days the symptoms abate, but there is usually some degree of nasal congestion for another ten days.

Prevention is difficult, and there is no specific treatment. The natural defenses of the body usually are capable of resolving the infection. Attention should be paid to avoiding further chilling of the body, exhausting activity, and late hours that can further lower the defenses and lead to complications.

Complications

Ear infection may develop because of blockage of the *Eustachian tube,* which leads from the back of the throat to the inner part of the ear. That complication is heralded by pain in the ear. Bronchitis and pneumonia may be recognized early by the development of cough and production of *sputum* (phlegm). *Sinusitis* develops when the sinus passages are obstructed so that the infected mucus cannot drain into the pharynx (as in postnasal drip). The pain develops near the sinus cavity involved. These complications can and should be treated with specific drugs, and, if they develop, a physician should be consulted.

Influenza

A number of other viruses cause respiratory illness similar to the common cold, but are much more severe in intensity and with frequently serious, and even fatal, complications. The best known member of the group is the *influenza* (flu) virus. It can cause mild symptoms that are indistinguishable from those of the common cold, but in the more easily recognizable form it is ushered in by fever, cough, and what physicians refer to as *malaise*—chills, muscle ache, and fatigue.

The symptoms of influenza appear quickly; they develop within hours and generally last in severe form from four to seven days. The disease gradually recedes over the following week. The severity of the local respiratory and generalized symptoms usually forces the influenza patient to stay in bed.

Not only is the individual case often severe, but an outbreak of influenza can easily grow to epidemic proportions, closing factories, schools, and hospitals in its wake. There have been 31 very severe *pandemics* (epidemics that sweep many countries) that have occurred since 1510. The most devastating of these pandemics was an influenza pandemic—the "Spanish Flu," which occurred in 1918-1919; it led to the deaths of 25 million worldwide. Rarely is death directly attributable to the influenza virus itself, but rather to complicating bacterial pneumonia or to the failure of previously weakened vital organs.

Flu Shots

Inoculation is fairly effective in preventing influenza, but it has to be renewed each year. Unfortunately, there are several different types of influenza virus, and a slightly different vaccine is needed to provide immunity to each type of infection. Each recent epidemic in the United States has been the result of a different strain, and although there had been several months' warning before the epidemics started, it was difficult to mass-produce a vaccine in time to use it before the epidemics developed.

Treatment

Once contracted, there is no cure for influenza, but the body's defenses are usually capable of destroying the virus if given the necessary time and if the defenses are not depressed by other illness. Fluids, aspirin, and bed rest help relieve the symptoms. Special attention should be paid to sudden worsening of fever after seeming recovery, or the onset of sputum production. For elderly people more intensive medical care is often necessary, including hospitalization for some.

Pneumonia

Pneumonia is an inflammation of the lungs caused primarily by certain bacteria, viruses, fungi, or by inhaling chemical irritants. The most common severe pneumonia is that caused by the *pneumococcus bacterium.*

Pneumonia can affect one or both lungs. It usually develops from inhaling infected mucus into the lower respiratory passages. The pneumococcus is often present in the nasal or throat secretions of healthy people, and it tends to be present even more often in the same secretions of an individual with a cold. Under certain conditions these secretions may be *aspirated,* or inhaled, into the lung. There the bacteria rapidly multiply and spread within hours to infect a sizable area.

In other cases, the organisms causing pneumonia enter the lungs from a nearby infection in the body; or through the bloodstream. As with the common cold, chilling and fatigue often play a role in this sequence. People with any chronic debilitating illness, as well as those age 65 or older and very young children, are at increased risk of developing pneumonia.

Symptoms

Pneumonia can develop very suddenly, especially some types of bacterial pneumonia. Symptoms include high fever, shaking chills, chest pain, and a very definite feeling of total sickness or malaise. Within hours, enough pus is produced within the lungs for the patient to start coughing up thick yellow or greenish sputum that often may be tinged or streaked with blood.

Before the development of antibiotics, the illness tended to last about seven days, at which time it would often suddenly resolve almost as quickly as it started. But it also could frequently lead to death or to serious complications, such as abscess formation within the chest wall, meningitis, or abscess of the brain. Because antibiotics are so effective in curing this illness today, physicians rarely see those complications.

Treatment

Pneumococcal pneumonia is treated with antibiotics such as penicillin and erythromycin. But antibiotics are effective only if the pneumonia has been caused by bacterium. There is no generally recommended treatment for viral pneumonia, but patients should be sure to get plenty of rest and increase their fluid intake; in some cases antiviral medications may be used. Most patients can be treated at home. Pneumonia caused by fungi is treated with antifungal drugs. Pneumonia caused by chemical irritants is treated with oxygen therapy and mechanical ventilation.

Prevention

There is no guaranteed way to prevent pneumonia. The advice to avoid chilling temperatures, overexertion, and fatigue when one has a cold is directed principally toward avoiding pneumonia. The elderly and debilitated become more susceptible when exposed to extremes of temperature and dampness.

A vaccine is available that protects against the most common varieties of pneumococcal pneumonia. It is recommended for the elderly and people with weakened immune systems or chronic disease.

Pneumonia is not really a contagious illness except in very special circumstances. Everyone carries the pneumococcus in our noses and throats, but we rarely have the constellation of circumstances that lead to infection. It is the added physical insults that allow pneumonia to take hold.

Other Kinds of Pneumonia

Many kinds of bacteria are capable of causing pneumonia and they do so in the same manner, via the inhalation of infected upper airway secretions. Some diseases, such as alcoholism, tend to predispose to certain bacterial pneumonias. Usually these are not as dramatic as those caused by the pneumococcus, but they may be much more difficult to treat and thereby can often be more serious.

Far less severe are the pneumonias caused by certain viruses or organisms called mycoplasmas that seem to be intermediate between a virus and a bacterium. The term *walking pneumonia* is often applied to this type, because the patient is often so little incapacitated that he may not be sick enough to stay in bed. These pneumonias apparently occur in the same way as the bacterial pneumonias, but the difference is that the infecting agent is not capable of producing such severe destruction. These pneumonias are usually associated with only mild temperature elevation, scant amount of sputum production, and fewer general body symptoms. Walking pneumonia should be suspected when coughing dominates the symptoms of a cold, especially if it turns from a dry or nonproductive cough to one that produces sputum. Antibiotic therapy tends to hasten recovery and prevent the development of bacterial pneumonia.

Pleurisy

Pleurisy develops when the *pleura,* the double membrane that lines the chest cavity and surrounds each lung, becomes inflamed. Infection is one of the most common causes of inflammation of the pleura. Pleurisy is almost always painful, the pain being felt on inhaling and exhaling but not when the breath is quietly held for a brief period. Chest pain should always receive the prompt attention of a physician and investigation of its cause. The same type of pain on breathing can often be mimicked by a strain of the chest wall muscles, but the difference can usually be determined by a physician's examination or a chest X ray.

Tuberculosis

At the turn of the century *tuberculosis* (TB) was the leading cause of death in the world. Today, more than 8 million new cases of TB occur worldwide every year. The World Health Organization estimates that the number will exceed 10 million by 2005. In the United States, TB had declined until the mid-1980s, due both to the discovery of antibiotics and to modern preventive measures. However, TB is still at the top of the list as the leading cause of death among infectious diseases worldwide. And it remains a very serious health problem, accounting for

40,000 new illnesses every year in the United States. In contrast to a disease like influenza, physicians already have the tools with which to eliminate tuberculosis. But many factors, primarily social, make that a very distant possibility.

Tuberculosis is caused by one specific type of bacterium. Certain ethnic groups seem particularly susceptible to the disease, but the reasons are unclear. The American Indian and the Eskimo are two susceptible groups. However, there is no recognized hereditary factor. The disease is different from many commonly known infections in several ways. Unlike pneumonia, tuberculosis is a chronic and painless infection, measured more in months than in days. Because of this pattern, it not only takes a long time to develop serious disease, but it also takes a long time to effect a cure.

Another very important difference between tuberculosis and many other infections is its ability to infect individuals without causing symptoms of illness, but then to lie dormant as a potential threat to that person for the rest of his life. The early stages of the disease do not produce any symptoms. Consequently a patient develops large areas of diseased tissue before he begins to feel sick. Screening procedures, therefore, are very important in detecting early disease in patients who feel perfectly healthy. Another is the skin testing of schoolchildren, which is carried out routinely in many communities today.

How Tuberculosis Spreads

Tuberculosis is contracted by inhaling into the lungs bacteria that have been coughed into the air by a person with advanced disease. It is, therefore, contagious, but not as contagious as measles, mumps, or chicken pox. Unlike those illnesses, it usually requires fairly close and prolonged contact with a tuberculous patient before the infection is passed on. Once the bacteria are inhaled, the body defenses are usually capable of isolating them into small areas within the tissues, thereby preventing any significant destruction or disease. However, though defenses are able to isolate the bacteria, they are not able to destroy all of them. Some bacteria persist in a state in which they are unable to break out and destroy tissue, but they always maintain the potential to do so at a time when the body defenses are impaired.

In about 20 percent of individuals the body defenses are not initially capable of isolating the tubercle bacilli. These individuals, mostly children, develop progressive tuberculosis directly following their initial contact. Others are successful in preventing actual disease at the time of initial contact, but they join a large group with the potential for active disease at some time in the future. Most of the new cases of active tuberculosis come from this second group; their defenses break down years after the initial contact and resultant infection.

Weight loss, malnutrition, alcoholism, diabetes, and certain other chronic illnesses are particularly likely to lead to deterioration of the defense mechanisms holding the tuberculosis organisms in check. Still other individuals develop active disease with no recognizable condition to account for the loss of defenses. In fact, the most likely age group to develop active disease as a result of breakdown of past infection is the 20- to 30-year-old group.

Once active disease has appeared it usually involves the chest, although it can develop anywhere in the body. There is gradual spread of inflammation within lung tissue until large areas are involved. Holes, or cavities, are formed as a result of tissue destruction. These contain large numbers of tuberculosis organisms and continue to enlarge as new tissue is destroyed at the edges. At any stage of this development organisms may find their way into the bloodstream and new foci of disease can spring up throughout the body. The sputum becomes loaded with organisms that are coughed into the air and go on to infect other individuals. The infected sputum from one area of the lung may gain access to other areas and cause development of diseased tissue there as well.

Treatment

Before the modern era of drug treatment all these events followed an inexorable course to death in 85 percent of people with active tuberculosis. Only a lucky few were able to survive as cured, usually because their disease was found at an early stage. That survival was often at the expense of years confined to a sanatorium. Because of its almost uniform outcome and the required separation from family and home, tuberculosis was formerly looked upon with quite as much dread as cancer is today.

The sanatorium rest cure of tuberculosis was first developed in the mid-nineteenth century at a time when the cause of the disease was unknown. In 1882, Robert Koch first demonstrated the tuberculosis organism, thereby proving the disease was an infection. As the twentieth century progressed, general public health measures helped limit the number of new cases, and new surgical procedures were developed to treat the disease. These measures were effective enough to arrest tuberculosis in another 25 percent of cases, brightening somewhat the dismal outlook of the past century.

But the discovery of specific antibiotics in the 1940s made the real difference in tuberculosis. Because of drug treatment, surgery is rarely resorted to today, although it still may be helpful in certain patients. Now patients with tuberculosis can face a relatively bright future without having to be hospitalized for prolonged periods or enduring periods of endless disability.

Tuberculosis Control

People still contract tuberculosis, and people still die from it. Two of the principal causes of death are delayed therapy and interruptions in therapy, the latter leading to the development of tuberculosis organisms that are unaffected by drugs. Both of these causes are often under the control of the patient. The first can be avoided by seeing a physician whenever one develops a cough that lasts more than two weeks, especially when it is not associated with the typical symptoms of a cold at the outset. The other symptoms of developing tuberculosis are also seen in other illnesses, and should always lead one to recognize that he is sick and needs to consult his physician. These symptoms are weight loss, loss of appetite, fever, and night sweats. When tuberculosis is diagnosed, the patient must follow carefully the directions regarding medication, which is always continued for a long time after the patient has regained his feeling of well-being.

There are other ways, however, to attack tuberculosis, even before one becomes sick. Once a person has had contact with tuberculosis, even though he usually does not develop active disease, he produces antibodies against the bacteria. A person with such antibodies can be recognized by injecting under the skin specially prepared material from dead tuberculosis bacteria, which gives rise to a reaction within the skin after two days. This material is called *tuberculin* and the test is known as the *tuberculin test.*

There are now many mass screening programs of tuberculin testing for schoolchildren, hospital personnel, and industrial groups. Those with positive skin test reactions are screened further for the presence of active disease. If they are found to be active cases, they are treated during what is usually an early and not very severe stage of the disease. The other people with positive tuberculin tests, without any evidence of active disease, are candidates for *prophylactic* (preventive) *therapy.* This therapy employs *isoniazid* (*INH*), the most effective of many drugs for the treatment of tuberculosis. INH does have many possible side effects. Treatment for six months to one year has been shown to reduce greatly the chance of future progress from the merely infected state to the state of active disease.

The goal of prophylactic therapy is chiefly to prevent the far more serious development of active disease. But in addition, by preventing disease before it develops, physicians can prevent the infection of others, since the typical patient with tuberculosis has already infected some of those living with him before he becomes ill and seeks medical attention. The surface has just been scratched in this regard, however, as there are estimated to be 25 million people in the United States who would demonstrate reactions to tuberculin tests. Many of these people have never been tested and are not aware of the potential threat within them.

In most foreign countries the tuberculosis problem is much more serious. An estimated 80 percent of the populations of the countries of Asia, Africa, and South America would show positive tuberculin skin tests, with the number of active cases and deaths being proportionately high.

Sarcoidosis

Sarcoidosis (or *Boeck's sarcoid*), a disease that affects black people more often than whites, has symptoms closely resembling those of tuberculosis and other diseases. The most obvious symptom is the formation of skin nodules, often of the face, but the nodules, called *granulomas* (small tumors composed chiefly of granulation tissue), commonly occur in many other places as well, especially in the lungs and lymph nodes. They can occur also in the liver, bones, eyes, and other tissues.

Although sarcoidosis occurs all over the world, it is more common in temperate regions. Men and women are about equally affected. The onset of the disease occurs usually in the third or fourth decade of life.

Diagnosis and Treatment

The disease is diagnosed by an examination of chest X rays, which will show the proliferation of nodules in the lungs. Surgical biopsy and microscopic examination of skin tissue or tissue from a lymph node is usually necessary to confirm the presence of the disease.

There is no specific treatment for sarcoidosis, and in spite of its similarities in some respects to tuberculosis, no connection between the two disorders has been established. Steroids are sometimes used to treat the skin lesions, but in many cases the skin nodules clear up eventually without any treatment. About half of the patients, however, do not recover completely, and the disease becomes chronic—though of varying severity. Ultimately the granulomas can change into fibrous scars that may pose serious threats to the patient, depending upon where the scarring occurs. Respiratory distress, heart failure, and glaucoma, for example, can result from tissue changes in the lungs, heart, and eyes, respectively.

Respiratory Diseases Caused by Fungi

Two fungal diseases affecting respiration are of great importance in particular regions of the United States. They are both caused by types of fungi capable of growing within mammalian tissue, thereby infecting and destroying it. Both cause chronic diseases very similar to tuberculosis and may lead to death, though that is a far less common outcome—even when untreated—than in tuberculosis.

The spores of the fungi are inhaled from the air, and the response of the body is similar to that in tuberculosis in that most people become merely infected (the spores being contained by body defenses) while a few develop progressive disease. The body also produces anitbodies, and consequently skin tests similar to the tuberculin test can identify infected individuals.

Histoplasmosis (named for a fungus called *histoplasma*) organisms are prevalent in the Midwest, generally in the areas of the Ohio, Mississippi, and Missouri rivers. Largely unknown prior to World War II, histoplasmosis has been studied extensively since. Local epidemics have brought it to public attention on several occasions. The fungus grows readily in soil containing large amounts of bird (chickens, pigeons, starlings) or bat excrement. One of the better ways to assure exposure is to clean out an old chicken coop. The concentration of organisms may reach such high levels in bat caves that entry by spelunkers may prove fatal. In contrast to tuberculosis, the amount of exposure seems to play a very important role in determining the extent of the disease. There also seem to be few cases of late breakdown (the rule in tuberculosis). Most people develop the active disease, if at all, at the time of their initial exposure.

Coccidioidomycosis (for *Coccidioides* fungus) also generates in the soil, in this case in California, the southwest United States, and Mexico. It grows best in hot, dry soil. The common names for this disease are *desert rheumatism* or *valley fever.* Infection and disease occur in a similar pattern to that of histoplasmosis. Skin testing of large population groups for both these fungi in the appropriate geographical areas indicates that the majority of exposed individuals quite adequately contain the initial infection and never develop any illness or active disease.

Because Americans travel into infected regions, these diseases are being seen more frequently in people who do not live where the fungi are found. Both conditions, fortunately, are often self-limited, even when active disease develops. For more severe cases there is a drug, *amphotericin-B,* which is quite effective; however, because it is also quite toxic to the patient, it must be given in progressive doses starting with a small initial dose, to permit the body's tolerance to build up. It is hoped that less toxic agents will be found in the future that will be just as effective against the fungus.

Allergic Respiratory Diseases

Hay fever (*allergic rhinitis*) and *asthma* are two very common allergic diseases of the respiratory tract. The two have much in common as to age at onset, seasonal manifestations, and causation. Hay fever involves the *mucosa,* or lining, of the upper respiratory tract only, whereas asthma is confined to the bronchial tubes of the lower respiratory tract. Physicians usually distinguish two main types of asthma, allergic and infectious. The infectious type of asthma resembles bronchitis, with cough and much wheezing as well. The discussion here will be confined to the allergic form of asthma.

In hay fever and asthma the allergenic substance causing the reaction is usually airborne, though it can be a food. In most cases the offender is pollen from a plant. The pollen is inhaled into the nostrils and alights upon the lining of the respiratory passages. In the allergic individual, antibodies react with the proteins in the pollen and cause various substances to be released from the tissue and blood cells in the immediate area. These substances, in turn, produce vessel enlargement in the area and an outpouring of mucus, plus certain irritating symptoms that result in a stuffy or runny nose and itchy eyes. The same reactions occur in the bronchial lining in asthma, but the substances released there also cause constriction of the bronchial muscle and consequent narrowing of the passages. This muscular effect and the narrowing caused by greatly increased amounts of mucus in the passages are both responsible for the wheezing in asthma.

Hay Fever

Hay fever is never a threat to life, but in severe cases it can upset one's life patterns immensely. For unknown reasons it is more common in childhood, where it is often seen in conjunction with eczema or asthma. The tendency to develop hay fever, eczema, and asthma is hereditary. The transmission of the hereditary factors is complex, so that within a family group any number of individuals or none at all may exhibit the trait.

Most people with hay fever have their only or greatest difficulty in the summer months because of the airborne pollens from trees, grasses, flowers, and molds that are prevalent then. The most notorious of all pollens is the ragweed pollen. This weed pollinates around August 15 and continues to fill the air until late September. In many cities an official pollen count is issued every day, and those with severe difficulty can avoid some trouble by staying outside as little as possible on high-count days. *Antihistamine* drugs are used to counteract the nasal engorgement in hay fever. These drugs counteract the effect of *histamine,* which is one of the major substances released by the allergic reaction.

Allergic Asthma

Allergic asthma is the result of the allergic reaction taking place in the bronchial mucosal lining rather than in the nasal lining. A person may suffer from both asthma and hay fever. The common inciting factors are pollens, hair from pets (especially cats), house dust, molds, and certain foods (especially shellfish). When foods are responsible, the reaction initially occurs within the bloodstream, but the major effect is felt within the lung, which is spoken of as the target organ.

Most allergic asthma is seen in children. Only the mildest cases of allergic asthma disappear at puberty. For those who continue to have difficulty after puberty, the role of infection as a cause for the asthma usually becomes more prominent. Allergic asthma attacks start abruptly and can usually be aborted rather easily with medication.

People with asthma are symptom-free much of the time. When exposed to high concentrations of pollen they begin wheezing and producing sputum. Wheezing refers to the high-pitched squeaking sound that is made by people exhaling through narrowed bronchi. Associated with the wheezing and sputum is a distinct sensation of shortness of breath that varies in severity according to the nature of the attack. Milder attacks of asthma often subside spontaneously, merely with relaxation. This is especially true when the wheezing is induced by nonspecific factors, such as a cloud of dust, cold air, or exercise. Asthmatic individuals have more sensitive air passages and they are more easily bothered by these nonspecific irritants.

Treatment

For more severe attacks of asthma there are several types of treatment. There are oral medications that dilate the bronchi and offset the effects of the allergic reaction. (Antihistamines, however, exert no effect on asthma and may even worsen the condition.) Also available are injectable medications, such as adrenaline, and sprays that contain substances similar to adrenaline and that can be inhaled. Any or all of these methods may be employed by the physician. During times of high exposure it is often helpful to take one of the oral medications on a regular basis, thereby avoiding minor episodes of wheezing.

A recently discovered remedy for asthma is particularly useful to persons—primarily infants and small children, who cannot swallow tablets. The remedy comes in capsules containing tiny pellets of the drug theophylline. Once the capsule is twisted open, the pellets can be sprinkled on soft foods, including strained baby food, applesauce, pudding, or hot or cold cereal. The pellets give relief for about 12 hours, long enough to protect children during sleep.

The best therapy for asthma and hay fever is avoidance of the allergen responsible for attacks. Obviously, cats and certain foods can be avoided more readily than pollens and other airborne substances. The first requisite, however, is to identify the offender. The most important method of identification is the patient's medical history. Sometimes the problem is easy, as when the patient states that he only has trouble during the ragweed season. At other times a great amount of detective work may be required. Skin testing is used to complement the history. The skin test merely involves the introduction under the skin (usually within a tiny scratch) of various materials suspected of being allergens. If the individual has antibodies to these substances he will form a hive at the site of introduction. That he reacts does not necessarily mean that his asthma is due to that test substance, because many people have reactions but no hay fever or asthma. The skin test results need to be interpreted in the light of the history of exposure. If the substance so identified cannot be avoided, then hyposensitization may prove useful. This form of treatment is based on the useful fact that the human body varies its ability to react depending upon the degree and the frequency of exposure. In a hyposensitizing program small amounts of pollen or other extract are injected frequently. Gradually the dose of extract is increased. By this technique many allergic individuals become able to tolerate moderate exposure to their offending material with few or no symptoms. Hyposensitization does not succeed in everyone, but it is usually worth attempting if other approaches are unsuccessful. For more information see Ch. 21, *Allergies and Hypersensitivities*.

Other Respiratory Diseases

SARS (Severe Acute Respiratory Syndrome)

Severe Acute Respiratory Syndrome, or *SARS*, is a contagious respiratory disease. It is caused by a coronavirus (SARS-CoV). It is spread by the coughing and sneezing of infected persons.

Symptoms typically appear 2-7 days after an infection occurs. Most persons infected will have a high fever, cough, and difficulty breathing. Other symptoms may include headache, chills, muscle aches, and diarrhea. Many persons infected with SARS develop pneumonia. Once a person is suspected of having SARS, they should seek immediate medical attention. They will likely be isolated to prevent further spread of the disease.

There is no cure for SARS, and treatment generally addresses the pneumonia symptoms. Most persons infected with SARS begin recovering a week after they first began exhibiting symptoms, but SARS can result in death.

13

Lung Disease

Two present-day problems of major proportions are not diseases in themselves, but both are detrimental to health. These are smoking and air pollution. The former is a habit that, in some users, has results as serious as those produced by narcotics or alcohol addiction. Knowledge of air pollution has grown with the increased public awareness of our environment. It is quite clear that there are many serious consequences produced by the products with which we foul our air. Both tobacco and air pollution are controllable: one by individual will, the other by public effort.

Smoking

About 50 million Americans smoke, and the vast majority of these people smoke cigarettes. This discussion will therefore center on cigarette smoking. In the 1960's, approximately half the adult men and one third of adult women in the United States smoked. In 1964, the first U.S. Surgeon General report on smoking outlined the health hazards of smoking. Since that time, continued efforts to educate the public about the dangers of smoking have helped reduce the number of smokers, and by 2000 only about one quarter of adult men and women in the United States smoked. With the realization that secondhand exposure to cigarette smoke is also a health hazard, smoking has been banned in many public buildings and vehicles.

Dangers of Smoking

Scientists know much about the ways in which smoking produces health dangers. As they burn, cigarettes release more than 4,000 different sub-

Lungs

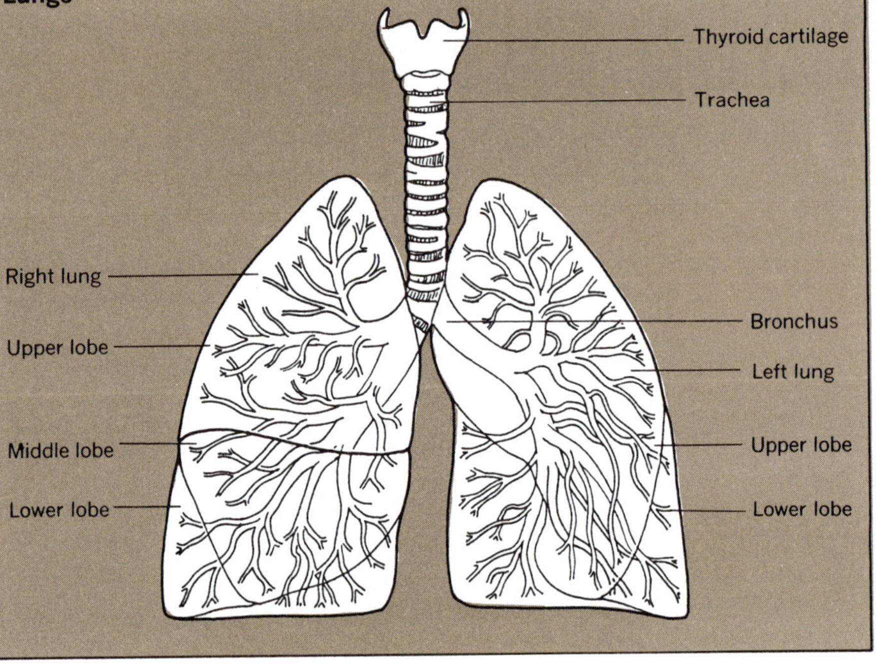

stances into the atmosphere. Carried in the cigarette smoke, these substances enter the smoker's lungs or simply dissipate in the air. Three of the substances, carbon monoxide, "tar," and nicotine, are the primary threats to health.

Smoking has "mainstream" effects on the smoker who inhales. But there are "sidestream" effects as well. For example, persons who habitually breathe the smoke from others' cigarettes may be inhaling higher concentrations of possibly harmful chemicals than the smokers themselves. These nonsmokers may experience such unpleasant symptoms as watery eyes and headaches. If they have lung or heart diseases, suffer from asthma or some allergies, or wear contact lenses, the nonsmokers may find that their symptoms are worsening.

Some of the direct effects of breathing tobacco smoke suggest its capacity for producing disease in the smoker. Smoking lowers skin temperature, often by several degrees, principally through the constricting effect of nicotine on blood vessels. Carbon monoxide levels rise in the blood when a person is smoking. Even a single cigarette may impair somewhat the smoker's ability to expel air from the lungs. Adverse changes in the activity of several important chemicals in the body can be demonstrated after smoking.

Smoking has been strongly implicated in bronchitis and emphysema, lung and other cancers, heart disease, and peripheral vascular disease. Cigarette smoking causes more "preventable" deaths in the United States than any other single factor. Of the five leading causes of deaths in the United States, cigarette smoking is related to four—heart disease, cancer, stroke, and chronic lung disease. According to the U.S. Surgeon General, cigarette smoking is responsible for more than 400,000 deaths in the United States each year and will result in death or disability in half of all regular smokers. The direct medical costs for treating smoking-related illness is more than $75 million; indirect economic costs are estimated to be as large.

Smoking by parents also affects their children. Studies have association parents' smoking with an increased frequency of colds, ear infections, and lower respiratory infections in children, as well as a worsening of asthma symptoms in asthmatic children.

A Cause of Cancer

Cigarettes contain more than 60 cancer-causing chemicals, many of which are released into the smoke of a burning cigarette. Cigarette smoking is known to cause cancers of the lungs, larynx, esophagus, mouth, and bladder. It is also known to contribute to cancers of the cervix, pancreas, and kidneys. Of all cancers, lung cancer takes more American lives (approximately 150,000) than any other type of cancer. Of these deaths, more than 80 percent are attributable to cigarette smoking. In addition, breathing secondhand smoke is estimated to cause more than 3,000 deaths from lung cancer among nonsmokers.

Other cancers related to cigarette smoking account for approximately 30,000 American deaths.

Heart Disease

Cigarette smoking is the single most important risk factor for the development of heart disease among young men and women. It greatly increases the risk in a person who has other risk factors for heart disease, such as obesity or high blood cholesterol. A smokers' risk of a heart attack is more than twice that of a nonsmoker. Cigarette smoking both increases blood pressure and the tendency for blood to clot. In the United States, smoking has been implicated in more than 100,000 deaths from heart disease each year—up to 30 percent of all deaths from heart disease.

Studies have shown that the smoker who refuses to give up smoking after a heart attack, to a significant degree, is inviting a second attack. But the smoker who quits would, after some 15 years, lower the risk of heart disease to about that of a nonsmoker.

Women and Smoking

Women were once thought to be less susceptible to smoking-related diseases than men. When the earlier studies were conducted, women had simply not been smoking as long as men had, or in such numbers. As the picture changed, so did the statistics. Between 1960 and 1990, deaths from lung cancer among women increased by more than 400 percent.

Women who smoke when they are pregnant are more likely to give birth to low-weight babies. Low birth weight carries an increased risk of infant death and is associated with a variety of health disorders in infants.

The Dose-Response Relationship

The number of cigarettes an individual smokes is one of the determinants of eventual health damage even though individual susceptibility is also important. Thus a dose-response relationship exists between smoking and disease. The more a person smokes, the sooner the smoker is likely to suffer health consequences. Nevertheless, when a person quits smoking, many of the health consequences of smoking begin to reverse themselves.

Breaking the Smoking Habit

Obviously, the best way not to develop a smoking habit is never to start smoking. Unfortunately, young people are continuing to join the smoking ranks at a rapid rate. The large majority of smokers begin smoking before the age of 21. It is typically difficult to convince teenagers of the hazards of smoking. They are generally healthy, suffer less from fatigue, headaches, breathlessness, and other immediate effects of smoking, and they often feel the need to smoke to fint in with their peers. Once they start, however, it is not long before they become addicted.

The addiction to cigarettes is very real. Though it may seem to be more a psychological dependency than a physical addiction, the nicotine in cigarettes is a very addictive and powerful drug. For most people, therefore, it is a big challenge to stop smoking. One obastacle consists of the reactions caused by the need for nicotine in the person who is stopping smoking. Such reactions, called withdrawal symptoms, very from person to person and include symptoms other than just a craving for a cigarette. Some people who stop smoking become jittery and sleepless, have difficulty concentrating, or develop an increased appetite. Another obstacle to quitting consists of overcoming the habits and routines the person has associated with smoking.

Steps for quitting successfully typically begin with making specific preparations for quitting. These preparations may include identifying reasons to quit and setting a date for quitting. Another important step is enlisting the support and encouragement of family, friends, and coworkers.

Programs for helping a smoker quit are provided at many hospitals, health centers, and clinics. In addition to providing counseling and support, they can provide medical guidance for various medications that are available—

some through prescription only—to help quit smoking. These medications include various kinds of nicotine medications (such as nicotine gum, nasal sprays, and patches) that provide small doses of nicotine to help overcome the urge to smoke.

Despite all efforts, many individuals who would like to stop smoking fail. The best advice for them is to keep trying. Continued effort will at least tend to decrease the amount of smoking and often leads to eventual abstinence, even after years of trying. For prospective quitters it is important to remember that cigarette smoking is an acquired habit, and that the learning process can be reversed. The problem most people have is too little knowledge of the dangers and too much willingness to believe that disease and disability only strike other people, not them.

Air Pollution

While 50 million Americans pollute the air they breathe individually with cigarettes, all 280 million of us collectively pollute the atmosphere we all breathe. Some people are obviously more to blame than others, but air, water, and land pollution is a disease of society and can be solved only through a concerted effort by the whole society. As we have become more urbanized, the problem of pollution has grown. At times, it has reached what many consider to be crisis proportions in our large cities and even in some of our smaller ones.

We have had ample warning. In 1948 a killer smog engulfed Donora, Pennsylvania, killing 20 persons and producing serious illness in 6,000 more. In 1952 a lingering smog over London was blamed for 4,000 deaths in a few weeks. New York City has had several serious encounters with critical smog conditions that have accounted for many illnesses and deaths. The exteriors of many buildings in our cities are showing signs of vastly increased rates of decay due to the noxious substances in the air. It is estimated that air pollution costs the United States more than $10 billion a year in damage, illness, and in other ways. Even if all this loss of life and property were not a result it would obviously be more pleasant to live in a clean atmosphere than in a foul one.

Emphysema and Bronchitis

Emphysema and chronic bronchitis are diseases that involve the whole lung. They can be of varying severity, and both are characterized by the gradual progression of breathlessness.

Because chronic bronchitis is almost invariably associated with pulmonary emphysema, the combined disorder frequently is called *obstructive-airway disease.* The disease involves damage to the lung tissue, with a loss of normal elasticity of the air sacs (*emphysema*), as well as damage to the *bronchi,* the main air passages to the lungs. In addition, chronic bronchitis is marked by a thickening of the walls of the bronchi with increased mucus production and difficulty in expelling these secretions. This results in coughing and sputum production.

The condition known as *acute bronchitis* is an acute process generally caused by a sudden infection, such as a cold, with an exaggeration of bronchitis symptoms. If a spasm of the bronchi occurs, accompanied by wheezing, the ailment is called infectious or nonallergic asthma.

Obstructive-airway disease is very insidious, and characteristically people do not, or will not, notice that they are sick until they suddenly are very sick. This is partly because of chronic denial of the morning cough and breathlessness, but also because we are fashioned in such a way as to have great reserve strength in our organs. As the disease progresses one starts using up his reserve for exertion. Because most people's life styles allow them to avoid exertion easily, the victim of this disease may have only rare

Bronchitis and Emphysema

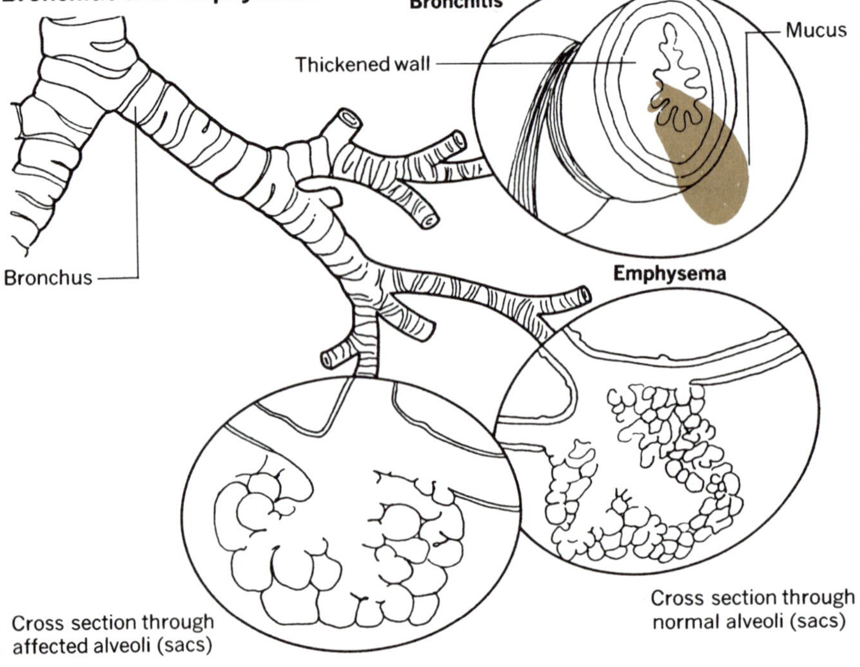

chances to notice his breathlessness. Then, suddenly, within a period of a few months he becomes breathless with ordinary activity because he has used up and surpassed all his reserve. He goes to a physician thinking he has just become sick. Usually this event occurs when the patient is fifty to seventy years old, and little can be done to correct the damage. The time for prevention was in the previous 30 years, when elimination of smoking could have prevented much or all of the illness.

Chronic cough and breathlessness are the two earliest signs of chronic bronchitis and emphysema. A smoker's cough is not an insignificant symptom. It indicates that very definite irritation of the bronchi has developed and it should be attended to early. Along with the cough there is often production of phlegm or sputum, especially in the morning, because of less effective emptying of the bronchial tree during the relatively motionless period of sleep. Another early manifestation of disease is the tendency to develop chest infections along with what would otherwise be simple head colds. With these chest infections there is often a tightness or dull pain in the middle chest region, production of sputum and sometimes wheezing.

Treatment

Once emphysema or bronchitis are diagnosed there are many forms of therapy that can help. Stopping smoking is the most important measure, and will, in itself, often produce dramatic effects. The more bronchitis the patient has, the more noticeable the effect, as the bronchial irritation and mucous production decrease, cough lessens, and a greater sense of well-being ensues. The emphysema component does not change, as the damage to the air sacs is irreversible, but the progression may be greatly slowed. If chest infections develop they can be treated with antibiotics.

For more severe disease a program of breathing exercises and graded exertion may be beneficial. When these people develop heart trouble as a result of the strain on the heart, a treatment to strengthen the heart is rewarding. For those with the most advanced stage of the disease, new methods of treatment have been devised in recent years. One of the most encouraging is the use of controlled oxygen administration, treatment that can sometimes allow a patient to return to activity from an otherwise helpless bed-and-chair existence. But it must be remembered that all these measures produce little effect if the patient continues to smoke.

Medication

Antibiotics and inoculations are used to fight respiratory infections such as influenza or pneumonia that may pose a particular danger to a person with emphysema or bronchitis.

Bronchodilators help relax and

open up narrowed airways. They are applied with devices called inhalers. Bronchodilators used to treat emphysema and bronchitis include anticholinergics, such as ipratropium bromide; beta$_2$-agonists, such as albuterol; and theophylline or aminophylline. Corticosteroids, such as prednisone, are used to control inflammation of the airways in the lungs. They are typically applied with a metered-dose inhaler.

Protein therapy, consisting of weekly applications of a protein called alpha$_1$-antitrypsin, is used to treat an inherited form of emphysema caused by a lack of the protein.

Oxygen Treatment

Oxygen treatment is used to raise the oxygen level in the blood, helping relieve shortness of breath. Some patients require only occasional supplemental oxygen; others need it on a continuous basis. Oxygen can be provided through the use of stationary or portable devices. The most common stationary device for oxygen delivery is a concentrator, which extracts oxygen from the air. Portable units use containers filled with compressed oxygen gas or with liquid oxygen.

Surgery

In severe cases, lung-reduction surgery is used. In this type of surgery 20 to 30 percent or more of the diseased lung is removed and the remaining parts of the lung are joined together. As a result air can move into and out of the remaining part of the lung more efficiently and the stress on the diaphragm is reduced. In yet other severe cases, a lung transplant is used to completely replace a diseased lung with a healthy lung from a deceased donor.

Smoking and Obstructive Diseases

The problems encountered by patients with obstructive lung disease do not encompass merely that disease alone. Because of their smoking history these patients are also prone to develop lung cancer. All too often a person with a potentially curable form of lung cancer is unable to undergo surgery because his lungs will not tolerate the added strain of surgery. Patients with obstructive lung disease are also more prone to pneumonia and other infectious pulmonary conditions. When these develop in the already compromised lung, it may be impossible for the patient to maintain adequate oxygen supply to his vital tissues. If oxygen insufficiency is severe and prolonged enough, the patient eventually dies from pulmonary failure.

Despite the emphasis placed on smoking as the predomiant factor for the development of obstructive lung disease, there are people with the disease who have never smoked. For many of these individuals there is no known cause for their disease. However, a group of younger people with obstructive disease has been found to be deficient in a particular enzyme. (Enzymes are agents that are necessary for certain chemical reactions.) Individuals with this deficiency develop a particularly severe form of emphysema, become symptomatic in their third or fourth decade, and die at a young age. They may not smoke, but if they do, the disease is much more severe. Just how the enzyme deficiency leads to emphysema is not clear, but a great amount of research is being conducted on this new link to try to learn more about the causes of emphysema.

The Pneumoconioses

Pneumoconiosis is a chronic reaction of the lung to any of several types of inhaled dust particles. The reaction varies somewhat but generally consists of initial inflammation about the inhaled particle followed by the development of scar tissue. The pneumoconioses develop predominantly from various occupational exposures to high concentrations of certain inorganic compounds that cannot be broken down by the cells of the body. The severity of the disease is proportional to the amount of dust retained in the lung.

Silica is the most notorious of these substances. People who work in mining, steel production, and any occupation involved with chipping stone, such as manufacturing monuments, are exposed to silica dust. Many of the practices associated with these occupations have been altered over the years because of the recognition of the hazard to workers. Other important pneumoconioses involve talc and asbestos particles, cotton fibers, and coal dust. Coal dust has gained wide attention in recent years with the heightened awareness of *black lung,* a condition seen in varying degrees in coal miners. The attention has resulted in a federal black lung disease law under which more than 135,000 miners have filed for compensation.

Although there are individual differences in reaction to the varied forms of pneumoconiosis, the ultimate hazard is the loss of functioning lung tissue. When enough tissue becomes scarred, there is interference with oxygenation. Those people with pneumoconiosis who smoke are in great danger of compounding their problem by adding obstructive disease as well.

Prevention

Once the scarring has taken place there is no way to reverse the process. Therefore, the answer to the pneumoconioses is to prevent the exposure. Attention to occupational diseases in the United States has lagged about 30 years behind Europe, so that we are just now beginning to show concern about certain industrial practices condemned as hazardous in many European countries in the 1940s. New lung diseases caused by inhaled substances are discovered every year, and more will undoubtedly be found in the future. People in industries in which there is exposure to industrial dust should be aware of the potential danger and should be prepared to promote the maintenance of protective practices and the investigation of new ideas and devices. Where masks have been supplied, the workers should wear them, a practice too often neglected.

Pulmonary Embolism

Pulmonary embolism is a condition in which a part of a blood clot in a vein breaks away and travels through the heart and into the pulmonary circulatory system. Here the vessels leading from the heart branch like a tree, gradually becoming smaller until finally they form *capillaries,* the smallest blood vessels. Depending on its size, the clot will at some point reach a vessel through which it cannot pass, and there will lodge itself. The clot disrupts the blood supply to the area supplied by that vessel. The larger the clot, the greater is the area of lung that loses its blood supply, and the more drastic the results to the patient.

This condition develops most commonly in association with inflammation of the veins of the legs (*thrombophlebitis*). People with varicose veins are particularly susceptible to thrombophlebitis. Because of constrictions produced by garters or rolled stockings, or just sitting with crossed legs for a long time, the sluggish blood flow already present is aggravated, and a clot may form in a vessel. Some people without varicose veins can also develop clots under the same conditions. The body often responds to the clot with the reaction of inflammation, which is painful. However, when there is no inflammatory response, there is no warning to tell that a clot has formed. In either situation there is always a chance that a piece may break off the main clot and travel to the lung. Of recent concern in this regard are studies that appear to link oral contraceptives with the incidence of clotting, thereby leading to pulmonary embolism. The number of women affected in this way by the use of oral contraceptives is small, but enough to be of concern.

The symptoms of pulmonary embolism are varied and may be minor or major. Most common are pleurisy—marked by chest pain during breathing—shortness of breath, and cough with the production of blood. Once the pulmonary embolism is diagnosed the treatment is simple in the less severe cases, which are the majority. But in cases of large clots and great areas of lung deprived of blood supply there may be catastrophic effects on the heart and general circulation.

Prevention

Certain preventive measures are worthwhile for all people. Stockings should not be rolled, because that produces a constricting band about the leg that impairs blood flow and predisposes to clot formation. Especially when taking long automobile or airplane rides one should be sure to stretch the legs periodically. Individuals with varicose veins or a history of thrombophlebitis should take these precautions more seriously. People who stand still for long periods during the day should wear elastic support stockings regularly and elevate their feet part of the day and at night.

When considering the use of oral contraceptives the physician must weigh the risks of developing clots from the drug against the psychological, social, and physical risks of pregnancy. The risk from oral contraceptives is lessened if the woman does not have high blood pressure. Any persistent pain in the leg, especially in the calf or behind the knee, deserves the attention of a physician. Anyone with varicose veins or anyone taking oral contraceptives should be especially attentive to these symptoms.

Pneumothorax

Another less common lung condition is spontaneous *pneumothorax* or collapse of a lung. This most commonly occurs in the second and third decade of life and presents itself with the sudden development of pain in the chest and breathlessness. The collapse occurs because of a sudden leak of air from the lung into the chest cavity.

The lung is ordinarily maintained in an expanded state by the rigid bony thorax, but if air leaks out into the space between the thorax and the lung, the lung collapses. This condition can be very serious and the patient needs to be observed to be sure that the air leak does not become greater with further lung collapse.

Treatment

Often a tube has to be placed in the chest, attached to a suction pump, and the air pumped out from the space where it has collected. When the air is removed the lung expands to fill the thoracic cage again. Some individuals tend to have several recurrences. Because the reason for the collapse is poorly understood, there is no satisfactory method of preventing these recurrences except by surgery. This is rarely required. In a person with a proven propensity for recurrence it is usually advisable to open the chest and produce scarring of the lung surface so that it becomes fixed to the thoracic cage. Although it is usually successful, even this procedure does not always solve this bothersome problem.

14

Diseases of the Endocrine Glands

Glands are organs that produce and secrete substances essential for normal body functioning. There are two main types of glands: the *endocrine* and the *exocrine*. The endocrines, or *ductless,* glands send their secretions directly into the bloodstream. These secretions, which are biochemically related to each other, are called *hormones*. The exocrines, such as the sebaceous or sweat glands, the mammary (or milk) glands, and the lachrymal (or tear) glands, have ducts that carry their secretions to specific locations for specific purposes.

The exocrine glands are individually discussed elsewhere in connection with the various parts of the body where they are found. This section is devoted to diseases of the ductless glands, which include:

- The *pituitary,* which controls growth and the activity of the adrenal, thyroid, and sex glands
- The *thyroid,* which controls the rate of the body's chemical activity or metabolism
- The *adrenals,* which affect metabolism and sex characteristics
- The *male gonads* or testicles and the *female gonads* or ovaries
- The *parathyroids,* which regulate bone metabolism

Unlike the exocrine glands, which can function independently of one another, the endocrines form an interrelated system. Thus a disorder in one of them is likely to affect the way the others behave. Glandular disorder can sometimes be anatomical, but it is usually functional. Functional disease can result in the production and release of too little or too much of a particular secretion.

When too much of a hormone is being secreted, the prefix *hyper-* is used for the condition, as in *hyperthyroidism*. When too little is being secreted, the prefix *hypo-* is used, as in the word *hypofunction,* to indicate that a gland operates below normal.

Abnormalities of the endocrine glands that cause changes in their functioning are responsible for a wide variety of illnesses. These illnesses are almost always accompanied by symptoms that can be recognized as distinctly abnormal. Prompt and accurate diagnosis can usually prevent the occurrence of irreversible damage. For many people with glandular disorders, treatment may have to be lifelong. They can feel well and function almost normally, but they must follow a program of regulated medication taken under a physician's supervision.

The Endocrine Glands

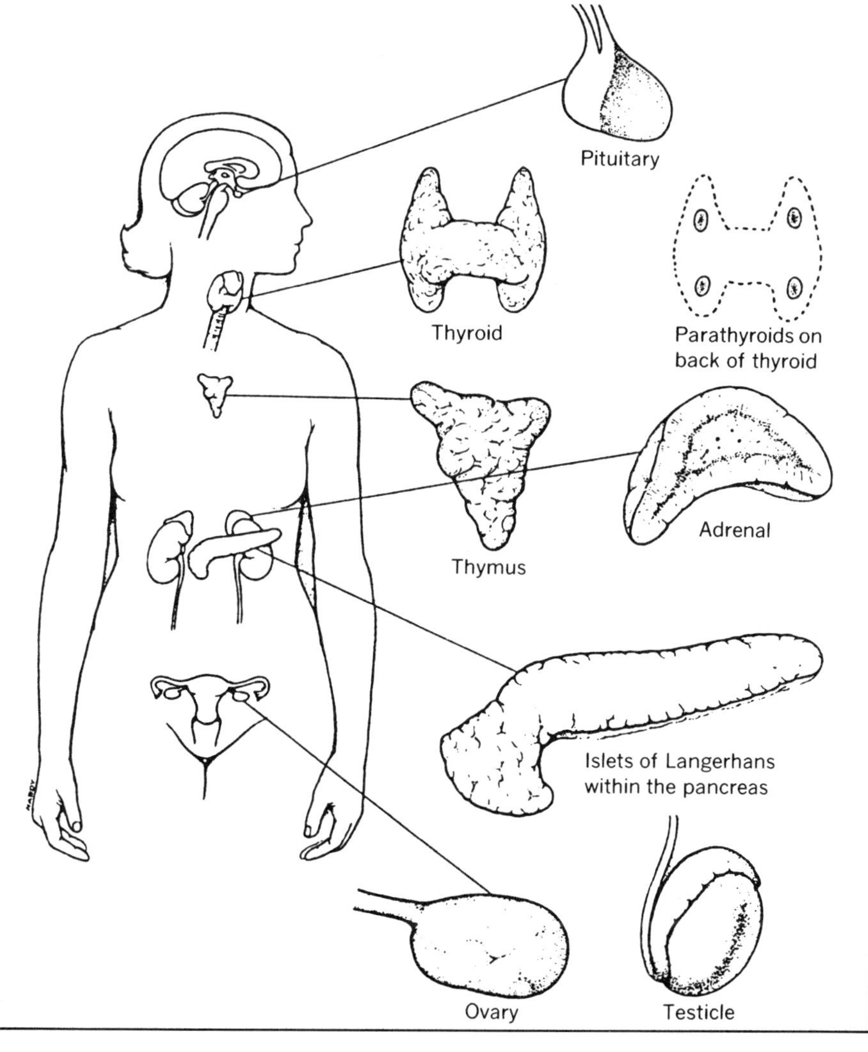

Anterior Pituitary Gland

The anterior pituitary gland, also called the *hypophysis,* is located in the center of the brain. It produces two types of secretions: a growth hormone and hormones that stimulate certain other glands.

The anterior pituitary gland is subject to neurochemical stimulation by the *hypothalamus,* a nearby part of the brain. This stimulation results in the production of the hormones that promote testicular and ovarian functioning, and does not occur normally until around 12 years of age in girls and 14 in boys. The beginning of this glandular activity is known as the onset of *puberty.*

Puberty is sometimes delayed for no apparent reason until age 16 or 17. Because the hypothalamus is affected by emotional factors, all of the endocrine glands governed by the anterior pituitary can also be affected by feelings. Psychological factors can therefore upset the relationships in the glandular system and produce the physical symptoms of endocrine disorders.

Pituitary Gland

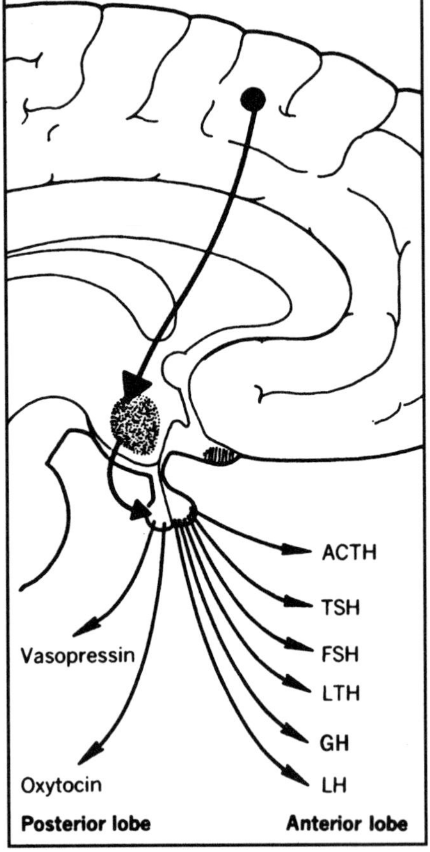

The Pituitary Gland

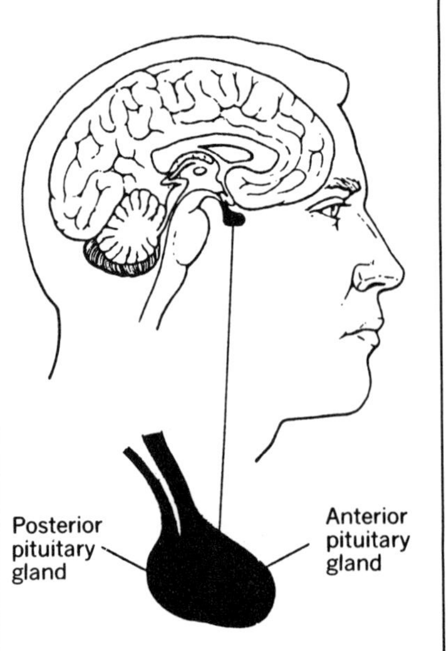

It is extremely rare for the anterior pituitary to produce too much or too little of its hormones, but sometimes hypofunction may follow pregnancy because of thrombosis or changes in the blood vessels.

A truly hypofunctioning anterior pituitary gland can cause many serious disturbances: extreme thinness, growth failure, sexual aberration, and intolerance for normal variations in temperature. When appropriate diagnostic tests determine the deficiency, the patient is given the missing hormones in pill form.

Absence of the growth hormone alone is unknown. Most cases of *dwarfism* result from other causes. However, excess production of the growth hormone alone does occur, but only rarely. If it begins before puberty when the long bones are still growing, the child with the disorder will grow into a well-proportioned giant. When it begins after puberty, the head, hands, feet, and most body organs except the brain slowly enlarge. This condition is called *acromegaly.* The cause of both disorders is usually a tumor, and radiation is the usual treatment.

The thyroid, adrenal cortex, testicles, ovaries, and pancreatic glands are target glands for the anterior pituitary's stimulating hormones, which are specific for the functioning of each of these glands. Therefore, a disorder of any of the target organs could be caused either by an excess or a deficiency of a stimulating hormone, creating a so-called *secondary disease.* There are various tests that can be given to differentiate primary from secondary disorders.

The Thyroid Gland

The thyroid gland is located in the front of the neck just above its base. Normal amounts of *thyroxin,* the hormone secreted by the thyroid, are necessary for the proper functioning of almost all bodily activities. When this hormone is deficient in infancy, growth and mental development are impaired and *cretinism* results.

Hypothyroidism

In adulthood, a deficiency of thyroxin hormone is caused primarily by a lack of sufficient iodine in the diet or by autoimmune factors. In *hypothyroidism,* the disorder resulting from such a deficiency, the metabolic rate is slower than normal, the patient has no energy, his expression is dull, his skin is thick, and he has an intolerance to cold weather.

Treatment consists of increasing the amount of iodine in the diet if it is deficient or giving thyroid hormone medication. Normal metabolic functioning usually follows, especially if treatment is begun soon after the symptoms appear.

Hyperthyroidism

An excess amount of thyroid hormone secretion is called *hyperthyroidism.* It causes physical fatigue but mental alertness, a staring quality in the eyes, tremor of the hands, weight loss with increased appetite, rapid pulse, sweating, and intolerance to hot weather.

Long-term treatment is aimed at decreasing hormone production with the use of a special medicine that inhibits it. In some cases, part of the gland may be removed by surgery; in others, radiation treatment with radioactive iodine is effective.

Hyperthyroidism may recur long after successful treatment. Both hypothyroidism and hyperthyroidism are common disorders, especially in women.

Other Thyroid Disorders

Enlargement of part or all of the thyroid gland occurs fairly often. It may be a simple enlargement of the gland itself caused by the lack of iodine, as in *goiter,* or it may be caused by a tumor or a nonspecific inflammation. Goiter is often treated with thyroxin, but it is easily prevented altogether by the regular use of iodized table and cooking salt. Treatment of other problems varies, but surgery is usually recommended for a tumor, especially if the surrounding organs are being obstructed.

The Adrenal Glands

The adrenals are paired glands located just above each kidney. Their outer part is called the *cortex.* The inner part is called the *medulla* and is not governed by the anterior pituitary. The cortex produces several hormones that affect the metabolism of salt, water, carbohydrate, fat, and protein, as well as secondary sex characteristics, skin pigmentation, and resistance to infection.

An insufficiency of these hormones can be caused by bacterial infection of the cortex, especially by *meningococcus;* by a hemorrhage into it; by an obstruction of blood flow into it; by its destruction because of tuberculosis; or by one of several unusual diseases.

In one type of sudden or acute underfunctioning of the cortex, the patient has a high fever, mental confusion, and circulatory collapse. Unless treated promptly, the disorder is likely to be fatal. When it persists after treatment, or when it develops gradually, it is called *Addison's disease* and is usually chronic. The patient suffers from weakness, loss of body

The Adrenal Glands

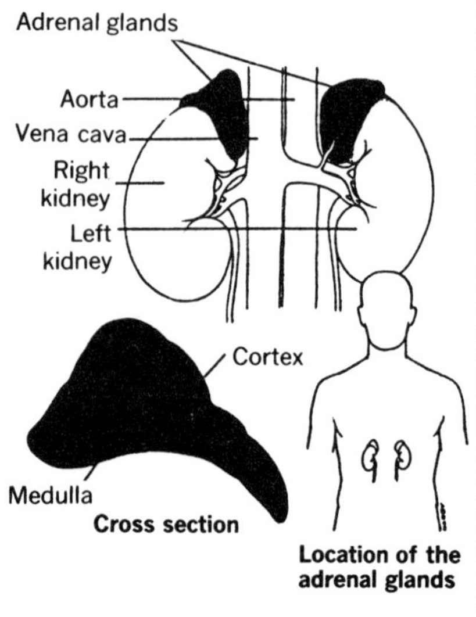

Adrenal Glands

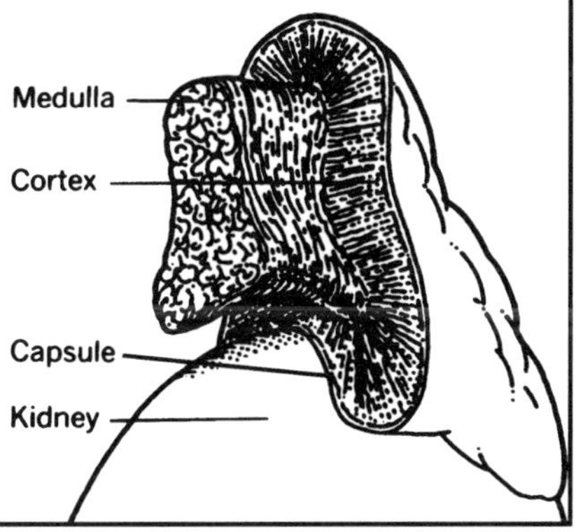

hair, and increased skin pigmentation. Hormone-replacement treatment is essential, along with added salt for as long as hypofunction persists.

The formation of an excess of certain cortical hormones (i.e., hormones produced in the adrenal cortex)—a disorder known as *Cushing's syndrome*—may be caused by a tumor of the anterior pituitary gland, which produces too much specific stimulating hormone, or by a tumor of one or both of the adrenal glands. It is a rare disease, more common in women, especially following pregnancy. Symptoms include weakness, loss of muscle tissue, the appearance of purple streaks in the skin, and an oval or "moon" face.

Treatment involves eliminating the overproducing tissue either by surgery or irradiation and then replacing any hormonal deficiencies with proper medication.

An excess of certain other cortical hormones because of an increase in cortical tissue or a tumor can result in the early onset of puberty in boys, or in an increase in the sexuality of females of any age. Surgical removal of the overproducing tissue is the only treatment.

The Adrenal Medulla

The medulla of the adrenal glands secretes two hormones: *epinephrine* (or *adrenaline*) and *norepinephrine*. Although they contribute to the proper functioning of the heart and blood vessels, neither one is absolutely indispensable. Disease caused by hypofunction of the medulla is unknown. Hyperfunction is a rare cause of sustained high blood pressure. Even more rarely, it causes episodic or paroxysmal high blood pressure accompanied by such symptoms as throbbing headache, profuse perspiration, and severe anxiety. The disorder is caused by a tumor effectively treated by surgical removal. Cancer of the adrenal medulla is extremely rare and virtually incurable.

Changes in hormone production can be caused by many intangible factors and are often temporary disorders. However, persistent or recurrent symptoms should be brought to a physician's attention. The accurate diagnosis of an endocrine disease depends on careful professional evaluation of specific laboratory tests, individual medical history, and thorough examination. No one should take hormones or medicines that affect hormone production without this type of evaluation, since their misuse can cause major problems.

Male Sex Glands

The male sex glands, or *gonads,* are the two testicles normally located in the *scrotum.* In addition to producing sperm, the testicles also manufacture the male hormone called *testosterone.* This hormone is responsible for the development and maintenance of secondary sex characteristics as well as for the male *libido,* or sexual impulse. Only one normal testicle is needed for full function.

Testicular Hypofunction

Hypofunction of one or both of the testicles can result from an abnormality in prenatal development, from infections such as mumps or tuberculosis, from injury, or from the increased temperature to which undescended testicles are exposed.

When hypofunction occurs before puberty, there is failure in the development of secondary sex characteristics. The sex organs do not enlarge; facial, pubic, and armpit hair fails to appear; and the normal voice change does not occur. Fertility and libido also fail to develop. A person with this combination of abnormalities is called a *eunuch.*

If the disorder is secondary to anterior pituitary disease, it is called *Froehlich's syndrome.* When it occurs after puberty, the body changes are less striking, but there may be a loss of fertility and libido. The primary disease is usually treated by surgery, and testosterone may be given. If the disorder is secondary to anterior pituitary disease, the gonad-stimulating hormone should be administered.

Testicular hypofunction is rare because it results only when both testicles are damaged in some way. Although mumps may involve the testicles, it is rarely the cause of sterility, even though this is greatly feared. Even so, everyone should be immunized against mumps in infancy.

It is advisable to wear an appropriate athletic supporter to protect the testicles when engaged in strenuous athletics or when there is a possibility that they might be injured. However, nothing that restricts scro-

The Gonads

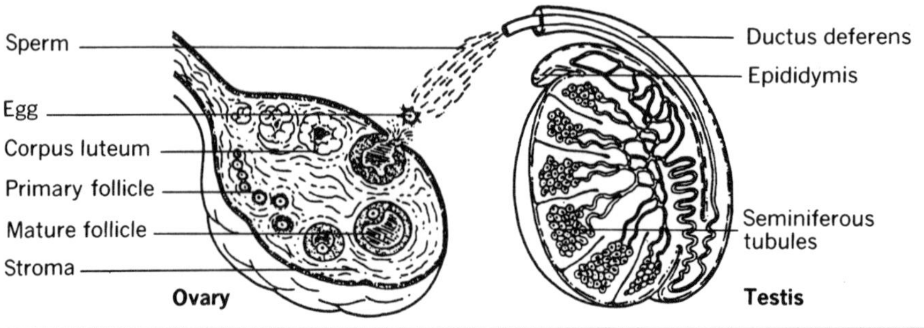

tal movement should be worn regularly, since movement is essential for the maintenance of constant testicular temperature.

A sudden decrease in sexual drive or performance may be caused by disease, trauma, or emotional factors. In certain cases administering male hormones may relieve the condition. However, a decrease in sexual drive is one of the natural consequences of aging. It is not a disease and should not be treated with testosterone.

Testicular Hyperfunction

Testicular hyperfunction is extremely rare and is usually caused by a tumor. Before puberty, the condition results in the precocious development of secondary sex characteristics; after puberty, in the accentuation of these characteristics. Such a tumor must be removed surgically or destroyed by irradiation.

Cancer can develop in a testicle without causing any functional change. It is relatively uncommon. When it appears, it shows up first as a painless enlargement. The cancer cells then usually spread quickly to other organs and have a fatal result. Prompt treatment by surgery and irradiation can sometimes arrest the condition.

Because an undescended testicle may become cancerous, it should be repositioned into the scrotum by surgery or removed.

Female Sex Glands

The female gonads are the *ovaries,* situated on each side of and close to the uterus or womb. In addition to producing an *ovum* or egg each month, they manufacture the female hormones *estrogen* and *progesterone,* each making its special contribution to the menstrual cycle and to the many changes that go on during pregnancy. Estrogen regulates the secondary sex characteristics such as breast development and the appearance of pubic and axillary hair.

The periodicity of the menstrual cycle depends on a very complicated relationship between the ovaries and the anterior pituitary. Birth control pills, most of which contain estrogen and progesterone, interrupt this relationship in such a way that no ovum is produced and pregnancy therefore should not occur.

Changes in normal ovarian hormone function create problems similar to changes in normal testicular hormone function, except of course for the female–male differences. In general, the diseases responsible for these changes are the same in males and females. However, changes in female hormone function are very often caused by emotional stress or by other unspecific circumstances.

Ovarian Hypofunction

Hypofunction of the ovaries may cause failure to menstruate at all or with reasonable regularity. A disruption of the menstrual cycle after puberty is an indication that something is wrong. A reduction or complete loss of fertility may accompany the disorder.

Both menstrual and infertility problems should be evaluated by a trained specialist, preferably a gynecologist, to determine their cause. If it should be hormonal deficiency, treatment may consist of hormone replacement therapy. In many cases, however, effective treatment consists of eliminating the emotional stress that has affected the stimulation relationship between the anterior pituitary and the ovaries, thereby inhibiting hormone production. Occasionally, hormone treatment for infertility causes several ova to be produced in the same month, increasing the possibility of a multiple pregnancy.

Menopause

All women eventually develop spontaneous ovarian hypofunction. This usually happens between the ages of 40 and 55. It is medically known as the *climacteric* and is commonly known as *menopause*. When menopause happens before the age of 40, it is called *premature menopause*.

Menopause is a naturally occurring process that usually lasts one to three years. During this time, menstrual periods become irregular, levels of the hormones estrogen and progesterone decrease, and egg production becomes infrequent. Menopause is completed when a woman no longer produces eggs and menstruation has ceased completely.

There are both physical and psychological aspects to menopause that affect every woman; these symptoms, however, vary. Many women, for example, experience "hot flashes" (a sudden rise in skin temperature). Some women may have them only once or twice. Other women may have them daily and be physically and emotionally upset by them. Physicians may prescribe estrogen replacement or progestin-estrogen replacement therapy to reduce some of the symptoms of menopause. A woman and her physician should discuss the risks and benefits of any hormone replacement therapy to decide if it is appropriate for her.

Ovarian Hyperfunction

Hyperfunction of the ovaries after puberty is one cause of increased menstrual flow during or at the end of each cycle. This is called functional bleeding and is caused by excess estrogen. The disorder is treated with progesterone, which slows down estrogen production. In cases where this treatment fails, it is sometimes necessary to remove the uterus by an operation

The Pancreas and the Islets of Langerhans

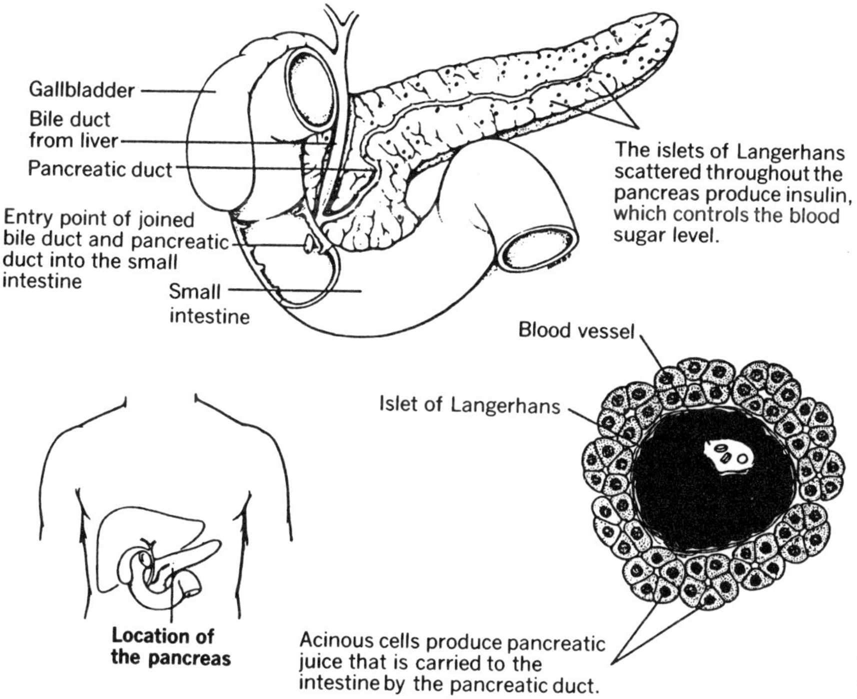

called a *hysterectomy.*

Some diseases of the ovaries, such as infections, cysts, and tumors, do not necessarily cause functional changes, but they may call attention to themselves by being painful, or a physician may discover them during a pelvic examination. Treatment may be medical, surgical, or by irradiation, depending on the nature of the disorder. See Ch. 25, *Women's Health,* for fuller treatment of ovarian and other disorders affecting women.

A rather common cause of short-lived ovarian pain is connected with *ovulation,* which occurs about 14 days before the next expected menstrual period. This discomfort is called *mittelschmerz,* which is German for "middle pain," and can be treated with aspirin or any other simple analgesic.

The Pancreas

The pancreas, a combined duct and endocrine gland, is to some extent regulated by the anterior pituitary. See Ch. 15, *Diabetes Mellitus,* for a discussion of the pancreas and diabetes.

The Pancreas and the Islets of Langerhans

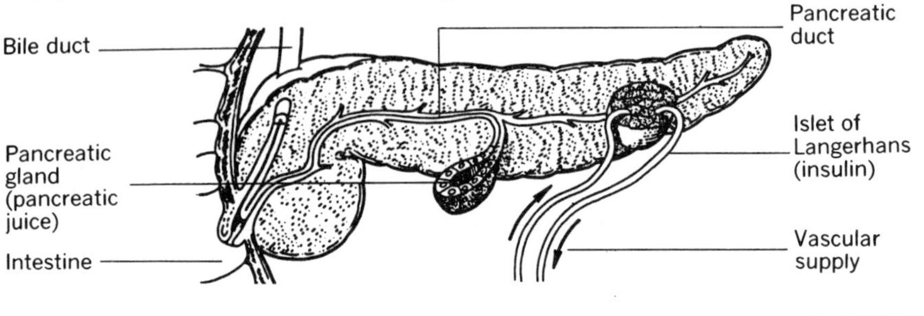

Posterior Pituitary Gland

The posterior lobe of the pituitary gland, the parathyroid glands, and the adrenal medulla are not governed by the anterior pituitary gland. The posterior pituitary produces a secretion called *antidiuretic hormone* which acts on the kidneys to control the amount of urine produced. A deficiency of this hormone causes *diabetes insipidus,* which results in the production of an excessive amount of urine, sometimes as much as 25 quarts a day. (A normal amount is about one quart.) The natural consequence of this disorder is an unquenchable thirst. It is an extremely rare disease, the cause of which is often unknown, although it may result from a brain injury or tumor. Treatment involves curing the cause if it is known. If not, the patient is given an antidiuretic hormone.

The Parathyroid Glands

The parathyroid glands are located in or near the thyroid, usually two on each side. They are important in the regulation of blood calcium and phosphorus levels and therefore of bone metabolism. Hypofunction of these glands almost never occurs except when they have been removed surgically, usually inadvertently during a thyroid operation. In underfunctioning of the parathyroids, blood calcium levels fall and muscle spasm results. The patient is usually given calcium and replacement therapy with parathyroid hormone to correct the disorder.

Hyperfunction is rare and is slightly more common in women. A benign tumor, or *adenoma,* is the usual cause. The amount of calcium in the blood rises as calcium is removed from the bones, which then weaken and may break easily. The excess calcium is excreted in the urine and may coalesce into kidney stones, causing severe pain. Treatment for hyperfunction of the parathyroids consists of surgical removal of the affected glands.

15

Diabetes and Other Autoimmune Diseases

The Structure of the Immune System

The immune system is what protects us from different types of disease. When an invading bacteria, virus, or other antigen enters the human body, a network of cells move in to attack and destroy the invading substance. This may happen without any side effects to the infected person, or the person may develop side effects from the battle between the immune system and the invader.

Blood cells known as macrophages roam through the body looking for foreign elements. When they find one, they digest it and produce something called peptides. These peptides serve as a marker that identifies the invading substance.

White blood cells (lymphocytes) then bind to the marker to "learn" the shape. The white blood cells seek out more of the substance to destroy it, while sending out a signal to the immune system to build up more forces. A result of this buildup is an increased white blood cell count, which is why doctors test blood to see if any infection is present. If you have an elevated white blood cell count, your immune system has detected an invading infection.

One type of white blood cell, the b-lymphocyte, secretes antibody proteins. The proteins work to destroy the invading antigen. Another type, T-lymphocytes, are white blood cells that "read" the markers and alert the immune system to the presence of an infection. T cells can also destroy invading bodies. There are two types of t cells: the helper T and the killer T.

Antibodies are just what the word sounds like, they are cells designed against a foreign body: anti-body. Alter a specific antibody is built up in the blood, some cells always remain to identify the invader more rapidly the next time the infection strikes. With viral infections, once the body knows the shape, it will eliminate the virus before it can make the person sick. Measles and mumps are illnesses that you can only get once because the body learns to attack those cells after the first exposure. Colds, flus, and other common illnesses occur over and over because there are so many strains of them. You do not have the same type of cold virus twice. One single white cell can produce 10 million antibodies every hour. At that speed, a recognized virus doesn't have a chance to survive in your system and make you sick.

This system of defense from infections, viruses, toxins, and other contaminants is extremely important to human survival. Without an immune system, you would not survive for very long. Babies born without functioning immune systems have to be kept in sterile rooms to protect them. The simplest infection can spread and kill a person if there is no counterattack from within the body.

Autoimmune Diseases

Autoimmune diseases are created when the human body stops recognizing one internal part as its own. It fails to recognize the "self" cells and attacks them as if they were foreign bodies. In normal immune system development, white cells are run through a test before leaving the thymus gland. If they fail to distinguish between foreign cells and self cells, they are destroyed. It is this process which keeps the healthy body from releasing an immunological army that could destroy all cells it encounters. In autoimmune diseases, the immune system stops recognizing a very specific part of the body and proceeds to destroy it. Medical researchers are still investigating why this happens and possible preventive measures.

Types of Autoimmune Diseases

Some of the most recognized autoimmune diseases include:

- Addison's disease
- anemia (pernicious)
- Crohn's disease
- diabetes mellitus
- glomerulonephritis
- Goodpasture's syndrome
- Graves' disease
- Hashimoto's thyroiditis

- hemolytic anemia
- lupus erythematosus (systemic)
- multiple sclerosis
- myasthenia gravis
- pemphigus
- rheumatoid arthritis
- scleroderma
- Sjögren-Larsson syndrome
- thrombocytopenic purpura

The area attacked can vary. In diabetes mellitus, the T cells attack the pancreas, destroying the organ's ability to produce insulin. Without insulin, the body cannot break down sugar. If left unchecked, the sugar amounts will reach dangerous levels in the blood and eventually cause death.

In multiple sclerosis, the immune system attacks the long nerve fibers (white matter) of the nervous system. Lesions appear in the brain, and loss of nerve function results. The loss can be the ability to feel things with one's hands, the ability to control the legs while walking, muscle weakness, blurred vision, and assorted other functions.

Each of the autoimmune diseases attacks a different site, or attacks the same sites differently. It is estimated that more than 8 million people in the United States suffer from an autoimmune disease.

Although there is a genetic link for autoimmune diseases, it is not solely through inheritance that someone gets the disease. People with two parents with the disease may not develop the disease, and others with no family history of autoimmune disease have been known to develop one. In identical twins, most autoimmune diseases occur less than 50 percent of the time in both twins.

Managing Autoimmune Diseases

Scientists are studying what turns the autoimmune disease on. The possibilities include the patient having a previous infection, unusual levels of stress, weight gain, or high hormonal levels. It could also be a combination of these factors.

An autoimmune disease does not progress smoothly. There are periods of rapid decline, and periods of remission where the disease is not as influential on the body. The care that the patient takes with following doctor's orders can help in alleviating some, but not all, of the symptoms.

The diseases vary as well from individual to individual. Some patients with diabetes mellitus will live relatively normal, healthy lives for decades with almost no side effects from the disease besides dependence on insulin. Other patients, even under strict diet and insulin monitoring, may suffer from many of the side effects such as neuropathy (death of the nerves in the arms and legs), blindness, and kidney failure. Why patients' reactions vary like this is not understood.

It is essential, though, that anyone with an autoimmune disease understand what behaviors and habits are harmful and avoid them. For a diabetic, controlling one's diet is essential. Although it requires constant monitoring, no diabetic can avoid the strict attention to dietary needs that diabetes requires. Ignoring the diet rules can kill a diabetic in days.

For people with lupus and psoriasis, stress increases the severity of the disease. Because the nerves release peptides that increase the body's immune response during periods of stress, the effect or the disease becomes worse during stressful times. Patients with stress-enhanced diseases may have to take meditation courses, change jobs, and practice daily relaxation exercises to lower their stress level.

Systemic lupus erythematosus is capable of attacking any human tissue. For reasons unknown to scientists, it is almost exclusively a disease that affects females. Only 10 percent of the sufferers are male. The disease attacks a variety of areas in the body, and the attacks differ from patient to patient. The most common areas, though, are the joints, kidneys, and the brain. It also undergoes periods of remission, but anxiety over having another attack can actually trigger another attack. Optimism about the disease's course by the patient can improve the patient's outlook.

Graves' disease also affects more women than men, but not as disproportionately as lupus. Graves' is one of several autoimmune diseases that affects the thyroid. It increases the hormone that regulates the metabolism, making weight gain a common side effect.

There are usually support and awareness groups for autoimmune disease sufferers. Check in your phone book for a local affiliation, and check with your physician. He or she can put you in contact with an organization that will assist you with information and encouragement. Since your mental attitude is very important in the treatment of the disease, it is in your best interest to take care of your spirits as well as your body.

Early detection

If you have a blood relative with an autoimmune disease, you should familiarize yourself and your family with the early symptoms of the disease. If there are tests that can be run (most of these diseases have simple blood tests), then you should discuss with your physician how often you should be tested for the disease. Ask about family testing and at what age your children should start getting tested.

With some of these diseases, science is developing some preventative treatments that may help keep a child from developing the disease. For example, diabetes specialists have several test groups in place to check different preventative measures. If one works it may become available to the general population.

Your strongest weapon is information. Know what to look for, what to expect, and be active in getting medical checks for the diseases for which you and your family are at risk. Avoid the things (like weight gain) that may increase your chances of getting an autoimmune disorder, and maintain general good health.

Diabetes mellitus (DM)

Diabetes has been known for several thousand years. Late in the nineteenth century, when diabetes was well recognized as an abnormality in carbohydrate metabolism (the ability to burn sugar), several scientists discovered that the experimental removal of certain cells, the islets of Langerhans, from the pancreas, produced diabetes in dogs. This observation led to the 1921 discovery and isolation of naturally produced insulin. Insulin is a hormone produced by the islets of Langerhans. Injection of insulin into the bodies of people with diabetes proved to be the first and, to this day, the most effective means of treating the disease.

Until injectable insulin was developed, death occurred within a year or two of the onset of the disease, and usually within weeks or months of development of the symptoms. With injectable insulin, the life expectancy rose dramatically.

An early pioneer in the treatment of diabetes with insulin was Dr. Elliott Joslin of Boston. Dr. Joslin realized that the diabetic patient needed to have a full understanding of his disease so that he could take care of himself. He knew that the diabetic, with the chronic abnormality of a delicate and dynamic metabolic process, could not be cared for successfully solely by knowledgeable physicians. The patient and his family had to be informed about the disease and be active in the day-to-day management of diabetes.

In many ways this marked the beginning of what has become patient-management of illness. It is important for every type of illness and injury, but it is essential to the welfare of patients with chronic illness.

Characteristics of Diabetes

The fundamental problem in diabetes is the body's inability to metabolize glucose (burn sugar), fully and continually. This is a vital process in creating body cell energy. Glucose is a chemical derivative of carbohydrates in food after they have been digested. Carbohydrates are mostly from plants. They may come in the form of starches (such as corn), sucrose (regular sugar), and fructose (fruit sugars). All natural sweeteners, including honey, are forms of sugar. Nonnatural sweeteners such as Equal, Sweet and Low, and others are not sugar and do not affect the body the same way.

Glucose is stored under normal conditions in the form of glycogen, an animal starch, in the liver and muscles for use later as energy fuel. It is reconverted to glucose and burned by the body when energy is needed.

Insulin

Insulin is necessary for both the storage and reconversion of glucose. The metabolic failure to burn sugar may occur because of an insufficiency of insulin, an inability of the body to respond to the normal triggers for producing insulin, or for a combination of those reasons. In any event, the failure to metabolize glucose results in an abnormal, and unhealthy, accumulation of sugar in the bloodstream.

This failure to break down sugar resembles starvation in its effect. A starved person eats no food, and the diabetic eats food but is unable to gain the benefits of the food because the body is unable to break the food down into a usable form. Eventually the body will start to digest fat, protein, and muscle cells from the body to maintain the energy level. This causes a rise in acid level in the blood which, when left untreated, will cause coma and death. Before insulin was

Injection of Insulin Dose

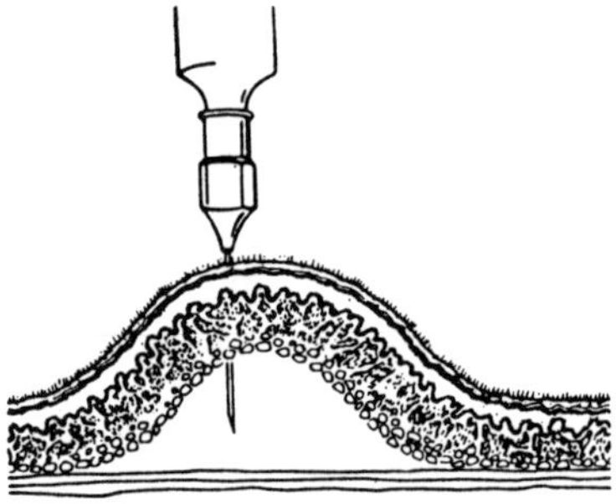

1. Wipe site of injection with cotton swab dipped in alcohol.
2. With one hand, pinch up skin at injection site. Place syringe perpendicularly to the skin and quickly insert needle for its entire length in order to insure injection of sufficient depth *(see illustration)*. The more rapidly the needle is inserted, the less the pain will be. Stainless steel needles are preferred.
3. Inject insulin dose.

Sites of Insulin Injections

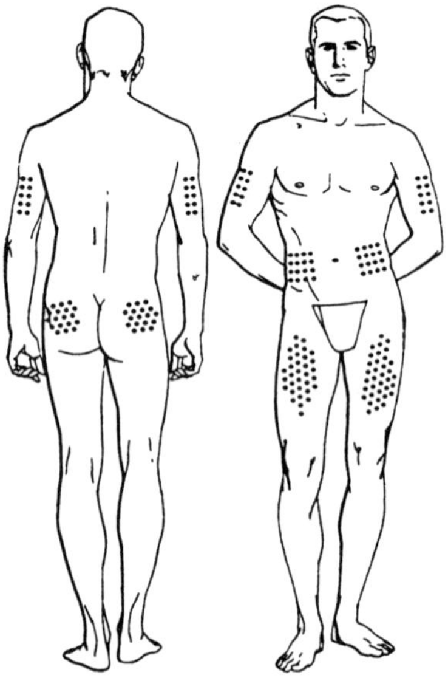

It is important to change the site of injection daily for best absorption of insulin.

discovered, this was why diabetics died.

For most of the 20th century, insulin was prepared commercially in the United States from beef or pork pancreas. There were difficulties from this because of allergic reactions in some patients. Patients who required insulin injections but were allergic to it also had to use steroids and other immune suppressing substances to keep the allergic reaction down. This made them more susceptible to other infections.

Researchers developed an insulin drug that is manufactured with an synthetic duplicate of human genes. Unlike animal insulins, Humulin, the first consumer health product made with DNA, can be produced in unlimited quantities. It has far fewer side effects and is less costly to produce. Research continues to refine and improve the quality of injectable insulin. The effort is to get insulin to match the body's natural insulin as closely as possible in both genetic structure and the speed with which it interacts with sugar.

Insulin is given by injection, usually subcutaneously (under the skin), because the stomach acids will destroy it, if it is swallowed. Insulin comes in several versions, classified by the speed with which it works. Fast-acting insulin usually follows meals. Slow-acting insulin is for evening, and periods between meals. A combination may be administered.

How insulin doses are determined

A diabetic's basic insulin dose initially has to be established by the physician, according to several factors. The severity of the disease, the general level of exercise, the general quantity of food eaten, and the general health of the patient all play a role in determining insulin needs. This is part of the reason for hospitalizing a patient after he or she is diagnosed with diabetes.

Once the dose has been established, the quantity of insulin has to be assessed before every injection. This is done through blood testing and an analysis of the expected activity level to follow the injection and the expected food consumption. The diabetic undergoes training for all these evaluations during his or her hospital stay.

Blood testing

The methods of testing blood have become much more easy and accurate in the past 10 years. A simple pinprick to a finger for a small drop of blood is all that is needed to get an accurate blood reading. Electronic monitors are available that read the blood sample automatically. If a patient cannot afford an electronic sampler, financial assistance may be available through the American Diabetics Association.

After a five-year study, it was determined that the most effective method of testing and determining insulin levels in diabetics was to test blood three to four times daily. At least once a week the diabetic should waken in the middle of the night to test blood levels. With this close monitoring of the blood sugar levels, peaks in sugar or insulin levels are less extreme, and the diabetic can avoid some of the deterioration that high sugar levels can cause.

Understanding Diabetes

There are two types of diabetes, insulin dependent and noninsulin dependent. Except for the symptoms, they are unrelated.

Noninsulin dependent diabetes

In noninsulin dependent diabetes, the patient's pancreas stops producing insulin, or produces insulin intermittently. Although the reasons for the pancreatic shutdown are unknown, the suspicion is there is undue stress on the pancreas. Triggers for noninsulin dependent diabetes are weight gain (including pregnancy), bad diet, lack of exercise, and general unfitness. Patients with noninsulin dependent diabetes can usually be treated by an oral tablet to boost insulin production and a change in diet and behavior. Patients with extreme stress on the pancreas may have to take injectable insulin. This disease is not assumed to be inherited, although the similar body build and lifestyle of parent and child will make the offspring of a noninsulin dependent diabetic more prone to developing the disease.

Pregnancy-induced diabetes, commonly called gestational diabetes, is usually the result of the stress on the body from carrying the developing fetus. In most women, the disease ends soon after the pregnancy. In some cases, though, the woman will develop insulin-dependent diabetes after the pregnancy. The first course of treatment in pregnant women is usually to control diet. If that is unsuccessful, or the pancreas production of insulin is too low, either pills or injections may be used.

Noninsulin dependent diabetes can occur at any age, but is most common in older adults.

Insulin dependent diabetes

Often referred to as juvenile onset diabetes, diabetes mellitus, and type I diabetes, all are the autoimmune form of diabetes. The disease can develop at any age; it is as common to develop in a 20-year-old as in a 40-year-old. There are no age restrictions for developing diabetes.

By the time a patient experiences symptoms, the area of insulin production in the pancreas has been nearly destroyed by the body's immune system. It is suspected that the initial immune attack on the pancreas can start as early as one year before any symptoms are experienced.

The warning signs of diabetes are excessive thirst, excessive urination, a sweet smell to the breath, and fatigue and lightheadedness. Other possible symptoms can include unexplained weight loss (sometimes rapid), extreme hunger, and disorientation. You can have one or more of these symptoms. But it is unlikely you will have all of them.

If at any point in your life you experience any one of the symptoms you should consult your doctor immediately. There are very simple blood and urine tests to determine if you have excessive sugar levels.

If it is determined that your sugar level is high, it is probable that you will be hospitalized immediately. One reason for this is to get you into a controlled environment where your food intake, sugar levels, and urine can be monitored regularly and frequently for several days. The other and more important reason is that excessive sugar levels in the blood are damaging to the kidneys, eyes, and circulatory system, and can cause death in a matter of days if left untreated.

Once you are in the hospital, you will be trained in giving yourself insulin injections, monitoring your diet, and decreasing your sugar consumption. There is nothing complicated about the diet or the insulin amounts. The blood sugar monitoring devices are quick, accurate, and easy to use. The insulin injections are painless once you learn how to do them. The difficult part for most patients is changing their diet. This takes understanding, determination, and will power. But it is essential that the patient follow the diet guidelines.

Diabetic side effects

The most important side effects to familiarize yourself with are sugar reactions and shock, and insulin reactions and shock. They are caused by either excessive sugar or excessive insulin.

Sugar reaction and shock

Sugar shock is triggered when the insulin in the body is not sufficient to break down the sugar. The excess sugar begins travelling through the blood stream. Since the body is unable to digest the sugar without insulin present, the body must turn to another source of energy. Ketone levels build when the body begins to break down fat cells for energy. The byproduct of the ketones is an acid buildup in the blood.

The earliest stage of the problem is called diabetic ketosis; a slightly later stage is called diabetic acidosis.

The symptoms of this are the same as the onset of diabetes, because the same thing happened when the patient was first diagnosed—early diabetic ketosis or acidosis was setting in. The symptoms are: excessive urination, excessive thirst, disorientation, weight loss, dry and hot skin, and fatigue. Call your physician immediately if you experience any of these symptoms.

When the blood gets too acidic, the body goes into shock. If the patient is left untreated, he or she will go into a coma. This occurs several days after diabetic ketosis starts. The unconscious patient will have deep, labored breathing, and a fruity odor to his or her breath.

Sugar shock resembles an insulin reaction, although they can be distinguish from each other. If you find a diabetic in a coma and you do not know the cause, assume the cause is an insulin reaction and treat him initially with sugar. This will give immediate relief to an insulin reaction but will not significantly affect sugar shock.

Diabetic acidosis and sugar shock occur for many reasons. The patient does not take his insulin or oral drugs for several days. He may take too little insulin. He may overeat or underexercise for a number of days. Illness can change the patterns of exercise and diet; the patient may need to change doses of insulin. In any case, the patient should be brought to a hospital immediately, where he or she may be admitted for further observation.

Insulin reaction and shock

Insulin reactions are caused when the quantity of sugar is insufficient to burn up the insulin in the blood. When there is not enough sugar, the blood sugar level falls, and the brain is deprived of an essential source of energy. This was commonly known as hypoglycemia, although the term is not currently used in medicine.

Insulin shock can be brought on by excessive insulin injection, excessive exercise, or undereating. Stomach viruses that cause vomiting and diarrhea need to be especially monitored in diabetics because the illnesses change the amount of sugar being absorbed by the body. Less insulin is usually required than normal.

The first sign of an insulin reaction is usually mild hunger. Sweating, dizziness, palpitations, shallow breathing, trembling, mental confusion, strange behavior, and loss of consciousness follow rapidly. The symptoms will appear fairly quickly. There is much less time to treat insulin reactions and shock than there is to treat sugar shock. Insulin reactions should always be treated as an immediate medical emergency.

Diabetics who use insulin should always have sugar or quick dissolving candy on hand for treating insulin reactions. They must learn to recognize the early symptoms of increased insulin levels.

If you find a diabetic unconscious, give sugar to him or her immediately, then call an ambulance. Some shocks need to be treated with intravenous glucose. Notify the medical team immediately that the patient is a diabetic.

Medical bracelets

Because immediate treatment can be lifesaving with a diabetic, it is important that the diabetic have some identification on him or her *at all times* explaining that he or she suffers from diabetes. If the patient loses consciousness, this ID can save his or her life. Your physician or pharmacist can help you get an ID piece to wear.

Long-term side effects

Long-term side effects are caused by sugar crystals passing through small tubes of the circulatory system. If the sugar crystals are larger than the tubes, as is the case with capillaries, then the tubes are scratched, torn or destroyed by the sugar.

This damage can cause plaque to build up on the inside of the arteries, leading to atherosclerosis and heart disease. It can cause scarring and hemorrhaging in the kidneys, leading to kidney failure and kidney disease. It can cause hemorrhaging in the back of the eyes because of tears to the capillaries and reduction of blood flow to the hand and feet, because of tears in the capillaries that provide blood to the extremities.

This lack of blood flow makes healing take longer, and infections become more likely. With reduced blood flow, the body cannot battle the infection as well, so infections are likely to be worse. Blisters won't heal as well, and scratches and cuts, particularly on the feet, are likely sources of infections.

Since the blood flow to the extremities is reduced, the nerves are not as well nourished and may begin to die off in the hands and feet. This causes unusual sensations and pain as it happens and leads to numbness in the extremities.

With reduced feeling, the diabetic is less likely to notice the small injuries, making him or her even more prone to infections. Particular care must be paid to the condition of hands and feet, and daily visual checks should be made of hands and feet to make sure no injuries go undetected. Catching injuries early helps immeasurably in preventing serious infection.

The diabetic is at risk of losing arms and legs because of the eventual decreased blood flow to the limbs. As nerve impulse is lost from these regions, the body is unable to recognize when an injury occurs. This becomes a problem for the diabetic because exercise is an important part of the daily health care for the disease. So, the diabetic must consider the types of exercise he or she will do with some care.

Early in the disease, these concerns are minimal, since there is still strong nerve response from the limbs. However, as the disease progresses, it may become important to reassess the types of athletics the patient is involved in. Diabetics should consider swimming over running, since there is less impact on the limbs in non-weight-bearing exercise.

Even with good management, there is some chance that the diabetic may lose eyesight, limbs, or kidney functions. Many years ago, these were considered end-stage complications of diabetes. This is no longer the case. Disease management has allowed diabetics to undergo amputations and still survive years after the surgery. With the improvement of prosthetic devices, the ability to lead normal lives is maintained. Laser surgery for retinal hemorrhaging in the eyes has improved the treatment of eye disease in diabetics. And improved dialysis allows patients regular treatment without the discomfort that was previously associated with dialysis.

Improvements in treatment and management occur regularly, with occasionally dramatic results. Research in autoimmune diseases, and particularly diabetes, is enhancing the understanding of and the treatment of the disease.

Long-term treatment

With diabetes and other autoimmune diseases, long-term treatment is a team effort. You, as the sufferer, have an equally important role in the management of your disease as the physician has. You are responsible for the day-to-day actions that increase or decrease the controllable elements that affect your disease. These controls are as essential to the course of the disease as any medical effort your doctor will provide.

So, if diet is an important element to disease management, then you should approach it with the same seriousness that you expect the doctor to approach your treatment. If you are to reduce stress in your life, then do it. Arguing about the importance, the feasibility, or the difficulty of making these changes helps no one, and only puts off the tasks you have to do.

The medical treatment of these diseases will change dramatically over the next several years. Autoimmune diseases are an area of intensive medical study, and the methods for treatment will improve as medical experts learn more about the disease. If you join a support group, are active in researching medical information about your disease, and develop a good relationship with your doctor, this should provide you with the resources to keep up-to-date on new treatments of autoimmune diseases. You are your strongest advocate. It is up to you to make sure you know everything there is to know about your treatment.

16

Diseases of the Eye and Ear

Most people never experience any impairment of the senses of smell, taste, and touch. But it is indeed lucky and unusual to reach old age without having some problems connected with sight or with hearing or both.

The Eyes

All sensations must be processed in the brain by a normally functioning central nervous system for their proper perception. In addition, each sensation is perceived through a specific sense organ. Thus, sight is dependent on at least one functioning eye.

The eye is an optical system that can be compared to a camera, because the human lens perceives and the retina receives an image in the same way that a camera and its film does. Defects in this optical system are called errors in refraction and are the most common type of sight problem.

Myopia

Nearsightedness or *myopia* is a refractive error that causes faraway objects to be seen as blurred and indistinct. The degree of nearsightedness can be measured by testing each eye with a Snellen Test Chart. Normal vision is called 20/20. This means that at 20 feet the eye sees an image clearly and accurately.

Eyesight of less-than-normal acuity is designated as 20/50 or 20/100 and so on. This means that what the

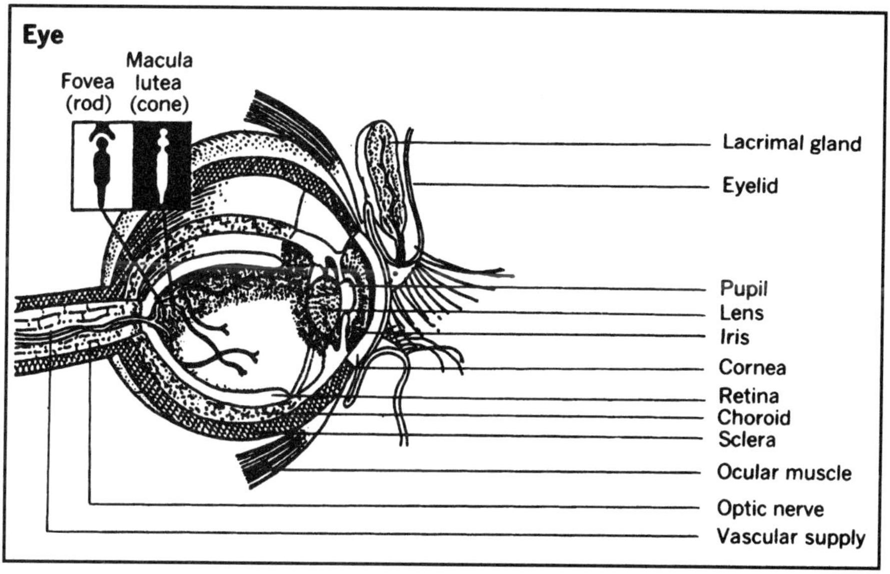

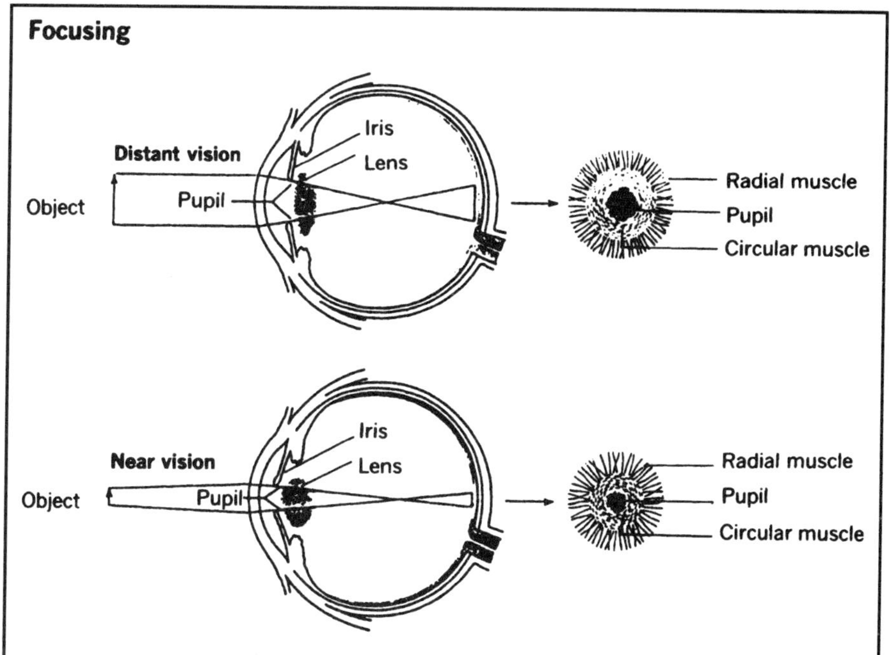

When viewing a distant object (more than 20 feet away), the lens flattens and the pupil dilates, allowing more light to enter the eye. The pupil is dilated by the action of the outer radial muscles of the iris, which contract and thus stretch the previously contracted circular muscles. When viewing a near object, the lens becomes more oval and the pupil contracts as more light enters the eye. This prevents overstimulation of the retina. The pupil is reduced in size by the contraction of the inner circular muscles, which serve to stretch the previously contracted radial muscles.

deficient eye can see accurately at a distance of 20 feet or less, the normal eye can see accurately at 50 or 100 feet.

Myopia, the most common of all refractive errors, results from an elongation of the eyeball that prevents images from being focused on the retina. Myopia usually develops between the ages of 6 and 15. Prescription eyeglasses or contact lenses can correct the refractive error.

Other corrective measures involve physically altering the shape of the cornea. In radial keratotomy, the cornea is flattened through surgical cuts in order to change the way light is bent by the eye. This technique is rarely performed, as it severely weakens the cornea. A revolutionary alternative to radial keratotomy is laser surgery. A laser beam trims and sculpts the cornea in seconds.

Farsightedness and Astigmatism

The opposite of myopia is *hyperopia,* or farsightedness, which results from a shortening of the eyeball. The two conditions may be combined with *astigmatism,* in which vertical and horizontal images do not focus on the same point, mainly because of some abnormality of the front surface of the cornea. Corrective lenses and laser surgery can correct all of these deficiencies.

Presbyopia

A fourth refractive error combines with the other three to make up about 80 percent of all visual defects, It is known as *presbyopia,* or "old sight," and results from an inability of the lens to focus on near objects. Almost everyone is affected by presbyopia some time after the age of 40, because of the aging of the lens itself or the muscles that expand and contract it. Presbyopia can be easily corrected with corrective lenses.

All these conditions represent variations in the sight of one or both eyes from what is considered the norm. Because factors such as seating distance from a school blackboard, the size of print, and the distance at which signs must be read are all based on what is considered to be normal vision, eye defects are handicaps, some mild and some severe.

Many people can function normally without glasses if their visual impairments are minor. But because uncorrected refractive errors can cause headaches and general fatigue as well as eye aches and eye fatigue, they should receive prompt medical attention.

Color Blindness

Color blindness is a visual disorder that occurs in about eight percent of men but is extremely rare in women. It is hereditary, and it usually involves an inability to differentiate clearly between red, green, and blue. It is a disorder for which there is no known treatment or cure at the present time.

Glaucoma

Glaucoma is a serious problem that affects many people who are over 40. It is caused not only by the aging process, but also and more importantly by anatomical changes inside the eye that prevent the normal drainage of fluid. These changes increase the pressure inside the eye, and this pressure causes further anatomical changes that can lead to blindness.

Glaucoma may begin with occasional eye pain or blurred vision, or it may cause no symptoms for years, only to be discovered at an eye examination. Glaucoma is among the leading causes of blindness, and routine eye exams every two to four years after age 40 and every one to two years after age 65 are generally recommended. The test is quick, easy, and painless. Early treatment can reduce the likelihood of any loss of sight.

Macular Degeneration

Macular degeneration is a disease in which the central, macular, area of the retina is impaired, causing flawed central vision. This disease affects mainly the elderly and is, in fact, the most common cause of legal blindness and poor vision in adults age 60 and over.

There are two types of macular degeneration. In *atrophic,* or *dry,* macular degeneration, the macula area of the retinal tissue deteriorates, causing gradual vision loss. The dry type is the most common. It does not usually produce severe vision loss. In the *exudative,* or *wet,* type of macular degeneration, retinal blood vessels rupture and leak fluids beneath the macula. The wet type can cause visual distortions and rapid and severe vision loss. Both types are usually painless.

Although macular degeneration does not affect side, or peripheral, vision, it can be devastating because it impairs central vision, which is needed to see what is directly in front of one.

Macular degeneration's cause is unknown. It is thought to have a hereditary component as it sometimes runs in families. Contributing factors may include cigarette smoking, some circulatory difficulties, long-term exposure to certain forms of light (particularly ultraviolet light and blue light), and low blood levels of certain vitamins and minerals.

There is no treatment for dry macular degeneration, but some cases of wet macular degeneration can be treated with laser surgery to seal off ruptured blood vessels. Certain patients with recent vision loss may be eligible for macular translocation surgery, which involves shifting the fovea (the central area of the macula) and sealing off certain blood vessels. Special eyeglasses that improve peripheral vision can also be prescribed.

Early diagnosis and treatment are key to preventing vision loss. Some doctors recommend having a thorough eye examination every year after age 50.

Cataracts

Another serious eye problem is the development of *cataracts.* These are areas in the lens that are no longer transparent. The so-called *senile cataract* is common among elderly people because of degenerative changes in the lens. The condition causes varying degrees of loss of vision which are readily noticed by the patient. If the vision is reduced a great deal, the entire lens can be removed surgically and appropriate glasses or contact lenses can be provided.

Detached Retina

Among the most serious eye disorders is the condition known as *separated* or *detached retina.* It occurs when fluid from inside the eye gets under the retina (the inner membrane at the back of the eye, on which the image is focused) and separates it from its bed, thus breaking the connections that are essential for normal vision. The most common cause of the detachment is the formation of a hole or tear in the retina. However, the condition may also develop following a blow to the head or to the eye, or because of a tumor, nephritis, or high blood pressure.

The symptoms of the onset of retinal separation are showers of drifting black spots and frequent flashes of light shaped like pinwheels that interfere with vision. These disturbances are usually followed by a dark shadow in the area of sight closest to the nose.

A retinal detachment is treated by surgical techniques in which the accumulated fluid is drained off and the hole in the tissue is sealed. About 60 percent of all cases are cured or considerably improved after surgery. The earlier the diagnosis, the more favorable is the outcome. Proper postoperative care usually involves several weeks of immobilization of the head so that the retinal tissue can heal without disturbance.

Trauma

Like any other part of the body, the eye can be injured by a major accident or *trauma,* although it is somewhat protected by the bones surrounding it. Trauma can cause most of the problems previously described. In addition, small objects can get into the eye easily, and particles of soot and other wind-borne dirt can cause great discomfort. The tearing that results from the irritation usually floats foreign substances away, but occasionally they have to be removed by an instrument.

When a particle in the eye or under the eyelid is not easily dislodged and begins to cause redness, it should be removed by someone qualified to do so. The eye should never be poked at or into by untrained hands.

Leaving contact lenses in the eye for too long can cause discomfort that lasts for quite a while even after they have been taken out. Bacterial or viral infections of the outer surface of the eye such as *conjunctivitis* or *pinkeye,* or of the eyelids, are quite common and should be treated by a physician if they are extensive or chronic.

Contact Lenses

Contact lenses, which are fitted directly over the iris and pupil of the eye in contact with the cornea (the tissue covering the outer, visible surface of the eye), are preferred by some people for the correction of vision defects. In some cases of severe astigmatism or nearsightedness, or following cataract surgery, contact lenses can be more effective and comfortable than eyeglasses. But the chief reason for their popularity has been cosmetic. They are practically invisible.

Hard contact lenses adhere to the eye by suction; a partial vacuum is created between the inner surface of the lens and the outer surface of the eyeball.

Soft plastic contact lenses are *hydrophilic* (literally, water-loving) and adapt their shape to the shape of the moist cornea, to which they adhere. Thus they are relatively easily fitted, and patients seldom experience discomfort in adjusting to them. It is virtually impossible for dust particles to get under them. Many ophthalmologists, however, advise that the soft lens be sterilized daily.

The soft lens has proved valuable in the treatment of some eye disorders. But it often leads to problems among wearers. It may scratch or tear, for example, and generally it has

Contact Lens Insertion

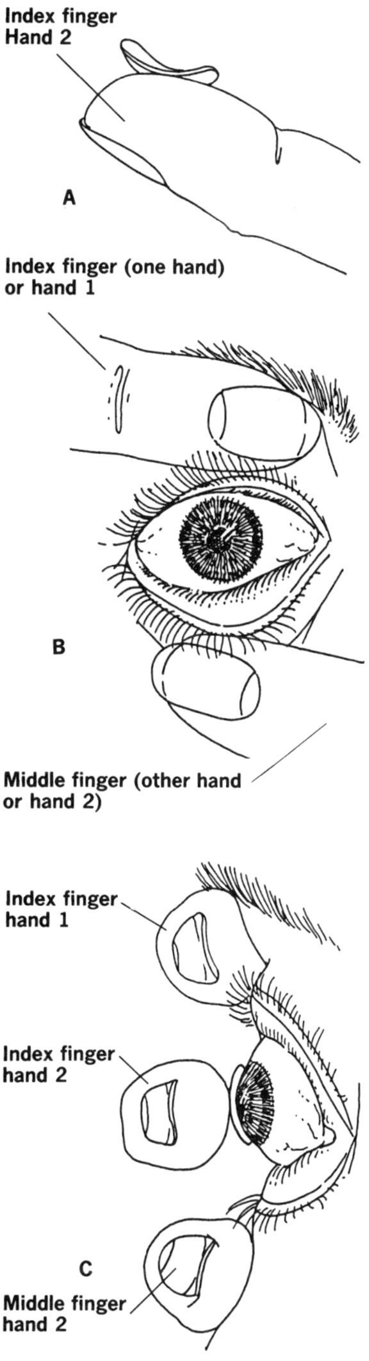

been limited to the correction of certain kinds of nearsightedness and farsightedness.

Extended wear lenses (EWLs) were introduced in the 1970s. Made of soft plastic like the older lenses, but thinner and more porous, they could be worn as long as 30 days. But wearing EWLs too long was found to cause such problems as scarring of the cornea; neurovascularization, the growth of tiny blood vessels that can cloud the vision and in extreme cases threaten the wearer's sight; the development of microcysts during sleep; and bacterial infections of the eye or eyelid, such as *Acanthamoeba keratitis.*

Disposable lenses and cosmetic contacts appeared in the late 1980s. Worn for a week and then discarded, disposable lenses reduce the danger of keratitis and other infections. But they cost about 50 percent more than the regular EWLs. Cosmetic contacts simply change the color of the eyes. Disposables should not be worn longer than prescribed, and cosmetic lenses should not be shared to prevent the spread of eye diseases and other infections. Clean the lenses according to instructions and seek medical help quickly if problems arise.

Diseases That Affect Vision

In addition to the various disorders involving only the eye, there are a number of generalized diseases that affect vision. Among these are arteriosclerosis, diabetes mellitus, and hypertension or high blood pressure, which often cause abnormalities in the blood vessels of various parts of the eye. These abnormalities can lead to tissue changes that cause the patient to see spots or to notice that his vision is defective.

Diseases of the brain, such as multiple sclerosis, tumors, and abscesses, although rare, can result in double vision or loss of lateral or central vision. Any sudden or gradual changes in vision should be brought to a physician's attention promptly, since early diagnosis and treatment is usually effective and can prevent serious deterioration.

The Ears

The ear, like the eye, is a complicated structure. Its major parts consist of the auditory canal, middle ear, and inner ear. Hearing results from the perception of sound waves whose loudness can be measured in decibels and whose highness or lowness of pitch can be measured by their frequency in cycles per second.

Sound waves usually travel through the auditory canal to the eardrum or *tympanic membrane,* vibrating it in such a way as to carry the vibrations to and along the three interlocking small bones in the middle ear to the inner ear. Here the vibra-

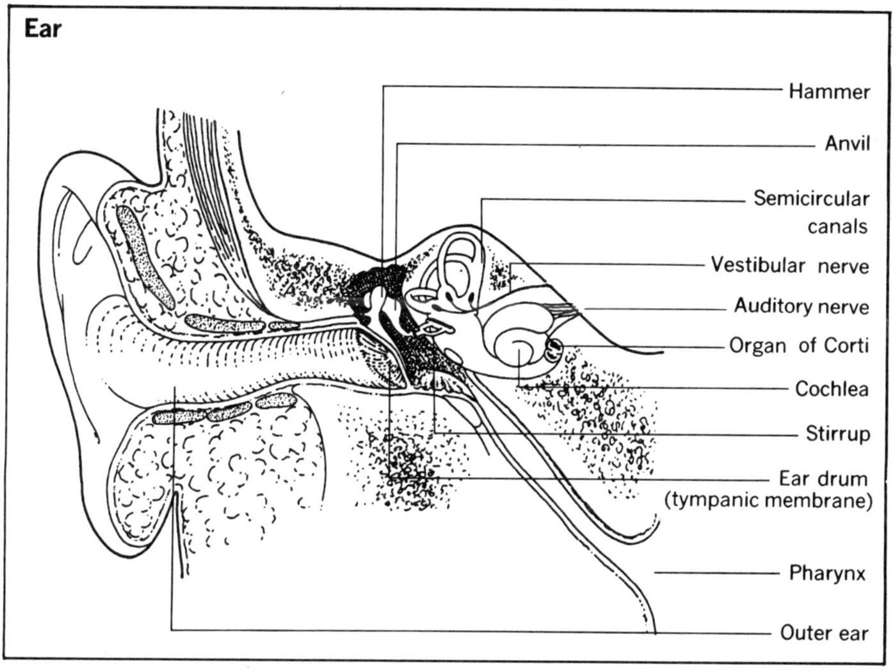

tions are carried to the auditory nerve through a fluid-filled labyrinth called the communicating channel.

An abnormality at any of these points can produce a hearing deficiency. Normal hearing means the ability to hear the spoken voice in a relatively quiet room at a distance of about 18 feet. How well a person hears can be tested by an audiometer, which measures decibels and frequency of sound.

Wax Accumulation

A very common cause of hearing deficiency is the excessive accumulation of wax in the auditory canal, where it is continually being secreted. When the excess that blocks the passage of sound waves is removed—sometimes by professional instrumentation—hearing returns to normal. Anyone whose hearing is temporarily impaired in this way should avoid the use of rigid or pointed objects for cleaning out the accumulated wax.

Infection

Infections or other diseases of the skin that lines the auditory canal can sometimes cause a kind of local swelling that blocks the canal and interferes with hearing. Although such a condition can be painful, proper treatment, usually with antibiotics, generally results in a complete cure.

A major cause of hearing deficiency acquired after birth is recurrent bacterial infection of the middle ear. The infecting organisms commonly get to the middle ear through the *Eustachian tube,* which connects the middle ear to the upper throat, or through the eardrum if it has been perforated by injury or by previous infection.

The infection can cause hearing loss, either because it becomes chronic or because the tissues become scarred. Such infections are usually painful, but ever since treatment with antibiotics has become possible, they rarely spread to the mastoid bone as they used to in the past.

Disorders Caused by Pressure

The Eustachian tube usually permits the air pressure on either side of the eardrum to equalize. When the pressure inside the drum is less than that outside—as occurs during descent in an airplane or elevator, or when riding through an underwater tunnel, or during skin diving—the eardrum is pushed inward. This causes a noticeable hearing loss or a stuffy feeling in the ear that subsides as soon as the pressure equalizes again. Yawning or swallowing usually speeds up the return to normal.

When the unequal pressure continues for several days because the Eustachian tube is blocked, fluid begins to collect in the middle ear. This is called *serous* (or *nonsuppurative*) *otitis media* and can cause permanent hearing damage.

Eustachian tube blockage is more commonly the result of swelling around its *nasopharyngeal* end because of a throat infection, a cold, or an allergy. Nose drops help to open up the tube, but sometimes it may be necessary to drain the ear through the eardrum or treat the disorder with other surgical procedures.

Otosclerosis

A very common cause of hearing loss that affects about 1 in 200 adults—usually women—is *otosclerosis.* This disorder is the result of a sort of freezing of the bones in the middle ear caused by an overgrowth of tissue. Only one ear may be involved, but the condition does get progressively worse. Although heredity is an important factor, the specific cause of otosclerosis is unknown. In some cases, surgery can be helpful.

Injury

A blow to the head, or a loud noise close to the ear such as the sound of a gunshot or a jet engine, especially when repeated often, can cause temporary and sometimes permanent hearing defects. Anyone who expects to be exposed to damaging noise should wear protective earmuffs. Injury to the auditory nerve by chemicals or by medicines such as streptomycin can also cause loss of hearing.

Ringing in the Ears

Sometimes people complain of hearing noises unrelated to the reception of sound waves from an outside source. This phenomenon is called *tinnitus* and occurs in the form of a buzzing, ringing, or hissing sound.

It may be caused by some of the conditions described above and may be relieved by proper treatment. In many cases, however, the cause is unknown and the patient simply has to learn to live with the sounds and ignore them.

Impairment of Balance

The *labyrinths* of the inner ear are involved not only in hearing but also in controlling postural balance. When the labyrinths are diseased, the result can be a feeling of *vertigo* or dizziness. This sensation of being unable to maintain balance is quite different from feeling lightheaded or giddy.

Vertigo can be an incapacitating disorder. Sometimes it is caused by diseases of the central nervous system such as epilepsy or brain hemorrhage, but more often it is caused by inflammation due to infection of the labyrinth. It can be sudden and recurrent as in *Ménière's disease,* or it may be gradual and nonrecurrent. It is sometimes accompanied by vomiting or hearing loss.

Deafness

Deafness at birth or in a very young baby is an especially difficult problem, because hearing is necessary for the development of speech. Although the deafness itself may be impossible to correct, its early recognition and management can usually prevent the development of muteness.

Many communities now have special schools for deaf children, and new techniques and machines are constantly being devised to help them learn how to speak, even if imperfectly. Any doubt about an infant's ability to hear should therefore be brought to a physician's attention immediately.

Deafness at birth can be caused by a maternal infection such as rubella (German measles) during pregnancy.

Hearing Aids

Hearing loss that cannot be treated medically or surgically can often be compensated for by an accurately fitted hearing aid. This device, which comes in many sizes, shapes, and types, converts sound waves into electrical impulses, amplifies them, and reconverts them into sound waves. A hearing aid can be placed in the ear canal, the outer ear, behind the ear, or it can be attached to the body and linked to the ear with wiring. See under "Hearing Loss" in Ch. 6, *The Later Years,* for further information about hearing aids.

17

Diseases of the Urinogenital System

The parts of the urinogenital tract that produce and get rid of urine are the same for men and women: the kidneys, ureters, bladder, and urethra. To understand some of the problems that can arise from diseases of the urinary tract, it is necessary to know a few facts about the anatomy and function of these parts.

The two kidneys are located on either side of the spinal column in the back portion of the abdomen between the last rib and the third lumbar vertebra of the spine. They are shaped like the beans named after them but are considerably larger.

Their function is to filter and cleanse the blood of waste substances produced in the course of normal living and, together with some other organs, to maintain a proper balance of body fluids. The kidneys do this job by filtering the fluid portion of the blood as it passes through them, returning the necessary solids and water to the bloodstream, and removing waste products and excess water, called *urine*. These products then flow into the *ureters*, the ducts that connect the kidneys and bladder.

The *bladder* holds the urine until voiding occurs. The duct from the bladder to the urinary opening is called the *urethra*. In the male, it passes through the penis; in the female, in front of the anterior wall of the vagina.

Symptoms of Kidney Disorders

Normal kidney function can be disrupted by bacterial or viral infection, by tumors, by external injury, or by congenital defects. Some of the common symptoms that may result under these circumstances are:

- *Anuria:* inability to produce or void urine
- *Dysuria:* pain, often of a burning quality, during urination
- Frequency: abnormally frequent urination, often of unusually small amounts
- Hesitancy: difficulty in starting urination
- Urgency: a very strong urge to urinate, often strong enough to cause loss of urine
- *Oliguria:* reduced production of urine
- *Polyuria:* voiding larger than normal amounts of urine
- *Nocturia:* frequent voiding at night
- *Hematuria:* voiding blood in the urine

Because any of these symptoms may indicate a disease of the urinary tract, their appearance should be brought to the attention of a physician without delay.

Kidney Failure

Kidney failure can occur gradually—either from kidney disease or as a secondary condition resulting from another disease—or suddenly, as from an infection.

Acute Kidney Failure

The sudden loss of kidney function over a period of minutes to several days is known as acute kidney failure. It may be caused by impairment of blood supply to the kidneys, by severe infection, by nephritis (discussed below), by poisons, and by various other conditions that injure both kidneys.

The body can function adequately throughout a normal life span with only one healthy kidney, but if both are impaired sufficiently over a short period of time, there will be symptoms of acute kidney failure: production of a decreased amount of urine (*oliguria*) sometimes with blood in it; fluid retention in body tissues, a condition known as *edema;* increasing fatigue and weakness; nausea and loss of appetite.

If damage to the kidneys has not been too severe, the patient begins to have a *diuresis,* or greater than normal urine output. When this happens—usually after one or two weeks of reduced urine output—he is kept on a restricted diet and reduced fluid intake after recovery until normal kidney function returns.

Causes

Heredity is rarely a factor in acute kidney failure, although people born with one kidney or with congenital defects of the urinary tract may lack the normal reserve capacity to prevent it. It is also unusual for external injury

Urogenital Systems

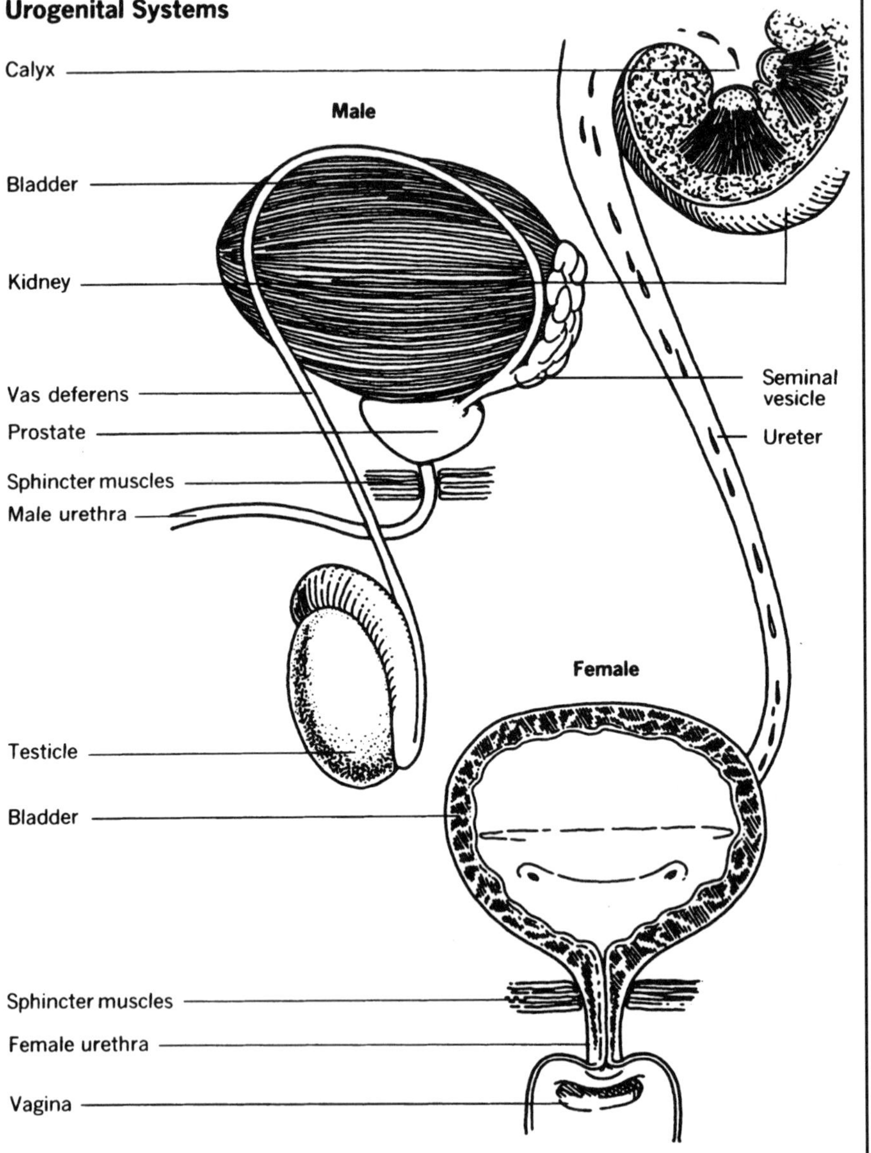

to result in a loss of function in both kidneys. However, severe internal shock accompanied by a reduction of blood flow to the kidneys can cause acute kidney failure.

Prevention and Treatment

Acute kidney failure can occur at any age. Prevention hinges on the proper control of its many causes. About 50 percent of patients with this disease may succumb to it; in cases of severe kidney failure involving widespread destruction of tissue, mortality may be almost 100 percent.

When acute kidney failure occurs as a complication of another serious illness, its prevention and treatment are usually managed by physicians in a hospital. If the patient is not already under a physician's supervision when he has the characteristic symptoms, he should immediately be brought to a medical facility for diagnosis and treatment.

Chronic Kidney Failure and Uremia

Many progressive kidney diseases can eventually lead to a group of symptoms called *uremia.* Other diseases, such as severe high blood pressure, diabetes, and those leading to widespread damage of kidney tissue, can also cause uremia.

In this condition, as in acute kidney failure, waste products and excess fluid accumulate in the body and cause the symptoms of chronic kidney failure. Certain congenital defects in the urinogenital system such as *polycystic kidney disease,* in which cysts in the kidneys enlarge slowly and destroy normal kidney tissue, may lead to uremia. Hereditary diseases such as hereditary nephritis may cause chronic

The Nephron

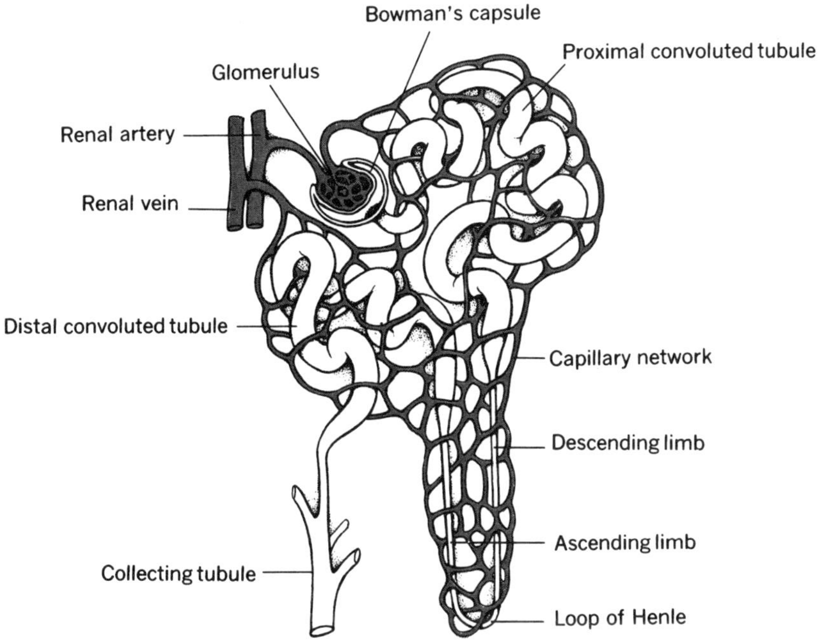

The nephron is a microscopic unit that filters out certain products from the blood. Useful products are reabsorbed by the capillary network. The waste product (urine) is carried to the collecting tubule and emptied into the renal pelvis.

kidney failure, but this is uncommon. Injury is also rarely the cause of uremia.

Although kidney failure is more common in older people because of their decreased capacity to respond to stress, uremia can occur at any age if kidney damage is severe. The onset of uremia may be so gradual that it goes unnoticed until the patient is weak and seems chronically ill. Voiding unusually large amounts of urine and voiding during the night are early symptoms.

Sleepiness and increasing fatigue set in as the kidney failure progresses, and there is a loss of appetite accompanied sometimes by nausea and hiccups. As the disease gets more serious, increasing weakness, anemia, muscle twitching, and sometimes internal bleeding may occur. High blood pressure is another characteristic symptom. Because of fluid retention, there will often be marked signs of facial puffiness and swelling of the legs.

Kidney damage that leads to chronic kidney failure is irreversible, and the outlook for the victim is poor. When the kidneys have become so damaged that they fail to work, there are two treatment options: *dialysis* and kidney transplantation.

Dialysis

If a transplant is not done, the normal work of the kidneys must be replaced by mechanical means using a procedure called dialysis. There are two types of dialysis, *hemodialysis* and *peritoneal dialysis*. Patients also follow a special diet to reduce waste buildup.

Hemodialysis

This procedure cleans and filters the blood, ridding the body of harmful wastes and extra salts and fluids. It controls blood pressure and restores the body's chemical balance. This is done using a filter called a *dialyzer*—in essence, an artificial kidney. The filter is hooked up to a machine that pumps the patient's blood through the filter. The blood is drawn through one set of tubes connected to the patient and is returned to the body through another set. Patients are awake and can read, write, talk, sleep, or watch television.

Hemodialysis is usually done three times a week and lasts two to four hours per session. It can be done either at a clinic, where nurses or trained technicians perform the procedure, or at home by the patient and a partner. Home hemodialysis is possible with patients who, with the partner, can be relied upon to perform the procedure as required after they have received special training.

Peritoneal Dialysis

This procedure, like hemodialysis, removes extra water, wastes, and chemicals from the body. It uses the lining of the abdomen, called the peritoneal membrane, to filter the blood.

A cleansing solution called *dialysate* is sent through a tube to the abdomen, where it takes on waste materials that come through the peritoneal membrane. A few hours later, the dialysate is drained away, together with the wastes it contains. The procedure is then repeated. There are three types of peritoneal dialysis, each using a different time frame and different equipment. Depending on the type of peritoneal dialysis used, sessions may take several hours each and take place several times a day; they may be performed overnight during sleep; or they may be done several times a week for up to 24 hours at a time. More information is available from the National Kidney and Urologic Diseases Information Clearinghouse, 3 Information Way, Bethesda, MD 20892-3560; (301) 654-4415.

Dialysis

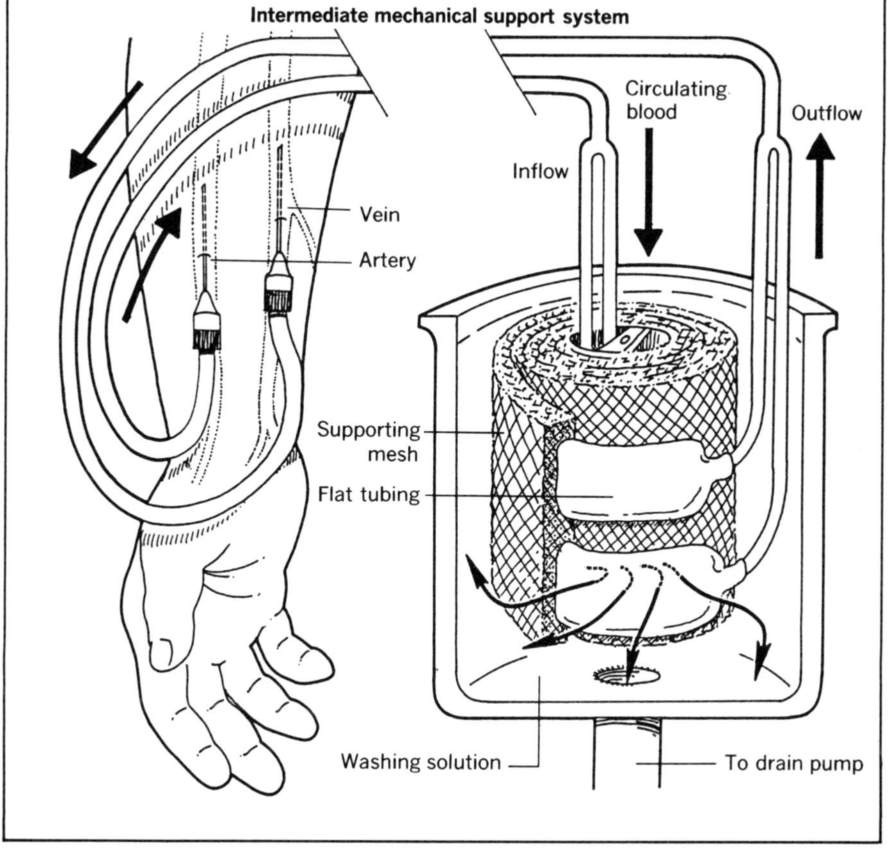

Kidney Transplant Surgery

Some people suffering from kidney disease may benefit greatly from the surgical transplant of a donor's kidney. The donor kidney may be taken from a live relative or from someone recently deceased. The organ is removed from the donor's abdomen, usually flushed with a salt solution, and then reattached to a large artery and vein in the recipient's abdomen and to his ureter.

The successfully transplanted kidney functions just as the patient's own did when he was healthy, removing wastes and excess fluids from his bloodstream and excreting the resulting urine through the bladder. The recipient of a kidney transplant must take special medication to prevent the rejection of the newly installed organ by his own body tissues. With proper medical care, recipients have lived for many years with their transplanted organs.

Medicare Coverage

Medicare coverage is now available for a part of the costs of kidney transplant surgery for those under 65 as well as those over 65. This coverage includes hospital charges for costs incurred by the donor. For details of this coverage, see your local social security office or write for the free booklet, *Medicare Coverage of Kidney Dialysis and Kidney Transplant Services,* published by the Social Security Administration.

Nephritis

Nephritis is a disorder characterized by inflammation of the *glomeruli* of the kidneys. The glomeruli are tiny coiled blood vessels through which the liquid portion of the blood is filtered as it enters the outer structure of the kidneys. There are about one million of these tiny blood vessels in each kidney. The fluid from the blood passes from them into many little ducts called *tubules.* Water and various substances are secreted into and absorbed from the liquid in the tubules. The final product of this passage of filtered fluid from the glomeruli through the tubules to the ureters and then to the bladder is urine. It contains the excess fluid and waste products produced by the body during normal functioning.

When the glomeruli become inflamed, the resulting disease is called *glomerulonephritis.* There are several forms of this disease. One type is thought to be caused by the body's allergic reaction to infection by certain streptococcal bacteria. Another type sometimes accompanies infection of the valves of the heart. The relationship between glomerulonephritis and strep infections is not fully understood at present, and the same may be said for nephritis, which is associated with allergic reaction to certain drugs and to heart valve infections.

Glomerulonephritis may occur ten

days to two weeks after a severe strep throat infection. For this reason, any severe sore throat accompanied by a high fever should be seen and diagnosed by a physician. Prompt treatment with antibiotics may decrease the possibility of kidney involvement.

Nephritis Symptoms

The inflammation and swelling of the glomeruli cause a decrease in the amount of blood that the kidney is able to filter. As a result of the slowing down of this kidney function, the waste products of metabolism as well as excess fluid accumulate in the body instead of being eliminated at the normal rate.

In a typical case, a person will develop a severe sore throat with fever and a general feeling of sickness. These symptoms will disappear, but after one or two weeks, there will be a return of weakness and loss of appetite. The eyes and the face may become puffy, the legs may swell, and there may be shortness of breath—all because of the retention of excess fluid in the body. The amount of urine is small and the color is dark brown, somewhat like coffee. Abdominal pain, nausea, and vomiting may occur, always accompanied by fatigue. In most cases, the blood pressure increases, leading to headaches.

Although there is a hereditary type of nephritis, the more common types of the disease have other causes. When the disease is suspected, the physician examines a specimen of urine under microscope and looks for red blood cells. These cells, which usually do not pass through the walls of the normal glomerulus in large numbers, do pass through the damaged walls of the inflamed blood vessels characteristic of nephritis. Evidence of decreased kidney function is also found by special blood tests.

Nephritis occurs in all age groups. Children under ten have an excellent chance of recovery, about 98 percent. In adults, from 20 to 50 percent of the cases may be fatal or may progress to chronic nephritis, which often leads to uremia and death.

Treatment

It is absolutely essential for anyone with a streptococcal infection, which may lead to acute glomerulonephritis, to receive prompt and proper treatment. Penicillin is considered the most effective antibiotic at present.

Once acute nephritis is present, the treatment consists of bed rest, some fluid restriction, and protein restriction if kidney failure occurs. If there is a total loss of kidney function, a specially restricted diet is prescribed. Complete lack of urine output—*anuria*— may last as long as ten days, but the patient can still make a full recovery if the treatment is right. Usually a gradual return of kidney function occurs over a period of several months.

Nephrosis

The *nephrotic syndrome,* commonly referred to as *nephrosis,* is a disease in which abnormal amounts of protein in the form of *albumin* are lost in the urine. Albumin consists of microscopic particles of protein present in the blood. These particles are important in maintaining the proper volume of fluids in the body, and they have other complicated functions as well. The loss of albumin in the urine affects the amount that remains in the blood, and it is this imbalance, together with other body changes, that results in the retention of excess fluid in the tissues, thus causing facial puffiness and swelling of the legs.

The disease is caused by damage to the glomeruli, but at the present time the exact nature of the damage is uncertain. It may be caused by an allergic reaction, by inflammation, or it may be a complication of diabetes. The nephrotic syndrome may also appear because of blood clots in the veins that drain the kidneys.

Although the disease is more common among children than among adults, it may affect a person of any age. The main symptom is painless swelling of the face, legs, and sometimes of the entire body. There is also loss of appetite, a tired, rundown feeling, and sometimes abdominal pain, vomiting, and diarrhea.

Recovery from nephrosis varies with age. More than 50 percent of child patients are completely free of kidney ailments after the first attack. Adults are more likely to develop some impairment of kidney function, or the disease may become chronic, with accompanying high blood pressure. In some people, protein loss may continue over the years, although the kidneys function in an apparently normal manner without any visible symptoms.

Treatment

Treatment of the nephrotic syndrome has been greatly helped by the use of the adrenal hormones known as *steroids.* The treatment is effective for about two-thirds of child patients and for about one-fourth to one-third of adults. Some patients may relapse after therapy is completed, sometimes years after such therapy has been discontinued. For this reason, steroids are sometimes continued after initial treatment but in reduced dosage, to avoid some of the unpleasant side effects such as acne and facial swelling.

Unlike the dietary treatment for uremia, a high protein diet is used with nephrotic patients so that the protein loss can be replaced. Salt intake is usually restricted because salt contributes to fluid retention and may cause high blood pressure or heart failure. If fluid retention doesn't respond to steroid treatment, other medicines called *diuretics,* which increase urinary output, are used.

Anyone with unusual swelling of the face, limbs, or abdomen should see a physician promptly. Even though the swelling is painless, it may be the first sign of the onset of a serious kidney problem.

Infection in the Urinary Tract

Infection in the urinary tract is a common disorder that can be serious if the kidneys themselves are involved.

Cystitis

Infection of the bladder is called *cystitis.* The symptoms include a burning sensation when urine is passed, the frequent need to urinate, occasionally blood in the urine, and sometimes difficulty in starting to urinate. Cystitis is rarely accompanied by high fever.

The problem may be recurrent and is more usual with women than men, probably because the female urethra is shorter and closer to the rectum, permitting bacteria to enter the bladder more easily. These bacteria multiply in the urine contained in the bladder, causing irritation to the bladder walls and producing the symptoms described above.

Cystitis should be treated promptly because the infection in the bladder can easily spread to the kidneys, with serious consequences. Treatment usually consists of antibiotics after urine analysis and culture have determined the type of bacteria causing the infection. Cystitis and other kidney infections are especially common during pregnancy because of the body changes that occur at this time. Cystitis can be serious, and must be diagnosed and treated promptly to avoid complications.

Other Causes of Infection

Infection of the bladder and kidneys may occur because of poor hygiene in the area of the urethra, especially in women. It is also caused by some congenital defects in the urinary tract or by the insertion of instruments used to diagnose a urinary problem.

Sometimes bacteria in the bloodstream can settle in and infect the kidneys. Patients with diabetes seem to be more prone to urinary infections—indeed to infections generally—than other people. Any obstruction to the flow of urine in the urinary tract, such as a kidney stone, increases the possibility of infection in the area behind the obstruction. Damage to the nerves controlling the bladder is another condition that increases the chances of infection in that area.

Pyelonephritis

Infection in the kidneys is called *pyelonephritis.* Although it sometimes occurs without any symptoms, a first attack usually causes an aching pain in the lower back, probably due to the swelling of the kidneys, as well as nausea, vomiting, diarrhea, and sometimes severe pain in the front of the abdomen on one or both sides, depending on whether one or both kidneys are involved. Fever may be quite high, ranging from 103° F to 105° F, often accompanied by chills.

Although the symptoms of pyelonephritis may disappear in a few days without treatment, bacterial destruction of the kidney tissue may be going on. This silent type of infection may eventually disrupt normal kidney function and result in a chronic form of the disease, which in turn can lead to uremia. If the disease is not halted before this, it can be fatal.

Anyone with symptoms of acute pyelonephritis must have prompt medical attention. To diagnose the disease properly, the urine is analyzed and the number and type of bacteria in the urine are determined. The disease is brought under control by the right antibiotics and by administering large amounts of fluids to flush out the kidneys and urinary tract, thus decreasing the number of bacteria in the urine. In its chronic form the disease is much more difficult to cure because bacteria that are lodged deep in the kidney tissue do not seem to be susceptible to antibiotics and are therefore almost impossible to get rid of.

Kidney Stones

Another cause of infection in the bladder and kidneys is obstruction in the urinary tract by *kidney stones.* These stones, crystallizations of salts that form in the kidney tissue, may be quite small, but they can grow large enough to occupy a considerable part of one or both of the kidneys. The smaller ones often pass from the kidney through the ureters to the bladder, from which they are voided through the urethra. However, obstruction of the flow of urine behind a kidney stone anywhere in the urinary tract usually leads to infection in the urine. This type of infection may lead to attacks of acute pyelonephritis.

Removal of Stones

Kidney stones must be removed unless they cause no symptoms of infection. Removal may be accomplished by flushing out the urinary tract with large fluid intake, by surgical methods, or by lithotripsy, a method of dissolving the stones with electrical shock waves so that the fragments can be flushed out of the body. Any accompanying infection may be treated with antibiotics. A drug, *potassium citrate,* may also be used to keep kidney stones from forming. See "Urinary Stones" in Ch. 20, *Surgery.*

Why kidney stones form in some people and not in others is not clearly understood. Because of metabolic disorders, certain substances may build up in the body. The increased excretion of these substances in the urine as well as excessive amounts of calcium in the blood may encourage kidney stone formation. People who have gout are also likely to develop them.

Renal Colic

Sometimes the formation and passage of stones cause no symptoms. However, when symptoms do occur with the passage of a kidney stone, they can be uncomfortably severe. The pain that results from the passage of a stone through the ureter, referred to as *renal colic,* is usually like an intense cramp. It begins in the side or back and moves toward the lower abdomen, the genital region, and the inner thigh on the affected side. The attack may last for a few minutes or for several hours. Sometimes bloody urine may be passed accompanied by a burning sensation.

Kidney stones are more likely to form in middle-aged and older people than in young ones. A history of stones is sometimes found in several generations of a family, since the metabolic disorders encouraging their formation have a hereditary basis.

Treatment for an acute attack of

Kidney Stones

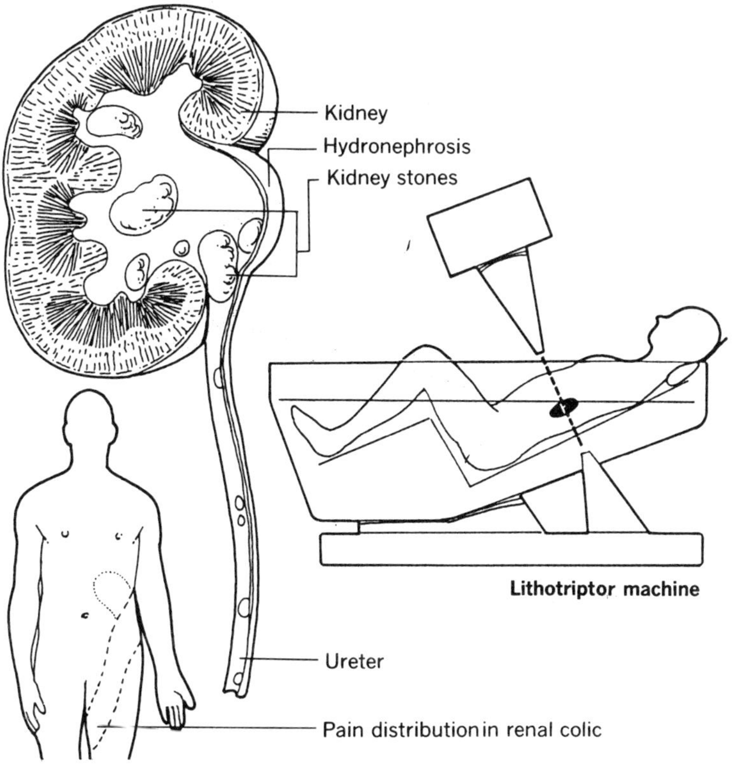

renal colic usually relieves the pain several hours after the patient has taken medication and fluids. If they are not promptly treated, kidney stones may lead to serious infection and eventual impairment of function.

Tumors of the Urinary Tract

Benign and malignant tumors of the kidney are not common problems. However, anyone with pain in the midback, blood in the urine, or a mass in the abdomen should have the symptoms diagnosed. If a malignant tumor is discovered early enough, it can be removed with the affected kidney, and normal function can be maintained by the healthy kidney that remains.

Malignant kidney tumors are most often found in children or adults over 40, and more often in men than in women. A tumor of any type can usually be diagnosed by X-ray studies. Where this technique is inadequate, an operation is necessary to search for the suspected growth. About one-fourth of all patients with a malignant kidney tumor live for more than ten years after surgery.

A malignant tumor of the bladder is a serious problem because it obstructs kidney drainage and may cause death from uremia. The main symptom is the painless appearance of blood in the urine, although sometimes a burning sensation and a frequent need to urinate are also present. Treatment usually includes surgical removal of the bladder followed by radiation treatment of the affected area to destroy any malignant cells that remain after the operation.

Some malignant bladder tumors grow very slowly and do not invade the bladder wall extensively. Surgical treatment for this type, called *papillary tumors,* is likely to be more successful than for tumors of the more invasive kind.

The Prostate Gland

The *prostate gland,* which contributes to the production of semen, encircles the base of the male urethra where it joins the bladder. When it begins to enlarge, it compresses the urethra and causes difficulty in voiding. Urination may be difficult to start, and when the urine stream appears it may be thinner than normal.

Because urine may remain in the bladder, there is the possibility of local infection that may spread to the kidneys. If the kidneys become enlarged because of this type of obstruction, a condition of *hydronephrosis* is said to exist. This disease can cause impaired kidney function and lead to uremia.

Benign Prostatic Enlargement

Enlargement of the prostate gland occurs in about half the male population over 50, and the incidence increases with increasing age. The condition is

Prostate Location

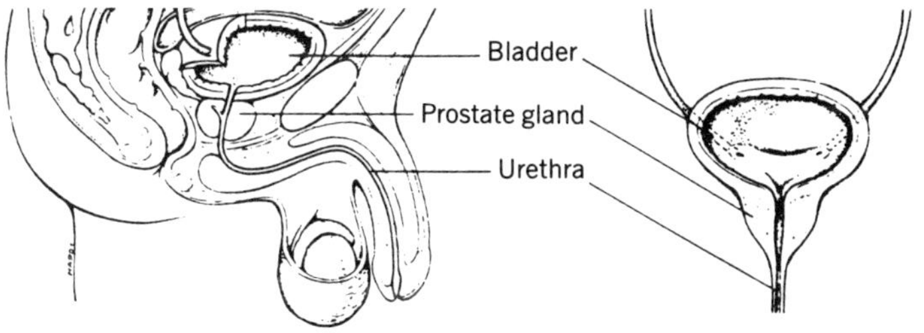

called *benign prostatic enlargement* and must be treated surgically if sufficient obstruction is present. For temporary relief, a catheter can be inserted into the bladder through the urethra, allowing the urine to drain through the catheter and out of the body. If surgery is necessary, the entire prostate may be removed or only that part of it that surrounds the urethra.

Symptoms of benign prostatic enlargement are quite distinctive: increased difficulty in voiding; an urge to continue to urinate after voiding has been completed; burning and frequent urination, caused in part by infection from urine retained in the bladder.

The cause of benign prostatic enlargement is thought to be a change during the aging process in the hormones that affect prostate tissue, but the exact nature of the change and its effect is not clear. It is likely that hormone-containing medicines will eventually be developed that will prevent or reverse prostate tissue growth.

Prostate

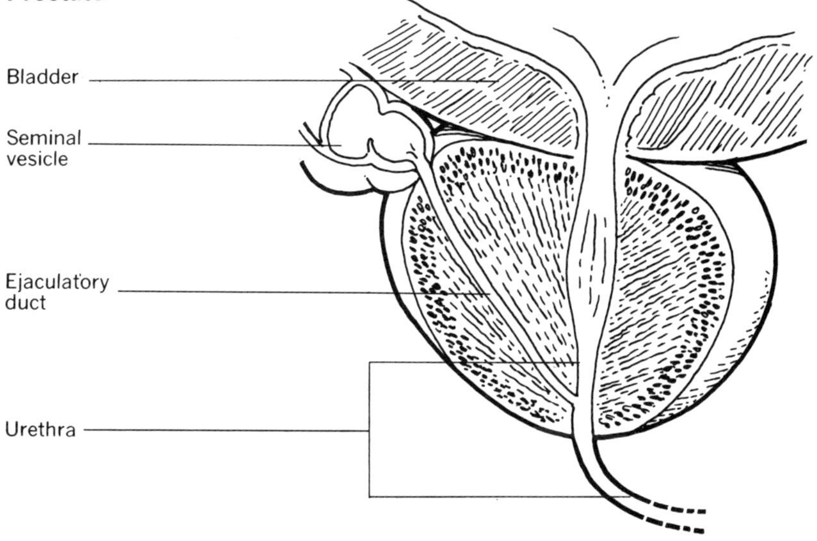

Acute Prostatitis

Acute prostatitis occurs typically in young men. Symptoms include pain on urinating, sometimes a discharge of pus from the penis, pain in the lower back or abdomen indicating a tender and enlarged prostate, and fever. It is caused by a bacterial infection and usually responds promptly to antibiotics.

Cancer of the Prostate

Cancer of the prostate is a common type of malignancy in older men. It accounts for about 10 percent of male deaths from cancer in the United States. The disease may be present without any symptoms or interference with normal function and is therefore difficult to diagnose. A very high proportion of men over 80—probably more than 50 percent—has been found to have had cancer of the prostate at autopsy.

When symptoms are present, they are likely to be the same as those of benign prostatic enlargement. The disease can be diagnosed only by a biopsy examination of a tissue sample taken from the prostate during surgery. If malignancy is found, the gland is surgically removed when feasible to do so; the testes are sometimes removed too so that the level of male hormones in the body is lowered.

Male hormones increase the growth of malignant prostate tissue, but because female hormones slow it down, they may be administered after a diagnosis of prostate malignancy. If the tumor has spread to bone tissue, radiation treatment of the affected areas may slow down cancerous growth and relieve pain.

Men over 50 should have a rectal examination and a prostate-specific antigen blood test once a year, since tumors of the prostate and benign prostatic enlargement can often be diagnosed early in this way.

Urinary Incontinence

Urinary incontinence, or the involuntary release of urine, is a highly treatable disorder of the urinogenital system. Controlled urination is a complex, synchronized process coordinated by the central nervous system involving the kidneys, the bladder, the urethra and the muscles of the pelvic floor and abdominal wall. Urine from the kidneys flows into the bladder, where it is stored until nerves in the spinal cord indicate that it is full. When this occurs, the muscles of the bladder contract in a reflex action and squeeze the urine into the urethra. In toilet training, the brain learns to control this reflex action by tightening the muscles of the pelvic wall and refusing release until an appropriate time. Disruption of nearly any part of this system can cause incontinence. Neurological problems affecting the central nervous system, infections of the genital or urinary systems, and anatomical abnormalities all can cause urinary incontinence in adults. Sometimes, though, no known cause can be discovered.

Contrary to popular myth, urinary incontinence is not the inevitable consequence of aging and is almost always treatable. A wide range of techniques including behavior modification, medication and surgery can improve or cure most cases.

Behavioral techniques, being the easiest and safest to administer, are usually tried first. These techniques involve bladder training and exercise of the pelvic muscles and bladder sphincter. Done at home, exercises such as Kegel exercises require a certain amount of practice and commitment, as it often takes several months to strengthen the relevant muscles. Medications are also available which relax the bladder or contract the muscles of the sphincter and pelvic wall. These medications can have undesirable side effects. Finally, surgery can tighten the pelvic muscles or create a vaginal "hammock" or support for the urethra to prevent it from prematurely releasing urine. A doctor should be consulted for a complete diagnosis and individualized treatment program.

Sexually Transmitted Diseases

The name of Venus, the Roman goddess of love, is preserved in the term *venereal disease* because they are transmitted by sexual contact. But today the broader phrase *sexually transmitted disease* (STD) is more commonly used to refer to both venereal and other diseases that may be passed from one person to another during sexual activity. STDs include some diseases, among them *acquired immunodeficiency syndrome,* or AIDS (see "AIDS" in Ch. 19, *Other Diseases of Major Importance*), that had not been identified as separate disorders until the 1970s or 1980s.

Sexually transmitted diseases were spreading at epidemic rates by the middle 1980s. Because all are contagious by definition, and can often cause serious complications, the symptoms should be treated without delay. At least two of the STDs, AIDS and genital herpes, or herpes simplex type II, are incurable. Some drugs and medications can, however, ameliorate specific symptoms of both diseases.

Except for pelvic inflammatory disease (PID), a serious complication among women, STDs afflict both men and women. Of the 11 most common STDs, chlamydia is the most prevalent. Public health officials believe the disease has spread because it has no obvious symptoms and victims can live for years without realizing they have it.

AIDS

Although not strictly speaking an STD or a disease of the urinogenital tract, the fact that acquired immunodeficiency syndrome (AIDS) is commonly transmitted sexually merits its inclusion in this section. Because the disease may be transmitted by intravenous needles that are shared by drug abusers as well as through sexual contact and contaminated blood, it cannot strictly be called an STD.

The disease strips the body of its acquired immunity against infections and certain cancers and leaves its victims susceptible to a variety of opportunistic infections. These include a rare form of pneumonia and Kaposi's sarcoma, a rare type of cancer. AIDS is uniformly fatal.

A virus called the *human immunodeficiency virus* (HIV) causes AIDS. Researchers speculate, however, that more than one virus may be the causative agent in AIDS. Exposure to the disease does not mean that a person will inevitably contract AIDS. About 5 to 10 percent of HIV-positive individuals develop AIDS symptoms rapidly during the first years of infection. About the same proportion may be infected with HIV for 15 or more years without progressing to AIDS.

Symptoms and Diagnosis

The symptoms of AIDS are common to various other illnesses. Because these symptoms can be related to other illnesses, diagnosis is even more difficult. The symptoms include night sweats, diarrhea, fatigue, rapid weight loss, swollen lymph nodes, fever, and loss of appetite. The symptoms may appear from one month to ten years or more after infection.

The ELISA (enzyme-linked immunosorbent assay), or HIV antibody test is used to detect the presence of antibodies to the AIDS virus in blood. Laboratories also use the Western Blot test to verify positive ELISA test results. Physicians also use the HIVAG-1 test to detect the AIDS virus and monitor its development. In 1996, a viral load test was approved that can identify the minutest evidence of HIV in the blood. This test, used in conjunction with tests that monitor white blood cell counts, enables physicians to more closely monitor the progression of the virus. Two home tests for HIV, Confide and Home Access Express Test, have recently been approved by the FDA. They allow people to take a blood sample at home, mail it to a laboratory for testing, and learn within days if they have tested positive for HIV. Those with positive tests receive the news from counselors, who give them information on medical treatment and long-term counseling.

Treatment

Although AIDS remains a fatal, incurable disease, a new class of drugs called protease inhibitors can reduce the presence of HIV in the blood to undetectable levels when taken in combination with nucleoside analogs such as AZT, dd1, ddC, d4T, and 3TC. Protease inhibitors include indinavir, nelfinavir, ritonavir, and saquinavir; others are being developed. An effective treatment regimen that combines these drugs is called highly active antiretroviral therapy (HAART). Even though the new drugs have brought tremendous relief to many patients, they have not been shown to work for everyone, they sometimes have serious side effects, and they are so expensive that they are inaccessible to the developing world, where HIV is spreading the fastest.

Chlamydia

Chlamydia is a bacterial infection that can cause sterility in men and women and is the leading sexually transmitted disease in the United States. Most women with the disease have no obvious symptoms. For that reason, physicians suggest that sexually active women undergo tests for chlamydia at least once a year. The disease is spreading more rapidly than any other STD.

Persons at highest risk of contracting chlamydia are under 35 years of age. A bacterium, *Chlamydia trachomatis,* causes the disease, which is spread to adults during sexual contact and to babies of infected mothers during birth. Complications affect both sexes: both men and women may become infertile, and women may have pregnancy problems that could kill a fetus. In some cases the disease may be fatal for the mother. Babies infected during birth may develop infections of the eyes, ears, or lungs.

Diagnosis

A new diagnostic technique has led to the hope that chlamydia can be brought under control. The technique, *antigen detection testing,* is a relatively simple and painless laboratory procedure.

Symptoms that indicate the possibility of chlamydia may or may not appear. Men may experience a discharge from the penis or a burning sensation while urinating. Women may have vaginal itching, bleeding between menstrual periods, and chronic abdominal pain. The symptoms may appear two to four weeks after infection.

Treatment

Even though chlamydia is spreading more rapidly than other STDs, it ranks among the lesser STD threats. Treatments involve drug therapies with tetracycline or doxycycline. Erythromycin has also been used successfully. The drugs usually take effect in about seven days. The partner of a person who is undergoing treatment for chlamydia should also be treated.

Gonorrhea

The second most common STD, *gonorrhea,* has afflicted humankind for centuries. Gonorrhea, caused by the bacteria gonococcus, lives in the mucous membranes of the body, including the vagina, rectum, throat, or hollow of the cheek. Cervical, penile, or rectal gonorrhea are contracted through intercourse; oral sex may lead to throat gonorrhea. Women may acquire gonorrhea in a single contact with an infected male; but men face only about a 20 to 40 percent risk of contracting the disease from a female.

Untreated, gonorrhea can lead to various complications. Women can suffer from pelvic inflammatory disease. In relatively unusual cases gonococci can enter the bloodstream and cause blood poisoning. The babies of infected mothers may be born blind. Gonococci settling in joints may cause arthritis. Very rarely the disease leads to *endocarditis,* an inflammation of the lining of the heart, or to *meningitis,* an inflammation that destroys the membrane surrounding the brain and spinal cord.

Except for PID, men experience most of the basic symptoms of untreated gonorrhea. Thus male problems can range from back pains to sterility.

Diagnosis

Two tests, gram stain and culture, are used to diagnose gonorrhea. Women are cautioned against douching before a visit to a physician or public health clinic; nor should self-treatment with antibiotics be attempted. In either case diagnosis may become more difficult.

Gonorrhea is more difficult to detect in women than in men. As many as four out of five women infected with cervical gonorrhea may not realize for days or weeks that they have the disease. When symptoms do appear, they include vaginal discharges and discomfort when urinating. These symptoms, appearing three to eleven days after exposure, may become steadily worse. Urinating may become extremely painful. With rectal gonorrhea, burning sensations, bleeding or mucous discharges may accompany defecation. Approximately nine of ten males know within a week to ten days that they have been infected. Male symptoms are, commonly, a puslike discharge from the penis and a burning sensation while urinating.

Treatment

Penicillin is the most effective treatment for gonorrhea. For persons allergic to penicillin, physicians usually prescribe tetracycline or erythromycin in oral doses. All three drugs are effective in most cases.

Researchers believe the possibility that they will find a vaccine for gonorrhea is strong. Experimental vaccines have been successfully tested on laboratory animals.

Genital Herpes

Genital herpes, or herpes simplex type II, is transmitted by physical—usually sexual—contact. The virus is one of the herpes viruses that also cause shingles, mononucleosis, or chicken pox. The disease is transmitted through skin-to-skin contact with herpes sores or the secretions of an infected person. The virus enters the body through the mucous membranes of the genitals, mouth, or anus.

The first attack of genital herpes usually occurs one to two weeks after exposure. Sores may appear; the afflicted person may have difficulty urinating or defecating. The symptoms usually disappear in ten days to three weeks, but for most herpes victims a recurrence can be expected within six months. Later attacks may be milder, but the disease is incurable and can be transmitted even when no symptoms are visible.

Stress and depression, authorities say, can trigger herpes attacks. Women suffering from the disease face increased risks of cervical cancer. They may also pass the virus to babies during delivery. So exposed, the babies may die within a few weeks; some newborns are deformed, blind, or mentally handicapped. Because of the danger that the herpesvirus poses to newborns, women with genital herpes should alert their obstetricians so that delivery can be by caesarian section. By avoiding vaginal mucous membranes, the infant will not be exposed to the virus.

Diagnosis

Physicians can usually diagnose herpes by visual examination while the characteristic sores are evident. A physician may also take a herpes culture from the base of the lesion.

Treatment

While no cure for genital herpes exists, the drug acyclovir has been found to reduce the severity of the flareups. Acyclovir is applied as a topical ointment, usually for initial outbreaks. In an oral form the drug alleviates subsequent attacks. The oral preparation has been reported to be effective in about seven cases out of ten.

Whether treated or not, later outbreaks of herpes are generally shorter and less severe than the first. Physicians agree that acyclovir effects improvement in the majority of cases, but some reserve judgment concerning the drug's long-term effects.

Trichomoniasis

A type of leukorrhea, *trichomoniasis* is caused by the *Trichomonas vaginalis,* an organism that causes an irritating itching condition in women. Men usually have no symptoms. The organism, a parasite, favors warm, moist areas, such as genital tissues; but some experts believe it can sometimes survive in damp cloths, douching syringes, towels, around toilet seats, on beaches, and around swimming pools. Thus the disease can, it is believed, be spread without sexual contact.

Complications can follow trichomoniasis. Women victims experience discomfort and pain. Chronic infection, according to some researchers, may make a woman more susceptible to cervical cancer. Constant irritation of the cervix is said to produce such susceptibility.

Diagnosis

The trichomoniasis leukorrhea consists of a yellow to green frothy discharge. The itching that accompanies the infection tends to begin or worsen immediately after a menstrual period. Some women report a burning sensation when they urinate. In diagnosis the physician uses a test similar to a Pap smear (see "Pap Smear" in Ch. 25, *Women's Health*), made with a specimen taken from the vagina. Under a microscope the trichomonas organisms are easy to identify because they are pear-shaped and have three to five whiplike tails.

Treatment

Several drugs are available for treating trichomoniasis. They include tablets taken orally and suppositories inserted in the vagina. Most commonly prescribed is metronidazole. Cures may be effected quickly. One dose of two grams (eight 250 mg tablets) may be adequate for both the victim and his or her partner. The oral medication may, however, be continued for weeks or months if the infection resists the drug.

Trichomoniasis victims have reported such side effects as nausea, depression, and hives. Because many persons are allergic to metronidazole, physicians may suggest the use of vaginal douches made up of vinegar and water, or of vaginal suppositories. The latter relieve trichomoniasis symptoms, but do not cure the disease.

Venereal Warts

Venereal warts, also called *genital warts,* may be painless but they can be serious and thus require medical attention. If left untreated, researchers say, venereal warts can increase the risk of penile cancer in men and cervical cancer in women. A pregnant woman with these growths may transmit the virus to her infant during delivery. Warts may then develop in the newborn's windpipe, causing later breathing problems.

The *human papilloma viruses* cause venereal warts, which may appear in a variety of places in the pubic area. The growths are usually small pink bumps, but they can grow together to resemble tiny cauliflowers. In most cases, the growths itch and produce a foul-smelling discharge.

Diagnosis

A physician can usually diagnose venereal warts from their external appearance. To make certain that the warts are not syphilis growths, however, the physician may take a biopsy. A tiny part of the wart is removed for study under a microscope. The papilloma virus can then be identified.

Women with external venereal warts may also have the growths on the cervix. A Pap test is required for detection of these internal warts.

Treatment

The drug podophyllin can be used in solution to remove venereal warts. The solution is painted on the growths, left for six hours, then washed off. The warts usually disappear within a few days. The treatment may have to be repeated several times. If any wart cells remain, the problem will most likely recur.

Podophyllin is not effective in all cases. Where it cannot achieve a cure, other methods, including surgery, may have to be attempted. Among these other methods, which are not always successful, are freezing and burning of the growths. Some studies have indicated that the hormone interferon can prevent recurrences of the disease. Interferon therapy may, however, produce such flulike side effects as fatigue and fever.

Syphilis

Historically, syphilis has ranked among mankind's chief health scourges. Modern medicine has brought it largely under control, but it can still be life-threatening.

Syphilis strikes men about three times as often as women. Approximately half of the male victims are homosexuals. A spiral-shaped bacterium called *Treponema pallidum* causes the disease. Transmittal takes place during sex with a person in the infectious stage in which open sores or rashes are typical symptoms. The *Treponema* bacteria fill the sores and in infecting another person invade the mucous membranes of the genitals, mouth, or rectum. The *spirochete,* or spiral bacterium, succumbs to heat, dryness, ordinary antiseptics, or even soap and water. But it can tolerate cold and survive freezing.

Stages

Unless it is treated early, syphilis progresses from a primary to secondary and sometimes tertiary stages. In the primary stage, the victim may have a painless chancre, or ulcer, that may be small, single, or multiple and that may look like any common skin ulcer. The reddish-brown ulcers generally appear between ten days and three months after exposure to the disease, with a typical incubation time of three weeks.

The secondary and latent stages of syphilis can lead to serious complications unless treatment is undertaken. A month to six weeks after the first ulcers appear, secondary lesions may develop, taking the form of a rash or almost any other kind of skin eruption. The lesions may appear on the trunk of the body, on the face, the arms and legs, or the palms of the hands and soles of the feet. The lesions may or may not itch, and they may not appear at all. The victim may, however, experience fevers and flu symptoms as well as hair loss. A latent stage of many years' duration follows untreated secondary syphilis. In this stage only a blood test can reveal the presence of the bacteria in the body.

If still untreated, late or tertiary-stage syphilis follows the secondary and latent stages in about one case in four. Tertiary syphilis involves the gradual destruction of the central nervous system, the heart, the bones,the liver, the stomach, or other organs. The bacteria can cause paralysis, convulsions, heart failure, insanity, and even death. Attacking the circulatory system, syphilis can cause an *aneurysm,* dilated section, of the aorta just above the heart. The blood flow to the heart is reduced; a ruptured aneurysm can produce a fatal hemorrhage. While gummas, rubbery syphilitic tumors inside organs, may respond to antibiotics in the late stage of syphilis, damage to the heart valves and arteries may be irreversible.

General Paresis

Permanent tissue damage to the brain and nerves can result from syphilitic invasion of the central nervous system; this the chronic, progressive form of syphilis known as *general paresis*. The damage occurs gradually, and early symptoms may include headaches, a tendency to forget things, or difficulty in concentrating. Mental effects may progress from memory loss to psychotic symptoms of delusions of grandeur.

Tabes Dorsalis

Late syphilis involving deterioration of the sheaths of spinal nerves (demyelination) and other destructive changes in the spinal cord is known as *tabes dorsalis*. The patient may become uncoordinated in movement. Tremors of the hands and fingers may be noticed, as well as tremors of the lips and tongue. Vision may be affected, and sensory effects can range from sharp sudden pains to a loss of feeling. The patient may lose control of bladder function or the ability to walk.

Congenital Syphilis

The latent syphilitic condition is not uncommon, and it is a period of great danger to the fetus if an infected woman, especially a recently infected woman, becomes pregnant at this time. The fetus can acquire syphilis through the placenta and be born with congenital syphilis. Or it can be stillborn or die shortly after birth. Some of the signs of syphilis in an infant born with the congenital form of the disease are similar to those of secondary syphilis. Others are very different, more closely resembling tertiary syphilis. Because of the hazards to the child, most physicians test the mother's blood for the presence of the spirochete during the first three months of pregnancy and during the last three months; syphilis acquired during pregnancy is especially likely to affect the fetus. Treatment of the mother has the added benefit of treating the fetus. Treatment begun before the eighteenth week of pregnancy will prevent syphilis from developing; treatment begun after the eighteenth week will cure the fetus of syphilis.

Diagnosis

Because the symptoms of syphilis may appear sporadically or not at all, and because they so closely resemble the symptoms of other diseases, diagnosis usually calls for a blood test. If a chancre has developed, the physician may take a scraping from the lesion and order a special microscopic examination.

Treatment

Long-lasting penicillin, given by intravenous injection, usually cures syphilis. But the disease can, as noted, cause irreversible damage if allowed to spread unchecked. For persons who are allergic to penicillin, physicians may prescribe tetracycline or erythromycin. Both are effective as treatments.

Pelvic Inflammatory Disease

Pelvic inflammatory disease (PID) is a serious complication of STDs. It affects women as a result of infection from a number of diseases including chlamydia and gonorrhea. To produce PID, a disease has to progress to the point where it leads to inflammation and abscesses of a victim's Fallopian tubes, ovaries, and pelvis.

One woman in about seven who contract PID becomes infertile. On the average, three of four women experiencing attacks of the disease will be unable to conceive.

Diagnosis and Treatment

Physicians can diagnose PID by conducting abdominal and pelvic examinations as well as various laboratory tests.

Antibiotics are prescribed in some cases. In more severe cases, surgery may be necessary. The surgery usually results in infertility.

Lymphogranuloma Venereum

This disease, also known as LGV and *lymphogranuloma inguinale,* is a venereal disease that produces a primary lesion like a small blister, which ruptures to form a small ulcer. It is caused by a virus that is spread by sexual intercourse, although sexual contact is not necessary for transmission of the disease. It can be acquired by contact with the fluid excreted by a lesion.

The primary lesion usually appears in the genital area within one to three weeks after contact with an infected person. It may appear only briefly or be so small as to go unnoticed. But the disease spreads to neighboring lymph nodes, where the next sign of the disorder appears 10 days to a month later. The swelling of the lymph nodes (forming *buboes*) is often the first symptom to be noted by the patient; the lymph nodes become matted together and hard, forming channels (or *fistulas*) through which pus drains to the surface of the skin. Enlargement of the lymph nodes may produce painful swelling of the external genitalia. The lymph-node involvement may spread to the anal region, leading to rectal constriction and painful bowel movements.

Diagnosis and Treatment

Because the lesions of lymphogranuloma venereum may resemble those of syphilis, chancroid, or certain nonvenereal diseases, physicians usually make a number of tests to determine whether or not the condition is, in fact, LGV. Therapy includes administration of antibiotics and sulfa drugs for a period of about a week to a month, depending on the severity of the infection.

Chancroid

Chancroid, or *soft chancre,* is a venereal disease transmitted by a bacterium that causes a tender, painful ulcer. The ulcer, which may erode deeply into the tissues, follows the formation of a primary pustule at the site of infection. The pustule appears within five days after contact with an infected person. While essentially a venereal disease, like other venereal diseases it is transmissible without sexual intercourse. Physicians, for example, have been known to develop a soft chancre on a finger after examining an infected patient.

Diagnosis and Treatment

Physicians usually do tests to make sure that the lesion is not a syphilitic chancre. Although the disease can spread from the genital region to other parts of the body, the soft chancre generally is self-limiting. Therapy consists of administration of sulfa drugs or tetracycline.

Granuloma Inguinale

Granuloma inguinale, also called *granuloma venereum,* is not the same, in spite of the similarity in name, as lymphogranuloma venereum. The former is an insidious, chronic venereal disease that produces lesions on the skin or mucous membrane of the genital or anal regions. The first sign of the infection may be a painless papule or nodule that leaves an ulcer with a reddish granular base. If untreated, the lesions tend to spread to the lower abdomen and thighs. In time, the sores produce a sour, pungent odor.

Treatment

Antibiotics such as streptomycin and tetracycline are prescribed. Relapses may occur and cure may be slow, especially in cases of long standing.

External Venereal Maladies

The two conditions described below, one related to viruses and one a parasitic infestation, may generally be considered sources of discomfort and disfigurement rather than threats to general health. Both of these STDs are transmissible by other means besides sexual contact.

Molluscum Contagiosum

A viral disease transmitted during sexual intercourse is known by the medical term *molluscum contagiosum.* The disease can also be transmitted by ordinary person-to-person contact, as between members of a family or children in a classroom. The virus causes raised lesions containing a waxy white material. The lesions, which may be very small or as large as an inch in diameter, occur on the skin or mucous membranes, commonly in the anal or genital area but sometimes on the face or torso. The lesions may last for several months or several years, then disappear spontaneously, or they may be removed by medications or surgery.

Pubic Lice

Infestations of pubic lice constitute a unique kind of venereal disease. Pubic lice, known popularly as crabs, are a species somewhat larger than body and head lice but still almost invisible to the naked eye. These whitish, oval parasites usually remain in the hair of the anal and genital regions, but they may sometimes be found attached to the skin at the base of any body hair, including eyelashes and scalp. A very few pubic lice in the anal and genital areas can cause intense irritation and itching. The itching results in scratching which, in turn, produces abrasions of the skin. The lice may also produce patches of bluish spots on the skin of the inner thighs and lower abdomen. Another sign of their presence is the appearance of tiny brown specks deposited by the lice on the inside of undergarments.

Pubic lice are commonly spread by sexual contact, but they can be acquired from toilet seats, clothing, towels, bedclothes, combs, or any article of intimate use. Creams or ointments containing various parasiticides are available for disinfestation. They are applied every night for several nights, but overuse should be avoided because of the danger of injury to the tender tissues of the genital and anal region. Some physicians recommend soaking the infested part of the body several times daily in a mild solution of potassium permanganate. Lice on the eyebrows and eyelashes may have to be removed individually with a pair of tweezers. Treatment must be repeated after one week to kill the nits (eggs) that have hatched since the first treatment. Clothing and other contaminated materials must be cleaned to prevent reinfestation.

Complications of an infestation of pubic lice include intense itching (known medically as *pruritus*) and secondary infections from scratching. These may require special medical care and administration of antibiotics, corticosteroid creams, or other appropriate remedies.

18

Cancer

Cancer has always figured uniquely in the diseases of humankind. For centuries people spoke of it only in whispers, or not at all, as if the disease were not only dreadful but somehow shameful as well. Today, the picture is changing rapidly. More than half of those diagnosed with cancer will reach the important five-year survival landmark. Having no evidence of cancer for five years or more is the definition of being cured of it. Also, much of the mystery that cloaked the disease has dissipated.

Of course, cancer remains a formidable enemy. Cancer is one of the leading causes of death in the United States; it causes nearly one in four deaths. About 1.4 million new cases of cancer are diagnosed annually in the United States, and more than 500,000 people die of it each year. The National Institutes of Health estimate that cancer costs society more than $100 billion annually in direct medical costs and loss of productivity.

But in context, the picture is not as bleak as it might seem. At the beginning of the twentieth century, survival from cancer was relatively rare. At the end of the 1930s, the five-year survival rate was one in five or lower. Ten years later it had shot up to one in four, and in the mid-fifties to one in three. By 2000, 4 of every 10 persons in the United States who were diagnosed with cancer survived. Improvements in survival rates will come with improved detection methods and preventive measures. The survival rate for some of the more widespread cancers has leveled off despite the best efforts of physicians to devise better forms of treatment.

Scientists have identified certain risk factors that increase the chances of developing cancer. Avoiding these factors is well-advised. They include tobacco use, sun exposure, excessive alcohol consumption, estrogen therapy, radiation exposure, exposure to certain industrial agents, such as asbestos and vinyl chloride, and diets high in fats or smoked, salt-cured, or nitrite-cured foods. Conversely, many doctors believe that a high-fiber diet that includes daily consumption of vegetables and foods high in vitamins A and C may decrease the risk of cancer.

Considerable progress is being made on many fronts in the war

Normal cells

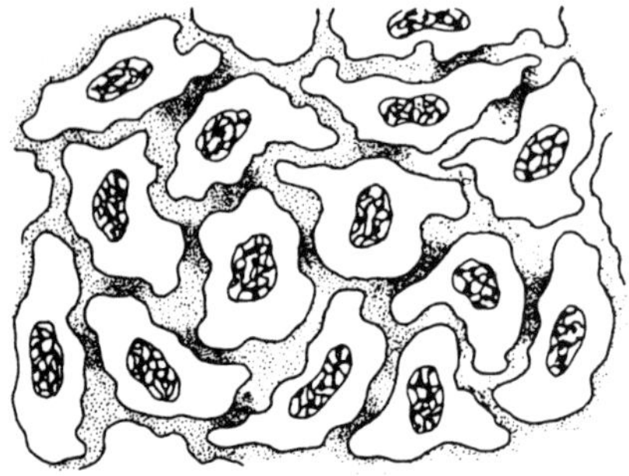

1. Cell surface bonding is strong.
2. Cells remain in place.
3. Electrical voltage level is high.
4. Cells divide at a low rate.

Malignant cells

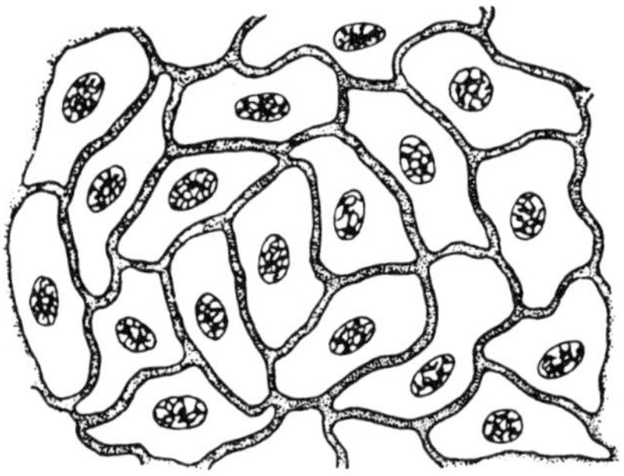

1. Cell surface bonding is very weak.
2. Cells spread and invade normal tissue.
3. Electrical voltage level is low.
4. Cells divide at a rapid pace.

against cancer. It ranges from advances in early detection to breakthroughs in treatment. Between the mid-1950s and early 1990s, for example, the death rate from cervical cancer—which used to be one of the most common causes of death in American women—declined by 74 percent, mostly because of the widespread use of the Pap test, which can detect the disease at an early stage. At the same time, children with acute lymphocytic leukemia, which used to be invariably fatal in weeks or months, have benefited from new therapies. The probability of an extended remission or cure was more than 75 percent in the mid-1990s; it was just 5 percent in 1960. Similar advances in the treatment of a cancer of the lymph system called *Hodgkin's disease* have improved from the five-year survival rate from 25 percent at the end of World War II to about 80 percent today.

What is Cancer?

Cancer would surely be easier to detect and treat if it were a single entity with a single simple cause. But it is not. Experts agree that there are more than 100 different kinds of cancer. They have different causes, originate in different tissues, develop for different reasons and in different ways, and demand vastly different kinds of treatment.

Nevertheless, all cancers have one element in common—abnormal cell behavior; specifically, uncontrolled and unregulated cell growth. Somehow in cancer cells, the normal mechanism whereby cells stop dividing ceases to work. This uncontrolled growth can then displace and injure nearby normal cells. Scientists believe this process starts because the genes in those cells have been damaged by either external factors (such as exposure to radiation) or by internal factors (such as inherited genetic mutations).

Initial Stages

The cancer may start with just one or a few cells somewhere in the body that undergo a change and become malignant, or cancerous. The cells divide and reproduce themselves, and the cancer grows.

Most cancers arise on the surface of a tissue, such as the skin, the lining of the uterus, mouth, stomach, bowel, bladder, or bronchial tube in the lung, or outside a duct in the breast, prostate gland, or other site. The cancer grows from a microscopic clump to a visible mass, then begins to invade underlying tissues. As long as the cells remain in one mass, however, the cancer is said to be localized.

Later Stages

At some later phase, in a process called *metastasis,* some of the cancer cells split off and are swept into the lymph channels or bloodstream to other parts of the body. They may be captured for a while in a nearby lymph node (a stage called *regional involvement),* but unless the disease is arrested, it will invade the rest of the body, with death the almost certain result. Some cancers grow with a malevolent rapidity; some are comparatively dormant. Some respond to various therapies, such as radiation therapy; others do not. About half of the known types of cancers are incurable at any stage. Of the remaining half, it is obviously imperative to diagnose and treat them as early as possible.

How Cancers Are Classified

The cancers described above, arising in *epithelial* (covering or lining) tissue, are, as a group, called *carcinomas.* Another class of malignant tumors, similar in most basic respects, is the *sarcomas,* which originate in connective tissue, such as bones and muscles. A third group of cancers—*leukemia* and *lymphomas*—includes diseases of the blood-forming organs and the lymphatic system, respectively, and does not produce tumors. They arise and spread in a basically different way.

What Causes Cancer?

In its battle with cancer, medical science devotes constant attention to a search for factors in our environment that can produce cancer in human beings. They include a large number of chemical agents such as those in tobacco smoke. Other factors include asbestos fibers and other occupational chemical hazards; ionizing radiation such as that from X rays, nuclear bombs, and sunlight; injury or repeated irritation; metal or plastic implants; flaws in the body's immune reaction; genetic mistakes; parasites; and—many scientists believe—viruses.

Scientists have also discovered that certain substances in the environment which by themselves may not stimulate the growth of a cancer can be dangerously activated to become carcinogenic by the presence of one or more substances. Each of these potential cancer-causing agents is called a *co-carcinogen.* It is possible that some *co-carcinogens* are present in ordinary fruits and vegetables, in certain food additives, and in such other substances as the synthetic estrogen diethylstilbestrol (DES). For more information on DES, see Ch. 25, *Women's Health.*

Cancer's Seven Warning Signals*

1. Change in bowel or bladder habits.
2. A sore that does not heal.
3. Unusual bleeding or discharge.
4. Thickening or lump in breast or elsewhere.
5. Indigestion or difficulty in swallowing.
6. Obvious change in wart or mole.
7. Nagging cough or hoarseness.

If you have a warning signal, see your doctor without delay.

*from the American Cancer Society

Major Forms of Cancer

The following material includes discussions of the major forms of cancer with the exception of those cancers that affect women only. For additional information on many kinds of tumors for which surgery might be indicated, see also Ch. 20, *Surgery.*

Breast Cancer

See under *Women's Health,* Ch. 25.

Lung Cancer

Lung cancer kills more Americans than any other cancer. More people die of lung cancer than of breast, prostate, and colon cancers combined. Lung cancer makes up about 13 percent of all new cancers. The average age of those diagnosed with lung cancer is 60. It is rarely diagnosed in people under age 40. The one-year survival rate for this disease is about 41 percent. The five-year survival rate is about 14 percent. Early diagnosis and treatment before the cancer has spread raises the five-year survival rate to about 40 percent.

Symptoms

Although some early lung cancers do not show up on X-ray film, they are the ones that usually produce coughing as an early symptom. For this reason, any cough that lasts more than two or three weeks—even if it seems to accompany a cold or bronchitis—should be regarded as suspicious and investigated in that light. Blood in the sputum is another early warning sign that must be investigated immediately; so should wheezing when breathing. Later symptoms include shortness of breath, pain in the chest, fever, and night sweats.

Detection

If many lives could be saved by preventing lung cancer in the first place, others could be saved by early detection. By the time most lung cancers are diagnosed, it is too late even for the most radical approach to cure—removal of the affected lung. Experts estimate that up to five times the present cure rate could be achieved if very early lung cancers could be spotted. They therefore recommend a baseline chest X-ray for everyone over age 40.

Causes

Lung cancer is one of the most preventable of all malignancies. Most cases, the majority of medical experts agree, are caused by smoking cigarettes. The U.S. Public Health Service has indicted smoking as "the main cause of lung cancer in men." Even when other agents are known to produce lung cancers—uranium ore dust or asbestos fibers, for example—cigarette smoking enormously boosts the risk among uranium miners and asbestos workers. Smoking accounts for about 90 percent of all lung cancer.

It is known that the lungs of some cigarette smokers show tissue changes before cancer appears, changes apparently caused by irritation of the *bronchi*—the large air tubes in the lung. Physicians believe these changes can be reversed before the onset of cancer if the source of the irritation—smoking—is removed. This is why a heavy smoker who has been puffing away for many years but then stops smoking has a better chance of avoiding lung cancer than one who continues smoking.

Until recently, the evidence linking cigarette smoking and lung cancer was purely statistical, although overwhelming. No one had succeeded in producing lung cancer in laboratory animals by having them ingest smoke. However, lung cancer has been introduced in dogs specially trained to inhale cigarette smoke, as reported by the American Cancer Society.

Cigarette smoking has also been implicated in other kinds of lung disease, including the often-fatal emphysema, and in cardiovascular diseases. To any sensible person, then, the options would seem clear: If you don't smoke, don't start. If you do smoke, stop. If you can't stop, cut down, and switch to a brand low in tars and nicotine—suspected but not proved to be the principal harmful agent in cigarette smoke.

Colon-Rectum Cancer

Cancer of the colon (large intestine) and rectum is the second leading cause of cancer-related deaths in the United States. Each year it claims an estimated 48,000 lives, and produces about 107,0000 new cases—more than any other kind of cancer except skin cancer. It afflicts men and women about equally. The five-year survival rate from this form of cancer, usually after surgery, is about 90 percent where the cancer was localized and about 65 percent where there was regional involvement. The death rate from colon and rectum cancer has decreased significantly over the past 20 years due to, among other factors, improved treatments and earlier diagnosis.

Symptoms

It is important, then, to be alert to the early symptoms of these cancers. Cancers of the colon often produce changes in bowel habits that persist longer than normal. The change may be constipation or diarrhea, or even both alternating. Cancers of the colon also often produce large quantities of gas, which cause abdominal discomfort ranging from a feeling of overfullness to pain, intermittent at first then coming as regular cramps.

Both colon cancer and rectal cancer may also cause bleeding. Sometimes such bleeding is evidenced in the stool or on the tissue (the most frequent first sign of rectal cancer); but if the bleeding is slight and occurs high enough up in the colon, it may not be visible at all. After a period of weeks, however, the persistent bleeding causes anemia in the patient.

All such symptoms should be investigated promptly. Unfortunately, many persons tend to ignore them. Chronic constipation, for example, or gas, is easy to dismiss for the nuisance that it usually is. Even rectal bleeding, which demands immediate medical consultation, is often ignored by hemorrhoid sufferers, who fail to realize that hemorrhoids and cancer, though unrelated, can and sometimes do exist in the same persons at the same time.

Detection

For these reasons, the key to successful and early diagnosis of colon and rectum cancer lies in making examination of the colon and rectum a part of the regular annual health checkup.

Common screening and diagnostic procedures include the digital rectal exam, in which the doctor uses a gloved finger to examine the lower part of the rectum for polyps. This is a painless test that can be done in the doctor's office. The fecal occult blood test checks for blood in a stool sample. In the flexible sigmoidoscopy test, a thin, lighted tube is inserted through the anus to examine the rectum and the sigmoid (about the last 2 feet of the colon). In the barium enema test, barium, serving as a contrast dye, is inserted into the bowel via an enema. The barium coats the lining of the large intestine and when an X-ray is taken, creates a clear visualization of the entire large intestine. Many doctors recommend having a digital exam and a fecal occult blood test annually after age 40. A flexible sigmoidoscopy test should be had at age 45 and every three to five years thereafter.

Therapy

The primary treatment for colon-rectum cancer is surgical removal of the affected part of the bowel. Adjacent portions and related lymph nodes may also be removed, and if the surgeon sees that the cancer is widespread, he or she may have to perform extensive surgery. This may require creation of a *colostomy*—a temporary or permanent opening in the abdominal wall through which solid wastes may pass. Although this method of voiding the bowels is somewhat inconvenient at first, most colostomy patients adjust to it very easily and lead perfectly normal, active, and healthy lives. An organization for colostomy patients called the United Ostomy Association keeps up with current information on diet, colostomy equipment, and other problems the members have in common.

If the cancer is at an early stage and is small and localized, it may, in some cases, be removed during a colonoscopy or by using surgical techniques (laparoscopic) that require only very small incisions.

Radiotherapy is sometimes used before the operation (occasionally to make surgery possible) and sometimes afterward to treat recurrence of the cancer. Various chemical agents have been found useful in treating colon-rectum cancer that has spread to the lymph nodes or more widely.

Skin Cancer

With as many as one million new cases occurring annually, skin cancer is the largest single source of malignancy in the United States. Since 1980, the number of cases of malignant melanoma, the most deadly form of skin cancer, has risen by more than 90 percent.

Experts believe that many cases of skin cancer could be prevented if more people avoided exposure to the sun. Ultraviolet radiation in sunlight not only burns and dries the skin; it also is thought to suppress the human immune system and thus contribute indirectly to skin problems. Long and continued exposure to the sun has been associated with cataracts as well as with skin aging and wrinkling.

Symptoms

Persons with skin problems should report promptly to their physicians any new growths or sores that refuse to heal, or changes in warts or moles. Pimples that itch and recur may also be symptoms of skin cancer.

Therapy

Most skin cancers remain localized. They can usually be removed by excisional surgery, with an electric needle, by laser surgery, or by cryosurgery (freezing). Radiation therapy and chemotherapy may also be used.

Causes

Scientists point to the ultraviolet radiation in sunlight as the primary cause, with ultraviolet-B (UV-B), the shorter wavelength band, as the more dangerous. But dermatologists recommend that ultraviolet-A (UV-A), used often in high-intensity sunlamps and tanning beds, be avoided as well. While UV-A is spread more evenly throughout the day, UV-B is largely concentrated around midday.

Fair-skinned individuals who burn readily, rather than tan, are more vulnerable to radiation-caused cancer than darker-skinned persons. Geographic location is also important. Skin cancer occurs more frequently in the southern belt of states, particularly in the sunny Southwest.

Kinds

Of the three primary kinds of skin cancer, two are both common and relatively curable. These are basal-cell and squamous-cell types.

Doctors recommend thorough examination of one's own skin, all over the body, on a regular basis. Report any changes to your physician. Your doctor should also check your skin during examinations.

A *melanoma* is a malignant tumor that may arise from a mole. The moles may begin as flat, soft, brown, and hairless protrusions, but they can change suddenly into darker, larger growths that itch and bleed. They can also metastasize, spreading cancer cells to other parts of the body through the bloodstream and the lymphatic system.

Unlike other types of skin cancer, melanomas may grow in skin areas not usually exposed to the sun, such as the feet, in the genital area, or under the belt or collar. Chronic irritation from tight clothing is one suspected cause.

Oral Cancer

Cancers of the mouth and lips strike an estimated 30,000 persons in the United States each year and kill a shocking 8,000. Shocking because anyone with the aid of a mirror and a good light can see into his mouth and therefore spot even very small cancers early in their development.

Symptoms

Any sore, lump, or lesion of the mouth or lips should be regarded as suspicious if it does not heal. A physician or dentist should then be consulted without delay. Other symptoms may include repeated bleeding in the mouth, lumps in the mouth, persistent mouth pain or numbness, or persistent changes in the look or feel of the mouth's soft tissues.

Detection

After discussion of any signs or symptoms, your doctor will usually take a small sample of the skin cells suspected of being cancerous. The cells will be screened and if cancer is detected, you will probably have to undergo further testing to see if the cancer has spread, and, if so, how far. Additional tests may include X rays, computed tomography (CT), magnetic resonance imaging (MRI), and ultrasound imaging.

Therapy

Oral cancers are treated by surgical removal or by irradiation.

Causes

A number of factors increase the risk of oral cancer. They include tobacco use, exposure to ultraviolet light (for lip cancer); sharp or rough-edged teeth or improperly fitted, irritating dentures; leukoplakia (white patches on the tongue or on the insides of the cheek); and excessive consumption of alcohol.

Ovarian and Uterine Cancer

See under *Women's Health*, Ch. 25.

Stomach Cancer

Before World War II, cancer of the stomach was the most common type of cancer among men and women in the United States. The death rate from stomach cancer in the 1930s was about 30 per 100,000 population. In recent years, stomach cancer has declined in proportion to other forms of the disease, such as lung, breast, and uterine cancer. However, stomach cancer is still a significant health problem because detecting it in its early stages, when treatment is more successful, is problematic.

Today, men are more likely to have stomach cancer than are women. Most persons found to have stomach cancer are in their 60s or 70s. One of the disease's mysterious incidental factors is its peculiar geographical distribution. Among the countries with high rates of occurrence are Japan, Chile, Costa Rica, Poland, and Hungary.

Symptoms

The most common early symptom is microscopic bleeding that can be detected only by examining the stools for blood. Stomach cancer seems to develop slowly and insidiously, with initial symptoms that may be disregarded by the patient because they mimic ordinary gastric distress. The patient may experience a distaste for foods, particularly meats, and display a slow but progressive loss of weight. There may be sensations of fullness, bloating, or pain after meals. The same symptoms may be noted between meals and be aggravated by eating. The pain may vary from intermittent stomachaches to intense pain that seems to extend into the patient's back. The patient also experiences fatigue or weakness and anemia, and, as the cancerous condition progresses, may have periods of vomiting. The vomitus is dark, much like the color of coffee grounds, and there may be other signs of bleeding in the patient's stools.

Detection

X rays of the stomach and examination of the stomach interior by gastroscopy usually locate and define the cancerous area; they may also reveal another cause of the symptoms, such as a peptic ulcer. During the physical examination, the physician may find a tissue mass and tenderness in the stomach area. A variety of laboratory tests will be performed and they will usually show signs of anemia from blood loss, the presence of blood in a stool sample, and the level of hydrochloric acid in the stomach; a lack of hydrochloric acid is found in more than half the stomach cancer patients. A biopsy study of the suspected tissue will usually be performed, as will computed tomography (CT) scan, which is used to see if the cancer has spread.

Therapy

Unfortunately, because of the insidious nature of stomach cancer, the disease becomes easier to diagnose as it progresses. By the time cancer has been confirmed, the most expedient form of treatment is surgery to remove the affected area of the stomach. If the cancer is small and has not spread by metastasis to lymph nodes in the region, the chances are relatively good that the patient will experience a full recovery.

Your doctor may also give you cancer-fighting drugs (chemotherapy). These may be given before surgery to reduce tumor size, or after surgery to destroy any cancer cells that may remain. Radiation treatment using X rays may also be used before or after surgery to kill cancer cells. Radiation may also be used in conjunction with chemotherapy.

Occasionally, a stomach tumor is found to be noncancerous. The tumor may be a polyp, a leiomyoma (a growth consisting of smooth muscle tissue), or a *pseudotumor* (false tumor), such as an inflammatory fibroid growth. Such benign tumors produce symptoms ranging from gastric upset to internal bleeding and should be removed by surgery.

Causes

Many possible factors have been suggested as causes of stomach cancer. These include a diet high in foods that have been preserved using the processes of smoking, pickling, salting, or drying. These foods contain relatively high amounts of nitrites and nitrates, which can be converted into carcinogenic substances in the stomach. Additional risk factors include alcohol abuse, smoking, and the presence in the stomach of *Helicobacter pylori* bacteria, a common cause of ulcers.

The widespread use of refrigeration has been offered as an explanation for the declining incidence of stomach cancer, since refrigeration reduces the need for chemical food preservatives.

Medical epidemiologists have also found that genetic factors may play a role in the development of stomach cancer. Statistical analysis of large population studies of stomach cancer shows a tendency for the disease to occur in persons with blood type A, or with below-normal levels of hydrochloric acid in the stomach, or with inherited variations in the stomach lining. There also seems to be a good possibility that stomach cancers evolve from noncancerous changes in the stomach lining, as from polyps or peptic ulcers.

Bladder Cancer

As a stomach cancer, the incidence of cancer of the bladder occurs more frequently in men than in women. In the United States, it is the fourth leading cause of cancer in men and the eighth leading cause in women.

Bladder cancer appears at an annual rate of more than 50,000 new cases each year in the United States and causes more than 12,000 deaths annually.

While the rate of bladder cancer has steadily risen over the last few decades, understanding of the disease has also increased and survival rates are higher now than in the past.

As with most cancers, early detection greatly increases the chances of successful treatment with the fewest side effects.

Symptoms

In its early stages, there are often no signs or symptoms.

A change in bladder habits is among the first signs of bladder cancer. The change might be the presence of pain while urinating, a noticeable difficulty in urinating, or a difference in the frequency of urination.

Another symptom of the disease is the appearance of blood in the urine. The degree of blood coloration is not necessarily related to the severity of the cancer; any sign of blood in the urine should be investigated. Nor should the absence of pain be allowed to minimize the seriousness of urinary bleeding as a symptom of a diseased bladder. Even without pain, the presence of blood can indicate a problem such as obstruction to the urinary flow that can lead to uremia, a toxic condition caused by retention of urinary waste products in the system.

Additional symptoms may include urinary incontinence, pain or tenderness in the abdomen, anemia, tiredness, and weight loss.

Detection

Cancer of the bladder is frequently diagnosed from common signs and symptoms, particularly the appearance of blood in the urine. A laboratory examination of the patient's urine may also reveal the presence of cancer cells that have been washed out of the bladder. The disease can be detected by an intra*venous pyelogram*—a kind of X-ray picture made by filling the urinary system with a fluid that makes tissue details appear in sharp contrast—and by examination of the membrane lining the bladder. The bladder lining may be examined by surgical biopsy or by *cystoscopy,* the viewing of the interior of the bladder by means of a device inserted in the urethra—or both.

Examination of the bladder lining is needed to determine the type and size of tumor that may be the cause of the symptoms. One type, called a *papillary tumor,* or *papilloma,* is relatively harmless and usually does not invade the wall of the bladder as does the more dangerous type, sometimes described as a solid lesion. The degree of invasion of the bladder tissues by the infiltrating mass determines the type of treatment recommended. However, any tumor found in the lining of the bladder must be removed, because the papillary type can progress into a solid lesion if not treated.

Therapy

Treatment depends upon the size and type of growth, the location of the tumor, and so on. Surgical excision of cancerous tissue is usually the most effective treatment. Chemotherapy, using drugs to destroy cancer cells, may be used before or after surgery. Usually, two or more drugs are used together, and they are either inserted into the bladder directly or administered intravenously. Radiation therapy also may be used by either inserting radioactive materials directly into the bladder or by administering X rays externally.

In advanced cases of bladder cancer, the bladder may be removed and its function performed by the construction of a substitute organ from other tissues or by the relocation of the upper ends of the ureters at other urine-collecting points.

Causes

The leading cause of bladder cancer is cigarette smoking. Certain carcinogenic chemicals accumulate in smokers' urine and over time damage the bladder lining.

Occupational factors have been associated with cancer of the bladder since 1895, when it was discovered that persons who worked with aniline chemical dyes were among those most likely to develop the disease. The incidence of the disease among chemical workers was found to be 30 times greater than that of the general population. The aniline dye workers developed bladder cancer at an average age 15 years younger than among the general population. The effect of the chemical dyes was verified by the development of cancer in the bladders of laboratory animals exposed to the dyes. Many other chemicals have been found to cause bladder cancer. In addition, exposure to arsenic has been found to increase the risk of bladder cancer.

Besides the influence of industrial environmental factors, bladder cancer is associated with *schistosomiasis,* a disease occurring in Africa, Asia, South America, and other regions. Schistosomiasis develops after bathing or wading in water infested by a blood fluke. The organisms penetrate the skin and migrate to the intestines or urinary bladder, producing an inflammation that eventually leads to cancer. See Ch. 19, *Other Diseases of Major Importance,* for a fuller description of the disease.

Cancer of the Prostate

Cancer of the prostate is the most common cancer among American men. About 30,000 men die of prostate cancer each year. The incidence increases with advancing age from the fifth decade of life, when prostatic cancer cells are found in nearly 25 percent of all men examined, to age 80, when 50 percent of the men have been found to have cancer cells in their prostate glands. Fortunately, while an American man has about a 30 percent chance of developing prostate cancer, he has only a 3 percent chance of dying of it.

Symptoms

In its early stages, prostate cancer, unfortunately, often does not produce symptoms. However, because the prostate encircles the urethra, which is the outlet from the bladder, any prostatic problem can cause such problems as increased frequency of urination, difficulty or discomfort in urinating, weak urine flow, blood in the urine, or dull pain in the lower pelvic area.

Detection

A digital rectal exam, during which a doctor inserts a gloved finger into the rectum in order to examine the prostate, should be a regular part of a physical examination for men over the age of 40. If the physician feels a lump or hardened area, further tests are ordered. About half of such lumps and nodules are caused by fibrosis, calcium deposits, or other noncancerous bodies.

A blood test for prostate specific antigen (PSA), has brought a 600 percent increase in the diagnosis of new cases of prostate cancer since the mid-1980s. The test indicates high levels of an enzyme produced by the prostate gland, revealing both potentially lethal cancers and slow-growing tumors that may never threaten life. Some doctors recommend having the PSA test annually after age 50. Additional tests include a biopsy of the prostate gland, various analyses of a man's urine for any abnormalities, and a transrectal ultrasound, in which a probe is inserted into the rectum. It emits sound waves that are used to create an image of the prostate gland.

Treatment

Each patient must consider a variety of complex issues such as his overall state of health, life expectancy, the degree and aggressiveness of the cancer, and expectations concerning full sexual capacity. The most common treatments for prostate cancer are surgery, radiation, and hormone therapy. They are frequently combined. Older men, or those in poor health, whose prostate cancer is detected at an early stage through the PSA test, may choose watchful waiting as a treatment. In watchful waiting, men must undergo frequent examination and testing to evaluate the cancer; cancer grows so slowly in older men that death is likely to be from other causes. Frequent testing is important.

In the event of an aggressive tumor, radical prostatectomy is advised. This surgical removal of the prostate and possibly the nearby lymph nodes is thought to offer the highest cure rate for those with cancer still confined to the gland. Surgeons try not to affect the nerves and muscles that control sexual functioning and urination. Possible risks include some bladder control problems and erectile dysfunction (impotence).

Radiation therapy uses X rays to kill cancer cells. It is another option for patients whose cancer has spread beyond the prostate. This therapy has the same risks as radical surgery—incontinence and impotence—but is considered less effective in producing a permanent cure.

Another option is hormone therapy, which consists of either an orchectomy, the surgical removal of the testicles, or using drugs to disrupt the normal production of male hormones or to block the entry of the hormones into cancer cells. This is because male sex hormones, particularly testosterone, can stimulate cancer cell growth. Hormonal therapy can slow the development of or shrink tumors.

Causes

The causes of prostate cancer are not completely understood, but certain risk factors for developing the disease have been identified. The chance of developing prostate cancer increases with age. It is more common among African-Americans than among white Americans. Prostate cancer may have a genetic component; it has been shown that having a father or brother with prostate cancer increases a man's risk of getting the disease. A diet high in fat also seems to increase the risk of developing the disease.

Cancer of the Kidney

Cancer of the kidneys is most likely to occur in people between the ages of 50 and 70. More than 30,000 Americans are diagnosed with kidney cancer annually. About 12,000 die of it annually. The exact causes of adult kidney cancer are unknown. The main types of kidney cancer are renal cell carcinoma, transitional cell cancer, and Wilms' tumor.

Renal Cell Carcinoma, Transitional Cell Cancer, and Wilms' Tumor

Renal cell carcinoma is the most common type of kidney cancer in adults. It usually starts in cells lining the renal tubules of the kidney—small tubes that filter the blood and help produce urine. Transitional cell cancer usually starts where the kidney and the ureter (the tube through which urine flows from the kidneys into the bladder) meet. Wilms' tumor occurs primarily in children. It is very rare in adults. Most children with Wilms' tumor are diagnosed before age 7.

Symptoms

Signs or symptoms of all types of kidney cancer are rare in their early stages. The most common signs of kidney cancer in its later stages are back pain and blood in the urine, which may be visible upon urination or may be visible only under a microscope.

Other less common symptoms may include weight loss, intermittent fever, fatigue, pain in other body parts, a lump in the kidney area, and an overall feeling of poor health.

Detection

Children with Wilms' tumor usually have no symptoms. Wilms' tumor is detected most often through physical examination of the child's abdomen.

Doctors usually obtain a patient's medical history and perform a general physical exam. He or she may also thoroughly palpate the abdomen for unusual masses. Blood and urine tests may be performed as well.

If cancer is suspected, the doctor usually orders tests that produce images of the kidneys and surrounding organs. These imaging tests may include: an intravenous pyelogram, wherein a dye is injected into the body and a series of X rays are taken as the dye moves through the kidneys and surrounding tissue; an ultrasound exam, which uses the measurement of the motions of sound waves to create images of internal organs; an arteriography, which takes X rays of blood vessels around the kidneys as injected dye moves through them. Magnetic resonance imaging and computed tomography scans are two additional imaging methods that may be employed. A biopsy, in which a sample of kidney tissue is examined under a microscope for cancer cells, is done if test results have indicated the presence of cancer.

Treatment

Surgery is the chief treatment for cancer of the kidneys. A simple nephrectomy removes only the kidney, partial nephrectomy removes only the cancerous tissue from the kidney, and a radical nephrectomy removes the entire kidney, the adrenal gland, nearby lymph nodes, and surrounding tissue.

In the procedure called arterial embolization, the main blood vessel leading to the kidney is injected with a material that will block it. This deprives the tumor of oxygen and slows its growth.

Radiation treatment using X rays may also be used to kill cancer cells. Radiation may also be used in conjunction with chemotherapy, in which cancer-fighting drugs are administered. These treatments may be administered before surgery to reduce tumor size or after surgery to destroy any cancer cells that may remain.

Immunotherapy, also called biological therapy, may also be used. This involves administration of substances designed to stimulate the body's own immune system to battle diseases including cancer. Administering hormones to slow cancer cell growth is used in some patients with advanced tumor growth.

Cancer of the Pancreas

Pancreatic cancer is the fourth leading cause of deaths due to cancer in women and men. It is most likely to develop after the age of 40, and approximately four-fifths of all cases occur after age 60. The exact cause of pancreatic cancer is unknown, but it has been determined that those who smoke develop pancreatic cancer at higher rates than those who do not. Cancer of the pancreas is usually fatal because it spreads rapidly and is rarely detected in its early stages

Symptoms and Detection

Symptoms of pancreatic cancer include digestive disorders, such as abdominal pain, nausea, diarrhea, loss of appetite, and perhaps severe constipation, as well as back pain. Abdominal distress may improve or worsen after eating and pain may increase when the patient lies on his back. The back pain that the patient experiences is often relieved by standing or bending forward. Pancreatic cancer patients will suffer pronounced weight loss, jaundice, and general bodily discomfort that comes and goes. Another sign of this cancer is a sudden onset of diabetes in an adult who is not overweight and does not have a family history of diabetes.

Pancreatic cancer is one of the most difficult cancers to diagnose because the pancreas is hidden by other organs in the body and early symptoms of this disease are vague. There are many tests that may be performed to detect this cancer. Ultrasound, a CT scan, or an MRI may be administered to image the abdomen and check for the presence of tumors. An endoscopy may be performed in which a physician examines and tests the pancreas by passing a tube down a patient's throat, through the stomach, and into the small intestine. A dye is injected through the tube into the common bile duct and the area is X-rayed. A biopsy may also be performed in which a fine needle is inserted into the pancreas or the liver to obtain tissue samples.

Therapy

Surgery is the usual treatment recommended for cancer of the pancreas; the precise location of the tumor within the pancreas may determine the exact surgical procedure to be undertaken. Surgical removal of the tumor has a more hopeful outcome if located at the head of the pancreas; cancers in the body or tail of the pancreas usually are not detected until the disease has spread to other parts of the body. Radiation therapy and chemotherapy are not as effective in the treatment of pancreatic cancer as in other organs, but are used frequently in treating certain stages of the disease. It is important that survivors of pancreatic cancer undergo frequent checkups, since pancreatic cancer can recur within one to three years. Any recurrence of symptoms should be reported immediately to the family physician.

Cancer of the Liver

Cancer of the liver is commonly found to be the result of metastasis from other parts of the body. Cancers that originate in the liver account for less than 2 percent of the cancers reported in the United States and occur more frequently in men than in women. Cancer of the liver is usually fatal.

Symptoms and Detection

In its early stages, liver cancer rarely produces any symptoms. Weakness, weight loss, and pain in the upper abdomen or right side of the chest are among the symptoms of liver cancer. A fever apparently unrelated to any infection also may mark the onset of liver cancer.

An enlarged liver with masses of abnormal tissue may be detected by an examining physician. Laboratory tests usually reveal alterations in metabolism that are associated with changes in the liver cells caused by the cancer growth. Imaging tests, such as a computerized tomography (CT) scan or an ultrasound, are usually also performed. A biopsy test of the abnormal liver tissue may confirm the presence of cancer. A more direct approach is to perform exploratory surgery for examination of the liver.

Therapy and Causes

If the tumor is located during exploratory surgery and the area can be excised, part of the liver is removed. Chemotherapy may also be used. Radiation therapy, injection of alcohol directly into tumors, which dries them out, and the use of electric current to destroy cancerous cells are other treatment options.

While the exact cause of primary liver cancer is unknown, a large proportion of cases is associated with cirrhosis of the liver. In recent years, some types of liver cancer have been traced to exposure of industrial workers to chemicals known to be carcinogenic. The high incidence of primary liver cancer in Asia and Africa is related to *aflatoxins* (molds) in grains and legumes, such as peanuts.

Secondary cancers of the liver are the result of primary cancer in other body areas; the liver is vulnerable to metastasis from cancers in every organ except the brain because of the pattern of blood circulation that carries cancer cells through the body.

Cancer of the Brain

Cancers in the brain tissue frequently are the result of metastasis from other body organs. They travel through the bloodstream, primarily from cancers of the lung, kidney, gastrointestinal tract, and breast. They become implanted in both the cerebrum and cerebellum, and, although there is wide distribution of the cancer cells, they are clustered mainly near the surfaces of the brain tissues. Primary brain tumors are more common among children than among adults; in children, other cancer sites are not likely to have had time to develop to the stage of metastasis required for the transmission of malignant cells to the brain.

A cancer that seems to originate in the brain tissues is known as *glioblastoma multiforme,* a malignant growth that may strike at any age but is more likely to occur during middle age. The glioblastoma may develop in nearly any part of the brain structure, including the brain stem, and spread extensively into a large tumorous mass.

Symptoms

Symptoms of brain cancer may include headache, dizziness, nervousness, depression, mental confusion, vomiting, and paralysis. The symptoms sometimes are interpreted as those of a psychiatric disorder, and treatment of the organic disease may be postponed until too late.

Detection

Diagnosis may be difficult, and the physician must evaluate the symptoms in terms of other findings from laboratory tests, X rays, and other techniques. The following imaging tests are commonly used: computerized tomography, magnetic resonance imaging, and angiograms. In some cases, cancer cells may be detected in samples of spinal fluid.

Therapy

Treatment of brain cancers usually requires surgery, radiation, chemotherapy, or some combination of the three. Treatment depends upon the type of tumor, its location, and other factors. Whether or not the brain tumor is a true cancer is not as important as early treatment; any abnormal tissue growth in the brain causes destructive pressure against vital tissues and their functions.

Cancer of the Larynx

Cancer of the larynx is chiefly a disease of men, afflicting many more men than women. It is not one of the major types of cancer, with about 12,000 new cases appearing each year in the United States. About 70 percent involve tumors on the vocal cords and are classed as *intrinsic* cancers of the larynx. The remainder of the cases involve tissues originating outside the vocal cords and are designated as *extrinsic.*

Symptoms

One of the first symptoms of intrinsic cancer of the larynx is hoarseness. Later the patient loses the ability to speak and has difficulty breathing. The same series of symptoms occurs in cases of extrinsic cancer except that there is an initial period of pain or discomfort in the throat before hoarseness begins. *Adenopathy,* or swelling of the lymph nodes in the area, also may be an early symptom of extrinsic cancer of the larynx.

Detection

Diagnosis of cancer of the larynx is relatively simple because the throat's interior can be examined by a physician and tissue samples can be removed for biopsy study. Detection of extrinsic cancer may be complicated by the fact that it is more likely to metastasize than intrinsic forms.

Therapy

In early cases of intrinsic cancer, or for small lesions that appear in the middle of the vocal cords, radiation may be the therapy of choice.

Surgery may be required for more serious cases, with radiation treatments before or after surgery, or both. The surgery, called a *laryngectomy,* may involve partial or total removal of the larynx. If a partial laryngectomy is performed, an effort is made to save as much of the vocal cords as possible. The voice will be changed after surgery, but it will be functional. The respiratory tract will be preserved. When total laryngectomy is required, the entire larynx is removed and lymph nodes may be removed if they are likely to have cancer or are proven to have cancer. This procedure is called a *neck dissection.* A new trachea is constructed by plastic surgery to permit normal or nearly normal respiration.

Chemotherapy, the use of cancer-fighting drugs, may also be prescribed.

Thyroid Cancer

Cancer of the thyroid gland is relatively uncommon. In United States about 15,000 women and 5,000 men are diagnosed with thyroid cancer annually. Treatment for thyroid cancer is highly effective.

Symptoms

These include rapid growth of the thyroid gland, hoarseness, paralysis of the nerves in the larynx, and enlarged lymph nodes in the neck and surrounding area. Diagnosis is aided by the rate at which suspected areas of cancer in the thyroid gland absorb radioactive iodine; the pattern of radioactive uptake helps pinpoint tissue abnormalities.

Therapy

Treatment may include surgery to remove the cancer in part of the surrounding tissue, plus removal of lymph nodes that may contain cancer cells that have metastasized from the thyroid tumor. In addition, other lymph nodes that are in the path of drainage from the thyroid gland may be removed. Surgery usually is more successful in young patients than in older patients. Radiation sometimes is used, either from an external source or by injection of large doses of radioactive chemicals. Additional treatments include chemotherapy, hormone treatment, and application of radioactive iodine, which kills thyroid cells.

Causes

The exact causes of thyroid cancer are unknown. A number of risk factors, however, have been identified. These include exposure of children and young adults to radiation therapy of the head and neck region and a family history of thyroid cancer.

Hodgkin's Disease

Hodgkin's disease is one of the *lymphomas*—cancers of the lymphatic system. It occurs most commonly among young adults, although it can appear at any age. Men are more likely to be victims than are women.

Symptoms

One of the first symptoms of Hodgkin's disease is a painless enlargement of a lymph node, usually in the area of the neck. The enlarged lymph nodes usually are firm and rubbery at first. The patient may experience a severe and persistent itching for several weeks before the first enlarged lymph node appears.

Other symptoms may include shortness of breath, fever, weight loss, anemia, and some pressure or pain as the disease progresses and nerve tissue becomes involved. Gradually, the lymph nodes that originally were separate and movable become matted and fixed, and sometimes inflamed. Over a period of months to years, the disease spreads to other parts of the body.

Therapy

Hodgkin's disease is ordinarily confirmed by removal of an affected lymph node for biopsy study. If the disease is limited to one or two localized areas the usual therapy is radiation treatments. Surgical excision of the nodes may be employed in special cases, as when a mass of nodes threatens a vital organ. But intense radiation exposure is generally more effective than surgery. Radiation treatments when properly applied may have a high cure rate. In cases where the disease has spread over a large area of the body, the treatment of choice may be chemotherapy. Doctors may employ any combination of these therapies.

Causes

The cause of Hodgkin's disease is unknown. Because of the fever and other symptoms associated with the disorder, and because it appears to occur more frequently among members of the same family or community than in the population as a whole, it has been suggested that Hodgkin's disease is a viral disease that has a malignant effect on the human lymphatic system.

Leukemia

Leukemia is cancer of the blood-forming tissue, including the lymph system and bone marrow. Because leukemia involves blood cells circulating through the body rather than a fixed mass of tissue, leukemia is sometimes not considered a true cancer. However, leukemia cells, when studied under a microscope and in cell cultures, behave like cancer cells found in tumors.

There are at least ten different kinds of blood cells that have been identified with various forms of the disease, which is why it frequently is referred to as leukemias. In addition, there are both acute and chronic forms of leukemia, such as *acute granulocytic leukemia* and *chronic lymphocytic leukemia,* named after the particular kind of white blood cells that are most affected.

Leukemia affects the blood forming tissues, such as the bone marrow, resulting in an overproduction of white blood cells. The incidence by age group varies according to the specific type of leukemia, however; one variety of acute granulocytic leukemia can occur at any age, but chronic lymphocytic leukemia usually does not appear before the age of 40. Men are more likely than women to be the victims of one of the various forms of leukemia.

Symptoms

Common symptoms of all leukemias include fever, weight loss, fatigue, bone pain, anemia as expressed in paleness, and an enlarged spleen or masses under the skin caused by an accumulation of leukemic cells. There may be skin lesions and a tendency to bleed. Infections may become more common and less responsive to treatment because of a loss of the normal blood cells needed to resist disease.

Detection

Diagnosis of leukemia from early symptoms may be difficult because they resemble those of mononucleosis and other infections. Biopsies of bone marrow and careful blood studies usually identify the disease.

Therapy

Treatment usually is directed toward reducing the size of the spleen and the number of white cells in the blood, and increasing the level of blood hemoglobin to counteract the effects of anemia.

Chemotherapy is the primary treatment for leukemia. It uses drugs to kill leukemia cells. A single drug or a combination of drugs may be used.

In a bone marrow transplant, cancerous bone marrow is replaced with cancer-free marrow. For the replacement marrow, some of the patient's bone marrow will have been saved and cleared of leukemic cells or a compatible donor is found.

A number of chemical agents have been found to be effective in treating leukemia. These include interferon-alfa, an antiviral agent that helps stop the spread of leukemic cells. It also helps strengthen the immune system. Cladribine is a drug used to treat a form of chronic leukemia called hairy cell leukemia. This type of leukemia is characterized by cells in the bone marrow, liver, and spleen being covered by hair-like projections, as well as by enlargement of the spleen. Cladribine kills leukemic cells.

Another treatment option is a stem-cell transplant. Healthy stem cells (those able to produce new cells) are harvested from the patient. After receiving radiation or chemotherapy, the healthy stem cells are re-injected, which increases the number of healthy cells in the bloodstream. Stem-cell transplant has a lower risk of infection than does bone marrow transplant.

Another treatment method involves using cell-specific antibodies to kill leukemic cells. These antibodies are removed from the patient's body and are multiplied in a laboratory. This greater amount of antibodies is then put back into the patient's body.

Radiation therapy uses high-energy rays such as X rays to injure cancerous cells and slow or stop their growth.

Retinoic acid prompts white blood cells to return to the normal patterns of growth and death that leukemia disrupts.

Causes

There is no general theory about the cause of leukemia. Animals are known to be susceptible to a form of leukemia transmitted by virus, but there is no solid evidence that human leukemias are caused by viral infections. Survivors of nuclear explosions as well as persons exposed to large doses of X rays have developed leukemia at a higher-than-normal rate than other people. There is evidence that at least one type of acute leukemia may be a result of an inherited genetic defect.

Other Cancers

Lymphosarcoma

Another of the cancers that involve the lymphatic system is called *lymphosarcoma*—a malignant lymphoma that tends to metastasize in lymphatic tissue. The most common first symptom is a swelling of the lymph nodes, and the diagnosis and treatment are similar to those of Hodgkin's disease. Lymphosarcoma can occur at any time and in any part of the body where there is lymphatic tissue, including the gastrointestinal tract, the tonsils, the tongue, or the nasopharynx area.

Reticulum-Cell Sarcoma

The lymphomas also include *reticulum-cell sarcoma.* (A sarcoma is a malignant tumor in the connective tissue. Reticulum cells are a particular kind of connective tissue.) The disease is marked by the invasion of normal tissue by increased numbers of reticulum cells or fibers. As in the treatment of leukemia, it is important to know which of the various types of cancer has affected the lymphatic system, because each of the lymphomas responds to a different therapeutic routine.

Myeloma and Multiple Myeloma

Myelomas, once considered rare but now reported in increasing numbers, are cancerous growths that seem to originate in the bone marrow. The average age at onset is about 65. Men are twice as likely as women to be victims of myelomas.

The disease is marked by bone destruction, mainly in the pelvis, ribs, and spine. The bones break easily, sometimes causing collapse of the spinal column and pressure on the spinal cord. There also may be anemia, kidney damage, and changes in the blood chemistry. When the myelomas occur at numerous sites in the bone marrow throughout the body, the disease is known as *multiple myeloma.*

Treatment

Various methods of treating lymphomas have evolved despite serious difficulties. Lymphomas appear in many different forms, and can change form in the process of spreading to another part of the body. Different types may be found in a single lymph gland.

Despite these difficulties, many chemotherapeutic agents have been found useful in treatment of lymphomas.

A number of drugs have been used in various combinations in the treatment of lymphomas. In addition to drug therapy, methods of treating lymphomas include irradiation therapy, or radiotherapy, and a combination of drugs and radiotherapy, and in extreme cases surgery is attempted to remove lymphoma.

19

Other Diseases of Major Importance

This chapter discusses a number of diseases of major importance that are not dealt with elsewhere: acquired immune deficiency syndrome (AIDS), a disease characterized by a defect in the body's natural immune system; plague, of great historical importance but fortunately now uncommon in the United States; three infectious diseases—Hantavirus, tularemia and Rocky Mountain Spotted Fever; and seven tropical diseases that afflict millions of people in the warmer regions of the world and that occasionally occur elsewhere: malaria and yellow fever, leishmaniasis, trypanosomiasis, filariasis, schistosomiasis, and leprosy.

AIDS

First reported widely in 1981, AIDS has become a priority of the U.S. Public Health Service. Researchers isolated the virus, the *human immunodeficiency virus* (*HIV*), that causes AIDS. Persons with AIDS (PWAs) are susceptible to a variety of unusual or rare illnesses called *opportunistic diseases.* These include *Pneumocystis carinii* pneumonia (PCP); Kaposi's sarcoma; thrush, or *Candida albicans*; dementia (AIDS dementia complex or ADC); herpes simplex; and meningitis.

Groups at highest risk of contracting AIDS include homosexual and bisexual men and intravenous drug users; hemophiliacs; prostitutes and their clients; heterosexuals with multiple partners in areas where HIV infections are highest; and recipients of multiple blood transfusions from areas where the disease was common between 1983 and 1985. Evidence suggests that the HIV virus may also be affecting more and more young people, particularly runaways, and migrants and refugees. In "passive transmission," a mother can pass AIDS to her child before or during birth.

Increasingly, medical authorities view AIDS as a disease with which victims may live for years. However, no treatment has successfully restored the immune system of an AIDS patient to normal functioning.

Symptoms

Once infection with HIV occurs, the human body produces antibodies in response to the virus's invasion of the bloodstream. The symptoms that can follow may resemble those of flu or even the common cold. Symptoms may include swollen glands, or enlarged lymph nodes in the neck, armpits, or groin; night sweats; fever; unexplained rapid weight loss; chronic, unexplained diarrhea; fatigue; loss of appetite, bruises that don't heal, and abnormal bleeding.

Prevention

To prevent the spread of AIDS, the U.S. Public Health Service has recommended that persons at risk of contracting the disease should:

- Not donate blood or plasma, sperm, body organs, or other tissues
- Limit sexual contacts and be assertive with sexual partners about engaging only in safe sexual practices
- Not engage in sexual acts in which exchange of body fluids, including semen, takes place
- Refrain from sharing toothbrushes, razors, or other implements that could be contaminated with blood
- Limit drug use, if a drug user; do not share needles, and do not leave needles or other drug paraphernalia where others might find and use them.

Additionally, women should avoid or postpone pregnancy if they have tested positive to antibodies to AIDS, or if they are a sexual partner of a man with a positive antibody test.

The Public Health Service has reported no evidence indicating that the AIDS virus can be transmitted through casual kissing or other social contacts. But persons who have had positive antibody tests should tell their physicians and dentists about the test results. There has been no risk of contracting AIDS through blood donations or transfusions since the introduction of blood-screening procedures in 1985.

Testing and Treatment

Contrary to past scientific opinion, the HIV virus does not lie dormant for long periods of time in the human body. The virus multiplies almost from the moment of infection, replicating quickly to counter the defense of the human immune system. Rigorous early treatment with a combination of powerful drugs usually delays the appearance of full-blown symptoms.

A blood test called the *ELISA* (enzyme-linked immunosorbent assay) test has been developed to detect the presence of antibodies to the AIDS virus in human blood. The test has helped to eliminate nearly all questionable blood and plasma from the nation's blood supply, but it has not helped to diagnose individuals. Laboratories have also used the Western Blot test to verify positive results from ELISA. The HIVAG-1 test is the first test designed to help physicians detect the AIDS virus and to monitor its development in the human body. A rapid screening test, the Recombigen HIV-1 Latex Agglutination test, can detect AIDS virus antibodies in five to thirty minutes. There are also home test kits available.

In recent years, AIDS has been successfully treated with a new class of drugs called protease inhibitors, which are used in combination with the nucleoside analogs AZT, dd1,ddC, d4T, and 3TC. Protease inhibitors are indinavir, nelfinavir, ritonavir, and saquinavir, and others are being developed. This new treatment does not work for everyone, and the drugs are very expensive and have serious side effects. However, in many patients the treatment reduces the pressence of HIV in the blood to almost undetectable levels. Despite the success of this treatment, it is the conclusion of most researchers that the HIV virus cannot be completely eradicated once a person has been infected.

Other drugs used to treat AIDS-related diseases include nevirapine, alpha-interferon, foscarnet and ganciclovir, trimetraxate, and aerosolized pentamidine.

Hantavirus pulmonary syndrome (HPS)

Hantavirus is contracted by breathing in traces of urine, feces, and saliva of infected rodents, especially deer mice. Direct contact with broken skin or mucous membranes, as well as rodent bites, have also caused the infection. This respiratory disease triggers an overreaction by the body's immune system, creating high counts of white blood cells that flood the air sacs of the lungs, hindering oxygen intake and causing suffocation and death in nearly half of those afflicted.

Symptoms and Treatment

Hantavirus pulmonary syndrome has been particularly difficult to detect because its symptoms—fever, cough, muscle aches, and sometimes vomiting and diarrhea—resemble that of the common flu. Hantavirus can be distinguished from the flu by its lack of sore throat, runny nose, and the rapid escalation of respiratory difficulties. Death may occur in days if symptoms go untreated. No vaccine exists. Doctors treat with antibiotics and mechanical ventilators to stop the buildup of fluid in the lungs.

Prevention

Exposure to Hantavirus can be prevented by avoiding the disruption of rodent burrows and nests, by using appropriate respiratory devices when cleaning buildings in high-rodent areas, and the eradication of rodent populations. Those exposed to high risk conditions, who come down quickly with flu-like symptoms, should seek medical care.

Plague

Bubonic plague, is transmitted to humans through direct or indirect contact with animals. At least three great epidemics of bubonic plague have been recorded, including the Black Death of the 14th century, when the disease claimed at least 50 million lives. While recent cases of the plague in North America have been relatively rare, cases still occur in the western United States. Increased outdoor activity in those areas has resulted in a higher incidence of the disease among humans in recent years.

Symptoms

The infection is transmitted from animals to man through the bite of a flea carrying the disease organism. Symptoms usually develop in several days but may take as long as two weeks after the flea bite. The victim experiences chills and fever, with the temperature rising above 102° F. He may experience headaches, a rapid heart beat, and difficulty walking. Vomiting and delirium also are among the symptoms of plague. There may be pain and tenderness of the lymph nodes, which become inflamed and swollen; the enlarged lymph nodes are known as *buboes,* a term that gives its name to the type of plague involved. The buboes occur most frequently in the legs and groin because these are the most frequent sites for flea bites.

The site of the flea bite may or may not be found after the symptoms develop. If present, it may be marked by a swollen, pus-filled area of the skin.

Diagnosis of plague can be confirmed by laboratory tests that might include examination of the bacteria taken in samples from buboes or other diseased areas of the body, inoculation of laboratory animals with suspected disease organisms, and studies of the white blood cells of the patient.

Complications can include pneumonia and hemorrhages, with bleeding from the nose or mouth or through the gastrointestinal or urinary tracts, and abscesses and ulcerations. The pneumonic form of plague can be transmitted from one person to another like colds or other infectious diseases; in other words, plague organisms are spread by being exhaled by one person and inhaled by another.

Treatment and Prevention

As in other infectious diseases, early treatment is most effective. Antibiotics are administered every day for a period of one to two weeks, and buboes are treated with hot, moist applications. The buboes may be drained if necessary after the patient has responded to antibiotic medications. Antibiotics have reduced the fatality rate from plague infections from a high of 90 percent to a maximum of about 10 percent. Vaccines are available but are of limited and temporary value. Prevention requires eradication of rats and other possibly infected rodents (some 200 species are known to carry the disease), use of insecticides to control fleas, and avoidance of contact with wild animals in areas where plague is known to exist. Domestic animals also should be protected from contact with possibly infected wild animals.

Tularemia

An infectious disease known as *tularemia,* sometimes called *rabbit fever,* is transmitted from animals to humans who come in contact with the animal tissues. It also can be transmitted through the bites of ticks or flies or by drinking contaminated water. Like the plague-disease organism, tularemia can be transmitted by inhalation of infected particles from the lungs of a diseased person, although such occurrences are rare.

Symptoms

Within a couple of days to perhaps two weeks after exposure to the tularemia germ, the patient develops chills and a fever with temperatures rising to 103° F. or higher. Other symptoms include headache, nausea and vomiting, extreme weakness, and drenching sweats. Lymph nodes become enlarged and a pus-filled lesion develops at the site of the infection. Usually only one pustular papule develops on a finger or other skin area, marking the point of the insect bite or contact with infected animal tissues; but there may be several such sores in the membranes of the mouth if that is the point of infection. It is not uncommon for the eyes or lungs to become involved.

Laboratory tests, along with a record of contact with wild animals or game birds, eating improperly cooked meats, being bitten by deer flies or ticks, or drinking water from ponds or streams, usually helps verify the cause of the symptoms as tularemia. In some cases the contact with the disease organism can be made through bites or scratches of infected dogs or cats, but most frequently the disease of humans originates through handling of the meat or fur of wild animals or by camping or hiking in areas where the disease is endemic.

Treatment

Treatment includes bed rest and administration of antibiotics. Adequate fluid intake is important and oxygen may be required. Aspirin usually is given also, to relieve headache and muscle aches. Hot compresses are applied to the enlarged lymph node areas; it may be necessary to drain the swollen, infected nodes. If the disease is complicated by pneumonic tularemia or infection of the eye, the patient usually is hospitalized. Success of the therapy depends upon early and adequate treatment. The disease is rarely fatal when properly treated with antibiotics, but it can be lethal if the symptoms are ignored. Anyone who develops the symptoms of tularemia after handling wild animals or being exposed to biting insects or contaminated water in rural or rugged country should seek immediate medical help.

Hunters, campers, hikers, and others venturing into the great outdoors should protect their bodies against invasion by ticks by wearing long-sleeved shirts and long trousers with cuffs securely fastened. Regular checks should be made of the scalp, groin, and armpits for ticks. Any ticks found should be detached quickly and the bite area cleansed with soap and water, followed by an alcohol cleansing. If the head of the tick breaks off, it can be removed by the same techniques used to remove a splinter from the skin. Raw water from ponds and streams should be boiled or disinfected with chemicals before using. Rubber gloves should be worn while dressing the meat of wild game or birds, and the meat should be thoroughly cooked. On the positive side, once the disease occurs, the recovered patient develops immunity to tularemia.

Rocky Mountain Spotted Fever

The name of an increasingly common tick-borne disease, *Rocky Mountain spotted fever,* is misleading, because humans are most likely to become infected in regions far from the Rocky Mountains. The disease, also known as *tick fever,* has become most prevalent in rural and suburban areas of the southern and eastern United States. It is caused by a rickettsial organism transmitted by a tick bite. Wild rodents are a reservoir of the infected ticks that carry the disease.

Symptoms

Rocky Mountain spotted fever may be relatively mild or dangerously severe. The symptoms of headache, chills, and fever may begin suddenly and persist for a period of two or three weeks. Fever temperatures may reach 104° F and may be accompanied by nausea and occasional vomiting. Headaches have been described in some cases as excruciating, with the pain most intense along the forehead. Muscles of the legs, back, and abdomen may ache and feel tender. The most serious cases seem to develop within a few days after a tick bite; milder cases usually are slower to develop. A rash usually develops a few days after the onset of other symptoms and is most likely to be concentrated on the forearm, ankles, feet, wrists, and hands. If untreated, Rocky Mountain spotted fever symptoms may abate in two weeks, but the infection can be fatal, particularly in persons over the age of 40.

Treatment

Treatment includes administration of antibiotics and, in some cases, steroid hormones. Careful nursing care and adequate intake of protein foods and liquids also are needed.

Preventive measures are similar to those recommended to guard against tularemia. Wear adequate protective clothing that forms a barrier against tick invasion of the skin surfaces, check the scalp and other hairy body areas regularly for ticks, and remove and destroy any ticks found. In addition, ground areas known to be inhabited by wood ticks should be sprayed with an effective insecticide safe for humans; insect repellents also should be applied to clothing and exposed skin surfaces when venturing into wooded or brushy areas. Ticks may become attached to dogs and other animals and care should be used in removing them from the pets, because the disease organism can enter the body through minor cuts and scratches on the skin. A vaccine is available for protection of persons who are likely to use possibly infested tick areas for work or recreation. Immunity usually is established by two inoculations, about a month apart, and booster shots as needed.

Tropical Diseases

Most people living in the temperate climates of North America and Europe are spared the ravages of some of the most lethal and debilitating diseases known to mankind. They include malaria, which probably has killed more people than any other disease in history, yellow fever, leishmaniasis, trypanosomiasis, filariasis, schistosomiasis, and leprosy.

While many persons probably have never heard of some of these diseases and at least a few doctors might have trouble in diagnosing the symptoms, they affect hundreds of millions of people each year and could pose a threat to persons living in any part of the world. They are generally classed as tropical diseases, but so-called tropical or exotic diseases have been prevented from spreading into temperate regions partly because of alert medical care and preventive measures by public health experts. Malaria, for example, has been found as far north as the Arctic Circle and as far south as the tip of South America. At one time, it was a disease of epidemic proportions in such northern cities as Philadelphia and London. These diseases have altered the course of history, ending the life of Alexander the Great as he tried to conquer the world, thwarting Napoleon's plans to retake Canada from the English, defeating French efforts to build the Panama Canal, and contributing to the black-slave trade between Africa and the Americas.

The major tropical diseases are caused by a variety of organisms, including viruses, protozoa, and worms. Some are transmitted by insect bites, some by contact with contaminated water, and others, like leprosy, are spread by means that remain a mystery despite centuries of medical experience with millions of cases of the disease. Space does not permit detailed discussion of all tropical diseases; only those regarded by medical authorities as among the most significant to world health are described in this chapter.

Malaria

Malaria, one of the most common diseases in the world, gets its name from the Italian word for "bad air" because of an ancient belief that a mysterious substance in the air was the cause of the ailment. It is now known that the disease is caused by any of at least four parasites carried by Anopheles mosquitoes. According to the World Health Organization (WHO), malaria causes more than 300 million acute illnesses and at least one million deaths annually. Ninety percent of deaths due to malaria occur in Africa, mostly among young children. The disease was relatively rare in the United States until the 1960s, when hundreds of cases began to appear among military personnel who apparently contracted the disease in southeast Asia but did not develop symptoms until they returned to the United States. The disease later occurred in soldiers who had never left the United States. It was apparently transmitted by domestic Anopheles mosquitoes that had become infested with the malaria parasites.

How Malaria Is Transmitted

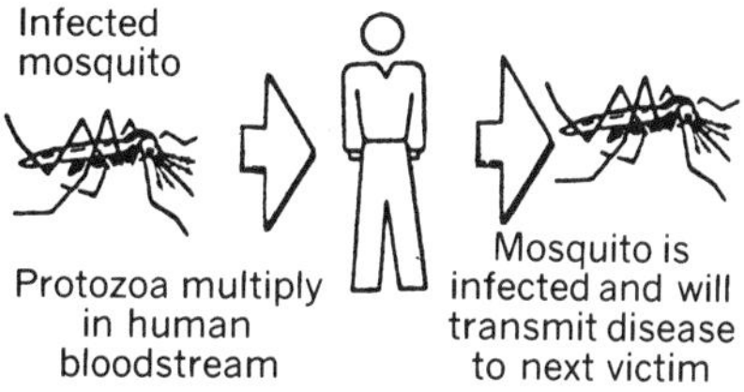

A mosquito infected with malaria protozoa bites a human. The protozoa produce daughter cells within the human bloodstream. These cells are transmitted to another mosquito that bites the infected human. This mosquito will infect the next human it bites, thus perpetuating the malaria cycle.

Symptoms

The symptoms of malaria differ somewhat among various patients because the four known kinds of plasmodia, or protozoa, that cause the infection do not produce the same specific effects. However, the general symptoms common to all forms of malaria are fever, chills, headache, muscle pains, and, in some cases, skin disorders such as cold sores, hives, or a rash. A malaria attack may begin with a severe chill that lasts from twenty minutes to an hour, followed by a fever lasting from three to eight hours with temperature rising to more than 104° F. The fever usually is accompanied by profuse sweating, and the afflicted person is left exhausted by the cycle of chills and fever. The attacks become more or less successively milder, less frequent, and more irregular, and finally cease, although there may be relapses.

One kind of malarial organism seems to cause attacks that occur every other day, while another type produces attacks that appear quite regularly on every third day; still another type of malaria plasmodium seems to cause a fever that is continuous. While the liver seems to be a favored target organ, other body systems can be involved, with related complications. If the organism reaches the brain, the patient may suffer convulsions, delirium, partial paralysis, or coma. If the organism invades the lungs, there may be coughing symptoms and blood-stained sputum. In some cases, there may be gastrointestinal symptoms with abdominal pain, vomiting, or diarrhea.

Medical examination of malaria patients frequently reveals signs of anemia, an enlarged spleen, liver abnormalities, and edema, or swelling because of fluid accumulation. Blood studies may show the malaria parasites in the blood, damaged red blood cells, and an abnormal white blood cell count. The four species of malaria organism are distinctive enough to be identified in laboratory tests.

Treatment

Treatment includes administration of antimalarial drugs such as quinine, chloroquine, or primaquine. Newer antimalarial drugs are sometimes used in combinations because of the development of drug-resistant strains of the organism in South America and Asia. There is no vaccine that protects against malaria.

Causes

The protozoa that cause malaria are carried by the Anopheles mosquito, but humans are the intermediate host. This means that both infected humans and infected mosquitoes are needed to continue the life cycle of the organism. The disease therefore can be controlled if Anopheles mosquito populations are eradicated and humans are not carrying the protozoa in their blood. When these organisms get into human blood, they invade the red blood cells and multiply until the blood cells rupture to release offspring called *daughter cells*. When the mosquito bites a human for a blood meal, the daughter cells enter the mosquito stomach, where they complete their life cycle and migrate to the mosquito's salivary gland to be injected into the next human, and so on. It takes from ten days to six weeks following a mosquito bite for the first malaria symptoms to develop, the time differences varying with the species of protozoa involved. The malaria mosquito in recent years has developed resistance to insecticides, and areas of infestation have spread in some countries where irrigation for farming has been expanded.

Yellow Fever

Yellow fever, which sometimes produces symptoms similar to those of malaria, also is transmitted by a mosquito. But yellow fever is a virus disease carried by the Aedes mosquito. Yellow fever also can be harbored by other animals, while the malaria organism that affects humans is not transmitted between humans and lower animals. Like malaria, yellow fever has in past years spread deeply into North America with cases reported along the Gulf Coast, the Mississippi River Valley, and as far north as Boston. A vaccine is available for protection against yellow fever.

Leishmaniasis

Leishmaniasis is similar to malaria in that the disease organisms are protozoa transmitted to humans by an insect bite, but the insect in this case is the sandfly. There are several forms that leishmaniasis can take. The kind considered most lethal, with a mortality rate of up to 95 percent of untreated adults, is known as *kala-azar,* a term derived from the Hindi language meaning "black disease." Kala-azar also is known as *black fever, dumdum fever,* and *visceral leishmaniasis*. It occurs from China through Russia and India to North Africa, the Mediterranean countries of Europe, and in parts of Central and South America. Kala-azar has appeared in the United States in cases contracted overseas.

Symptoms

The symptoms may not appear for a period of from ten days to more than three months after the bite of a sandfly, although the disease organism may be found in blood tests before the first symptoms occur. Symptoms include a fever that reaches a peak twice a day for a period of perhaps several weeks, then recurs at irregular intervals while the patient experiences progressive weakness, loss of weight, loss of skin color, and a rapid heartbeat. In some cases, depending upon the type of infection, there may be gastrointestinal complaints and bleeding of the mucous membranes, particularly around the teeth. There also can be edema, an accumulation of fluid in the tissues that conceals the actual loss of body tissue. Physical examination shows an enlarged spleen and liver plus abnormal findings in blood and urine tests.

American Cutaneous Leishmaniasis

The American cutaneous form of leishmaniasis usually begins with one or more skin ulcers resulting from sandfly bites, with the skin of the ear the target site of the insect in many cases. The skin lesion may enlarge, with or without secondary infection by other disease organisms, and spread into the lymphatic system of the body. From the lymph system, the infecting protozoa may invade the mouth and nose, producing painful and mutilating skin ulcers and other destructive changes in the tissues. Bacterial infections and respiratory problems can lead to the death of the patient. In some areas of Central and South America, more than 10 percent of the population suffer from the disfiguring effects of leishmaniasis. Diagnosis usually is confirmed by medical tests that identify the leishmaniasis organism in the patient's tissues.

Old World Cutaneous Leishmaniasis

A milder form, sometimes known as Old World cutaneous leishmaniasis, occurs from India westward to the Mediterranean countries and North Africa. An ulcer appears at the site of a sandfly bite, usually several weeks after the bite, but it heals during a period of from three months to a year. A large pitted scar frequently remains to mark the site of the ulceration, but the invading organism does not spread deeply into the body tissues as in the severe types of leishmaniasis.

Treatment

Therapy for leishmaniasis cases includes administration of various medications containing antimony, along with antibiotics for the control of secondary infections. Bed rest, proper diet, and, in severe cases, blood transfusions also are advised.

Causes

The leishmaniasis organisms injected into the human body by the sandfly bite multiply through parasitic invasion of the tissue cells, particularly blood cells that usually resist infection. They may invade the lymph nodes, spleen, liver, and bone marrow, causing anemia and other symptoms. In populated areas, sandflies can be eradicated by insecticides. Unfortunately, rodents and other wild and domestic animals serve as a reservoir for the leishmaniasis protozoa and tend to perpetuate the disease in rural and jungle areas with warm climates.

Trypanosomiasis

Trypanosomiasis is a group of diseases caused by similar kinds of parasitic protozoa. The diseases, which include two kinds of African *sleeping sickness* and *Chagas' disease* of Central and South America, affect about 10 million people. The sleeping-sickness forms of trypanosomiasis are transmitted by species of the tsetse fly, while Chagas' disease is carried by insects known as *assassin bugs* or *kissing bugs.* Besides affecting humans, the trypanosomiasis organisms infect other animals, including cattle, horses, dogs, and donkeys, and have impeded agricultural and rural development across one-third of the continent. According to the World Health Organization, the African land devastated by trypanosomiasis contains large fertile areas capable of supporting 125 million cattle, but domestic animals cannot survive the infestation of tsetse flies.

Sleeping Sickness

The two kinds of African sleeping sickness, Gambian and Rhodesian, are similar. Gambian, or mid-African, sleeping sickness is transmitted by a tsetse fly that lives near water; Rhodesian, or East African, sleeping sickness is carried by a woodland species of tsetse fly that uses antelopes as a reservoir of the infectious organism. The most likely victims of tsetse fly bites are young men, probably because they are more likely to be exposed to the insects.

Symptoms

The symptoms of trypanosomiasis infections from tsetse fly bites can vary considerably according to various factors, such as the general health of the victim. A small area of inflammation, called a *chancre,* appears at the site of the tsetse fly bite about two days after the incident; some patients complain of pain and irritation in the area around the bite for several weeks, but others have no symptoms. Then, for a period of perhaps several months, episodes of fever occur, with temperatures rising to 106° F. The bouts of fever may be accompanied by skin rashes, severe headaches, and heart palpitations. Loss of appetite and weight follow, along with insomnia, inability to concentrate, tremors, and difficulty in speaking and walking. There also may be signs of anemia and delayed reaction to a painful stimulus. Eventually, the protozoa can invade the central nervous system, producing convulsions, coma, and death.

Sleeping sickness, which may progress gradually, gets its name from the appearance of the patient, who develops a vacant expression and drooping eyelids, along with blurred speech, general lethargy, and occasional periods of paralysis.

Gambian and Rhodesian Varieties

A major difference between the Gambian and Rhodesian forms of African sleeping sickness is that the Rhodesian variety, which has similar symptoms, is more acute and progresses more rapidly than the Gambian. The fevers are higher, weight losses greater, the disease more resistant to treatment, and the span of time from first symptoms to death much shorter. Even with intensive treatment, Rhodesian sleeping sickness patients have only a 50–50 chance of survival, while 90 to 95 percent of the Gambian sleeping sickness patients recover when properly treated for the disease.

Treatment

Several chemotherapeutic agents are available for treatment of Gambian and Rhodesian sleeping sickness; they include suramin, pentamidine, and tryparsamide given by injection. Good nutrition, good nursing care, and treatment of secondary infections are additional therapeutic measures.

Chagas' Disease

Chagas' disease, or American trypanosomiasis, is a primary cause of heart disease from Mexico through much of South America. The protozoan infection is rare in the United States, but cases have been reported. The first symptoms may be edema of the face. The accumulation of fluid occurring in the area of the eyelids, conjunctivitis, hard reddish nodules on the skin, along with the fever and involvement of the heart, brain, and liver tissues. The assassin or kissing bugs by which the disease is spread tend to bite the face, especially around the lips or eyelids, accounting for the swelling of those facial areas. The bite may be painful, or if the victim is sleeping at the time, it may not be noticed at all.

Symptoms

The protozoa multiply rapidly at the site of the bug bite, frequently producing symptoms resembling those of leishmaniasis—intermittent fever, swollen spleen, and enlarged liver, after signs of an insect bite. After several days, the trypanosomiasis organisms spread from the site of infection into other tissues, especially the heart and brain, where they cause tissue destruction, inflammation, and often death.

Treatment

There is no specific treatment for Chagas' disease, and, except for experimental drugs, most therapeutic measures are intended to treat the symptoms.

Like the African sleeping sickness forms of trypanosomiasis, the American type can involve reservoirs of wild and domestic animals; the disease has been found in cats and dogs as well as in opossums and armadillos. Persons traveling in endemic areas should use preventive measures that are appropriate, such as insect sprays and repellents. Efforts to eradicate large areas of insects carrying the trypanosomiasis organisms have been futile; in some instances it has been found to be more effective to move villages away from the insects than to try to remove the insects from the villages.

Filariasis

The species of mosquitoes that transmit malaria and yellow fever, diseases caused by protozoa and viruses, also transmit *filariasis,* caused by a parasitic worm—a nematode or roundworm. Filariasis affects 300 million people living in tropical and subtropical areas of the world. The worm invades the subcutaneous tissues and lymph system of the human body, blocking the flow of lymph and producing symptoms of inflammation, edema, abscesses, and, in one form of the disease, blindness. Filariasis is not unknown to Americans; some 15,000 soldiers contracted the disease during World War II fighting in the Pacific Theater, and cases have been reported along the Carolina coast area. But most of the victims of filariasis live in a region extending from Africa through Asia to the islands of New Guinea and Borneo.

Symptoms

Symptoms of filariasis can develop insidiously during an incubation period that may last from three months to a year after infection. There can be brief attacks of a low-grade fever, with chills and sweating, headache, nausea, and muscle pain. The patient also may feel sensitive to bright lights. Signs and symptoms more specifically related to filariasis are the appearance of red, swollen skin areas with tender spots that indicate the spread of the threadlike worms through the lymphatic system. Most likely sites for the first signs of filariasis are the lymph vessels of the legs, with later involvement of the groin and abdomen, producing the swollen lower frontal effect known as *elephantiasis.* Diagnosis of the disease is confirmed by finding the tiny worms in the lymph; the infecting organism also may be found in blood tests, but only at certain times. The worms of one form of the disease are only 35 to 90 millimeters long in the adult stage, and those of a second type of the disease are only half that size. Larvae, or embryos, of the worms may be only 200 microns (one-fifth of a millimeter) in size.

Treatment

An oral medication, diethylcarbamazine, is available to kill the larvae in the system; the drug has only limited value in destroying the adult worms. The drug is taken orally for three weeks, but courses may have to be repeated over a period of two years because relapses can occur. Other therapeutic measures include bed rest during periods of fever and inflammation, antibiotics to control secondary infections, and, occasionally, surgery to remove damaged tissues that may interfere with normal working activities following recovery.

Onchocerciasis

The type of filariasis that causes blindness is transmitted by a species of blackfly that introduces or picks up the worm larvae while biting. As in mosquito-transmitted filariasis, the worms work their way through the skin to the lymphatic system but tend to migrate to eye structures. Blackfly filariasis, also called *onchocerciasis,* occurs most frequently in Africa and from southern Mexico to northern South America. More than one million cases of onchocerciasis have been found in the upper basin of the Volta River of Africa, with thousands of patients already blinded by the infection.

Loiasis

A third variation of filariasis is called *loiasis.* It is carried from man to monkey or from monkey to man by a biting fly. The larvae develop into adult worms that migrate under the skin and sometimes through the eye. Migration of a worm through the skin causes swelling, irritation, and redness. The disease is treated with drugs to kill the larvae, as well as by antihistamines and, occasionally, surgery to remove the adult worms.

Control of filariasis requires eradication of the flies and mosquitoes that transmit the parasitic worms and perhaps the wild animals that can serve as reservoirs. As in the examples of other tropical diseases, it frequently is easier to separate the humans from the areas infested by the insects than to eradicate the insects.

Schistosomiasis

A worm of a different sort—the trematode, a flatworm of the class *Trematoda,* which includes the flukes—is responsible for *schistosomiasis.* This disease occurs in various forms in Africa, Asia, South America, and the Caribbean, including Puerto Rico. About 200 million people are infected with schistosomiasis, also called *bilharziasis*.

Life Cycle of the Fluke Parasite

The process of infection by one kind of fluke involves free-swimming larvae that penetrate the skin of a human who has entered waters containing the organism. The larvae follow the human bloodstream to the liver, where they develop into adult worms. The adult worms then move into the blood vessels of the host and lay eggs. Some of the eggs find their way into the intestine or urinary bladder and are excreted with the urine or feces of the host. If they find their way to fresh water, the eggs hatch and the released organisms find their way to the body of a snail. Inside the snail they multiply into thousands of new larvae over a period of one or two months, after which they return to the water and invade the skin of another human. In this manner the fluke worm continues its life cycle, infecting more humans who venture into the contaminated waters.

Symptoms

Skin rashes and itching, loss of appetite, abdominal discomfort, and diarrhea are among early symptoms of schistosomiasis infections. There also may be fever and generalized aches and pains. During a period of from one to two or more months after the initial infection, more severe symptoms may occur as a result of a growing number of adult worms and eggs in the body, which produce allergic reactions. Those symptoms may include diarrhea, abdominal pain, coughing spells, and high fever and chills. Medical examination may reveal a tender and enlarged liver plus signs of bleeding in the intestinal tract. Complications may result from obstruction by masses of worms and eggs or by rupturing of the walls of body organs during migration of the organisms. Diagnosis usually can be confirmed by examination of the victim's stools or of the lining of the rectum for the presence of eggs of the fluke worms.

Treatment

Therapy may consist of administration of antimony-based drugs, tartar emetic, measures to relieve the symptoms, and, when deemed necessary, surgery. In some cases, a medication may be administered to flush the eggs of the fluke worm through a specific part of the circulatory system during a surgical procedure in which a filter is inserted in a vein to trap the eggs; thousands of fluke worms can be removed by this technique. Some of the medications used in treating schistosomiasis can have serious side effects and are used cautiously. However, the alternative may be prolonged emaciation of the victim, with a bloated abdomen and early death by cancer or other causes related to the infection. The female fluke worm has been known to continue depositing eggs during a life span of 30 years, causing frequent recurrence of acute symptoms.

Other Forms of Schistosomiasis

There are several other forms of schistosomiasis that cause variations in symptoms. One kind involves the liver and central nervous system, resulting in death of the victims within as little as two years after infection. Another form seems to involve the urinary bladder, causing frequent, painful, and blood-tinged urination with bacterial infection as a complication.

Swimmer's Itch

A mild form of schistosomiasis is known by the popular name *swimmer's itch.* It can occur anywhere from Asia to South America and as far north as Canada and western Europe, affecting bathers in both fresh water and sea water. As in the severe forms of schistosomiasis, snails are the intermediate hosts, and wild animals and birds provide a reservoir of the organism. The effects are treated as a skin allergy, and shallow local waters used for swimming are treated with chemicals to eradicate the snails. Careful drying and examination of the skin after swimming in possibly infected waters can control to some degree the invasion of the skin by fluke larvae. A chemical skin cream that tends to repel fluke larvae also is available as a protective measure.

Leprosy

More than 10 million people are victims of *leprosy,* an infectious disorder also known as *Hansen's disease.* Although leprosy is more common in tropical regions, where up to 10 percent of some population groups may be affected, the disease also occurs in several northern countries, including the United States, where the disease is found in coastal states from California through Texas and Louisiana, and from Florida to New York. Ancient medical writings indicate that leprosy was known in China and India about 3,000 years ago but did not spread to the eastern Mediterranean until A.D. 500 or 600. Thus, the disease described in the Bible as leprosy probably was not the same disease known today by that name.

Symptoms

The manifestations of leprosy resemble those of several other diseases, including syphilis, sarcoidosis, and vitiligo, a skin disease marked by patches where pigmentation has been lost. The lesions of leprosy, which may begin as pale or reddish areas of one-half inch to three or four inches in diameter, appear on body surfaces where the temperature is cooler than other body areas. These cooler surfaces include the skin, nose and throat, eyes, and testicles. The lesions are followed gradually by a loss of feeling in the affected areas because of involvement of the nerve endings in those tissues. At first the patient may notice a loss of ability to distinguish hot and cold sensations in the diseased area. Then there may be a loss of tactile sensation. Finally, there is a loss of pain sensation in the affected tissues.

A case of leprosy may progress into one of two major forms, *tuberculoid leprosy* or *lepromatous leprosy,* or a combination of the two forms. The advanced symptoms can include more severe nerve damage and muscular atrophy, plus damage to body areas from burns and injuries that are not felt but that can become infected. Damage to nose tissues can lead to breathing difficulties and speech problems. Crippling and blindness may develop in untreated causes of leprosy, and death may occur as a result of secondary infections.

Treatment

A number of different sulfone drugs have been found effective against the mycobacterium that apparently causes leprosy, but the drugs also produce such side effects as fever and anemia. When intolerance to sulfones occurs, other medications are offered, including thiourea, mercaptan, and streptomycin. Steroid hormones are used to help control adverse reactions. In 1998, thalidomide was approved for treatment of lepromatous leprosy.

Causes

The disease organism, *Mycobacterium leprae,* or *Hansen's bacillus,* is believed to enter the skin or the respiratory system of the victim, probably during childhood. It is not highly infectious except under unusual circumstances, such as skin tattooing. Some medical scientists believe the infection may be transmitted through an insect bite, because the disease organism has been found in insects. However, the true process of leprosy infection remains unknown, and efforts to cultivate the mycobacterium in laboratory tissue cultures have been futile, although the disease can be induced in the footpads of experimental animals. Doctors have not found it necessary to isolate patients with the disease except during the period when treatments begin. Regular and thorough skin examinations of persons who have been in contact with leprosy patients and early detection and treatment of the disease by specialists are the recommended means of control.

20

Surgery

Surgery Today

Computer and video screens surround the operating table, their displays projecting larger-than-life sections of a patient's internal organs. Monitors beep and blip in the foreground as a surgical assistant quickly hands the surgeon his tools—two slender fiber-optic tubes, one equipped with telescopic lens, video camera and light source, the other fitted with a laser. The surgeon makes two tiny incisions in the patient's abdomen, each smaller than a dime, and then inserts the instruments. The telescopic lens and camera help the surgeon locate the organ. Watching his movements on the video screen, he uses the laser to first carefully cut away a lesion and then seal the organ where the cut was made. Even as the piece of tissue is being sent to the laboratory for biopsy, the patient's incisions have been stitched and covered with Band-Aids.

This scene is reenacted every day in hospitals across the country. New developments in techniques, instruments and knowledge have revolutionized the field of surgery, moving it into what once was considered only the realm of science fiction. Doctors routinely make microscopic incisions with beams of light, freeze cancerous cells with liquid nitrogen, and use computer-operated cameras to view the interior landscape of the body. While the range of surgical procedures remains vast, the procedures, themselves, have changed. For example, a patient undergoing surgery to remove his gall bladder previously faced an operation that sliced through the major muscles of the abdomen to reach the organ and then kept him in the hospital for a week with restricted physical activity for up to six weeks following the procedure. Today, the same patient would most likely undergo a laparoscopic cholecystectomy, a procedure in which surgeons make four tiny incisions in the abdomen and then insert delicate instruments and cameras that they manipulate from outside. In less than an hour, the diseased gall bladder is extricated through one of the incisions. After an overnight stay in the hospital followed by a week of rest, the patient is back to his normal activities.

Just when operations, such as open heart surgery, were becoming more and more complex, as well as risky, technological innovations simplified the field. Less invasive surgical techniques, new antibiotics and anesthesia, improved imaging techniques, and advances in preoperative management all have contributed to making the surgical experience of the average patient safer and less painful and his recovery time much quicker.

Surgical Innovations

Researchers and surgeons have begun to view the best surgical techniques as those that manage to dispense with the typical symbols of their craft—the knife and scalpel. Advanced technology is changing the way a surgeon plans and executes an operation.

Videoscope Surgery & Imaging Techniques

One of the primary reasons why overall health care has improved in the last decade is the development of slender, fiber-optic tubes, or *scopes*, that can be inserted deep inside the body through nearly invisible incisions. Fitted with cameras, telescopic lenses, and lights and hooked up to video screens, scopes enable surgeons to see images of a patient's internal organs, usually with greater clarity than if they were looking directly at the organ. The appeal of videoscope surgery to both surgeons and patients is simple; while it enables doctors to pinpoint the location and type of the problem they're facing, it dramatically reduces surgical trauma for the patient. Conventional "open" surgery results in high levels of stress to the patient's body. Surgeons must cut through skin, muscles, fat and, depending on the surgery, bone. The use of videoscopes dramatically lowers the number of conventional operations, especially in the area of exploratory surgery, in which surgeons perform an operation to discover the nature of a patient's problem. Some doctors predict that the day will come when making any kind of incision will be viewed as a failure.

Various scopes are named for the area of the body in which they are generally used. *Laparoscopes* are used in the abdomen, *arthroscopes* are applied to the joints, *thoracoscopes or endoscopes* are used in the chest, and *angioscopes* are used inside the walls of blood vessels.

Improved imaging techniques such as *computerized tomography (CT)* and *magnetic resonance imaging (MRI)* have also moved the science of surgery forward. The CT scan provides surgeons with cross-section X-ray images of the inside of the body. All of the organs can be seen and evaluated. The MRI, on the other hand, creates three-dimensional images of the body's interior using a magnetic field and radio waves instead of X rays. Using these improved methods, surgeons can narrow the scope of the procedure considerably and meticulously plan every aspect of the operation.

Laser Surgery

First used in eye surgery in the 1960s, laser technology is coming to be regarded as a conventional surgical technique. Laser surgeons are the new breed of surgeons and precision separates their tools from the traditional knife and scalpel. Without even cutting skin, a laser surgeon can often completely eradicate a problem with absolute precision even in the most inaccessible areas of the body. Lasers cause little, if any, trauma to the patient, thus offering less invasive, even noninvasive, solutions.

An acronym for **L**ight **A**mplification by **S**timulated **E**mission of **R**adiation, the laser is a precisely controlled light beam that is narrowly focused and then aimed at a target. In each laser, various frequencies of light are converted into an intense beam of single wavelength, or color. The color determines how the beam will interact with particular types of tissue, and it may vary for different kinds of surgery. Lasers may function continuously or in pulsed bursts. The type of laser determines the number of pulses per second, the duration of the pulses and whether the light will be used to cut through, vaporize, or seal tissue.

Various lasers take their names from the different substances that produce the beam.

The *carbon dioxide laser*, with a wavelength in the far infrared spectrum, penetrates tissue to a depth of only one millimeter. Carbon dioxide's ability to turn the body's water content into steam allows it to sear or cut tissue to a precisely controlled depth. It can seal blood vessels and nerve endings in a bloodless procedure. The carbon dioxide laser has been used widely to treat some types of cancer, gynecological disorders, and brain tumors.

The *argon laser*, functioning in the blue-green frequencies, reacts with the color red and penetrates the skin until it comes in contact with blood. Because it readily coagulates with blood in the operating area, the argon laser has been particularly useful in the fields of opthalmology, plastic surgery, and dermatology.

The *YAG laser*, with a wavelength in the near infrared spectrum, is used to cook or vaporize tissue that will then be removed from the body. The most invasive of all surgical laser devices, the YAG laser can penetrate 4 to 5 millimeters.

Dye lasers can be tuned to react to different wavelengths of light, simply by adding or diluting tint. The *free-electron laser*, also tunable, uses magnets to stimulate pulsed light from a stream of electrons.

The *excimer laser* breaks up intermolecular bonds and decomposes matter, allowing precise surgery through holes so small no stitches are necessary. When certain gases are stimulated and combined and then returned to a disassociated state, their electrons emit photons of light in ultraviolet wavelengths. For example, patients undergoing excimer laser surgery to repair corneal damage do not experience the thermal effects or shock waves of conventional lasers. Without even touching the cornea, the excimer vaporizes with cool UV light the molecular links that bond the tissue.

Microscopic Surgery

The development of microsurgery—surgery performed under the lens of a high-powered microscope—allows surgeons access to parts of the body that would otherwise be too small to see. Many tumors, formerly considered inoperable, now can be removed through microsurgery. Often the use of microscopes is paired with another innovative technology, such as the use of lasers, because what the surgeon can't see with the naked eye, he also can't cut with a scalpel. Using the microscope to locate and isolate a tumor, the surgeon can then destroy it with a laser beam. Microsurgery has frequently been used to eradicate-brain tumors with success.

Cryosurgery and Hypothermic Arrest

Precancerous skin conditions, such as acute keratosis, as well as skin cancers, are often treated with a procedure called cryosurgery. Liquid nitrogen, applied to the growth, freezes and kills the abnormal cells. Once the dead tissues thaws, it falls off or is easily removed. Anesthesia is usually not necessary in cryosurgery, but patients may experience pain after treatment. Scarring after cryosurgery may also occur.

The human body's vulnerability to extreme temperature fluctuations and how it has reacted in the past has provided surgeons and researchers with valuable information that they have used to develop new surgical techniques. The discovery that the human body can survive without circulation at very low temperatures arose from cases in which children who lost consciousness after hours of submersion in extremely cold water were later revived. After six to ten minutes without oxygen, brain cells begin to die. In a new, experimental procedure called *hypothermic arrest*, the body is cooled to approximately 40 degrees below normal, where it needs much less energy and the brain can actually survive for up to sixty minutes without oxygen. Hypothermic arrest has been used almost exclusively for brain surgery.

Surgery Classifications

Surgery is classified according to whether it is vital to life, necessary for continued health, or desirable for medical or personal reasons. Although there are many ways in which surgical procedures are classified, the following breakdown is one that is widely accepted among surgeons.

Emergency Surgery

Unpredictable events that result in the need for medical immediate attention are classified as emergency surgeries. An automobile accident, a fire, a violent crime, or even a sudden change in a chronic medical problem, like a perforated ulcer or a strangulated hernia, can create situations in which the life of the patient depends upon the time it takes to get the victim into the hands of a trained surgeon. Emergency surgery cases typically involve the treatment of gunshot and stab wounds, fractures of the skull and other major bones, severe eye injuries, or life-threatening situations, such as obstruction of the windpipe caused by choking on a piece of food.

Emergency surgery may be one of the most common routes for patients entering the operating room. Accident patients present tremendous challenges to surgeons, because emergency room patients frequently have multiple injuries involving several organ systems. Such victims are often unconscious or otherwise unable to communicate coherently about their injuries, and there may be little or no time to obtain medical histories or information about their blood types, allergies to medicines, etc.

When possible, vital information about the patient and the circumstances surrounding the injury or sudden need for surgery is obtained by medical personnel who question anybody who might provide one or more clues. Efforts to maintain life are begun even while blood samples are taken for laboratory analysis and X-ray photographs made of the chest, abdomen, and other body areas that may be involved. When life is in immediate peril, resuscitation, induction of anesthesia, and surgery might proceed simultaneously as soon as a diagnosis is made.

Urgent Surgery

Next in priority for the surgeon are cases in which an operation is vital but can be postponed for a few days. A person injured in an automobile accident but conscious and suffering a minor bone fracture may be classed as an urgent rather than emergency surgery case, and the delay would give surgeons and other medical personnel time to study X-rays carefully, evaluate blood tests and other diagnostic data, and otherwise plan corrective therapy while under less pressure. Kidney stones, an acute, inflamed gall bladder, or cancer of a vital organ are examples of urgent surgery.

Elective Surgery

Elective surgery is usually subdivided into three categories: required, selective, and optional.

Required Surgery

Physical ailments that are serious enough to need corrective surgery but that can be scheduled a matter of weeks or months in advance generally are designated as required surgery cases. Conditions such as a chronically inflamed gall bladder, cataracts, bone deformities, or diseased tonsils and adenoids would be examples of conditions that require surgery.

Selective Surgery

Selective surgery covers a broad range of conditions that are of no real threat to the immediate physical health of the patient but nevertheless should be corrected by surgery in order to improve his comfort and emotional health. Certain congenital defects such as cleft lip and cleft palate would be included in this classification, as well as removal of certain cysts and nonmalignant fatty or fibrous tumors.

Optional Surgery

Of the lowest priority are operations that are primarily of cosmetic benefit, such as removal of warts and other nonmalignant growths on the skin, blemishes of the skin, and certain cases of varicose veins. Optional surgery also includes various kinds of plastic surgery undertaken for cosmetic effect. Among popular types of plastic surgery are operations to reduce or enlarge the shape of female breasts, reshape the nose, correct protruding ears, remove bags under the eyes, decrease facial wrinkles.

Types of Surgery

Surgery is further divided according to the following groups of major operations.

Surgeries with the suffix *-ectomy* involve the partial or complete removal of an organ, the most common being the appendectomy.

Operations to restore, reconstruct or refigure body parts are denoted by the suffix *-plasty*; thus cosmetic surgery to reshape the nose is called rhinoplasty.

Surgeries with the suffix *-otomy* involve the perforation or incision of organs or tissue, as in radial keratotomy, laser surgery performed on the eye.

The Surgical Team

Most surgical operations are performed not by the surgeon alone, but by a surgical team. Depending upon the complexity of the surgical procedure involved, the surgeon may have one or more assistants working him. The assistants may be interns or hospital residents who participate in the operation as a part of the advanced training in surgical techniques, or they may be other surgeons who are specialists in a particular field. An abdominal surgeon or orthopedic surgeon, for example, may be assisted by a neurosurgeon if the operation is likely to require a special knowledge of the nervous system as it affects another organ system.

The Anesthetist

The anesthetist, who is also likely to be a physician, specializes in maintaining the proper degree of anesthesia in the patient, while also helping to maintain the body's life systems. In addition to making the patient unaware of pain during the operation—sometimes by making him unconscious, sometimes without affecting consciousness—the anesthetist must keep the muscles and nervous reflexes in a proper state for the type of surgery to be performed. Each of the various functions, muscle relaxation, for example, requires a different anesthetic drug. Their performance must be perfectly coordinated to prevent complications during the operation. Obviously, the anesthetist must prepare a different combination of drugs for a child, an elderly person, a pregnant woman in labor, or a man with heart disease.

Other Members of the Surgical Team

As noted earlier, there are occasions when several surgeons are working more or less simultaneously on an accident victim with injuries to multiple organ systems. In such cases of emergency surgery, a general surgeon may supervise and coordinate the work of the other surgeons. The Chief Operating Room Nurse supervises and coordinates the activities of the scrub nurses who assist the surgeon in the actual operation, and the supply and circulating nurses who aid the rest of the surgical team by making available as needed the various towels, drapes, sponges, sutures, instruments, and other equipment.

One or more of the nurses wear gowns and gloves that have been sterilized so they can work directly with the surgeon and hand him equipment or supplies that he requests. Such a nurse is called a *scrub nurse* because he scrubs his hands and arms for ten minutes before the operation, just as the surgeon does. Other nurses in the operating room who do not wear sterilized gowns and gloves are not permitted to handle equipment directly but may be permitted to pick up sterilized materials with an instrument that has been sterilized. One or more orderlies, who are responsible for lifting the patient and keeping the operating room in tidy condition, complete a surgical team.

Preoperative Procedures

Preparation of a patient for surgery involves a variety of procedures determined by the urgency of the operation, the anatomical area involved, the nature of the disease or injury requiring surgery, the general condition of the patient, and other factors. Emergency surgery of an accident victim in critical condition obviously requires a greatly accelerated pace of preparing the patient for the operating room; medical personnel may cut away the clothing of the victim in order to save precious minutes. An operation on the intestine, on the other hand, may require a full week of preparation, including the five or so days needed to evaluate laboratory tests and sterilize the bowel with drugs. However, most preop procedures, as they are commonly called, generally follow a similar pattern designed to insure a safe and sound operation. Even in a case of emergency surgery, certain information must be compiled to help guide the surgeon and other hospital staff personnel in making the right decisions affecting proper care of the patient during and after the operation.

Medical History

The medical history should reveal the general health of the patient and any factors that might increase the risk of surgery. Perhaps one of his parents or another close relative suffered from heart disease or diabetes; such facts might suggest a predisposition of the patient to problems associated with those disorders. The data should also show whether the patient has a tendency to bleed easily and whether he has been following a special diet, such as a sodium-restricted diet.

It is important that the patient reveal to his own physician, the surgeon, and the anesthetist, the names of any drugs or other medications used. It also is vital that the medical personnel have a complete record of any patient experiences, including allergic reactions to certain drugs, that might help predict drug sensitivities that could complicate the surgery. The simple fact that a patient suffers from asthma or hay fever might indicate that he may be more sensitive than other individuals to drugs that might be administered.

Allergic Reactions

Some patients are allergic to penicillin or other antibiotics. Others may be sensitive to aspirin or serums. Still others could be allergic to iodine, Merthiolate, or even adhesive tape. All of these factors, if they are known and if they apply to the patient about to undergo surgery, should be brought to the attention of the medical staff.

Medications Currently Being Used

Among medications routinely used by the patient that should be brought to the attention of the surgeon and anesthetist are insulin for diabetes, digitalis drugs for heart diseases, and cortisone for arthritis. Depending upon various factors relating to the individual case, the patient may be directed to continue using the medication as usual, change the size of the dose before or after surgery, or discontinue the drug entirely for a while.

A patient who has been taking certain sedatives or drinking alcohol beverages regularly for a prolonged period before surgery may begin to experience withdrawl symptoms or he may have developed a tolerance for the anesthetic used, which means that he would require a larger than usual dose to get the desired effect. A patient who has been using epinephrine-type eye drops for glaucoma may be asked to increase the dosage before surgery as an adjustment to one of the drugs used in conjunction.

Diuretics, tranquilizers, and anticoagulant drugs are among other medications commonly used by patients that could affect the manner in which a surgical procedure is carried out. Patients should take a sample of the medication or the pharmacist's label from a container of the medication to the hospital so the medical staff can verify the type of drug used.

Psychological Evaluation

Of increasing importance in recent years has been a psychological evaluation of the patient. Individuals with a past history of mental disease or patients whose complaints may be based on psychoneurotic factors may react differently to surgery than persons who could be described as psychologically well balanced. The preoperative interviews also may seek to obtain information about the patient's abuse of drugs or alcohol.

Physical Examination

In addition to the medical history evaluation, the surgeon will need vital information about the physical condition of the patient. This requires a complete physical examination, including a chest X ray, an electrocardiogram of the heart activity, a neurological examination, and a check of the condition of the blood vessels in various areas of the body. Other body areas may be checked as warranted by complaints of the patient or by the type of surgery to be performed. An examination of the rectum and colon may be suggested, for example, if the medical history includes problems related to the digestive tract. Adult women patients usually receive a Pap test and possibly a pelvic examination. Samples of blood and urine are taken for laboratory analysis, including blood typing in the event a transfusion is needed. The laboratory tests for older patients frequently are more detailed and may include an examination of a stool sample. Any or all of these tests can be conducted days or hours in advance of the surgery.

Additional blood and urine samples may be taken immediately after admission to recheck the body chemistry, and a brief physical examination may be made to make sure the patient does not have any open wounds or infections that might complicate the chances of recovery or introduce a dangerous strain of bacteria into the sterile environment of the operating room.

Legal Authorization

Before the preoperative preparations are complete, chances are good that a member of the hospital staff will make sure that the patient has signed a legal permit authorizing the operation. The permit describes the operation, special diagnostic or therapeutic procedure to be performed and it may be signed by a close relative or legal guardian if for some reason the patient is unable to take responsibility for this action. For example, a parent will be asked to sign a permit authorizing an operation on his child.

Exceptions may be made in cases of emergency surgery where the patient is unable to sign a permit and a relative or a guardian cannot be located in time. But there are in-house procedures of consultation among staff members who accept the responsibility. Laws regarding permission to perform surgery may vary locally.

Preop Meals

A light but adequate evening meal is served if the surgery is scheduled for the following morning, but no solid food is permitted for 12 hours before surgery. No fluids are allowed during the eight hours before surgery. Children and patients with certain diseases, such as diabetes, may be given special orders regarding nutrients.

Preparation of the Skin Area

The area of the skin around the surgery site is carefully prepared beginning the evening before the operation. A member of the hospital staff may assist or direct the cleaning of the area with soap and warm water. The cleaned skin area is usually scrubbed again in the operating room as further protection against possible infection.

Shaving

Whether or not the skin area is to be shaved depends upon the amount of hair present. If there is no hair, the tiny nicks or cuts made by a razor would constitute an unnecessary hazard of infection. Where hair is present, however, shaving is essential in order to make available a very clean skin surface. Also, it is important that no hair or hair fragments be close enough to the surgical incision to fall beneath the skin; the bit of hair beneath the skin could cause a serious infection after surgery.

Anesthetics and How They Are Used

Anesthesia is a word derived from ancient Greek, meaning "without perception," or a loss of sensation. During a major or minor operation, as in having a tooth extracted by a dentist, it is helpful to both the patient and the physician if there is a lack of sensation during the procedure. But eliminating pain isn't the only consideration in the choice of anesthetic and other drugs used in conjunction with it. The age of the patient, chronic ailments, the site of the operation, and the emotional status of the patient are among factors considered. If a patient has undergone surgery previously and had an adverse effect from a particular kind of anesthesia, this information would have an important influence on the choice of an alternative type of anesthetic.

For many types of surgery, the kind of anesthetic chosen may be the result of an agreement among the surgeon, the patient, and the anesthetist. Some patients, given a choice, would prefer to remain conscious during an appendectomy or hernia repair; others would rather not. The surgeon frequently recommends the use of a general anesthetic because the procedure may require more time than the patient can be comfortable with in an operating room situation. Therefore, patients should realize that when a surgeon recommends a general anesthetic for an operation in which a local or spinal anesthetic might be adequate, it is for their own welfare.

General Anesthetics

General anesthetics are those that produce "sleep," or unconsciousness, along with *analgesia,* or absence of pain. They also cause a kind of amnesia in that the patient remembers nothing that occurs during the period in which the anesthetic is effective. At the same time, general anesthetics produce a certain loss of muscle tone and reflex action. A general anesthetic, however, should not interfere significantly with such normal bodily functions as respiration and circulation, nor should it produce permanent damage to body tissues.

How They Work

General anesthetics cause the patient to fall into a kind of sleep state by depressing the central nervous system, an effect that is reversible and lasts only until the drug has been eliminated by the body tissues. The general anesthetic reaches the central nervous system rather quickly because it is introduced directly or indirectly into the bloodstream. The use of a gas to produce anesthesia is an indirect method of producing unconsciousness.

A gas-type anesthetic, such as nitrous oxide or cyclopropane, can be delivered under compression from tanks or cylinders, or it may be stored in the operating room as a liquid that is converted to a vapor, like ether or halothane. The compressed-gas anesthetics are administered with the help of an anesthetic machine. The liquid forms of gases may be dripped through a mask over the patient's face; or the liquid may be vaporized and directed to the patient by anesthetic equipment. Whether the source of the anesthetic is compressed gas or a volatile liquid, the purpose is the same: to get the anesthetic into the patient's lungs. There the gas enters the bloodstream through the walls of the blood vessels of the tiny sacs that make up the lungs.

Kinds of General Anesthetics

Nearly a dozen different kinds of gases are available as general anesthetics. Each has certain advantages and disadvantages and interacts differently with other drugs used by the patient. The effects of each on chronic diseases of the patient must be weighed. Some gases induce anesthesia more rapidly than others; some are tolerated better by patients. These are among the many factors that can determine which gas or mixture of gases might be selected by the anesthetist for a particular surgical procedure.

Intravenous Anesthetics

Not all general anesthetics come in the form of compressed gases or volatile liquids. Several commonly used general anesthetics are administered intravenously, by injection into the bloodstream. The group includes barbiturates, such as thiopental, and narcotics, such as morphine. Ketamine is a general anesthetic drug that can be injected into the muscles as well as into the bloodstream. The intravenous anesthetics may be used instead of the gaseous general anesthetics or in combination with them. Thiopental is often administered to a patient first, to bring on sleep quickly, after which an inhaled general anesthetic is applied. Like the gaseous general anesthetics, each of the injected general anesthetics has its own peculiarities and may have different effects on different individuals. The rate of recovery from thiopental anesthesia varies according to the ability of a patient's body tissue to eliminate the drug; narcotics can affect the patient's respiration; ketamine may produce hallucinations in some patients.

Regional Anesthetics

Regional anesthetics include *local anesthetics* and *spinal anesthetics.* They are more likely to be used than general anesthetics when the patient is ambulatory and the surgery involves removal of moles or cysts, plastic surgery, certain eye, ear, nose, and throat procedures, and certain operations such as hernia repair that generally are uncomplicated. Regional anesthetics also may be recommended by the surgeon for operations to correct disorders in the arms or legs.

The surgical procedure may require that the patient remain conscious so he can follow instructions of the surgeon in manipulating muscles or bones to test the function of a body part being repaired. In such cases, a regional anesthetic would be preferred; a regional also would be advised for a patient with severe heart or lung disease that might be complicated by the effects of a general anesthetic. A restless child, on the other hand, might be given a general anesthetic for a relatively minor operation, because the youngster would not be likely to remain motionless for the duration of the operation.

Topical Anesthetics

Regional anesthetics generally are administered by infiltration of a drug into the tissues involved or into the nerve trunks leading into the area of incision. A simple kind of regional anesthesia is the topical application of a substance to a sensitive membrane of a body organ. For example, the eye drops applied by an ophthalmologist may anesthetize a patient's eyes to make it easier for him to examine them. Topical anesthetics are not very effective when applied to the skin, which forms a tough barrier against most invasive substances, but they can effectively anesthetize the inner surfaces of the mouth, nose, throat, and other inner body surfaces. The anesthetic might be administered by sprays, gargles, or by direct application. Topical anesthetics commonly are used to prepare the throat and upper lung passages for examination with medical instruments.

Local Anesthetics

Local anesthetics, which are similar to those used by the dentist, are usually injected via a hypodermic needle into the tissues surrounding the area to be operated on. The injection of an anesthetic into the tissue area sometimes is referred to as a *field block.* A variation of this technique is the *nerve* or *plexus block,* in which a hypodermic needle is used to inject the drug into the region of one or more key nerve trunks leading to the site of the incision. Local anesthetics are not recommended by most surgeons if there is an inflammation or infection of the tissues around the surgery site. The drugs used for local anesthetics can lower the patient's resistance to the infection while at the same time the inflammation may reduce the effectiveness of the drug as a pain-killer.

Intravenous Administration

Sometimes a regional anesthetic is administered intravenously by injecting it into a vein that runs through the site of the surgery. The drug is confined to the area, such as an arm or leg, by applying a tourniquet about the limb. Because of the possible dangers in suddenly releasing a potent anesthetic drug into the general bloodstream after the operation is ended, the tourniquet is intermittently tightened and released to slow the flow to a mere trickle. A sudden release also would quickly end the pain-killing effect in the area of the incision.

Spinal Anesthetics

Spinal anesthesia is similar to a nerve or plexus block method of eliminating pain sensation in a region of the body, except that the nerves receive the drug at the point where they leave the spinal cord. The drugs may be the same as those used as local anesthetics. They are injected either by hypodermic needle or by catheter into tissues surrounding the spinal cord. Although there are several variations of spinal anesthesia—each involving the precise layer of tissue or space around the spinal cord which is the immediate target area of the injection—for all practical purposes the objective is the same. They are all intended to produce a lack of sensation in the spinal nerves along with a loss of motor function so there will be no movement of the body area to be operated on during surgery.

The spinal anesthetic may affect not only the targeted nerve system but neighboring spinal nerves as well, generally all the spinal nerves below the point of drug injection. For its purposes, spinal anesthesia can be a highly effective alternative to a general anesthetic. However, side effects are not uncommon. Severe headache is one of the most frequent complaints of patients. Temporary adverse effects can occur after use of other regional anesthetics as well and may be owing in part to individual allergic reactions to the drug used.

Care after Surgery

The last thing you may remember as a patient, before receiving a general anesthetic, is being wheeled into the operating room and lifted by hospital orderlies onto the operating table. You may not see the surgeon, who could be scrubbing for the operation or reviewing the information compiled on your case. The anesthetist and a few nurses may be in the operating room. You are feeling relaxed and drowsy because of the preanesthetic medications. A tube may be attached to your arm to drip an intravenous solution into a vein. The anesthetist may administer a dose of a drug such as sodium pentothal, a not unpleasant medication that brings on a deep sleep within a matter of seconds.

The Recovery Room

You will probably remember nothing after that point until you gradually become aware of the strange sounds and sights of a recovery room. The recovery room may contain a number of patients who have undergone surgery at about the same time, especially in a large hospital. Each is reclining in bed equipped with high railings to prevent a groggy, confused patient just recovering from a general anesthetic from falling onto the floor.

Nurses move briskly about the room, checking the conditions of the various patients. As each patient gains some awareness of the situation, a nurse puts an oxygen mask over his face and explains the purpose: to help restore the tiny air sacs of the lungs to their normal condition. During administration of the anesthetic, the air sacs can become dry and partially collapsed. The humidified oxygen mixture helps restore moisture to the inner surfaces of the lungs; by breathing deeply of the oxygen, the patient expands the air sacs to their normal capacity. Before the use of oxygen masks in the recovery room and deep-breathing techniques for patients recovering from the effects of an anesthetic gas, there was a much greater danger of pneumonia developing as a postoperative complication.

Nurses assigned to the recovery room are given a report on each patient arriving from the operating room and instructions about such matters as the position of the patient in the bed. One patient may have to lie flat on his back, another on his side, a third in a sitting position, and still another with the head lower than the feet. If the patient has received a general anesthetic, the nurses may be instructed to turn him from one side to the other at regular intervals until he is able to turn himself.

The patient's blood pressure, pulse, and respiration are checked at regular intervals by the recovery room nurses, who also watch for any signs of bleeding or drainage from the area of incision. The surgeon is notified immediately of any signs of complications. Because the recovery room usually is located next to the operating room, the surgeon can quickly identify complications and attend the problem without delay. Most surgical patients will remain in the recovery room for a few hours at the most, and when they appear to be able to manage somewhat on their own they are returned to their beds in the regular nursing area of the hospital.

The Intensive Care Unit

Critically ill patients or those with heart, lung, kidney, or other serious disorders usually are assigned to an intensive care unit where each bed may be isolated from the others in a glass booth designed to provide privacy and quiet during the recovery period. Patients can still be clearly observed from the central nursing station.

Patients in an intensive care unit are given continuous care by nurses. Electronic equipment is used to monitor pulse, blood pressure, heartbeat, and, when needed, brain function and body temperature. Other devices are available for making bedside measurements of bodily function and to obtain laboratory data such as blood chemistry without moving the patient from his bed.

Pain

Most surgical patients will be concerned about how much pain they will feel after leaving the operating room. It is not unusual to expect greater pain than is actually experienced; the incision may cause no more discomfort than the problem that required surgical therapy. Obviously, a minor operation will result in less painful discomfort than a major operation. Generally, the pain or discomfort associated with a surgical incision may last for one or two days, then subside over a period of perhaps three or four days. After that an occasional twinge may be felt in the area of the incision when shifting the body puts extra stress on the muscles or other tissues involved in the operation. During the hospital stay, medications will be available to help relieve any serious pain resulting from the operation.

Signs of Recovery or Complication

While the patient may be concerned about pain following surgery, the physicians and nurses are more likely to direct their attention toward other signs and symptoms that will help them to gauge the rate of recovery, such as the patient's body temperature, skin coloring, urine output, and his ability to cough. The health professionals are well aware that surgery, and drugs or anesthetics administered in conjunction with surgery, can be disruptive to normal bodily activities. A major operation is more likely to cause changes in the patient's physiology than a minor operation.

Vital Signs

Nurses can be expected to make regular checks of temperature, pulse, and respiration because these common measures of the body functions (sometimes called *vital signs*) can provide early-warning signals of possible post operative complications. A patient may have a temperature of 100° F. even after a major operation, but because of increased metabolic activity of the body following surgery, a slightly elevated thermometer reading is considered normal. The pulse and respiration also may be slightly above the patient's rate before surgery, but the mild change again is caused by the normal stress reaction of the body. However, a temperature rising above 100° F. and/or a significantly faster pulse or respiration rate suggests that a complication may have developed.

If a nurse seems interested in the patient's ability to cough, it is because the cough reflex helps the patient get rid of mucus accumulation in his lungs, especially after the use of a general anesthetic. If coughing is difficult, a plastic tube may be inserted into the patient's throat to help clear the breathing passages. Normal breathing can also be restored by steam inhalation, aerosol sprays of water or special medications, or positive pressure breathing equipment that forces air into the lungs. Failure to expand the air passages of the lungs leads to serious respiratory complications.

Urine output is also checked. This is just one more way of watching the rate of recovery of a patient and alerting the staff to any signs of complications. If for some reason the patient is unable to pass urine, a *catheter,* or plastic tube, is inserted into the bladder to drain it. The volume of urine drained is collected and measured.

The Incision Area

Some blood may accumulate under the skin in the area of the incision or in nearby tissues, causing a discoloration of the skin. But this effect is seldom a serious matter, and the discoloration gradually vanishes. In some cases of excess blood accumulation, the surgeon may simply remove one or two sutures and drain away the blood. Any continued bleeding about the incision would, of course, be a complication.

A more common complication is infection of the incision area by bacteria that enter the wound. An infection may develop any time from one day to one week after an operation. However, most postoperative infections of incision wounds are easily controlled by antibiotics, drainage, or natural defenses against disease. The surgeon or other physicians will make regular inspections of the incision during the first few days after surgery to make sure it is healing properly.

Postoperative Nourishment

A light meal may be offered the patient a few hours after surgery. The patient may or may not feel like eating, especially if he still feels a bit nauseated from the effects of a general anesthetic. At this stage fluid intake is probably more important, especially if the patient has not been allowed to have even a sip of water since the previous evening. If the surgery was not performed on the stomach or intestinal tract, a small amount of water or tea may be permitted within a few hours after the operation. It is unlikely in any case that the patient will feel a great desire for fluid, because intravenous solutions may have been dripping slowly into a vein since he entered the operating room. Intravenous solutions can satisfy hunger as well as thirst because they may contain proteins, carbohydrates, and essential vitamins and minerals dissolved in a finely formulated broth. Perhaps unnoticed by the patient, the amount of fluid intake will be routinely measured by members of the hospital staff.

Ambulation

Ambulation—getting the patient out of bed and moving about—is an important part of postoperative care. Experience has shown that recovery from surgery is more effective if the patient spends increasing amounts of time each day in simple physical activity. The degree of ambulation depends upon the magnitude of the surgery and the general physical health of the patient. But in a typical case of hernia surgery or an appendectomy, the patient may be asked, on the first or second day after the operation, to sit on the edge of his bed and dangle his legs for a while. On the second or third day, he may be allowed to walk about the room, and may in fact prefer to walk to the bathroom rather than use a bedpan or urinal. On the following day, he may walk up and down the halls with the help of a nurse or other hospital staff member.

Each patient is encouraged to handle the ambulation phase of recovery at his own pace, and there are few hard and fast rules. Of two persons entering the operating room on the same day for the same kind of elective surgery, one may feel like walking to the bathroom a few hours after surgery while the second may prefer to remain in bed and use a bedpan a week after surgery. The surgeon and attending physicians may encourage and in some cases even insist upon early ambulation, however, because it reduces the rate of complications.

Back at Home

Dressings used to cover the incision are changed regularly, as the incision is inspected once each day, more frequently if warranted. If the patient is anxious to be discharged from the hospital as early as possible, the surgeon may give him instructions for changing his own dressings. The surgeon will also outline a plan for recovery procedures to be followed after he leaves the hospital. The plan will include a schedule of visits to the surgeon's office for removal of stitches that may remain and a final inspection of the incision. The surgeon will also offer his advice on how the patient should plan a return to normal activities, including a return to his job and resumption of sports or recreational programs.

Special Diets

Proper foods are as important as proper medicines in helping a patient recover from surgery. Despite the common complaints about hospital meals, the nutrients that are provided in certain special diets for surgical patients are as carefully prescribed and prepared as are some medications that are served in pill or capsule form.

Surgical nutrition has become increasingly important in recent years because of an awareness by physicians that an operation, minor or major, is not unlike an organic disease that creates physiological stresses and a nutritional imbalance in the patient's body. To help compensate for alterations in the patient's physiology as it recovers from the effects of surgery, special diets may be ordered.

Bland Soft Diet

A bland soft diet frequently is ordered for patients who are unable to handle a regular diet but whose condition is not serious enough to require a liquid diet. The foods are selected because they are low in cellulose and connective tissue; they are bland, smooth, and easily digested. The choice of food, nevertheless, represents as great a variety as one might be served in a restaurant or at home, except for an absence of spices and other substances that would be stimulating to the gastrointestinal tract. Included in the surgical soft diet might be lean meat, fish, poultry, eggs, milk, mild cheese, cooked tender or pureed fruits and vegetables, refined cereals and breads with butter or margarine, plus gelatin desserts, puddings, custards, and ice cream.

Liquid Diet

Liquid diets for surgical patients may be prepared with or without milk. They are usually ordered for patients with impaired function of the gastrointestinal tract. A liquid diet without milk may include a cereal gruel made with water, clear bouillon or broth, gelatin, strained fruit juce, and coffee or tea. Liquid diets with milk are similar but may also include creamed soups, sherbets, ice cream, cereal gruel made with milk instead of water, cocoa and beverages of milk or cream. Beverage options permitted are tomato juice and some carbonated beverages such as ginger ale.

Diets Following Particular Kinds of Surgery

Peptic Ulcers

A special diet for peptic ulcer patients may include a half-and-half mixture of milk and cream, plus mashed potatoes, eggs, toast and butter, pureed vegetables, cottage cheese, rice, plain puddings and gelatin desserts. But meat soups, tea, coffee, raw vegetables, and fried foods are prohibited.

Rectal Surgery

Following rectal surgery, and other procedures in which it is necessary to prevent bowel movements for a period of several days, a low residue diet is ordered. A low residue diet (or *minimal residue diet,* as it is also called) might offer eggs, poached or boiled, rice, soda crackers, cereals made with water, butter, bouillon or clear broths, carbonated beverages, tea, coffee, and certain meats, including oysters, sweetbreads, and tender bits of beef or veal. An alternative low residue diet is the bland soft diet with all milk-containing items eliminated.

Gallbladder Surgery

Gallbladder surgical patients may expect a modified fat diet that eliminates as much as possible fats and gas-producing food items. It includes foods that provide protein and carbohydrate sources of energy to replace fats and includes primarily fish, poultry, lean cuts of beef, cottage cheese, cereal products and bread, and certain fruits and vegetables. However, foods prohibited are mainly pork products and fatty cuts of other meats, cream, chocolate, melons, apples, fried foods of any kind, onions, cabbage, turnips, cucumbers, radishes, green peppers, and dried beans and peas.

Restricted Salt Intake

Chronic heart failure patients and those with liver ailments or edema are placed on a low-sodium diet before and after surgery. The low-sodium diet is fairly simple in that it is prepared mainly with foods from which sodium or salt either is naturally absent or has been removed. Many salt-free or low-sodium foods are available commercially from manufacturers that also supply special dietetic foods for persons suffering from diabetes.

Fractures or Burns

Special consideration is given the diets of patients who are recovering from accidents that result in fractures or burns. Because of complex body responses to such injuries, there may be an abnormal loss of nitrogen from the tissues and a breakdown of muscle tissue, which is a rich source of nitrogen, an important component of protein. As a result, adequate amounts of protein need to be provided to surgical patients with burn injuries and broken bones.

Potassium Loss

Normal body stores of potassium also may be diminished during and immediately after surgery, but potassium can be replaced in the tissues by including in the meals adequate amounts of meats, fish, poultry, bananas, raisins, figs, dates, and prunes, as well as dried peaches and dried apricots. Prune, tomato, orange, and pineapple juices also are a rich source of potassium for postoperative patients.

Replacement of Water Losses

While water is not always thought of as a food, it is an important part of the gastronomic intake of the surgical patient; adequate amounts of water need to be provided the person recovering from an operation. The postoperative patient usually requires larger than normal amounts of water even though he may not feel inclined to help himself to as much fluid intake as he would at home or on the job. In addition to normal water losses through perspiration, urine, and breathing, there may be additional water losses through vomiting. Water replacement may be provided through sufficient amounts of fruit juices and other beverages offered during meals and between meals.

Apprehensions about Surgery

Most people feel anxious when faced with the need for surgery. This is to be expected. After all, a certain amount of anxiety normally accompanies any prolonged or incapacitating illness or infirmity. When surgery is the recommended therapy, it's natural for the patient to feel some anxiety about the surgery even if he's optimistic about a favorable result.

Factors That Reduce the Risk of Modern Surgery

Much of the risk of surgery these days is eliminated through the careful preoperative screening examinations reviewed earlier. A patient with a chronic disease who might have been a surgical risk a generation ago may have one or more options not available in past years, such as regional anesthetics that allow surgeons alternatives to general anesthetics that would be less than satisfactory. Antibiotics and other backup medications are available to control possible complications after surgery. Recovery room techniques and intensive care units with electronic monitoring of vital life systems provide added insurance of safe recovery. And, of course, surgeons today have the added experience of many millions of successful operations involving a range of procedures such as kidney and heart transplants, open heart surgery, and replacement of important organ parts with plastic substitutes. These and other procedures, including the implanting of electronic heart pacemakers, were beyond the dreams of surgeons of past years.

Surgery for the Older Patient

With the rapid increase in the proportion of older people in the population, the surgical patient is more likely to be an older person with problems associated with aging. An older man who underwent surgery to remove his prostate gland before World War II had a life expectancy of a few years after the operation. Today, such procedures in older men are considered routine cases with little or no effect on longevity. It is not unusual nowadays to find men and women in their 70s and 80s who have undergone five or six major operations since reaching the traditional retirement age and without any significant restrictions on their physical activities.

Part of the reason for the greatly improved outlook for surgery on older patients may be that older persons today are simply in better health because of the improved medical care available. Thus they are better surgical risks than their parents would have been at the same age. Advanced preoperative and postoperative care has also improved the outlook for the older patient. He may be admitted to the hospital a few days earlier than the younger patient for more intensive examinations, and he may remain a few days longer for postoperative care. Convalescence for the older patient may take longer, and in some instances the recovery may not be as complete as that of a younger person. But in general, modern surgical techniques are likely to offer a safe and effective therapy for people of advanced age with complaints that can be corrected by an operation.

In addition to the physical benefits, surgery may improve the mental capacity, personality, and sensitivity of older persons who had been depressed about a disorder before surgery. The patient who complained that he is no longer the person he used to be physically may have assumed that his medical problem was simply a result of growing old and overlooked the possibility that the complaint was due to a disease that might respond to treatment.

Surgery for the Child

A child, on the other hand, may have his own reasons to be apprehensive about the trip to a hospital for surgery. Most children seem to worry that the operation will hurt or that other procedures, such as taking a blood sample for testing, will be painful.

Telling the Truth

Many surgeons recommend that the child be told as realistically as possible, in terms he can understand, what can be expected. The youngster should not be given a sugar-coated story about the operation which might give the impression that he is embarking upon a happy adventure. At the same time, the child should not be frightened by suggestions that he may be given drugs to make him unconscious while he is strapped to a table so that strangely masked and gowned strangers can cut him open with sharp knives.

Children are more likely to appreciate surgery if they are told that a friendly person will help them go to sleep; that the operation will hurt a little but the pain will go away after a while; and that the operation will make them feel better or help correct a problem so they can be more active like other children. A small child should always understand that he may have to remain overnight at the hospital without his parents, but that he will have other adults to take care of him and there probably will be other children at the hospital to keep him company.

Common Surgical Procedures

In this section some of the more common surgical procedures are described. The operations discussed are organized by the system or region of the body with which they are concerned. The following areas are covered in this order:

- Male Reproductive System (for surgical procedures involving the female reproductive system, see Ch. 25, *Women's Health*);
- Urinary Tract;
- Abdominal Region;
- Oral Cavity and Throat;
- Ear Surgery;
- Eye Surgery;
- Chest Region;
- Vascular Surgery;
- Orthopedic Surgery; and
- Neurosurgery.

Many of the conditions treated in this chapter from a surgical point of view are also treated elsewhere, in the chapter devoted to diseases of the appropriate body system or organ; the reader is invited to turn to those chapters for additional information. For example, although heart surgery is discussed in this chapter, heart disease is treated in greater detail in Ch. 10, *Heart Disease.*

Male Reproductive System

Surgical procedures of the prostate, testis, scrotum, and penis are considered in this section. Undescended testicles and vasectomy are also among the subjects discussed.

Prostate Surgery

The prostate gland is a small cone-shaped object that surrounds the male urethra, the tube that carries urine from the urinary bladder to the penis. It is normally about one-half inch long and weighs less than an ounce. Ejaculatory ducts empty through the prostate into the urethra, and other ducts drain glandular secretions of the prostate into the urethra. Because of the intimate association of the prostate gland and the urinary tract, a disorder in one system can easily affect the other. A urinary infection can spread to the prostate and an abnormality of the prostate can interfere with the normal excretion of urine.

Enlargement of the Prostate

A relatively common problem is the tendency of the prostate to grow larger in middle-aged men. The gradual enlargement continues from the 40s on, but the symptoms usually go unnoticed until the man is in his 60s. At that point in life, the prostate may have become so enlarged that it presses on the urethra and obstructs the flow of urine from the neighboring bladder. The older man may experience various difficulties in emptying his bladder. He may have to urinate more frequently, and suddenly find himself getting out of bed at night to go to the bathroom. He may not be able to develop a urine stream of the size and force he had in earlier years. He may have trouble getting the stream of urine started and it may end in a dribble.

In addition to the somewhat embarrassing inconveniences caused by prostate enlargement, the urinary bladder may not drain properly and can eventually lose its own muscle tone needed for emptying. Residual urine in the bladder can become a source of infection, and backflow into the ureters can gradually affect those tissues and the kidneys. It has been estimated that 20 percent of all older men may need treatment of some kind, including surgery, for correcting this problem of the prostate gland.

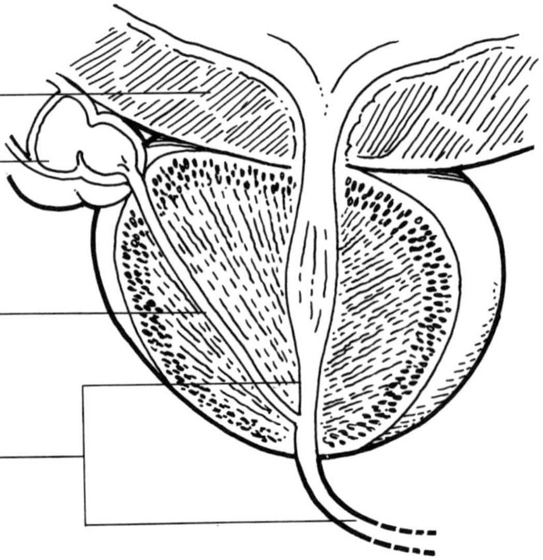

Factors Indicating the Need for Surgery

Factors that may decide in favor of surgical alteration of the prostate include residual urine in the patient's bladder; blood in the urine with evidence that the blood came from the prostate; the severity of the inconveniences associated with irregular urination; and complications such as the presence or threat of failure of the urinary bladder wall, bladder stone formation, and signs and symptoms of infection.

Surgical Methods

There are several methods of performing a *prostatectomy* (excision of all or part of the prostate) for relief of the symptoms of an enlarged prostate gland, a condition referred to as *benign prostatic hyperplasia* or *benign prostatic hypertrophy*. One method, called *transurethral resection*, requires insertion of an instrument into the urethra through the penis. The instrument, a *resectoscope*, uses a high-frequency electric current to cut away the tissue inside the gland. This technique does not require an external incision and requires a postoperative hospital stay of only a few days. In another method, an optical fiber is inserted into the prostate through the uretha and short blasts of laser energy destroy prostate tissue and produce shrinkage.

The other surgical methods involve *open surgery*, in which an incision is made in the pelvic or rectal area to make the prostate gland accessible so that its inner tissues can be removed.

Use of the various open surgery techniques depend upon such factors as where the incision should be made and the risks associated with the approaches. The incision is made either in the *perineum,* the region between the rectum and the testicles, or through the abdomen. Only a small percentage of patients experience complications or regrowth of the prostate tissues that produce a second enlargement problem. Impotence is not usually an aftereffect of the surgery, and a man's sex drive remains the same.

Infections of the Prostate

Infections of the prostate gland can involve obstruction of the urethra, but the problem usually can be resolved with medications and techniques other than surgery. An abscess, however, may require an incision to drain the prostate. Surgery may also be recommended for the treatment of stones, or calculi, that develop in the prostate and cause obstruction or contribute to infections.

Cancer of the Prostate

Cancer of the prostate may also occur, causing obstruction of the urinary flow or contributing to infection of the urinary tract. If examination, including biopsy studies, confirms the presence of cancer, the surgeon may recommend radical prostatectomy. In this procedure, an incision is made either through the lower abdomen or through the perineum to remove the entire prostate gland and surrounding tissues. Hormonal therapy, chemotherapy, and radiation treatments may also be administered.

Tumors of the Testis

Tumors of the testis occur most frequently in men between the ages of 18 and 35. Such a tumor appears as a firm and enlarged testis and usually causes no pain unless bleeding is involved as a symptom. Testicular tumors generally are malignant and spread rapidly to other parts of the body, including the lungs. The onset of the disorder can be so insidious that the patient may seek medical advice for a more obvious secondary problem, such as the apparent development of mammary glands on his chest, the result of disruption of his normal male hormonal balance.

Special laboratory tests and other examination techniques usually are required to determine which of several kinds of testicular tumors may be involved and the extent of the metastasis of the cancer cells to other body areas. If cancer of a testicle is confirmed, it is usually removed surgically. Some of the neighboring lymph nodes may also be removed. The surgical procedure usually is supplemented with chemotherapy, radiation therapy, or bone marrow transplantation. The chances for recovery after surgical removal of a testicular tumor depends upon the particular kind of cancer involved and how far the disease had progressed before medical treatment was begun.

Tumors of the Scrotum and Penis

Tumors of the scrotum and penis are relatively uncommon but do occur. Cancer of the scrotum is usually associated with exposure to cancer-causing chemicals. Boys who worked as chimney sweeps a century ago tended to develop cancer of the scrotum from body contact with soot in coal-burning fireplaces. Cancer of the penis occurs usually in men who have not been circumcised. In either type of cancer, the treatment usually requires removal of the affected tissues. This can mean castration in the case of scrotal cancer or amputation of a part or all of the penis, depending upon the extent of the cancerous growth. Surgery that requires removal of a part of the reproductive system can have a devastating psychological effect on a man, but the alternative is likely to be early death from the spread of cancer.

Undescended Testicles

About 10 percent of cases of tumors of the testis occur in men with an undescended testicle. Because the chances of a tumor developing in an undescended testicle are as much as 50 times greater than the incidence for the normal male population, the existence of an undescended testicle can warrant corrective surgery.

Ordinarily, the testicles descend from their fetal location in the abdomen into the scrotum about two months before birth. But in one case in 200 male births, a child is found with a failure of one or, less commonly, both testicles to descend properly into the scrotum. In addition to the risk of cancer, undescended testicles are associated with lack of fertility and other problems, such as hernias.

Cryptorchidism

In male babies and young boys, an undescended testicle sometimes can be encouraged to enter the scrotum by manipulation or administration of hormones. Many surgeons recommend that the developmental problem of undescended testicles, or *cryptorchidism,* be corrected before a child enters school, although the surgical procedure for correcting the situation can be postponed until adolescence or adulthood. The operation for correcting an undescended testicle is called *orchidopexy* and involves an incision in the groin to release the testicle and its attached cord from fibrous tissue holding it in the abdomen. The testicle may be brought directly down into the scrotum, where it may be anchored temporarily with a suture, or it may be brought down in stages in a series of operations to permit the growth and extension of blood supply to the testis. The original location of the undescended testicle determines which procedure is used.

Vasectomy

Vasectomy is a birth control technique that is intended to make a man permanently sterile. It does not involve the removal of any of the male reproductive system and does not result in a loss of potency or libido. A vasectomy is a relatively simple operation that can be performed in a physician's office in less than 30 minutes and requires only a local anesthetic. The operation is similar to but much less complicated than the procedure in which a woman may be sterilized by cutting or tying her Fallopian tubes. A vasectomy requires no hospitalization, and the man is able to return to work or other normal activities after a day or two.

How the Procedure Is Done

The vasectomy procedure requires a small incision, about one-half inch in length, on either side of the scrotum. The surgeon removes through the incision a short length of the *vas deferens,* the tube that carries spermatozoa from the testicles, and ties a piece of surgical thread at two points about an inch apart. Then a small piece of the vas deferens between the tied-off points is snipped out of the tube. The procedure is done on each side. With the ducts of the vas deferens cut and tied, sperm from the testicles can no longer move through their normal paths to the prostate, where they would become mixed with semen from the prostate and seminal vesicles and be ejaculated during sexual intercourse.

Vasectomy

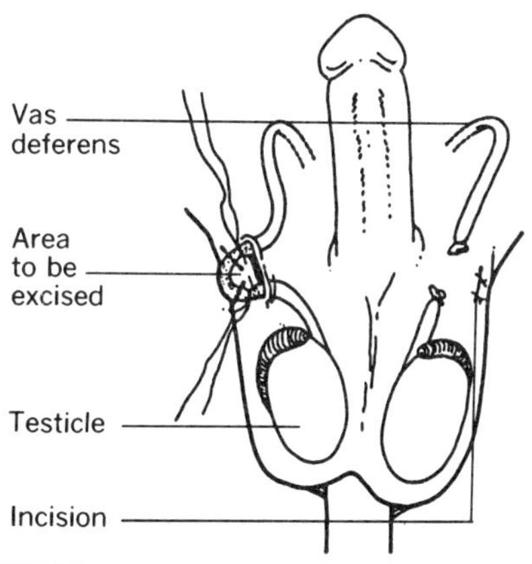

Sterility Is Usually Permanent

A vasectomy does not immediately render a man sterile. Sperm already stored in the seminal "pipeline" can still be active for a period of a month to six weeks, and a woman who has intercourse with a vasectomized man during that period can become pregnant. On the other hand, a man who undergoes a vasectomy should not expect that the severed ducts can be connected again should he want to become a father in the future. Sperm banks have been offered as a possible alternative for the man who might want to store some of his spermatozoa for future use, but there is little evidence that the sperm will remain fertile in a sperm bank for more than a year or 18 months. In rare cases, men who have undergone vasectomies have unintentionally become fertile again because of *canalization,* or creation of a new channel connecting the severed ends of the vas deferens; in one case the canalization occurred 8 years after the vasectomy was performed.

The vasectomy is regarded as an extremely safe operation, and complications are infrequent. Some swelling and discomfort are reported by a small percentage of men undergoing the operation. Steroid hormone drugs are sometimes administered to control these aftereffects.

Urinary Tract

Surgical procedures involving urinary stones and tumors of the bladder, ureter, urethra, and kidney are considered in this section. Also discussed are kidney cysts and conditions affecting the adrenal glands which might require surgery.

Urinary Stones

Most stones that occur in the urinary tract are formed in the kidneys, but kidney stones can travel to other areas, such as the ureters, and cause problems there. Various types of stones can develop in the kidneys from several different causes. A common cause is a metabolic disorder involving calcium, proteins, or uric acid. Other causes are infections or obstructions of the urinary tract, the use of certain drugs, such as diuretics, or vitamin deficiency.

Symptoms

Kidney stones seldom cause problems while they are forming, but movement of the stones irritates the urinary tract and can cause severe pain; the irritation of the tissues may cause bleeding that will ultimately show up in the urine. Other symptoms may indicate obstruction of the flow of urine, and infection. In some cases obstruction of a ureter can lead to failure of the kidney. X-ray techniques can usually verify the cause of the patient's symptoms and locate the urinary stone. Most stones cast a shadow on X-ray film, and by injecting special dyes into the urinary system, the degree of obstruction by a stone can be determined.

Ureter Stones

Most stones released by the kidney are small enough to pass through a ureter to the bladder and be excreted while urinating. But if a stone is large enough it can become lodged in a ureter, causing excruciating pain that may be felt both in the back and in the abdomen along the path of the ureter.

Ureter stones often can be removed by manipulation, using catheter tubes that are inserted through the bladder. If the stuck stone cannot be manipulated from the ureter, an operation in a hospital is required. However, the surgical procedure is relatively simple and direct. An incision is made over the site of the stuck stone, and the ureter is exposed and opened just far enough to permit removal of the stone. The operation is safe and requires perhaps a week in the hospital.

Kidney Stones

If the urinary stone is lodged in the kidney, the surgical procedure also is a relatively safe one although more complicated and requiring a longer hospital stay. The surgeon must work through skin and muscle layers to reach the kidney, then cut into the kidney if necessary to remove the stone. If the obstruction has been serious enough to impair normal kidney function or if infection has damaged the kidney tissue, the surgeon may elect to remove the affected kidney. Fortunately, the human body can get along fairly well with one good functioning kidney, so a *nephrectomy,* as the procedure is called, may not be as drastic a maneuver as the patient might imagine. If, on the other hand, the affected kidney has not been seriously damaged, the stone or stones can be removed with instruments or by the surgeon's fingers and the incision in the kidney sewed up so that it can resume its normal functions.

More modern techniques for removing kidney stones include two that hold promise of eliminating nearly all surgical methods. One involves the use of the lithotriptor, a machine that shatters the stones with an electrical shock wave. The wave is focused on the stones with the aid of a reflector and two sophisticated X-ray machines that "aim" the target beam. No surgery is required, and the patient is usually back at work within a week. A second means of attacking kidney stones is a drug, *potassium citrate,* which keeps the stones from forming. The drug actually corrects the metabolic disorders that cause the formation of kidney stones.

Vesical Stones

Occasionally, urinary stones are found in the neck of the bladder or in the bladder itself. They are called *vesical stones* and, depending upon their size and other factors, may be removed by several techniques, including use of a cystoscope inserted through the urethra. In some cases the stone can be broken into smaller pieces for removal. If it appears unlikely that the stone can be removed directly or by crushing it, the surgeon can make an incision directly to the bladder in a manner similar to the approach used in removing a stone from the ureter.

Bladder Tumors

About three-fourths of the tumors of the bladder occur in men past the age of 45. Although the specific cause of bladder tumors is unknown, physicians suspect that a cancer-producing chemical is involved. Several studies have found an association between the disease and cigarette smoking or occupations that require contact with organic chemicals used in making dyes. Tumors that appear in the female bladder are less likely to be cancerous than those that occur in the male bladder.

Symptoms and Diagnosis

The first symptom of bladder tumor is blood in the urine. The tumor itself may cause no pain, but an early complication could be an infection producing inflammation and discomfort in the region of the bladder. If the tumor blocks the normal flow of urine, the patient may feel pain or discomfort in the area of the kidneys; this condition is most likely to happen if the tumor is located at the opening of a ureter leading from a kidney to the bladder. An early examination of the bladder may fail to locate a small tumor, although X rays might show the growth as a bit of shadow on the film, and obstruction of a ureter could be seen. Nonetheless, examination of the interior of the bladder by a cystoscope is necessary to confirm the presence of the tumor. A biopsy can be made by removing a few tissue cells from the area in a manner quite like the procedure for making a Pap-smear test for possible cancer of the cervix in a female patient.

Treatment

Most early and simple cases of bladder tumor can be corrected by a procedure called *saucerization* by an instrument that removes the abnormal tissue, leaving a shallow wound that normally will grow over with healthy tissue cells. But a tumor that invades deeply into the wall of the bladder requires more radical therapy, such as surgery to cut away the part of the bladder that is affected by the growth. Radiation also may be employed to control the spread of tumor cells, particularly if laboratory tests indicate that the type of tumor cells involved are sensitive to radiation.

Surgical Procedure

If it is necessary to cut away a part of the bladder, the surgeon simply shapes a new but smaller organ from the remaining tissues. If a total *cystectomy* is required to save the life of the patient, the entire bladder is removed, along with the prostate if the patient is a man. When the bladder is removed, a new path for the flow of urine is devised by the surgeons, usually to divert the urine into the lower end of the intestinal tract.

Tumors of the Ureter or Urethra

Tumors of the ureter, above the bladder, or of the urethra, below the bladder, may begin with symptoms resembling those of a bladder tumor, although X rays might show the growth as a bit of shadow on the normal flow of urine. Treatment also usually requires removal of the affected tissues with reconstructive surgery as needed to provide for a normal flow of urine from the kidneys.

Kidney Tumors

Wilms' Tumor

Tumors of the kidney generally occur either in children before the age of eight or in adults over the age of 25. The type of tumor that affects children usually is the Wilms' tumor, one of the most common kinds of cancer that can afflict a youngster. The tumor grows rapidly and may be painful even though there may be no obvious signs of urinary tract disorder in the child's urine. The tumor frequently becomes so large that it appears as an abdominal swelling. A Wilms' tumor usually occurs only on one side of the body, but in a small percentage of the cases the disorder can develop in both right and left kidneys. Kidney function may continue normally during growth of the tumor, but cancerous cells from the tumor may be carried by the bloodstream to other parts of the body, by metastasis, causing the problem to spread to the lungs and other vital organs.

Treatment usually requires surgical removal of the affected kidney and radiation therapy; the tumor cells responsible for the growth are sensitive to radiation. The younger the child and the earlier treatment is started, the better are the child's chances for recovery from a Wilms' tumor.

Adult Kidney Tumor

The adult type of kidney tumor, which is more likely to affect men than women, may also appear as an enlarged abdominal mass. But, unlike the Wilms' tumor, the adult kidney tumor presents as an early symptom blood in the urine. Bleeding from the kidney may be painless. X-ray studies may show an enlarged and sometimes distorted kidney. The patient may have symptoms indicating metastasis of the tumor cells to the lungs, bones, or other body systems. Adult kidney tumors are almost always malignant.

Treatment usually requires nephrectomy, or surgical removal of the diseased kidney. Radiation therapy may be provided in addition to the surgery, although the kind of tumor cells involved in the adult type of kidney tumor usually are resistant to radiation. Chemotherapy also may be offered. The chances for complete recovery from a kidney tumor depend upon several factors, such as the location of the tumor in the kidney and the extent of metastasis of the cancerous cells to other organ systems.

Kidney Cysts

A cyst is a small pouch enclosed by a membrane; technically, the urinary bladder and gall bladder are cysts. But the cysts of medical disorders are small pouches or sacs filled with a fluid or viscous substance; they may appear on the skin, in the lungs, or in other body systems, such as the kidneys.

Symptoms

Kidney cysts produce symptoms that resemble the symptoms of cancer of the kidney; in a few cases kidney cysts are associated with tumors that cause bleeding into the cysts. In addition to the troublesome symptoms of flank pain and blood in the urine, untreated cysts can grow until they damage normal kidney tissue and impair the function of the organ's functions. Simple or solitary kidney cysts usually do not occur before the age of 40.

Diagnosis

X-ray techniques are made to determine the exact nature of kidney cyst symptoms, but in some cases exploratory surgery is recommended to differentiate a cyst from a tumor. The cyst is excised, frequently by cutting away the exposed wall of the growth. The chances of the cyst reforming are very slight.

Polycystic Kidney Disease

A different kind of kidney cyst disease, consisting of many small cysts, may be found in younger persons, including small children. The symptoms again may be flank pain and blood in the urine; examination may show some enlargement of the kidney. This form of the disease, sometimes called *polycystic kidney disease,* can be complicated by uremia and hypertension as the patient grows older. Treatment usually is medical unless the cysts interfere with urine flow by obstructing the upper end of the ureter. If the outlook for recovery through conservative treatment is poor, the surgeon may consider a kidney transplant operation.

Adrenal Glands

The adrenal glands are small hormone-producing organs that are located just above the kidneys. Although the combined weight of the two glands may be only one-fourth of an ounce, the adrenals affect a number of important body functions, including carbohydrate and protein metabolism and fluid balance. Surgery of the adrenal glands may be needed for the correction of various bodily disorders associated with oversecretion of the adrenal hormones; it may also be indicated to help control of cancer of the breast in women and cancer of the prostate in men.

Tumors of the Adrenal Glands

Tumors of the adrenal glands produce a disorder known as *primary hyperaldosteronism,* which is marked by symptoms of muscle weakness, hypertension, abnormally large outputs of urine, and excessive thirst. Another kind of tumor invasion of the adrenal glands can produce symptoms of hypertension with headaches, visual blurring, and severe sweating. Still another adrenal-related disorder, called *Cushing's syndrome,* tends to affect women under the age of 40. The symptoms may range from hypertension and obesity to acne, easy bruising, and *amenorrhea* (cessation of menstruation). Adrenal tumors may also alter secondary sex characteristics of men and women; they may result in body hair and baldness in women and increased sex drive in men.

Despite the tiny size of the adrenal glands, they are complex organs, and the varied disorders caused by tumors of the glands may depend upon the precise kind of tumor cells involved and the precise area of the glands affected by the tumor, as well as the interactions of the adrenal hormones with hormones from other glands, such as the pituitary, or master gland of the body, located at the base of the brain.

The Adrenal Glands

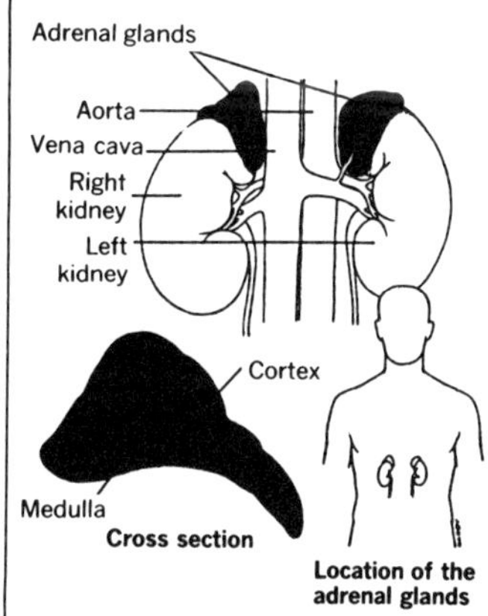

Preoperative Tests

Before adrenal surgery for correction of a disorder is begun, the surgeon may ask for detailed laboratory tests and other diagnostic information. A radioactive scan to help locate and identify the kind of tumor more precisely may be ordered. Women patients who have been using oral contraceptives usually have to discontinue use of "the pill" for two months or more, because the medication can interfere with laboratory studies of hormones in the bloodstream.

Long-Range Effects

Physicians handling the case also must evaluate the long-range effects of an adrenal gland operation because normal metabolism is likely to be disrupted by removal of the glands, if that should be necessary. Hormone medications usually are needed in such cases to replace the hormones normally secreted. An *adrenalectomy* (removal of an adrenal gland) sometimes is explained as the substitution of a controllable disease for a life-threatening disease that cannot be controlled by medical therapy. If only one of the adrenal glands must be removed, however, the patient may be able to recover and resume a normal life without the need for hormone medications.

Surgical Procedure

The surgical approach to the adrenal glands is similar to that used in kidney operations. The incision may be made through the abdomen or through the flank. The surgery may be primarily exploratory, or the surgeon may excise a part of a gland, an entire gland, or both glands, depending upon the extent of the disease, or upon other factors, such as the need to control cancers in other parts of the body.

Abdominal Region

This section discusses the following procedures or conditions: appendicitis, peptic ulcers, hiatus hernia, adhesions, cancer of the stomach and of the intestines, gallbladder surgery, inguinal hernia, and hemorrhoids.

Appendicitis

Inflammation of the appendix is one of the most common causes of abdominal surgery today, particularly among children. But appendicitis was not recognized as a disease until 1886, leading some doctors to believe that this digestive tract infection may be related to a change in eating habits that occurred within the past century. The vermiform appendix, the site of the inflammation, is a short, wormlike (or *vermiform*) appendage at the junction of the small and large intestines. Its function in humans is unknown; plant-eating animals have an appendix, but carnivorous animals, like cats, do not. Humans live quite well without an appendix, so it seems reasonable to have a diseased appendix removed.

Symptoms

The appendix can cause trouble if it becomes obstructed by a foreign body, a tumor, an infection, or other cause of inflammation. Pain is a common symptom; there may be two kinds of pain at the same time: one, localized on the lower right side of the abdomen, near the site of the appendix; the other, more generalized and colicky, of the kind sometimes associated with gas in the intestine. Some patients experience diarrhea or a constant urge to defecate, an effect attributed to irritation of the bowel by the abnormal activity of the appendix. Frequently there is loss of appetite, nausea and vomiting, and a fever.

The symptoms of appendicitis may begin suddenly, but frequently take from 6 to 18 hours to develop into a pattern typical of the disease, so most cases permit ample time for a doctor to examine the patient and make a diagnosis before the problem becomes critical. During the period that any symptoms suggest a possibility of appendicitis, the patient should avoid the use of any laxatives.

Ruptured Appendix

A potentially serious complication of untreated appendicitis is rupture of the appendix, which can produce a slightly different set of symptoms because of the onset of *peritonitis,* a dangerous inflammation of tissues outside the intestinal tract. The contents of the ruptured appendix leak into the body cavity, spreading the bacterial infection and irritating the lining (peritoneum) of the abdominal cavity. Diarrhea and a fever of more than 101° F. are frequently associated with a perforated or ruptured appendix. The colicky pain may disappear suddenly, because the internal pressure ends with perforation of the wall of the appendix, but it is quickly replaced by the pain of peritonitis. The severe pain of peritonitis usually is made worse by any body movement, including the abdominal muscle movement required for coughing or sneezing.

Appendicitis with perforation is much more common in older persons, perhaps because the early symptoms of colicky pain that younger people notice are not felt by older people, so the disease is not detected until it has reached an advanced stage. Appendicitis also requires special attention in pregnant women, because the enlarged uterus crowds and repositions segments of the intestinal tract and the potential threat grows more serious during the last trimester of pregnancy.

Surgical Procedure

Laboratory tests usually are checked before surgery proceeds if there is no evidence of perforation. The usual symptoms of appendicitis can be produced by a number of other ailments, and the symptoms may diminish with bed rest, time, and medications. However, appendicitis must be considered in any case of acute abdominal complaints, and many surgeons and physicians follow the rule of "When in doubt, operate." Surgery for appendicitis is fairly simple and safe if the appendix has not perforated. An incision is made in the lower right side of the abdomen, the connection between the end of the large intestine and appendix tied off with surgical thread, and the appendix cut away from the stump. The actual operation, if uncomplicated by peritonitis or other factors, may require only a few minutes. A hospital stay of a few days is usually required during which the diet is readjusted from nothing by mouth at first, to a liquid diet, then a soft diet, etc. Normal work activities usually can be resumed within two or three weeks after surgery. Complications other than those related to peritonitis are rare. In untreated cases involving peritonitis, however, the risk of complications is very high.

Peptic Ulcers

Peptic ulcers are sores on the stomach lining or the duodenum (the beginning of the small intestine). Peptic ulcers are common, affecting about 10 percent of the population at some time in life. Peptic ulcers in the stomach, are called *gastric ulcers*. In the duodenum, they are called *duodenal ulcers*. Ninety percent of the ulcer cases that require a physician's treatment are in the duodenum. Autopsy studies indicate that gastric ulcers may be as common as duodenal ulcers, but are frequently not detected during the individual's lifetime.

Causes

Peptic ulcers can be caused by bacterial infection, long-term use of nonsteroidal anti-inflammatory drugs (NSAIDs), such as ibuprofen and aspirin, or, more rarely, by cancerous tumors in the pancreas or stomach. Researchers believe the bacteria *Helicobacter pylori (H. pylori)* causes most peptic ulcers. Contrary to what was previously thought, peptic ulcers are not caused by stress or spicy foods.

Symptoms

A common symptom is a gnawing pain in the area of the stomach from 30 minutes to several hours after eating; the pain is relieved by food or antacid medications. The pain sometimes is likened to heartburn and may be described as radiating from the abdomen to the back. Some patients report the discomfort is more like a feeling of hunger or cramps; they may be awakened from sleep by discomfort, which may be relieved by a snack. Other symptoms include burping, bloating, and nausea. In severe cases there may be bleeding without any abdominal pain; bleeding occurs from erosion of the lining of the stomach or duodenum and penetration of blood vessels in those membranes.

Complications other than bleeding can include perforation of the wall of the stomach or duodenum by continued erosion, or inflammatory swelling and scarring by an ulcer at a narrow part of the digestive tract, causing an obstruction. A duodenal ulcer can erode into the head of the pancreas, which secretes its digestive juices into the small intestine in that area. The pain may then become more or less continuous regardless of efforts to relieve it with food or antacids.

Symptoms vary only slightly between duodenal and gastric ulcers. Gastric ulcer pain usually begins earlier after a meal, attacks generally last longer, and symptoms, including vomiting and loss of appetite, may be more severe than in duodenal ulcer. But because of the similarities, physicians usually rely on examination of the esophagus, stomach, and duodenum by inserting through the mouth an *endoscope,* a narrow lighted tube with a camera on its tip, laboratory tests, or X-ray studies to determine the precise location in the digestive tract of the peptic ulcer.

Treatment

The overwhelming majority of peptic ulcers heal within one to three months with the use of drug therapy. Because most peptic ulcers are caused by *H. Pylori* bacteria, they are usually treated with antibiotics to kill the bacteria. These antibiotics include amoxicillin, metronidazole, clarithromycin, and tetracycline. Doctors also strive to reduce the amount of acid in the digestive system by prescribing acid-suppressing drugs, which may be either H_2 blockers, such as cimetidine and nizatidine, or proton pump inhibitors, such as omeprazole and lansoprazole. A stomach-lining protector, such as sucralfate and bismuth subsalicylate, is usually also prescribed. Patients are usually treated with a combination of these drugs and with more than one antibiotic at a time.

Ulcers that don't heal in one to three months are called refractory ulcers. Not taking medications according to instructions and regular use of alcohol, tobacco, and NSAIDs can impede healing. In addition, some *H. pylori* are resistant to certain antibiotics. Refractory ulcers may also be due to an infection not caused by *H. pylori,* severe overproduction of stomach acid, or by other diseases of the digestive system, such as cancer or *Crohn's disease,* a chronic inflammation of the gastrointestinal tract. Peptic ulcers that don't heal within one to three months may require surgery.

Surgery for either duodenal or gastric ulcer is designed to reduce gastric acid secretion rather than simply to excise the ulcer from the normal digestive tract tissue. Operations for ulcers have become less invasive with the increasing use of *laparoscopes*—tiny, long tube-like instruments with cameras at their end that can be inserted through very small incisions. With this instrument, surgeons can see the field of operation through a video monitor.

One surgical approach, a *vagotomy,* involves cutting a part of the vagus nerve trunk that controls the secretion of stomach acid. There are several variations of vagotomy, each technique affecting a different portion of the vagus nerve distribution to the stomach.

A second surgical approach, called

antrectomy, involves cutting away the *antrum* portion of the stomach, which secretes a hormone that stimulates the secretion of digestive juices. A vagotomy is usually performed along with an antrectomy.

A third surgical method involves enlarging the pylorus, which is the opening into the duodenum and the small intestine. Called *pyloroplasty,* this procedure allows the stomach's contents to pass more easily from it.

Hiatus Hernia

The term *hiatus hernia* describes a diaphragmatic hernia or weakness in the diaphragm, the horizontal muscular wall separating the organs of the chest from the organs of the abdomen. A *hernia* is an abnormal protrusion of an organ or tissue through an opening. A *hiatus,* or opening, permits the esophagus to carry food from the mouth to the stomach. Blood vessels and nerves also pass through the diaphragm. The diaphragm is an important group of muscles for contracting and expanding the lungs, forcing air in and out of the lung tissues.

Hiatus hernias are rare in children, but as people grow older, the diaphragm muscles and associated tissues may weaken. Aided by a tendency toward obesity and the use of girdles or other tight garments, a portion of the stomach may be pushed through the opening designed by nature for use of the esophagus. Potential dangers of incarceration of the stomach include obstruction, strangulation, and hemorrhage with erosion of the stomach lining. In severe complications, the entire stomach along with intestines and other abdominal organs may be forced through the hiatus hernia into the chest area.

The most common kind of hiatus hernia is sometimes called *sliding hiatus hernia* from the tendency of the stomach to slide in and out of the thorax, or chest cavity, when the patient changes body positions or as a result of the pressure of a big meal in the gastrointestinal tract. Sometimes the herniated stomach does not move at all but remains fixed, with a significant portion of the stomach above the diaphragm. Hiatus hernia causes heartburn symptoms, including regurgitation of digested food and gastric acid from the stomach, especially when one is in a lying, straining, or stooping position. The effect also may be noticeable in a woman during pregnancy.

Hiatus Hernia

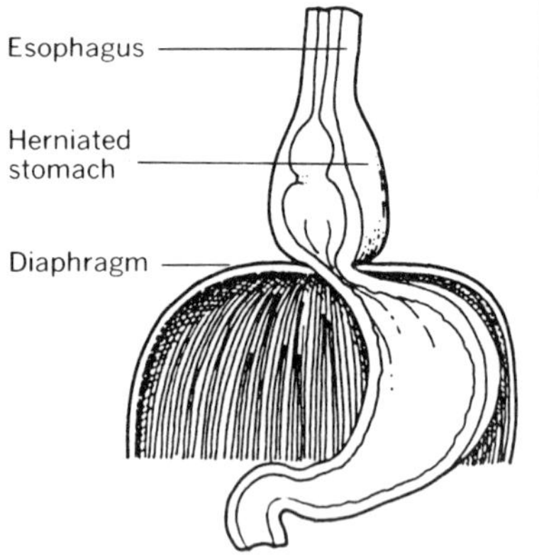

Nonsurgical Treatment

Many cases of hiatal hernia can be treated without surgery through a change of eating habits and the use of antacid medications. The patient may be advised to eat small amounts more frequently during the day with dietary emphasis on high-protein, low-fat foods. Some physicians recommend that patients use liquid antacid medications rather than antacid tablets or lozenges.

Surgical Treatment

When surgery is recommended to correct hiatus hernia, the repair may be performed either through the abdominal wall or through the chest. About three-fourths of the procedures are handled through abdominal incisions, because surgeons often find other abdominal problems that need to be corrected at the same time, such as peptic ulcers or gall bladder disease. The opening through the diaphragm is firmly closed with sutures to prevent upward movement of the stomach. The stomach and lower end of the esophagus may be anchored in place in the abdomen. The chances of recurrence are about one in ten, although some patients may continue to have a few of the symptoms of the disorder for a while after the hernia repair.

Adhesions

Adhesions may develop between various abdominal organs and the peritoneum, the membrane lining the abdominal cavity. The bowel may acquire adhesions that result in obstruction of the intestinal tract. Adhesions may form between the liver and the peritoneum or between the liver and the diaphragm. The symptoms may be pain or cramps in the area where tissues are literally stuck together; in more serious cases that involve bowel obstruction, symptoms may include constipation, vomiting, and distension of the abdomen. Adhesions do not show on X-ray film and can be difficult to diagnose unless the patient's medical history suggests a cause for the bands or filaments of tissues responsible for the adhesions.

Causes

The causes may be peritonitis, injury, infection, internal bleeding, or foreign objects. Adhesions occur after an operation, perhaps because of a bit of blood resulting from surgery or as a result of a speck of talc from the surgeon's glove or a fiber from a surgical drape which produces a foreign-body reaction, much like an allergic reaction, when it comes in contact with abdominal tissues. Disease organisms may enter the female abdominal cavity through the Fallopian tubes to produce adhesions, especially in the case of gonorrhea, which can escape early detection in women because of the lack of obvious symptoms.

Complications

Adhesions can cause complications, such as changing the position of the intestinal tract through twisting or otherwise distorting its path so that bowel movements are obstructed. If the involved portion of the intestine becomes so seriously damaged that it no longer functions properly, the surgeon may have to remove that section. Generally, when the surgeon is correcting the problem of adhesions, a relatively simple procedure of cutting away the tissue bands or filaments holding organs in abnormal ways, he inspects the organs to determine if they appear to be in good working order. That part of the operation may add 15 or 20 minutes to the time spent on an operating table, but it helps insure that the patient will not have to be returned soon for further surgery.

Cancer of the Stomach

There are several possible types of stomach tumors, but one kind, called *adenocarcinoma,* is one of the greatest killers of men over the age of 45. Although the incidence of stomach cancer in the United States has declined considerably since the end of World War II, the death rate from this problem in the United States alone is about 15,000 per year. In central and eastern Europe the incidence of stomach cancer is about four times, and in Japan seven times, that of the United States. Almost two-thirds of the stomach cancers develop near the pylorus, the opening from the stomach into the small intestine; only five percent involve the entire stomach area.

Symptoms

Symptoms include a feeling of heaviness rather than pain following a meal. The patient in many cases mysteriously loses his appetite for meat and begins to lose weight. There may be vague symptoms of an upset stomach, with some vomiting, especially if the tumor begins to obstruct the pylorus such that stomach contents cannot be emptied into the intestine. The vomitus usually is the color of coffee grounds, suggesting a loss of blood from the stomach lining because of the tumor, and the patient's stools also may be dark in coloration because of internal bleeding. The physician frequently can confirm his suspicions about the cause of the symptoms by laboratory analysis of a specimen of cells from the stomach, by X-ray studies of the stomach, or by an examination with a gastroscope that permits a direct view of the interior of the stomach. In some cases the physician will be able to feel an abnormal mass in the stomach by palpating the stomach area of the abdomen with his hands.

Treatment

Treatment is by cutting away the tumor and surrounding tissues that may be involved, including parts of neighboring organs. The lymph nodes in the region of the stomach are also removed. The remaining part of the stomach is used to build a new digestive organ, as in a case of partial gastrectomy for correcting a peptic ulcer problem. However, before beginning reconstructive surgery, the physician usually orders biopsy tests of the remaining tissues to make sure the new stomach will not be made of tissues in which tumor cells have spread. If the edges of the remaining stomach wall are found to contain tumor cells, the surgeon simply extends the area to be removed. As in subtotal gastrectomy for peptic ulcers, the remaining portion of the stomach may be connected directly to the upper portion of the small intestine, at the duodenum or the jejunum.

Meals are provided in the form of intravenous feedings for the first few days following surgery. Sips of water may be permitted on the second or third day after the operation with the amounts gradually increased to one or two ounces of water per hour as the new digestive system adjusts to fluid intake. Then soft or bland foods can gradually be taken orally in a half-dozen small feedings each day. It may take three or four months for the new stomach to distend and adjust to normal eating habits of the patient.

Postoperative Effects

Some patients may experience a variety of symptoms ranging from nausea to cramps and diarrhea while recovering from stomach surgery. The symptoms form what is known as the *dumping syndrome,* which occurs within a half hour after a meal, presumably by rapid distension of the upper portion of the small intestine as fluid rushes, or is dumped, into that part of the digestive tract from the new stomach. The effects can be controlled by a change of diet to eliminate starches and sugars, by delaying the intake of fluids until after the meal, by medications, and by training the patient to lie in a recumbent or semirecumbent position to lessen discomfort following a meal. The symptoms occur in only a small proportion of stomach surgery patients, and they usually diminish gradually during the period of recovery.

Cancer of the Intestines

Small Intestine

Tumors of the small intestine are not common, but they also are not rare. It has been estimated that less than five percent of all tumors of the gastrointestinal tract occur in the small intestine. Of tumors that do develop in this portion of the gastrointestinal tract, about 90 percent are benign, or noncancerous, growths. The symptoms of small intestine tumors may include bleeding, obstruction, and perforation of the intestinal wall. However, most tumors of the small intestine produce no symptoms at all. When tumors are found in the small intestine they usually are found at the same time in other parts of the body, and usually in a patient over 40 years of age, although the more malignant growths can occur in younger persons. Treatment of a cancer of the small bowel is by removing the affected section and administration of radiation therapy for certain kinds of cancerous tumors.

Large Intestine

Tumors of the large intestine, unlike those of the small bowel, account for a large proportion of cancers of the human body and for most of the malignant growths of the entire gastrointestinal tract. More than 40,000 deaths each year in the United States are a result of cancers of the colon and rectum portions of the large bowel. And about three-fourths of all large-intestine tumors develop near the rectal portion of the bowel, where, ironically, they should be easily available for detection during physical examination.

Tumors of the large intestine can be found in persons of any age, but they occur most frequently in patients who are of middle age or older, reaching a peak of incidence around the age of 65. Men are more likely to develop cancer of the rectum, but women are more frequently affected by cancer of the colon. While cancer of the large intestine tends to occur among members of the same families at a rate that is two or three times the normal incidence, it is believed that family environment factors, such as life style and diet, are the causative influences, rather than hereditary factors. People who develop cancer of the large intestine usually eat foods that are low in cellulose and high in animal fats and refined carbohydrates.

Bowel cancers appear to grow in size at a very slow rate, doubling about once every 20 months, so a number of years may elapse between the start of a bowel tumor and the appearance of signs or symptoms of cancer.

Symptoms

The location of the growth can influence the types of symptoms experienced. Cancer in the right colon may be found as an abnormal mass during a physical examination by a physician after complaints of fatigue and weakness and signs of anemia. The tumor can develop to a rather large size without producing signs of blood in the stools. Cancer in the left colon, by contrast, may be found after complaints of alternate periods of constipation and frequent urge to defecate, pain in the abdomen, and stools marked by dark and bright red blood. When the cancer is in the rectum, the patient may find blood mixed with the bowel movements but experience no pain in the early stages. Other symptoms of cancer of the large intestine may mimic those of appendicitis, hemorrhoids, peptic ulcer, or gall bladder disease.

As noted above, most cancers of the large bowel are close enough to the end of the intestinal tract to be observed directly by palpation or the use of fiberoptic instruments, such as a sigmoidoscope or colonoscope, which can be inserted into the rectum or colon. Biopsy samples can be removed for study and X-ray pictures taken after administration of a barium enema, which coats the bowel membrane in such a way that abnormal surfaces are clearly visible.

Surgical Procedures

Surgical procedures for treatment of cancer of the large intestine vary somewhat according to the location of the growth, but the objective is the same: to remove the affected portion and reconstruct the bowel so that normal digestive functions can resume. Radiation therapy and chemotherapy may be used in the treatment of certain advanced cases. When surgical treatment is begun soon after the first symptoms are diagnosed, the chances of curing cancer of the large bowel are very good.

If there are complications, such as obstruction of the portion of the large intestine, the surgery may be conducted in a series of stages over a period of several weeks. The several stages involve a colostomy procedure in which an opening is made in the wall of the abdomen to permit a portion of the intestinal tract to be brought to the surface of the body. After the complicating problem is treated and resection of the cancerous segment is completed, the colostomy is closed by sewing the open end of the bowel to the remaining portion and closing the opening in the abdomen.

Preoperative Steps

Some special preoperative measures are ordered for patients awaiting surgery for treatment of bowel cancer. They consist primarily of several days of liquid diets, laxatives, and enemas to make the interior of the intestinal tract as clean as possible. Other measures will be directed toward correction of anemia and compensation for possible loss of blood resulting from the cancer's invasion of bowel tissues.

Gallbladder Surgery

Gallbladder disease is one of the most common medical disorders in the United States. It has been estimated that more than 15 million Americans are affected by the disease and about 6,000 deaths a year are associated with it. The incidence increases at middle age; 1 of every 5 women over the age of 50 and 1 of every 20 men can expect to be treated for gallbladder symptoms. Approximately 1,000 people in the United States enter operating rooms each day for removal of gallstones, a primary cause of the symptoms of the disorder.

Gallstones

Gallstones generally are formed from crystals of cholesterol that gradually increase in size in the gallbladder; some, however, are formed from other substances, such as bile salts and breakdown products of red blood cells. Because they are very small in size, the stones may produce no symptoms at first. But as they grow in size they become more threatening and eventually can block the normal flow of bile from one of the bile ducts emptying into the intestine. Bile contains substances needed by the body to digest fats in the diet.

Symptoms

A common symptom of *chronic cholecystitis,* or gallstone disease, is a pain that appears suddenly in the upper abdomen and subsides slowly over a period of several minutes to several hours. The pain may occur after a meal or with no apparent relationship to meals. There can be tenderness in the upper right side of the body, with pain extending to the shoulder. The pain also can appear on the left side or near the center of the upper abdomen, producing misleading symptoms suggesting a heart attack. Nausea, heartburn, gas, indigestion, and intolerance to fatty foods are among other possible symptoms. The gallbladder attacks may occur frequently or there may be remissions (periods without symptoms) lasting for several months or years.

A careful and extensive physical examination, including X-ray studies of the gallbladder area, may be needed to confirm the presence of gallstones. Until recently, the most commonly used test was the oral cholecystogram (OCG), in which the patient swallowed an iodine-based "dye," or contrast agent. X rays taken about 12 hours after administration of the dye might or might not provide useful "pictures" of the gallstones. As a result, ultrasound has largely replaced X rays as a primary test for suspected gallstones.

Acute Cholecystitis

About three-fourths of the cases of acute cholecystitis are patients who have had previous attacks of gallstone disease. In the acute phase there is persistent pain and abdominal tenderness, along with nausea and vomiting in many cases and a mild fever. Complications may include perforation, or rupture, of the gallbladder, leading to peritonitis, or development of adhesions to neighboring organs such as the stomach or intestine.

Treatment

Surgical treatment of chronic or acute cholecystitis is basically an elective procedure that can be scheduled at a time convenient to the patient. But acute cases with complications may require emergency operations. The patient can usually be maintained, after surgery, on intravenous fluids and pain-killing medications.

In gallstone surgery, the abdomen is opened so that the surgeon can examine the gall bladder and the ducts leading from it for stones. The gallbladder may be freed of stones and a temporary drainage tube inserted, with an opening to the outside of the upper abdomen. But usually the surgeon removes the entire gallbladder in an operation called a *cholecystectomy*. The bile duct, which remains as a link between the liver and the small intestine, gradually replaces the gallbladder in function. Conventional cholecystectomies are rarely performed now. The less invasive laparoscopic cholecystectomy has almost completely replaced the conventional surgical removal of diseased gallbladders. In the innovative method, a laparoscope removes the entire gallbladder and any stones it contains. Using videoscope surgery, everything is neatly pulled through tiny incisions in the abdomen.

A number of alternatives to surgery have been developed. A gastroenterologist may use an endoscope on older patients or those in poor health. The endoscope, a tube inserted through the chest wall, enables the physician to view the gallbladder's duct area and to widen its opening so that small gallstones can slip through the small intestine. Using a small basket on the endoscope, the physician can sometimes catch and withdraw or crush the stones.

Other nonsurgical treatments include chemical preparations. Chenodeoxycholic acid, or chenodiol, has been given orally to dissolve smaller, floating cholesterol stones. But the drug has little effect against pigment stones or stones with a high calcium content, and can cause diarrhea as a side effect.

Among the most advanced techniques is *choledocholithotripsy,* a nonsurgical method using shock waves to destroy gallstones. Already in use as a method of shattering kidney stones, lithotripsy requires only a local anesthetic and the recovery period lasts only a few days. The physician uses a hollow tool—the lithotriptor—that is inserted through the patient's chest until it approaches the stones. With a foot switch, the physician then triggers a jolt of high-voltage, low-current electricity that shatters the stones.

In another advance, drugs have been utilized to dissolve gallstones. A drug called *methyl tertbutyl ether* (MTHE) has been found to break down gallstones as large as golf balls. Still partly experimental, the compound could replace most surgical operations for gallstones.

Inguinal Hernia

An inguinal hernia (hernia of the groin) can develop in either men or women at almost any age from infancy to late adult years. But the incidence of inguinal hernia is much more common in males. An inguinal hernia is one in which the intestinal tract protrudes through the opening of one of the inguinal rings on either side of the groin. In males, the inguinal rings are temporary openings through which the testicles descend into the scrotum before birth; in females, the openings permit the passage of a ligament supporting the ovary.

Causes

Normally, the inguinal rings are closed after the birth of the child. However, they may fail to close completely or the muscles and connective tissues may become stretched or weakened in later years to permit a portion of the abdominal contents, usually part of the intestine, to protrude. A number of factors can contribute to the development of a hernia, including physical strain from exercise or lifting, straining over a bowel movement, coughing spells, pregnancy, pressure of abdominal organs, or obesity.

Reducible and Irreducible Hernias

The hernia may be *reducible,* that is, the bulge in the abdominal wall may disappear when the body position is changed, as in lying down, only to reappear upon standing. An *irreducible* hernia does not allow the hernia sac contents to return to the abdominal cavity; an irreducible hernia also may be called *incarcerated,* a term aptly describing the hernia as being trapped. A serious complication is strangulation of the hernia contents, which usually involves obstruction of normal blood flow and resulting damage or destruction of the incarcerated intestines. A strangulated hernia may be life-threatening because of the possibility of gangrene in body tissues damaged by incarceration.

Inguinal Hernia

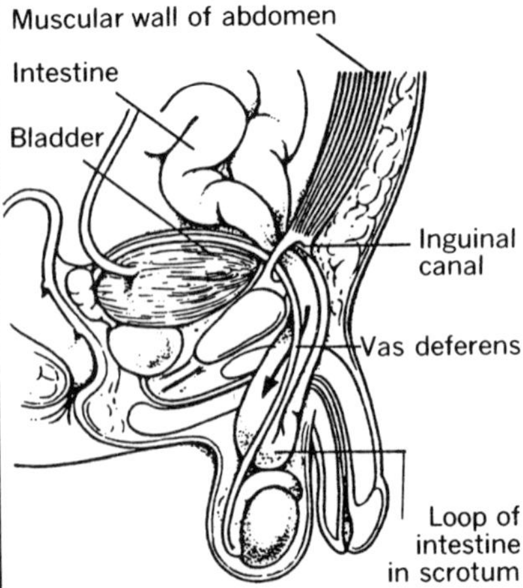

In this type of indirect hernia, a loop of small intestine has pushed through the weakened inguinal canal in the abdominal wall and descended into the scrotal sac.

Femoral Hernia

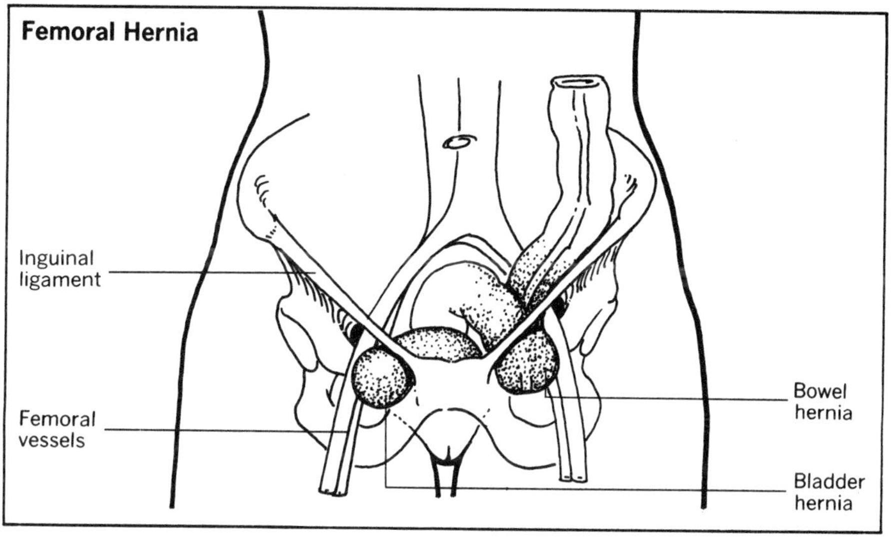

Surgical Procedure

Some hernias are called *direct*, some *indirect*, for purposes of medical records. These terms indicate to the surgeon specific layers of muscle and connective tissue that have been breached and are of no real significance to the patient, because the surgical repair procedures are essentially the same for either type. In the absence of complications, the operation is fairly simple and usually can be performed with either a general or a local anesthetic. An incision is made in the lower abdomen in the area of the hernia, the protruding organ is returned to its normal position, and the weakened or ruptured layers of muscle and connective tissue are repaired and reinforced to provide a strong internal wall that will hold the abdominal contents in place. In some cases the surgeon will use available tissues from the patient's own body in building a new wall against future hernias. The surgeon also may use a variety of materials, including silk, catgut, stainless steel, tantalum mesh gauze, or mesh screens made of plastics, in building a new barrier.

Recovery

The hospital stay for hernia repair is relatively brief, usually from three days to a week; some healthy children undergo surgery early in the morning and return home in the evening of the same day. The patient usually is instructed to avoid exercise or exertion for a couple of weeks and can return to work in a month to six weeks, depending upon the work load expected. Hernias tend to recur in only a small percentage of cases among adults and very rarely in children.

Femoral Hernia

About five percent of all hernias of the groin area are femoral hernias, with the hernia bulge appearing along the thigh. Femoral hernias occur about four times as frequently among women and usually appear in middle age. While a femoral hernia is not necessarily limited to obese patients, it is more likely to be associated with being overweight, and the movement of a bowel segment or the urinary bladder into the hernia frequently is preceded by a fat pad—a mass of fatty tissue. Femoral hernias are more prone to incarceration and strangulation than inguinal hernias. The surgical treatment of femoral hernias is similar to that used in the repair of inguinal hernias, although the incision may be made through the thigh in a few cases.

Hemorrhoids

Hemorrhoid, a term derived from Greek words meaning "blood flowing," refers to a system of arteries and veins that serve the rectal area. The medical problem known as *hemorrhoids,* or *piles,* is a tortuous enlargement of the hemorrhoidal veins, a problem similar to the varicose veins of the legs. Causes of the varicosities of the hemorrhoidal veins include the human peculiarity of standing and walking in an erect posture—animals that walk on all fours do not get hemorrhoids.

Women during pregnancies are particularly subject to hemorrhoidal problems because of the pressure on the veins of the lower body area. Other causes are constipation and straining at stool; diseases of the digestive tract resulting in anal infection; and cirrhosis of the liver, which obstructs blood flow and puts increased pressure on the hemorrhoidal veins.

Hemorrhoids

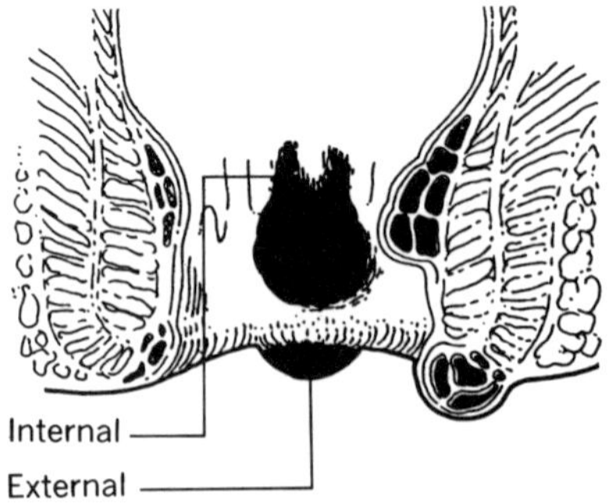

Symptoms

Symptoms usually include bleeding, which may stain the patient's clothing; irritation and discomfort, including itching, in the anal region; and occasionally pain with inflammation. Because rectal bleeding also can be a sign of a number of other diseases, the physician usually makes a thorough examination to rule out other possible causes, such as cancer or ulcerative colitis.

Treatment

If the hemorrhoids do not warrant surgery, medical treatments may be prescribed. *Prolapsed hemorrhoids* (veins that protrude from the anus) can be reduced by gentle pressure. Bed rest, warm baths, and medications are also a part of medical treatments. A type of injection chemotherapy sometimes is used to control bleeding and eliminate the varicosed veins.

Surgery can be used to excise all the affected tissues, and the disorder also can be treated by cryosurgery in which the hemorrhoids are destroyed by a probe containing supercold liquid nitrogen or carbon dioxide. The patient usually is able to recover and return to work within one or two weeks after surgical removal of the hemorrhoidal tissues.

Oral Cavity and Throat

This section discusses oral cancers, tonsils and adenoids, and surgery of the thyroid. For a discussion of cosmetic surgery of the face area, see "Plastic and Cosmetic Surgery" later in this chapter.

Oral Cancers

There are many potential problems of the mouth, or oral cavity, besides an occasional toothache. Surgical treatment frequently is needed to correct a disorder or to prevent a life-threatening situation from developing. Cancers of the lips, tongue, hard and soft palate, and other areas of the mouth, for example, affect about 25,000 people in the United States each year. Elsewhere in the world, the incidence varies considerably according to sex and location; the rate in Hong Kong for men is three times the figure for women, and the incidence of oral cancer for women in Hong Kong is nearly 10 times as high as that of women in Japan. Environmental factors such as tobacco and contact with chemical and physical agents have been suggested as causes, although one form of oral cancer, known as *Burkitt's lymphoma,* is believed to be transmitted by a mosquito-borne virus.

Cancer of the Lip

Oral cancers tend to occur after the age of 45. Some types of oral cancer, particularly when the lips are affected, are found most frequently in persons exposed to a great deal of sunlight. Farmers, sailors, and other outdoor workers develop such tumors around the age of 60, with the lesion appearing on the lower lip. Like other cancers, cancer of the lip may begin as a tiny growth, but, if untreated, can spread through neighboring tissues and eventually destroy part of the chin. Treatment may include both radiation therapy and surgical excision of the growth; if surgery is performed when the tumor is small, the scar is likewise small. Obviously, the larger the tumor is allowed to grow, the more difficult the treatment.

Cancer of the Cheek

Similarly, cancers that develop on the inner surface of the cheek usually can be excised and the wound closed with simple surgery if treatment is started early. If the cancer is allowed to grow before treatment, the surgery becomes more complicated with removal of tissues extending to the outer skin layers and repair of the wound with skin grafts. Radiation therapy also may be used to augment the surgical repair.

Cancer of the Mouth

Cancer of the floor of the mouth may be second only to lip cancer in rate of occurrence of oral cavity tumors; together they may account for half of the oral cavity cancers in the United States. A tumor of the floor of the mouth may involve the under surface of the tongue, the lower jawbone, and other tissues of the area. A small lesion detected early can be controlled in most cases by excision of the growth and radiation therapy.

Cancer of the Tongue

The tongue may be the site of cancerous growths beginning in the 30s of the patient's life, particularly if the individual is a heavy user of tobacco and alcohol and has been neglectful of proper oral hygiene, such as brushing the teeth regularly. If the growth is at the tip of the tongue rather than underneath or along the sides, the operation is easier and there is less chance that the normal function of the tongue will be impaired by removing the growth and surrounding tissue cells. Radiation therapy for cancer of the tongue sometimes involves the implantation of needles containing radium into the tongue. The procedure is done while the patient is under a general anesthetic. Tumors at the base of the tongue, as well as some growths on the floor of the mouth, sometimes are approached through an incision in the neck.

Other Surgery

Apart from cancers, surgery of the oral cavity may be needed to treat genetic defects, such as cleft lip and cleft palate, damage to tissues from injuries, and noncancerous tumors of the soft tissues, such as cysts.

Tonsils and Adenoids

Tonsils and adenoids are glands of lymphoid tissue lying along the walls near the top of the throat. The tonsils are located on the sides of the pharynx, or throat, near the base of the tongue. Unless an adult's tonsils are inflamed, they may not be easily visible to a physician or other person looking into the throat, but when inflamed and swollen they can be seen without difficulty. The adenoids are located higher in the pharynx and cannot be seen by looking into the back of the mouth without special instruments, because the palate, or roof of the mouth, blocks the view.

Tonsillitis

The function of the tonsils and adenoids apparently is that of trapping infectious organisms that enter the body through the nose and mouth. But sometimes the glands do such a good job of collecting infections that they lose their effectiveness, becoming enlarged and inflamed, a condition known as *tonsillitis*. The patient develops fever and sore throat and the breathing passages become obstructed. The infections can spread through the nearby Eustachian tubes to the ears, causing *otitis media* (inflammation of the middle ear), resulting in deafness. Disease organisms also can spread from the tonsils and adenoids to the kidneys, joints, heart, eyes, and other body areas. Many youngsters survive occasional bouts of tonsillitis, and the infections can be treated with antibiotics and medications to relieve pain and fever symptoms. But many surgeons recommend that the tonsils and adenoids be removed if tonsillitis occurs repeatedly.

Tonsillectomy

A *tonsillectomy* (removal of the tonsils) is not a complicated operation, but it usually is performed under a general anesthetic if the patient is a child. A local anesthetic may be used for an adult. The adenoids usually are removed at the same time; they consist of the same type of lymphoid tissue in the same general area, and adenoids develop similar problems from the same kinds of infectious agents. An overnight stay in the hospital may be required or it may be possible for the patient to have the tonsils and adenoids removed in the morning and be released from the hospital in the evening of the same day, after a few hours of postoperative rest under medical observation.

Preoperative and Postoperative Care

The patient may receive antibiotic medications two or three days prior to surgery and is instructed to avoid eating foods or drinking fluids for at least 12 hours before the operation. If the patient has a cold or other viral infection, the surgery may be delayed or postponed. Some surgeons also prefer to avoid tonsillectomy operations during the hay-fever season. If there is any evidence of bleeding after the patient is released, such as spitting blood, he is returned to the hospital and the surgeon is notified; the bleeding usually can be controlled without difficulty. The patient also returns for checkups a couple of weeks after the operation and again about six months later.

Adenoidectomy

In some cases, a surgeon may recommend an *adenoidectomy* (removal of the adenoids) without a tonsillectomy. This is particularly true when the patient suffers from recurrent ear infections and hearing loss. An adenoidectomy is a relatively simple operation performed under a local anesthetic when the patient is an adult or older teenager; a general anesthetic is preferred for younger patients.

The surgeon can reach the adenoid mass through the open mouth of the patient. The tissue grows on a palate ledge near the point where the nasal passage enters the back of the mouth cavity. Using a special instrument, the surgeon cuts away the adenoid tissue within a few minutes. A medicated pack is inserted into the postnasal area to help control bleeding and the patient is moved to a recovery room. The only aftereffects in most cases are a soreness in the postnasal area for a few days and, occasionally, a temporary voice change that is marked by a nasal tone while the wound heals.

Thyroid Surgery

The thyroid gland lies along the trachea, or windpipe, at a point just below the Adam's apple. Secretions of the thyroid gland are vital for metabolic activities of the body, and the gland's functions are closely orchestrated with those of other endocrine glands of the body. When the thyroid is less active than normal, mental and physical functions are slow and the patient gains weight. When the gland is overly active, body functions operate at an abnormally fast pace, with symptoms of weight loss, irritability, heart palpitations, and bulging eyes. Occasionally, lumps develop on the thyroid, requiring medical or surgical treatment. A lump on the thyroid gland may be a nodular, or nontoxic, goiter. Or it could be a tumor. A nodular goiter poses several threats: it can make the thyroid gland become overactive, it can press on the windpipe and cause hoarseness, or it can develop into a cancer. Some growths of the thyroid gland can be treated effectively with medications, radiation, or a combination such as radioactive iodine. However, when conservative forms of therapy no longer appear to control the condition, or when it is suspected that a thyroid growth may be a malignant cancer, surgical removal of the affected area is advised promptly.

Surgical Procedure

The operation itself is fairly simple. An incision is made through the skin folds of the neck, neck muscles beneath the skin are separated, and the affected portion of the gland is cut away. The neck and throat area may be sore and painful for a few days after the operation; within a few weeks the patient can resume normal activities. A thin scar remains at the line of incision, but it is usually partly concealed by skin folds of the neck.

The Thyroid Gland

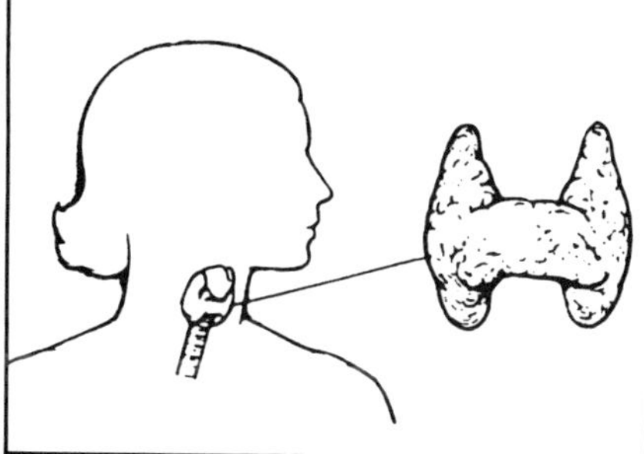

Ear Surgery

Surgical treatment of the ear usually is directed toward restoring the function of normal hearing which may have been lost or impaired by disease or injury. The eardrum, or tympanic membrane, can be perforated or ruptured by direct injury, by the shock waves of an explosion, or by an infection of the middle ear. Infection or injury also can disrupt hearing function by damaging the ossicles, a chain of tiny bones that transmit sound waves from the eardrum to the inner ear. Disease, aging effects, and exposure to loud noises can cause hearing loss or impairment.

Surgery of the ear usually involves working with the middle ear, the compartment between the eardrum and the inner ear, which contains the nerve endings that carry impulses to the auditory centers of the brain. The middle ear contains three ossicles, known by their common names of *hammer, anvil,* and *stirrup*—terms that suggest their functions in translating movements of air molecules into the vibrations the brain understands as sounds.

Otitis Media

One common disease of the middle ear is otitis media, which can occur by infection from a number of different kinds of organisms. Otitis media also can develop from secretions or fluids such as milk being forced into the ear through the Eustachian tube, particularly in infants who are fed while they are in a reclining position. The symptoms of otitis media are pain in the ear, fever, and loss of hearing; a small child may indicate the symptoms by crying and tugging at the ear.

Surgical Procedure

Many cases of otitis media respond to medical treatment, such as the use of antibiotics, but for patients who suffer severe pain or who have middle ears filled with pus, a surgical procedure called *myringotomy* is performed. "Myringotomy" means simply perforating the eardrum. But the operation usually is peformed in a hospital, under a local anesthetic, and with great care to avoid disturbing the ossicles or other ear structures beyond the eardrum. The middle ear is drained and the eardrum either heals spontaneously or can be subsequently repaired with a graft from the patient's own tissues.

Surgery to Correct Hearing Loss

Occasionally surgery is required to correct a conductive hearing loss involving the structures of the middle ear. Such problems happen more frequently among older persons because of abnormal tissue growths that in effect "freeze" the ossicles, so that they no longer work with normal flexibility. Ossicular disorders also can occur in younger persons, including children, because of congenital defects, injury, or repeated infections, as of otitis media. The exact procedure for restoration of hearing depends upon the type of disorder. If one of the ossicles has slipped out of position or has become rigidly attached to another structure, like the tympanic membrane, the tiny bones can be repositioned or freed from the tissues that may have immobilized them. It is not unusual for the surgeon, working in a space about the size of a pea and viewing his progress through a microscope, to literally take the middle ear structures apart, rebuild the organ with bits of plastic or metal shaped like the ossicles, and reconstruct the eardrum with tissue grafts. This kind of surgery is called *microsurgery*.

Inner Ear Disturbances

Disorders of the inner ear usually are treated with medications. Surgery in that area is seldom performed unless there is a great risk to the life of the patient. Little can be done to restore hearing loss caused by nerve deafness except with hearing aids; these are designed to pick up sounds on the affected side of the head and route the sounds by electronic circuitry to an area where they can be picked up by remaining functional auditory nerves.

Eye Surgery

Among common types of eye surgery are procedures for correcting eye muscles, glaucoma, cataracts, cornea and retina disorders. Operations on the eye muscles are intended to correct crossed eyes or similar problems in which the two eyes fail to work together.

Crossed Eyes

The condition technically known as *strabismus,* in which one eye drifts so that its position is not parallel with the other, is caused by a congenitally weak muscle. Infants often appear to have crossed eyes, but in most cases the drifting corrects itself by the time the baby is six months old. If the condition persists beyond that time, a physician should be consulted. He may recommend the use of an eye patch over the stronger eye so that the weaker one will be exercised. If this does not achieve the desired result, he may prescribe special glasses and eye exercises as the child gets older, so that there is no impairment of vision.

Corrective Surgery

If corrective surgery proves necessary after these measures, it is usually done before the child enters school. The operation is a simple one involving the muscle and not the inside of the eye itself. Each eye has six *extraocular* muscles—muscles originating outside the eyeball—to move the eye up, down, left, right, etc.; the surgeon lengthens or shortens these muscles, as may be required, to coordinate the eye movements. The operation is safe and requires only a brief hospital stay.

Amblyopia

If the lack of eye coordination is not corrected, a kind of blindness called *amblyopia* can result in one of the eyes. This condition occurs particularly in young children who depend upon the vision of one good eye; the function of the other eye is allowed to deteriorate. It has been estimated that about two million Americans have lost a part of their vision in this manner. Crossed eyes should receive professional attention early enough to prevent a permanent visual handicap.

Cataract

Cataract is a condition in which there is a loss of transparency of the lenses of the eyes. Each lens is made up of layers of cells naturally formed to focus a visual image on the retina at the rear of the eyeball. As a result of aging, or because of an injury to the eye, the lens may develop cloudy or opaque areas, or *cataracts,* that result in a blurring of vision. About five percent of the population of the United States have cataracts. Some physicians claim that anyone who lives long enough can expect to have cataracts, although age is not the only determining factor.

Surgical Correction

The condition can be corrected rather easily by several different kinds of surgical procedures. Among these, a relatively simple, advanced technique involves a microsurgery procedure called *extracapsular extraction* followed by implantation of a new lens. Using this method, the surgeon first makes a tiny incision in the cornea. Reaching through that incision, the surgeon then makes a circle of tiny cuts in the lens. The lens and its cataract are then drawn through the opening in the cornea. The back part of the lens remains in place to support the implant lens.

Extracapsular extraction requires only a local anesthetic injected into the facial muscles. Because the sutures are tiny, healing time can be as short as a few weeks.

In a second procedure, called *phacoemulsification,* or *phaco,* a small incision is made on the side of the cornea and a tiny probe is inserted into the eye. The probe then produces ultrasound waves that soften and dissolve the lens. The lens and its cataract are then removed by suction.

Laser surgery has also been used effectively following cataract lens replacements. The neodymium yttrium-aluminum garnet (Nd:YAG) laser has helped to clear part of the natural lens that was not removed, which sometimes becomes cloudy after surgery.

Deciding when to have cataract surgery may be difficult. To help you decide, the physician may use a potential acuity meter (PAM) to show what kind of vision you should have after a cataract is removed. The PAM projects a light beam that flashes a standard eye chart through tiny clear areas in the cataract. Because the beam hits your retina directly, you can read the chart without interference.

Lens implants normally effect greatly improved vision. But for optimum results most patients need to wear eyeglasses or contact lenses after the operation. Because implanted lenses cannot focus as your eye's natural lens does, you will probably need reading glasses. The artificial lenses may require some adjustments to compensate for visual illusions regarding distances and shapes, but the blurring caused by progressive blindness will have been eliminated.

Corneal Transplant

The cornea of the eye is a clear window of several cells in thickness at the very front of the eye. Although it is protected by the constant sweeping of the corneal surface by the eyelid and the washing of the surface by the tears, it is vulnerable to injury and infection, allergies, and metabolic disorders. The simple habit of rubbing the eyes can distort the shape of the cornea, changing the normal round shape to a cone shape. Eventually, a cornea may degenerate from wear and tear and become so clouded that the patient can no longer see clearly, if at all. However, since the 1930s, it has been possible to replace a clouded cornea with an undamaged cornea from a deceased person. Corneas are contributed by donors and stored in eye banks.

The overwhelming majority of corneal transplants are successful; the chances of success depend upon many factors, including the health of the remaining tissues of the original cornea.

Other Procedures

Another precedure used to treat certain problems of the cornea is called *phototherapeutic keratectomy* (PTK). In it, a laser is used to vaporize layers of diseased tissue and to smooth out surface irregularites that impair vision. New tissue can grow and replace the altered tissue. The laser enables great precision and the procedure has a very high success rate. Vision can reoccur rapidly and recovery usually takes only a few days.

Glaucoma

Glaucoma, a leading cause of blindness, is a disease caused by a failure of the fluid produced inside the eye to drain properly. The fluid, or *aqueous humor,* is produced in the anterior chamber of the eye, between the cornea and the lens. In a normal eye it drains through a duct at the base of the cornea at the same rate at which it is produced. But if the drainage system is obstructed, fluid buildup creates pressure backward through the eye. If untreated, such pressure can cause gradual blindness by crushing the nerves at the back of the eye.

Treatment

Some cases of glaucoma can be treated with medications that control the rates of fluid production and drainage. But when medications are no longer effective or when an acute attack occurs—with symptoms of severe eye pain sometimes accompanied by abdominal pain, nausea, and vomiting—immediate surgery is recommended. Several surgical procedures for the treatment of glaucoma are available; all are designed to release the fluid pressure in the eye. One common procedure involves cutting a small opening in the iris. Another technique is to insert a fine wire into the duct that normally drains the fluid and literally ream it open.

Other surgical and nonsurgical treatments for glaucoma are available. For example, laser surgery is effective for treating both open-angle and closed-angle glaucoma. In the former, the eye's internal drain system does not work properly, causing pressure to build up in the eye. In closed-angle glaucoma, fluid cannot pass properly from the front to the back of the eye, again producing dangerous pressure. A laser is usually used in treatment to burn a series of holes in the meshwork behind the eye's lens. This helps increase fluid drainage. Because marijuana has also been found to reduce pressure in the eye, manufacture of the chemical known as THC (delta-9-tetrahydrocannabinol), marijuana's key psychoactive ingredient, was authorized by the Food and Drug Administration in 1985 and begun in 1986. THC has also been used to relieve the nausea accompanying cancer chemotherapy and to slow the progression of multiple sclerosis.

An estimated 3 million people in the United States are afflicted by glaucoma, and the chances of developing it increase with age. Blacks over age 40 are at a higher risk of developing the disease than is the general population, and there is some evidence that the risk is hereditary. However, glaucoma also is easily preventable and controllable, because it usually develops slowly and can be detected during routine eye examinations in its early stages.

Retinal Detachment or Disease

Retinal detachment can result from bleeding in the retinal area, an injury, a change in the shape of the eyeball, or other causes. The surgical treatment to correct the problem usually is related to the specific cause. For example, if fluid or blood has accumulated behind the retina, it is drained away. Alternatively, pressure may be directed within the eyeball to push the retina back into its proper position. For some cases, such as those associated with *diabetic retinopathy,* a kind of retinal bleeding in diabetes patients, a laser beam is used to seal the blood vessels responsible for the tiny hemorrhages in the eye.

Chest Region

This section deals with surgery of the lungs and heart. For a discussion of cosmetic surgery of the chest area, as of the breast, see "Plastic and Cosmetic Surgery" later in this chapter.

The Lungs

Before the era of modern drugs such as antibiotics, lung disorders were the leading cause of death in the United States. Lung diseases are still relatively common. With every breath taken in, the lungs are vulnerable to damage from disease organisms, chemicals, and air pollutants, many of which did not exist 50 years ago when pneumonia and tuberculosis were among the greatest threats to human life. Because the lungs are not as sensitive to pain as some other organs, a respiratory disorder may develop insidiously with few or no symptoms. When pain is felt in the chest area, the source of the pain may be the chest wall, the esophagus, or the bronchial tubes that branch from the trachea into smaller units that distribute air through the lung tissues. Other symptoms of respiratory disease include coughing, shortness of breath, or sputum that contains blood.

Tuberculosis

Any of the signs or symptoms mentioned above could be associated with tuberculosis, which also can cause appetite loss, lethargy, and heavy perspiration, especially during the night. Tuberculosis is still one of the most common causes of death in the world, and new cases are found in the United States each year at a rate of 18 per 100,000 population. In addition, an estimated 35 million Americans are tuberculin-positive, indicating they have been in contact with the infectious organism but have developed an immune response to it. For an explanation of how tuberculosis is spread and of tests devised to check its spread, see "Tuberculosis" in Ch. 12, *Diseases of the Respiratory System.*

Surgical Treatment of Tuberculosis

A dozen different drugs are available for medical treatment of tuberculosis and several types may be taken in combination by a patient. Intensive treatment may require a hospital stay of several months and use of the drugs for at least 18 months. However, because of the adverse side effects of drugs, resistance of the bacterium to the drugs, and other reasons, surgery may be required. If one of the five lobes of lung tissue—the right lung has three lobes, the left lung two—has been severely damaged by tuberculosis, it may be removed by surgeons. In some instances, physicians may recommend that surgery be undertaken to allow one of the lungs to rest while it recovers from the infection. This is accomplished by crushing the phrenic nerve, under a local anesthetic, creating a partial paralysis of the diaphragm. Partial lung collapse also can be accomplished by removing parts of the ribs over the affected lung.

Lung Cancer

Cancer of the lung may appear with early symptoms of coughing, wheezing, or the appearance of blood in sputum; in about 10 percent of cases there is chest pain or shortness of breath. However, it is not unusual for the lung cancer patient to have no complaints of illness. Chest X rays during a routine physical examination may reveal the disease. In many cases, the cancer develops from metastases of cancers that have spread from other body systems. Medical therapy for lung cancer patients, including the use of radiation, is primarily for the purpose of relieving pain or other symptoms. The only effective cure is surgical excision of the affected lung tissue along with the nearby lymph nodes. Surgical treatment is most effective in young adults when the tumor has not invaded neighboring tissues, although the five-year survival rate for lung cancer is still poor.

Heart Surgery

Heart surgery procedures that are routine in many hospitals today were unheard of a generation ago. Since World War II, techniques have been devised to permit attachment of a heart-lung machine to the human

Coronary Bypass Surgery

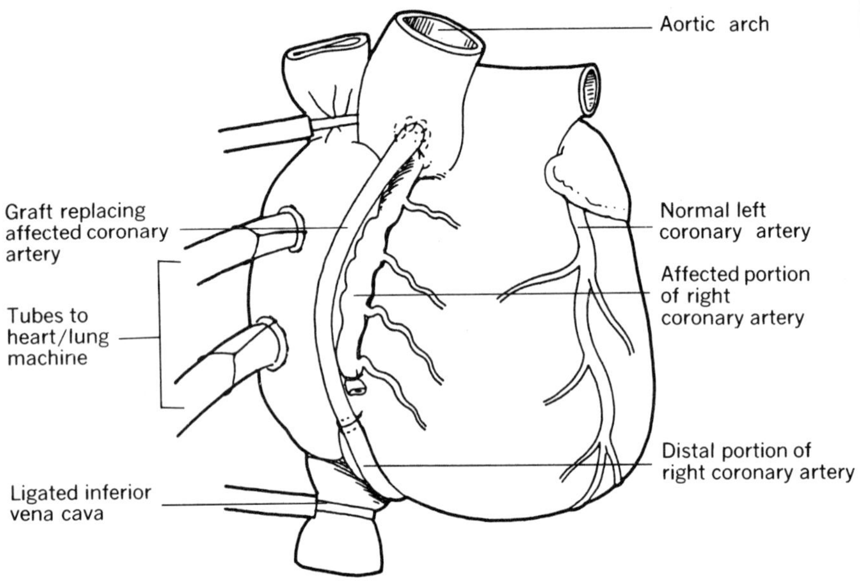

body so that the patient's blood can be circulated and refreshed with oxygen while the heart itself is stopped temporarily for surgery.

Heart Valve Repair

While the blood flow is shunted away from the heart, surgeons can replace a diseased heart valve that may have become calcified with deposits that keep it from closing normally. An artificial valve made of metal and plastic may be used to replace the patient's diseased mitral valve that no longer effectively controls the flow of blood from the left atrium to the left ventricle of the heart. Artificial valves also can be installed between the right chambers of the heart. In some cases, a diseased valve leaf may be repaired with a graft of tissue from the patient's body.

Installation of artificial heart valves has had a remarkably good record of success; some surgeons recommend the procedure over other techniques for treatment of heart valve diseases and report the operation has been well tolerated by patients over 70. While some activites may be restricted, life expectancy is increased for most patients, and they are able to have comfortable and more normal lives after such operations.

Septal Defect

Another kind of heart surgery is used to correct a septal defect. The right and left atria of the heart are separated by a septum, a wall of muscular tissue. A similar but much thicker septum separates the left and right ventricles. Occasionally, usually because of a birth defect, the septum does not close completely and blood flows from one side to the other through the opening in the heart wall. The problem is solved by putting the patient on a heart-lung machine while the heart is opened and the septum closed either by sewing the opening or by stitching into the septum a patch of plastic material.

Coarctation of the Aorta

An equally dramatic bit of heart surgery is used to correct a defect called *coarctation,* or narrowing, of the aorta, the main artery leading from the heart. This short, pinched section interferes with normal blood flow. If untreated, the patient may die of a ruptured aorta or heart failure. Treatment requires an operation in which the narrowed section of the aorta is cut away and the two normal-sized ends sewed together. In some cases, a piece of plastic material is sewed into the reconstructed aorta to replace the coarctated section.

Aortal-Pulmonary Artery Shunt

A comparatively simple bit of heart surgery is employed to correct a defect that occurs in some newborn children. Before birth, when the lungs are not needed because fresh blood is supplied from the placenta via the umbilical cord, the aorta is connected by a shunt to the pulmonary artery. After birth the shunt closes in most cases so the pulmonary artery can carry the blood from the heart to the lungs for oxygenation. In some children this shunt fails to close. To correct the defect and prevent heart failure, the surgeon opens the child's chest, ties off the open shunt, and cuts the ligated connection.

Aortal-Pulmonary Artery

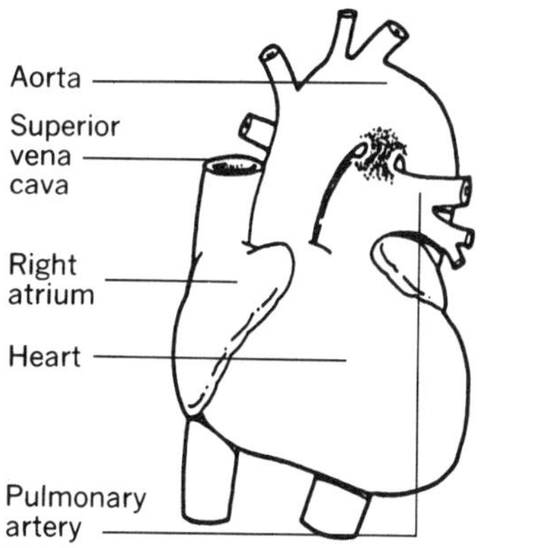

Vascular Surgery

This section consists of discussions of aneurysms, varicose veins, phlebitis, and intermittent claudication.

Aneurysm

When a blood vessel develops a balloonlike malformation the defect is called an *aneurysm.* A common complication of the aneurysm is that it may rupture if not treated. A ruptured aneurysm of a large blood vessel, or of a small blood vessel in a critical area such as the brain, can be fatal or severely disabling.

Surgical Procedures

If the aneurysm develops at a vital site such as the aorta, heroic surgical measures may be required to correct the problem. Before the important artery can be clamped off, the patient may have to be attached to a heart-lung machine and the body temperature lowered so as to reduce normal body functions to a minimum. After the aneurysm is removed, that section of the aorta may have to be replaced with a piece of plastic artery. Not all aneurysms require such complicated methods of repair; if the ballooning section of artery develops as a saclike appendage, it frequently can be tied off and removed while the relatively small opening between the blood vessel and the sac is sewed closed.

Surgical removal of an aneurysm is the only available treatment for the disorder. The surgery is much less complicated if the abnormal section of the blood vessel is replaced before it ruptures than after. When the patient has recovered from correction of the aneurysm, he can resume a rather active, normal life style.

Varicose Veins

Varicose veins can develop in many parts of the body. But they are most obvious and commonly a problem when they appear in the legs, especially in the *saphenous veins,* large veins that lie close to the surface of the skin.

Causes

The cause of varicose veins is a failure of tiny valves in the blood vessels to function properly, so that venous blood destined for the heart flows backward and forms pools that can make the veins distended, tortuous, and painful. Varicose veins are related to the erect posture of humans; the heart pumps blood through arteries to the extremities, but the return flow must fight the pull of gravity. Ordinarily, venous blood gets a boost up the legs by a pumping action of leg-muscle contractions. Valves in the legs are designed to let the blood move upward but are supposed to block any backward flow. People whose jobs require them to stand all day are among those likely to suffer from a breakdown of the normal functioning of the valves. Women who have had multiple pregnancies and obese individuals are also apt to develop varicose veins.

Ulceration

Varicose veins can cause ulcers in the lower leg near the ankle that bleed through the skin after an injury to the area.

Treatment

Most varicose veins require medical treatment only if complications develop, such as severe bleeding, which can be caused by injury to the vein. An ultrasound or an X-ray (venogram) may be performed to check for any problems.

Discomfort from varicose veins may be relieved by wearing support hose, by elevating the legs whenever possible, and by not standing or sitting in the same position for long periods of time.

Severe cases of varicose veins may require further treatment, such as *sclerotherapy,* injecting the vein with a solution that scars and closes the vein; *ligation,* the removal of the vein; or *vein stripping,* tying off the main veins and removing superficial veins. Laser surgery may be used in some cases to close smaller veins.

Complications of varicose veins include *varicose ulcers,* skin ulcers near the ankle; and *phlebitis,* inflammation and clotting in a vein.

Phlebitis

A problem related to varicose veins is *phlebitis,* a general term for inflammation of a vein. It tends to occur in veins in the lower limbs. Often, a clot (thrombus) forms that blocks blood flow through the vein. This condition, called thrombophlebitis, is potentially dangerous. The danger is that the clot will break loose—that is, become an *embolus*—and travel to the lungs, where it can obstruct a vital blood vessel, with serious or even fatal results. The obstructing clot is called an *embolism.*

Causes and Treatment

Causes of phlebitis can be injury, infection, poor circulation, or simply sitting for long periods of time. Medical therapy may include wet dressings and medications, especially anticoagulant drugs to thin the blood and reduce the chances of clot formations. Supportive bandages, leg exercises, and elevation of the legs may also be recommended.

Surgical Procedure

Surgery is reserved usually for cases in which medical therapy fails to control the risk of emboli forming. The surgical procedure is directed toward treatment of the deep vein that is the source of the phlebitis symptoms. The surgeon may open the vein to remove the clot, or a device can be inserted in the vein to strain out any clots that may form in the vein and travel toward the lungs. In some cases the surgeon may block the upward flow of blood from the affected vein, allowing other veins to assume that function. However, if other veins already have been stripped or ligated in the treatment of varicose veins, it is unlikely that a surgeon would occlude or block the flow of blood in a deep leg vein.

Intermittent Claudication

Intermittent claudication is lower leg pain caused by insufficient blood flow to exercising muscle. It is primarily a disease of aging, with gradual, progressive narrowing of the lumen (interior space) of the arteries by atherosclerosis. Atherosclerosis of the arteries occurs in other parts of the body, including the arms. Intermittent claudication is marked by muscle fatigue and pain when the leg muscles are used, as in walking. For those whose symptoms are relieved by rest, lifestyle modifications, such as stopping smoking and exercising more, can be very helpful. The condition may be relieved by drugs, particularly medications that help dilate the arteries, but in severe cases, surgery to alter the leg arteries is the solution.

Surgical Procedures

The surgeon may build a bypass artery by grafting a length of synthetic tubing into the affected blood vessel and around the area blocked by atherosclerotic narrowing. Sometimes surgeons use a piece of a vein from the patient's body to make a bypass artery; for example, a vein from the arm may be transformed into an artery for the leg. Another procedure involves simply removing the portion of the artery blocking the normal flow of blood.

Orthopedic Surgery

Orthopedics originally was the name given the subject of treating deformities in children; the original Greek term could be translated as "normal child." But the medical world now uses the word to describe treatment of the bones, muscles, joints, and associated tissues of the body's locomotion apparatus. Orthopedic surgery, therefore, might involve repair of a broken big toe, as well as treatment of a whiplash injury to the neck.

This section discusses disorders of the spine, including herniated (or "slipped") disk, fractures, and torn ligaments.

Slipped Disk

The spinal column, consisting of 33 stacked vertebrae, is a common source of problems that may require treatment. In addition to helping sup-

Herniated Disk

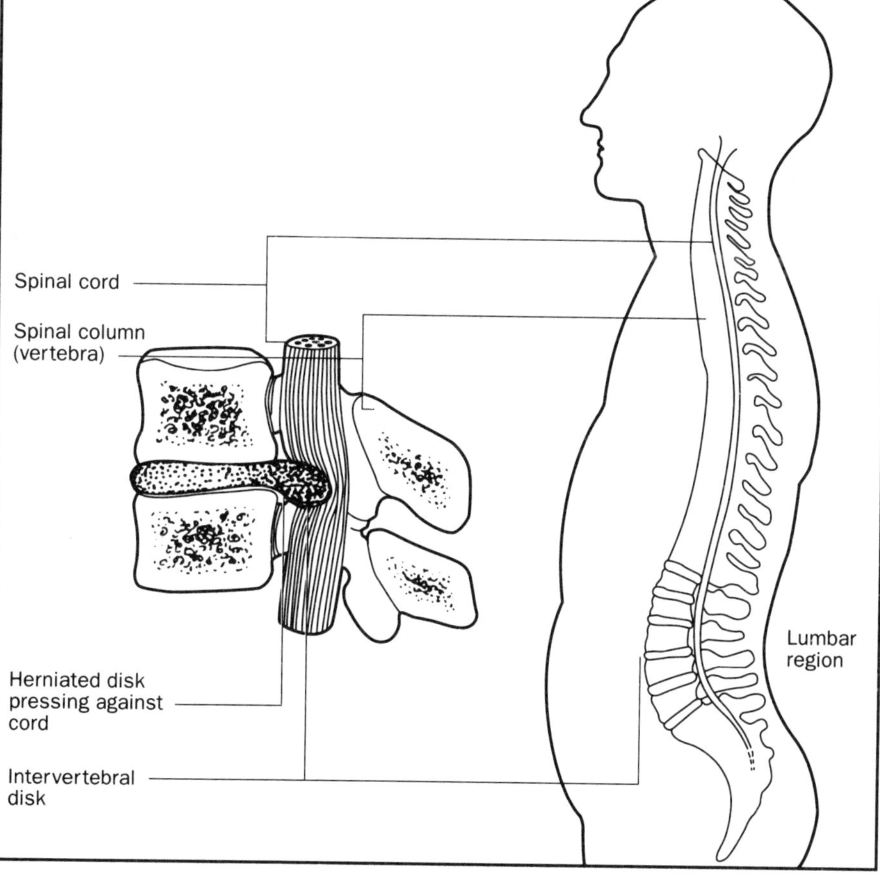

port the weight of the body above the hips, the vertebrae are subjected to a variety of twists, turns, and strains during a typical day. Much of the nearly continuous shock exerted on the spinal column is absorbed by the gel-like disks between the vertebrae.

Symptoms

Eventually, one of the disks may *herniate,* or slip out of place, causing pressure on a spinal nerve. The result can be severe pain that radiates along the pathway of the nerve as far as the lower leg. The pain may be accompanied by muscular weakness and loss of reflexes, even perhaps by a loss of feeling in part of the leg affected by a pinched or squeezed nerve. This condition, known popularly as a *slipped disk,* has symptoms of low back pain or leg pain that are similar to those of other disorders, such as intermittent claudication, arthritis, strained muscles, and prostatitis. Also, a herniated disk can occur near the top of the spinal column with symptoms of head

Spinal Fusion

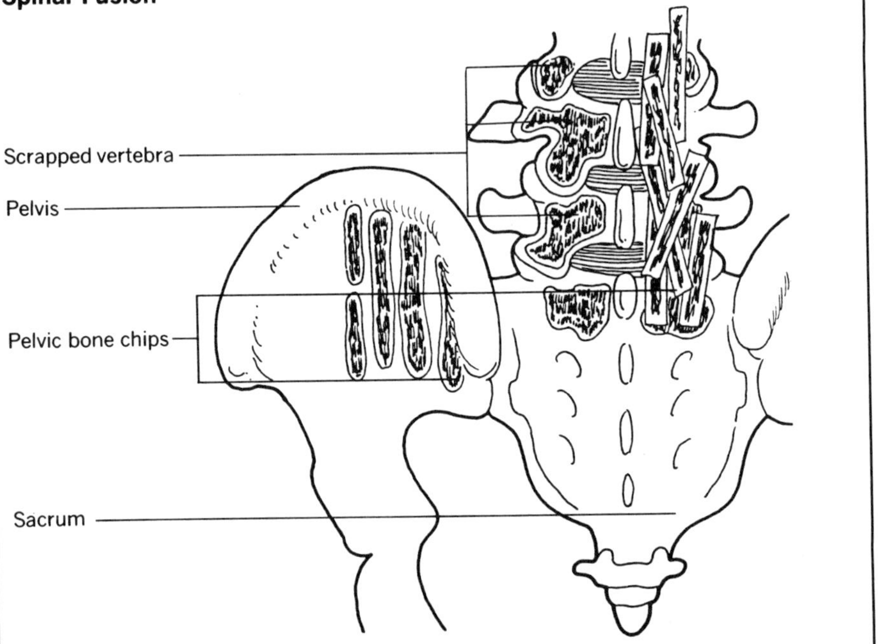

and neck-area pains. But more than 90 percent of herniated disk cases involve the lumbar region of the spinal column, in the lower back.

Diagnosis

Physicians usually can confirm a herniated disk problem by a technique called *myelography,* in which a dye is injected into the spinal canal and X-ray pictures taken. Another procedure, called *electromyography,* can help determine which nerve root is involved.

Treatment

Conservative measures generally are used at first to reduce the pain and other symptoms. They include bed rest on a hard mattress, medications, and sometimes the use of traction and back braces. If conservative therapy fails to correct the problem and the diagnosis has been well established by a myelogram, surgery may be advised to remove the herniated disk.

Spinal Fusion

The surgeon may recommend a procedure called *spinal fusion,* in which the edges of several of the vertebrae are roughened and a piece of bone from the pelvis grafted onto the roughened edges. The bone graft will fuse with the vertebrae and in effect make the several vertebrae a single bone. However, the fused vertebrae will not interfere noticeably with body movements after the fusion is completed, which takes about six months. The operation requires a hospital stay of from one to two weeks and the patient must wear a body cast for the first few weeks and then use a back brace for a period of possibly several months. The patient usually can return to work and resume some normal activities within a couple of months after the operation. Strenuous activity, however, is usually restricted after an operation on the spinal column.

Other Spinal Disorders

Spondylolisthesis

Spinal fusion surgery also may be used to correct two other kinds of spinal disorders. One disorder is known as *spondylolisthesis,* a condition in which one of the vertebrae slips out of alignment. Spondylolisthesis usually occurs at the bottom of the group of lumbar vertebrae, where that section of the spinal column rests on the sacrum.

Scoliosis

The other disorder is *scoliosis,* or abnormal curvature of the spinal column. If the case of scoliosis is mild and causes no severe symptoms, it may be treated with conservative measures such as braces and special exercises. Surgical treatment of scoliosis may involve not only spinal fusion but reinforcement of the spinal column with metal rods attached to the vertebrae to hold them in proper alignment.

Scoliosis

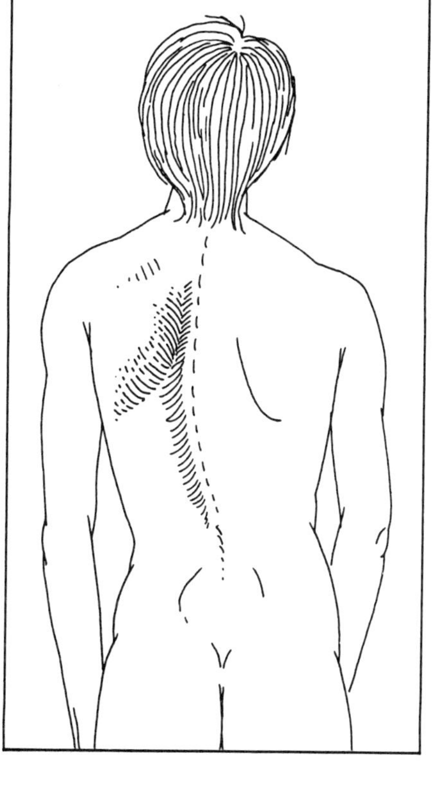

Disorders of the cervical portion of the spinal column, in the area of the neck, may cause symptoms similar to those of a herniated disk in the lower back. But there is pain in the neck and shoulders and weakness in the arms. Surgical treatment also is similar, with removal of a herniated disk portion or fusion of cervical vertebrae when conservative therapy, with bed rest, neck braces, and medications, does not prove helpful.

Fractures

Many fractures of the spinal column also are treated by fusion operations, use of casts, braces, bed rest, or traction, in addition to therapy directed toward the specific problem. Spinal fractures frequently are compression fractures of vertebrae caused by falling in a sitting or standing position or mishaps in which a bony process of a vertebra is broken. Spinal fractures that result in permanent damage to the spinal cord, with resulting paralysis, are relatively uncommon.

Reduction of Fractures

Fractures of the long bones of the arms and legs are treated by a method called *reduction,* the technique of aligning the broken ends of the bones properly so the healing process will not result in a deformity. Reduction also requires that the muscles and surrounding tissues be aligned and held in place by immobilizing them as the break heals.

If the break is simple enough, the limb can be immobilized by putting a plaster cast around the part of the involved limb after the fractured ends of the bone and associated tissues have been realigned. In complicated cases with a number of bone fragments resulting from the fracture and surrounding tissues in some disarray, the patient usually is given a general anesthetic while the surgeon recognizes the shattered limb like a player assembling pieces of a jigsaw puzzle. If some of the needed pieces are missing, the surgeon may fill the gaps with bone from a bone bank, although bank materials usually are not as effective in the healing process as pieces of the patient's own bones.

Use of Internal Appliances

A common technique of modern fracture surgery is the application of wires, screws, pins, metal plates, and other devices to provide internal fixation of a broken long bone during the healing process. Nails and pins may be used to fasten the fractured neck of a femur, the long bone of the upper leg, to the shaft of that bone. A steel rod may be driven through the shaft of a long bone to align the broken sections. Screws may be used to hold together bone ends of a fracture in which the break runs diagonally across the shaft. Screws also may be employed to hold a metal plate or strip of bone from the patient's own body across the break. The screws, nails, and other devices generally are well tolerated by the body and may be left in the bones indefinitely if they do not cause adverse reactions after the healing process is completed.

Traction

Traction frequently is employed to hold a limb in alignment while a fracture is healing. A clamp sometimes is placed at one end of the fractured limb and a weight attached by wires over a pulley is connected to the clamp. Depending upon the kind of fracture and type of traction prescribed, a system of several weights and pulleys may be rigged around the bed of a patient to fix the bone and related tissues in correct positions.

Torn Cartilage

Joints of the body can be vulnerable to damage from sudden twisting and turning actions, particularly when the force of the individual's body weight is added to the pressure on the joint. The effect of such forces on the knee joint can result in tearing of the half-moon-shaped cartilages that cushion friction of the upper and lower leg bones where they are joined. Sports fans are particularly aware of the vulnerability of the knee joint because of the high incidence of knee injuries to athletes, especially in football and basketball. Obese individuals are also particularly liable to develop cartilage problems in the knee.

Symptoms

When a cartilage of the knee joint is torn, the patient may feel pain and weakness in the area of the injury. Swelling usually occurs, and in more than half the cases the knee cannot be straightened, because it has become "locked" by the cartilage. There may be a remission of symptoms, but surgery frequently is required sooner or later.

Surgical Procedure

The surgeon makes an incision in the area of the kneecap and cuts away the torn cartilage. Full recovery takes several weeks after the first few postoperative days, during which the patient remains in bed with the affected leg elevated. Special exercises are required to overcome muscle weakness in the leg and to help the patient learn to use the leg with part of the cartilage cushion missing.

Neurosurgery

Neurosurgery may be employed to treat a wide assortment of disorders involving the nervous system, from the brain to nerve endings in the fingers and toes. Neurosurgery may involve treatment of epilepsy, Parkinson's disease, and psychiatric disorders, as well as herniated disks of the spinal column and aneurysms that affect the nervous system.

Causes of neurosurgical problems can be injury, tumors, infectious diseases, or congenital disorders.

This section includes discussions of trigeminal neuralgia, brain tumors, and head injuries.

Trigeminal Neuralgia

Trigeminal neuralgia is one of many types of pain that sometimes can be treated by surgery. The disorder, also known as *tic douloureux* or *facial neuralgia,* tends to develop in persons between 40 and 60 years of age, causing attacks of acute pain and muscular twitching in the area of the face containing branches of the trigeminal nerve. The painful attacks occur with no apparent reason but seem to be associated with certain stimuli, such as touch or temperature changes, at points around the face and mouth. During periods of attacks, the patient may avoid eating, shaving, or any other activity that might trigger a spasm of severe pain. But the pain attacks also may cease, with or without treatment, for three or four months, only to resume for weeks or months.

Treatment

Alcohol injections and medications may offer relief of symptoms, but when symptoms continue, surgery frequently is recommended. The operation consists of an incision to reach the root of the nerve and cut the divisions that appear to be involved with the painful symptoms. However, cutting the nerve can result in loss of feeling for the entire side of the face, including the cornea of the eye, so that the patient must wear special glasses to protect the cornea. An alternative procedure that is not always effective involves exposing the nerve root and rubbing it, a technique that seems to produce a temporary loss of sensation in the nerve fibers.

Brain Tumor

Brain tumors are popularly associated with neurosurgery skills. And while brain surgery requires great skill and knowledge of brain anatomy, which in itself is quite complicated, most brain tumor operations are conducted safely and successfully. Diagnosing, locating, and identifying a brain tumor are challenges faced by the physician before surgery begins. There are a dozen major types of brain tumors plus some minor types. The types of tumors tend to vary according to the age of the patient; the patient's age and the type of tumor may suggest where it develops.

Symptoms

Because brain tumors can cause organic mental changes in the patient, the symptoms of changed behavior can be mistaken for neurotic or psychotic disorders, with the result that a patient may spend valuable time receiving psychiatric treatment rather than surgical treatment; autopsies of

Brain Tumors

Frequent locations of common lesions

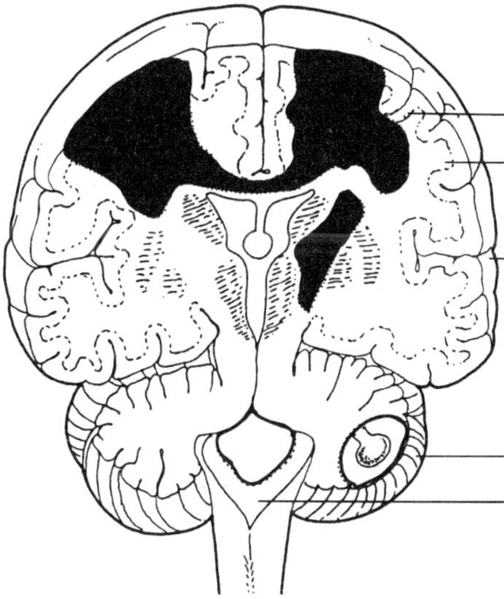

a significant number of patients who die in mental hospitals reveal the presence of brain tumors. In addition to mental changes, the person suffering from a brain tumor may complain of headaches, experience convulsions, or display signs of neurological function loss, such as abnormal vision.

Diagnosis

The specific signs and symptoms, along with X-ray studies, electroencephalograms, and other tests, help the physicians determine the site and extent of growth of a brain tumor. A recently developed technique called *CT scanning* (for *computed tomography*) aids the neurosurgeon by producing a series of X-ray pictures of the interior of the skull as if they were "slices" of the brain taken in thicknesses of about two-thirds of an inch. The detailed anatomical portrait of the patient's brain helps pinpoint the disorder and indicate whether it is a tumor or another kind of abnormality.

Surgical Procedure

The usual method of removing a brain tumor after it has been diagnosed and located is a procedure called a *craniotomy.* The entire head is shaved and cleaned to eliminate the possibility that a stray bit of hair might fall into the incision that is made in the scalp. After the scalp has been opened, a series of holes are drilled in a pattern outlining the working area for the surgeon; a wire saw is used to cut the skull between the drilled holes.

Removing the tumor is a delicate operation, not only because of the need to avoid damage to healthy brain tissue but because accidental severing of a blood vessel in the brain could produce a critical hemorrhage. The surgeon tries to remove the entire tumor, or as much of the tumor as appears possible without damaging vital brain tissues or blood vessels. All the various types of brain tumors are considered dangerous, whether malignant or benign, because within the rigid confines of the skull there is no opportunity for outward release of pressure. Therefore any growth may compress or destroy vital brain tissues if left untreated.

After the tumor is removed, the piece of skull removed at the start of the operation is replaced and the scalp flap is sewed in place. Radiation therapy may be administered for a month to six weeks after surgery to destroy any tumor tissue left behind or tumor cells that may have drifted into the spinal canal. Some tumors near the base of the brain may be treated effectively with radiation alone if the tumor cells are radiosensitive. Tumors of the pineal gland and the pituitary gland also may be treated with radiation.

Laser Surgery

In an alternative procedure, *laser neurosurgery,* a brain surgeon may use a laser beam to vaporize the tumor. The hair is removed from all or part of the skull; a section of the skull is removed with a power or hand saw after being marked out with tiny holes; and the surgeon then uses the laser to destroy the tumor. Typically, the surgeon may actually control two laser beams: a helium-neon type that guides the surgical work, and a carbon dioxide (CO_2) laser that does the vaporizing.

Because the "no-touch" CO_2 laser works slowly, an operation may require 10 or more hours. The laser beam can focus on and destroy one tumor cell at a time, targeting areas of tissue 1/50th the thickness of a human hair, or it can attack a number of cells in a group. The surgeon controls the electrical power that activates the beam with a foot pedal. In effect, the laser causes the tumor cells to heat up beyond the boiling point and then to explode into vapor. At the same time, the beam coagulates the tiny blood vessels that it passes through, preventing bleeding.

Head Injuries

Brain Hemorrhage

Head injuries, such as a blow to the head, can produce massive hemorrhages within the skull. As in the case of brain tumors, the expanding pool of blood within the skull gradually compresses the brain tissue and can result in death unless the problem is corrected. The damage of a brain hemorrhage can be insidious, with no immediate signs or symptoms of the problem until irreversible changes have occurred in the brain tissue. The patient may receive what may appear to be a minor head injury, for example, and not lose consciousness. Or he may be unconscious for a brief period, then recover and seem very alert. But gradually, over a period of hours or even days, neurological signs of disintegrating brain function appear.

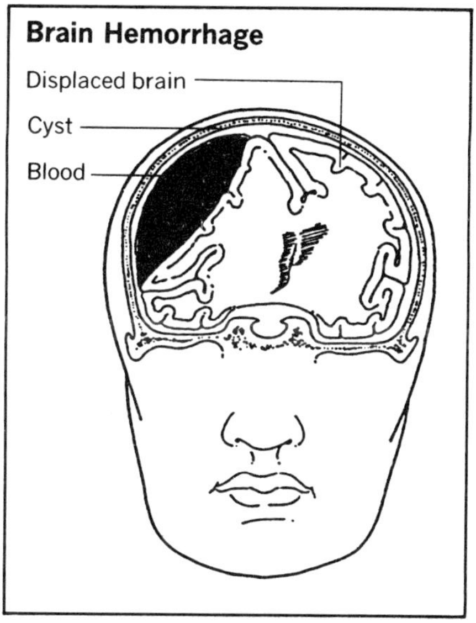

Treatment

The treatment requires a procedure similar to that used for removing brain tumors. An opening is made in the skull to remove the blood or blood clot and relieve pressure upon the brain tissues. The chances for full recovery depend somewhat upon the extent of brain damage caused by the hemorrhage before treatment.

Skull Fracture

Surgical treatment for a skull fracture may combine techniques of various other methods for fractures and brain injuries. The scalp is shaved and cleaned carefully so the surgeon can determine the extent of the injury and its location with respect to vital tissues under the skull. With the help of X rays and signs of neurological damage, the surgeon frequently can tell how severe the fracture may be and whether there is bleeding beneath the skull.

Treatment

If the skull appears to be intact but there are signs of a brain hemorrhage, the skull is opened to remove the blood or blood clot and relieve pressure on the brain. If the skull fracture is compound and depressed, or with skull fragments in the brain tissue, efforts also must be made to elevate the depressed bone section so it does not press on vital brain areas and to remove bits of bone or other foreign materials that may have entered the brain.

Surgeons frequently can rebuild a fractured skull by replacing missing bits of bone or adding appropriate synthetic materials such as a piece of metal plate. Full recovery depends upon such factors as the age of the patient and the severity of damage before treatment was started. Younger patients generally respond better to the repair procedures, but full recovery from a severe skull fracture may take as long as a year.

Aneurysm in the Brain

Aneurysms can develop in blood vessels of the brain, and like aneurysms in other parts of the body they can be corrected surgically. A ruptured aneurysm produces a brain hemorrhage. The condition is most likely to develop in people over the age of 30; in patients over 40, women are more likely than men to be victims of the disorder. The approach to repair of an intracranial aneurysm depends upon the condition of the patient and the location and size of the aneurysm, which frequently can be identified by X-ray pictures after an opaque dye has been injected into the bloodstream. The diseased blood vessel may be ligated, reinforced, or repaired, depending upon the conditions found by the surgeon after the aneurysm has been exposed and examined.

Plastic and Cosmetic Surgery

The use of surgical techniques for the correction of physical deformities is by no means a modern development. The practice goes back to ancient India, where as early as the sixth century B.C. Hindu specialists were reconstructing noses, reshaping ears, and grafting skin for reducing scar tissue.

Through the centuries, improvements in procedure and new types of operations became part of the common fund of information. During World War I, great technical advances were made when the Medical Corps of the United States Army created a special division of ***plastic surgery*** to treat the deformities caused by battle injuries. Today's plastic surgery is based on many of the procedures perfected then and during World War II.

Today, attention focuses not only on birth and injury deformities but on lesser irregularities as well. Surgeons in the field of ***cosmetic surgery*** perform such procedures as nose reconstruction, face lifting, reshaping of breasts, removal of fatty tissue from upper arms and legs, and the transplanting of hair to correct baldness. In the instance of hair transplants, hair follicles, commonly called plugs, are removed from dense areas of hair such as the side or back of the head and repositioned to bald areas. While largely effective, this surgery can be time-consuming, expensive, and painful.

There is no longer any reason for someone to suffer from the emotional and professional problems caused by abnormalities in appearance. No child should be expected to live with the disability of a cleft lip or crossed eyes. Anyone interested in undergoing any form of cosmetic surgery should stay away from so-called beauty experts, and deal only with a reputable surgeon or physician.

Some surgical specialists, called *plastic surgeons,* perform cosmetic or plastic surgery exclusively. Other surgeons and physicians, including general surgeons, dermatologists, ophthalmologists, and others, are qualified to do some kinds of plastic surgery, usually the techniques related to their particular specialties. The kind of surgery desired should first be discussed with the family doctor, who can then evaluate the problem and recommend a qualified surgeon to deal with it.

Before undergoing any kind of plastic surgery, the prospective patient should realize that it is neither inexpensive nor totally painless. Most cosmetic surgery is performed in hospitals, which means that in addition to the surgeon's fees there can be a bill for the anesthetist, use of the operating and recovery rooms, and the hospital stay itself. Also, because cosmetic surgery is often optional surgery—surgery not needed to ensure the patient's physical health—it may not be covered by a health-insurance policy.

Reshaping the Nose

Known technically as a *rhinoplasty,* the operation for the reconstruction of the nose is not only one of the oldest but also one of the most common forms of cosmetic surgery. Depending upon the demands of facial symmetry and individual taste, the nose can be shortened, straightened, narrowed, or even lengthened. If a nose deformity has caused breathing problems, the surgeon will take the correction of this into account in planning the reconstruction.

Barring accidents, most children's noses are perfectly adequate until they enter their teens, when the facial bones begin to take on the contours determined by inheritance. Teenagers are especially sensitive about their looks, but if nose surgery seems advisable, it is usually best to wait until the child is at least 14 or 15 years of age.

Cosmetic Breast Surgery

Breast Lifting

Breasts that sag even though they are not too large can be lifted to a more attractive contour by an operation that consolidates the tissue. The surgical procedure, called *mastopexy,* consists of removing strips of skin from the base of the breasts and bringing the rest of the skin together

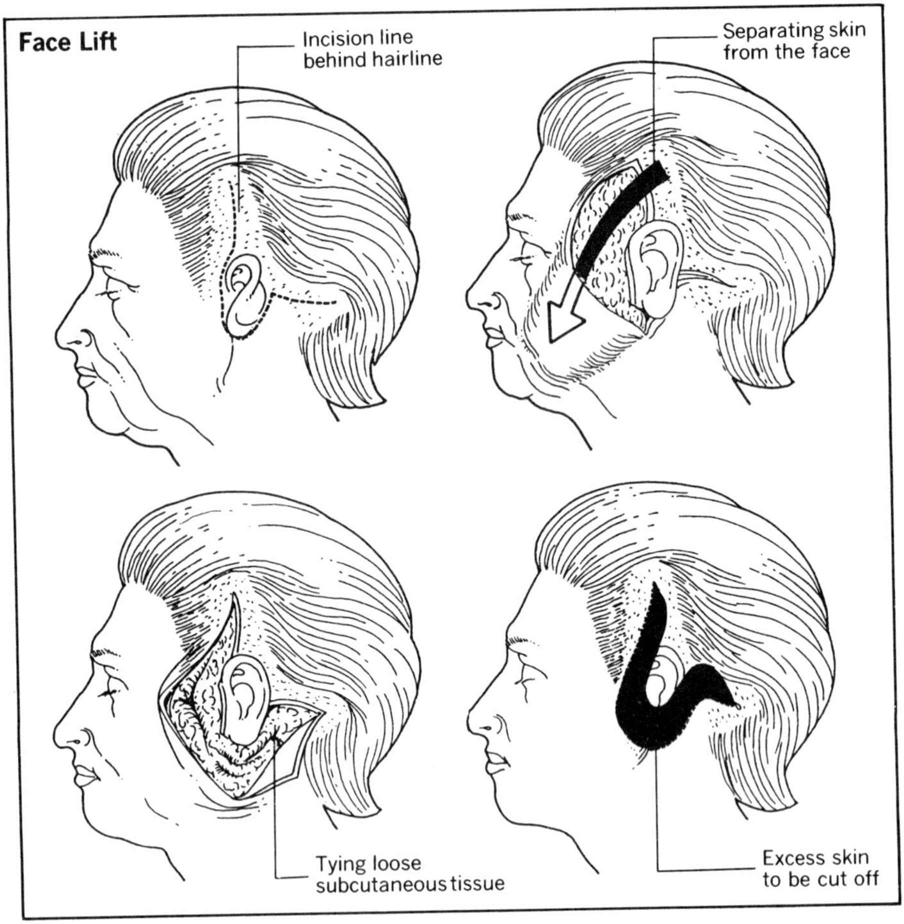

under tension so that it is tight enough to support the tissue in an upward position. The nipple is moved to a higher position.

Breast Reduction

In spite of all the publicity given to breast augmentation, most cosmetic surgery involving the breasts is concerned with reducing rather than enlarging them. Breast reduction is frequently undertaken not only to improve appearance but also for purposes of health and comfort.

The operation, called a *reduction mammoplasty*, is performed under either local or general anesthesia, depending on the extent of the reduction. The surgeon cuts out fatty tissue and skin and repositions the nipple to a higher placement. The incisions are positioned so that the scars will be hidden when the patient is wearing normal clothing.

Breast Enlargement

The techniques used in this operation, called *augmentation mammoplasty*, have changed over the years. Early operations to augment the size of the breasts involved the injection of paraffin, but this was soon abandoned as unsatisfactory. Experimentation with the use of various synthetic substances and of fatty tissue taken from the buttocks also gave poor results.

Breast implants containing silicone gel and inserted under the breast tissue were once the norm in augmentation surgery, but concerns developed regarding leakage of the gel into surrounding tissue and its subsequent migration to other parts of the body. Although no health complications were definitively linked to silicone implants, lawsuits against the manufacturers and public concern led to their being taken off the market almost entirely. Saline implants—salt water in a jacket made of silicone in a rubber-like form—are now the only kind available for cosmetic breast enlargement.

Liposuction

Excess fat can be removed by means of *liposuction*, also called *suction lipectomy*. The procedure is normally performed under general anesthesia. A blunt-tipped, hollow rod is inserted under the skin and moved through the fat tissue, suctioning out unwanted fat cells. Liposuction is most successful on the abdomen, hips, buttocks, and thighs.

Face Lift

Face lifting, or *rhytidoplasty*, is a form of cosmetic surgery designed to eliminate as far as possible signs of aging, such as wrinkles, pouches under the chin and eyes, and sagging tissue generally.

In deciding on the advisability of a face lift, a reputable surgeon will take into account the person's age, emotional stability, and physical condition. The main procedure involves tightening the skin after the surplus has been removed. The resulting scars are usually hidden in the hair and behind the ears. Those directly in front of the ears are visible only under very close scrutiny. Even after a face lift, however, the same wrinkles will eventually reappear, owing to the characteristic use of the individual's facial muscles.

Eyelids

The shape and size of the eyelids can be changed by an operation called a *blepharoplasty*. In this procedure, an incision is made in the fold of the upper eyelid, and excess skin and fat are removed. The technique can be used to correct congenital deformities, such as hanging upper eyelids that do not fully open. When a comparable incision is made below the lash line on the lower lid, the surgeon can remove the fat that causes bags under the eyes.

Ears

Surgery to correct protruding or overlarge ears is called *otoplasty.* Though it can be performed on adults, it is usually performed on children before they enter school, to prevent the psychological problems that often result from teasing. In the procedure, an incision is made behind the ear, cartilage is cut, and the ear is repositioned closer to the skull. Otoplasty can also build up or replace an ear missing because of a birth defect or accident.

Scar Reduction

Unsightly scars that are the result of a birth defect or an injury can usually be reduced by plastic surgery to thin hairlines. The procedure is effective only if there has been no extensive damage to surrounding areas of underlying tissue, as sometimes occurs in severe burns. The operation involves the removal of the old scar tissue, undermining the surrounding skin, and pulling it together with very fine stitches.

Uncommon Surgical Procedures

Organ Transplants

The ability to rebuild human bodies from the parts of other humans or from artificial organs is one of modern medicine's greatest accomplishments and one of its oldest dreams. Some of the most ancient documents, thousands of years old, tell of medical efforts to transplant organs, limbs, and other tissues to save lives or enable disabled persons to pursue normal activities. In the twentieth century, medical scientists discovered how to overcome a number of obstacles to the transplanting of organs, and today the transplantation of a variety of organs has become commonplace.

Tissue Compatibility

A major obstacle to organ transplants has been one of *histoincompatibility* (*histo* means "tissue"): the tissues of the person receiving the transplant tend to reject the tissues of the transplanted organs. The problem is quite similar to that of allergies or the body's reaction to foreign bodies, including infectious organisms. Each individual has a set of antigens that are peculiar to that person, because of genetic variations among different persons. The histoincompatible antigens are on the surfaces of the tissue cells. But in most cases the antigens on the cells of the transplanted organ do not match those of the person receiving the transplant, so the recipient's body in effect refuses to accept the transplant.

The major exception to this rule is found in identical twins, who are born with the same sets of antigens. The organs of one twin can be transplanted to the body of the other twin with a minimum risk of rejection. Antigens on the tissue cells of brothers and sisters and of the parents will be similar, because of the biological relationship, but they will not be as compatible as those of identical twins. Even less compatible are antigens of people who are not related.

Types of Grafts

There is virtually no problem in transferring tissues from one area to another of the same patient. Skin grafts, bone grafts, and blood-vessel transplants are commonly made with a patient's own tissues, which have the same antigens, as in spinal fusions, repair of diseased leg arteries, and so on. Tissue transplants within an individual's body are called *autografts.* Transplants of tissues or organs from one human to another are called *homografts,* or *allografts. Heterografts,* or *xenografts,* are tissues from one species that are transplanted to another; they offer the greatest risk of histoincompatibility and are used mainly as a temporary measure, such as covering a severely burned area of a person with specially treated pieces of pigskin. The heterograft will be rejected, but it will provide some protection during the recovery period.

Much of the experience of surgeons in handling tissue transplants between humans came from early experiments in skin grafting. It was found that histoincompatibility in transplants of skin appeared to sensitize the recipient tissues in the same way that allergy sensitivity rises. Thus, when a second skin graft from the same donor is attempted, the graft is rejected more rapidly than the first graft because of the buildup of antibodies from the first rejection. The same sort of rejection reaction can occur in transplants of kidneys, hearts, and other organs unless the problem of histoincompatibility is overcome.

Immunosuppressive Chemicals

In order to make the host body more receptive to an organ transplant, *immunosuppressive* chemicals are injected into the recipient's tissues to suppress their natural tendency to reject the foreign tissue. However, the technique of suppressing the immune response of the host tissues is not without hazards. By suppressing the natural rejection phenomenon, the transplant recipient is made vulnerable to other diseases. It has been found, for example, that persons who receive the immune response suppression chemicals as part of transplant surgery develop cancers at a rate that is 15 times that of the general population. Transplant patients also can become extremely vulnerable to infections, such as pneumonia.

Antigen Matching

The breakthrough in human organ transplantation was helped by the development of a system of matching antigens related to lymphocytes—a type of white blood cell—of the donor and recipient. At least a dozen lymphocyte antigens have been identified, and it is possible to match them by a process similar to matching blood factors of patients before making a blood transfusion. If all or most of the antigens of the donor tissue and the recipient match, the chances for a successful transplanting procedure are greatly enhanced.

Antigen matching is less important in some kinds of homografts, such as replacing the cornea of the eye. The cornea is a unique kind of tissue with no blood vessels, and therefore is unlikely to be invaded by antibodies of the recipient. Pieces of human bone also may be used in homografts with a minimum risk of rejection, although surgeons usually prefer to use bone from the patient's own body in repairing fractures and in other orthopedic procedures.

Types of Transplants

Cornea Transplant

Cornea transplants helped to pioneer the art of homografts. The first successful cornea transplants were made during the 1930s. In addition to the absence of rejection problems because of incompatible antigens, cornea transplants probably succeeded in the early days of homografts because only small pieces of the tissue were used.

Kidney Transplant

Kidney transplants began in the 1950s. Antigen typing was unknown at that time, but physicians had learned of the genetic factors of blood groups and found from experience that although kidney transplants from

Immunosuppressive Chemicals

In order to make the host body more receptive to an organ transplant, *immunosuppressive* chemicals are injected into the recipient's tissues to suppress their natural tendency to reject the foreign tissue. However, the technique of suppressing the immune response of the host tissues is not without hazards. By suppressing the natural rejection phenomenon, the transplant recipient is made vulnerable to other diseases. It has been found, for example, that persons who receive the immune response suppression chemicals as part of transplant surgery develop cancers at a rate that is 15 times that of the general population. Transplant patients also can become extremely vulnerable to infections, such as pneumonia.

Antigen Matching

The breakthrough in human organ transplantation was helped by the development of a system of matching antigens related to lymphocytes—a type of white blood cell—of the donor and recipient. At least a dozen lymphocyte antigens have been identified, and it is possible to match them by a process similar to matching blood factors of patients before making a blood transfusion. If all or most of the antigens of the donor tissue and the recipient match, the chances for a successful transplanting procedure are greatly enhanced.

Antigen matching is less important in some kinds of homografts, such as replacing the cornea of the eye. The cornea is a unique kind of tissue with no blood vessels, and therefore is unlikely to be invaded by antibodies of the recipient. Pieces of human bone also may be used in homografts with a minimum risk of rejection, although surgeons usually prefer to use bone from the patient's own body in repairing fractures and in other orthopedic procedures.

Types of Transplants

Cornea Transplant

Cornea transplants helped to pioneer the art of homografts. The first successful cornea transplants were made during the 1930s. In addition to the absence of rejection problems because of incompatible antigens, cornea transplants probably succeeded in the early days of homografts because only small pieces of the tissue were used.

Kidney Transplant

Kidney transplants began in the 1950s. Antigen typing was unknown at that time, but physicians had learned of the genetic factors of blood groups and found from experience that although kidney transplants from

Heart transplants have become increasingly successful. Hospitals are working to set up a better distribution system for donated hearts. Doctors are also making progress toward the development of an artificial self-contained heart.

Bone-Marrow Transplant

A bone marrow transplant is a procedure to replace bone marrow, which is at the center of bones and produces red blood cells. Transplantation may use a patient's own marrow saved before treatment or marrow from someone else. Bone-marrow transplant is most commonly used to treat leukemia and lymphoma. It is also used to treat brain tumors in children and neuroblastoma (a rare cancer that occurs most often in infants and children).

Other Kinds of Transplants

Surgeons also have experimented with varying success with human transplants of livers, lungs, and pancreas tissue. Lung transplant efforts have been hampered by infection, rejection, and hemorrhage. Because the lungs are exposed to pathogenic organisms in the environment, they are especially vulnerable to infections when the host tissues have been treated with immunosuppressive chemicals. Liver transplants are difficult to perform because of a lack of satisfactory donor organs and the complex circuitry of arteries, veins, and bile duct that must be connected to the recipient before the liver can begin to function.

Most major organ transplants are considered only in terms of a "last-ditch" effort to prolong the life of a patient who is critically ill. Although homografts are not always a perfect success and may lengthen a patient's life by only a few years, remarkable strides in these surgical techniques have been made over a relatively short period of time.

Reattachment of Severed Members

Because an individual's tissues present no histocompatibility problem with other parts of his own body, severed fingers and other members can be rejoined to the rest of the body if vital parts are not damaged beyond repair. For example, a fingertip can be severed when caught in a closed door of an automobile. If the severed part of the finger is saved and the patient is given immediate medical care, the finger usually can be rejoined and sutured in place with a very good chance of survival of the graft.

Rejoining a Severed Limb

One of the most dramatic cases of a rejoined limb in American medical annals involved a 12-year-old whose right arm was severed at the shoulder when he was crushed between a train and a tunnel wall in 1962. Railroad workers called an ambulance, and the boy, his severed arm still encased in his sleeve, was rushed to a hospital. The boy was given plasma by physicians who packed the severed arm in ice and flushed out the blood vessels of the arm with anticoagulant drugs and antibiotics. During three hours of surgery, the major veins and artery of the arm were carefully stitched to the vessels at the shoulder. For the next five hours, surgeons joined the bones, located the main nerve trunks and connected them to the nerve ends in the shoulder, and repaired the muscles. The boy was released from the hospital three weeks after the accident but returned for additional operations to connect various nerve fibers. That operation was a success, but similar attempts to rejoin severed arms of middle-aged men have failed despite heroic attempts by surgeons to restore the limbs as functioning parts of the body.

A Chinese factory worker suffered accidental amputation of his right hand when it was caught in a metal-punching machine, and was rushed to a hospital in Shanghai. Chinese medical reports of the case indicate that a procedure similar to the one used on the American boy was followed. Blood vessels were rejoined first to permit the flow of blood to tissues. This was followed by surgery to connect the tendons and main nerve trunks. The bones of the forearm, where the amputation occurred, were joined and held in place with metal plates and screws. Physicians reported that the graft was successful, and the patient, a 27-year-old man, was able to move his fingers again within three weeks after the accident.

Medical records indicate that major reattachments of severed limbs are still rare, although rejoined finger tips, ears, and other parts not involving main arteries, veins, or nerve trunks are not as uncommon.

The Complete Reference Guide to

MEDICINE AND HEALTH

The Complete Reference Guide to MEDICINE AND HEALTH

EDITED BY
Richard J. Wagman, M.D., F.A.C.P.
Assistant Clinical Professor of Medicine
Downstate Medical Center
New York, New York

Volume Three

FACTS ON FILE/NEW YORK

ISBN 0-8160-6144-0 (hardcover)

Printed in the United States of America

Editor

Richard J. Wagman, M.D., F.A.C.P.

Assistant Clinical Professor of Medicine

Downstate Medical Center

New York, New York

Contributors to The New Complete Medical and Health Encyclopedia

Consultant in Surgery

N. Henry Moss, M.D., F.A.C.S.
Associate Clinical Professor of Surgery
Temple University Health Sciences Center and Albert Einstein Medical Center;
Past President, American Medical Writers Association;
Past President, New York Academy of Sciences

Consultant in Gynecology

Douglass S. Thompson, M.D.
Clinical Professor of Obstetrics and Gynecology and Clinical Associate Professor of Community Medicine
University of Pittsburgh School of Medicine

Consultant in Pediatrics

Charles H. Bauer, M.D.
Clinical Associate Professor of Pediatrics and Chief of Pediatric Gastroenterology
The New York Hospital-Cornell Medical Center
New York, New York

Consultants in Psychiatry

Julian J. Clark, M.D.
Assistant Professor of Psychiatry

and

Rita W. Clark, M.D.
Clinical Assistant Professor of Psychiatry
Downstate Medical Center

Consulting Editor

Kenneth N. Anderson
Formerly Editor
Today's Health

Bruce O. Berg, M.D.
Associate Professor
Departments of Neurology and Pediatrics
Director, Child Neurology
University of California
San Francisco, California

D. Jeanne Collins
Assistant Professor
College of Allied Health Professions
University of Kentucky
Lexington, Kentucky

Anthony A. Davis
Vice President and Education Consultant
Metropolitan X-Ray and Medical Sales, Inc.
Olney, Maryland

Peter A. Dickinson
Editor Emeritus
Harvest Years/Retirement Living

Gordon K. Farley, M.D.
Associate Professor of Child Psychiatry
Director, Day Care Center
University of Colorado Medical Center

Arthur Fisher
Group Editor
Science and Engineering
Popular Science

Edmund H. Harvey, Jr.
Editor
Science World

Helene MacLean
Medical writer

Ben Patrusky
Science writer

Stanley E. Weiss, M.D.
Assistant Attending Physician, Renal Service
Beth Israel Hospital and Medical Center, New York

Jeffrey S. Willner, M.D.
Attending Radiologist
Southampton Hospital
Southampton, New York

Contents

Volume III

21

Skin and Hair

Not many people have perfectly proportioned faces and bodies, but practically anyone, at any age, can present an attractive appearance if skin is healthy-looking and glowing and hair is clean and shining. Healthy skin and hair can be achieved through good health habits, cleanliness, and personal grooming. Expensive skin-and-hair products may boost self-confidence, but they are a poor substitute for proper diet, exercise, enough sleep, and soap and water or cleansing creams.

The condition of skin and hair reflects a person's physical and emotional health. Of course, general appearance is determined not only by what is going on inside the body but also by outward circumstances, such as extremes of temperature or the use of harsh soaps. Appearance can also be altered temporarily by cosmetics and permanently by surgery.

The Skin

The skin is one of the most important organs of the body. It serves as protection against infection by germs and shields delicate underlying tissue against injury. Approximately one-third of the bloodstream flows through the skin, and as the blood vessels contract or relax in response to heat and cold, the skin acts as a thermostat that helps control body temperature. The two million sweat glands in the skin also regulate body temperature through the evaporation of perspiration. The many delicate nerve endings in the skin make it a sense organ responsive not only to heat and cold but also to pleasure, pain, and pressure.

Certain cells in the skin produce a protective pigmentation that determines its color and guards against overexposure to the ultraviolet rays of the sun. By absorption and elimination, the skin helps regulate the body's chemical and fluid balance. One of the miracles of the skin is that it constantly renews itself.

Structure of the Skin

The skin is made up of two layers. The outer layer, or *epidermis,* has a surface of horny, nonliving cells that form the body's protective envelope. These cells are constantly being shed and replaced by new ones, which are made in the lower or inner layer of the epidermis.

Underneath the epidermis is the *dermis,* the thicker part of the skin. It contains blood vessels, nerves, and connective tissue. The sweat glands are located in the dermis, and they collect fluid containing water, salt, and waste products from the blood. This fluid is sent through tiny canals that end in pores on the skin's surface.

The oil, or *sebaceous,* glands that secrete the oil that lubricates the surface of the skin and hair are also located in the dermis. They are most often associated with hair *follicles.*

Anatomy of the Skin

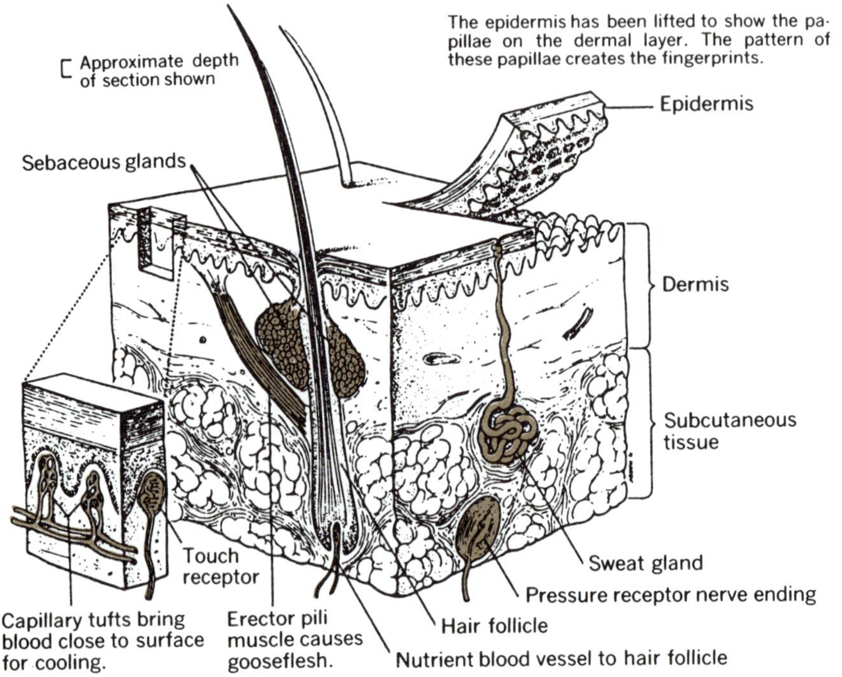

Hair follicles and oil glands are found over most of the body, with the exception of the palms of the hands and the soles of the feet.

The layer of fatty tissue below the dermis, called *subcutaneous* tissue, acts as an insulator against heat and cold and as a shock absorber against injury.

Skin Color

The basic skin color of each person is determined at birth, and is a part of his heritage that cannot be changed.

Melanin

There are four pigments in the normal skin that affect its color: melanin, oxygenated hemoglobin, reduced hemoglobin, and various carotenes. Of these, *melanin* is the most powerful. The cells that produce it are the same in all races, but there is wide variation in the amount produced, and wide variation in its color, which ranges from black to light tan. Every adult has about 60,000 melanin-producing cells in each square inch of skin.

Melanin cells also affect eye color. When the cells are deep in the eye, the color produced is blue or green. When they are close to the surface, the eye is brown. An *albino,* a person with no melanin, has eyes that appear pink, because the stronger pigment that ordinarily masks the blood vessels is lacking.

Hemoglobin

The pigment that gives blood its color, called *hemoglobin,* has the next greatest effect on skin color. When it is combined with oxygen, a bright red is the result, and this in turn produces the rosy complexion associated with good health in light-skinned people. When such people suffer from reduced hemoglobin because of anemia, they appear to be excessively pale. A concentration of reduced hemoglobin gives the skin a bluish appearance. Because hemoglobin has a weaker coloring effect than the melanin that determines basic skin color, these variations are more visible in lighter-skinned individuals.

Carotenes

The weakest pigments in the skin are the *carotenes.* These produce a yellowish tone that is increased by eating excessive amounts of carrots and oranges. In people with black or brown skin, excess carotene is usually masked by the melanin pigment.

Aging Skin

Skin appearance is affected by both internal and external factors. A baby's skin has a silken quality because it has not yet begun to show the effects of continued exposure to sun and wind. The skin problems associated with adolescence reflect the many glandular changes that occur during the transition to adulthood. As the years pass, the skin becomes the most obvious indicator of aging.

Heredity, general health, and exposure to the elements are some of the factors that contribute to aging skin. Because people with darker skin have built-in protection against the ravages of the sun, their skin usually has a younger appearance than that of lighter-skinned people of comparable age.

In general, the skin of an older person is characterized by wrinkles and shininess. It feels thinner when pinched because it has lost its elasticity and part of the underlying fat that gives firmness to a younger skin.

Constant exposure to sunlight is now thought to play a more important role in the visible aging of skin than the aging process itself. Such exposure also appears to be directly related to the greater frequency of skin cancer among farmers, sailors, and others who spend most of their working hours out of doors.

Care of the Skin

Healthy, normal skin should be washed regularly with mild soap and warm water to remove grease, perspiration, and accumulated dirt. For those with a limited water supply or inadequate bath and shower facilities, sponge baths are a good substitute if the sponge or washcloth is thoroughly rinsed as various parts of the body are washed. Many people feel that a shower is a much more efficient way of getting clean than a bath, since the bath water becomes the receptacle for the dirt washed from the body, instead of its being rinsed away.

No matter what method is used, all soap should be thoroughly rinsed off the skin after washing. Unless specifically prescribed by a physician, medicated or germicidal soaps should not be used, since they may be an irritant. Skin should be dried with a fluffy towel, and bath towels should never be shared. Hands should be washed several times a day, and fingernails kept clean.

Facial skin requires special care because of its constant exposure. The face should be cleaned in the morning and before bedtime. Some people may prefer to use a cleansing cream rather than soap and water. Everyone should avoid massaging soap into the skin, because this may cause drying.

Dry and Oily Skin

Both heredity and environment account for the wide variation in the amount of oil and perspiration secreted by the glands of different people. Also, the same person's skin may be oily in one part of the body and dry in another. Skin on the nose and chin tends to be the oiliest.

Dry Skin

This condition is the result of loss of water from the outer surface of the epidermis and its insufficient replacement from the tissues below. Some causes of the moisture loss are too frequent use of soap and detergents, and constant exposure to dry air. Anyone spending a great deal of time in air-conditioned surroundings in which the humidity has been greatly lowered is likely to suffer from dry skin.

To correct the condition, the use of soap and water should be kept to a minimum for those parts of the body where the skin is dry. Cleansing creams or lotions containing lanolin should be used on the face, hands, elbows, and wherever else necessary. If tub baths are taken, a bath oil can be used in the water or applied to the skin after drying. Baby oil is just as effective and much cheaper than glamorously packaged and overadvertised products. Baby oil or a protective lotion should also be used on any parts of the body exposed to direct sunlight for any extended length of time. Applying oil to the skin will not, however, prevent wrinkles.

Oily Skin

The amount of oil that comes to the surface of the skin through the sebaceous glands is the result not only of heredity but also of temperature and emotional state. In warm weather, when the skin perspires more freely, the oil spreads like a film on the surface moisture. Nonoily foundation lotions can be helpful in keeping the oil spread to a minimum, and so can frequent washing with soap and water. When washing is inconvenient during the day, cleansing pads packaged to fit in pocket or purse are a quick and efficient solution for both men and women.

Too much friction from complexion brushes, rough washcloths, or harsh soaps may irritate rather than improve an oily skin condition.

Deodorants and Antiperspirants

Sweat glands are present almost everywhere in the skin except for the lips and a few other areas. Most of them give off the extremely dilute salt water known as sweat, or perspiration. Their purpose is to cool the body by evaporation of water. Body odors are not produced by perspiration itself but by the bacterial activity that takes place in the perspiration. The activity is most intense in warm, moist parts of the body from which perspiration cannot evaporate quickly, such as the underarm area.

Deodorants

The basic means of keeping this type of bacterial growth under control is through personal cleanliness of both skin and clothing. Deodorant soaps containing antiseptic chemicals are now available. Though they do not kill bacteria, they do reduce the speed with which they multiply.

Underarm deodorants also help to eliminate the odor. They are not meant to stop the flow of perspiration but rather to slow down bacterial growth and mask body odors with their own scent. Such deodorants should be applied immediately after bathing. They are usually more effective if the underarm area is shaved, since the hair in this unexposed area collects perspiration and encourages bacterial growth.

Antiperspirants

Antiperspirants differ from deodorants in that they not only affect the rate of bacterial growth but also reduce the amount of perspiration that reaches the skin surface. Because the action of the chemical salts they contain is cumulative, they seem to be more effective with repeated use. Antiperspirants come under the category of drugs, and their contents must be printed on the container. Deodorants are considered cosmetics, and may or may not name their contents on the package.

No matter what the nature of the advertising claim, neither type of product completely stops the flow of perspiration, nor would it be desirable to do so. Effectiveness of the various brands differs from one person to another. Some may produce a mild allergic reaction; others might be too weak to do a good job. It is practical to experiment with a few different brands, using them under similar conditions, to find the type that works best for you.

Creams and Cosmetics

The bewildering number of creams and cosmetics on the market and the exaggerated claims of some of their advertising can be reduced to a few simple facts. Beauty preparations should be judged by the user on their merits rather than on their claims.

Cold Creams and Cleansing Creams

These two products are essentially the same. They are designed to remove accumulated skin secretions, dirt, and grime, and should be promptly removed from the skin with a soft towel or tissue.

Lubricating Creams and Lotions

Also called night creams, moisturizing creams, and conditioning creams, these products are supposed to prevent the loss of moisture from the skin and promote its smoothness. They are usually left on overnight or for an extended length of time. Anyone with dry skin will find it helpful to apply a moisturizer under foundation cream. This will help keep the skin from drying out even further, and protect it against the effects of air-conditioning.

Vanishing Creams and Foundation Creams

These products also serve the purpose of providing the skin with moisture, but are meant to be applied immediately before putting on makeup.

Rejuvenating Creams

There is no scientific proof that any of the "royal jelly," "secret formula," or "hormone" creams produce a marked improvement on aging skin. They cannot eliminate wrinkles, nor can they regenerate skin tissue.

Medicated Creams and Lotions

These products should not be used except on the advice of a physician, since they may cause or aggravate skin disorders of various kinds.

Lipsticks

Lipsticks contain lanolin, a mixture of oil and wax, a coloring dye, and pigment, as well as perfume. Any of these substances can cause an allergic reaction in individual cases, but such reactions are uncommon. Sometimes the reaction is caused by the staining dye, in which case a "nonpermanent" lipstick should be used.

Cosmetics and the Sensitive Skin

Anyone with a cosmetic problem resulting from sensitive skin should consult a *dermatologist,* a physician specializing in the skin and its diseases. Cosmetic companies will inform a physician of the ingredients in their products, and he or she can then recommend a brand that will agree with the patient's specific skin problems. The physician may also recommend a special nonallergenic preparation.

Eye Makeup

Eye-liner and mascara brushes and pencils—and lipsticks, for that matter—can carry infection and should never be borrowed or lent. *Hypoallergenic* makeup, which is specially made for those who get allergic reactions to regular eye makeup, is available.

Suntanning Creams and Lotions

Growing awareness that exposure to the sun may cause skin cancer (see "Skin Cancer" in Ch. 18, *Cancer*) has led to a demand for a variety of skin creams and lotions. The preparations protect the skin or speed the tanning process. Many of the "sunblocks" and "sunscreens" keep the ultraviolet radiation in sunlight from reaching the skin. They are adapted to six basic skin types, ranging from type 1, which burns easily and never tans, to types 5 and 6, which never burn and usually tan well.

Skin lotions and creams are rated according to a "sun protection factor" (SPF). Among the basic ratings are SPF 4, providing "moderate protection;" SPF 8, a "maximal" sunscreen; and SPF 15, with "ultra" protection. Other ratings range up to SPF 50. Some medical authorities question the need for sunscreens rated higher than 15 or 20. Food and Drug Administration ratings go only to SPF 15. Many newer sunscreens are greaseless, hypoallergenic, waterproof, or PABA-free. PABA, or para-aminobenzoic acid, is a sunscreen chemical that can irritate skin and stain clothing.

Sunscreen ratings indicate, in theory, how long the user can stay in the sun without burning. A lotion or cream with a rating of SPF 2 should allow users to remain exposed twice as long as they could with no protection at all. The Skin Cancer Foundation believes that persons who burn in the sun should uniformly wear an SPF 15 protective preparation.

Persons who want suntans have many products from which to choose. "Tanning accelerators" in lotion form speed up the tanning process. A pocket-sized "sun exposure meter" operated electronically alerts the user when overexposure may be taking place. The meter is programmed with the individual's skin type and SPF.

Tanning Pills

Case-studies have proven that tanning pills can cause serious medical problems, possibly resulting in death. Ailments include aplastic anemia (a decrease in the production of red blood cells), orange skin, headaches, weight loss, easy bruising, and increased fatigue. Treatment involves blood transfusion therapy. Physicians believe that the ingredient canthaxanthin is responsible for the disorders.

This drug is not approved as a prescription or an over-the-counter preparation by the Federal Drug Administration. Ultimately, this product serves no purpose, and it is best to avoid using it.

Hair

Hair originates in tiny sacs or follicles deep in the dermis layer of skin tissue. The part of the hair below the skin surface is the root; the part above is the shaft. Hair follicles are closely connected to the sebaceous glands, which secrete oil to the scalp and give hair its natural sheen. Hair grows from the root outward, pushing the shaft farther from the scalp.

Texture

Each individual hair is made up of nonliving cells that contain a tough protein called *keratin*. Hair texture differs from one part of the body to another. It also differs between the sexes, among individuals, and among the different races.

If an individual hair is oval in cross-section, it is curly along its length. If the cross-section is round, the hair is straight. Thick, wiry hair is usually triangular or kidney-shaped. The fineness or coarseness of hair texture is related to its natural color.

Curling

Anyone using a home permanent preparation should follow the instructions with great care: improper mixing, application, or exposure time could result in serious damage to the hair.

Electric curling irons are not safe, because they may cause pinpoint burns in the scalp that are hardly noticeable at the time but may lead to permanent small areas of baldness. The danger can be minimized, however, if instructions for use are followed exactly. It is especially important that the iron not be hot enough to singe the hair. Setting lotions used with rollers or clips have a tendency to dull the hair unless they are completely brushed out.

Straightening

The least harmful as well as the least effective way of straightening the hair temporarily is the use of pomades. They are usually considered unsatisfactory by women because they are too greasy, but are often used by men with short, unruly hair. Heat-pressing the hair with a metal comb is longer-lasting but can cause substantial damage by burning the scalp. The practice of ironing the hair should be discouraged, since it causes dryness and brittleness, with resultant breakage. Chemical straighteners should be used with great care, since they may cause serious burns. Special efforts must be made to protect the eyes from contact with these products.

Hair Color

In the same way that melanin colors the skin, it also determines hair color. The less melanin, the lighter the hair. As each hair loses its melanin pigment, it gradually turns gray, then white. It is assumed that the age at which hair begins to gray is an inherited characteristic and therefore can't be postponed or prevented by eating special foods, by taking vitamins, or by the external application of creams. The only way to recolor gray hair is by the use of a chemical dye.

Dyes and Tints

Anyone wishing to make a radical change in hair color should consult a trained and reliable hairdresser. Trying to turn black hair bright red or dark red hair to blond with a home preparation can sometimes end up with unwanted purplish or greenish results. When tints or dyes are used at home to lighten or darken the hair color by one or two shades, instructions accompanying the product must be followed carefully. Anyone with a tendency to contract contact dermatitis should make a patch test on the skin to check on possible allergic reactions. Hair should be tinted or dyed no more often than once a month.

Dye Stripping

The only safe way to get rid of an unwanted dye color that has been used on the hair is to let it grow out. The technique known as stripping takes all color from the hair and reduces it to a dangerously weak mass. It is then redyed its natural color. Such a procedure should never be undertaken by anyone except a trained beautician, if at all.

Bleaching

Hydrogen peroxide is mixed with a hair lightener to prebleach hair before applying blond tints. Bleaching with peroxide alone can cause more damage to the hair than dyeing or tinting it with a reliable commercial preparation, because it causes dryness, brittleness, and breakage.

General Hair Care

Properly cared for hair usually looks clean, shiny, and alive. Unfortunately, too many people mask the natural good looks of their hair with unnecessary sprays and "beauty" preparations.

Washing the Hair

Hair should be washed about once a week—more often if it tends to be oily. The claims made by shampoo manufacturers need not always be taken too seriously, since most shampoos contain nothing more than soap or detergent and a perfuming agent. No shampoo can restore the natural oils to the hair at the same time that it washes it. A castile shampoo is good for dry hair, and one containing tincture of green soap is good for oily hair.

Thorough rinsing is essential to eliminate any soap deposit. If the local water is hard, a detergent shampoo can be rinsed off more easily than one containing soap.

Drying the Hair

Drying the hair in sunlight or under a heat-controlled dryer is more satisfactory than trying to rub it dry with a towel. Gentle brushing during drying reactivates the natural oils that give hair its shine. Brushing in general is excellent for the appearance of the hair. Be sure to wash both brush and comb as often as the hair is washed.

Hair pomades should be avoided or used sparingly, since they are sometimes so heavy that they clog the pores of the scalp. A little bit of olive oil or baby oil can be rubbed into dry hair after shampooing. This is also good for babies' hair.

There is no scientific evidence that creme rinses, protein rinses, or beer rinses accomplish anything for the hair other than making it somewhat more manageable if it is naturally fine and flyaway.

Dandruff

Simple dandruff is a condition in which the scalp begins to itch and flake a few days after the hair has been washed. There is no evidence that the problem is related to germ infection.

Oiliness and persistent dandruff may appear not only on the scalp but also on the sides of the nose or the chest. In such cases, a dermatologist should be consulted. Both light and serious cases often respond well to prescription medicines containing tars. These preparations control the dandruff, but there is no known cure for it.

Nits

Head lice sometimes infect adults as well as children. These tiny parasites usually live on the part of the scalp near the nape of the neck, and when they bite, they cause itching. They attach their eggs, which are called *nits,* to the shaft of the hair, and when they are plentiful, they can be seen by a trained eye as tiny, silvery-white ovals. This condition is highly contagious and can be passed from one head to another by way of combs, brushes, hats, head scarfs, and towels. A physician can be consulted for information on effective ways of eliminating nits—usually by the application of chemicals and the use of a fine-tooth comb.

Baldness

Under the normal circumstances of combing, brushing, and shampooing, a person loses anywhere from 25 to 100 hairs a day. Because new hairs start growing each day, the loss and replacement usually balance each other. When the loss rate is greater than the replacement rate, thinning and baldness are the result.

The medical name for baldness is *alopecia,* the most common form of which is *male pattern baldness.* Dr. Eugene Van Scott, Professor of Dermatology of Temple University's Health Sciences Center, sums up the opinion of medical authorities on the three factors responsible for this type of baldness: sex, age, and heredity. Unfortunately, these are three factors over which medical science has no control.

Two drugs have been approved for regrowing hair: minoxidil and finasteride. Minoxidil, a topical solution, is available over the counter and is sold under the brand name Rogaine and as a generic drug. Approximately 25 percent of men and 20 percent of women using it experience some hair growth. Finasteride, a pill marketed as Prope-

Balding (Alopecia)

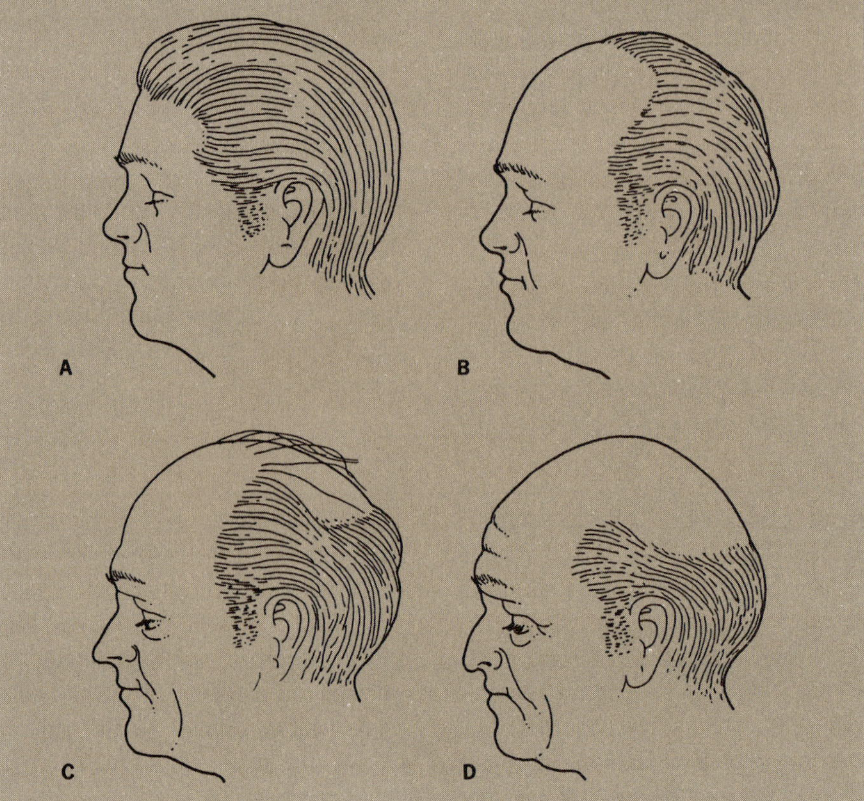

cia, was approved in 1997. More than 80 percent of men in trials experienced a slowing of hair loss and 60 percent grew new hair. Propeicia is available by prescription only.

Other forms of baldness may be the result of bacterial or fungal infections, allergic reactions to particular medicines, radiation, or continual friction. It has been suggested that stress from hair curlers or tight ponytails can cause loss of hair. These forms of baldness usually disappear when the cause is eliminated.

Although diet has very little to do with baldness, poor nutrition can result in hair that is dry, dull, and brittle enough to break easily. Any serious illness can lead to hair loss as well. It is thought that vitamin A taken in grossly excessive amounts can contribute to hair loss.

Women ordinarily lose some of their hair at the end of pregnancy, after delivery, and during the menopause, but regrowth can be expected in a few months.

A surgical procedure for treating male pattern baldness and baldness in women is called hair transplantation; it is discussed in Ch. 5, *The Middle Years*.

Hair Removal

Over the centuries and around the world, fashions in whiskers and beards come and go, but the average American male still subjects at least part of his face to daily shaving. Although feminine shaving practices are a more recent phenomenon, most American women now consider it part of good grooming to remove underarm and leg hair with a razor as often as twice a week. Shaving removes not only the dead skin cells that make up the protective layer of the body's surface but also some of the living skin underneath. Instead of being harmful, this appears to stimulate rather than damage new skin growth.

Male Shaving

The average beard grows about two-tenths of an inch a day. However, the density of male face hair varies a great deal depending on skin and hair color. In all races, the concentration is usually greatest on the chin and in the area between the nose and upper lip.

There is no proof that an electric razor is safer or better for all types of skin than a safety razor. Both types result in nicks and cuts of the living skin tissue, depending on the closeness of the shave.

Twice as many men prefer wet shaving to dry because the use of soap and hot water softens the hair stubble and makes it easier to remove. Shaving authorities point out that thorough soaking is one of the essentials of easy and safe shaving. Leaving the shaving lather on the face for at least two minutes will also soften whiskers a good deal.

The razor should be moistened with hot water throughout the process, and the chin and upper lip left for last so that the heavier hair concentration in these areas has the longest contact with moisture and lather.

Oily Skin

Men with oily skin should use an aerosol shaving preparation or a lather-type applied with a brush. These are really soaps and are more effective in eliminating the oils that coat the face hair, thus making it easier to shave.

Dry Skin

A brushless cream is advisable for dry skin, since it lubricates the skin rather than further deprives it of oil.

Ingrown Hairs

One of the chief problems connected with shaving is that it often causes ingrown hairs, which can lead to pore-clogging and infection. Hair is more likely to turn back into the skin if it is shaved against the grain, or if the cutting edge of the blade is dull and rough rather than smooth. Men with coarse, wiry, curly, rather than fine, hair may find that whisker ends are more likely to become ingrown than men with fine hair. The problem is best handled by shaving with the grain, using a sharp blade, and avoiding too close a shave, particularly in the area around the neck.

Shaving and Skin Problems

For men with acne or a tendency to skin problems, the following advice is offered by Dr. Howard T. Behrman, Director of Dermatological Research, New York Medical College:

- Shave as seldom as possible, perhaps only once or twice a week, and always with the grain.
- If wet shaving is preferred, use a new blade each time, and shave as lightly as possible to avoid nicking pimples.
- Wash face carefully with plenty of hot water to make the beard easy to manage, and after shaving, rinse with hot water followed by cold.
- Use an antiseptic astringent face lotion.
- Instead of plucking out ingrown hairs, loosen them gently so that the ends do not grow back into the skin.
- Although some people with skin problems find an electric shaver less irritating, in most cases, a wet shave seems best.

Female Shaving

Millions of American women regularly shave underarm and leg hair, and most of them do so with a blade razor. In recent years, various types of shavers have been designed with blade exposure more suited to women's needs than the standard type used by men. To make shaving easier and safer, the following procedures are recommended.

- Since wet hair is much easier to cut, the most effective time to shave is during or immediately following a bath or shower.
- Shaving cream or soap lather keeps the water from evaporating, and is preferred to dry shaving.
- Underarm shaving is easier with a contoured razor designed for this purpose. If a deodorant or antiperspirant causes stinging or irritation after shaving, allow a short time to elapse before applying it.
- Light bleeding from nicks or scrapes can be stopped by applying pressure to a sterile pad placed on the injured area.

Unwanted Hair

The technical word for excess or unwanted hair on the face, chest, arms, and legs is *hirsutism.* The condition varies greatly among different ethnic strains, and so does the attitude toward it. Women of southern European ancestry are generally hairier than those with Nordic or Anglo-Saxon ancestors. Caucasoid peoples are hairier than Negroid peoples. The sparsest amount of body hair is found among the Mongolian races and American Indians. Although heredity is the chief factor of hirsutism, hormones also influence hair growth. If there is a sudden appearance of coarse hair on the body of a young boy or girl or a woman with no such former tendency, a glandular disturbance should be suspected and investigated by a physician.

A normal amount of unwanted hair on the legs and under the arms is usually removed by shaving. When the problem involves the arms, face, chest, and abdomen, other methods of removal are available.

Temporary Methods of Hair Removal

Bleaching

Unwanted dark fuzz on the upper lip and arms can be lightened almost to invisibility with a commercially prepared bleach or with a homemade paste consisting of baking soda, hydrogen peroxide (bleaching strength), and a few drops of ammonia. Soap chips can be used instead of baking soda. The paste should be left on the skin for a few minutes and then washed off. It is harmless to the skin, and if applied repeatedly, the hair will tend to break off as a result of constant bleaching.

Chemical Depilatories

These products contain alkaline agents that cause the hair to detach easily at the skin surface. They can be used on and under the arms, and on the legs and chest. However, they should not be used on the face unless the label says it is safe to do so. Timing instructions should be followed carefully. If skin irritation results, this type of depilatory should be discontinued in favor of some other method.

Abrasives

Devices that remove hair from the skin surface by rubbing are cheap but time-consuming. However, if an abrasive such as pumice is used regularly, the offending hairs will be shorter with each application. A cream or lotion should be applied to the skin after using an abrasive.

Waxing

The technique of applying melted wax to the skin for removal of excess facial hair is best handled by an experienced cosmetician. The process involves pouring hot wax onto the skin and allowing it to cool. The hairs become embedded in the wax, and are plucked out from below the skin surface when the wax is stripped off. Because this method is painful and often causes irritation, it is not very popular, although the results are comparatively long-lasting.

Plucking

The use of tweezers for removing scattered hairs from the eyebrows, face, and chest is slightly painful but otherwise harmless. It is not a practical method for getting rid of dense hair growth, however, because it takes too much time.

Permanent Hair Removal by Electrolysis

The only permanent and safe method of removing unwanted hair is by *electrolysis.* This technique destroys each individual hair root by transmitting electric current through fine wire needles into the opening of the hair follicle. The hair thus loosened is then plucked out with a tweezer. The older type of electrolysis machine uses galvanic current. The newer type, sometimes called an *electrocoagulation machine,* uses modified high-frequency current. In either case, the efficiency and safety of the technique depends less on the machine than on the care and skill of the operator.

Because the process of treating each hair root is expensive, time-consuming, and uncomfortable, it is not recommended for areas of dense hair growth, such as the arms or legs. Before undertaking electrolysis either at a beauty salon or at home, it would be wise to consult a dermatologist about individual skin reaction.

Nails

Fingernails and toenails are an extension of the epidermis, or outer layer of the skin. They are made of elastic tissue formed from keratin, the substance that gives hair its strength and flexibility.

Some of the problems associated with fingernails are the result of too much manicuring. White spots, for example, are often caused by too much pressure at the base of the nail when trying to expose the "moon"—the white portion that contains tissue not yet as tough as the rest of the nail.

To ensure the health of toenails, feet should be bathed once a day and the nails cleaned with a brush dipped in soapy water. Shoes should fit properly so that the toenails are not subjected to pressure and distortion. To avoid ingrown toenails, trimming should be done straight across rather than by rounding or tapering the corners.

Splitting

Infection or injury of the tissue at the base of a fingernail may cause its surface to be rigid or split. Inflammation of the finger joints connected with arthritis will also cause nail deformity. For ordinary problems of splitting and

Nail Anatomy

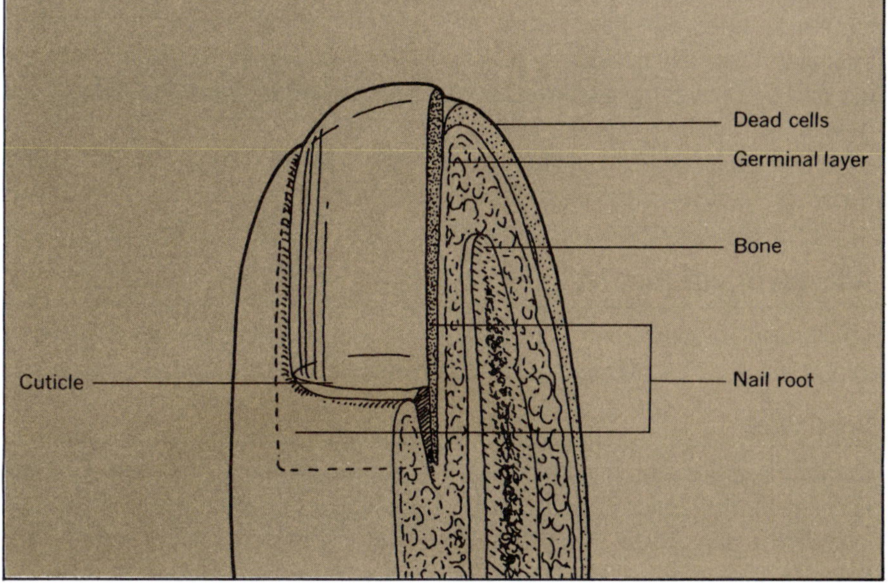

peeling, the nails should be kept short enough so that they don't catch and tear easily. For practical purposes, the top of the nail should not be visible when the palm is held about six inches from the eye. As the nails grow stronger, they can be grown longer without splitting.

Brittleness

This condition seems to be caused by such external factors as the chemicals in polish removers, soaps, and detergents. It is also a natural consequence of aging. Commercial nail-hardening preparations that contain formaldehyde are not recommended, because they are known to cause discoloration, loosening, or even loss of nails in some cases.

Nail damage can be reduced by wearing rubber gloves while doing household chores. Hand cream massaged into the skin around the nails will counteract dryness and lessen the possibility of hangnails. Although nail polish provides a shield against damage, it should not be worn all the time, particularly if the nail is polished right down to the base; this prevents live tissue from "breathing."

Disorders of the Skin

The skin is subject to a large number of disorders, most of which are not serious even though they may be temporarily uncomfortable. A disorder may be caused by one or another type of allergy; by excessive heat or cold; or by infection from fungi, bacteria, viruses, or parasites. Many skin ailments are caused or aggravated by emotional disturbances.

The symptoms and treatment of the more common disorders are discussed in the following pages. Any persistent change in skin condition should be brought to the attention of a physician.

Allergies and Itching

Itching and inflammation of the skin may be caused by an allergic reaction, by exposure to poisonous plants, or by a generalized infection.

Dermatitis

Dermatitis is the term used for an inflammation of the skin. The term for allergic reactions of the skin resulting from surface contact with outside agents is *contact dermatitis.* This condition is characterized by a rash and may be brought out by sensitivity to cosmetics, plants, cleaning materials, metal, wool, and so on. Other forms of dermatitis can be caused by excesses of heat or cold, by friction, or by sensitivity to various medicines. Dermatitis is usually accompanied by itching at the site of the rash.

Poison Ivy

This common plant, unknown in Europe but widespread everywhere in the United States except in California and Nevada, produces an allergic reaction on the skin accompanied by a painful rash and blisters. Some people are so sensitive to it that they are affected by contact not only with the plant itself but with animal fur or clothing that might have picked up the resin weeks before.

A mild attack of poison ivy produces a rash and small, watery blisters that get progressively larger. The affected area of the skin becomes crusty and dry, and after a few weeks, all symptoms vanish. If the exposed area is thoroughly washed with cold, running water immediately after contact, the poison may not penetrate the skin.

If the symptoms do develop, they can be relieved with applications of over-the-counter medications such as Domeboro or calamine lotion. If the symptoms are severe, and especially if the area around the eyes is involved, a physician should be consulted. He may prescribe an application or an injection of cortisone.

The best way to avoid the unpleasantness of a poison ivy attack is to learn to recognize the plant and stay away from it. Children especially should be warned against putting the leaves and berries in their mouths.

Poison oak and poison sumac produce somewhat the same symptoms and should also be avoided.

Under no circumstances should these plants be burned to eliminate them, because the inhaling of the contaminated smoke even from a distance can cause a serious case of poisoning. The application of special sprays, if the instructions are followed carefully, will get rid of the plants without affecting people or the neighborhood greenery.

Hives

These are large, irregularly shaped swellings on the skin that burn and itch. The cause is unknown, but allergic reactions to certain foods and medicine or to insect bites have been suggested as possible causes. The swellings of hives usually disappear within a day or so, but they can be very uncomfortable while they last. The itching and burning can often be relieved by applying cold water and a calamine solution. However, some people are sensitive to cold and develop wheals when subjected to intense cold. Commercial preparations containing surface anesthetics are seldom effective and may cause allergic reactions.

If the outbreak of hives can be traced to a specific food, such as shellfish or strawberries, the food should be eliminated from the diet. If a medicine such as penicillin or a sulfa drug is the cause, a physician should be told about the reaction.

Eczema

This condition is an allergic reaction that produces itching, swelling, blistering, oozing, and scaling of the skin. It is more common among children than among adults and may sometimes cover the entire body, although the rash is usually limited to the face, neck, and folds of the knees and elbows. Unlike contact dermatitis, it is likely to be caused by an allergy to a food or a pollen or dust. Advertised cures for eczema cannot control the cause and sometimes make the condition worse. A physician should be consulted if the symptoms are severe, particularly if the patient is an infant or very young child.

Itching

The technical name for the localized or general sensation on the skin that can be relieved by scratching is *pruritus*. Itching may be caused by many skin disorders, by infections, by serious diseases such as nephritis or leukemia, by medicines, or by psychological factors such as tension. A physician should always be consulted to find the cause of persistent itching, because it may be the symptom of a basic disorder. Repeated scratching may provide some relief, but it can also lead to infection.

Anal Pruritus

If itching in the anal area is so severe that only painful scratching will relieve it, the condition is probably *anal pruritus*. It is often accompanied by excessive rectal mucus that keeps the skin irritated and moist. This disorder is most commonly associated with hemorrhoids, but many other conditions, such as reactions to drugs, can cause it. Anxiety or tension can also contribute to it. Sitz baths with warm water are usually recommended. Every effort should be made to reduce scratching and to keep the anal skin clean and dry. Cortisone cream may be prescribed in persistent cases.

Skin Irritations and Weather

Extremes of weather produce local inflammations and other skin problems for many people.

Chapping

In cold weather, the sebaceous glands slow down the secretions that lubricate the skin, causing it to become dry. When dry skin is exposed to wintry weather, it becomes irritated and is likely to crack, particularly around the lips. Chapped skin is especially sensitive to harsh soaps. During such periods of exposure, the skin can be protected with a mild cream or lotion. A lubricating ointment should be used on the lips to prevent them from cracking. Children who lick their lips continually no matter what the weather can benefit from this extra protection. Chapped hands caused by daily use of strong soaps and detergents can be helped by the use of a lubricating cream and rubber gloves during housework.

Frostbite

Exposure to extreme cold for a prolonged period may cause freezing of the nose, fingers, toes, or ears, thus cutting off the circulation to the affected areas. Frostbitten areas are of a paler color than normal and are numb. They should not be rubbed with snow or exposed to intense heat. Areas should be thawed gradually, and a physician should be consulted for aftercare in extreme cases.

Chilblain

A localized inflammation of the skin called *chilblain* is common among people who are particularly sensitive to cold because of poor circulation. Chilblain may occur in the ears, hands, feet, and face, causing itching, swelling, and discoloration of the skin. Anyone prone to chilblain should dress protectively during the cold weather and use an electric pad or blanket at night. Affected parts should not be rubbed or massaged, nor should ice or extreme heat be applied directly, since these measures may cause additional damage. Persistent or extreme attacks of chilblain should be discussed with a physician.

Chafing

This condition is an inflammation of two opposing skin surfaces caused by the warmth, moisture, and friction of their rubbing together. Diabetics, overweight people, and those who perspire heavily are particularly prone to chafing. Chafing is accompanied by itching and burning, and sometimes infection can set in if the superficial skin is broken. Parts of the body subject to chafing are the inner surfaces of the thighs, the anal region, the area under the breasts, and the inner surfaces between fingers and toes.

To reduce the possibility of chafing, lightweight clothing should be worn and strenuous exercise avoided during hot weather. Vaseline or a vitamin A and D ointment may be applied to reduce friction. In general, the treatment is the same as that for diaper rash in infants. If the condition becomes acute, a physician can prescribe more effective remedies.

Prickly Heat

This skin rash is usually accompanied by itching and burning. It is caused by an obstruction of the sweat ducts such that perspiration does not reach the surface of the skin but backs up and causes pimples the size of a pinhead. If the obstruction is superficial, the pimples are white; if it is deeper, they are red. The condition can be brought on by other minor skin irritations, by continued exposure to moist heat, such as a compress, or by exercise in humid weather. Infants and people who are overweight are especially prone to prickly heat.

The discomfort can be eased by wearing lightweight, loose-fitting clothing, especially at night, and keeping room temperature low. Alcoholic beverages, which tend to dehydrate the body, should be avoided. Tepid baths and the application of cornstarch to the affected skin areas will usually relieve itching. If the rash remains for several days, a physician should be consulted to make sure it does not arise from some other cause.

Calluses and Corns

As a result of continued friction or pressure in a particular area, the skin forms a tough, hard, self-protecting layer known as a *callus*. Calluses are common on the soles of the feet, the palms of the hands, and, among guitarists and string players, on the tips of the fingers. A heavy callus that presses against a bone in the foot because of poorly fitted shoes can be very painful. The hard surface can be reduced somewhat by the use of pumice, or by gently paring it with a razor blade that has been washed in alcohol.

Corns are a form of callus that appear on or between the toes. They usually have a hard inner core that causes pain when pressed against underlying tissue by badly fitted shoes. A hard corn that appears on the surface of the little toe can be removed by soaking for about ten minutes and applying a few drops of ten percent salicylic acid in collodion. The surface should be covered with a corn pad to reduce pressure, and the corn lifted off when it is loose enough to be released from the skin. Anyone suffering from a circulatory disease and particularly from diabetes should avoid home treatment of foot disturbances. Those with a tendency to callus and corn formations should be especially careful about the proper fit of shoes and hose. A *chiropodist* or *podiatrist* is a trained specialist in foot care who can be visited on a regular basis to provide greater foot comfort.

Fungus Infections

Fungi are plantlike parasitic growths found in the air, in water, and in the soil. They comprise a large family that includes mushrooms, and are responsible for mildew and mold. Only a small number cause disease.

Ringworm

This condition is caused not by a worm but by a group of fungi that live on the body's dead skin cells in those areas that are warm and damp because of accumulated perspiration. One form of ringworm attacks the scalp, arms, and legs, especially of children, and is often spread by similarly affected pets. It appears as reddish patches that scale and blister and frequently feel sore and itchy. Ringworm is highly contagious and can be passed from person to person by contaminated objects such as combs and towels. It should therefore be treated promptly by a physician. Ringworm can best be prevented by strict attention to personal cleanliness.

Athlete's Foot

Another form of ringworm, *athlete's foot,* usually attacks the skin between the toes and under the toenails. If not treated promptly, it can cause an itching rash on other parts of the body. Athlete's foot causes the skin to itch, blister, and crack, and as a result, leaves it vulnerable to more serious infection from other organisms. The disorder can be treated at home by gently removing the damaged skin, and, after soaking the feet, thoroughly drying and dusting between the toes with a medicated foot powder. Some of the powder should be sprinkled into shoes. If the condition continues, a fungicidal ointment can be applied in the morning and at night. Persistent cases require the attention of a physician.

Scabies

An insectlike parasite causes the skin irritation called *scabies,* otherwise known as "the itch." The female itch mite burrows a hole in the skin, usually in the groin or between the fingers or toes, and stays hidden long enough to build a tunnel in which to deposit her eggs. The newly hatched mites then work their way to the skin surface and begin the cycle all over again. There is little discomfort in the early period of infestation, but in about a week, a rash appears, accompanied by extreme itching, which is usually most severe at night. Constant scratching during sleep can lead to skin lesions that invite bacterial infection.

Scabies is very contagious and can spread rapidly through a family or through a community, such as a summer camp or army barracks. It can also be communicated by sexual contact.

Treatment by a physician involves the identification of the characteristic tunnels from which sample mites can be removed for examination. Hot baths and thorough scrubbing will expose the burrows, and medical applications as directed by the physician usually clear up the condition in about a week.

Bacterial Infections

The skin is susceptible to infection from a variety of bacteria. Poor diet and careless hygiene can lower the body's resistance to these infectious agents.

Boils

These abscesses of the skin are caused by bacterial infection of a hair follicle or a sebaceous gland. The pus that accumulates in a boil is the result of the encounter between the bacteria and the white blood cells that fight them. Sometimes a boil subsides by itself and disappears. Sometimes the pressure of pus against the skin surface may bring the boil to a head; it will then break, drain, and heal if washed with an antiseptic and covered with a sterile pad. Warm-water compresses can be applied for ten minutes every hour to relieve the pain and to encourage the boil to break and drain. A fresh, dry pad should be applied after each period of soaking.

Anyone with a serious or chronic illness who develops a boil should consult a physician. Since the bacteria can enter the bloodstream and cause a general infection with fever, a physician should also be consulted for a boil on the nose, scalp, upper lip, or in the ear, groin, or armpit.

Carbuncles

This infection is a group of connected boils and is likely to be more painful and less responsive to home treatment. Carbuncles may occur as the result of poor skin care. They tend to occur in the back of the neck where the skin is thick, and the abscess tends to burrow into deeper tissues. A physician usually lances and drains a deep-seated carbuncle, or he may prescribe an antibiotic remedy.

Impetigo

This skin infection is caused by staphylococcal or streptococcal bacteria, and is characterized by blisters that break and form yellow crusted areas. It is spread from one person to another and from one part of the body to another by the discharge from the sores. Impetigo occurs most frequently on the scalp, face, and arms and legs. The infection often is picked up in barber shops, swimming pools, or from body contact with infected people or household pets.

Special care must be taken, especially with children, to control the spread of the infection by keeping the fingers away from infected parts. Bed linens should be changed daily, and disposable paper towels, as well as paper plates and cups, should be used during treatment. A physician should be consulted for proper medication and procedures to deal with the infection.

Barber's Itch

Sycosis, commonly called *barber's itch,* is a bacterial infection of the hair follicles of the beard, accompanied by inflammation, itching, and the formation of pus-filled pimples. People with stiff, curly hair are prone to this type of chronic infection, because their hair is more likely to curve back and reenter the skin. The infection should be treated promptly to prevent scarring and the destruction of the hair root. In some cases, physicians recommend antibiotics. If these are not effective, it may be necessary to drain the abscesses and remove the hairs from the inflamed follicles. During treatment, it is best to avoid shaving, if possible. If one must shave, the sterilization of all shaving equipment and the use of a brushless shaving cream are recommended.

Erysipelas

An acute streptococcal infection of the skin, *erysipelas* can be fatal, particularly to the very young or very old, if not treated promptly. One of its symptoms is the bright redness of the affected areas of the skin. These red patches enlarge and spread, making the skin tender and painful. Blisters may appear nearby. The patient usually has a headache, fever, chills, and nausea. Erysipelas responds well to promptly administered antibiotics, particularly penicillin. The patient is usually advised to drink large amounts of fluid and to eat a nourishing, easily digested diet.

Viral Infections

The most common skin conditions caused by viruses are cold sores, shingles, and warts, discussed below.

Cold Sores

Also called fever blisters, *cold sores* are technically known as *herpes simplex.* They are small blisters that appear most frequently in the corners of the mouth, and sometimes around the eyes and on the genitals. The presumed cause is a virus that lies dormant in the skin until it is activated by infection or by excessive exposure to sun or wind. There is no specific cure for cold sores, but the irritation can be eased by applying drying or cooling agents such as camphor ice or cold-water compresses. Recurrent cold sores, especially in infants, should be called to a physician's attention.

Recent studies have shown that a variety of the herpes simplex virus called HSV-II (for herpes simplex virus-Type II) can be a serious danger to the fetus of a pregnant woman. For a discussion of this condition, see Ch. 25, *Women's Health.* The variety that causes cold sores is called Type I.

Shingles

Shingles are caused by a infection of nerve tissue caused by the *varicella-zoster virus,* the same virus that causes chicken pox. The infection produces small, painful blisters that appear on the skin along the path of the affected nerve—usually on one side of the chest or abdomen. Shingles typically occur in people more than 50 years of age or in people who have compromised immune systems.

Before the blisters appear, some people experience headache, fever, nausea, chills, pain, or itching sensations. Once the blisters are evident, they are painful and itchy, and may take from three to five weeks to dry up and disappear.

Shingles can be treated with aspirin to relieve pain; and with antiviral medications, such as acyclovir, famcyclovir, and valacyclovir, to lessen the severity and to shorten the duration of an attack.

Warts

These growths are caused by a virus infection of the epidermis. They never become cancerous, but can be painful when found on the soles of the feet. In this location, they are known as *plantar warts,* and they cause discomfort because constant pressure makes them grow inward. Plantar warts are most likely to be picked up by children because they are barefooted so much of the time, and by adults when their feet are moist and they are walking around in showers, near swimming pools, and in locker rooms. Warts can be spread by scratching, by shaving, and by brushing the hair. Because warts can spread to painful areas, such as the area around or under the fingernails, and because they may become disfiguring, it is best to consult a physician whenever they appear.

In many ways, warts behave rather mysteriously. Warts may disappear without any treatment at all. Sometimes, when warts on one part of the body are being treated, those in another area will disappear. The folklore about "witching" and "charming" warts away has its foundation in fact, because apparently having faith in the cure, no matter how ridiculous it sounds, sometimes brings success.

There are several more conventional ways of treating warts. Depending on their size and the area involved, electric current, dry ice, or various chemicals may be employed. A physician should be consulted promptly when warts develop in the area of the beard or on the scalp, because they spread quickly in these parts of the body and thus become more difficult to eliminate.

Sebaceous Cysts

When a sebaceous gland duct is blocked, the oil that the gland secretes cannot get to the surface of the skin. Instead, it accumulates into a hard, round, movable mass contained in a sac. This mass is known as a *sebaceous cyst.* Such cysts may appear on the face, back, ears, or in the genital area. A sebaceous cyst that forms on the scalp is called a *wen,* and may become as large as a billiard ball. The skin in this area will become bald, because the cyst interferes with the blood supply to the hair roots.

Some sebaceous cysts just disappear without treatment. However, those that do not are a likely focus for secondary infection by bacteria, and they may become abscessed and inflamed. It is therefore advisable to have cysts examined by a physician for possible removal. If such a cyst is superficial, it can be punctured and drained. One that is deeper is usually removed by simple surgical procedure in the physician's office.

Acne

About 80 percent of all teenagers suffer from the skin disturbance called *acne.* It is also fairly common among women in their twenties. Acne is a condition in which the skin of the face, and often of the neck, shoulders, chest, and back, is covered to a greater or lesser extent with pimples, blackheads, whiteheads, and boils.

The typical onset of acne in adolescence is related to the increased activity of the glands, including the sebaceous glands. Most of the oil that they secrete gets to the surface of the skin through ducts that lead into the pores. When the surface pores are clogged with sebaceous gland secretions and keratin, or when so much extra oil is being secreted that it backs up into the ducts, the result is the formation of the skin blemishes characteristic of acne. Dirt or makeup does not cause acne.

The blackheads are dark not because they are dirty but because the fatty material in the clogged pore is oxidized and discolored by the air that reaches it. When this substance is infected by bacteria, it turns into a pimple. Under no circumstances should such pimples be picked at or squeezed, because the pressure can rupture the surrounding membrane and spread the infection further.

Although a mild case of acne usually clears up by itself, it is often helpful to get the advice of a physician so that it does not get any worse.

Cleanliness

Although surface dirt does not cause acne, it can contribute to its spread. Therefore, the affected areas should be cleansed with a medicated soap and hot water twice a day. Hair should be shampooed frequently and brushed away from the face. Boys who are shaving should soften the beard with soap and hot water. The blade should be sharp and should skim the skin as lightly as possible to avoid nicking pimples.

Creams and Cosmetics

Nonprescription medicated creams and lotions may be effective in reducing some blemishes, but if used too often, they make the skin dry. They should be applied according to the manufacturer's instructions and should be discontinued if they cause additional irritation. If makeup is used, it should have a nonoily base and be completely removed before going to bed.

Forbidden Foods

Although acne is not caused by any particular food, it can be made worse by a diet overloaded with candy, rich pastries, and fats. Chocolate and cola drinks must be eliminated entirely in some cases.

Professional Treatment

A serious case of acne, or even a mild one that is causing serious emotional problems, should receive the attention of a physician. He or she may prescribe antibiotics, usually considered the most effective treatment, or recommend sunlamp treatments. A physician can also be helpful in dealing with the psychological aspects of acne that are so disturbing to teenagers.

Psoriasis

Psoriasis is a noncontagious chronic condition in which the skin on various parts of the body is marked by bright red patches covered with silvery scales. The areas most often affected are the knees, elbows, scalp, and trunk, and less frequently, the areas under the arms and around the genitals.

The specific cause of psoriasis has not yet been discovered, but it is thought to be an inherited abnormality in which the formation of new skin cells is too rapid and disorderly. In its mild form, psoriasis responds well to a variety of long-term treatments. When it is acute, the entire skin surface may be painfully red, and large sections of it may scale off. In such cases, prompt hospitalization and intensive care are recommended.

Conditions That Can Bring On an Outbreak

The onset or aggravation of psoriasis can be triggered by some of the following factors:

- bruises, burns, scratches, and overexposure to the sun
- sudden drops in temperature—a mild, stable climate is most beneficial
- sudden illness from another source, or unusual physical or emotional stress

- infections of the upper respiratory tract, especially bacterial throat infections and the medicines used to cure them

Treatment

Although there is no specific cure for psoriasis, these are some of the recommended treatments:

- controlled exposure to sunlight or an ultraviolet lamp
- creams or lotions of crude coal tar or tar distillates, used alone or in combination with ultraviolet light
- psoralen and ultraviolet light (PUVA), a combined systemic-external therapy in which a psoralen drug is taken orally before exposure to ultraviolet light
- systemic drugs, such as methotrexate, which can be taken orally
- steroid hormone medications applied to the skin surface under dressings

Pigment Disorders and Birthmarks

The mechanism that controls skin coloration is described above under "Skin Color." Abnormalities in the creation and distribution of melanin result in the following disorders, some of which are negligible.

Freckles

These are small spots of brown pigment that frequently occur when fair-skinned people are exposed to the sun or to ultraviolet light. For those whose skin gets red rather than tan during such exposure, freckles are a protective device. In most cases, they recede in cold weather. A heavy freckle formation that is permanent can be covered somewhat by cosmetic preparations. No attempt should be made to remove freckles with commercial creams or solutions unless supervised by a physician.

Liver Spots

Flat, smooth, irregularly placed markings on the skin, called *liver spots,* often appear among older people, and result from an increase in pigmentation. They have nothing to do with the liver and are completely harmless. Brownish markings of similar appearance sometimes show up during pregnancy or as a result of irritation or infection. They usually disappear when the underlying cause is eliminated.

Liver spots are permanent, and the principal cause is not aging but the accumulated years of exposure to sun and wind. They can be disguised and treated in the same way as freckles. A liver spot that becomes hard and thick should be called to a physician's attention.

Moles

Clusters of melanin cells, called *moles,* may appear singly or in groups at any place on the body. They range in color from light tan to dark brown; they may be raised and hairy or flat and smooth. Many moles are present at birth, and most make their appearance before the age of 20. They rarely turn into malignancies, and require medical attention only if they become painful, if they itch, or if they suddenly change in size, shape, or color.

There are several ways of removing moles if they are annoying or particularly unattractive. They can be destroyed by the application of an electric needle, by cauterizing, and by surgery. A mole that has been removed is not likely to reappear. The hairs sometimes found in moles can be clipped close to the surface of the skin, or they can be permanently removed. Hair removal often causes the mole to get smaller.

Vitiligo

Vitiligo is an autoimmune disease in which the body's white cells attack its pigment cells, causing a loss of pigment in the skin. About 1 percent of the U.S. population suffers from this condition, which can appear any time up to middle age and is believed to be inherited. Vitiligo can occur anywhere on the body, from small spots to large patches, but the nose, hands, feet, and genital area are the most common areas affected.

There is no cure for vitiligo, but it can be treated with drugs and exposure to ultraviolet A radiation. The condition itself is not physically painful, but many vitiligo sufferers, particularly dark-skinned persons, experience emotional pain and embarrassment.

Birthmarks

About one-third of all infants are born with the type of birthmark called a*hemangioma,* also known as a vascular birthmark. These are caused by a clustering of small blood vessels near the surface of the skin. The mark, which is flat, irregularly shaped, and either pink, red, or purplish, is usually referred to as "port wine stain." There is no known way to remove it, but with cosmetic covering creams, it can usually be successfully masked.

The type of hemangioma that is raised and bright red—called a strawberry mark—spontaneously disappears with no treatment in most cases during early childhood. If a strawberry mark begins to grow rather than fade, or if it begins to ulcerate, a physician should be promptly consulted.

See Ch. 18, *Cancer,* for a discussion of skin cancer; see Ch. 3, *The Teens,* for a discussion of adolescent skin problems; see Ch. 23, *Aches, Pains, Nuisances, Worries,* for further discussion of minor skin problems.

22

The Teeth and Gums

Although a human baby is born without teeth, a complete set of 20 *deciduous,* or baby, teeth (also called *primary teeth*) already has formed within the gums of the offspring while it still is within the mother's womb. The buds of the permanent or secondary teeth are developing even before the first baby tooth appears at around the age of six months. The baby teeth obviously are formed from foods eaten by the mother. Generally, if the mother follows a good diet during pregnancy, no special food items are required to ensure an adequate set of deciduous teeth in the baby.

It takes about two years for the full set of deciduous teeth to appear in the baby's mouth. The first, usually a central incisor at the front of the lower jaw, may erupt any time between the ages of three and nine months. The last probably will be a second molar at the back of the upper jaw. As with walking, talking, and other characteristics of infants, there is no set timetable for the eruption of baby teeth. One child may get his first tooth at three months while another must wait until nine months, but both would be considered within a normal range of tooth development.

The permanent teeth are never far behind the deciduous set. The first permanent tooth usually appears around the age of six years, about four years after the last of the baby teeth has erupted. As the baby teeth gradually fall out, they are replaced by permanent teeth. The chart below shows the usual ages for the appearance and shedding of baby teeth.

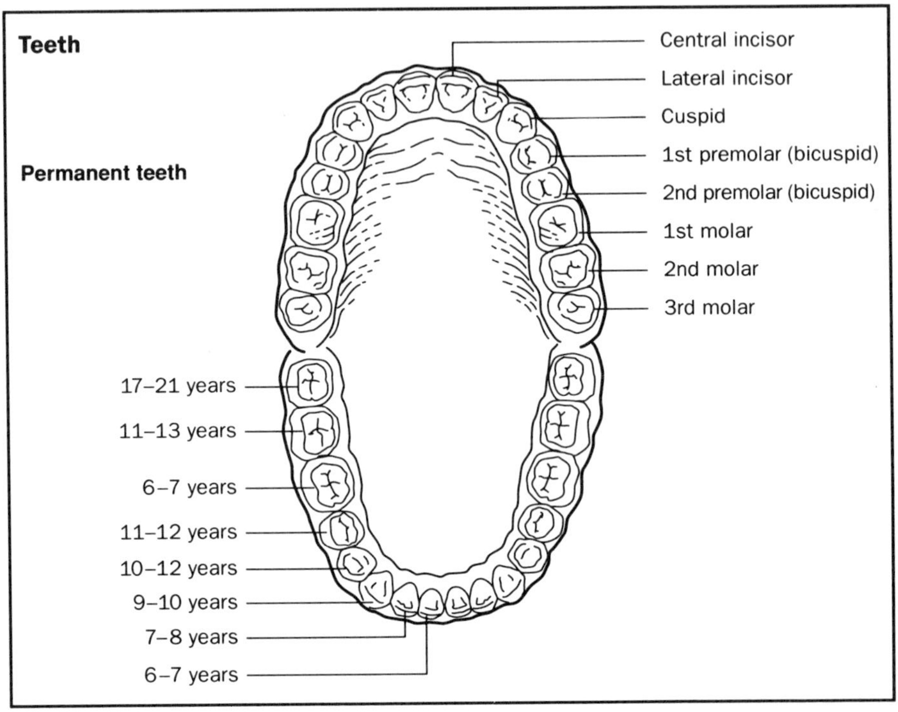

UPPER JAW		
central incisor	8-12 mos	6-7 yrs
lateral incisor	9-13 mos	7-8 yrs
canine (cuspid)	16-22 mos	10-12 yrs
first molar	13-19 mos	9-11 yrs
second molar	25-33 mos	10-12 yrs

LOWER JAW		
central incisor	6-10 mos	6-7 yrs
lateral incisor	10-16 mos	7-8 yrs
canine (cuspid)	17-23 mos	9-12 yrs
first molar	14-18 mos	9-11 yrs
second molar	23-31 mos	10-12 yrs

Types of Teeth

The permanent teeth number 32. In advancing from deciduous to permanent teeth, the human gains six teeth in the lower jaw, or ***mandible,*** and six in the upper jaw, or ***maxilla,*** of the mouth. In general, each kind of tooth appears first in the lower jaw. The usual ages for the appearance of the permanent teeth are as follows:

	LOWER	UPPER
incisors	6-8 yrs	7-9 yrs
cuspids	9-10 yrs	11-12 yrs
bicuspids	10-12 yrs	10-12 yrs
first molars	6-7 yrs	6-7 yrs
second molars	11-13 yrs	12-13 yrs
wisdom teeth	17-21 yrs	17-21 yrs

An *incisor* is designed to cut off particles of food, which is then pushed by muscles of the tongue and cheeks to teeth farther back in the mouth for grinding. The front teeth, one on each side, upper and lower, are central incisors. Next to each central incisor is a lateral incisor.

A *cuspid* is so named because it has a spear-shaped crown, or *cusp*. It is designed for tearing as well as cutting. Cuspids sometimes are called *canine teeth* or *eyeteeth;* canine teeth owe their name to the use of these teeth by carnivorous animals, such as dogs, for tearing pieces of meat. There are four cuspids in the mouth, one on the outer side of each lateral incisor in the upper and lower jaws.

Bicuspids sometimes are identified as *premolars*. The term "bicuspid" suggests two cusps, but a bicuspid may in fact have three cusps. The function of the bicuspids is to crush food passed back from the incisors and cuspids. The permanent set of teeth includes a total of eight bicuspids.

The *molars,* which also number eight and are the last teeth at the back of the mouth, are the largest and strongest teeth, with the job of grinding food. The third molars, or wisdom teeth, are smaller, weaker, and less functional than the first and second molars.

Structure of the Tooth

The variety of shapes of teeth make them specialized for the various functions in preparing food for digestion—biting, chewing, and grinding. All varieties, however, have the same basic structure. Each tooth has a crown (the part of the tooth visible above the gum line) and a root, which is embedded in a socket in the jaw.

Enamel

The outer covering of the crown is *enamel,* the hardest substance in the human body. Enamel is about 97 percent mineral and is as tough as some gemstones. It varies in thickness, with the greatest thickness on the surfaces that are likely to get the most wear and tear.

Enamel begins to form on the first tooth buds of an embryo at the age of about 15 weeks, depending upon substances in the food eaten by the mother for proper development. Once the tooth has formed and erupted through the gum line, there is nothing further that can be done by natural means to improve the condition of the enamel. The enamel has no blood supply, and any changes in the tooth surface will be the result of wearing, decay, or injury.

While the health and diet of the mother can affect the development of tooth enamel in the deciduous teeth, certain health factors in the early life of a child can result in defective enamel formation of teeth that have not yet erupted. Some infectious or metabolic disorders, for example, may result in enamel pitting.

Dentin

Beneath the enamel surface of a tooth is a layer of hard material—though not as hard as enamel—called *dentin,* which forms the bulk of a tooth. The dentin forms at the same time that enamel is laid down on the surface of a developing tooth, and the portion beneath the crown of the tooth probably is completed at the same time as the enamel. However, the dentin, which is composed of calcified material, is not as dense as the enamel; it is formed as myriad tubules that extend downward into the pulp at the center of the tooth. There is some evidence that dentin formation may continue slowly during the life of the tooth.

Cementum

The *cementum* is a bonelike substance that covers the root of the tooth. Though harder than regular bone, it is softer than dentin. It contains attachments for fibers of a periodontal ligament that holds the tooth in its socket. The periodontal ligament serves as a kind of hammock of fibers that surround and support the tooth at the cementum surface, radiating outward to the jawbone. This arrangement allows the tooth to move a little while still attached to the jaw. For example, when the teeth of the upper and lower jaws are brought together in chewing, the periodontal ligament allows the teeth to sink into their sockets. When the teeth of the two jaws are separated, the hammocklike ligament permits the teeth to float outward again.

Pulp

The cavity within the dentin contains the *pulp.* There is a wide pulp chamber under the crown of the tooth and a pulp canal that extends from the

Structure of Tooth

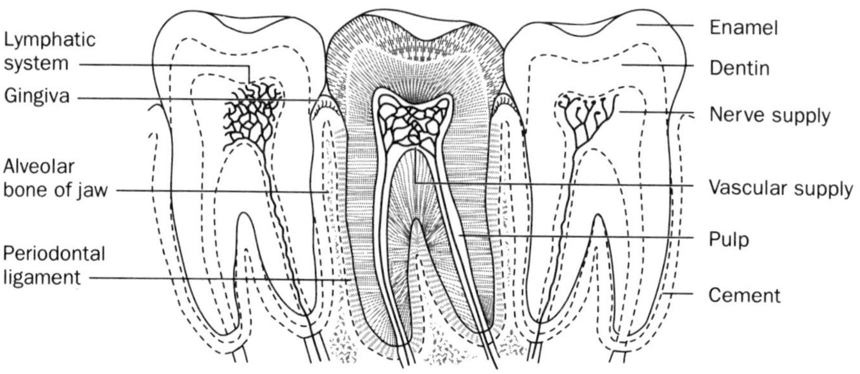

chamber down through the root or roots. Some teeth, such as the molars, may contain as many as three roots, and each of the roots contains a pulp canal.

The pulp of a tooth contains the nerve fibers, lymphatic vessels, blood vessels, and connective tissue. Although the blood supply arrangement is not the same for every tooth, a typical pattern includes a dental artery entering through each passageway, or *foramen,* leading into the root of a tooth. The artery branches into numerous capillaries within the root canal. A similar system of veins drains the blood from the tooth through each foramen. A lymphatic network and nerve system also enter the tooth through a foramen and spread through the pulp, as branches from a central distribution link within the jawbone. The nerve fibers have free endings in the tooth, making them sensitive to pain stimuli.

Supporting Structures

The soft, pink gum tissue that surrounds the tooth is called the *gingiva,* and the bone of the jaw that forms the tooth socket is known as *alveolar bone.* The gingiva, alveolar bone, and periodontal ligaments sometimes are grouped into a structural category identified as the *periodontium.* Thus, when a dentist speaks of periodontal disease, he is referring to a disorder of these supporting tissues of the teeth. The ailment known as *gingivitis* is an inflammation of the gingiva, or gum tissue around the teeth.

Care of the Teeth and Gums

Years ago, loss of teeth really was unavoidable. Today, thanks to modern practices of preventive dentistry, it is possible for nearly everyone to enjoy the benefits of natural teeth for a lifetime. But natural teeth can be preserved only by daily oral-hygiene habits and regular dental checkups.

The Dental Examination

Dental checkups should begin in early childhood and continue throughout adult life. A child should see a dentist at the age of two or two-and-a half, once all the primary teeth have emerged. Children who require special attention in treating dental problems can benefit from seeing a pedodontist, a dentist who specializes in the care of children. After the permanent teeth have become established, the dentist should be visited every six months, or at whatever intervals the dentist recommends for an individual patient who may need more or less care than the typical patient.

The dentist, like the family physician, usually maintains a general health history of each patient, in addition to a dental health history. He examines each tooth, the gums and other oral tissues, and the *occlusion,* or bite. A complete set of X-ray pictures may be taken on the first visit and again at intervals of perhaps five to seven years. During routine visits, the dentist may take only a couple of X-ray pictures of teeth on either side of the mouth; a complete set of X rays may result in a file of 18 or 20 pictures covering every tooth in the mouth.

X rays constitute a vital part of the dental examination. Without them the dentist cannot examine the surfaces between the teeth or the portion of the tooth beneath the gum, a part that represents about 60 percent of the total length of the tooth. The X rays will reveal the condition of the enamel, dentin, and pulp; any impacted wisdom teeth; and the alveolar bone, or tooth sockets. Caps, fillings, abscessed roots, and bone loss resulting from gum disease also are clearly visible on a set of X rays.

Other diagnostic tests may be made, such as a test of nerve response. Sometimes the dentist will make an impression of the teeth, an accurate and detailed reverse reproduction, in plaster of paris, plastic impression compound, or other material. Models made from these impressions are used to study the way the teeth meet. Such knowledge is often crucial in deciding the selection of treatment and materials.

After the examination, the dentist will present and explain any proposed treatment. After oral restoration is completed, the dentist will ask the patient to return at regular intervals for a checkup and *prophylaxis,* which includes cleaning and polishing the teeth. Regular checkups and prophylaxis help prevent periodontal diseases affecting the gum tissue and underlying bone. Professional cleaning removes hard deposits that trap bacteria, especially at the gum line, and polishing removes stains and soft deposits.

Dental Care in Middle Age

Although periodontal disease and cavities—called *dental caries* by dentists—continue to threaten oral health, two other problems may assume prominence for people of middle age: replacing worn-out restorations, or fillings, and replacing missing teeth. No filling material will last forever. The whitish restorations in front teeth eventually wear away. Silver restorations tend to crack and chip with age because they contract and expand slightly when cold or hot food and drinks come in contact with them. Even gold restorations, the most permanent kind, are subject to decay around the edges, and the decay may spread underneath.

If a needed restoration is not made or a worn-out restoration is not replaced, a deep cavity may result. When the decay reaches the inner layer of the tooth—the dentin—temporary warning twinges of pain may occur. If the tooth still is not restored, the decay will spread into the pulp that fills the inner chamber of the tooth. A toothache can result from inflammation of the pulp, and although the pain may eventually subside, the pulp tissue dies and an abscess can form at the root of the tooth.

Dental Care During Pregnancy

It may be advisable for a pregnant woman to arrange for extra dental checkups. Many changes take place during pregnancy, among them increased hormone production. Some pregnant women develop gingivitis (inflammation of the gums) as an indirect consequence of hormonal changes. A checkup by the dentist during the first three months of pregnancy is needed to assess the oral effects of such changes, and to make sure all dental problems are examined and corrected. Pregnant women should take special care to brush and floss their teeth to minimize these problems.

Infection

To avoid the problem of toxic substances or poisons circulating in the mother's bloodstream, all sources of infection must be removed. Some of these sources can be in the mouth. An abscessed tooth, for example, may not be severe enough to signal its presence with pain, but because it is directly connected to the bloodstream it can send toxic substances and bacteria through the mother's body, with possible harmful effects to the embryo.

It is during pregnancy that tooth buds for both the deciduous and permanent teeth begin to form in the unborn child. If the mother neglects her diet or general health care during this period, the effects may be seen in the teeth of her child.

Maintaining Good Oral Hygiene

Fluoridation

Among general rules to follow between dental checkups are using fluorides, maintaining a proper diet, and removing debris from the teeth by brushing and by the use of dental floss. Fluorides are particularly important for strengthening the enamel of teeth in persons under the age of 15. Many communities add fluorides to the water supply, but if the substance is not available in the drinking water, the dentist can advise the patient about prescription fluoride rinses and treatments. Studies show that fluoride keeps teeth and gums healthy for older adults as well as for children and teenagers.

Dental sealants are also used in the prevention of tooth decay. The dentist brushes a plastic protective coating on the chewing surfaces of the back teeth, creating a barrier against food particles and bacteria. Since sealants can prevent up to 80 percent of all cavities, the American Dental Association recommends this treatment for all children.

Diet

Although a good diet for total health should provide all of the elements needed for dental health, several precautions on sugars and starches should be added. Hard or sticky sweets should be avoided. Such highly refined sweets as soft drinks, candies, cakes, cookies, pies, syrups, jams, jellies, and pastries should be limited, especially between meals. One's intake of starchy foods, such as bread, potatoes, and pastas, should also be controlled. Natural sugars contained in fresh fruits can provide sweet flavors with less risk of contributing to decay if the teeth are brushed regularly after eating such foods. Regular chewing gum may help remove food particles after eating, but it deposits sugar; if you chew gum, use sugarless gum.

Because decay is promoted each time sugars and other refined carbohydrates are eaten, between-meals snacks of sweets should be curtailed to lessen the chances of new or additional caries. Snack foods can be raw vegetables, such as carrots or celery, apples, cheese, peanuts, or other items that are not likely to introduce refined carbohydrates into the mouth between meals.

Brushing

Brushing the teeth is an essential of personal oral hygiene. Such brushing rids the mouth of most of the food debris that encourages bacterial growth. Brush with a fluoride toothpaste at least twice a day, more often if your dentist recommends it. A complete cleaning of brushing and flossing should take three to five minutes.

There is no one kind of toothbrush that is best for every person. Most dentists, however, recommend a brush with soft end-rounded or polished bristles. The size and shape of the brush should allow you to reach every tooth. Replace your toothbrush every three or four months, sooner if the bristles become worn, frayed or splayed. A hard, brittle brush can injure the gums. An interdental brush, a small brush tip at the end of a handle, is useful for cleaning between widely spaced teeth, between a tooth and an artificial crown or a bridge, or any tooth surface that is hard to reach.

Although several different methods may be used effectively, the following is the technique most often recommended. Brush the outside, inside, and chewing surfaces of the teeth with short, gentle strokes. Hold the brush with the bristle tips angled against the gum line at 45 degrees. Use a slight side-to-side motion. Brush the outside surface of each tooth before proceeding to the next tooth. Use the same technique on the inside surface of each tooth as well. For the hard-to-brush inside surfaces of the front teeth hold the handle of the brush in front of the mouth and apply the tip in an up-and-down motion. Next, carefully brush the chewing surfaces, or tops, of the back upper and lower teeth. Then brush the tongue to remove food particles and bacteria.

Some people prefer electric toothbrushes, which require less effort to use than ordinary toothbrushes. These are available with two basic motions—up and down and back and forth. Your dentist may advise which kind best serves an individual's needs and proper use of equipment. Some dentists point out that back-and-forth brushing applied with too much pressure can have an abrasive effect on tooth enamel because it works against the grain of the mineral deposits. The American Dental Association also evaluates electric toothbrushes and issues reports on the safety and effectiveness of various types.

Flossing

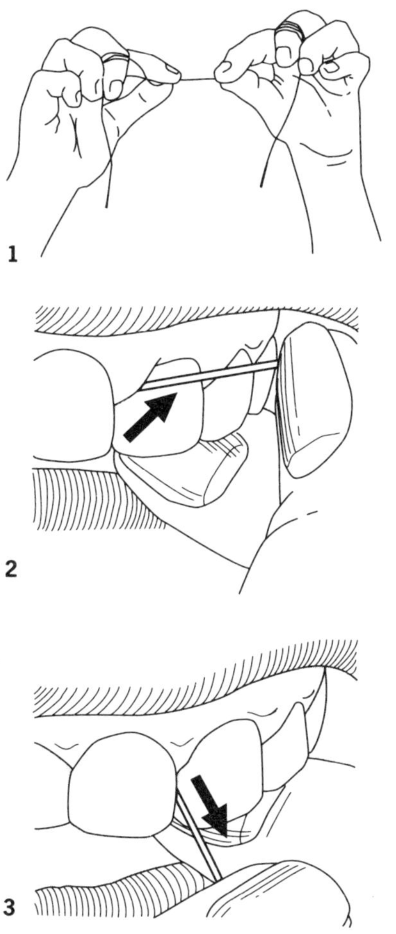

1. Wrap floss several times around middle fingers and pull center section taut between thumbs or index fingers.
2. Insert floss between teeth and gently slide back and forth against every tooth. Work floss into the space between tooth and gumline.
3. To remove, pull floss gently downward along the angle of the tooth. Snapping it in and out may cause gum irritation.

Removing Debris with Dental Floss

Brushing often does not clean debris from between the teeth. But plaque and food particles that stick between the teeth usually can be removed with dental floss. A generous length of floss, about 18 inches, is needed to do an effective job. The ends can be wrapped several times around the first joint of the middle finger of each hand. Using the thumbs or index fingers, the floss is inserted between the teeth with a gentle, sawing, back-and-forth motion. Then it is slid gently around part of a tooth in the space at the gum line and gently pulled out; snapping the floss in and out may irritate the gums. After brushing and flossing, the mouth should be rinsed with water. A mouthwash is unnecessary, but it may be used for the good taste it leaves in the mouth.

The dentist may recommend the use of an oral irrigating device as part of dental home care. These units produce a pulsating stream of water that flushes food debris from between teeth. They are particularly useful for patients wearing orthodontic braces or for those who have had recession of the gums, creating larger spaces between the teeth.

People who want to see the areas of plaque on their teeth can chew a *disclosing tablet,* available at most pharmacies, which leaves a harmless temporary stain on plaque surfaces. Some dentists recommend the use of disclosing tablets about once a week so that patients can check on the effectiveness of their tooth-cleaning techniques.

Dental Care in Emergencies

If a tooth is knocked out, you should immediately rinse the tooth gently in water to remove dirt or debris. Then place the tooth back in its socket. If reinsertion isn't possible, place the tooth in a cup of milk or water since it is important not to let the tooth dry out. Then see a dentist or go to a hospital emergency room immediately. Studies show that if a tooth is placed back into its socket within 30 minutes of being knocked out, there is a 50 percent chance of saving the tooth.

If a tooth is pushed out of place (inward or outward) but not knocked out of its socket, gently clean any dirt or debris from the injured area with warm water. Push (but do not force) the tooth back into place and hold it in the socket with a moist tissue or gauze. Go to a dentist or emergency room immediately.

When you have a toothache, rinse your mouth thoroughly with warm water to clean out food particles. Use dental floss to remove any food that might be wedged between the teeth. Take an aspirin or other pain reliever to help dull the ache. An over-the-counter medication containing benzocaine can be applied to the tooth. See your dentist as soon as possible.

Tooth Decay

In addition to wear, tear, and injury, the major threat to the health of a tooth is tooth decay, or *caries*. Tooth decay and gum diseases are the leading causes of tooth loss. Tooth decay is caused by the bacteria that are normally present in the mouth and in the foods we eat. The bacteria digest the sugars and starches in the particles of food that remain in the mouth and begin to produce harmful acids within 20 minutes after eating. Although saliva and the actions of the tongue generally wash away some of the harmful material, decay will occur in places where bacteria and food particles accumulate and remain undisturbed.

The bacteria and acids build up in the mouth and become part of *plaque*, a sticky, transparent substance that forms a film over the surface of the teeth. Plaque forms on a continuous basis, which is the reason teeth must be flossed and brushed daily. Plaque can grow between the teeth and gums and irritate the soft tissues that support the teeth. The acids in plaque can eat through tooth enamel, creating a cavity. Plaque that is not removed combines with minerals in the saliva and hardens into a rough-textured substance called *tartar*, or *dental calculus*. Tartar can only be removed with a professional cleaning.

Other Causes of Decay

Bacterial acid is not the only way in which the tooth enamel may be damaged to permit the entry of decay bacteria. Certain high-acid foods and improper dental care can erode the molecules of enamel. Temperature extremes also can produce cracks and other damage to the enamel; some dental scientists have suggested that repeated exposure to rapid temperature fluctuations of 50° F, as in eating alternately hot and cold foods or beverages, can cause the enamel to develop cracks.

Complications of Tooth Decay

Tooth decay occurs gradually. It begins on the tooth's outer enamel surface where plaque has formed. The initial stage of tooth decay is usually painless and often goes unnoticed. Once decay activity breaks through the hard enamel surface, the bacteria can attack the dentin. Because the dentin is about 30 percent organic material, compared to 5 percent in the enamel layer, the decay process can advance more rapidly there. If the tooth decay is not stopped at the dentin layer, the disease organisms can enter the pulp chamber, which contains sensitive nerve endings. The decay can produce an acute inflammation, or abscess, which, if unchecked, can spread to adjoining teeth or other parts of the body. Osteomyelitis, an infection of the bone and bone marrow, and endocarditis, an inflammation of the lining of the heart, are among diseases in other parts of the body that can begin with untreated tooth decay.

Periodontal disease, described below, is another possible complication of tooth decay.

Treatment of Tooth Decay

The portion of a tooth invaded by decay is called a *cavity;* it may be compared to an ulcer that develops because of disease in soft tissues. In treating the decay process, the dentist tries to prevent further destruction of the tooth tissue. The dentist also tries to restore as much as possible the original shape and function of the diseased tooth. The procedure used depends on many factors, including the surfaces affected (enamel, dentin, etc.) and the tooth face and angle involved, as well as whether the cavity is on a smooth area or in a pit or fissure of the tooth surface.

The decayed portions of the tooth are removed with various kinds of carbide burrs and other drill tips, as well as with hand instruments. The dentist may also use a caries removal system that reduces or eliminates drilling. In this system two solutions are combined in one liquid and squirted in a pulsating stream onto the decayed area. The stream does not harm gums or healthy teeth; rather, it softens the caries so that it can easily be scraped away. Used, generally, in conjunction with rotary or hand instruments, the "squirt" system may make anesthesia unnecessary.

In other cases an anesthetic may be injected for the comfort of the patient. The dentist usually asks whether the patient prefers to have an anesthetic before work commences. In the cleaning process, an effort is made to remove all traces of diseased enamel or dentin, but no more of the tooth material than is necessary.

The cleaned cavity is generally filled in a layering procedure. The layers of liners and bases used before insertion of the filling are determined by the depth of the cavity and other factors. If pulp is exposed, special materials may be applied to help the pulp recover from the irritation of the procedure and to form a firm base for the amalgam, inlay, plastic resin, or other restorative substance that becomes the filling.

Tooth Extraction

When it becomes necessary to remove a diseased, damaged, or malpositioned tooth, the procedure is handled as a form of minor surgery, usually with administration of a local anesthetic to the nerves supplying the tooth area. However, there is no standard routine for extraction of a tooth, because of the numerous individual variations associated with each case. The dentist usually has a medical history of the patient available, showing such information as allergies to drugs, and medications used by the patient that might react with those employed in oral surgery. Because the mouth contains many millions of bacteria, all possible precautions are taken to prevent entry of the germs into the tooth socket.

The condition of the patient is checked during and immediately after tooth extraction, in the event that some complication develops. The patient is provided with analgesic (pain killing) and other needed medications, along with instructions regarding control of any postoperative pain or bleeding. The dentist also may offer special diet information with suggested meals for the recovery period, which usually is quite brief.

Root Canal Therapy

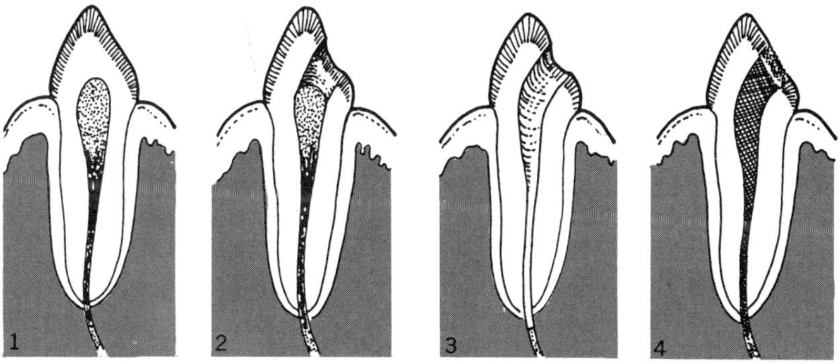

(1) The first step of root canal, or removal of the nerve of a tooth, begins with examining the infected pulp to determine its vitality. (2) The depth of the root is measured by X ray and, after administering local anesthetic, the dentist extracts the pulp with drill or hand instrument marked to indicate when the end of the root has been reached. (3) When the entire pulp and nerve have been removed the canal is sterilized to prevent infection. (4) After filling the tooth with silver or a tough plastic substance known as *gutta-percha,* or sometimes a combination of both, the dentist then caps the tooth.

Dry Socket

Severe pain may develop several days after a tooth has been extracted if a blood clot that forms in the socket becomes dislodged. The condition, commonly called *dry socket,* can involve infection of the alveolar bone that normally surrounds the roots of the tooth; loss of the clot can expose the bone tissue to the environment and organisms that produce *osteitis,* or inflammation of the bone tissue. Dry socket may be treated by irrigating the socket with warm salt water and packing it with strips of medicated gauze. The patient also is given analgesics, sedatives, and other medications as needed to control the pain and infection.

General anesthetics are sometimes necessary for complicated oral surgery. In such cases, there are available dental offices or clinics that are as well equipped and staffed as hospital operating rooms.

Endodontic Therapy

Tooth extraction because of caries is less common today than in previous years, although an estimated 25 million Americans have had all of their teeth removed. Modern preventive dentistry techniques of *endodontics* now make it possible to save many teeth that would have been extracted in past decades after the spread of decay into the pulp canal. The procedures include *root canal therapy, pulp capping,* and *pulpotomy.*

Root Canal Therapy

Once the tooth has fully developed in the jaw, the nerve is not needed, so if the pulp is infected, the nerve as well as the pulp can be removed. Only minor effects are noticeable in the tooth structure after the pulp is removed, and the dentist compensates for these in filling the tooth after root canal therapy.

Briefly, the procedure of root canal work begins by examination and testing of the pulp viability. The pulp may be tested by heat, cold, or an electrical device called a *vitalometer,* which measures the degree of sensation the patient feels in a tooth. If the pulp is dead, the patient will feel no sensation, even at the highest output of current.

After the degree of vitality in the pulp has been determined, a local anesthetic is injected and the dentist begins removing the pulp, using rotary drills and hand instruments. By means of X-ray pictures, the dentist measures the length of the root, which may be about one and a half times the length of the crown. Stops or other markers are placed on the root excavation tools to show the dentist when the instrument has reached the end of the root. The canal is then sterilized and filled with gutta-percha—a tough plastic substance—silver, or a combination of the two, and a cap is added.

Pulp Capping

Pulp capping consists of building a protective cover, or cap, over the exposed pulp with layers of calcium hydroxide paste, which is covered by zinc oxide and topped with a firm cement.

Pulpotomy

A pulpotomy procedure involves removal of the pulp in the pulp chamber within the crown of the tooth, while leaving the root canal pulp in place. The amputated pulp ends are treated and a pulp-capping procedure is used to restore the crown of the tooth.

Periodontal Disease

It is important in the middle years of life and later to continue good oral-hygiene habits and the practice of having regular dental checkups. Studies have found that after the age of 50 more than half the people in America have periodontal disease. At the age of 65, nearly everybody has this disease.

The Course of the Disease

Periodontal disease is an infection of the tissues surrounding and supporting the teeth. This includes the gums (gingiva), connective tissue (period-

Periodontal Disease

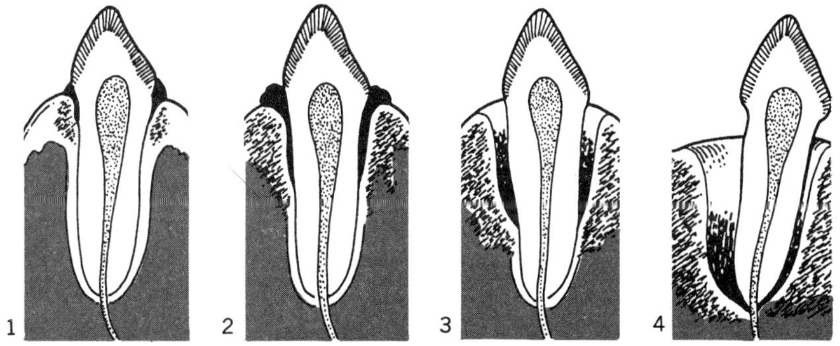

(1) If allowed to build up at the gumline, deposits of plaque and calculus result in damage to the gum tissues (periodontal disease). (2) As gums become increasingly irritated and inflamed, they may bleed easily and begin to recede from the tooth itself. (3) Untreated, the inflammation spreads to the roots of the teeth. Bacteria and particles of food lodge in the pockets between tooth and gums, aggravating the condition. (4) A tooth held by the diseased gum loses most of its bony support structure, causing it to loosen and move out of position. Eventually, such teeth may need to be extracted.

ontal ligament), and tooth sockets (alveolar bone). It is caused by plaque, a sticky, colorless film of bacteria that constantly forms on the teeth. If plaque isn't removed each day by brushing and flossing, it hardens and turns into tartar, or calculus. The toxins (poisons) produced by the bacteria in plaque and tartar irritate the gums.

Gingivitis, an inflammation of the gums, is the mildest form of periodontal disease. At first there is a slight redness and swelling of the gum tissue around one or more teeth. Later the redness and swelling become more pronounced and the gums tend to bleed easily. Bleeding that occurs during flossing or toothbrushing is one of the earliest signs of periodontal disease. Gingivitis is reversible with professional treatment and with good home oral care.

Periodontitis, also called *pyorrhea*, is an advanced stage of gum disease. Symptoms include persistent bad breath; receding and shrinking gums; loose or separating teeth; a hypersensitivity to hot, cold, or sweet foods or beverages; and a change in the way your teeth fit together when you bite.

Periodontitis occurs when plaque and tartar extend below the gum line. The gums separate from the teeth, forming pockets that fill up with more plaque and bacteria. As the disease progresses, the bacteria weakens the bone supporting the teeth and the affected teeth begin to loosen and drift from their normal position. Finally, if the disease is left untreated, the teeth may be lost.

Another form of periodontal disease is an acute infection called *trench mouth*. It is also known as *necrotizing gingivitis* or *Vincent's infection*. The condition is very painful and is characterized by profuse bleeding at the slightest pressure or irritation. The affected areas become inflamed and develop blisters. A grayish-yellow membrane covers the infected areas and unpleasant breath odor is usually present. Other parts of the mouth, such as the insides of the cheeks and the tonsils, sometimes become infected. The disease was given the name trench mouth during World War I, when soldiers living in trenches contracted the disease. The infection is associated with poor oral hygiene and poor nutrition.

Causes

The accumulation of bacterial plaque and tartar between the gums and teeth is the chief cause of most periodontal diseases. If plaque is not removed daily by brushing and flossing, bacteria produce infections that destroy the supporting tissues around the teeth, including the bone.

Other factors can contribute to the development of gum disease. The hormonal changes that occur during puberty and pregnancy can make the gums more susceptible to bacterial infection. Poor nutrition and a diet rich in sugar-containing foods and beverages can increase the risk of gum disease. People who use tobacco products are more likely to get periodontal diseases and suffer from the more severe forms. Diseases such as leukemia or AIDS lower resistance to infection and can make gum disease more severe or harder to control.

Bruxism

Bruxism—the nervous habit, often unconsciously done, of clenching and grinding the teeth—can contribute to the development of periodontal disease. Bruxism frequently occurs during sleep.

Malocclusion

Another contributing cause to periodontal disease is repeated shock or undue pressure on a tooth because of *malocclusion,* or an improper bite. This effect accelerates damage to the tooth and gum structure during such simple activities as biting and chewing.

Treatment

Periodontal treatment may include a variety of techniques ranging from plaque removal to oral surgery. Early periodontal disease, when the beginnings of gum recession are seen, is treated by nonsurgical deep cleaning around the teeth below the gums. This procedure, called *scaling and root planing,* removes tartar and bacteria from tooth surfaces. As a result, the surfaces of the teeth become smoother both above and below the gum line, making it difficult for bacteria to attach themselves to the tooth.

In advanced periodontal disease dentists need to perform a surgical procedure, such as flap surgery or a gum tissue graft. Flap surgery involves pulling back gum tissue and cleaning both the infected side of the root and the bottom of the periodontal pocket. Then the flap is sutured back in place. Gum tissue grafts involve surgically removing a small piece of healthy gum tissue from the mouth, transferring it to receded gum tissue, and suturing it in place.

Guided tissue regeneration is another surgical treatment. It is a technique for regenerating periodontal ligament and bone. A mesh-like barrier is placed around the tooth root. The barrier keeps the gum tissue away from underlying ligaments and bone and leaves space for the ligaments and bones to grow.

After periodontal treatment, the patient should visit the dentist for a professional teeth cleaning every three or four months to maintain good oral health.

Dental Implants & Dentures

If it becomes necessary to have some teeth removed, they should be replaced as soon as possible with dental implants, a bridge, or partial or full dentures.

Why Missing Teeth Must Be Replaced

Most patients show some concern over the replacement of natural teeth with dentures, associating the loss of teeth with old age in the same way that others resist wearing eyeglasses or using a hearing aid. Millions of persons of all ages have improved their eating, speaking, and physical appearance by obtaining attractive and well-fitted dental implants or dentures. Also, each tooth functions to hold the teeth opposite and on either side in place. Missing teeth would mean shifting teeth and a host of other problems. For example, food particles could lodge in the spaces created by the shifting teeth, followed by the formation of plaque and the development of periodontal disease, resulting in the loss of additional teeth.

Dental Implants

Dental implants, or *osseointegration,* are an effective alternative to ordinary dentures because they serve as substitutes for natural tooth roots that rely on the jawbone for support. Implants are capable of supporting dentures or replacing individual teeth or bridges.

Although physicians have been experimenting with dental implants for centuries, researchers only recently developed the most advanced version of the implant using titanium, whose primary advantage is that bone tissue actually fuses to it.

An implant consists of a small post

Partial Denture

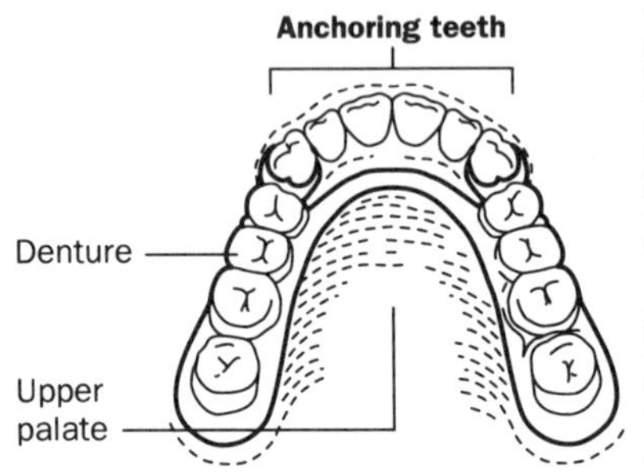

that protrudes from the gum tissue and is anchored either in the jaw bone (endosseous) or fitted directly over the jaw bone (subperiosteal). Prosthetic teeth are attached to the posts. These prosthetic teeth can be permanent or removable; cleaning and care depends upon the type.

Because it is a surgical procedure that can take up to three visits over a period of three to six months, most implant surgery occurs in two stages. First, the general dentist or oral surgeon implants the metal "roots" and then, in a second surgery, attaches the metal posts with the prosthetic teeth.

Not everyone is a candidate for implants. You must have healthy gums and an adequate amount of jawbone to secure the implant. You must be in general good health and not have a disease or condition, such as diabetes, that would interfere with the healing process after surgery. Meticulous oral hygiene is essential once you have an implant. Failing to brush, floss, and care properly for implants can lead to gum inflammation and bone loss. Consult with your dentist to determine if this procedure is compatible with your dental problems.

Fitting of Dentures

Modern techniques and materials of construction and the skill of modern dentists should assure well-fitting, natural-looking dentures. The dentist selects the tooth shade and shape that are best for an individual's face size, contours, and coloring. No one, however, has perfectly arranged, perfectly white natural teeth. Tooth coloring depends upon genetic factors and changes as one grows older.

Bridges and Partial Dentures

Several different types of dental appliances may be constructed to fill empty spaces. Some, such as dental bridges, may be cemented to the remaining natural teeth. Others, such as complete sets of dentures, are removable.

A bridge may be made entirely of gold, a combination of gold and porcelain, or combinations of gold and porcelain and other materials. If there is a sound natural tooth on either side of the space, an artificial tooth (or *pontic*) may be fused to the metal bridge. The crown retainer on either side of the pontic may then be cemented to crowns of the neighboring natural teeth.

If there are no natural teeth near the space created by an extracted tooth, a partial denture may be constructed to replace the missing teeth.

This appliance usually fastens by a clasp onto the last tooth on each side of the space. A bar on the inside of the front teeth provides stability for the partial denture. A "Maryland bridge," a fixed partial denture, eliminates the need for crowns to anchor false teeth.

A removable partial denture should be taken out and cleaned with special brushes whenever the natural teeth are brushed. Your dentist should check bridges and partial dentures periodically to make sure they have not become loosened. A loose clasp of a partial denture can rock the teeth to which the device is attached, causing damage and possible loss.

New materials have brought bonding into more common use as an alternative to crowning and for cosmetically restoring chipped, malformed, stained, or widely spaced teeth. In the bonding process the dentist applies first liquid plastic and then thin layers of tooth-colored materials known as composite resins and laminate veneers. The layers are sculpted and polished.

Complete Dentures

Before a full set of removable dentures is constructed, the dentist determines whether there are any abnormalities in the gum ridges, such as cysts or tooth root tips that may have to be removed. If the gums are in poor condition, treatments may be needed to improve the surfaces of the ridges on which the dentures will be fitted. The dentist may also have to reconstruct the bone underlying the gums—the alveolar ridge. Human bone "harvested" from another part of the patient's body was used in such reconstruction for decades but has been replaced by ceramic materials such as arehydroxylapatite and beta tricalcium phosphate.

The dentist now makes an impression of the patient's mouth. Tooth and shade choices are discussed. Several other appointments may be arranged before the new dentures are delivered to the patient, either for "try-ins" of dentures as they are being constructed or for adjustments after completion of the set.

Although dentures do not change with age, the mouth does. Therefore, it is necessary for the denture-wearer to have occasional check-ups during which the dentist examines oral tissues for irritation and determines how the dentures fit with respect to possible changing conditions of the mouth, and if a replacement should be recommended. The dentist also seeks to correct any irritations of the oral tissues of the mouth and polishes the dentures, making them smooth and easier to clean between check-ups.

Care of Dentures

Dentures should be cleaned daily with a denture brush and toothpaste; each night at bedtime dentures should be removed and soaked for seven or eight hours in a denture cleaner or in water. To avoid breaking them during the brushing process, fill a wash basin with water and place it under the dentures while they are being cleaned; if they are dropped, the dentures will be cushioned by the water. A harsh abrasive that could scratch the denture surface should not be used. Scratches allow stains to penetrate the surface of the dentures, creating permanent discoloration.

The use of adhesives and powders is only a temporary solution to ill-fitting dentures. In time, the dentist may rebuild the gum side of the denture to conform with the shape of the patient's gum ridge. The patient should never try to make his own changes in the fit of dentures. Rebuilding the gum side of the dentures, or relining, as it is called, usually begins with a soft temporary material if the patient's gums are in poor condition, and requires several appointments over a period of two or three weeks while the gum tissues are being restored to good health.

Orthodontics

Orthodontics is a term derived from the Greek words for straight, or normal, teeth. Straight teeth are easier to keep clean and they make chewing food more efficient. There also is a cosmetic benefit in being able to display a smile with a set of straight teeth, although many dentists consider the cosmetic aspect of orthodontics as secondary to achieving proper occlusion, or bite.

Causes of Improper Bite

Orthodontic problems can be caused by hereditary factors, by an infectious or other kind of disease, by the premature loss of primary teeth, by the medications used in treatment, or by individual factors such as injury or loss of permanent teeth. A person may have congenitally missing teeth resulting in spaces that permit drifting of neighboring teeth or collapse of the dental arch. Or he may develop extra (supernumerary) teeth resulting from an inherited factor. The supernumerary teeth may develop during the early years of life while the deciduous teeth are in use. A supernumerary tooth may force permanent teeth into unnatural positions.

Nutritional disorders can also affect the development of jaws and teeth, while certain medications can cause abnormal growth of gingival, or gum, tissues, resulting in increased spaces between the teeth.

Teeth that erupt too early or too late, primary teeth that are too late in falling out when permanent teeth have developed, and habits such as grinding of the teeth, thumb-sucking, or pushing the tongue against the teeth are among other factors that can result in *malocclusion,* or improper bite, and the need for orthodontic treatment.

Diagnosis of Orthodontic Problems

Each child should visit a dentist before the eruption of the permanent teeth for an examination that may determine the need for orthodontic treatment. Because there are many genetic and other influences that help shape the facial contours and occlusion of each individual, there are no standard orthodontic procedures that apply to all children. The dentist may recommend what treatment, if any, would be needed to produce normal occlusion and when it should begin; some dentists advise only that necessary procedures for correcting malocclusion be started before the permanent set of teeth (excluding wisdom teeth) has become established, or around the age of 12 or 13. However, there are few age limits for orthodontic care, and increasing numbers of adults are receiving treatment today for malocclusion problems that were neglected during childhood.

In the normal or ideal occlusion positions of the teeth, the first and second permanent upper molars fit just slightly behind the same molars of the lower jaw; all of the teeth of the upper jaw are in contact with their counterparts of the lower jaw. In this pattern of occlusion, all of the biting surfaces are aligned for optimum use of their intended functions of cutting, tearing, or grinding.

There are numerous variations of malocclusion, but generally, in simple deformities, the teeth of the upper jaw are in contact with lower jaw teeth once removed from normal positions. Other variations include an *open bite,* in which the upper and lower incisors do not contact each other, or *closed bite,* in which there is an abnormal degree of overlapping (*overbite*) of the front teeth.

Diagnosis is made with the help of X-ray pictures, photographs of the face and mouth, medical histories, and plaster models of the patient's teeth and jaws. The plaster models are particularly important because the dentist can use them to make experimental reconstructions without touching an actual tooth of a patient. For example, the dentist can remove one or more teeth from the plaster model and reorganize neighboring teeth in the jawbones to get an accurate representation of the effects of extracting teeth or forcing teeth into different developmental situations.

Orthodontic Appliances

Once a plan of orthodontic treatment has been determined by the dentist, he may choose from a dozen or more types of bands, braces, or other orthodontic appliances, some removable and some nonremovable, for shaping the teeth and jaws of the patient. A typical orthodontic appliance may include small curved strips or loops of metal, ceramic, or plastic cemented to the surfaces of the teeth as anchors for arch wires that pass around the dental arch. Springs and specially designed rubber bands, called elastics, are sometimes used to bring about alignment of the two jaws, or to align teeth within a dental arch.

In addition to the appliances that are attached to and between the upper and lower dental arches, the dentist may prescribe the use of an elastic tape device with a strap that fits around the back of the patient's neck and is attached also to the arch wire inside the mouth, thus providing a force from outside the mouth to bring teeth into alignment.

Orthodontic appliances are custom-designed and built for the individual patient. This requires several rather long sessions or one all-day session in the dental chair while the appliance is being organized and properly anchored. Thereafter, the patient must return at regular intervals spaced a few weeks to a month apart so the dentist can make adjustments in the appliance, determine if any of the bands have pulled away from tooth surfaces, and prevent plaque from building up in places that the braces may make impervious to brushing.

The patient, meanwhile, must follow a diet that prohibits sticky foods or items that may damage the appliance or any of its parts. A conscientious program of oral hygiene, including regular cleaning by the dentist or hygienist, also is necessary because, as indicated above, it is more difficult to do a thorough job of cleaning the teeth when orthodontic appliances are in the mouth.

Orthodontic Appliance

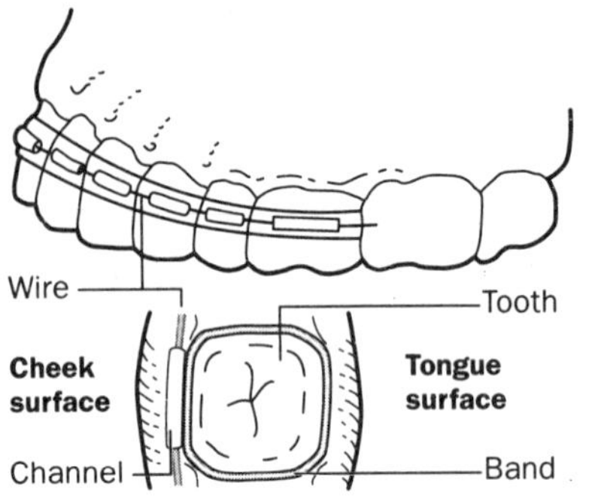

Orthodontics for Adults

Although orthodontic treatment originally was applied only to children, adults are undergoing treatment with increasing frequency to correct a variety of facial and dental disorders. Receding chins, buck teeth, sunken cheeks, sunken mouths, and other abnormalities have been treated successfully in adults beyond the age of 40. Orthodontists have observed that adult patients usually are more patient and cooperative during the long periods of treatment than youngsters.

The upper age limit for orthodontic work has not really been established, but doctors at the National Institute of Dental Research believe it is possible to treat adult patients with protrusion of the upper jaw and related disfigurements until the age of 70. This is possible because the upper jaw does not completely unite with the frontal bone of the skull, according to the experts, until after the

Improper Bite

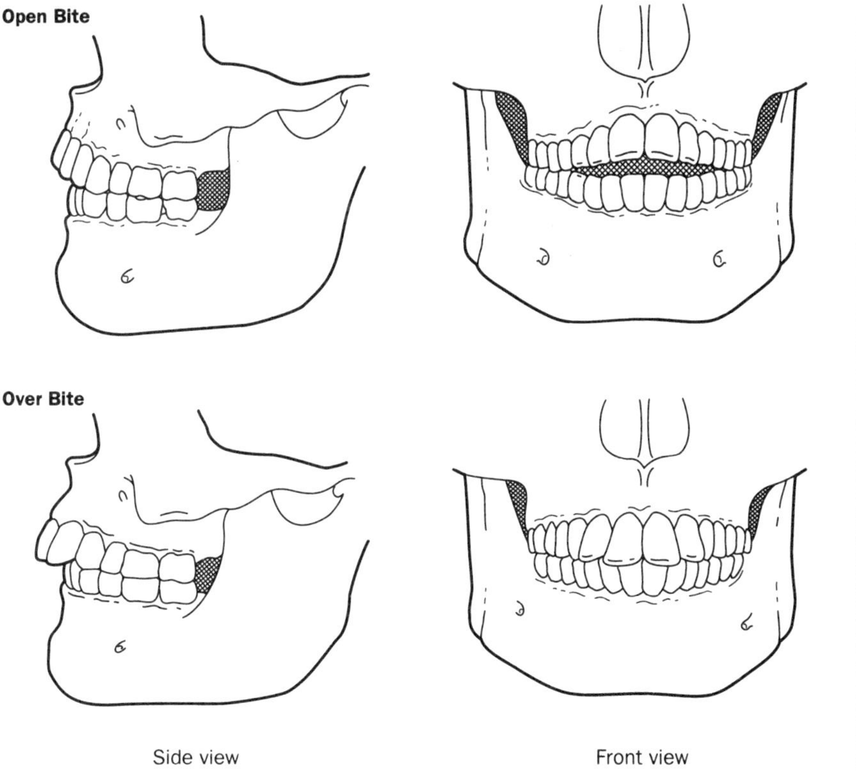

age of 70 in most people.

Orthodontic treatments can be relatively expensive and involve many visits to a dentist's office over a long period of time. Any parent of a prospective patient or a responsible older patient seeking orthodontic work for himself should have a frank discussion with the dentist regarding the time and money to be invested in the corrective procedures before making an agreement to begin the work. In nearly every case some arrangement can be made for covering the costs of dental work that is vital to the health and welfare of a patient.

TMD: Temporomandibular Disorder

The temporomandibular joints connect both sides of the lower jaw (mandible) to the temporal bone of the skull. Ligaments, tendons, and muscles attached to and surrounding the joints control the up-and-down and side-to-side movement of the jaw. Temporomandibular (jaw) disorders, formerly called temporomandibular joint (TMJ) syndrome, include problems with the jaw joints and the muscles that control chewing and talking.

TMD symptoms include pain or tenderness in the jaw muscles; pain that radiates to the face, neck, or shoulders; clicking, popping, or grating noises in a jaw joint when opening or closing the mouth; locking or limited movement of the jaw. There is typically no single cause of temporomandibular disorders. A severe injury to the jaw or dislocation of the jaw joint can cause TMD. Some experts believe that anxiety and stress can lead to *bruxism* (the clenching and grinding of teeth at night), which can cause muscle spasms and pain. Malocclusion (an improper bite) and arthritis in a jaw joint may contribute to TMD.

TMD symptoms should be evaluated by a dentist or physician. In most cases the problems causing TMD pain are temporary and simple treatment is all that is needed to relieve discomfort. Simple remedies a dentist may suggest include eating soft, nonchewy foods; avoiding extreme jaw movements, such as wide yawning and gum chewing; applying hot or cold compresses to the chewing muscles along the sides of the face; and taking aspirin or other anti-inflammatory medication.

The dentist may prescribe a mouth guard that is worn over the teeth while sleeping. The guard can reduce bruxism and ease muscle tension and joint stress. Other conservative treatments include biofeedback and relaxation therapies, muscle-relaxant medications, and physical therapy. Surgery and other permanent changes to the mouth or jaw are usually not necessary and may make TMD discomfort worse.

23

Aches, Pains, Nuisances, Worries

And Other Things You Can Live With But Could Get Along Very Well Without

None of the variety of discomforts discussed in this chapter is a laughing matter. The best thing about most of them is that they will pass, given your commonsense attention, or will disappear if you follow your physician's advice. This includes taking the medications prescribed by your physician exactly as directed. In a few cases, such as allergies or gout, long-term drug therapy may be necessary on a self-supervised basis, once treatment has been established by a physician. Of course, when symptoms of any kind persist or get worse, you should waste no time in seeking a professional diagnosis.

There may be somebody, somewhere, who has never felt rotten a day in his life. But most of us are not so fortunate. Among the most common nuisance ailments are:

- upper respiratory infections
- allergies
- occasional headaches
- backaches
- weight problems
- weather discomforts
- disturbances of normal sleep patterns
- aching feet
- indigestion

The unpleasant feeling associated with any of these common disorders can almost always be banished with a modicum of care and thought. For example, allergic reactions to particular foods can be curtailed by identifying the offending food and avoiding it.

Self-diagnosis and self-discipline can often enable one to cope with weight problems. A backache may be cured by attention to posture, or adjusting your office chair. A sensible approach to clothing and exposure can often do away with weather discomforts.

For many minor disorders and discomforts, particularly those caused by stress, massage may be the answer. Massage is a process that is at least 3,000 years old and has been used to help relieve tension, increase muscle tone, improve blood and oxygen circulation, and aid major body functions. Massage has also helped alleviate aches and pains resulting from exercise, improve posture, and increase joint flexibility. Among the disorders for which massage should not be used are osteoporosis, varicose veins, inflamed joints, herniated discs, tumors, and some cardiovascular problems.

Massage invariably involves kneading, manipulation, and methodical pressure on various body parts. The process should never be painful. The three kinds of massage in most common use are Swedish, a pleasant, muscle-kneading procedure; Shiatsu, or "acupressure," which depends on finger and hand pressure on so-called energy meridians in the body; and reflexology, a system that calls for pressure on various points of the foot.

When symptoms do not respond to self-help—as when sporadic difficulty in sleeping burgeons into a string of near-sleepless nights, or when abdominal pain you interpret as indigestion is intense or frequent in spite of avoiding rich or heavy foods, it's time to see a physician.

The Common Cold and Upper Respiratory Infections

Common cold is the label attached to a group of symptoms that can be caused by one or more of some 20 different viruses. Colds are considered highly contagious, but some physicians think that people don't entirely catch others' colds—in a sense they catch their own. While the viruses that carry the infection are airborne and practically omnipresent, somebody in good health is usually less susceptible to a cold than someone who is run down. Both environmental factors (such as air pollution) and emotional ones (such as anxiety or depression) seem to increase susceptibility.

Symptoms

Symptoms differ from person to person and from cold to cold with the same person. Generally, a cold starts with sneezes, a running nose, teary eyes, and a stuffed head. Sometimes the nasal membranes become so swollen that a person can breathe only through the mouth; sometimes the senses of smell and taste simply disappear. The throat may be sore; a postnasal drip may cause a constant cough when the person is lying down at night.

When these symptoms are acute and are accompanied by fever and aching joints, the illness is usually referred to as influenza or “the flu.” There are many different viruses that cause influenza, and new ones are always turning up. Unfortunately, there is as yet no medicine that can cure either a cold or a flu attack, although many people do get relief from symptoms by taking various cold remedies. Antibiotics are sometimes prescribed by doctors to prevent more serious bacterial diseases, such as pneumonia, from developing, but antibiotics are not effective against the cold viruses.

Treatment

Some people can get away with treating a cold with contempt and an occasional aspirin, and go about their business. Others are laid low for a few days. If you are the type who is really hit hard by a cold, it isn’t coddling yourself to stay home for a couple of days. In any event, a simple cold usually runs its course, lasting anywhere from a few days to two weeks.

Discomfort can be minimized and recovery speeded by a few simple steps: extra rest and sleep, drinking more liquids than usual, and taking aspirin as needed. Sucking on zinc gluconate lozenges within 24 hours of the first sign of a cold may help lessen the duration of a cold, although this has not been proven definitively. Antihistamine preparations or nose drops should be avoided unless specifically prescribed by a physician.

A painful sore throat accompanied by fever, earache, a dry, hacking cough, or pains in the chest are symptoms that should be brought to the attention of a physician.

Prevention

A person typically becomes infected with a cold by touching his or her eyes or nose after touching a surface—or another person’s hand—that is contaminated with the cold virus. Since cold viruses can live for hours on hands and surfaces, one of the most effective defenses against catching a cold is to avoid touching your face and to wash your hands frequently, particularly after being in public places, before and after using the bathroom, and after blowing your nose. Taking large doses of vitamin C, a practice favored by some people, has not been scientifically proven to help prevent or cure a cold.

Inoculation against particular types of viruses is recommended by many physicians in special cases: for pregnant women, for the elderly, and for those people who have certain chronic heart and lung diseases. Flu shots are effective against a particular virus or viruses for a limited period.

Allergies

Discomforts of various kinds are considered allergies when they are brought on by substances or conditions that ordinarily are harmless. Not too long ago, perturbed allergy sufferers would say things like:

"I can't use that soap because it gives me hives."

"Smelling roses makes me sneeze."

Nowadays, such complaints are commonly recognized as indications of allergies.

Symptoms

Allergic symptoms can range from itching eyes, running nose, coughing, difficulty in breathing, welts on the skin, nausea, cramps, and even going into a state of shock, depending upon the severity of the allergic individual's response. Almost any part or system of the body may be affected, and almost anything can pose an allergic threat to somebody.

Allergens

Substances that trigger an allergic reaction are called *allergens.* The system of an allergic individual reacts to such substances as if they were germs, producing ***antibodies*** whose job it is to neutralize the allergens. But the body's defense mechanism overreacts: in the process of fighting off the effects of the allergens, various chemicals, particularly ***histamines,*** are dumped indiscriminately into the bloodstream. It is the overabundance of these "good" chemicals that causes the discomforts associated with allergies.

Allergens are usually placed in the following categories:

- Those that affect the respiratory tract, or ***inhalants,*** such as pollens, dust, smoke, perfumes, and various airborne, malodorous chemicals. These bring on sneezing, coughing, and breathing impairment.
- Food substances that affect the digestive system, typically eggs, seafood, nuts, berries, chocolate, and pork. These may cause not only nausea and diarrhea but also hives and other skin rashes.
- Medicines and drugs, such as penicillin, or a particular serum used in inoculations.
- Agents that act on the skin and mucous membranes, such as insecticides, poison oak, and poison ivy, particular chemical dyes, cosmetics, soaps, metals, leathers, and furs.
- Environmental agents, such as sunlight or excessive cold.
- Microbes, such as particular bacteria, viruses, and parasites.

Treatment

In general, approaches to treatment for allergies fall into three categories:

removing or avoiding as many allergens from the environment as possible; using creams, inhalers, pills, and other medications to control the symptoms; and undergoing immunotherapy (allergy shots) to reduce the allergic response. The type of treatment selected often depends on test findings that indicate what is causing the allergic reaction; the tests may produce such identification quickly or they may have to be continued for weeks or months before the allergen is finally tracked down.

As soon as the source of the allergen is identified, the obvious course is to avoid it, if possible. Avoidance may not, however, be possible. Few persons can avoid breathing pollen in the spring and fall. Giving up a house pet may be almost as difficult, but may be necessary as a health or comfort measure.

New medications that control the symptoms of allergies have been marketed in recent years. Newer antihistamines, for example, relieve allergic reactions but do not cause the drowsiness associated with earlier medications. Other medicines that have been used to treat allergies include adrenaline, ephedrine, and cortisone. Aerosol drugs may be used to attack specific symptoms. Some, for example, may be inhaled to treat the linings of the nose and throat.

In addition to histamines, other body chemicals are released during an allergy "attack." Researchers have found that these chemicals include leukotrienes. Consequently, antileukotrienes have been tested as medications.

Direct or specific immunotherapy constitutes the third approach to treatment of allergy. The shots are effective in reducing allergic responses. A person with a substance allergy receives increasing amounts of the substance over a period of years. For example, a person who is allergic to insect stings receives injections of the particular insect's venom.

A life-threatening allergic reaction calls for emergency treatment, usually with adrenalin. Physicians suggest that persons with very intense food allergies or who are allergic to insect stings should carry special kits that include an adrenalin-filled syringe. The allergy victims administer the medication to themselves in case of *anaphylaxis*—an acute, life-threatening response (see "Allergic Shock" in Ch. 31, *Medical Emergencies*).

Persons subject to severe, disabling allergy attacks by a known allergen should also carry a card describing both the allergen and the allergic reactions. Detailed information on the latest developments in allergy treatment is available from the Asthma and Allergy Foundation of America, 1233 20th Street, NW, Suite 402, Washington, DC 20036, (800) 727-8462. See also Ch. 24, *Allergies and Hypersensitivities.*

Headaches

The common headache is probably as ancient as primitive man. The headache, a pain or ache across the forehead or within the head, may be severe or mild in character, and can last anywhere from under half an hour to three or four days. It may be accompanied by dizziness, nausea, nasal stuffiness, or difficulty in seeing or hearing. Headaches occur when nerves in the head and neck are stimulated, which can have many causes. A headache is sometimes a symptom of a physical or emotional disorder.

Causes

Headaches in today's modern world can arise from any of a number of underlying causes. These include excessive drinking or smoking, lack of sleep, hunger, drug abuse, and eyestrain. Eyestrain commonly results from overuse of the eyes, particularly under glaring light, or from failure to correct defective vision.

Treatments for headaches are as varied as the causes of headaches. Diagnosis may take some time, but if you suffer from severe or chronic headaches, it is important to consult your doctor. Headaches may point to an underlying problem, such as high blood pressure.

Headaches that are non-debilitating may be treated with analgesics such as aspirin or ibuprofen. Debilitating headaches such as tension, migraine, or cluster headaches can be treated with prescription drugs if your doctor advises it.

Chronic headaches should be diagnosed so the sufferer does not have to always depend on medication to treat the problem. Long-term solutions may include meditation, relaxation exercises, and exercise to reduce tension and stress. Dietary changes such as eliminating chocolate, caffeine, cheese, alcohol, sugar, or other products may also help.

Migraine

Migraine is an often recurring, particularly severe, intense kind of headache. An attack may last several days and necessitate bed rest. Dizziness, sensitivity to light, and chills may accompany a migraine headache.

The exact cause of migraine is unknown, but researchers suspect a hereditary link, since the majority of migraine patients have one or more close relatives with migraine.

Migraine headaches can be caused by changes in body hormone balances, sudden body temperature changes, bright light or noise, shifts in barometric pressure, alcohol and drug use, or by a combination of these triggers.

For chronic migraine sufferers, keeping a daily journal of food consumed, activities done, emotional status, and (for women) menstrual cycles, may help provide an indication of why migraines occur.

Migraines can be avoided by eliminating any apparent triggers. The fluctuation in estrogen is believed to be a major cause of migraines. Some foods bring on headaches only during certain times of the menstrual cycle. Hormone replacement therapy, some types of birth control pills, and menopause may increase incidence of migraines, although menopause may also end migraines in women who had them for years.

Tension Headaches

Tension headaches are characterized by a painful pressure in the head. Such headaches can be caused by stress, depression, or poor posture and should be treated with analgesics such as aspirin and ibuprofen, a massage or a cold shower. Tension headaches can occur at any time; you can even wake up with one. The best long-term treatment is learning to reduce or manage the stress in your life.

Cluster Headaches

Cluster headaches cause pain around a specific area of the head, and eye tearing, nasal stuffiness, and a burning sensation on the side of the head affected. The headaches usually last only a few hours but are usually described as excruciating. These headaches usually occur after a person has fallen asleep and typically affect men and heavy smokers. Since the pain is resistant to over-the-counter medicine, cluster headaches can be treated with corticosteroids, such as prednisone, or inhaling 100 percent oxygen.

Backaches

"Oh, my aching back" is probably the most common complaint among people past the age of 40. Most of the time, the discomfort—wherever it occurs, up or down the backbone—can be traced to some simple cause. However, there are continuous backaches that have their origin in some internal disorder that needs the attention of a physician. Among the more serious causes are kidney or pancreas disease, spinal arthritis, and peptic ulcer.

Some Common Causes

Generally a backache is the result of strain on the muscles, nerves, or ligaments of the spine. It can occur because of poor posture, carelessness in lifting or carrying heavy packages, sitting in one position for a long time in the wrong kind of chair, or sleeping on a mattress that is too soft. Backache often accompanies menstruation, and is common in the later stages of pregnancy. Emotional tension can also bring on back pain.

Prevention

In general, maintaining good posture during the waking hours and sleeping on a hard mattress at night—if necessary, inserting a bed board between the mattress and bedsprings—are the first line of defense against backaches. Anyone habitually carrying heavy loads of books or groceries, or even an overloaded attaché case, should make a habit of shifting the weight from arm to arm so that the spine doesn't always get pulled in one direction. Workers who are sedentary for most of the day at a desk or factory table should be sure that the chair they sit in provides firm support for back muscles and is the right height for the working surface.

Treatment

Most cases of simple backache respond to rest, aspirin, and the application of heat, applied by a hot water bottle or heating pad. In cases where the pain persists or becomes more acute, a physician should be consulted. He may find that the trouble is caused by the malfunctioning of an internal organ, or by pressure on the sciatic nerve (*sciatica*). With X rays he may also locate a slipped disk or other abnormality in the alignment of the vertebrae of the spine. See "Back Pain and Its Causes" in Ch. 7, *Diseases of the Skeletal System.*

Weight Problems

A few people can maintain the weight that is right for their body build without ever having to think about it. However, most experts believe that just about half the people in the United States may be risking shorter lives because they are too heavy. By one estimate, approximately one out of five American men and one out of four American women are 10 percent or more overweight, a group that may be called the borderline obese.

There is no longer any reasonable doubt that, if you are overweight, you have statistically a greater chance of high blood pressure, diabetes, and *atherosclerosis* (lumpy deposits in the arteries). And because atherosclerotic heart disease alone accounts for 20 percent of deaths among adults in the United States, it is understandable why physicians consider weight truly a national problem.

Causes

In practically all cases, weighing too much is the result of eating too much and exercising too little. In many cases, the food eaten is of the wrong kind and leisure time is used for riding around in a car rather than walking, or for watching television rather than playing tennis.

Many people like to think that they weigh too much only because they happen to like good food; but the real explanations may be considerably more complicated. In some cases, overeating has been found to have emotional sources: feelings of inadequacy; the need to compensate for a lack of affection or approval, or an unconscious desire to ward off the attention of the opposite sex. Psychological weight problems of this kind can be helped by consulting a psychiatrist or psychologist.

Treatment

There are many overweight people who merely need the support and encouragement that come from participating in a group effort, and for them, joining one of the various weight-control organizations can be extremely beneficial in taking off extra pounds and keeping them off.

Permanent results are rarely achieved by crash diets, faddish food combinations, or reducing pills. Not only are such solutions usually temporary; they may actually be harmful. See "Weight" in Ch. 27, *Nutrition and Weight Control,* for further information about weight problems.

Weather Discomforts

Using good sense about clothing, exercise, and proper diet is probably our best protection against the discomforts caused by extremes of temperature. Sometimes circumstances make this exercise of good sense impossible, with unpleasant but rarely serious results, if treatment is promptly administered. Following are some of the more common disorders resulting from prolonged exposure to excessive heat or cold, and what you can do to alleviate them.

Heat Cramps

In a very hot environment, a person may drink great quantities of water while "sweating buckets" of salty perspiration. Thus, the body's water is replaced, but its salt is not. This salt–water imbalance results in a feeling of faintness and dizziness accompanied by acute stomach cramps and muscle pains in the legs. When the symptoms are comparatively mild, they can be relieved by taking coated salt tablets in five-to-ten-grain doses with a full glass of tepid or cool—not iced—water. Salt tablets along with plenty of fluids should be taken regularly as a preventive measure by people who sweat a great deal during hot weather.

Sunburn

If you have not yet been exposed to much sun, as at the beginning of summer, limit your exposure at first to a period of 15 to 20 minutes, and avoid the sun at the hours around midday even if the sky is overcast. Remember, too, that the reflection of the sun's rays from water and beach sand intensifies their effect. Some suntan lotions give effective protection against burning, and some creams even prevent tanning; but remember to cover all areas of exposed skin and to reapply the lotion when it's been washed away after a swim.

Treatment

A sunburn is treated like any other burn, depending upon its severity. See "Burns" in Ch. 31, *Medical Emergencies*. If there is blistering, take care to avoid infection. Extensive blistering requires a physician's attention.

Heat Exhaustion

This condition is different from heatstroke or sunstroke, discussed below. Heat exhaustion sets in when large quantities of blood accumulate in the skin as the body's way of increasing its cooling mechanism during exposure to high temperatures. This in turn lowers the amount of blood circulating through the heart and decreases the blood supply to the brain. If severe enough, fainting may result. Other symptoms of heat exhaustion include unusual pallor and profuse cold perspiration. The pulse may be weak, and breathing shallow.

Treatment

A person suspected of having heat exhaustion should be placed in a reclining position, his clothing loosened or removed, and his body cooled with moist cloths applied to his forehead and wrists. If he doesn't recover promptly from a fainting spell, smelling salts can be held under his nose to revive him. As soon as he is conscious, he can be given salt tablets and a cool sugary drink—either tea or coffee—to act as a stimulant. Don't give the patient any alcoholic beverages.

Sunstroke or Heatstroke

Sunstroke is much more of an emergency than heat exhaustion and requires immediate attention. The characteristic symptom is extremely high body temperature brought on by cessation of perspiration. If hot, dry, flushed skin turns ashen gray, a physician must be called immediately. Too much physical activity during periods of high temperature and high humidity is a direct contributing cause.

Treatment

See "Heatstroke" in Ch. 31, *Medical Emergencies,* for a description of the emergency treatment recommended for this condition.

Chapped Skin

One of the most widespread discomforts of cold weather is *chapped skin.* In low temperatures, the skin's sebaceous glands produce fewer oils that lubricate and protect the skin, causing it to become dry. Continued exposure results in reddening and cracking. In this condition, the skin is especially sensitive to strong soaps.

Treatment

During cold, dry weather, less soap should be used when washing, a bath oil should be used when bathing, and a mild lotion or creme should be applied to protect the skin from the damaging effects of wind and cold. A night cream or lotion containing lanolin is also helpful, and the use of cleansing cream or oil instead of soap can reduce additional discomfort when cleansing chapped areas. The use of a colorless lip pomade is especially recommended for children when they play out of doors in cold, dry weather for any length of time.

Chilblain

A *chilblain* is a local inflammation of the skin brought on by exposure to cold. The condition commonly affects people overly sensitive to cold because of poor circulation. When the hands, feet, face, and ears are affected, the skin in these areas itches and burns, and may swell and turn reddish blue.

Treatment

The best way to avoid chilblains is to wear appropriate clothing during cold weather, especially warm socks, gloves, and ear coverings. The use of bed socks and a heating pad at night is also advisable. Once indoors, cold, wet feet should be dried promptly, gently, and thoroughly. Rubbing or massaging should be avoided, because these can cause further irritation. People who suffer from repeated attacks of chilblains should consult a physician for diagnosis of circulatory problems.

Frostbite

Frostbite is a considerably more serious condition than chilblains, because it means that a part or parts of the body have actually been frozen. The fingers or toes, the nose, and the ears are most vulnerable. If frostbitten, these areas turn numb and pale and feel cold when touched. The dangerous thing about frostbite is that pain may not be a warning. If the condition is not treated promptly, the temperature inside the tissues keeps going down and eventually cuts off blood circulation to the overexposed parts of the body. In such extreme cases, there is a possible danger of gangrene.

Treatment

In mild cases, prompt treatment can slowly restore blood circulation. The frozen parts should be rewarmed *slowly* by covering them with warm clothing or by soaking them in lukewarm water. Nothing hot should be applied—neither hot water nor a heating pad. Nor should the patient be placed too close to a fireplace or radiator. Because the affected tissues can be easily bruised, they should not be massaged or rubbed. If you are in doubt about restoring circulation, a physician should be called promptly or the patient taken to a hospital for emergency treatment.

Sleep and the Lack of It

Until rather recently, it was assumed that sleep was the time when the body rested and recovered from the activities of wakefulness. Although there is still a great deal to learn about why we sleep and what happens when we are sleeping, medical researchers have now identified several different phases of sleep, all of them necessary over the long run, but some more crucial than others.

How much sleep a person needs varies a great deal from individual to individual; and the same individual may need more or less at different times. Children need long periods of unbroken sleep; the elderly seem to get along on very little. No matter what a person's age, too little sleep over too long a time leads to irritability, exhaustion, and giddiness.

Insomnia

Almost everybody has gone through periods when it is difficult or impossible to fall asleep. Excitement before bedtime, temporary worries about a pressing problem, spending a night in an unfamiliar place, changing to a different bed, illness, physical discomfort because of extremes of temperature—any of these circumstances can interfere with normal sleep patterns.

But this is quite different from *chronic insomnia,* when a person consistently has trouble falling asleep for no apparent reason. If despite all your commonsense approaches insomnia persists, a physician should be consulted about the advisability of taking a tranquilizer or a sleeping pill. Barbiturates should not be taken unless prescribed by a physician.

The Vulnerable Extremities

Aches and pains in the legs and feet occur for a wide variety of reasons, some trivial and easily corrected, others serious enough to require medical attention. Those that originate in such conditions as arthritis and rheumatism can often be alleviated by aspirin or some of the newer prescription medications.

Gout

Gout, which is usually a metabolic disorder, is a condition that especially affects the joint of the big toe, and sometimes the ankle joint, causing the area to become swollen, hot, and acutely painful. Although the specific cause of gout is not yet clearly understood, the symptoms can be alleviated by special medication prescribed by a physician. An attack of gout can be triggered by a wide variety of causes: wearing the wrong shoes, eating a diet too rich in fats, getting a bad chill, surgery in some other part of the body, or chronic emotional anxiety, as well as the use of certain medicines, such as diuretics ("waterpills"). See also "Gout" in Ch. 7, *Diseases of the Skeletal System.*

Fallen Arches

Fallen arches can cause considerable discomfort because the body's weight is carried on the ligaments of the inside of the foot rather than on the sole. When the abnormality is corrected by orthopedic shoes with built-in arches for proper support, the pressure on the ligaments is relieved. A physician rather than a shoe salesman should be consulted for a reliable diagnosis. In some cases, the physician may also recommend special exercises to strengthen the arch.

Flat Feet

Flat feet can usually be revealed by a simple test—making a footprint on level earth or hard-packed sand. If the print is solid rather than indented by a curve along the big-toe side of the foot, the foot is flat. Aching ligaments in the area of the instep are often a result, but can be relieved by proper arch supports inside the shoes. Corrective arch supports are particularly important for young children, for anyone who is overweight, and for anyone who has to stand a great deal of the time.

Blisters

Although blisters are sometimes a sign of allergy, fungus infection, or sunburn, they most commonly appear on the feet because of the friction of a shoe or of hosiery that does not fit properly. A *water blister* is a collection of lymph that forms inside the upper level of the skin; a *blood blister* goes down deeper and contains some blood released from broken capillaries. A normal amount of walking in shoes and hosiery that fit comfortably—neither too loose nor too tight—rarely results in blisters. When blisters do appear, it is best to protect them from further friction by the use of a sterile bandage strip.

Treatment

A blister that causes acute pain when one is walking can be treated as follows: after cleaning the area with soap and water, pat it dry and swab it with rubbing alcohol. Sterilize the tip of a needle in a flame, let it cool a little, and then puncture the edge of the blister, absorbing the liquid with a sterile gauze. The loose skin can be removed with manicure scissors that have been sterilized by boiling for ten minutes. The surface of raw skin should then be covered with an adhesive bandage. This procedure is best done before bedtime so that healing can begin before shoes are worn again.

If redness appears around the area of any blister and inflammation appears to be spreading, a physician should be consulted promptly.

Bunions

A *bunion* is a deformation in the part of the foot that is joined by the big toe. The swelling and pain at the joint is caused by inflammation of the *bursa* (a fluid-filled sac) that lubricates the joint. Although bunions often develop because of wearing shoes that don't fit correctly, they most frequently accompany flat feet. Pain that is not too severe can be relieved by the application of heat; the condition may eventually be cured by doing foot exercises recommended by a physician, who will also help in the choice of correct footwear. A bunion that causes acute pain and difficulty in walking can be treated by a simple surgical procedure.

Calluses

A *callus* is an area of the skin that has become hard and thick as a result of constant friction or pressure against it. Pain results when the callus is pressed against a nerve by poorly fitting shoes. A painful callus can be partially removed by rubbing it—very cautiously—with a sandpaper file or a pumice stone sold for that purpose. The offending shoes should then be discarded for correctly fitted ones. Foot care by a podiatrist is recommended for anyone with recurring calluses and corns (see below), and especially for those people who have diabetes or any disorder of the arteries.

Corns

A *corn* is a form of callus that occurs on or between the toes. When the thickening occurs on the outside of the toe, it is called a *hard corn;* when it is located between the toes, it is called a *soft corn*. The pain in the affected area is caused by pressure of the hard inside core of the corn against the tissue beneath it. The most effective treatment for corns is to wear shoes that are the right size and fit. Corns can be removed by a podiatrist, but unless footwear fits properly, they are likely to return.

Treatment

To remove a corn at home, the toes should be soaked in warm water for about ten minutes and dried. The corn can be rubbed away with an emery file, or it can be treated with a few drops of 10 percent salicylic acid in collodion, available from any druggist. Care should be exercised in applying the solution so that it doesn't reach surrounding tissue; it is highly irritating to normal skin. The area can then be covered with a corn pad to relieve pressure. This treatment may have to be repeated several times before the corn becomes soft enough to lift out. Diabetics or those suffering from any circulatory disorder should never treat their own corns.

Bursitis

Bursitis is a pain and swelling in a joint caused when the bursa, a sac-like cushion between the bones and tendons, becomes worn or torn from constant use.

Forms of bursitis include: housemaid's knee, characterized by a swollen kneecap that has become inflamed by injury or constant pressure; bunions, where the joint of the big toe is swollen and inflamed by poorly fitting shoes; and weaver's bottom, where the bursa around the pelvic girdle become damaged from long periods of sitting on hard surfaces.

Bursitis can be treated by resting the inflamed joint, applying heat, taking an anti-inflammatory drug, such as aspirin or ibuprofen, or getting a corticosteroid injection or antibiotic therapy. For chronic bursitis, surgery may be required, and physical therapy to repair the joint may follow treatment.

Tendinitis

Tendinitis is inflammation of a tendon, and tenosynovitis is inflammation of the tendon sheath from injury. These problems tend to occur together. The tendon becomes injured by excessive or unusual use, such as a weekend athlete might experience, or from extreme strain on the tendon by overexertion in lifting, carrying, or moving something heavy. The tendon may also be injured by repetitive movement. The areas most susceptible to tendon injuries are the shoulder, hips, hamstrings, ankles, and heels.

Tendinitis can be treated with aspirin or ibuprofen, corticosteroid injections, elevating the injured limb and applying ice, and using a sling. Tendinitis can be avoided by doing warm-up exercises before engaging in an athletic activity, and by not overexerting.

If the pain is persistent, you should seek professional medical advice. Because rest and then gradually increased exercise of the injured area is required, your doctor will have to help you develop a plan for recovery.

Carpal tunnel syndrome

Carpal tunnel syndrome is caused when a median nerve, which provides feeling in the wrist, thumb and fingers, is compressed and becomes swollen and inflamed. The result is a painful stiffness of the hand, wrist, or fingers. The pain also can reach an arm or shoulder.

The debilitating condition is caused by repetitive motion caused by overusing the wrist. It typically affects people who type, such as secretaries and reporters, and is common among carpenters, meat cutters, gymnasts, and supermarket checkers. Water retention and weight gain in pregnant women often causes them to develop carpal tunnel syndrome which disappears after the baby is born.

Treatments include halting the activity that caused the syndrome, performing the activity differently, and using a splint to keep the wrist from bending while it heals. Anti-inflammatory drugs are also used. In severe cases, a carpal tunnel sufferer may be injected with corticosteroid drugs or undergo surgery to cut the bandlike ligament that is pressing on the median nerve.

Unnecessary delays in treating carpal tunnel may cause loss of function, although the condition need not reach such a stage.

The Exposed Integument

Common skin and scalp annoyances such as rashes, itches, dandruff, excessive perspiration, and infections of various kinds (such as athlete's foot and ringworm), as well as acne, wrinkles, and baldness, are discussed in Ch. 21, *Skin and Hair.*

Splinters

If lodged superficially in the hand, a splinter will usually work its own way out, but a splinter of no matter what size in the sole of the foot must be removed promptly to avoid its becoming further embedded by pressure and causing infection. The simplest method of removal is to pass a needle through a flame; let the needle cool; then, after the skin surface has been washed with soap and water or swabbed with alcohol, press the point of the needle against the skin, scraping slightly until the tail of the splinter is visible and loosened. It can then be pulled out with tweezers that have been sterilized in boiling water or alcohol.

Hangnails

Hangnails are pieces of partly living skin torn from the base or side of the fingernail, thus opening a portion of the underskin to infection. A hangnail can cause considerable discomfort. It should not be pulled or bitten off; but the major part of it can be cut away with manicuring scissors. The painful and exposed area should then be washed with soap and water and covered with a sterile adhesive bandage. Hangnails are likely to occur when the skin is dry. They can therefore be prevented by the regular use of a hand cream or lotion containing lanolin.

"Normal" Disorders of the Blood and Circulation

Almost everybody is bothered occasionally by minor disturbances of the circulatory system. Most of the time these disturbances are temporary, and in many cases where they are chronic they may be so mild as not to interfere with good health. Among the more common disturbances of this type are the following.

Anemia

Anemia is a condition in which there is a decrease in the number of red blood cells or in the hemoglobin content of the red blood cells. *Hemoglobin* is the compound that carries oxygen to the body tissues from the lungs. Anemia in itself is not a disease but rather a symptom of some other disorder, such as a deficiency of iron in the diet; excessive loss of blood resulting from an injury or heavy menstrual flow; infection by industrial poisons; or kidney or bone marrow disease. A person may also develop anemia as a result of hypersensitivity (allergy) to various medicines.

In the simple form of anemia, caused by a deficiency of iron in the diet, the symptoms are rarely severe. There may be feelings of fatigue, a loss of energy, and a general lack of vitality. Deficiency anemia is especially common among children and pregnant women, and can be corrected by adding foods high in iron to the diet, such as liver, lean meat, leafy green vegetables, whole wheat bread, and dried peas and beans.

If the symptoms persist, a physician should be consulted for diagnosis and treatment. For more information on anemia, see "Diseases of the Blood" in Ch. 9, *Diseases of the Circulatory System.*

Varicose Veins

Varicose veins are veins that have become ropy and swollen, and are therefore visible in the leg, sometimes bulging on the surface of the skin. They are the result of a sluggish blood flow (poor circulation), often combined with weakened walls of the veins themselves. The condition is common in pregnancy and occurs frequently among people who find it necessary to sit or stand in the same position for extended periods of time. A tendency to develop varicose veins may be inherited.

Even before the veins begin to be visible, there may be such warning symptoms as leg cramps, feelings of fatigue, or a general achiness. Unless the symptoms are treated promptly, the condition may worsen, and if the blood flow becomes increasingly impeded, ulcers may develop on the lower area of the leg.

Treatment

Mild cases of varicose veins can be kept under control, or even corrected, by giving some help to circulation, as follows:

- Several times during the day, lie flat on your back for a few minutes, with the legs slightly raised.
- Soak the legs in warm water.
- Exercise regularly.
- Wear lightly reinforced stockings or elastic stockings to support veins in the legs.

If varicose veins have become severe, a physician should be consulted. He or she may advise injection treatment or surgery. See also "The Inflammatory Disorders" in Ch. 9, *Diseases of the Circulatory System.*

Chronic Hypertension

Hypertension, commonly known as *high blood pressure,* is a condition that may be a warning of some other disease. In many cases, it is not in itself a serious problem and has no one underlying specific cause: this is called *functional, essential,* or *chronic hypertension.* The symptoms of breathing difficulty, headache, weakness, or dizziness that accompany high blood pressure can often be controlled by medicines that bring the pressure down, by sedatives or tranquilizers, and in cases where overweight is a contributing factor, by a change in diet, or by a combination of these.

More serious types of high blood pressure can be the result of kidney disease, glandular disturbances, or diseases of the circulatory system. Acute symptoms include chronic dizziness or blurred vision. Any symptoms of high blood pressure call for professional advice and treatment. See "Hypertensive Heart Disease" in Ch. 10, *Heart Disease.*

Tachycardia

Tachycardia is the medical name for a condition that most of us have felt at one time or another—abnormally rapid heartbeat, or a feeling that the heart is fluttering, or pounding too quickly. The condition can be brought on by strong feelings of fear, excitement, or anxiety, or by overtaxing the heart with sudden exertion or too much exercise. It may also be a sign of heart disease, but in such cases, it is usually accompanied by other symptoms.

The most typical form of occasional rapid heartbeat is called *paroxysmal tachycardia,* during which the beat suddenly becomes twice or three times as fast as it is normally, and then just as suddenly returns to its usual tempo. When the paroxysms are frequent enough to be disturbing and can be traced to no specific source, they can be prevented by medicines prescribed by a physician.

Nosebleed

Nosebleeds are usually the result of a ruptured blood vessel. They are especially common among children, and among adults with high blood pressure. If the nosebleed doesn't taper off by itself, the following measures should be taken: the patient should be seated—but not lying down—clothing loosened, and a cold compress placed on the back of the neck and the nose. The soft portion of the nostril may be pressed gently against the bony cartilage of the nose for at least six minutes, or rolled wads of absorbent cotton may be placed inside each nostril, with part of the cotton sticking out to make its removal easier. The inserted cotton should be left in place for several hours and then gently withdrawn.

Fainting

Fainting is a sudden loss of consciousness, usually caused by an insufficient supply of blood and oxygen to the brain. Among the most common causes of fainting are fear, acute hunger, the sight of blood, and prolonged standing in a room with too little fresh air. Fainting should not be confused with a loss of consciousness resulting from excessive alcohol intake or insulin shock. A person about to faint usually feels dizzy, turns pale, and feels weak in the knees.

Treatment

If possible, the person should be made to lie down, or to sit with his head between his knees for several minutes. Should he lose consciousness, place him so that his legs are slightly higher than his head, loosen his clothing, and see that he gets plenty of fresh air. If smelling salts or aromatic spirits of ammonia are available, they can be held under his nose. With these procedures, he should revive in a few minutes. If he doesn't, a physician should be called.

Troubles Along the Digestive Tract

From childhood on, most people are occasionally bothered by minor and temporary disturbances connected with digestion. Most of the disturbances listed below can be treated successfully with common sense and, if need be, a change in habits.

The Mouth

The digestive processes begin in the mouth, where the saliva begins chemically to break down some foods into simpler components, and the teeth and the tongue start the mechanical breakdown. Disorders of the teeth such as a malocclusion or poorly fitted dentures that interfere with proper chewing, should promptly be brought to the attention of a dentist.

Inflammation of the Gums

Also known as *gingivitis,* inflammation of the gums is caused by the bacteria that breed in food trapped in the spaces between the gums and the teeth. The gums become increasingly swollen, may bleed easily, and be sore enough to interfere with proper chewing. The condition can be prevented by cleaning the teeth thoroughly and frequently, which includes the use of dental floss or the rubber tip on the toothbrush to remove any food particles lodged in the teeth after eating. Because gingivitis can develop into the more serious condition of *pyorrhea,* persistent gum bleeding or soreness should receive prompt professional treatment. See Ch. 22, *The Teeth and Gums.*

Canker Sores

Canker sores are small ulcers inside the lips, mouth, and cheeks. Their specific cause is unknown, but they seem to accompany or follow a virus infection, vitamin deficiency, or emotional stress. They may be additionally irritated by citrus fruit, chocolate, or nuts. A canker sore usually clears up in about a week without special treatment. A bland mouth rinse will relieve pain and, in some cases, speed the healing process.

Coated Tongue

Although a coated tongue is commonly supposed to be a sure sign of illness, this is not the case. The condition may occur because of a temporary lack of saliva.

Glossitis

Glossitis, an inflammation of the tongue causing the tongue's surface to become bright red or, in some cases, glazed in appearance, may be a symptom of an infection elsewhere in the body. It may also be a symptom of anemia or a nutritional deficiency, or it may be an adverse reaction to certain forms of medication. If the inflammation persists and is accompanied by acute soreness, it should be called to a physician's attention.

Halitosis or Bad Breath

Contrary to the millions of commercial messages on television and in print, bad breath cannot be cured by any mouthwash, lozenge, spray, or antiseptic gargle now on the market. These products can do no more than mask the odor until the basic cause is diagnosed and cured. Among the many conditions that may result in bad breath (leaving out such fleeting causes as garlic and onions) are the following: an infection of the throat, nose, or mouth; a stomach or kidney disorder; pyorrhea; respiratory infection; tooth decay; improper mouth hygiene; and excessive drinking and smoking. Anyone who has been made self-conscious about the problem of bad breath should ask his physician or dentist whether his breath is truly offensive and if it is, what to do about it.

Gastritis

Gastritis, one of the most common disorders of the digestive system, is an inflammation of the lining of the stomach that may occur in acute, chronic, or toxic form. Among the causes of *acute gastritis* are various bacterial or viral infections; overeating, especially heavy or rich foods; excessive drinking of alcoholic beverages; or food poisoning. An attack of acute gastritis may be severely painful, but the discomfort usually subsides with proper treatment. The first symptom is typically sharp stomach cramps, followed by a bloated feeling, loss of appetite, headache, and nausea. When vomiting occurs, it rids the stomach of the substance causing the attack but usually leaves the patient temporarily weak. If painful cramps persist and are accompanied by fever, a physician should be consulted about the possibility of medication for bacterial infection. For a few days after an attack of acute gastritis, the patient should stay on a bland diet of easily digested foods, taken in small quantities.

Toxic Gastritis

Toxic gastritis is usually the result of swallowing a poisonous substance, causing vomiting and possible collapse. It is an emergency condition requiring prompt first aid treatment and the attention of a physician. See "Poisoning" in Ch. 31, *Medical Emergencies.*

Chronic Gastritis

Chronic gastritis is a recurrent or persisting inflammation of the stomach lining over a lengthy period. The condition has the symptoms associated with indigestion, especially pain after eating. It can be caused by excessive drinking of alcoholic beverages, constant tension or anxiety, or deficiencies in the diet. The most effective treatment for chronic gastritis is a bland diet from which caffeine and alcohol have been eliminated. Heavy meals should be avoided in favor of eating small amounts at frequent intervals. A tranquilizer or a mild sedative prescribed by a physician may reduce the tensions that contribute to the condition. If the discomfort continues, a physician should be consulted about the possibility of ulcers. See Ch. 11, *Diseases of the Digestive System.*

Gastroenteritis

Gastroenteritis is an inflammation of the lining of both the stomach and the intestines. Like gastritis, it can occur in acute or toxic forms as a result of food poisoning, excessive alcohol intake, viral or bacterial infections, or food allergies. Vomiting, diarrhea, and fever may be more pronounced and of longer duration. As long as nausea and vomiting persist, no food or fluid should be taken; when these symptoms cease, a bland, mainly fluid diet consisting of strained broth, thin cereals, boiled eggs, and tea is best. If fever continues and diarrhea doesn't taper off, a physician should be called.

Diarrhea

Diarrhea is a condition in which bowel movements are abnormally frequent and liquid. It may be accompanied by cramps, vomiting, thirst, and a feeling of tenderness in the abdominal region. Diarrhea is always a symptom of some irritant in the intestinal tract; among possible causes are allergy, infection by virus or bacteria, accidentally swallowed poisonous substances, or excessive alcohol. Brief attacks are sometimes caused by emotions, such as overexcitement or anxiety.

Diarrhea that lasts for more than two days should be diagnosed by a physician to rule out a more serious infection, a glandular disturbance, or a tumor. Mild attacks can be treated at home by giving the patient a light, bland diet, plenty of fluids, and the prescribed dosage of a kaolin-pectin compound available at any drugstore.

Constipation

Many people have the mistaken notion that if they don't have a bowel movement every day, they must be constipated. This is not necessarily so. From a physician's viewpoint, constipation is determined not by an arbitrary schedule of when the bowel should be evacuated but by the individual's discomfort and other unpleasant symptoms. In too many instances, overconcern and anxiety about bowel movements may be the chief cause of constipation.

The watery waste that results from the digestion of food in the stomach and small intestine passes into the large intestine, or colon, where water is absorbed from the waste. If the waste stays in the large intestine for too long a time, so much water is removed that it becomes too solid and compressed to evacuate easily. The efficient removal of waste material from the large intestine depends on wavelike muscular contractions. When these waves are too weak to do their job properly, as often happens in the elderly or the excessively sedentary, a physician may recommend a mild laxative or mineral oil.

Treatment

Constipation is rarely the result of an organic disorder. In most cases, it is caused by poor health habits; when these are corrected, the disorder corrects itself. Often, faulty diet is a major factor. Make sure that meals contain plenty of roughage in the form of whole-grain cereals, fruit, and leafy green vegetables. Figs, prunes, and dates should be included from time to time. Plenty of liquid intake is important, whether in the form of juices, soups, or large quantities of water. Scheduling a certain amount of exercise each day strengthens the abdominal muscles and stimulates muscle activity in the large intestine. Confronting the sources of worries and anxieties, if necessary with a trained therapist, may also be helpful.

An enema or a laxative should be considered only once in a while rather than as regular treatment. The colon should be given a chance to function properly without relying on artificial stimulation. If constipation resists these commonsense approaches, the problem should be talked over with a physician.

Hemorrhoids

Hemorrhoids, commonly called *piles,* are swollen veins in the mucous membrane inside or just outside the rectum. When the enlargement is slight, the only discomfort may be an itching sensation in the area. Acute cases are accompanied by pain and bleeding. Hemorrhoids are a very common complaint and occur in people of all ages. They are usually the result of straining to eliminate hard, dry stools. The extra pressure causes a fold of the membranous rectal lining to slip down, thus pinching the veins and irritating them.

Because hemorrhoids may be a symptom of a disorder other than constipation, they should be treated by a physician. If neglected, they may bleed frequently and profusely enough to cause anemia. Should a blood clot develop in an irritated vein, surgery may be necessary.

Treatment

Advertised cures should be avoided because they are not only ineffective but can cause additional irritation. Laxatives and cathartics, which may temporarily solve the problem of constipation, are likely to aggravate hemorrhoids.

If pain or bleeding becomes acute, a physician should be consulted promptly. Treatment can be begun at home. Sitting for several minutes in a hot bath in the morning and again in the evening (more frequently if necessary) will provide temporary relief. Preventing constipation is of the utmost importance.

Anal Fissure

This is a condition in which a crack or split or ulcerated place develops in the area of the two anal sphincters, or muscle rings, that control the release of feces. Such breaks in the skin are generally caused by something sharp in the stool, or by the passage of an unusually hard and large stool. Although discomfort often accompanies a bowel movement when there is a fissure, the acute pain typically comes afterward. Healing is difficult because the injured tissue is constantly open to irritation. If the condition persists, it usually has to be treated by a minor surgical procedure. Intense itching in this area is called *anal pruritis.*

Minor Ailments in the Air Pipes

In addition to all the respiratory discomforts that go along with the common cold, there are various other ailments that affect breathing and normal voice production.

Bronchitis

Usually referred to as a chest cold, *bronchitis* is an inflammation of the bronchial tubes that connect the windpipe and the lungs. If bronchitis progresses down into the lungs, it can develop into pneumonia. Old people and children are especially susceptible to acute bronchitis. The symptoms include pain in the chest, a feeling of fatigue, and a nagging cough. If the infection is bacterial, it will respond to antibiotics. If it is viral, there are no specific medicines. The attack usually lasts for about ten days, although recovery may be speeded up with bed rest and large fluid intake.

Chronic Bronchitis

Chronic bronchitis is a condition that may recur each winter, or may be present throughout the year in the form of a constant cough. The condition is aggravated by smoking and by irritants such as airborne dust and smog. The swollen tissues and abnormally heavy discharge of mucus interfere with the flow of air from the lungs and cause shortness of breath. Medicines are available that lessen the bronchial phlegm and make breathing easier. People with chronic bronchitis often sleep better if they use more than one pillow and have a vaporizer going at night.

Coughing

Coughing is usually a reflex reaction to an obstruction or irritation in the trachea (windpipe), pharynx (back of mouth and throat), or bronchial tubes. It can also be the symptom of a disease or a nervous habit. For a simple cough brought on by smoking too much or breathing bad air, medicines can be taken that act as sedatives to inhibit the reflex reaction. Inhaling steam can loosen the congestion (a combination of swollen membranes and thickened mucus) that causes some types of coughs, and hot drinks such as tea or lemonade help to soothe and relax the irritated area. Constant coughing, especially when accompanied by chest pains, should be brought to a physician's attention. For a discussion of whooping cough and croup, see the respective articles under the "Alphabetic Guide to Child Care" in Ch. 2, *The First Dozen Years.*

Laryngitis

Laryngitis is an inflammation of the mucous membrane of the larynx (voice box) that interferes with breathing and causes the voice to become hoarse or disappear altogether. This condition may accompany a sore throat, measles, or whooping cough, or it may result from an allergy. Prolonged overuse of the voice, a common occupational hazard of singers and teachers, is also a cause. The best treatment for laryngitis is to go to bed, keep the room cool, and put moisture into the air from a vaporizer, humidifier, or boiling kettle. Don't attempt to talk, even in a whisper. Keep a writing pad within arm's reach and use it to spare your voice. Drinking warm liquids may help to relieve some of the discomfort. If you must go out, keep the throat warmly protected.

Chronic laryngitis may result from too many acute laryngitis attacks, which can cause the mucous membrane to become so thick and tough that the voice remains permanently hoarse. The sudden onset of hoarseness that lasts for more than two weeks calls for a physician's diagnosis.

Hiccups

Hiccups (also spelled *hiccoughs*) are contractions of the diaphragm, the great muscle responsible for forcing air in and out of our lungs. They may be brought on by an irritation of the diaphragm itself, of the respiratory or digestive system, or by eating or drinking too rapidly. Common remedies for hiccups include sipping water slowly, holding the breath, and putting something cold on the back of the neck. Breathing into a paper bag is usually effective because after a few breaths, the high carbon dioxide content in the bag will serve to make the diaphragm contractions more regular, rather than spasmodic. If none of these measures helps, it may be necessary to have a physician prescribe a sedative or tranquilizer.

The Sensitive Eyes and Ears

Air pollution affects not only the lungs but the eyes as well. In addition to all the other hazards to which the eyes are exposed, airborne smoke, chemicals, and dust cause the eyes to burn, itch, and shed tears. Other common eye troubles are discussed below.

Sty

This pimplelike inflammation of the eyelid is caused by infection, which may be linked to the blocking of an eyelash root or an oil gland, or to general poor health. A sty can be treated at home by applying clean compresses of hot water to the area for about 15 minutes at a time every two hours. This procedure should cause the sty to open, drain, and heal. If sties are recurrent, a health checkup may be indicated.

Pinkeye

Pinkeye, an acute form of *conjunctivitis,* is an inflammation of the membrane that lines the eyelid and covers the eyeball, causing the eyes to become red and the lids to swell and stick together while one is sleeping. The condition may result from bacterial or viral infection—in which case it is extremely contagious—or from allergy or chemical irritation. A physician should be consulted.

Conjunctivitis can be treated by washing the eyes with warm water, drying them with a disposable tissue to prevent the spread of infection, and applying a medicated yellow oxide of mercury ophthalmic ointment (as recommended by your physician) on the inner edges of the lids. This should be done upon rising in the morning and upon retiring at night. The eyes should then be closed until the ointment has spread. Apply compresses of hot water three or four times a day for five-minute periods.

Eyestrain

Eyestrain—with symptoms of fatigue, tearing, redness, and a scratchy feeling in the eyelids—can be caused by a need for corrective glasses, by a disorder of the eye, or by overuse of the eyes. One of the most common causes of eyestrain, however, is improper lighting. Anyone engaged in close work, such as sewing or miniature model building, and at all times when reading, should have light come from behind and from the side so that no shadow falls on the book or object being scrutinized. The light should be strong enough for comfort—not dazzling. Efforts should be made to avoid a shiny or highly polished work surface that produces a glare. To avoid eyestrain when watching television, be sure the picture is in sharp focus; the viewer should sit at least six feet from the screen; and see that the room is not in total darkness.

Ear Infections

Ear infections related to colds, sore throats, or tonsillitis can now be kept from spreading and entering the mastoid bone by the use of sulfa drugs and other antibiotics. Any acute earache should therefore be called to a physician's attention promptly. Aspirin, in adults, can be taken for temporary relief from pain; holding a heating pad or a hotwater bottle to the affected side of the face may also be helpful until proper medication can be prescribed.

Earwax

An excessive accumulation of earwax can cause pain and interfere with hearing. A small wad of cotton should be used to gently clean the ear canal, and sharp objects such as hairpins and matchsticks should never be used.

Hardened earwax can be softened by a few drops of hydrogen peroxide. Sometimes a doctor may have to flush out earwax that is deeply imbedded.

Ear Blockage

A stopped-up feeling in the ear can be caused by a cold, and also by the change in air pressure experienced when a plane makes a rapid descent. The obstruction of the eustachian tube can usually be opened by swallowing hard or yawning.

Ringing in the Ear

The general word for a large variety of noises in the ear is *tinnitus*. Tinnitus can be ringing, buzzing, or other low level continual sounds. Everyone experiences some form of ear ringing on occasion, such as after listening to loud music or noise. However, chronic noise is symptomatic of other problems. Tinnitus can be caused by tension in the jaw muscle from stress, grinding of the teeth, or structural problems with the jaw. It can also be caused by high blood pressure, infections, or as a reaction to chemicals, such as nicotine. If you experience continual or chronic ringing, you should discuss it with your physician.

Tinnitus is treated by avoiding excessive noise, masking irritating ear noises with music or amplified sounds from a hearing aid or cleaning ear wax out of ears. A doctor's opinion should also be sought to determine if the ringing is caused by an inner ear infection. Avoiding caffeine, nicotine and alcohol also helps.

The Path from the Kidneys

Cystitis

Cystitis is the general term for inflammation of the bladder caused by various types of infection. It is more common in women than in men. Infecting microbes may come from outside the body by way of the urethra, or from some other infected organ, such as the kidney. When the bladder becomes inflamed, frequent and painful urination results.

Cystitis may also occur as a consequence of other disorders, such as enlargement of the prostate gland, a structural defect of the male urethra, or stones or a tumor in the bladder. Although there is no completely reliable way to prevent cystitis, some types of infection can be prevented by cleansing the genital region regularly so that the entrance of the urethra is protected against bacterial invasion. Cystitis is usually cured by medicines prescribed by a physician. For a detailed discussion of cystitis and related conditions affecting women, see "Disorders of the Urinary System" in Ch. 25, *Women's Health.*

Prostatitis

Prostatitis is an inflammation of the prostate gland (present in males only), caused by an infection of the urinary tract or some other part of the body. It may occur as a result of venereal infection. The symptoms of painful and excessive urination generally respond favorably to antibiotics. *Acute prostatitis* is less common: the patient is likely to have a high fever, as well as a discharge of pus from the penis. These symptoms should be brought to a physician's attention without delay.

Excessive Urination

A need to empty the bladder with excessive frequency can be merely a nuisance caused by overexcitement or tension, or it can be the sign of a disorder of the urinogenital system. A physician should be consulted if the problem persists.

The All-Important Feet

The *podiatrist* is the specialist who treats foot problems. Causes of foot ailments range from lack of cleanliness to ill-fitting shoes and overindulgence in athletic activities (see "Care of the Feet" in Ch. 5, *The Middle Years,* "The Vulnerable Extremities" in Ch. 23, *Aches, Pains, Nuisances, Worries*).

An ache, pain, or other disorder of the foot can be particularly annoying because it usually hampers mobility. A severe problem can keep a person bedridden, sometimes in the hospital, for substantial periods of time. As humans, we move about on our feet. They deserve the best of care from us, as their owners, and from the podiatrist in case a serious problem arises.

Podiatry, the science of foot care, has become more and more important as Americans have taken to athletics and exercises of various kinds. Most of these activities require the use of the feet. Increasing numbers of persons in the adult years are also taking up walking, jogging, or running as diversions or exercises.

Podiatrists believe that some persons "walk old"—they give the appearance, by the way they walk, of greater age than their chronological years. Others "walk young," or walk normally. Those who walk old may be inviting foot problems, and a fact of podiatric science is that every foot problem has its reflection in another part, or other parts, of the body.

By contrast, good foot and body posture often suggests that the owner of the feet enjoys good health in other parts of the body. Foot care may in effect help other body parts to function better. Because many problems with parts of the body remote from the feet make good foot posture and normal walking difficult or impossible, individuals with diverse problems, such as back pains, sometimes go to a podiatrist for treatment. The back pain may disappear when the feet have been brought into good working order.

Diabetes and the Feet

"Care" for the feet of diabetics means prevention. The diabetic tries to keep his feet so healthy that he avoids major problems. He knows that diabetes affects blood circulation, and that the leg and foot are extremely vulnerable to circulatory problems. Where blood cannot reach a limb or member, gangrene becomes a possibility.

Foot Care

What kind of care serves the diabetic best? Effective care means that the diabetic takes steps quickly to treat such problems as abrasions or ulcers that refuse to heal. Other conditions that warn of possible future problems are dry skin, numbness, and dry or brittle nails. Ulcers that appear in the skin of the foot and that appear to have roots in deeper layers of tissue serve as danger signals. Such ulcers may appear on the site of an injury, cut, or scratch. A physician will usually prescribe medication, dietary adjustments, or other measures.

Ulcers may result from neglect of a corn or callus. But such neglect itself indicates the risks that diabetics incur: they may neglect to have a foot problem such as a corn treated because their disease has, over time, reduced the sensitivity of their feet. They may lose much of their ability to feel pain, heat or cold, or stress in the foot. Because of such problems, diabetics generally follow certain rules of foot care, including the following:

- Give the feet a daily examination for cuts, bruises, or other abnormalities
- Use only prescribed medications in caring for the feet—and avoid over-the-counter preparations

- Visit a podiatrist regularly, as often as once a month, and avoid medical "treatment" of one's own feet or even cutting one's own toenails
- Wash the feet daily in warm, not hot, water and dry them carefully, including the area between the toes
- Use a gentle lubricant on the feet after washing and drying—and never go barefoot
- Avoid the use of items of clothing that may interfere with circulation, including wraparound garters and support hosiery
- Avoid "holey" socks, darned socks, or anything else that may irritate the soles of the feet and
- Avoid constrictive boots or shoes

Jogging and Running

The podiatrist usually tries to learn about a patient's work, his hobbies and sports, and other facts before undertaking treatment. In particular, the podiatrist asks whether the patient runs or jogs or takes part in other strenuous exercises. With such background information, he or she can suggest appropriate treatment.

A podiatrist will advise runners or joggers on the kind of footwear that would be best—especially if problems have been encountered or may be expected. Shoe inserts may be custom-designed if needed. The podiatrist may also advise runners and joggers to run on softer surfaces rather than cement. Jogging or running "in place," without forward movement, is to be avoided if possible; even when jogging inside the home or apartment, the jogger should move from room to room.

Podiatrists point out that even the more serious knee and ankle problems incurred in running and jogging can be treated. "Jogger's ankle," pain resulting from too much jogging and the attendant strain, can be controlled if the jogger will use moderation. Beginning joggers in particular should start slowly and gradually increase their level of participation. Runners' knee problems may be cured in many cases by treatment that enables the feet to carry the weight of the body properly. In part, the treatment requires practice in throwing the body weight onto the balls of the feet, not on the inner sides of the feet. The remainder of the body, including the knees, can be kept in proper alignment with the feet if the weight falls where it should.

Podiatrists also advise runners, joggers, and others taking part in sports to make certain *all* their clothing and equipment are appropriate. That applies especially in skiing, ice-skating, and other sports requiring extensive foot use.

With proper equipment, including good shoes, and a moderate approach, runners and joggers can avoid physical difficulties that could require podiatric care. These others include fallen arches; corns, calluses, and bunions.

24

Allergies and Hypersensitivities

Allergy is a broad term used to describe an unusual reaction of the body's tissues to a substance that does not have a comparable effect on the majority of other persons. Each year, more than 50 million Americans experience an allergic, or hypersensitive, reaction to one or more substances that are known to precipitate such reactions. Such substances, known as *allergens,* include a variety of irritants, among them mold spores, pollens, animal dander, insect venoms, and dust mites. Some individuals are allergic to substances in soap, which produce a skin irritation. Others may react to the smell of a rose by sneezing. Still others react to allergens in foods with an outbreak of hives, diarrhea, or other symptoms.

How Allergens Affect the Body

Depending on the severity of an individual's sensitivity and response, allergic symptoms can range from itching eyes, a runny nose, sneezing, coughing, difficulty in breathing, and skin welts to nausea, cramps, and even going into a state of shock. Almost any part or system of the body can be affected, and almost anything can act as an allergen and potentially cause an allergic reaction.

The Role of Antibodies

The system of an allergic individual reacts to allergens in the way it would react to an invading disease organism: by producing proteins in the blood called *antibodies,* whose job is to neutralize the allergen. In the process of fighting off the effects of the allergen, the body's defense mechanism may overreact by releasing a chemical mediator, *histamine,* indiscriminately into the bloodstream. It is the overabundance of this protective chemical that causes the discomforts associated with allergies.

At the same time, the antibodies can sensitize the individual to the allergen. Then, with each new exposure to the allergen, more antibodies are produced. Eventually the symptoms of allergy appear whenever the allergen is encountered. Most allergic reactions, including hay fever, asthma, gastrointestinal upsets, irritant contact dermatitis, and hives, are of the type just described; their effect is more or less immediate. A second type, known as the delayed type, seems to function without the production of antibodies; allergic contact dermatitis is an example of the delayed type.

Eosinophils

Some individuals are sensitive to only one known allergen, but others are sensitive to a variety of substances. Persons who suffer acute allergic reactions have abnormally high levels of a type of white blood cell called *eosinophil.* The eosinophil contains an enzyme that may have some control over the allergic reaction, and varying degrees of the enzyme's efficiency appear to account for individual differences in the severity of allergic reactions.

Allergic Symptoms in Children

Many of the common allergies appear during the early years of life. It has been estimated that nearly 80 percent of the major allergic problems begin to appear between the ages of 4 and 9. Heredity is a factor in determining the presence of allergies in children. Allergic youngsters may have nasal speech habits, breathe through the mouth, have coughing and wheezing spells, or rub their eyes, nose, and ears because of itching. A not uncommon sign of allergic reaction in a child may be dark circles under the eyes caused by swelling of the mucous membranes to such an extent that blood does not drain properly from the veins under the lower eyelids. Nose twitching and mouth wrinkling also are signs that a youngster has allergic symptoms.

Common Allergens

The allergens responsible for so many unpleasant and uncomfortable symptoms take a variety of forms too numerous and sometimes too obscure for any book to enumerate. Discussed below are some of the more common types of allergens.

Foods

Approximately 200 deaths per year are caused by food allergies. Food allergies are most commonly found in very young children. Although nearly any food substance is a potential allergen for certain sensitive individuals, those most frequently implicated are cow's milk, orange juice, and eggs, all considered essential in a child's diet. However, substitute foods are almost always available. Vitamins tablets and many natural foods contain vitamin C, or ascorbic acid, found in orange juice. All of the essential amino acids and other nutrients in cow's milk and eggs also can be obtained from other food sources, although perhaps not as conveniently packaged for immediate use. Other common food offenders are chocolate, pork, shellfish, nuts, and berries. Some people are allergic to the gluten in wheat, rye, and oats, and products made from those grains.

Inhaled Allergens

Allergens also may affect the respiratory tract, bringing on sneezing, coughing, and breathing impairment. The substances involved can include pollens, dust, mold spores, smoke, perfumes, and various airborne chemicals.

Mold Spores

A person can become allergic to a certain mold by inhaling the spores, or reproductive particles, of fungus. Mold spores are a primary cause of seasonal allergic *rhinitis.* Rhinitis is an inflammation of the mucous membrane of the nose. Mold spores, when inhaled through the nose, trigger a reaction in cells of the tissues beneath the mucous membranes that line the nasal passages. This, in turn, leads to the symptoms of allergy. Because they are small, mold spores can evade the natural protective mechanisms of the nose and upper respiratory tract to reach the lungs and bring on an allergic reaction in that site. Usually, this leads to the buildup of mucus, wheezing, and difficulty in breathing associated with asthma.

Less frequently, inhaling mold spores can result in skin lesions similar to those of eczema or chronic hives. In all but the very warmest areas of the United States, molds are seasonal allergens, peaking from July to late summer. But unlike pollens, molds do not disappear with the killing frosts of autumn. Actually, frost may help increase the activity of molds, which thrive on dying vegetation produced by cold temperatures.

Dust and Animal Hair

House dust (dust mites) and cat and dog hair (dander) are also responsible for respiratory allergies in many peopie. Asthma attacks are often triggered by contact with these substances. In the United States, dust mite populations usually peak in July and August. Mite allergen levels stay high through December and are lowest in late spring. Some dust mite-sensitive people experience more severe symptoms during the winter.

Nonorganic Allergens and Smog

An example of respiratory allergy caused by nonorganic allergens is a complaint known as "meat wrappers' asthma," which results from fumes of the price-label adhesive on the polyvinyl chloride film used to package foods. The fumes are produced when the price label is cut on a hot wire. When the fumes are inhaled, the result is burning eyes, sore throat, wheezing and shortness of breath, upset stomach, and other complaints. Studies show that exposure to the fumes from the heat-activated label adhesive for as little as five minutes could produce airway obstruction in food packagers.

Another source of respiratory allergy is the photochemical smog produced by motor vehicle exhaust in large city areas. The smog is composed of hydrocarbons, oxides of nitrogen, and other chemicals activated by the energy of sunlight. When inhaled in the amounts present along some of the nation's expressways and thoroughfares, the smog has been found to impair the normal function of membranes in the lungs.

Drugs

Medicines and drugs, such as penicillin, or serums used in inoculations, can cause allergic reactions. Penicillin is a common cause of drug allergy, and penicillin allergy is a more common cause of death than food allergy. The National Institutes of Health has calculated that just three common drugs—penicillin, sulfonamides, and aspirin—account for as much as 90 percent of all allergic drug reactions. The allergic reactions include asthmatic symptoms, skin rash, shock, and other symptoms similar to tissue reactions to other allergens.

Insect Venom

About 1 to 3 percent of the general population has had a serious allergic reaction from stings of insects such as bees, fire ants, yellow jackets, wasps, or hornets. A single sting to a sensitive person may lead to a serious drop in blood pressure, shock, and possibly death. There are more than 50 reported fatalities a year, and experts suspect that other deaths occur as a result of insect stings but are listed as heart attacks, stroke, or convulsions. Self-injecting epinephrine (adrenaline) is the recommended treatment for severe allergic reactions to insect venom.

Sensitivity tests of persons who might be acutely allergic to insect stings have been difficult to develop, because allergic individuals reacted in the same way as nonallergic persons to skin tests performed with extracts from insect bodies. More recently, physicians have found that using pure insect venom produces a reaction that determines whether a person is allergic to the sting. Medical scientists also have isolated the major allergen in an insect venom for use in diagnosing and treating patients who are particularly sensitive to stings.

Skin Allergies

Allergies affecting the skin take many forms, the most common being eczema, urticaria (hives), angioedema (swelling of the subcutaneous tissues), irritant contact dermatitis, and allergic contact dermatitis. Among the most common causes are foods, cosmetics, fabrics, rubber, metals, plants (such as poison ivy) and flowers, plastics, insecticides, furs and leather, jewelry, and many industrial chemicals. Studies of patients who seem to be especially sensitive to skin allergies show that they have higher than average amounts of a body protein called *immunoglobulin E* in their systems.

Allergic contact dermatitis usually is distinguished by skin swelling, itching, hives, or blisters. The area affected is usually the skin that comes in direct contact with the allergen, so a watch band allergy response will appear as a band around the wrist where the watchband touches the skin.

Allergic contact dermatitis reactions are not immediate; reactions tend to occur 14 to 28 hours after contact.

Poisonous Plants

Poison ivy, poison oak, and poison sumac contain an extremely irritating oily resin, called *urushiol,* that sensitizes the body; repeated contact seems to increase the severity of the allergic reactions. About 50 percent of the population who come in contact with the resin will experience a severe form of dermatitis, and up to 10 percent will be temporarily disabled by the effects. Exposure to the resin may come from direct contact with the plant, from contact with other objects or animals that have touched the plant, or from inhaling smoke from the burning plant.

Cosmetics and Jewelry

A wide variety of cosmetics and jewelry can cause allergic reactions through skin contact. Even jewelry that is presumably pure gold can contain a certain amount of nickel that can produce a mild reaction, causing a skin discoloration. Chemical activity resulting from perspiration in the area of jewelry contact sometimes contributes to the allergic reaction. Among cosmetics that may be involved in allergic reactions are certain permanent-wave lotions, eyelash dyes, face powders, permanent hair dyes, hair-spray lacquers, and skin-tanning agents. Of course, not all persons are equally sensitive to ingredients known to be allergens, and in most cases, a similar product with different ingredients can be substituted for the cosmetic causing allergic reactions. For more information on skin allergies, see "Disorders of the Skin" in Ch. 21, *Skin and Hair.*

Environmental Hypersensitivities

Environmental agents such as sunlight, heat, excessive cold, and pressure are known to produce allergy-like reactions in certain individuals. Exposure to cold, for example, can result in hives and may even lead to a drop in blood pressure, or to fainting, severe shock, and sometimes death. Research into the causes of hypersensitivity to cold has shown that cold urticaria, or hives, results from a histamine released from body tissues as they begin to warm up after a cold stimulus. Extremely high histamine levels coincide with episodes of very low blood pressure, the cause of fainting.

Although reaction of the body tissues to the invasion of microbes, such as bacteria, viruses, and other microorganisms, generally is not considered an allergic situation, the manner in which the body musters its defenses against the foreign materials is essentially the same as the way the antibodies are mobilized to neutralize other allergens. Thus, there is a similarity between infectious diseases and allergies.

Temporary Allergies

Occasionally, a change in the body's hormonal balance may trigger a hypersensitivity to a substance that previously had no effect on the individual. Pregnant women are especially susceptible to temporary allergies, which almost always disappear after childbirth. On the other hand, some women during pregnancy experience complete relief from allergies that had plagued them since childhood.

People who suffer from seasonal allergies, such as hay fever, often have heightened allergic reactions to dust, animal dander, and even certain foods, such as chocolate and pineapple, during the season when ragweed pollen or other airborne allergens are plentiful.

Diagnosis of Allergies

Some allergic reactions are outgrown; some don't develop until adulthood; some become increasingly severe over the years, because each repeated exposure makes the body more sensitive to the allergen. In many instances, the irritating substance is easily identified, after which it can be avoided. In other cases, it may take a long series of tests before the offending allergen is tracked down.

Medical History

If a person suspects he may have an allergy, he should first consult a physician, who will determine whether the patient should be referred to an allergy specialist. The physician or allergist will first take a complete medical history and check the patient's general health. Not infrequently, the source of an allergy can be found by general questioning about the patient's lifestyle. For example, the reaction may occur only immediately after the patient eats seafood. Or a patient may have an apparently chronic allergy but be unaware that it may be related to daily meals that include milk and eggs. A patient who keeps several cats or sleeps every night with a dog in the bedroom may not realize that an asthmatic condition actually is an allergic reaction to dander from the fur of the animal.

The history taken by the physician will include questions about other known allergies, allergies suffered by other members of the family, variations in symptoms according to the weather, time of day, and season of the year. The symptoms may be related to a change in working conditions or, if resulting from house dust, for example, the symptoms may diminish during periods of outdoor exercise. A person sensitive to cold may unwittingly exacerbate the symptoms with cold drinks, while another person who is sensitive to heat may not realize that symptoms can be triggered by hot drinks but relieved by cold drinks.

Skin Testing

If the patient is referred to an allergy specialist, the allergist will continue tracking down the suspected allergen by conducting skin tests.

Scratch Test

Based on information in the medical history of the patient and the allergist's knowledge of molds, pollens, and other airborne allergens in the geographical area, the allergist will conduct what is called a *scratch test.*

A diluted amount of a suspected allergen is applied to a small scratch on the patient's arm or back. If the results of the scratch test are inconclusive, a more sensitive test may be tried.

Intracutaneous Test

In the *intracutaneous,* or *intradermal* test, a very small amount of the suspected allergen is injected into the underlayer of skin called the *dermis.* The intracutaneous test also may be used to verify the results of a positive scratch test. With either test, a positive reaction usually consists of a raised reddish welt, or *wheal.* The welt should develop within 15 or 30 minutes if that particular allergen is the cause of the symptoms.

Culture Plates

If the allergen has been identified, or if the allergist still suspects a substance in the environment of the patient despite negative or inconclusive tests, the patient may be given a set of culture plates to place around his home and office or work area. If the allergen has been identified, the culture plates can help the physician and patient learn where his exposure to the substance takes place. If the allergen is not known, the cultures may pick up samples of less common allergens that the specialist can test.

Mucosal Test

Another kind of approach, the *mucosal test,* sometimes is used by allergists when skin tests fail to show positive results despite good evidence that a particular allergen is the cause of symptoms. The allergist using the mucosal test applies a diluted solution of the suspected allergen directly to the mucous membranes of the patient, usually on the inner surface of a nostril or by aerosol spray into the bronchial passages. In some cases, the allergic reaction occurs immediately and medication is administered quickly to counter the effects. Because of the possibility of a severe reaction in a hypersensitive patient, the mucosal test is not employed if other techniques seem to be effective.

Relief from Allergies

Other Tests

Allergists have other ways to test for allergies. They can, for example, use the *prick test,* a kind of skin test in which a physician or nurse pricks the skin as many as 30 or 40 times. On each pricked spot a drop of a watery solution is dropped; the solution contains a small amount of one allergen. A red welt appears on the spot within 15 to 30 minutes if the patient is allergic. Using another approach, an *elimination diet,* an allergist may specify a diet that omits certain foods for stated periods. Improvement in the patient's condition while avoiding certain foods usually indicates that the individual has an allergy to that food.

A variation of the prick test involves injection of small amounts of food in solution under the skin or application of the solution under the tongue. If the injection or drops provoke reactions, an allergy is indicated.

Avoidance

For a patient sensitive to a particular type of allergen, such as molds, complete avoidance of the substance can be difficult, but some steps can be taken to avoid undue exposure. For example, the mold allergy sufferer should avoid areas of his home, business, or recreational places that are likely spots for mold spores to be produced. These would include areas of deep shade or heavy vegetation; basements; refrigerator drip trays; garbage pails; air conditioners; bathrooms; humidifiers; dead leaves or wood logs; barns or silos; breweries, dairies, or any place where food is stored; and old foam, rubber pillows, and mattresses.

Medication

To supplement avoidance measures, the allergist may prescribe medications that will significantly reduce or relieve the irritating symptoms of the allergic reaction. Antihistamines, corticosteroids, and a drug called cromolyn sodium are among medications that may be prescribed, depending upon the nature and severity of the patient's reactions to the allergen.

Immunotherapy

If avoidance measures and medications do not control the symptoms effectively, the allergist may suggest *immunotherapy* ("allergy shots"). Immunotherapy consists of injections of a diluted amount of the allergen, a technique similar to that used in the skin tests. The objective of immunotherapy is to cause the immune system to become less sensitive to the allergen. It is thought that the incremental increases of the allergen may cause the production of an antibody that reduces the allergy symptoms when the allergen is encountered in the future.

A small amount of a very weak extract is injected once or twice a week at first. The strength of the extract is gradually increased, and the injeclions are given less frequently as relief from the symptoms is realized. The injections are continued until the patient experiences complete relief of the symptoms for a period of two or three years. However, some people may have to continue the injections for longer time spans. Even though the treatments may relieve the symptoms, they may not cure the allergy.

Identification Cards

Any person subject to severe disabling allergy attacks by a known allergen should carry a card describing both the allergic reaction and the allergen. Detailed information can be obtained from the Asthma and Allergy Foundation of America, 1233 20th Street, NW, Suite 402, Washington, DC 20036, (800) 727-8402. See also "Allergic Respiratory Diseases" in Ch. 12, *Diseases of the Respiratory System,* and "Asthma Attack" in Ch. 35, *Medical Emergencies.*

25

Women's Health

The special health matters that are related to a woman's reproductive system belong to the branch of medicine known as *gynecology*. *Obstetrics* is a closely related specialty associated with pregnancy and childbirth. The distinction is something of a technicality for most patients, since obstetricians usually are quite capable of handling gynecological cases and vice versa. The practice of obstetrics and gynecology is commonly combined in a medical service identified by the contraction *Ob-Gyn*. However, there are medical matters that are specifically concerned with female reproductive organs and related tissues but have little to do with obstetrics. For a discussion of obstetrics, see "Infertility, Pregnancy, and Childbirth" in Ch. 4, *The Beginning of a Family*.

The Gynecological Examination

What should a woman expect on her first visit to a gynecologist? First, the gynecologist will interview her, asking about her family, her medical history, and any fears or apprehensions she may have about her personal health. The woman's answers and comments are written into her medical records for future reference. The information can contain important clues that may help in diagnosing any present or future disorders.

A sample of urine and a sample of blood are usually obtained for laboratory tests. During the ensuing physical examination, the woman lies on a special examination table with her feet in metal stirrups and her knees apart. A nurse will be present to assist the doctor. While she is in the *lithotomy position,* the woman's abdomen will be palpated for lumps or other abnormalities. The breasts also will be palpated for possible lumps. Then an external inspection of the vulva and surrounding areas is made by the physician, followed by internal inspection, in which a speculum is used to spread apart the sides of the vagina so that the cervix is exposed. A digital examination (using the fingers) is made of the walls of the vagina and rectum and the neighboring tissue areas, in a search for possible growths or other abnormal conditions. And a sample of cells and secretions from the cervix is taken for a Pap-smear test.

In addition to the examination of the breasts and reproductive system, the gynecologist usually conducts a general physical examination, recording information about height, weight, blood pressure, heart and lung condition, and so on. The routine physical examination, like the medical history, provides additional clues that, when added to the results of the examination of the breasts and reproductive system, will give a complete picture of the patient's gynecological health.

Following the examination, the gynecologist discusses his appraisal of the woman's condition and answers questions. He will discuss whatever treatment she needs. Medications can be explained at this time, including reasons why certain drugs can or should not be taken. If any surgery or further testing is recommended, those aspects of the health picture also should be discussed in some detail. Any important information that might be misunderstood or forgotten should be jotted down for future reference.

Results of some laboratory tests and the Pap smear are not usually available for several days. But the physician or nurse will contact the patient when the results are available and advise if she should return in the near future for follow-up testing. The American Cancer Society and the American College of Obstetricians and

The Female Reproductive System

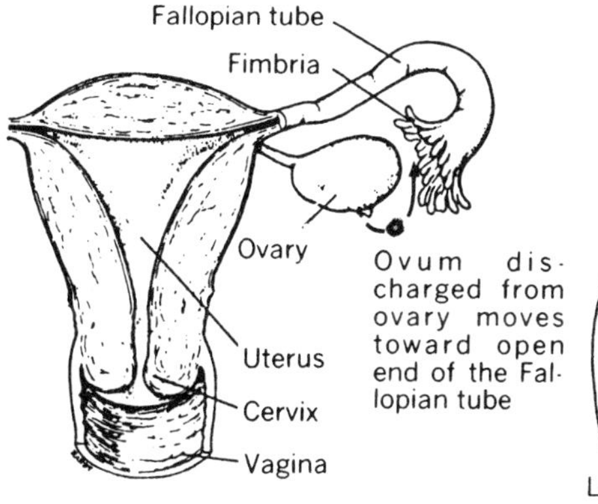

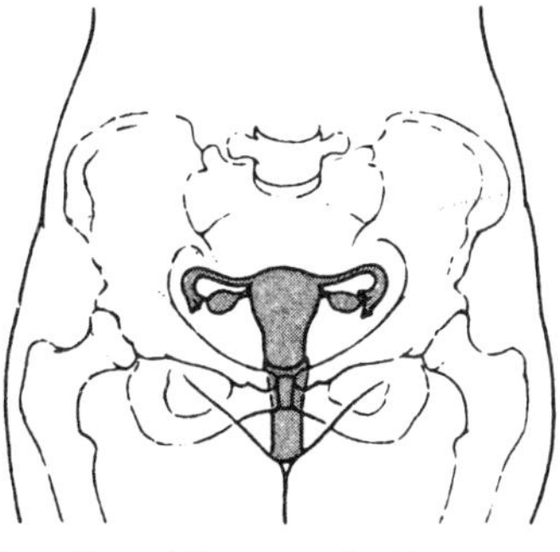

Location of the reproductive organs

Gynecologists agree (1) that all women should have their first Pap smear when they become sexually active or at age 18, whichever occurs first; (2) that every woman should have a yearly Pap smear for the following two years; and (3) that later tests should be administered at the physician's discretion if the first three Pap smears are negative. The woman also should discuss arrangements for future checkups or Pap smear tests rather than wait until signs or symptoms of a serious disorder warrant an immediate visit.

Menstrual Disorders

Among the health concerns of women that specifically belong to gynecology are menstrual disorders. Normally, the first menstrual period (menarche) occurs about age 12 or 13, or sometimes earlier or later. Periods are generally irregular for the first year or two, and then they tend to recur at intervals of 24 to 32 days. Each period begins about two weeks after ovulation, or the release of an egg cell (ovum) from the ovary—unless, of course, the ovum happens to be fertilized in the interval and pregnancy interrupts the whole process.

The menstrual flow, which lasts from three to seven days, is composed mainly of serum, mucus, and dead cells shed from the lining (endometrium) of the uterus. The loss of blood is minimal, usually from two to four ounces. The volume of flow, as well as the time schedule, tends to be fairly regular for most women. When one's menstrual pattern varies noticeably from the expected pattern, and in the absence of pregnancy, it may be a sign of a physical or emotional disorder.

Amenorrhea

Failure to menstruate is called *amenorrhea.* Amenorrhea is a natural effect of pregnancy and of nursing a baby. In an older woman, it may be a sign of menopause. But if a nonpregnant or nonnursing woman after menarche and before menopause (say between the ages of 17 or 18 and 52) fails to menstruate for two or more periods, she should bring it to the attention of a doctor—unless, of course, she has undergone a hysterectomy or other surgical or medical treatment that eliminates menstruation.

Primary Amenorrhea

When menarche has not occurred by the age of 16 or 17, the absence of menstruation is called *primary amenorrhea.* In such a case, a physical examination may show that an imperforate hymen or a closed cervix is obstructing the flow of menses, or a congenital defect may be interfering with menstruation. In almost all cases, menarche can be started with a bit of minor surgery, by treatment of any existing systemic disease, or by the injection of sex hormones; or it will start spontaneously later.

Secondary Amenorrhea

When menstrual periods cease after menarche, the condition is known as *secondary,* or *acquired, amenorrhea.* Secondary amenorrhea may involve missing a single menstrual period or many periods in consecutive months. Among possible causes of interrupted menstruation are certain medications, drugs of abuse, emotional stress, normal fluctuations in ovarian activity in the first few years after menarche, and a number of organic diseases. Medicines that can disrupt normal menstrual activity include tranquilizers and other psychotropic (mind-affecting) drugs that apparently influence hormonal activity in the brain centers, amphetamines, and oral contraceptives. When a particular medication is found to be the cause of amenorrhea, the medical treatment may be judged to be more important than maintaining normal menstrual cycles. When the use of oral contraceptives is followed by amenorrhea for six or more months, normal menstrual activity may resume eventually, but it can often be started sooner by a prescribed medication. Among drugs of abuse known to cause amenorrhea are alcohol and opium-based drugs.

Just as the mind-altering effects of psychotropic drugs involve the hypothalamus and pituitary glands in the brain, which control the hormones that regulate menstrual functions, emotional stress seems to have a parallel influence on the incidence of amenorrhea. *Anorexia nervosa,* a disorder associated with emaciation resulting from an emotional disturbance, also can result in an interruption of menstruation.

Other factors contributing to secondary amenorrhea are measles, mumps, and other infections; cysts and tumors of the ovaries; changes in the tissues lining the vagina or uterus; premature aging of the ovaries; diabetes; obesity; anemia; leukemia; and Hodgkin's disease. In many cases, normal or near-normal menstrual function can be restored by medical treatment, such as administration of hormones, or by surgery, or both. In one type of amenorrhea, marked by adhesion of the walls of the uterus, curettage (scraping of the uterus) is followed by insertion of an intrauterine contraceptive device (IUD) to help hold the uterine walls apart.

Menorrhagia

Almost the opposite of amenorrhea is *menorrhagia,* an excessive menstrual flow. The causes of menorrhagia are as varied as those associated with amenorrhea. They include influenza and other infectious diseases, emotional stress, polyps of the cervical or uterine tissues, hypertension, congestive heart failure, leukemia, and blood coagulation disorders. Menorrhagia may occur during the early stages of a young woman's reproductive life soon after reaching puberty, and medical treatment may be necessary to control the excessive loss of blood. In some cases, dilation and curettage is recommended in addition to the administration of hormones and other medications, such as iron tablets to correct anemia resulting from the loss of red blood cells.

Dilation and Curettage

Dilation and curettage, generally referred to as *D and C,* is a procedure in which the cervix is dilated and the cavity of the uterus is cleaned out by a scooplike instrument, a curette. The same procedure is sometimes used to abort an embryo or to remove a tumor or a polyp.

Although it takes only a few minutes to perform a D and C, the procedure is done in a hospital while the patient is anesthetized. There is no afterpain, only a dull discomfort in the lower pelvic region similar to menstrual awareness.

A physical examination is usually made to determine if there are tumors anywhere in the reproductive organs. Except where tumors are found to be a causative factor, most women will resume normal menstrual cycles after treatment of menorrhagia with medications and D and C. For women beyond the age of 40, the physician may recommend a hysterectomy to prevent recurrence of excessive menstrual blood loss.

Polymenorrhea and Metrorrhagia

These medical terms refer to two other ways in which menstrual periods may depart from typical patterns. *Polymenorrhea* is abnormally frequent menstruation, so that menstrual periods occur at intervals of less than 21 days. This short interval may be the natural established pattern for some women. If it is not, the cause may be physical or emotional stress. *Metrorrhagia* is marked by menstrual bleeding that occurs erratically at unpredictable times. It may be the result of a cyst in the lining of the uterus, a tumor in the reproductive tract, polyps, or some hormonal imbalance, including a disorder of the thyroid gland.

Dysmenorrhea

Abdominal or pelvic pain occurring just before or along with the onset of menstruation is known as *dysmenorrhea.* The symptoms include severe colicky abdominal cramps, backache, headache, and, in some cases, nausea and vomiting. As with amenorrhea, there are two general types of dysmenorrhea, primary and secondary.

Primary Dysmenorrhea

This type includes all cases in which no organic disorder is associated with the symptoms, which are presumed to be a result of uterine contractions and emotional factors. More than 75 percent of all cases are of this type. Primary dysmenorrhea generally begins before age 25, but it may appear at any time from menarche to menopause. It frequently ends with the birth of the first child.

Since primary dysmenorrhea by definition occurs in the absence of organic disease, the diagnosis can be made only after a careful medical history is compiled and a special study of the reproductive organs is made to ensure that no disorder has been overlooked. In some cases, oral contraceptives may be prescribed because of the effect such drugs have in suppressing ovulation; the contraceptives prevent the natural production of the hormone progesterone, which is responsible for certain tissue changes associated with the discomfort of dysmenorrhea. Analgesic drugs to relieve pain and medications that help to relax muscles may be prescribed. Medication is often less beneficial, however, than emotional support—including the easing of any stress at home, school, or work, and reassurance about the worries sometimes associated with menstruation.

Secondary Dysmenorrhea

This condition comprises all menstrual pain that is a result of or associated with an organic disease of the reproductive organs, such as endometriosis, to cite just one example. Secondary dysmenorrhea can occur at any age.

Premenstrual Syndrome

Premenstrual syndrome (PMS) has emerged in recent years as a major challenge to the medical profession. PMS clinics have begun to offer specialized counseling, physical examinations, and treatment for women unable to cope with the disorder. Treatment regimens or therapies range from aspirin to large doses of sex hormones, diet programs, and exercise.

A group of related symptoms, PMS involves both psychological and physical changes. Among the psychological are lethargy, tension, irritability, depression, and feelings of aggression. The physical signs may include headache, bloating, asthma, and more exotic problems, such as recurrent herpes or hives. In all, more

Ovarian Cycle

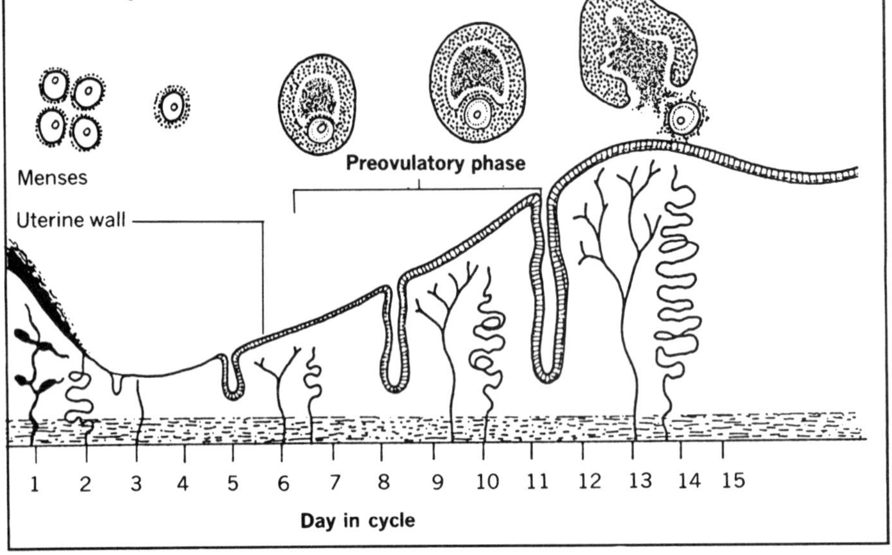

than 300 different symptoms have been attributed to PMS.

The symptoms, gynecologists warn, should become "disturbing" before they are labeled PMS. Restlessness, minor cramps, and other premenstrual problems may indicate that menstruation is about to start but do not necessarily point to PMS. Such minor problems are called *menstrual molimina.* Cramping and other painful conditions occurring during menstruation are referred to as *dysmenorrhea* (see above).

Of the many treatments for PMS, none has proved uniformly effective. This is because the cause or causes of PMS are not totally understood. Most commonly, physicians believe the disorder represents some basic imbalance in the major female hormones, estrogen and progesterone. Thus one treatment calls for administration of "natural" progesterone to correct the supposed imbalance.

Another common treatment suggested for PMS is vitamin B_6, although the treatment remains partly experimental. Some researchers and physicians, however, have reported disturbing neurological side-effects.

Other theories and treatments exist. Some physicians who have studied PMS and its symptoms believe *prolactin,* a pituitary hormone that stimulates milk secretion, and PMS are associated. A diet and nutrition theory has evolved out of findings that some women report improvement after going on a hypoglycemic diet.

Treated over a substantial period, PMS victims often find that diagnostic tests combined with diet and exercise regimens and vitamin therapy bring good results. If such initial attempts fail, the physician may prescribe medications. In all cases of PMS, according to researchers, psychological support for the sufferer may be important to treatment effectiveness.

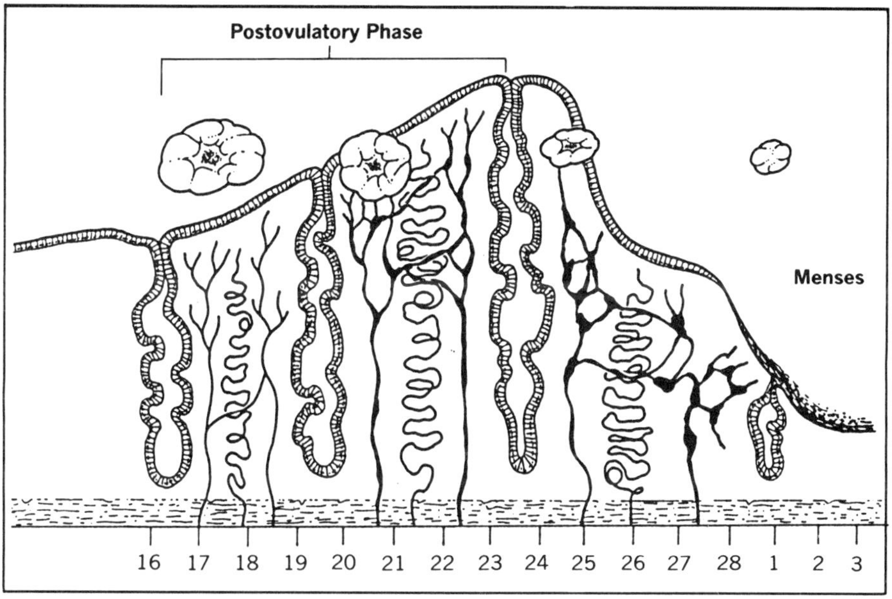

Minor Menstrual Problems

Blood Clots

There is not usually any cause for alarm if blood clots are expelled during menstruation. Ordinarily, the menstrual flow is completely liquefied, but a few clots tend to appear when the flow is profuse. However, if many clots appear and the flow seems excessive, medical advice is recommended, since these conditions may be a sign of fibroid tumors in the uterus.

Oral Contraceptives

Women on combination birth-control pills can expect to see a changed menstrual pattern. The flow becomes slighter than before and very regular. For a discussion of oral contraceptives, see "Birth Control" in Ch. 4, *The Beginning of a Family.*

Odor

The menstrual flow of a healthy woman generally has a mild odor that develops when it is exposed to the air or to the vulva. Some women are concerned about this odor, although it usually is not offensive. When it is, it tends to be associated with inadequate bathing. Detergents are added to some commercial tampons and pad products, and special deodorants have been developed to mask the odor. However, such materials produce allergic reactions in some women, and they can have the unfortunate effect of masking an odor that may be the sign of an abnormal condition.

Onset of Menopause

Menstrual irregularities almost always precede the natural cessation of menstrual function. For a full discussion of menopause, see Ch. 5, *The Middle Years*.

Postmenopausal Bleeding

Bleeding that occurs after the final cessation of menstrual activity should be seen as an urgent signal to seek medical advice. The bleeding may be painless or painful and may range from occasional spotting that is brownish or bright red to rather profuse bleeding that continues for several days or more. The various signs and symptoms should be noted carefully because they can help suggest to a physician the possible cause of bleeding. Bleeding after the menopause is often a sign of cancer of the cervix or the lining of the uterus, but there is a wide variety of other possible causes, including polyps, ulcers, hypertensive heart disease, an ovarian tumor, or infection. In many cases, the problem can be treated by dilation and curettage or withdrawal of any hormone medications, such as estrogens prescribed for menopausal symptoms, or both. In these cases, if D and C and treatment and discontinuance of hormone therapy fail, the physician may advise a hysterectomy.

Infections of the Reproductive Tract

Vaginal and other reproductive tract infections are among the most common gynecological problems, and among the most stubborn to treat successfully.

Leukorrhea

A whitish, somewhat viscid discharge from the vagina, which is known medically as *leukorrhea,* may be quite normal, especially if it is not continual but occurs only intermittently—prior to menstruation, for example, or associated with sexual excitation. It may also be increased when oral contraceptives are used.

Constant leukorrhea, on the other hand, often is a symptom of an abnormality. Leukorrhea resulting from disease can occur at any age. It is generally associated with an infection of the lower reproductive tract. The discharge may occur without any discomfort, but in some cases there is itching, irritation, and *dyspareunia*—or painful intercourse.

Laboratory tests of vaginal secretions may be needed to help identify the precise cause of the discharge. Leukorrhea can result from vaginal ulcers; a tumor of the vagina, uterus, or fallopian tubes; gonorrhea; or infection by any of various disease organisms of the vulva, vagina, cervix, uterus, or tubes. It may also result from an abnormality of menstrual function, or even emotional stress.

Treatment, of course, depends on the cause. If the discharge is because of an infection, care must be taken to avoid being reinfected or transmitting the disease organism through sexual contact or possibly contaminated underclothing, etc.

Moniliasis

Moniliasis, also known as *candidiasis,* is an infection by a yeastlike fungus that invades mucous membrane and sometimes skin in various parts of the body. Inside the mouth, the organism causes thrush, most commonly in babies. When the organism invades the vaginal area, it causes a scant white discharge of a thick consistency resembling that of cottage cheese. There is itching, burning, and swelling of the labial and vulvar areas. The symptoms tend to worsen just before the menstrual period. The occurrence of the disease is thought by some researchers to be fostered by oral contraceptives. Antibiotic therapy may increase the moniliasis organism because it destroys many of the benign organisms that regularly share the same environment.

Moniliasis is treated with suppositories, creams, and other medications. The woman's partner should be treated at the same time to prevent a cycle of reinfection because the fungus will otherwise spread to the genital tissues of the man.

Trichomoniasis

A type of leukorrhea that consists of a copious yellow to green frothy and fetid discharge is caused by infection by the *Trichomonas* organism. The organism causes an irritating itching condition that tends to set in or worsen just after a menstrual period. The condition is diagnosed by a test similar to a Pap smear, made with a specimen taken from the vagina. Trichomonas organisms, if present, are easy to identify under a microscope;

they are pear-shaped protozoa with three to five whiplike tails.

The organism favors warm, moist areas, such as genital tissues, but it can also survive in damp towels and washcloths, around toilet seats, and on beaches and the perimeters of swimming pools. Thus it can spread from one member of a family to other members and from one woman to other women. *Trichomoniasis* is not technically a venereal disease, but it can be transmitted by sexual contact. When one partner is infected with trichomoniasis, both must be treated at the same time and a condom must be worn during intercourse.

Several drugs are available for treating trichomoniasis, including tablets taken orally and suppositories inserted in the vagina. The tablets are taken for ten days, then an examination is made to determine if any *Trichomonas* organisms are still present. Medication may be continued for several months if the infection resists the drug—studies show that the organism appears to survive in about 10 percent of treated cases.

Herpes Simplex Virus Type 2

Herpes is acquired by contact with the mucous membranes of an infected person. The mucous membrane of the mouth and lips, the genitals, or the rectum may be affected. The causative agent is known as *herpes simplex virus Type II,* or *HSV-II.* It is similar to but not the same as the virus that causes fever blisters, or cold sores, which is Type *I* (HSV-I). The virus is associated with some spontaneous abortions. If the mother has blisters at the time of delivery, the virus can be transmitted to the baby as he or she passes through the vagina. The central nervous system, including the brain, may be damaged by the virus if the baby becomes infected. To avoid exposure to the virus, a caesarian delivery is recommended.

Symptoms

Patients with their first HSV-II infection usually complain of intense itching, painful blisterlike eruptions, and ulcerated patches with a discharge. Other symptoms may include genital pain and vaginal bleeding. Fever, swelling, difficult urination, and a general feeling of ill health and lack of appetite may accompany the infection.

Symptoms may subside after a few weeks, but recurrences are common, though they are less painful and of shorter duration. There is no known cure for the viral infection.

Treatment

No drug has been found to attack the viruses while they are "hibernating" in cells at the base of the spine. But one antiviral drug, *acyclovir,* has been found to reduce recurrent outbreaks and to block flareups for up to several months. Taken orally in pill form, acyclovir is ingested daily. Some patients can stop taking acyclovir and still have no further flare-ups. Researchers have discovered that the capsules kill or neutralize the herpes viruses only when they are active. Because of evidence that the virus may be related to the subsequent development of cervical cancer, women sufferers should have Pap-smear tests at intervals of six months instead of the usual twelve.

Pelvic Inflammatory Disease

Pelvic inflammatory disease, or PID, is on the increase in the female population. Commonly caused by bacteria from other diseases such as chlamydia or gonorrhea, PID may go for years without detection. Frequently symptomless, PID infects and destroys the interior of the reproductive system. It attacks the fallopian tubes and uterine lining, leaving permanent scarring. The increase in the number of ectopic pregnancies (fallopian tube pregnancies) is believed to stem from the increase in women who have scarring from PID. The increase in sterility in the population is also linked directly to PID scarring.

One is seven women in the United States has been infected with PID. Treatment for both partners involves antibiotics to kill the bacteria, and treatment of any original disease that may have caused it. Douching should be avoided if PID is suspected. Symptoms include abdominal tenderness or pain, vaginal discharge, or dull ache or twitching in the uterine cavity.

Blood tests and cultures for chlamydia or other diseases should be done. Two-thirds of PID cases are from sexual transmission. If left untreated, PID can cause sterility, miscarriage, ectopic pregnancy, blood infection, and eventually death.

Disorders of the Urinary System

Both men and women are subject to disorders of the urinary system. There are, however, a few disorders that affect women chiefly or women only, for reasons related to anatomical structure. See also Ch. 17, *Diseases of the Urinogenital System.*

Inflammation of the Bladder

Any inflammation of the bladder is known medically as *cystitis*. Factors such as urinary tract stones, injury, and obstructions to the normal flow of urine can aggravate or cause cystitis in either sex. Cystitis resulting from infectious organisms, however, is much more common in women than in men. This is understandable in view of the relative shortness of the female urethra—the tube through which urine is discharged from the bladder and through which infectious organisms can reach the bladder from the outside. In addition, the anus and the vagina, both of which may frequently be sources of infection, are situated relatively close to the external opening of the female urethra.

In women generally, the symptoms of cystitis may include a burning sensation around the edges of the vulva. There is usually a frequent urge to urinate and difficulty or pain (*dysuria*) associated with urination. Urinary retention and dehydration, which are generally under the control of the individual, can contribute to the spread of infection once it begins. The lining of the urinary bladder is relatively resistant to infection by most microorganisms as long as the normal flow of liquids through the urinary tract is maintained. In cases that do not yield quickly to copious fluid intake, there are medications that may be prescribed to cure the infection. Where urinary frequency or difficulty is accompanied by the appearance of blood in the urine, a physician should be consulted immediately.

Honeymoon Cystitis

One type of cystitis tends to occur mostly in young women during the first few weeks of frequent sexual activity, to which it is attributed. Sexual activity may result in swelling of the urethra and the neck of the bladder, making urination difficult. The inflammation of these tissues can in turn make them more susceptible to infection. A treatment recommended specifically for honeymoon cystitis is to drink large quantities of water or other fluids and to empty the bladder before and after engaging in sexual intercourse. Adequate lubrication, such as K-Y Jelly™ or a water-soluble product, is also important. Medical care should be sought if the condition persists.

Urethral Disorders

The urethra is perforce involved in the inflammation of cystitis because it is the route by which infectious organisms reach the bladder. In addition, there are disorders that are essentially confined to the urethra.

Urethral Caruncle

Urethral caruncle is a rather uncommon urinary tract disorder that tends to be confined to women after the menopause. A *caruncle* (not to be confused with *carbuncle*) is a small, red, fleshy outgrowth. It may be visible near the opening of the urethra. A caruncle growing from the cells of the urethra may be a sign of a bacterial infection, a tumor, or any of several other possible conditions. Symptoms may include vaginal bleeding, pain, tenderness, painful sexual intercourse (dyspareunia), a whitish, viscid discharge, and difficulty in urinating. A physician should be consulted when such symptoms are present. A tissue biopsy and Pap smear may be taken to diagnose the condition. Caruncles are easily treated and of no long-term consequence.

Urethral Diverticulum

Another disorder of the urethra is a *urethral diverticulum,* or outpocketing of the urethra. The problem can be caused by a developmental malformation, an injury, inflammation, a cyst, a urinary stone, or a venereal disease. Stones are a common cause, and in some patients there may be more than one diverticulum. The symptoms may include discomfort and urinary difficulty, as well as dyspareunia. The disorder can be diagnosed with the help of X-ray photographs of the region of the urethra and bladder after they have been filled with a radiopaque substance that flows into any diverticula that may be present.

Treatment of a urethral diverticulum includes antibiotics to stop infection, medications to relieve pain and discomfort, and douches. In some cases, surgery is needed to eliminate the diverticula.

Structural Anomalies

Various kinds of injury may be sustained by the female reproductive system and other abdominal organs, chiefly as a result of childbearing. The structural damage can generally be repaired by surgical measures.

Fistula

An abnormal opening between two organs or from an organ to the outside of the body is known as a *fistula.* Fistulas may involve the urinary and reproductive systems of a woman. Damage to the organs during pregnancy or surgery, for example, can result in a fistula between the urethra and the vagina, causing urinary incontinence. A similar kind of fistula can develop between the rectum and the vagina as a result of injury, complications of pregnancy, or surgery. Disorders of this sort must be repaired surgically.

Prolapsed Uterus

The uterus normally rests on the floor of the pelvis, held in position by numerous ligaments. Damage to the ligaments and other supporting tissues causes the uterus to descend, or *prolapse,* into the vagina. There are various degrees of prolapse, ranging from a slight intrusion of the uterus into the vagina to a severe condition in which the cervix of the uterus protrudes out of the vaginal orifice. Prolapse of the uterus resembles a hernia but is not a true hernia, because the opening through which the uterus protrudes is a normal one.

Backache and a feeling of heaviness in the pelvic region may accompany the condition. Many women complain of a "dragging" sensation. An assortment of complications may involve neighboring organ systems; bleeding and ulceration of the uterus are not uncommon. Coughing and straining can aggravate the symptoms.

Like the various types of hernia, a prolapsed uterus does not improve without treatment but tends instead to worsen gradually. The only permanent treatment is surgical repair. In mild cases, a woman may get relief from symptoms through exercises intended to strengthen the muscles of the pelvic region. Supporting devices,

Prolapsed Uterus

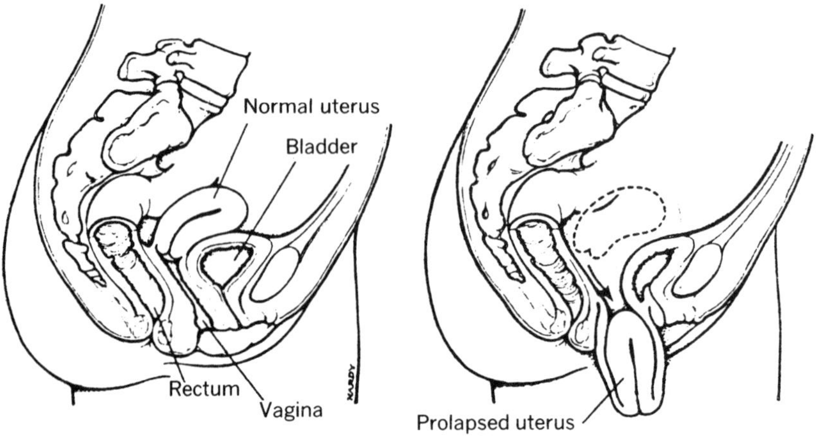

such as an inflatable, doughnut-shaped pessary, are available as temporary methods of correcting a prolapse. Preventive exercises may be recommended for childbearing women who want to avoid weakened muscles and ligaments leading to prolapse.

Tipped Uterus

The uterus may be out of its normal position without being prolapsed. A malpositioned uterus may be "tipped" forward, backward, or otherwise be out of alignment with neighboring organs. A malpositioned uterus may cause no symptoms, or it may be associated with dysmenorrhea or infertility. If a malpositioned uterus causes pain, bleeding, or other problems, the condition can be corrected surgically, or a pessary support may relieve the symptoms. Displacement of the uterus occasionally is the result of a separate pelvic disease that requires treatment.

Hernias of the Vaginal Wall

The wall of the vagina may be ruptured in childbirth, especially in a mul-

Hernias of the Vaginal Wall

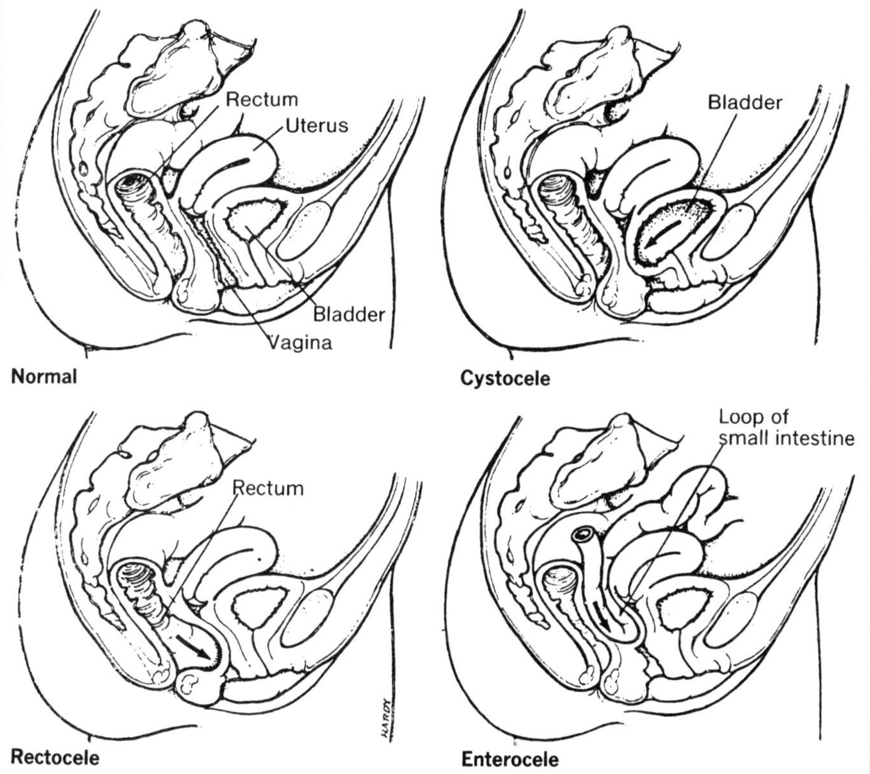

tiple delivery or birth of a larger-than-average baby. The kind of hernia depends on the exact site of the rupture and what organ happens to lie against the vaginal wall at that point. The condition may be further complicated by a prolapsed uterus. Careful examination of the patient and X-ray pictures may be necessary to determine whether just one or several of the urinary, reproductive, and gastrointestinal organs in the pelvic cavity are involved.

Cystocele

Cystocele is a hernia involving the bladder and the vagina. Structurally, part of the bladder protrudes through the wall of the vagina. The symptoms, in addition to a feeling of pressure deep in the vagina, may be urinary difficulties, such as incontinence, a frequent urge to urinate, and inability to completely empty the bladder. Residual urine in the bladder may contribute to infection and inflammation of the bladder. Treatment includes surgery to correct the condition, pessaries if needed to support the structures, and medications to control infection.

Rectocele

A hernia involving the tissues separating the vagina and the rectum, behind the vagina, is called a *rectocele.* The symptoms are a feeling of fullness in the vagina and difficulty in defecating. Enemas or laxatives may be needed to relieve constipation because straining, or even coughing, can aggravate the condition. Surgery is the only permanently effective treatment. Special diets, laxatives, and rectal suppositories may be prescribed pending surgery.

Enterocele

A herniation of the small intestine into the vagina is called an *enterocele.* Some of the symptoms are similar to those of other hernias involving the vaginal wall, and in addition, a patient with an enterocele may experience abdominal cramps shortly after eating. An enterocele can be dangerous, as well as uncomfortable, because a segment of the small bowel can become trapped and obstructed, requiring emergency surgery.

Varicose Veins

Varicose veins of the vulva, vagina, and neighboring areas are another possible effect of pregnancy, although the legs are more often affected. Obesity, reduced physical activity during pregnancy, and circulatory changes associated with pregnancy can contribute to the development of varicose veins. The symptoms generally are limited to discomfort, although there can be bleeding, particularly at the time of childbirth. Varicose veins that occur in the vulva and vagina during pregnancy and cause discomfort can be treated surgically during the early months of pregnancy. Some drugs and supportive therapy can be used to help relieve symptoms. But many physicians recommend that surgical stripping of veins be delayed until after the pregnancy has been terminated. A complication of untreated varicose veins can be development of blood clots in the abnormal blood vessels. For a discussion of varicose veins of the legs during pregnancy, see "Leg Cramps and Varicose Veins" in Ch. 4, *The Beginning of a Family.*

Varicose Veins

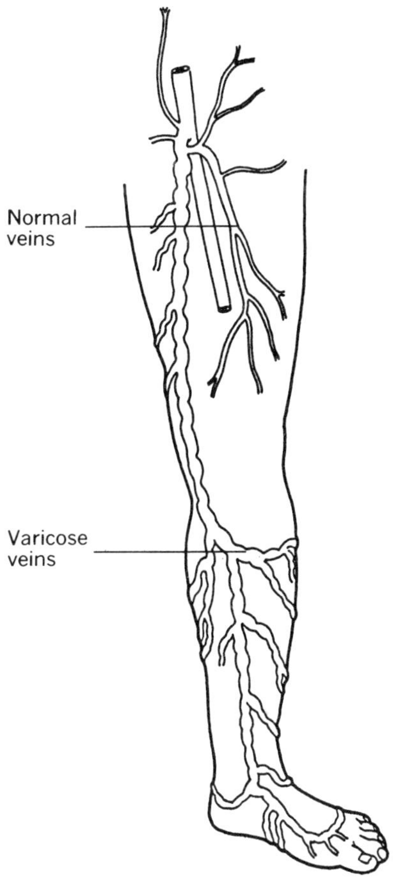

Benign Neoplasms

The word *neoplasm* refers to any abnormal proliferation of tissue that serves no useful function. There are numerous kinds of neoplasms but just two main groups—cancerous, or *malignant;* or noncancerous, or *benign.* In ordinary speech the word *benign* suggests some positive benefit, but a benign neoplasm, though noncancerous, may in fact be harmful to health or at least worrisome. Benign neoplasms that are of particular concern to women are discussed below.

Cysts

A *cyst* is a sac containing a gaseous, fluid, or semisolid material. (Certain normal anatomical structures, like the urinary bladder, are technically known as cysts—hence the term *cystitis* for inflammation of the bladder.) Abnormal, or neoplastic, cysts can develop at several sites within the urinary and reproductive systems.

Vaginal Cysts

A cyst may develop in a gland at the opening of the vagina as a result of infection with a venereal or other disease. Such a cyst can block the flow of secretions from the gland and produce swelling and pain. Dyspareunia, or painful intercourse, is sometimes a symptom. A vaginal-gland cyst usually is treated with antibiotics and hot packs. In some cases, it may be necessary for a physician to make an incision to drain the cyst.

Ovarian Cysts

Cysts in the ovaries may be caused by a malfunction of physiological process or by a pathological condition. Some pathological cysts are malignant. The cysts in the ovaries generally are filled with fluid that may range in color from pale and clear to reddish brown, depending upon the source of the fluid. Some cysts are too small to be seen with the naked eye, whereas others may be four or five inches in diameter when symptoms begin to cause discomfort. There are several different kinds of ovarian cysts.

Follicular Cyst

A *follicular,* or *retention,* cyst is a physiological cyst and is one of the most common types. It develops in an old follicle in which an ovum for some reason has failed to break out of its capsule during the ovulation process. Ordinarily, the contents of such a follicle are resorbed, but sometimes a cyst develops. It rarely grows larger than about two inches in diameter. It may rupture but usually disappears after a few months. The symptoms may include pain with some uterine bleeding and dyspareunia. Treatment consists of warm douches, analgesics, and hormone therapy designed to restore normal ovarian activity. If the symptoms persist or the cyst continues to increase in size, or if serious complications occur, the physician may recommend exploratory surgery.

Occasionally such cysts, whether or not they rupture, produce symptoms that mimic those of appendicitis, with severe abdominal pain. The abdomen may become so tender that a physician cannot palpate the organs in order to distinguish between an ovarian cyst and appendicitis, particularly if the right ovary is involved. The symptoms occur at the time that ovulation would be expected. If the physician cannot be certain that the cause of the abdominal pain is indeed a cyst, for which surgery is not needed, he may recommend surgery anyway—just to be on the safe side.

Multiple follicular cysts, involving the ovaries on both sides (*bilateral polycystic ovaries*) can result in a syndrome (or group of symptoms) that includes infertility, obesity, and abnormal growth of body hair. All of these effects are related to a disruption of normal sex-hormone activity; they generally occur in young women, from teenagers to those in their 20s. The therapy includes both medical and surgical efforts to restore normal menstrual function, a diet to control obesity, and the use of various depilatory techniques to remove unwanted body hair.

Corpus Luteum Cyst

This kind of cyst may develop in the ovary following ovulation or during the early part of a pregnancy. The corpus luteum is a small, temporary gland that forms in the empty follicle after the ovum has been released from the ovary. Its function is to produce the hormone progesterone, which is important in preparing the endometrium, the lining of the uterus, to receive a fertilized ovum. The corpus luteum, however, also can be overproductive of a brownish fluid that fills the former follicular space, causing it to swell to a diameter of two or three inches. The cyst causes symptoms of pain and tenderness and may also result in a disruption of normal menstrual cycles in a woman who is not pregnant.

Most corpus luteum cysts gradually decrease in size without special treatment, except to relieve the symptoms. There may, however, be complications, such as torsion, or painful twisting of the ovary, or a rupture of the cyst. A ruptured corpus luteum cyst can result in hemorrhage and peritonitis, requiring immediate surgery.

Chocolate Cyst

So called because of their brownish-red color, chocolate cysts consist of misplaced endometrial tissue growing on the ovary instead of in its normal position lining the uterus. Chocolate cysts are among the largest of the ovarian cysts, ranging up to five or six inches in diameter. They cause symptoms associated with a variety of disorders of the reproductive system, including infertility, dyspareunia, and dysmenorrhea. Surgery usually is a favored method of therapy, the precise procedure depending upon the amount of ovarian tissue involved. A small chocolate cyst can be cauterized, but a large cyst may require removal of a portion of the ovary. See also "Cancer of the Ovary" later in this chapter.

Cysts of the Breast

Cysts are noncancerous tissues masses that may form in the milk glands or the ducts leading from the glands. They are caused by imbalances in ovarian hormones and they tend to develop in women of all ages and tend to disappear once women reach menopause. The cysts tend to fluctuate in size, often enlarging just before or during menstruation. Pain and tenderness are usually present, although painless cysts are sometimes discovered only when a woman examines her breasts for possible lumps. Cysts may be almost microscopic in size or as large as an inch or more in diameter. It is not uncommon for more than one cyst to occur at the same time in one breast or both.

A medical examination is recommended when any kind of lump can be felt in the breast tissue. This is particularly important for women who have passed menopause. The physician frequently can determine whether a lump is a result of a cyst or cancer by the patient's history and by physical examination, especially when repeated at intervals of several weeks. Mammography and ultrsound are used to confirm the diagnosis.

Women who are troubled by breast cysts may be helped by wearing a good brassiere at all times, even during sleep, to protect tender areas. The only medications available are those that relieve pain and discomfort—symptoms that usually subside when the menopause is reached.

Other Noncancerous Masses

A benign lump in the breast can be caused by either a fat deposit or an abscess. A fatty mass frequently forms if an injury to the breast damages adipose tissue. Because of a similarity of the symptoms to those of breast cancer, a biopsy is usually required to distinguish the lesion from a cancer. The involved tissue may in any case be removed surgically.

An abscess of the breast as a result of an infection, although a rare problem, may produce a lump that requires treatment with antibiotic medications or by an incision to drain the pus. Breast infections leading to abscesses are most likely to occur in nursing mothers but can also develop in women who are not lactating. When an infection develops in a breast being used to nurse a baby, nursing has to be discontinued temporarily while the infection is treated. See also "Cancer of the Breast" later in this chapter.

Polyps

A *polyp* is a strange-looking growth, even for an abnormal growth of tissue. It has been described as having the appearance of a tennis racket or a small mushroom. Polyps are found in many parts of the body, from the nose to the rectum. Usually they are harmless. But a polyp can result in discomfort or bleeding and require surgical excision. Although polyps generally are not cancerous, it is standard procedure to have the polyp tissue, like any excised tissue, tested in the laboratory. If malignant cells accompany a polyp, they are usually found at the base of the growth, which means that some of the tissue around the polyp must be excised along with the growth itself. Once a polyp is removed it does not grow again, although other polyps can occur in the same region.

Cervical Polyp

Polyps in the cervix are not uncommon, occurring most frequently in the years between menarche and menopause. A cervical polyp may be associated with vaginal bleeding or leukorrhea; the bleeding may occur after douching or sexual intercourse. In some cases, the bleeding is severe. Cervical polyps can usually be located visually by an examining physician and removed by minor surgery.

Endometrial Polyp

Endometrial polyps, which develop in the lining of the uterus, usually occur in women who are over 40, although they can develop at any age after menarche. They are frequently the cause of nonmenstrual bleeding. They tend to be much larger than polyps that grow in other organs of the body: an endometrial polyp may be rooted high in the uterus with a stem reaching all the way to the cervix. Such a polyp is usually located and removed during a D- and C- procedure. As in the case of a cervical polyp, the growth and a bit of surrounding tissue are studied for traces of cancer cells.

Benign Tumors

Tumors are rather firm growths that may be either benign or malignant. In practice, any tumor is regarded with suspicion unless malignancy is ruled out by actual laboratory tests. Even a benign tumor represents a tissue abnormality, and if untreated can produce symptoms that interfere with normal health and activity.

Fibromas

Among the more common of the benign tumors is the *fibroma,* commonly known as a *fibroid tumor,* composed of fibrous connective tissue. About one of every 20 ovarian tumors is a fibroma, and a similar growth in the uterus is the most common type of tumor found in that organ. Fibromas also occur in the vulva.

Ovarian Fibroma

Ovarian fibromas are usually small, but there are instances in which they have grown to weigh as much as five pounds. A large fibroma can be very painful and produce symptoms such as a feeling of heaviness in the pelvic area, nausea, and vomiting. The growth may crowd other organs of the body, causing enlargement of the abdomen and cardiac and respiratory symptoms. The only treatment is surgical removal of the tumor, after which there is usually a quick and full recovery.

Uterine Fibroma

Fibroid tumors of the uterus can also grow to a very large size, some weighing many pounds. Like ovarian fibromas, they can press against neighboring organs such as the intestine or the urinary bladder, producing constipation or urinary difficulty. More commonly, there is pain and vaginal bleeding, along with pelvic pressure and enlargement of the abdomen. It is possible in some cases for a fibroid tumor to grow slowly in the uterus for several years without causing serious discomfort to the patient. If the tumor obstructs or distorts the reproductive tract, it may be a cause of infertility.

Treatment of fibroid tumors varies according to their size, the age of the patient and her expectations about having children, and other factors. If the tumor is small and does not appear to be growing at a rapid rate, the physician may recommend that surgery be postponed as long as the tumor poses no threat to health. For an older woman, or for a woman who does not want to bear children, a hysterectomy may be advised, especially if symptoms are troublesome. If the patient is a young woman who wants to have children, the physician is likely to advise a *myomectomy,* a surgical excision of the tumor, since a fibroid tumor of the uterus can cause serious complications during pregnancy and labor. It can result in abortion or premature labor, malpresentation of the fetus, difficult labor, and severe loss of blood during childbirth. While fibroid tumors of the uterus are not malignant, special tests are made of the endometrial tissue as part of any myomectomy or hysterectomy to rule out the possibility that cancer cells may be involved in the disorder.

Endometriosis

Endometriosis is the medical term for a condition in which endometrial tissue, the special kind of tissue that lines the uterus, grows in various areas of the pelvic cavity outside the uterus. Endometrial cells may invade such unlikely places as the ovaries (the most common site), the bladder, appendix, Fallopian tubes, intestinal tract, or the supporting structure of the uterus. The external endometrial tissue may appear as small blisters of endometrial cells, as solid nodules, or as cysts, usually of the ovary, which may be four inches or more in diameter, like the chocolate cysts of the ovaries. Such a mass of sometimes tumorlike endometrial cells is called an *endometrioma.*

The misplaced endometrial tissue causes problems because it goes through menstrual cycles just as the endometrium does within the cavity of the uterus. The endometrial tissue proliferates after ovulation and may cause almost constant pain, wherever it is located, for a few days before the start of menstruation. The symptoms subside after the menstrual flow begins. The effects may include dyspa-

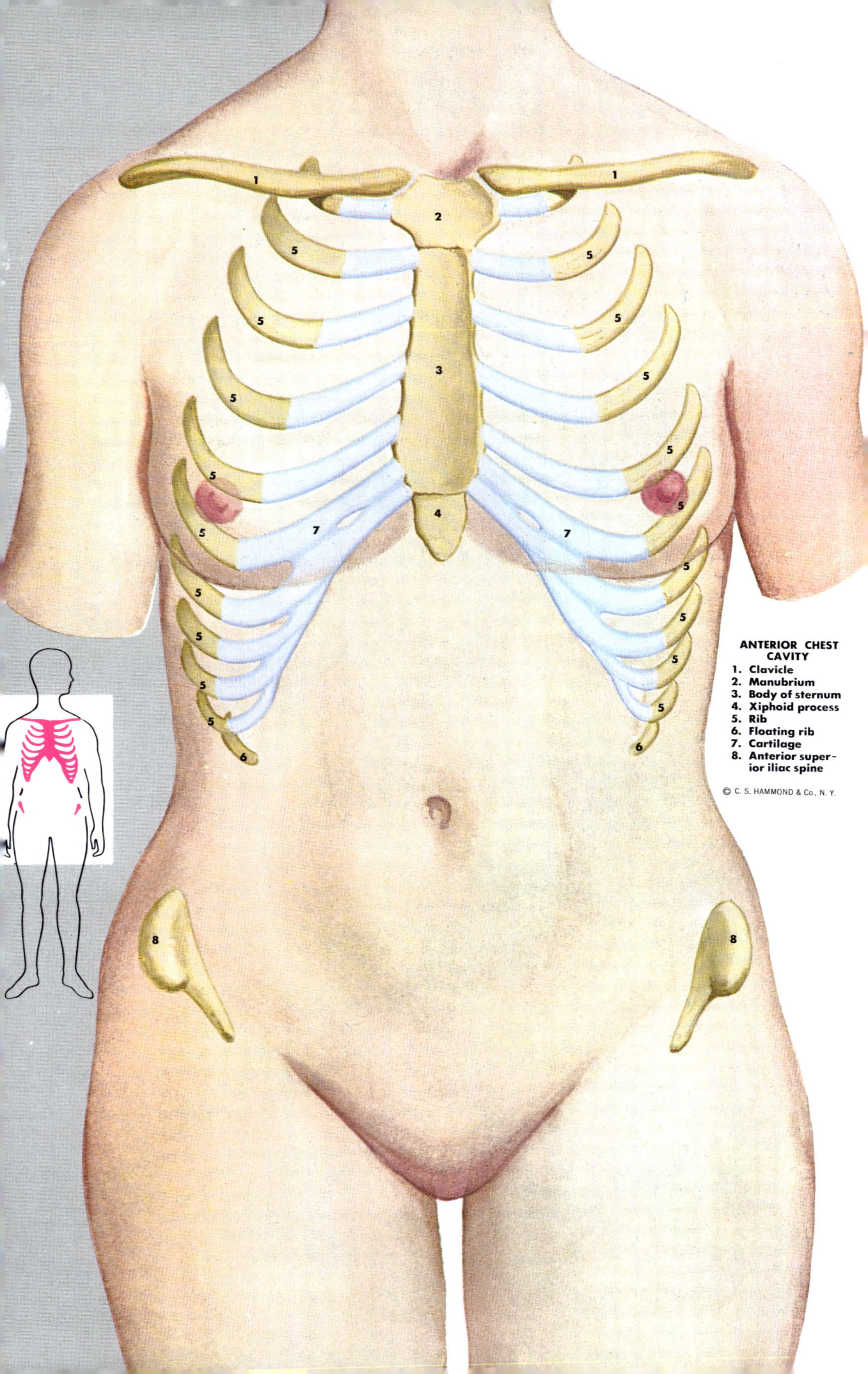
ANTERIOR CHEST CAVITY
1. Clavicle
2. Manubrium
3. Body of sternum
4. Xiphoid process
5. Rib
6. Floating rib
7. Cartilage
8. Anterior superior iliac spine
© C. S. HAMMOND & Co., N. Y.

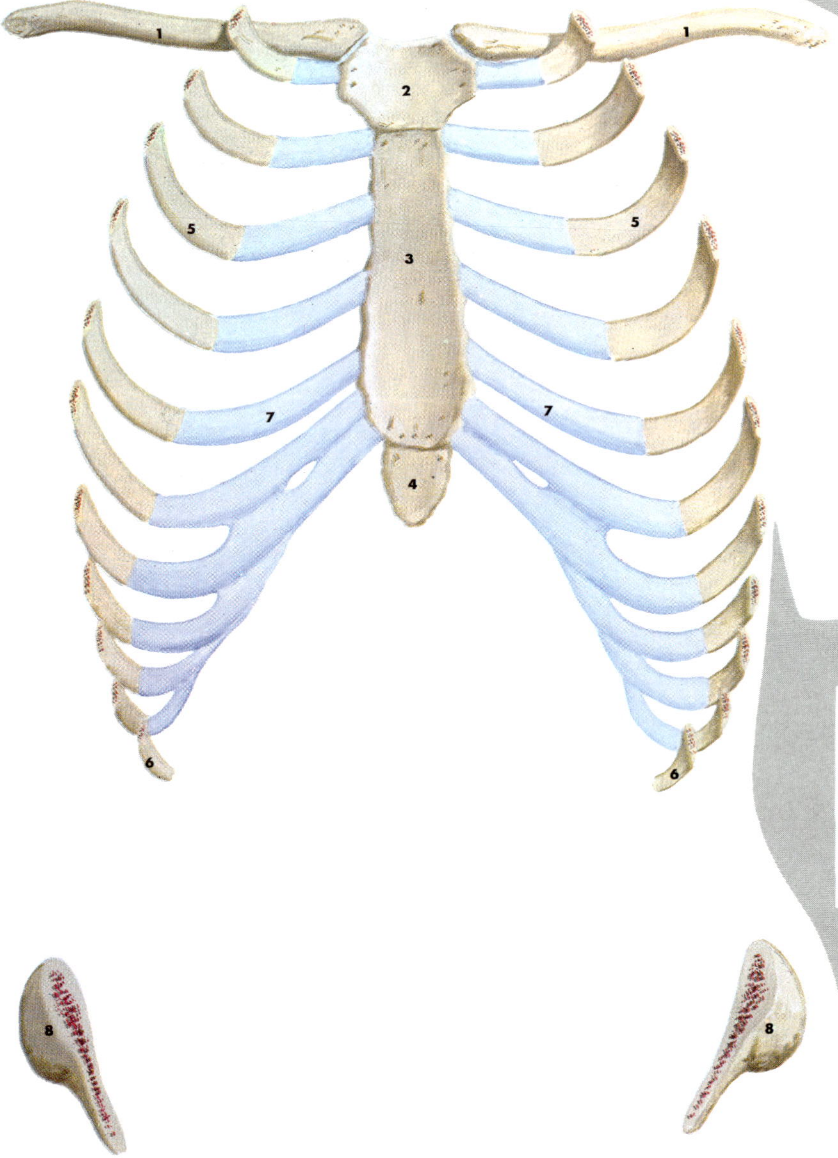

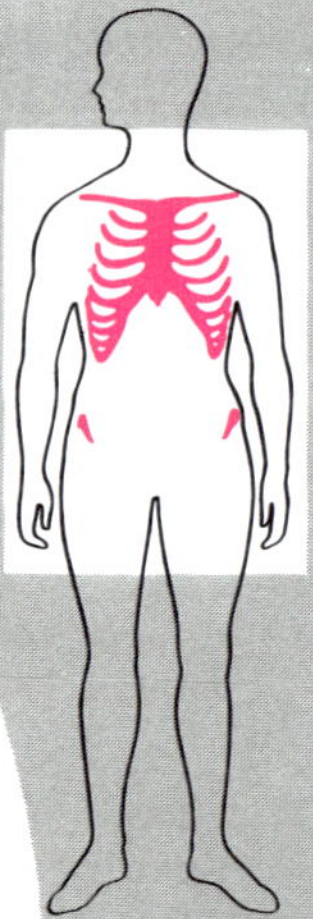

POSTERIOR INTERIOR CHEST CAVITY

1. Clavicle
2. Manubrium
3. Body of sternum
4. Xiphoid process.
5. Rib
6. Floating rib
7. Cartilage
8. Anterior superior iliac spine

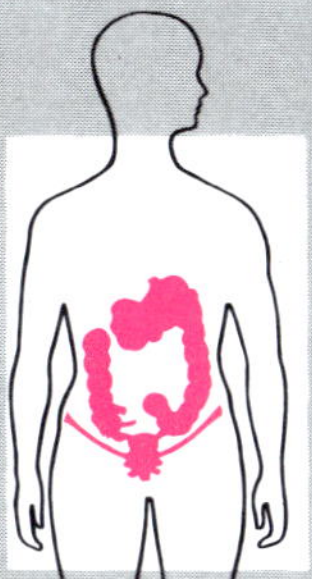

ANTERIOR STOMACH, COLON, AND ORGANS OF REPRODUCTION

23. Esophagus
24. Stomach (cardia)
25. Stomach (fundus)
26. Stomach (body)
27. Stomach (pylorus)
28. Duodenum
31. Ileum
32. Ileocolic junction
33. Caecum
34. Ascending colon
36. Descending colon
37. Sigmoid colon
39. Vermiform appendix
40. Taenia coli
45. Spleen
49. Superior mesenteric artery
50. Superior mesenteric vein
51. Pancreas (head)
52. Pancreas (tail)
80. Bladder
81. Urachus
82. Pubic symphysis
83. Inguinal ligament
100. Uterus
102. Vagina (cross section)
103. Fallopian tube
104. Ostium of fallopian tube
105. Ovary

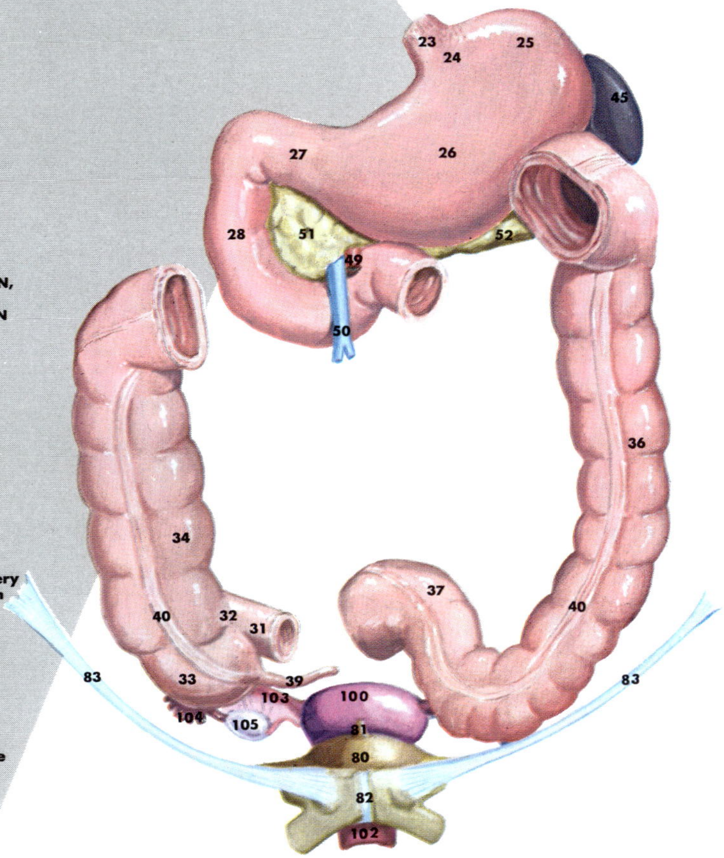

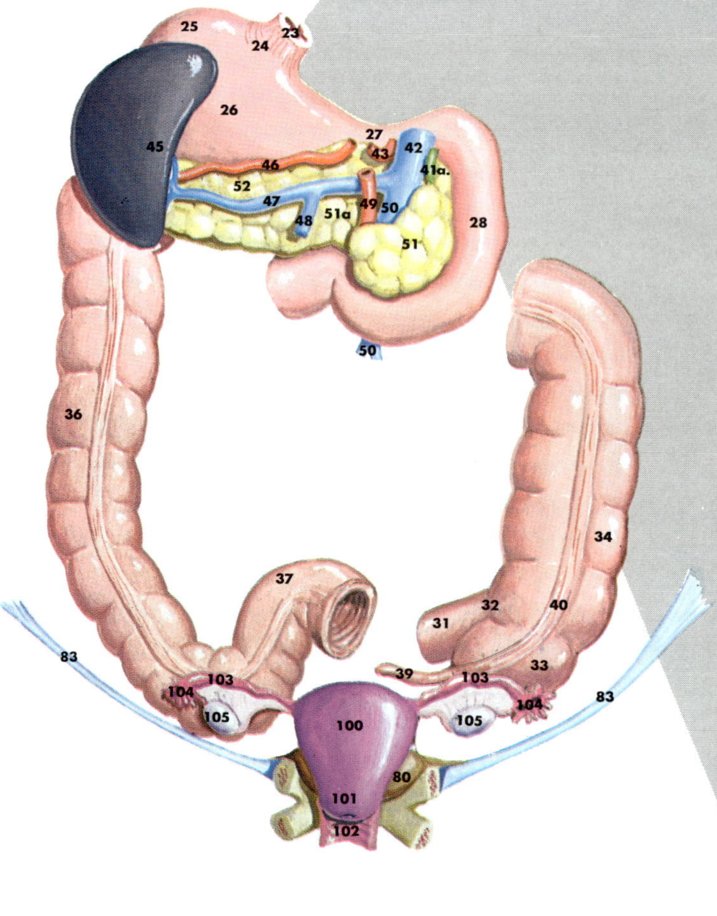

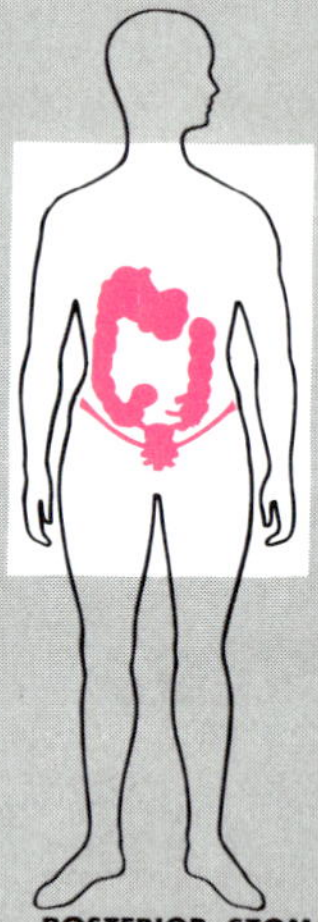

POSTERIOR STOMACH, COLON, AND ORGANS OF REPRODUCTION

23. Esophagus
24. Stomach (cardia)
25. Stomach (fundus)
26. Stomach (body)
27. Stomach (pylorus)
28. Duodenum
31. Ileum
32. Ileocolic junction
33. Caecum
34. Ascending colon
36. Descending colon
37. Sigmoid colon
39. Vermiform appendix
40. Taenia coli
41. Cystic duct
41a. Common bile duct
42. Portal vein
43. Hepatic artery
45. Spleen
46. Splenic artery
47. Splenic vein
48. Inferior mesenteric vein
49. Superior mesenteric artery
50. Superior mesenteric vein
51. Pancreas (head)
51a. Pancreas (body)
52. Pancreas (tail)
80. Bladder
83. Inguinal ligament
100. Uterus
101. Cervix
102. Vagina (cross section)
103. Fallopian tube
104. Ostium of fallopian tube
105. Ovary

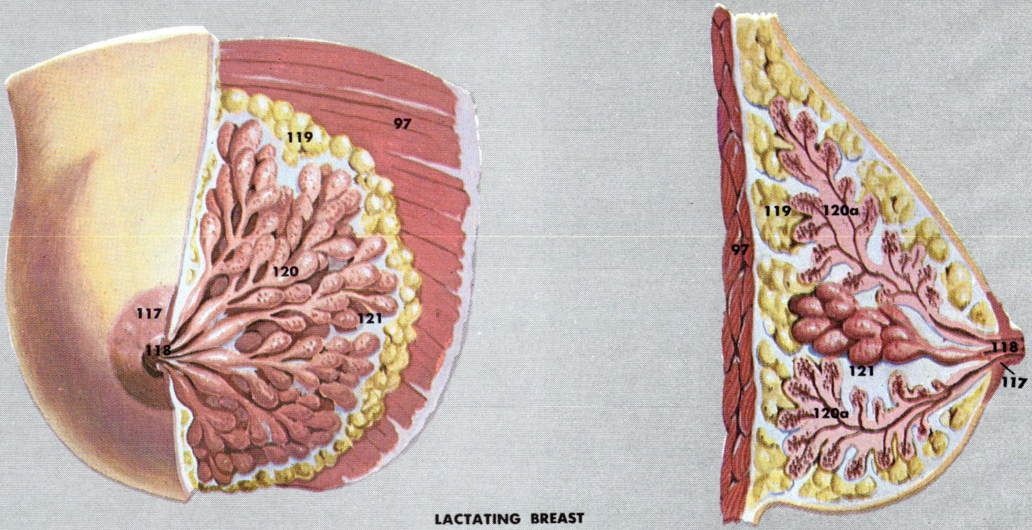

LACTATING BREAST

97. Pectoralis major muscle
117. Areola
118. Nipple
119. Fat
120. Lactiferous (milk producing) glands and ducts
120a. Cross section of gland and duct
121. Tissue separating and supporting glandular tissue

STRUCTURE OF THE MAMMARY GLANDS

The mammary glands are composed of three major elements:

1. Their skin covering and special structures (nipple, areola).
2. The lactiferous glands or functional units of the breast.
3. The supporting structures, the connective tissue "ligaments" and the fat tissue that makes up the mass of the breast.

The breast is supported by the "suspensory ligaments." These are anchored to the sheet of connective tissue surrounding the pectoralis major muscle, and extend in a complex network separated by the fat tissue outward to the skin. The lactiferous glands are buried in the supporting tissues and empty outward onto the surface of the nipple. These glands at first are very small and clustered just beneath the nipple and areola. In pregnancy they enlarge and push downward into the mass of the breast causing it to enlarge in turn. The enlargement continues through the period of breast feeding, following which the glands gradually grow smaller and the entire breast returns to normal size.

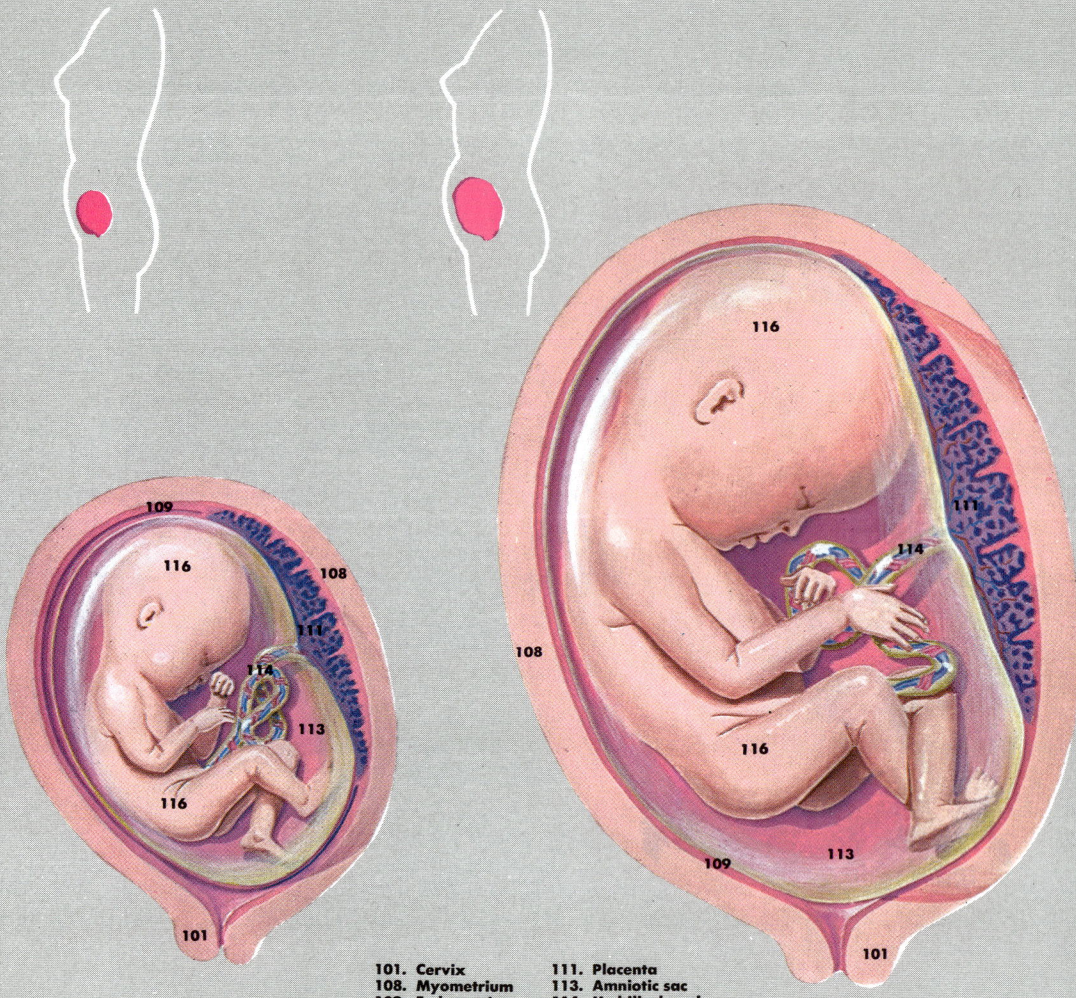

101. Cervix
108. Myometrium
109. Endometrium
111. Placenta
113. Amniotic sac
114. Umbilical cord
116. Fetus

THE FETUS AT 3 1/2 AND 6 MONTHS

Most of the definitive development of the fetus occurs during the first 3½ months, and the remaining 5½ months is primarily concerned with gradual increase in size and maturation of organs already begun. The fetus receives all of its nourishment through the placenta and umbilical cord. There is no direct contact between fetal and maternal blood in the placenta. During its entire development, the fetus floats in a fluid (amniotic fluid) contained within a sac (the amniotic sac) attached to the placenta. This sac is in turn surrounded by the uterine cavity, the endometrium and the muscle or myometrium of the uterus.

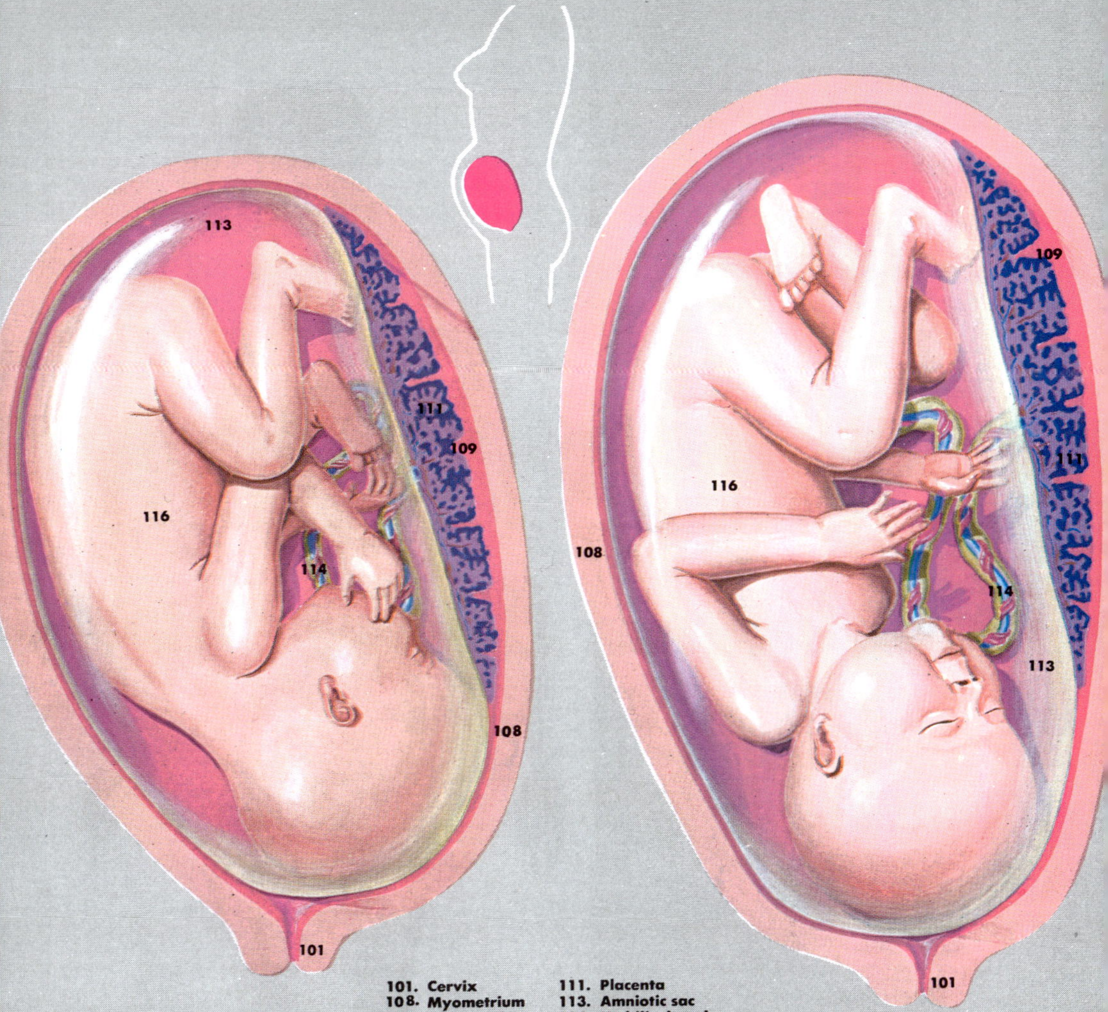

101. Cervix
108. Myometrium
109. Endometrium
111. Placenta
113. Amniotic sac
114. Umbilical cord
116. Fetus

THE FETUS AT 8 AND 9 MONTHS

Until birth, the fetus is surrounded by the amniotic sac and fluid, and attached to the placenta by the umbilical cord. The fetus continues to increase in size and the uterus stretches to accommodate it. Usually before the eighth month the fetus assumes a head-downward position. At birth, the amniotic sac ruptures, the fluid escapes, and the child is slowly pushed out of the uterine cavity by the contractions of the myometrium. Shortly after birth of the child, the placenta is similarly expelled having been detached from the endometrium.

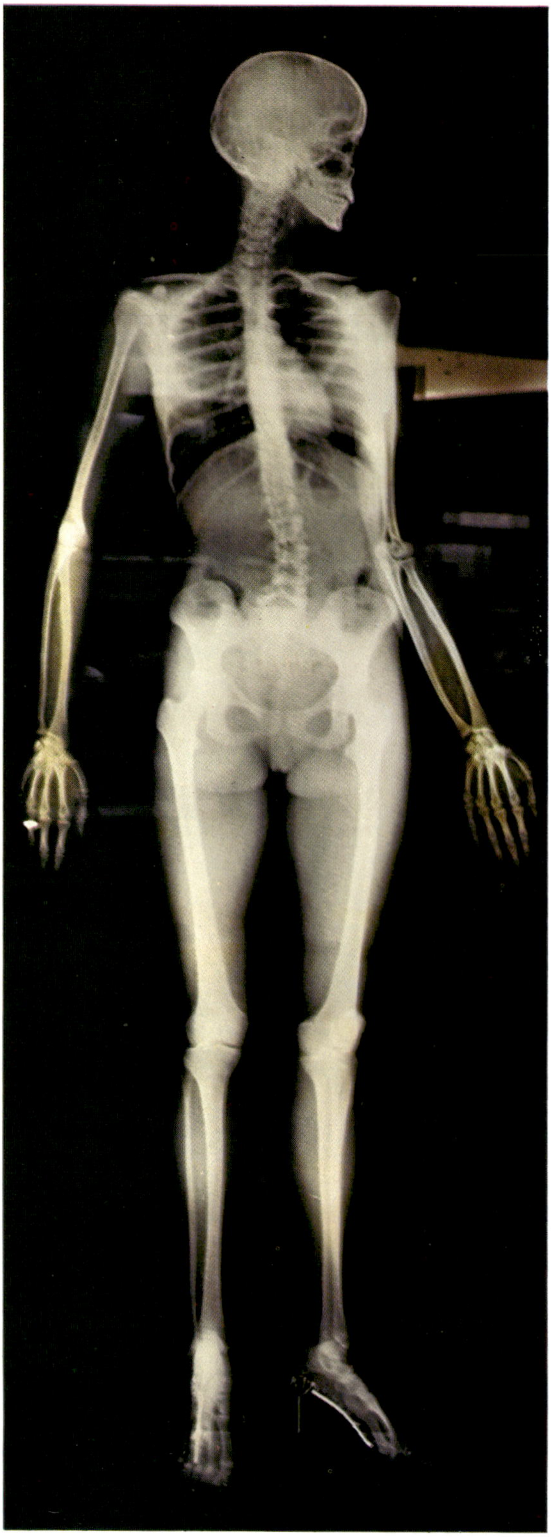

X-RAY OF THE HUMAN BODY
SHOWING THE
BONE STRUCTURE

reunia, rectal bleeding, backache, and generalized pain in the pelvic region as sensitive tissues throughout the pelvic cavity are irritated by monthly cycles of swelling and bleeding.

Because infertility is associated with endometriosis, which can become progressively worse, young women who want to bear children are sometimes encouraged to begin efforts to become pregnant as early as possible if they show signs or symptoms of the disorder. Treatment includes hormone medication and surgery to remove the lesions of endometriosis or the organ involved. For patients with extensive spread of endometrial tissue outside the uterus, the physician may recommend removal of one or both ovaries. Destruction of the ovaries surgically or by radiation therapy may be employed to eliminate the menstrual cycle activity that aggravates the symptoms of endometriosis. These procedures cause sterility and premature menopause, but some women prefer this to the discomfort of endometriosis. The hormone therapy inhibits the ovulation phase of the menstrual cycle. Without ovulation, the endometrial tissue does not proliferate. For this reason, pregnancy often eliminates or eases the symptoms of endometriosis during parturition and for a period of time thereafter.

Dyspareunia

Dyspareunia, or painful intercourse, is often associated with endometriosis and is attributed to irritation of nerve fibers in the area of the cervix from the pressure of sexual activity. There are many other possible causes of painful intercourse, some functional and some organic in nature. In addition to endometriosis, the problem may be owing to a vaginal contracture, a disorder involving the muscles of the pelvic region, inflammation of the vagina or urethra, prolapsed or malpositioned uterus, *cervicitis* (inflammation of the cervix), or a disorder of the bladder or rectum. A cause of dyspareunia in older women may be a degeneration of the tissues lining the vagina, which become thin and dry. Temporary therapy for dyspareunia may include water-soluble lubricants, anesthetic ointments, steroid hormones, analgesics, and sedatives. In appropriate cases, surgery is effective in correcting an organic cause of painful sexual intercourse. Functional or psychogenic (of psychological origin) causes of dyspareunia usually require psychological counseling for the patient and her sexual partner.

Backache

Still another effect of endometriosis that can suggest other disorders is backache. When endometrial tissue invades the pelvic region, there may be a fairly constant pain in the back near the tailbone or the rectum. Usually the backache subsides only after the cause has been eliminated. Temporary measures include those advised for other kinds of backache: sleeping on a firm mattress, preferably reinforced with a sheet of plywood between springs and mattress; application of dry heat or warm baths; sedatives to relieve tension, and analgesics to relieve the pain.

A backache that radiates down the back and into a leg, following the path of a sciatic nerve, can be the result of a disorder of the ovaries or uterus. An ovarian cyst or infection of the Fallopian tubes can produce a backache that seems to be centered in the lumbosacral area of the spinal column. Such backaches, sometimes called gynecologic backaches, tend to occur most frequently during a woman's childbearing years and more often affect women who have had several children than women who have not been pregnant. Tumors also can produce backache symptoms. X-ray pictures, myelograms, and laboratory studies may be required in order to rule out the possibilities that the back pain may be caused by a tumor, a herniated or "slipped" disk, or a deformity of the spinal column that might have been aggravated by one or more pregnancies. Most backaches, however, relate to poor posture or muscle tension. Anxiety or other kinds of emotional stress can aggravate the symptoms. See also "Backaches" in Ch. 23, *Aches, Pains, Nuisances, Worries,* and "Back Pain and Its Causes" in Ch. 25, *Women's Health.*

Cancers of the Reproductive System

Cancer of the Cervix

The cervix of the uterus is the ninth most common site of cancers affecting women. As compared with all cancers of the reproductive organs of women, it rates third, after uterine cancer and ovarian cancer. It has been estimated that about 13,000 cases of cervical cancer are found among American women each year, and approximately 4,500 deaths every year are a result of this disease.

The number of cases of preinvasive cervical cancer is down because of the increased number of women who undergo regular gynecological examination. When cancer is diagnosed early, the survival rate increases tremendously for the patient.

The actual causes of cervical cancer are still unknown. Current medical thinking suggests that there is no causal relationship between cervical cancer and the use of oral contraceptives.

Preinvasive Stage

The earliest signs of cervical cancer tend to appear between the ages of 25 and 45. At this early, *preinvasive* stage, the cancer is described as *in situ*—confined to its original site. If the cancer is not treated at this stage, the disease spreads and becomes a typical invasive cancer within five to ten years. Signs of bleeding and ulceration usually do not appear until this has occurred. However, because of the relatively slow growth of cervical cancer in the early stage, the disease usually can be detected by a Pap smear test before it becomes invasive.

Invasive Cancer

Cancer that has spread beyond the cervix is far more difficult to treat. Surgery, radiation or chemotherapy, and regular examinations to catch any recurrence of cancer will probably be necessary. It is unusual for anyone to develop invasive cancer without knowing it, if she has undergone regular, routine pelvic exams.

Diagnostic Methods

Pap Smear Test

The *Pap smear* test (named for Dr. George Papanicolaou, who developed the technique in 1928) is a quick and simple method of detecting cancerous cells in secretions and scrapings from mucous membrane. It requires the collection of small samples of cells from the surface of the cervix and from the cervical canal. Such samples are obtained by inserting a plastic spatula or a brush-tipped tube into the vagina, into which a speculum has been placed previously. The device is scraped gently over the area of the cervix. The physician may collect also a sample of vaginal secretions, which may contain possibly cancerous cells not only from the cervix but from the ovaries and uterus as well. (This is the only way a Pap smear test can be done if a woman has had a complete hysterectomy and has no cervix.) All cell samples are placed (smeared) on microscope slides and treated with a chemical preservative. The slides are sent to a laboratory for study and a report is made to the examining physician, usually within a few days, on the findings.

Results from the Pap smear are reported as: normal, inadequate sampling, showing infection, or showing cell abnormalities. Except for the normal results, Paps will be done again to ensure accuracy. No one should wait more than six months for a follow-up reading on an infectious diagnosis and treatment. For all others, follow-up should be immediate. Cell abnormalities are divided into at least three categories: low-grade lesions (noncancerous), high-grade lesions (noncancerous), and cancer.

Other Diagnostic Tests

When a report of positive findings is returned by the laboratory, the physician immediately arranges for further studies. These involve examination of the cervix visually by a special microscopic technique known as *colposcopy,* and the removal of small tissue samples. These studies are usually done in a physician's office. In some cases a biopsy is necessary. The biopsy sample is taken when possible from the same location on the cervix as the Pap smear that resulted in positive findings. The Loop Electrosurgical Excision Procedure (LEEP) is a method of combining the biopsy and the excision of the diseased tissue. An electrified loop removes the abnormal tissue from the cervix. The small circle that is removed can then be examined for signs of cancer. The electrical charge of the loop cauterizes the cut to prevent infection and bleeding. Treatment ordinarily is not started until all of the studies have verified that there is cancer in the tissues of the cervix; other disorders, such as cervicitis, venereal infection, and polyps, can mimic symptoms of cervical cancer.

Therapy

The kind of treatment recommended for a case of cervical cancer generally depends upon several factors, such as the stage of cancer development and the age and general health of the patient. For a young woman who wishes to have children despite cancer *in situ,* which is limited to the cervix, surgeons may excise a portion of the cervix and continue watching for further developments with frequent Pap smears and other tests. The treatment of choice for cervical cancer in the early stage, however, is surgical removal of the body of the uterus, as well as of the cervix—a procedure called a *total hysterectomy.* This is the usual treatment for women over the age of 40 or for those who do not wish to have children. Sometimes more extensive surgery is necessary.

Radiation treatment may be advised for women who are not considered to be good surgical risks because of other health problems. Radiation may be recommended along with surgery for women with advanced cervical cancer in order to help destroy cancer cells that may have spread by metastasis to other tissues.

The five-year cure rate for cervical cancer is about 99 percent when treatment is started in the early, preinvasive stage. The chances of a cure drop sharply in later stages, but the five-year cure rate is still as high as 65 percent if treatment is started when the cancer has just begun to spread to the vagina or other nearby tissues.

Cancer of the Body of the Uterus

Cancer of the body of the uterus, or *endometrial cancer,* is more common than cancer of the cervix. Uterine cancer is the most common type of cancer of the reproductive organs. Cervical cancer primarily affects women before middle age; uterine cancer occurs more frequently among women beyond the menopause, with its highest rate occurring among women between the ages of 50 and 70. Survival rate for cancer of the uterus is high, with 82 percent living 5 years after diagnosis. Risk factors for uterine cancer include obesity, diabetes, and ovarian cysts. Other potential risks are for women who have taken estrogen-only pills for menopausal symptoms and women who have taken tamoxifen for breast cancer.

Diagnostic Methods

Early symptoms usually include bleeding between menstrual periods or after menopause, and occasionally a watery or blood-stained vaginal discharge. Most patients experience no pain in the early stages, although pain is a symptom in advanced uterine cancer or when the disease is complicated by an infection. Unfortunately, there is no simple test, like the Pap smear for cervical cancer, that provides a good diagnostic clue to the presence of endometrial cancer. The Pap smear does occasionally pick up cells sloughed off by the endometrium, and laboratory tests can tell if they might be malignant. The best chance for early diagnosis is for a woman to report to her gynecologist or physician any signs of abnormal bleeding between periods, or postmenopausal bleeding. Unusual bleeding should be followed up by the doctor with examination of the uterine lining.

A physician who is suspicious of symptoms of endometrial cancer must depend upon direct methods to confirm or rule out the disease. The usual method is a dilatation and curettage (D and C), during which a small sample of uterine lining will be removed for biopsy, or a sample may be withdrawn by suction (aspirated) from the uterine cavity. The cervix is dilated (opened) and the uterine lining scraped with a curette. Aspiration can be done in the physician's office with local anesthesia of the cervix or with no anesthesia. There is little or no discomfort following aspiration.

Therapy

If the diagnostic D and C is done when the abnormal bleeding associated with uterine cancer first begins, the chances of a cure are very good. The first step, if the general health of the patient permits surgery, is complete removal of the uterus, ovaries, and fallopian tubes—a procedure called a *radical hysterectomy.* Radiation may also be administered to control the spread of cancer cells.

A hysterectomy should not affect a woman's normal sexual activity. Sexual relations usually can be resumed about six to eight weeks after the operation, or when the incision has healed. If the incision is made through the pubic region or vagina, there should be little or no visible scar. See "Family Planning," in Chapter 4.

Estrogen and Cancer

There is a higher incidence of cancer of the uterus among women who have tumors of the ovary that produce estrogen, as well as among women whose menopause begins later than the usual age (and hence who have produced estrogen naturally for a longer-than-usual period). Because of the statistical associations between uterine cancer and estrogen-producing tumors, as well as other factors, the American Cancer Society has cautioned that physicians should exert "close supervision of women on estrogen, with an awareness that sustained use [of estrogens] may stimulate dormant factors in the body and lead to development of endometrial cancer." For women who are prescribed estrogen for menopause, it is recommended that the estrogen be given in combination with a synthetic progestin. Unopposed estrogen increases the growth of cancerous tumors already present, and is suspected of increasing the risk of new cancer growths.

Among the conditions for which estrogen has been prescribed for women of middle age and beyond are uncomfortable effects of menopause, such as itching and irritation caused by dryness of the vagina, and what is commonly referred to as "hot flashes." See *The Middle Years,* Ch. 5, "Menopause" for more information.

Diethylstilbestrol

An estrogenlike synthetic compound has definitely been implicated in the development of a type of cancer, *adenocarcinoma,* which primarily affects epithelial tissue. The synthetic hormone known chemically as *diethylstilbestrol* (DES) or stilbestrol was taken for the most part in the late 1940s and through the 1960s by pregnant women for the treatment of such complications as bleeding and threatened miscarriage. Around 1971, physicians became aware that some of the daughters whose mothers had taken DES during their pregnancy had developed an unusual cell formation in vaginal tissue, vaginal and cervical cancers, and some anatomical abnormalities. Cancers have been discovered in daughters as young as seven years of age. An unknown but substantial number of women in the United States alone received DES while pregnant, but approximately 1 in 1000 have been found to be afflicted with cervical or vaginal cancers. The National Cancer Institute has urged that all mothers and daughters who may have been exposed to DES during the mother's pregnancy arrange to be examined by a physician for possible effects of the drug.

The use of DES for pregnant women has been discontinued, although the compound is still available for treating certain cases of breast cancer and menopausal symptoms in nonpregnant women.

Cancer of the Ovary

Ovarian cancer is the fifth most common type of cancer in women, with an average of 21,000 new cases each year. It is second to uterine cancer in the number of cases of cancer of the reproductive system. It has, however, a much lower survival rate. Because of the difficulty in diagnosing ovarian cancer, the cancer is more likely than other forms to go unchecked until it has spread to other areas of the body. Less than 2 in 5 women will survive five years after diagnosis. There are several different kinds of malignant tumors of the ovary; some originate in the ovaries and others are caused by cells that have metastasized from a cancer at some other site, such as the uterus.

There are no age limits for cancer of the ovary, although most cases are detected in women between 50 and 70. A physician at a routine pelvic examination may notice a lump or other abnormal growth in the abdominal region. The symptoms reported by patients usually include abdominal discomfort or digestive problems, possibly because ovarian cancers often grow large enough to press on neighboring organs and cause urinary difficulties, constipation, or other digestive disorders. A clue is given in some cases by endometrial bleeding as a result of abnormal hormone production by the affected ovary. However, the more common kinds of ovarian cancers do not produce hormones. Occasionally, cancer cells from an ovarian tumor will be found in a Pap smear sample. But there are no direct, simple tests for cancer of the ovary.

Treatment for ovarian cancer varies with the individual case. As with cancer at other sites, surgery is generally necessary. The extent of the surgery depends upon the type of lesion and other factors. In an advanced case of an older woman, total hysterectomy along with removal of the ovaries and fallopian tubes would be the treatment of choice. But if the patient is a young woman and the cancer is not extensive, the surgeon may excise the affected ovary and leave the remainder of the reproductive system intact. Radiation and chemotherapy are commonly applied in addition to surgery. The most important risk factor is having relatives who have had ovarian cancer. If a mother, grandmother, or sibling have been diagnosed with ovarian cancer, then the woman is recommended to undergo regular blood tests to check for malignancy. Let your doctor know if you have a family history of ovarian cancer.

Cancer of the Breast

Breast cancer remains the most common of cancers affecting women, killing more women that any other kind of cancer, except lung cancer. About 150,000 women in the United States develop breast cancer each year, and 35 percent die of the disease. The cause of breast cancer is still unknown.

Prevention

The best prevention is education, mammography screening, self-examinations, and the monitoring of high-risk patients. Women whose female relatives have had breast cancer are more likely to be victims than women from families in which breast cancer is not present. Two genes, BRCA1 and BRCA2, have accounted for at least 80 percent of the breast cancer in women with a significant family history of the disease, but 80 percent of the women who develop breast cancer have no family history. High risk patients are defined as women who do not have children or who do not have them before their 30s; women who reach menopause later than normal; women who began menstruating earlier in life than normal. It should be noted that the increased risk is minimal. Also, women with ovarian tumors and women who use supplementary estrogen have been shown by some studies to be at increased risk, while the process of having many children and nursing them, which suppresses estrogen hormone activity, is associated with a decreased risk of developing breast cancer. However, 55 percent of the diagnosed cases are for women who have no known risk factors.

Cancer of the breast is generally not found before the age of 30 and the incidence peaks around the age of 55. There is a second period after the age of 65 when the incidence of breast cancer rises again.

Breast cancer usually begins in the ducts of the milk glands or lobules of the breast. The first noticeable sign is a lump in the breast. The lump may occur anywhere in the breast, but the most common site is the upper, outer quadrant. Most lumps are not usually cancerous, but a biopsy must be performed to check the tissue involved.

A small tumor half an inch in diameter is large enough to be detected during careful self-examination. The lump generally causes no pain; pain is rarely associated with early breast cancer. If the tumor is allowed to grow unchecked, it may cause pulling of the skin from within. The breast may flatten or the skin may dimple or the nipple may sink, tilt, or flatten. Less frequently, the tumor begins in a duct near the nipple, causing irritation of the skin of the nipple and a moist discharge. In such cases a scab eventually forms at that site. In time, cancer cells spread to the nearby lymph nodes and the danger of metastasis to any part of the body becomes very serious.

Detection of Breast Cancer

Fortunately, breast cancer can be treated effectively if it is detected early enough. Some 95 percent of breast cancers are discovered by the patient when she notices a lump. In all too many cases the discovery is made by chance and the lump may be quite large.

The cure rate for breast cancer could be greatly improved if all women made a routine of monthly self-examination and then consulted a physician immediately if they found the least indication of a thickening or a lump. Most such lumps are benign, but it is most important that the ones that are malignant be identified without delay.

The American Cancer Society and the National Cancer Institute recommend that every woman follow a prescribed method of self-examination just after the menstrual period, continuing every month after the menopause. The procedure (see illustration) should only take a few minutes and consists of carefully looking at and feeling the breasts. For more information, contact the American Cancer Society at (800) ACS-2345.

In recent years, methods of early detection have been refined to the point that tumors once undetectable can now be detected before any lump becomes palpable. As many as 80 percent of women diagnosed with early stages of breast cancer can be treated with a lumpectomy, the removal of underarm lymph nodes, radiation, and perhaps chemotherapy.

Mammography

Mammography is a low-dose X ray developed specifically for examination of breast tissue. A tumor shows up on a mammogram as an opaque spot because of mineral concentrations associated with the growth. However, mammography cannot determine whether a tumor is benign or malignant or if the opaque spot on the film is because of some other mineral-rich tissue rather than a tumor. Physicians use mammography and ultrasound as diagnostic tools.

Recommendations for when to seek clinical breast examinations and mammograms are as follows:

- Women 20 years of age and over should perform a breast self-examination every month.
- Women between 20 and 39 years of age should have a physical examination of the breast every three years, performed by a physician, physician assistant, nurse, or nurse-practitioner.
- Women 40 and over should have a physical examination of the

Self-examination of the Breasts

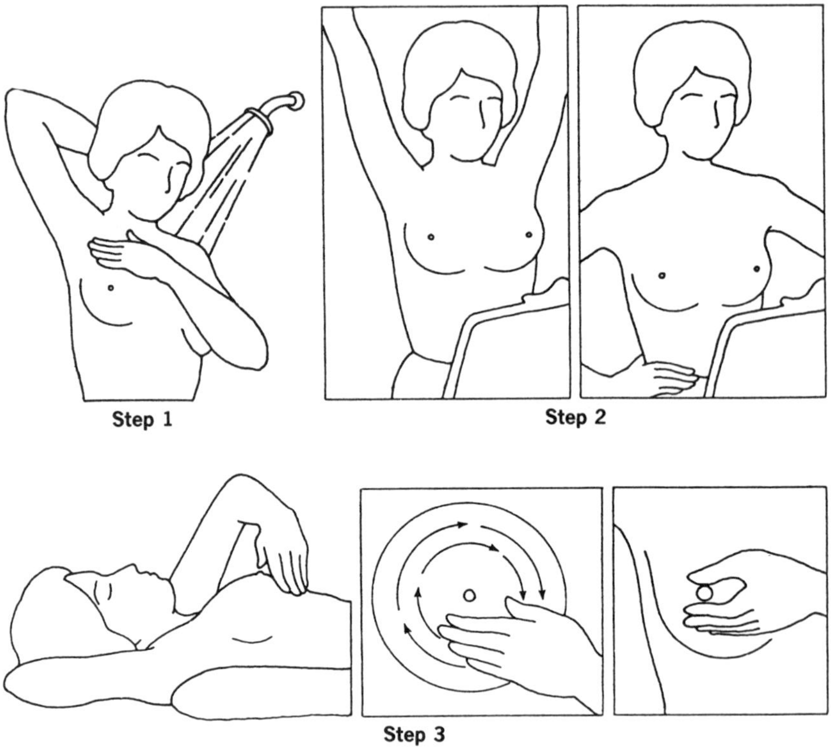

Self-examination of the breasts as recommended by the American Cancer Society. *(Step 1)* Examine breasts during a shower or bath; hands glide easier over wet skin. With fingers flat, move the left hand gently over every part of the right breast, then the right hand over the left breast. Check for any lump, hard knot, or thickening. *(Step 2)* Before a mirror, inspect the breasts with arms at the sides, then with arms raised. Look for any changes in the contour of each breast, a swelling, dimple of skin, or changes in the nipple. Then rest palms on hips and press down firmly to flex the chest muscles. Left and right breasts will not match exactly—few women's breasts do. But regular inspection will show what is normal for you. *(Step 3)* While lying down with a pillow or folded towel under the right shoulder and with the right hand behind the head, examine the right breast with the left hand. With fingers flat, press gently in small circular motions around an imaginary clock face. Begin at 12 o'clock, then move to 1 o'clock, and so on around back to 12. A ridge of firm tissue in the lower curve of each breast is normal. Next, move in an inch toward the nipple and keep circling to examine every part of the breast, including the nipple. This requires at least three more circles. Then repeat the procedure slowly on the left breast with the pillow under the left shoulder and left hand behind the head. Notice how the breast structure feels. Finally, squeeze the nipple of each breast gently between thumb and index finger. Any discharge, clear or bloody, should be reported to a physician immediately.

breast every year, performed by physician, physician's assistant, nurse, or nurse-practitioner.

- Women 40 years of age and older should have a mammogram every year.

Most insurance companies will pay for yearly mammograms; others pay for biannual mammogram exams. Some states require insurance companies by law to pay for at least one exam. Check with your insurance company about their policy. Medicare covers mammograms for women over the age of 65.

Screening Mammograms

Screening mammography is performed on women with no symptoms in order to detect the very early stages of breast cancer. Screening mammography for women in their forties has been shown to reduce breast cancer deaths in that age group by as much as 44 percent.

Diagnostic Mammograms

Diagnostic mammograms are performed on women who currently have a breast problem such as a lump or nipple discharge, a history of breast cancer, or an area of concern seen in a previous screening mammogram. This diagnostic X ray looks more closely at the problem in the breast by utilizing a wide variety of X-ray views.

Scheduling a Mammogram

If you have regular periods, you should consider scheduling your mammogram seven to ten days after the beginning of your period, when the breasts are less tender. If your periods are irregular, you can schedule a mammogram at any time of the month. Bringing along any previous mammogram films as comparisons between your old films and your current exam will facilitate early detection of the disease.

Ultrasound

Ultrasound depends on sound waves that vibrate at frequencies beyond the range of human hearing; transmitted into the breast, ultrasound can distinguish between lumps that are cystic and fluid-filled—and therefore benign—and those that are solid. Small calcium deposits, which are one of the first signs of breast cancer, are not visible by ultrasound.

Biopsy

When a physician believes there is good evidence of a cancer in a breast as a result of mammography or ultrasound, the next step is a biopsy study. An entire nodule of breast tissue is removed for microscopic examination of the cells. The methods for extraction depend entirely upon the size of the tumor or lesion—whether or not it is large enough to be felt, and also on whether or not the entire tumor or lesion is to be removed. If, for example, the lesion is palpable, that is, the physician can feel it, and it is known to be cancerous, then the patient undergoes what is called a ***surgical biopsy.*** The patient is transferred to a surgery room where the physician surgically removes the entire lesion. Like most surgical procedures, some scarring is to be expected. If the lesion is viewable only by mammogram or ultrasound, then the radiologist performs a *needle localization.* Using a mammogram or ultrasound as a guide, the radiologist inserts a wire into the breast precisely where the lesion or tumor is located. The patient is transferred to a surgery room where the surgeon extracts the tumor, using the wire as his guide.

If the physician merely wants to sample either breast cells or tissue, several methods are available. In a *stereotactic core biopsy,* usually performed by a radiologist, a specially designed needle is used to draw out a tissue sample. Potentially cancerous cells are sampled in a similar procedure known as *fine needle* aspiration, which is routinely performed by both physicians and radiologists. Scarring is minimal, if at all, in both of these methods.

In each of the procedures discussed above, microscopic examination of the extracted specimen follows.

The Two-Step Procedure

Because of the psychological and physical problems associated with breast cancer, the test and operation can take place in two separate stages. In many cases, though, it may be necessary or more expedient to perform both operations on the same day.

Presurgical Staging involves the administration of various tests that are carried out before any breast surgery. These tests show whether or not the cancer has already spread (or metastasized) to parts of the body other than the breast and local lymph node regions. Staging is widely regarded as a necessary procedure in all cases of breast cancer.

A two-step procedure involves other choices. Where the biopsy is to be carried out separately, the patient may ask to have it done under local anesthesia, as an outpatient. If a general anesthetic appears preferable, the patient may have to spend a night in the hospital. But the *diagnostic biopsy*—involving removal of the tumor or portions of it—and any breast surgery can still be performed separately. After a biopsy specimen is removed, the specimen may be subjected to an estrogen-receptor assay. The assay tells the surgeon whethor or not the cancer depends on the female hormone estrogen for its growth. That information provides a clue to possible future treatment.

Following the biopsy, the pathologist reports on whether or not the specimen is positive or negative for cancer. If the finding is positive, precise information will usually be given on the type of cancer and where it is located in the breast. The patient may want to obtain a second opinion on the permanent-section pathology report and slides from another pathologist.

Breast Cancer Surgeries

Until recently, radical mastectomy was the usual procedure for breast

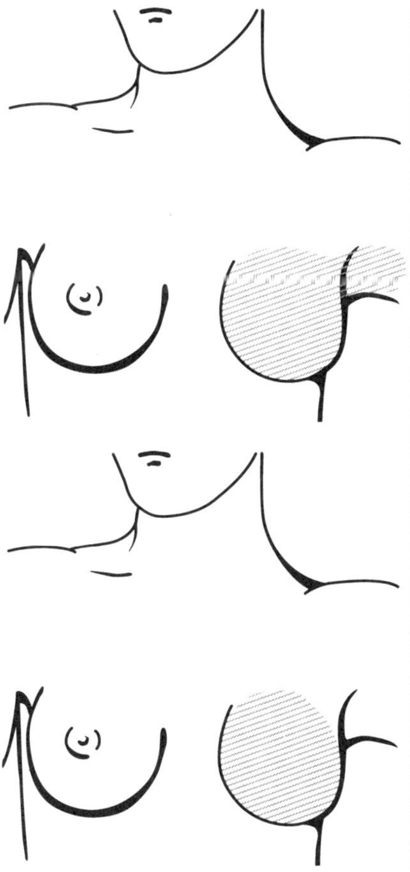

The striped areas show the tissue removed in a radical *(above)* and a simple *(below)* mastectomy, including the axillary lymph nodes in the former case.

cancer treatment. Today, it's rarely performed. The type of surgery is determined by the type and size of the cancerous growth, the risk of further growth, and other factors. Depending upon the seriousness of the case and the procedure recommended by the surgeon and the pathologist, the patient may decide to remove just the breast tissue, leaving the skin (with the exception of the nipple) for reconstructive surgery, to remove the skin tissue as well, or to remove breast tissue and tissue from around the breast area.

A *lumpectomy*, also known as *segmental mastectomy*, is the solution to a great percentage of breast cancer cases, particularly those that are diagnosed early. In a lumpectomy, only the cancer and surrounding tissue are removed. Generally, no reconstructive surgery is necessary and a lumpectomy is usually followed by some combination of radiation therapy and chemotherapy. A common misconception is that radiation and chemotherapy are "either/or" treatments. In general, a patient must have radiation and may or may not undergo chemotherapy.

Other types of breast surgeries include the following:

- Modified radical mastectomy: the underlying muscle stays intact while the breast, lymph nodes and surrounding muscle are removed.
- Simple mastectomy: the breast tissue is removed, but the surrounding muscles and lymph nodes remain.
- Radical mastectomy: the breast, lymph nodes and surrounding muscle are entirely removed. Studies indicate it was no more successful than a lumpectomy or a modified radical mastectomy, yet left the patient deformed and with a very high risk of developing lymphodema (severe arm swelling).

Survival rates depend as much on timely use of pre- and postoperative radiotherapy and postoperative chemotherapy as on the type of operation, but the surgery type can determine the length of the recovery period.

Some surgeries allow reconstruction of the breast either during or after a mastectomy, usually using artificial material to create a breast to match the natural one.

Radiation

Radiation is used in conjunction with breast-sparing surgery or with large tumors that were treated by mastectomy. It is also used in cases where the cancer recurred or metastasized and as a pain-reliever for patients suffering pain to the bone. Treatments are typically given five days a week for five to seven weeks. A "booster" treatment may follow completion of the initial series of treatments. Consult your physician for a complete list of expected side effects.

Chemotherapy

Adjuvant (auxilliary) chemotherapy is given in addition to surgery and radiation. Typically, chemotherapy is administered if a patient has a large tumor, or if the patient's lymph nodes are involved, or if the patient is in the high-risk category for recurrence or distant metastasis. The preference is to avoid treating a postmenopausal patient with chemotherapy, but there are many instances in which chemotherapy is unavoidable. Postmenopausal women may be given tamoxifen, an antiestrogen drug, or may undergo chemotherapy, anyway.

Hormone therapy

Less toxic than chemotherapy, hormone treatments are normally given to those women whose cancer has not spread to the underarm nodes and whose tumors were hormone-dependent. This is especially the case if a patient is postmenopausal. For these women tamoxifen would also be a standard treatment if the cancers had spread to the lymph nodes.

Prophylactic Mastectomy

A *prophylactic*, or preventive, mastectomy is the removal of an entire breast, or both breasts (total mastectomy), when there is no known breast cancer. In this case, it is not necessary to remove any lymph nodes. Prophylactic mastectomy is an *elective* surgery (that is, while you may choose to have it done, it is not *required*). A woman might consider this option to lessen the risk of developing breast cancer if she has a strong family history of breast cancer or if certain forms of benign breast problems have lead to several biopsies, but it is considered drastic and by many, unnecessary.

Prophylactic mastectomy is controversial because there is no guarantee that it will prevent breast cancer. In rare cases, breast cancer has developed in the scar of the mastectomy. Most doctors prefer to closely observe high-risk patients rather than perform such drastic surgery.

Before taking this irreversible step, women should discuss the mastectomy, reconstructive surgery, possible complications, and postoperative care with their physician and the plastic surgeon who will perform the reconstructive surgery. A second medical opinion, and consultation with a genetic counselor, who, through testing, may be able to provide new or more complete information concerning their risk for breast cancer, is also advised. Patients should also be mindful that reconstructed breasts will not have the same physical appearance as normal breasts.

Women opting for prophylactic mastectomies need to be aware that they will be second-guessed by friends, health care advocates, and even some physicians, who consider this type of mastectomy senseless and barbaric. Many women who have the surgery feel that their decision has allowed them to live a life less crippled by fear, worry, and frequent medical tests and procedures.

Breast implants

Breast implants for reconstruction are the same types used for cosmetic breast enlargement. There are two basic types: silicone-gel and saline filled. The saline sacs duplicate the natural breast's shape. The sac is inserted under the skin and then filled slightly larger than the final size. After the skin has adjusted to the enlarged sac, some of the liquid is drained to give the breast a natural sag, in most cases closely matching the remaining breast.

Although silicone-gel implants have been widely discouraged for cosmetic use since 1992, they are still considered an important rehabilitation option for women with breast cancer or women with premalignant conditions requiring mastectomies, according to the American Cancer Society. The silicone implant is carefully inserted under the skin tissue and the body forms a scar tissue seal around the sac.

Reactions to silicone-gel implants may include side effects such as hardening of scar tissue around the implant, ruptured silicone sacs, and obscured diagnostic X rays. The link between silicone and diseases of the immune system is still under study. In addition, implants also may block the results of mammographic X rays. However, studies show that implants do not increase the risk of breast cancer or cancer in other parts of the body.

According to the United States Food and Drug Administration, women should only consider removing implants if they are experiencing difficulties. Women should have periodic exams to check for ruptures. Those who want implants for cosmetic purposes should know the importance of detecting early cancer through mammography and the chance of having results obscured by implants.

Preventing and Surviving Rape

Precautions

Although the majority of rape attacks take the victim by surprise, there are precautions that women may take to avoid potentially dangerous situations.

Precautions on a Date

- Make sure you tell someone where you are going and what time you expect to be back.
- Don't become intoxicated, since your reaction to any potentially dangerous situation will be slower.
- Be aware of drugs known as date-rape drugs. They cause disorientation, unconsciousness, and memory loss, allowing the person who has given you the drug to rape you. And, because they are odorless and have no taste, you should take precautions against anyone slipping the drug into your drink.
- Don't bring a man home or go home with him, or go to a secluded spot with him.
- Don't depend solely upon him for a ride home. Be prepared to call a cab, friend, or relative for a ride in case you feel uncomfortable being with him.
- Even if you have known someone for a while, you should still be cautious about any indications of extreme jealousy, possessiveness, or anger.

Overall Precautions

- Keep all entrances to your home well lit. All doors and windows should be locked. Keep your window shades down at night.
- Use a peephole to confirm the identity of all visitors before opening a door.
- Walk assertively, maintaining a brisk stride and upright posture. Stay alert. Be ready to react, if necessary.
- Many schools, businesses, apartment buildings, and parking facilities will provide you with a security guard or other escort. Request an escort if you are uneasy about going alone.
- When possible, avoid deserted areas. Park in well-lit areas. When walking, use well-lit routes.
- Have your keys out and ready to use, before you reach your car or

home. Once there, get in and lock the doors immediately.

- If you are being followed, go into the nearest place of business or ring the nearest doorbell. If you are in your car, try to drive to the nearest police station or a well-lit, populated area.

Most importantly, heed your own instincts. Many victims of crime report having "gut feelings" that something was wrong just prior to being attacked. If you feel uneasy or in danger, try to remove yourself from a situation before anything happens.

Surviving the Rape Attack

- Talk to the rapist: this may allow you to stall for time until someone else comes by, or you might be able to calm your attacker and avoid rape.
- Tell the rapist you are meeting someone or expecting someone to come by soon.
- Try to disgust your attacker by inducing yourself to vomit, urinate, defecate, or expel gas.
- Scream. Yell "fire" since many potential rescuers are hesitant to respond to a cry for "police." If there is a fire alarm nearby, set it off.
- Use any sharp object you have available—keys, a pen or pencil, your fingernails—and aim for the attacker's eyes, Adam's apple, ears, or temples.
- Kicking or hitting the attacker's groin or throat may disable him temporarily and provide you with time to escape.

If a Rape Occurs

A woman who has been raped may face a long period in which recovery and normal living seem impossible. Authorities say that what a victim does after experiencing rape may make the transition to normal living easier while also protecting her against recurring health problems.

Talk With Someone

Sharing the events of the rape with a friend, relative or counselor will be painful and difficult, but talking about it will help you cope with the many levels of pain and fear you will probably experience. Rape counselors are among the persons best equipped to handle the emotional needs of a woman who has been raped. The person confided in should be able to go to the police station with you, provide support, make sure your rights are protected, and listen sympathetically to your story.

If you have been raped, and do not have anyone close to turn to, contact one of the Rape Crisis Centers listed at the end of the chapter.

Going to the Hospital

A person that has been raped should go as soon as possible to a hospital and undergo the pelvic and other examinations that physicians administer in such cases. If the woman goes to the hospital immediately, she should not wash herself or change clothes. A shower can remove valuable medical evidence. The pelvic examination is designed to find evidence of abrasions or internal damage, and for collection of any semen left by the rapist. Physicians will also examine for any of the rapist's hair, blood, skin, or semen. Any such evidence may be important in court later, if opting to file a police report.

The hospital visit has other purposes. A physician can also administer preventive injections for sexually transmitted diseases and, if desired, an antipregnancy medication. The latter medication must be taken within three days if it is to be effective.

Reporting to the Police

Failure to report a rape immediately or after a few days probably means the rapist will not be apprehended, unless the identity of the rapist is known. Even so, many rapes go unreported simply because most victims cannot face the added trauma of being questioned in detail. The woman who does report to the police should do so as soon as possible. But reporting late is better than not reporting at all. Reporting a rape does not mean that the victim has to press charges later.

Rape Crisis Centers

Rape crisis centers operate in most communities. Staffing at the centers often include rape victims who devote time to helping other victims. To find help, you can call the Rape, Abuse & Incest National Network (RAINN): 1-800-656-HOPE. It is a national 24-hour toll-free hotline for survivors of sexual assault. By reading the area code and prefix of the caller's telephone number, the hotline automatically routes the call to the rape crisis center nearest the caller. Each call is confidential. Every center participating in the network provides counseling and support.

26

Physicians and Diagnostic Procedures

Many people dislike going to the doctor; many fear going to the hospital. And many are overwhelmed by the enormity of the health care industry; much of its costs and procedures seem incomprehensible to us and out of control. Too often, these people put off seeing a doctor until they develop a debilitating problem. Yet many people overlook the one very important way they can alleviate some of their anxiety over their own medical care: choosing a doctor. Having a doctor you trust and with whom you can communicate well not only makes it more likely that you will make appointments for regular checkups, tests, and immunizations, but you will feel comfortable reporting any symptoms that may be the first signs of serious illness, many of which, when diagnosed early, can be treated successfully.

Your Primary Care Physician

Your primary care physician is your regular doctor, the person you see for checkups, and the first person you call when signs of illness appear. More than likely, he or she will be a *general practitioner* or a *family practitioner,* but may also be an *internist* or other specialist (see below). In selecting a primary care physician you should try to get a few recommendations from other patients, doctors, nurses, or hospital workers. Don't hesitate to make an appointment for an informational interview to meet the doctor in person and ask any questions about his or her methods, background, and philosophy that may be important to you.

Another important thing to check is the doctor's training—how much and from where. Check the American Medical Association's *The Directory of Medical Specialists* and other such directories in the library to find out whether the doctor has graduated from a fully accredited medical school and where he or she received further training.

In addition, remember that good communication is often the key to good health care. Make sure your doctor understands your questions and concerns and make sure you understand your doctor's answers and instructions. Don't hesitate to ask why you're being given a particular medication, or what the purpose is of any tests that are recommended. There are alternatives to some medications, and many tests are very expensive and not always necessary. If you are ever uncomfortable with what your doctor has ordered, seek a second opinion; your doctor should be happy to recommend someone. If not, find out why.

General Practitioner

All doctors must complete four years of schooling at an approved medical school, receive one year of postgraduate training in a supervised clinical setting, and pass a state board examination to become licensed to practice medicine. At this point in his or her training a doctor qualifies as a *general practitioner.* Like the stereotypical old-time country doctor, they treat just about everything from warts to measles, set broken bones, deliver babies, and dispense antibiotics and painkillers.

Family Practitioner

The general practitioner has largely been replaced by the *family practitioner.* Family practitioners must complete a three-year residency that covers certain aspects of internal medicine, pediatrics, obstetrics, and orthopedics, and then pass an exam. They treat the same things that general practitioners treat.

Osteopath

A doctor of osteopathy (D.O.) or *osteopath* has similar qualifications as a doctor of medicine. Osteopathy was founded by Andrew Taylor Still (1828-1917) on the principle that the body possesses a natural ability both to defend itself against disease and to heal itself. Osteopaths place great emphasis on the importance of normal body mechanics and on the use of the hands for detecting and correcting problems.

Medical Specialties

Among the major specialties are the following:

Allergy and Immunology: *Allergists* and *immunologists* specialize in the treatment of allergic and immunologic diseases.

Anesthesiology: An *anesthesiologist* decides which type of anesthesia will be used, administers it during surgery, and monitors its effects after surgery.

Dermatology: A *dermatologist* diagnoses and treats diseases of the skin, hair, and nails.

Emergency Medicine: An *emergency medicine specialist* practices emergency medicine in a trauma center.

Family Practice: The role of the *family practitioner* is discussed above.

Gastroenterology: A *gastroenterologist* diagnoses and treats disorders of the digestive system and of the liver.

Internal Medicine: An *internist* specializes in the diagnosis and nonsurgical treatment of diseases. Subspecialties of internal medicine include: *cardiology,* the study of diseases of the heart; *endocrinology,* the study of diseases of the glands; *gastroenterology; hematology,* the study of blood and blood-forming tissues; *infectious diseases; medical oncology,* the study of tumors; *nephrology,* the study of disorders of the kidneys; *pulmonary diseases,* the study of disorders of the lungs and respiratory system; and *rheumatology,* the study of connecting and supporting tissues.

Neurological Surgery: The *neurological surgeon* deals with the diagnosis, treatment, and surgical management of disorders and diseases of the brain, spinal cord, and nervous systems.

Neurology: A *neurologist* diagnoses and treats disorders of the brain and nervous system as well as of the muscles.

Nuclear Medicine: The *nuclear medicine specialist* is concerned with the use of radioactive material in the diagnosis and treatment of disease.

Obstetrics and Gynecology: An *obstetrician* specializes in the treatment of pregnant women and delivers babies. A *gynecologist* specializes in the treatment of women and their particular diseases, especially the reproductive system. Often, physicians specialize in both areas.

Ophthalmology: An *ophthalmologist* specializes in the medical and surgical treatment of the eye. Ophthalmologists also treat eye diseases.

Orthopedic Surgery: An *orthopedist* diagnoses, treats, and surgically corrects disorders and injuries of the bones, joints, muscles, cartilage, and ligaments.

Otorhinolaryngology: An *otorhinolaryngologist* treats disorders of the ears, nose, and throat.

Pathology: A *pathologist* investigates the course and causes of diseases.

Pediatrics: A *pediatrician* specializes in all medical aspects of child care. Subspecialties of pediatrics include: *pediatric cardiology, pediatric endocrinology, pediatric hematology/oncology, neonatal/perinatal medicine,* and *nephrology.*

Physical Medicine and Rehabilitation: A *physiatrist* deals with restoring either the full or partial use of body parts that have been injured or diseased, or have been defective at birth.

Plastic Surgery: A *plastic surgeon* repairs defects of the skin and underlying tissue. The plastic surgeon also performs surgery sought purely for cosmetic reasons.

Psychiatry: A *psychiatrist* treats behavior disorders, often with psychotherapy, but also with drugs.

Radiology: A *radiologist* specializes in the use of radiant energy such as X rays to diagnose and treat disease.

Surgery: A *general surgeon* specializes in the diagnosis and surgical treatment of a wide range of diseases, although most surgeons choose to specialize further.

Urology: A *urologist* diagnoses and treats disorders of the urinary-tract organs, and in men, problems of the reproductive system.

The Physical Examination

One of the first questions many people have about the physical exam is "How often should I have one?" Visits for infants from birth to 18 months are typically scheduled at 2, 4, 6, 15, and 18 months. Visits for children from 2 to 18 are typically scheduled once a year. Visits for individuals aged 19 to 65 are recommended every 1 to 3 years, for most people beginning on the low side (every 3 years) and progressing to every year as one approaches age 65. After age 65 annual visits are recommended.

A typical physical examination will include a careful health appraisal by an examining physician, including a detailed health history of the patient and study of the patient's body appearance and functions.

The patient's *medical history* is important because the physician needs to know any medical problems the patient may have had in the past, including operations or pregnancies, medications the patient is allergic to or is currently taking, and any incidence of family illnesses that may make the patient more susceptible to such things as heart disease or cancer.

After the medical history has been recorded or updated, the physician may begin a general inspection of the patient's body, beginning with the head and neck and working down to the feet. The physician looks for possible deformities, scars or wounds, pulsations, or throbbing areas. Bruises, areas of skin peeling or flaking, areas of heavy skin pigmentation or loss of pigmentation, hair distribution, perspiration or goose bumps, firmness or slackness of the skin, warts, calluses, and other features are noted.

The physician usually checks the

Stickpin Blood Collection

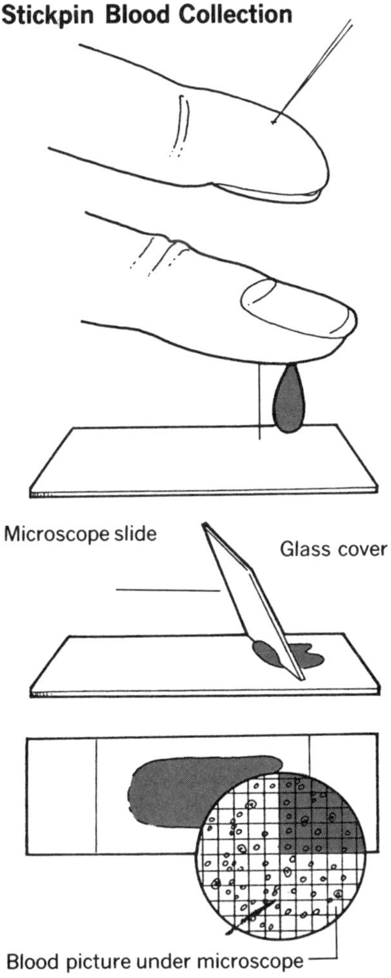

exterior of the body by a method known as *palpation,* which means feeling with the fingers and hands. Rough vibrations from a disorder in the respiratory system, the trembling sensation of blood encountering an obstruction, or the grating feeling of a bone deformity can be detected during palpation. In addition to palpation, the physician may apply *percussion,* or tapping, of certain body areas. Tapping the chest, for example, gives the physician some information about the condition of the lungs. A related technique, *auscultation,* involves listening to sounds within the body through a stethoscope. During percussion, the physician listens for changes in sounds that range from resonance over hollow spaces to dullness over solid or muscular areas. Lack of resonance over a normally resonant area of the lung might indicate fluid, pneumonia, or perhaps an abnormal mass. Percussion may also give the first sign of enlargement of organs, such as the liver, heart, or spleen. During auscultation, the physician listens for abnormal breathing sounds as the air rushes in and out of the lungs. Abnormal breathing sounds can indicate specific aberrations in lung function. In auscultation of the heart, the physician listens for extra heartbeats, rubbing sounds, the rumbling noises of a heart murmur, or the sounds of normally functioning heart valves opening and closing.

The physician may also use the stethoscope to listen to sounds beyond the chest area. He or she may listen to the sounds of blood flowing through vessels of the neck, bowel sounds through the wall of the abdomen, and the subtle noises made by joints, muscles, and tendons as various limbs are moved.

Weight, height, blood pressure, and pulse rate are also checked as part of any routine examination. There can be a wide variation in these readings from individual to individual, but drastic changes for a given person may signal a health disorder.

Common Screening Tests

A variety of tests may be given in a routine physical exam, depending on the patient's age, family history, and current state of health. Some of the following tests will be done each time the patient visits the doctor and some are necessary only when specific complaints or concerns are raised or when an individual reaches a certain age or risk category. Your doctor should explain any new test to you.

Blood Pressure and Pulse Rate

The patient's blood pressure and pulse rate are checked on every office visit. Blood pressure is measured with a *sphygmomanometer* and a stethoscope. The sphygmomanometer is attached to an inflatable cuff, which is wrapped around the upper arm; a rubber bulb is used to inflate the cuff and increase pressure in it so that it can control the blood flow in the arm. The physician locates the pulse with the stethoscope and increases the cuff pressure until the pulse (heartbeat) can no longer be heard. Then the physician slowly deflates the cuff and lets the reading on the gauge fall gradually until he hears the first beat of the heart. The reading on the gauge at that point is recorded as the *systolic pressure*. The physician continues to relax the pressure in the cuff and watches for the reading at the point where the thumping of the heart disappears again. That number is recorded as the *diastolic pressure*.

The doctor checks a patient's pulse rate to find out if the heart is beating normally. The pulse is the rhythmic expansion of the arteries that takes place after each heart beat. The pulse rate is the number of pulsations of an artery per minute. The normal pulse rate for a person at rest varies from as little as 50 for elderly people to as much as 100 for children.

Eyes, Mouth, and Ears

Inspection of the eyes is usually done with the aid of an *ophthalmoscope*, with which the physician can see the retina at the back of the eye. Distended retinal veins may be a sign of a variety of disorders, including diabetes or heart disease; signs of hardening of the arteries also may be observed in the eyes before other indications are found elsewhere. The condition of retinal blood vessels may also signal the development of hypertension.

A device called an *otoscope* is inserted in the outer ear to examine the external auditory canal and eardrum. The condition of the tongue, teeth, and gums can reveal much about the health of the individual.

Cholesterol Measurement

An elevated blood cholesterol level is an important risk factor for coronary artery disease. For most people a blood cholesterol level above 200 mg/dl should be cause for concern, indicating a need for further tests and perhaps a change in life-style.

Blood cholesterol levels are measured by withdrawing a small amount of blood—usually from the arm—to be analyzed in a lab. The result is given in terms of milligrams of cholesterol per deciliter of blood. It's a good idea to have your blood cholesterol checked at age 25 and then once every 3 to 5 years thereafter.

Blood Tests

Complete Blood Count

A Complete Blood Count (CBC) provides the physician with more information than any other single laboratory screening procedure. Four common measurements are taken from it:

Hemoglobin concentration. Hemoglobin is the chemical substance that transports oxygen through the bloodstream to all the cells of the body. This measurement determines the amount of hemoglobin per unit volume of blood.

Red blood cell count. This test measures the number of red cells per cubic millimeter of blood. A low red blood cell count may indicate anemia, as well as be a potential early warning sign for leukemia, kidney malfunction, internal bleeding, or sickle cell anemia.

Hematocrit. The hematocrit measures the ratio of red blood cells to the plasma in the blood. Like the hemoglobin concentration and the red blood cell count, the hematocrit can indicate anemia, and all three tests are generally given in order to help diagnose the specific type and cause of anemia.

White blood cell count. This test measures the number of white cells per cubic millimeter of blood. A high white blood cell count can indicate an infection, a major injury, or even leukemia. A low count can be a sign of poor diet, certain infections, or another type of leukemia. If taken in the presence of a fever, the white blood cell count can help distinguish between a bacterial and a viral infection.

Blood Glucose

The glucose test determines the amount of sugar in the blood. Individuals who experience symptoms of diabetes mellitus (such as excessive thirst or urination), hypoglycemia (lightheadedness or fainting), or who are pregnant will most likely be given a blood glucose test. A very high level of blood sugar can indicate diabetes, while a very low level can indicate hypoglycemia. In either case or in border-line cases an *oral glucose tol-*

erance test is given. This test requires that the individual fast for 12 to 14 hours before the test. The patient is then given a concentrated sugar solution to drink, and blood is drawn at regular intervals over the next several hours. This test has replaced the urine test for sugar.

Blood Urea Nitrogen (BUN) and Blood Creatinine

Blood urea and creatinine are products of protein metabolism. A high level of either in the blood means that the kidneys are not filtering them properly from the blood, possibly because of kidney damage.

Blood Electrolytes

The four blood electrolytes are sodium, potassium, chloride, and bicarbonate, and they play important roles in the blood pH, the cells' water balance, and kidney function. Most often this test is given to patients who are taking diuretics, those with liver, kidney, or heart disease, or those who may be experiencing dehydration or excessive vomiting or diarrhea.

Urinalysis

The urinalysis is a simple and important test that can indicate much about a person's overall health and identify potential problems, such as kidney disease, diabetes, and urinary tract infections. For a routine urinalysis a sample can be taken at any time of day, although the physician may specify the first morning's urine, or may give special instructions about food and water intake before taking the urine sample.

Urinalysis includes a specific gravity test (a test to measure the extent to which solids are concentrated in the urine as an indication of how well the kidneys are conserving the body's fluids) and a pH test (a test to measure the acidity of the urine as an indication of how well the kidneys are able to remove acid wastes).

There are also tests for the presence of glucose (sugar), protein, blood, and bilirubin (a substance produced in the liver from the breakdown of old blood cells); none of these substances is normally found in the urine. The presence of glucose is an indication of diabetes; protein in the urine is associated with diabetes, hypertension, and other diseases; blood in the urine can indicate many problems including kidney stones, cysts, infection, and cancer; the presence of bilirubin suggests a problem in the liver or bile ducts. The presence of bacteria or of a large number of white blood cells is typically an indication of a urinary tract infection.

Routine blood work and a urinalysis are simple, common tests that can catch many potential problems early. When abnormalities exist, other, more specific—and often more expensive—tests are required for confirmation before treatment can begin. Given the fact that any test can give a false result, whether through human error or through individual variations, the question of whether or

Electrocardiogram

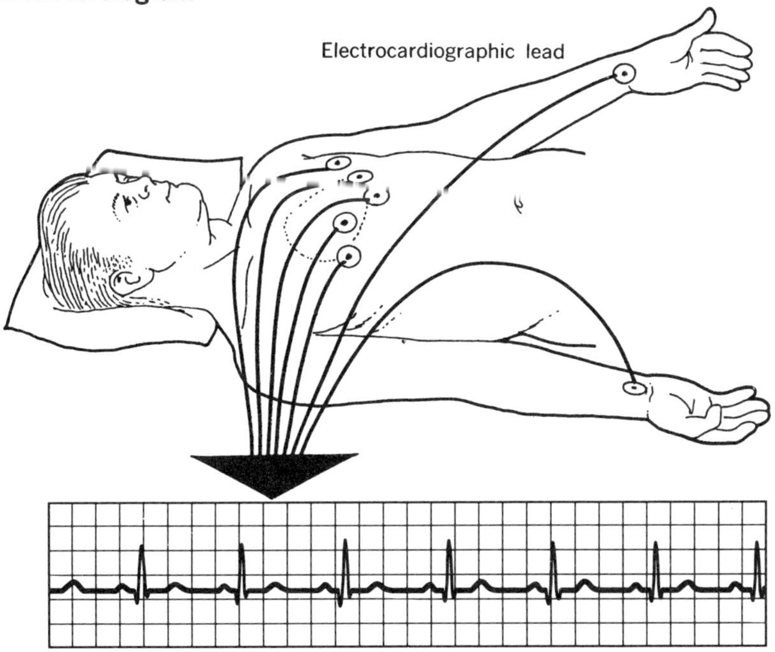

not individuals should have these tests is a much-debated point in the medical community and one best discussed with one's primary care physician.

Electrocardiogram

The electrocardiogram (ECG or EKG) measures heart activity by detecting the electrical activity in the heart. Electrodes attached to the chest, neck, arms, and legs record the pathway of electrical impulses through the heart muscle and record these impulses as tracings on special graph paper. The test is simple and safe, and takes five to ten minutes to perform.

The purpose of the EKG is to detect heart disorders or blockages in the coronary arteries. A normally beating heart produces basically the same pattern of waves in all people. Variations in this pattern can indicate a number of potential problems: irregular heart rhythms, damage to the heart muscle, enlargement of the heart's chambers, mineral imbalances in the blood. The EKG can also reveal whether the patient has had, or is having, a heart attack.

This test is not foolproof, however, and can produce false results. Some people with normal EKGs have heart trouble, and the graph may show abnormalities where none exists.

EKGs are usually a routine part of a physical checkup after age 40; before that age, patients are recommended to have at least one EKG to use for comparison later.

Cancer Screening Test

Carcinoembryonic antigen (CEA), a substance normally found only in fetuses, may indicate the presence of certain cancers when found at elevated levels in adults. This test is typically used in patients who have been treated for such cancers as colon/rectal, breast, lung, ovarian, pancreatic, and stomach to check for possible recurrence of the disease.

Mammogram

A *mammogram* is an X ray of the breast done to locate breast tumors and cysts. To date, it is the only screening exam that can find small tumors before they can be felt and when they have the greatest chance of being cured. It is estimated that yearly mammograms for women over 40 could lead to a one-third reduction in the number of deaths from breast cancer.

The patient must remove all clothing from the waist up and stand with the breast placed on a small shelf that extends out from the machine. The patient is then guided forward so that the edge of the shelf presses into the chest just below the breast. A compression device is brought down onto the breast, and pressure is applied for less than 30 seconds. This is the most uncomfortable part of the test, as much pressure is necessary in order to get the most detailed picture possible and use the least amount of radiation. Eliminating caffeine and foods that tend to cause water retention two weeks prior to the exam makes the breasts less sensitive.

The American Cancer Society recommends that women aged 40 and older have a mammogram every year.

For more information and a comparison of diagnostic and screening mammograms, see *Women's Health*, Ch. 25, "Cancer of the Breast."

Pap Smear

The *pap smear* tests for cervical cancer by the microscopic examination of cells from the vaginal walls and cervix. Although it is not infallible this test detects 95 percent of cervical cancers; it is an important aid in the detection of this disease at a stage when it is often without symptoms and it is still curable.

The procedure can be done any time except during the menstrual period. The patient undresses from the waist down and lies down on her back with her legs spread apart and her feet in special stirrups. The physician inserts a lubricated *speculum* into the vagina and opens it to expose the cervix and its os (mouth). The doctor then inserts a small applicator through the speculum and rubs it gently against the cervix and sometimes the os. The applicator is removed and rubbed onto a glass slide (the smear). The speculum is then removed.

The first pap smear should be done when a woman turns 18 or becomes sexually active (whichever occurs first), and should be followed by pap smears for 2 consecutive years. Providing these tests are negative and there are no risk factors present, tests can be done less frequently at the discretion of one's doctor, although an annual pap smear for women between 25 and 60 is common.

Prostate Tests

Cancer of the prostate is a leading cause of death in men over 50. If detected early, prostate cancer can usually be cured. It can often be detected by digital rectal examination (DRE), a routine procedure in which the doctor inserts a gloved finger into the rectum and feels the prostate gland. Another test measures blood levels of the prostate-specific antigen (PSA), a protein produced in the prostate that may be elevated when cancer is present.

Occult Blood Test

Colon cancer is the second most common form of cancer in the United States. An early warning sign of colon cancer is blood in the stool. It is called *occult,* or hidden, blood because it cannot be detected by sight. It is recommended that everyone over age 50 be tested for occult blood annually.

Usually, stools are tested for occult blood at home with the help of a self-test kit. The test calls for smearing cards with stool samples collected over several days. The samples are sent to a lab to be tested for hidden blood. If blood is detected, further diagnostic tests, including a colonoscopy (a visual examination of the entire colon), may be ordered.

Sigmoidoscopy

Another procedure for detecting colon cancer is *sigmoidoscopy,* the use of a tubular scope called a sigmoidoscope to examine the lower segment of the large intestine. The purpose of this test is to detect tumors in the rectum and colon. To ensure a clean lower bowel, the patient must follow a special diet—typically an all-liquid diet—for several days prior to the test, use laxatives the night before, and take an enema on the day of the test. The patient puts on a hospital gown and lies on the left side with the knees drawn up to the chest. A thin, lubricated tube is inserted into the rectum and slowly advanced along the large intestine. The tube contains optical filaments through which light can pass and transmit images to a microscope or monitor for the doctor to view. It may also contain small instruments that enable the doctor to take tissue samples. Air may be forced through the tube to expand the intestine, which can cause a feeling of discomfort. The procedure takes from 15 to 30 minutes. The American Cancer Society recommends a baseline sigmoidoscopy for everyone at age 50 (or 40 if there is a family history of colon cancer) and once every three years after that.

Sexually Transmitted Diseases

The prevalence of sexually transmitted diseases (STDs), such as syphilis, gonorrhea, chlamydia, genital herpes, and AIDS makes regular tests for these diseases in sexually active people who are not in monogamous relationships vitally important. Tests are typically blood tests or swab tests and should be done every year or two.

Tuberculosis

Tuberculosis is normally tested for with a simple *skin test.* The forearm is either pricked with a small device with four prongs or a subcutaneous injection is used. In either case, the patient is asked to check the area after 48 to 72 hours for signs of redness, raised bumps, or swelling.

Stress Test

Stress tests are often given to older people who are about to begin an exercise program. During this test, the heart's activity is monitored with an electrocardiogram (EKG) while the patient exercises on a treadmill or stationary bicycle. The procedure is usually done in a physician's office or a local hospital. It is a trouble-shooting test designed to reveal problems that a resting EKG does not. At rest, an EKG may indicate that the heart is receiving sufficient oxygen; but with exertion, as the heart's workload increases, the exercise stress test may reveal signs of an inadequate oxygen supply to certain areas of the heart muscle. The most common cause of this condition is a narrowing of coronary arteries due to a buildup of plaque. Thus the stress test can help identify an abnormality that might otherwise go undetected until a person is exercising and unexpectedly experiences chest pain. A routine stress test is often recommended at age 45, and as early as 35 if the patient has at least one risk factor for coronary artery disease. Risk factors include smoking, obesity, hypertension, and elevated cholesterol levels.

Chest X ray

The *chest X ray* was once a routine part of the physical exam. Its expense, potential danger, and limited results in the absence of symptoms has made it less popular. (An individual X ray in and of itself is not harmful, but because exposure to radiation is cumulative throughout your life, a series of

X rays over a lifetime can result in increased risk of cancer.) A chest X ray produces a picture that includes the heart and lungs. It can be useful in identifying certain heart problems, and is also used to detect lung cancer.

If you are advised to have a chest X ray, you will be asked to remove all clothing from the waist up and to wear a gown. Depending on the particular area to be X rayed, you will either sit, stand, or lie down. Generally two or three exposures are taken for each area targeted.

Immunizations

Nearly everyone knows the importance of having their children immunized, but many people may not realize that it is important for adults to have regular immunizations as well. When a patient is immunized, he or she receives a shot of modified microbes (bacteria or viruses) or toxins. Although not strong enough to actually give the patient the disease, the dose of microbes does stimulate the patient's own immune system to build up antibodies against the disease, thus making him or her immune to future exposures. Vaccines do wear off, however, and it is best to keep a record of all immunizations and receive scheduled booster shots.

Diphtheria

Diphtheria is spread by airborne bacteria that release toxins that can attack the heart and other internal organs. Adults should receive a booster shot every ten years.

Tetanus

Tetanus is spread by bacteria that enter the body through a contaminated wound. Adults should receive a booster shot (often combined with the diphtheria shot) every ten years. If you sustain a contaminated wound, your doctor may recommend a tetanus booster is you have not had one in 5 years.

Influenza

The risk of death from the *flu* increases with age, and people over 65 are strongly advised to receive annual flu shots in the fall. In 1976 about 500 cases of a rare paralytic condition called Guillain-Barre syndrome were associated with a swine flu vaccine. No influenza vaccines since have been associated with the development of Guillain-Barre.

Pneumococcal Pneumonia

A vaccine is available that offers protection against the 23 strains of bacteria that cause about 80 percent of pneumococcal diseases in the United States. All adults age 65 and older should receive the pneumonia vaccine on an annual basis, as should younger adults with chronic cardiopulmonary disorders, diabetes, renal disease, liver disease, blood diseases, cancers, and diseases that suppress immunity such as HIV infection.

Those at risk of death from influenza should also be immunized with the pneumonia vaccine, but only once. Because it may increase adverse side effects, repeat or booster shots of the vaccine are not recommended.

Measles and Mumps

Many people born after 1957 have not had and have not been immunized against *measles* and *mumps* and thus are particularly susceptible to these diseases. In addition, those vaccinated between 1963 and 1967 may have gotten a short-lasting killed-virus vaccine and should be revaccinated. Anyone born between 1957 and 1967 should be revaccinated unless 1) they had a case of measles confirmed by a physician's diagnosis, 2) they are immune, as demonstrated by a blood test, 3) they have a record of receiving live vaccine no earlier than their first birthday.

Hepatitis A

Hepatitis is an inflammation of the liver, usually caused by a virus infection. Hepatitis A is the most common form of the disease. It is transmitted mainly by contaminated food or water. Symptoms include fever, nausea, vomiting, and jaundice.

There is a safe and effective vaccine available to people at high risk for the disease and to travelers to countries where hepatitis A is endemic.

Hepatitis B

Like the HIV virus that causes AIDS, hepatitis B is spread through blood contact with virus-infected body fluids; the most common form of transmission is sexual contact. However, hepatitis B is much more contagious than the HIV virus and is the leading cause of cirrhosis and cancer of the liver. Half of those infected with hepatitis B never develop symptoms, and thus become unwitting chronic carriers of it. Vaccination is strongly recommended, especially for those with a high risk of infection, such as health care workers, sexually active persons with multiple partners, intravenous drug users, hemodialysis patients, newborns with infected mothers, and residents and staff of institutions for the mentally retarded.

Children

The standard immunizations for children are 1) combined vaccines for diphtheria, pertussis, and tetanus (DPT); 2) a series of polio vaccinations combining inactivate poliovirus vaccine (IPV) followed by oral, attenuated poliovirus vaccine (OPV); 3) vaccines for measles, mumps, and rubella (MMR); 4) hemophilus influenza type B conjugate vaccine (HIB). The Centers for Disease Control recommends the following schedule:

- 2 months: DPT, IPV, HIB
- 4 months: DPT, IPV, HIB
- 6 months: DPT and HIB
- 12 months: DPT, OPV, HIB, TB test, MMR
- 4 to 6 years: DPT, MMR, and OPV

Hepatitis B and chicken pox vaccines are also available.

Other Diagnostic Tests

If a definite diagnosis cannot be made on the basis of the medical history, preliminary physical exam, and routine diagnostic tests, more specialized tests may be required. What follows is a description, grouped by body system, of some of the other diagnostic tests.

Tests for Mental Disorders

When a physician suspects that a patient has a mental disorder, the physician must first rule out the possibility that the symptoms are caused by a physical illness. After physical disorders have been ruled out, mental-status tests may be administered. These include the Rorschach inkblot test, the Thematic Apperception Test, the Minnesota Multiphasic Personality Inventory, and the Wechsler Adult Intelligence Scale. These tests are used to diagnose various psychological and psychiatric disorders, including depression, paranoia, anxiety, psychopathy, and schizophrenia.

The Skeletal System

The skeletal system includes the bones and cartilage, and the specialist who handles problems of the skeletal system is the orthopedic surgeon. Disorders of the nervous system and joints often overlap skeletal problems and may necessitate tests by a neurologist or rheumatologist.

X rays are the most important diagnostic tool for special investigations of the bones. They can reveal a hairline fracture of a major bone, a bony deposit, or abnormal alignment.

Synovial aspiration, or a *synovial fluid exam,* involves the withdrawal of a tiny amount of synovial fluid with a needle inserted into a joint. The laboratory analysis of the fluid can help diagnose such problems as gout and some forms of arthritis.

MRI, or *magnetic resonance imaging,* is a way of creating an image of a body part by taking advantage of the way protons behave in a magnetic field when exposed to a radio-frequency pulse: the way they line up and the form of the radiowave that they emit produces the image. The patient lies down on a table, and a surface coil is applied. The surface coil

The Human Skeleton

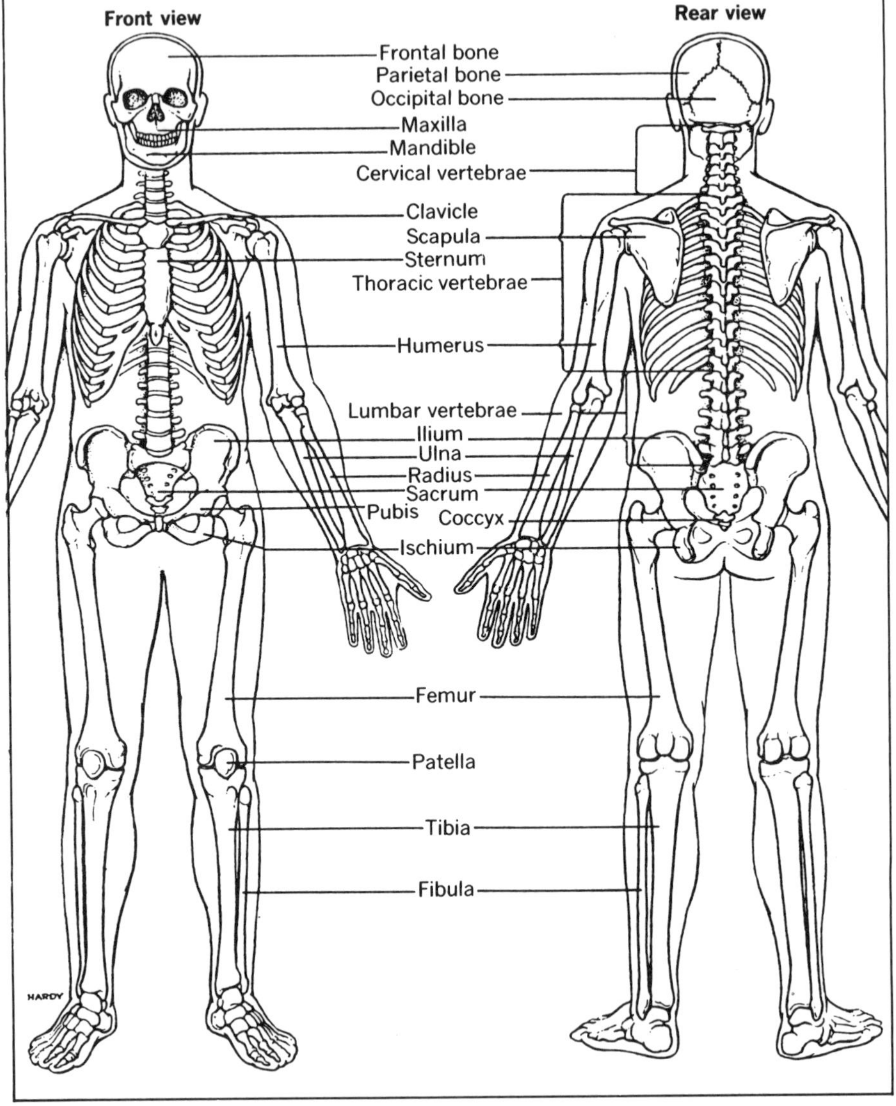

is the device that emits the radiofrequency pulse. The patient's heartbeat and respiration are monitored, usually by a small band placed around a finger. Next, the table moves the patient so that the area to be examined is inside the magnet. The magnet is in the form of a tunnel and may make some people feel claustrophobic. At this point the noise level increases and may be uncomfortable. Several images are taken, with the table moving slightly between each. MRI is safer than X rays because there is no exposure to ionizing radiation; however, pregnant women and people with implanted stimulatory devices, such as pacemakers, should not have MRI performed.

Nuclear imaging involves the injection, swallowing, instillation, or inhalation of a *radioactive isotope* (a marker, or tracer) of a substance that is naturally absorbed by the organ or tissues that need observation. A camera sensitive to the radiation emitted by the isotope is then used to create an image that shows the location of the material within the body. Two uses of this technique for skeletal exams are the bone scan and the bone density test. These tests are more sensitive than X rays and can often identify a problem months before it shows up on the X ray. They are used when the X ray comes back normal, but symptoms persist.

In the *bone scan* the patient receives an injection of an isotope that is taken up by bone tissues. Scanning begins two to four hours later. Either the entire body or just the part under observation is imaged. Injuries, infections, and tumors can all be located with this technique.

The *bone density test* is used to diagnose osteoporosis, the decrease in bone density that is the major cause of fractures in the elderly. The most accurate bone-density test is dual-energy X-ray absorptiometry (DXA), which uses low doses of radiation—less than is used in an X ray—to measure bone density. The test is painless and safe and can be performed in 5 to 15 minutes.

Ultrasonography is most often employed in skeletal exams to determine whether a "lump" or "bump" is solid or fluid-filled. Ultrasonography follows the same principle that applies to sonar: Sound waves emitted by a transducer are directed at a particular part of the body; they bounce back, and are translated into an image. Tissues, bones, water, air— all vary consistently in the way they reflect the sound wave, thus making possible the interpretation of the reflected image.

Arthroscopy is a way of seeing inside the body by using an arthroscope, an optical instrument equipped with lenses and lights that is inserted in a small opening. The area most often studied by this method is the knee.

The Muscles and Joints

The human body has more than 600 muscles of various sizes and shapes, all of them attached to the skeletal system. They enable us to move as they contract. The joints are the spaces between two coupled bones that allow the bones to move in more than one direction. Muscles and joints are the domain of the rheumatologist.

The synovial fluid exam, X rays, MRI, nuclear imaging, and ultrasonography described under the skeletal system are used to examine the muscles and joints as well. When there is a problem with muscle control, inability to relax a muscle, or weakness in commonly used muscles, another test that may be ordered is the *electromyogram.* This test measures a muscle's electrical potential, which should be zero if the muscle is relaxed. An electrode is attached to the skin over the target muscle and another electrode, in the form of a small needle, is inserted in the muscle. Lead wires from the two electrodes are attached to a monitor, and measurements of the muscle's electrical activity are made while the patient contracts and relaxes it. This test helps determine whether the problem is with the muscle itself or with the nerves controlling it (in which case an electroneurogram is in order).

Joints are prone to stiffness and damage from swelling of the surrounding bursa and tendons. X rays and MRIs will detect damage to the bursa and tendons.

Skin

The dermatologist specializes in treating skin disorders. Many problems specific to the skin can be diagnosed by physical examination and questioning of the patient.

Skin tests are commonly done on allergy sufferers to determine what they are allergic to. In a *prick test* the forearm is cleansed and a drop each of up to 35 different solutions is placed in rows on the arm. The doctor then takes a small needlelike object and pricks the center of each drop. After 15 minutes any of the solutions to which the patient is allergic will produce a slight swelling much like a mosquito bite. A *scratch test* is similar; a small scratch is made on the arm and the drop is applied. In the *intradermal test* the solution is injected. A *patch test* is done when the patient has a rash, probably caused by something that touches the skin. Patches of possible allergens are placed on the back, and the patient returns in two days for a reading.

Sores that refuse to heal; changes in the shape, color, and texture of warts or moles; and blemishes that bleed or itch are all considered symptoms of skin cancer and should be checked by your doctor. These skin eruptions are usually removed entirely and a biopsy is performed on the tissue. They can be cut out (excised) or removed with an electric needle or laser.

The Nervous System

The brain, spinal cord, and network of nerves make up the nervous system. The neurosurgeon and the neurologist are the specialists.

In a *spinal tap,* or *spinal fluid exam,* the doctor inserts a needle into the lower back and removes a small amount of spinal fluid, which is then examined in the lab. The test may cause severe headaches; it is used to diagnose infections, brain hemorrhages, tumors, polio, meningitis, and other conditions. *Myelography* is a similar study, much more painful, in

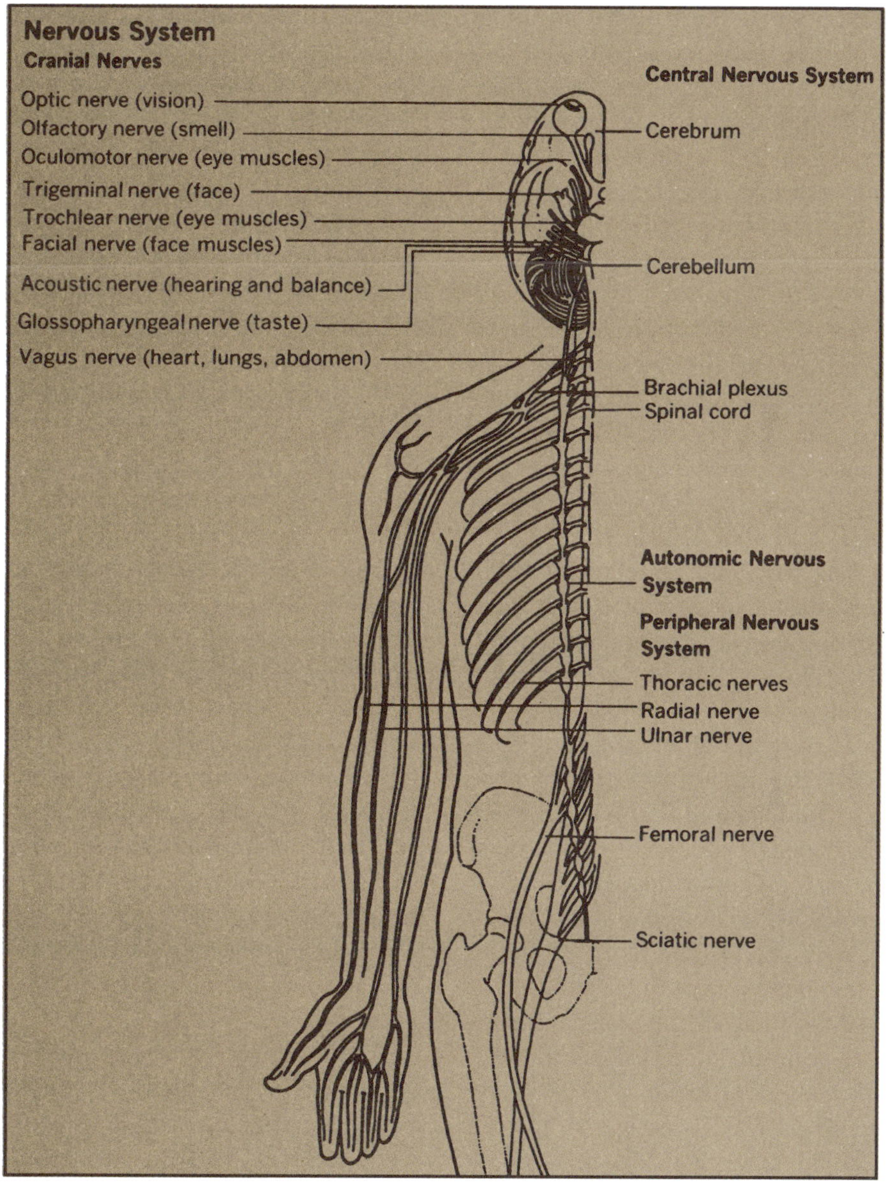

which a small amount of spinal fluid is removed, dye injected in its place, and X rays are taken while the patient lies on a table. Slipped disks, some types of arthritis, and different types of tumors are commonly diagnosed this way, although the use of MRI (see skeletal system) and computerized axial tomography (CT) are also used and are often done first.

The CT exam is a noninvasive procedure that produces a series of X-ray images showing "slices" of the targeted body part. For the exam, the patient lies on a table (called a gantry) which is then moved into the machine. Several exposures are taken, with the table moving slightly between each. For some studies it is necessary to inject a special dye, which can cause mild discomfort. Some people experience a claustrophobic reaction while inside the machine. CT is about 100 times more sensitive than conventional X rays and is used to detect calcium deposits, tumors, cysts, and abscesses. Because of its sensitivity to tissue density, it can sometimes distinguish benign from malignant tumors.

The *brain scan* continues to be an important diagnostic tool. This radioisotope study of the brain is used to detect tumors, hemorrhages, stroke, or blood vessel abnormalities.

The brain scan involves the injection in the arm of a radioactive isotope and the scanning of the brain by either a single-photon emission computed tomography camera (SPECT) or a positron emission tomography camera (PET). The SPECT scanner uses gamma rays to create images and the PET scanner uses positrons (a type of subatomic particle found in the nucleus of an atom) to create images. The PET scan is able to read through different depths of tissue, so problems deeply buried in the brain can be detected without surgery.

When the blood supply to the brain is limited by the blocking of the carotid arteries (a condition known as transient ischemic attack, or TIA), momentary loss of brain function can occur and can eventually lead to a stroke. Thus examining the carotid arteries is important if the patient has symptoms or significant risk factors. This can be done by X ray or by ultrasound. In the ultrasound test two techniques are generally used. The first creates images (called duplex) and the second measures the rate and quality of blood flow (called Doppler). Both involve the gentle movement of the transducer slowly over each side of the neck. The procedure takes about 30 minutes.

Patients who have experienced TIA, stroke, or vertigo may undergo *ocular plethysmography* (OPG) to detect narrowing of the ophthalmic artery. The patient is seated in a chair with a headrest, blood pressure is taken in each arm, and EKG leads are placed on the chest. Anesthetic drops are placed in each eye. The technologist then places tiny plastic cups into the corner of each eye. The cups are attached to wire leads connected to the machine. The patient is instructed to keep the eyes wide open. The machine then produces a slight suction on each eye and measures its pressure.

When epilepsy is suspected, following certain head injuries, or when the patient is experiencing confusion, sleep problems, and even impotence, an *electroencephalograph* (EEG) may be ordered. The patient sits in a chair while a technologist attaches 16 to 22 electrodes to his or her head. EKG leads are also placed on the chest. The patient then lies down and may even fall asleep. The technologist may instruct the patient to open and close both eyes while a strobe light flashes. The test takes about two hours.

The electromyogram was discussed under the section on muscles. If the muscle is not the problem, the nerves connected to it may be and a *nerve conduction study,* or *electroneurogram,* is ordered. This test measures the speed of the electrical impulse across a nerve and the speed of the muscle's response to it. Electrodes are affixed to the skin over the target muscle. The target nerve is then given a mild electric shock. The electrode over the muscle measures both the time between the shock and the response (the muscle will twitch) and the intensity of the response. The corresponding nonaffected muscles are also tested for comparison. There is no hazard, and the shock feels like a mild sting or burn.

The Circulatory System

The cardiologist specializes in diseases of the heart and circulatory system. Coronary artery disease is the most common form of heart disease and involves the blocking of the arteries to the heart. There can also be problems with the heart muscle itself, problems with the heart valves, or congenital problems resulting from birth defects.

The electrocardiogram and the stress test have already been discussed. Nuclear imaging, ultrasound, and X rays are also used to detect coronary artery disease. In order to detect exactly how blocked the arteries are and determine the necessary correctional procedure, an *angiograph,* or *angiogram,* is done.

The angiograph begins with the insertion of a special needle in a major artery (usually in the groin). A sudden spurt of blood indicates correct positioning. A wire is then inserted through the needle, which stops the bleeding. The wire is advanced to the target area, and the needle is removed. A catheter is then slid over the wire and is advanced to the target area. The wire is then withdrawn. The next step is the injection of a special dye to the target area. To prevent its being diluted it must be injected at high velocity and in large quantity. For most people the injection is extremely uncomfortable, with some reporting severe pain, a feeling of heat, headache, chest pain, or dizziness. The next step involves the rapid imaging of the target area, usually by a series of X-ray pictures. Often different views are needed of the targeted area, which means that the catheter must be repositioned and the dye reinjected. Once the pictures are finished the catheter is slowly removed and pressure is applied to the hole to seal the artery. The pressure involved is intense and lasts for 10 to 15 minutes. Because it is necessary for the patient to be conscious during the procedure, the entire process may cause extreme anxiety, which in turn increases the risk of heart attack. The patient is normally given a sedative to help relieve the anxiety. An overnight stay in the hospital following the procedure is routine. *Venography* is a sim-

The Circulatory System

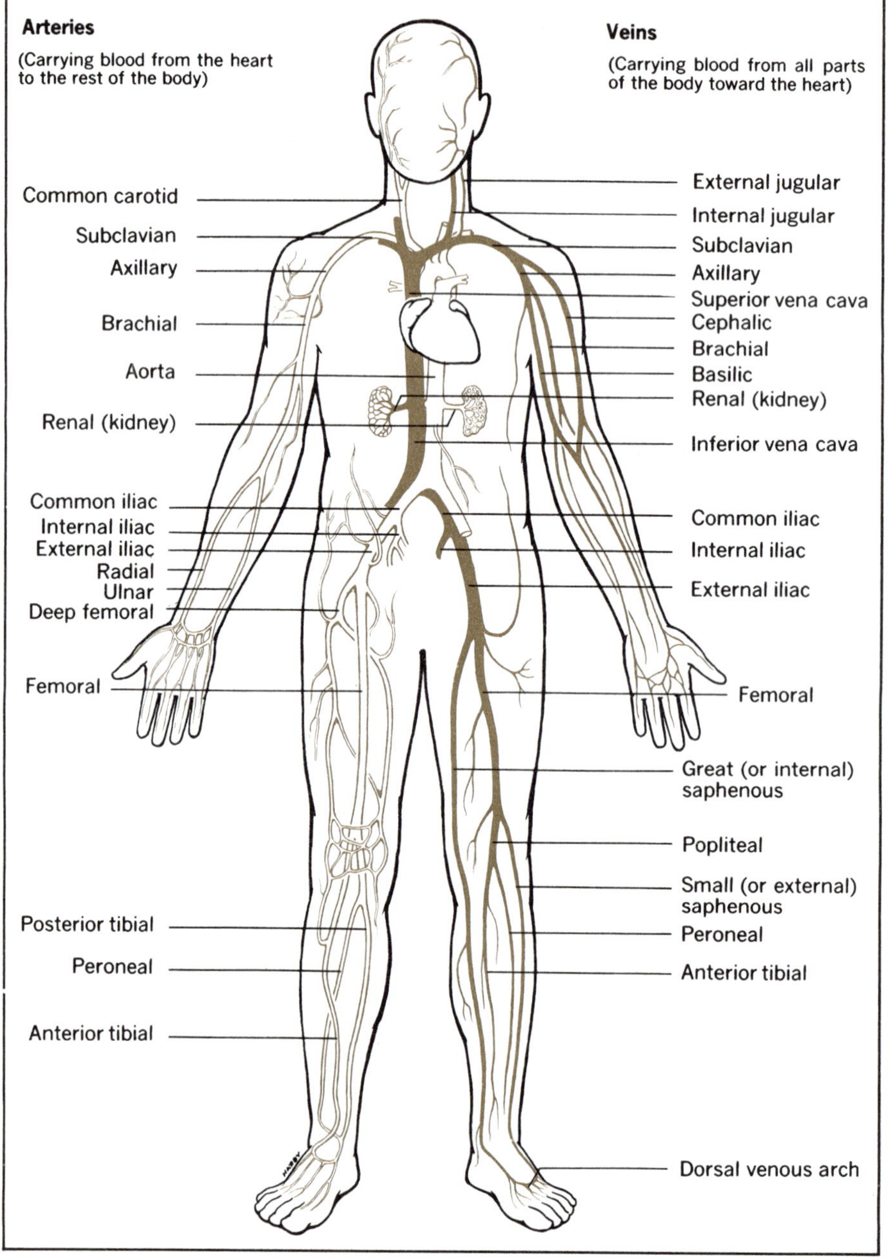

ilar study of the veins.

Not all people who experience sudden and severe chest pain are having a heart attack. A technique called *infarct detection* can confirm the diagnosis of heart attack. Normally per-

The Heart

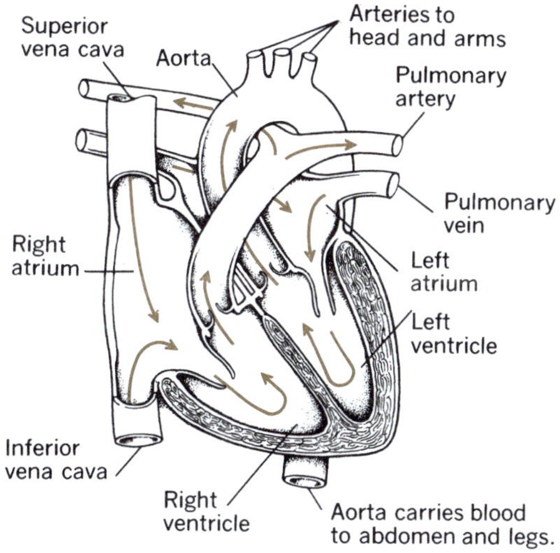

Septal Defects

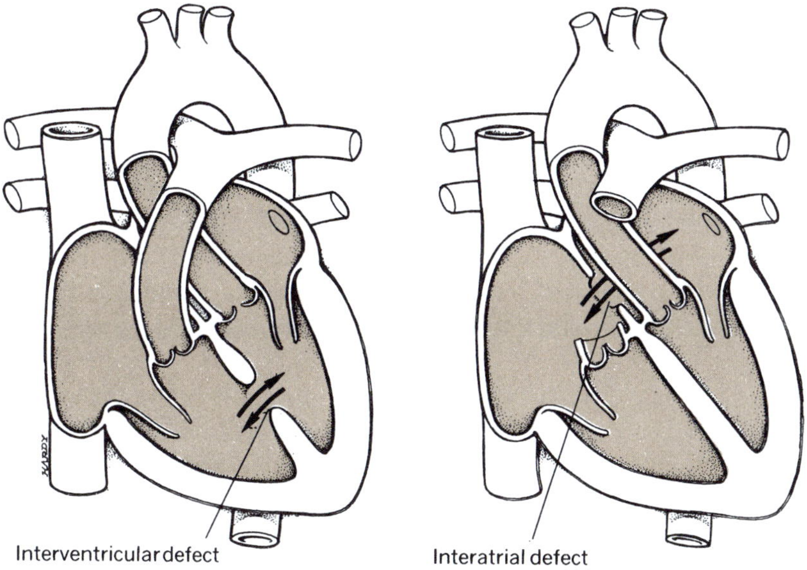

A normal heart in cross section *(top)*, shows the circulation of the blood. An interventricular defect *(bottom left)* allows blood to pass directly between the left and right ventricles. An interatrial defect *(bottom right)*, with the aorta seen in cross section over the left atrium, allows blood to pass freely between the two atria. Any septal defect interferes with the effectiveness of the pumping action of the heart.

formed within the first 12 to 24 hours after the onset of the pain, the test involves the injection of an isotope (thallium-201) into a vein. The patient is then positioned under a gamma-ray camera and an image is created of the heart that will make evident any occluded (blocked) vessels. A similar nuclear imaging process is used to obtain information about the heart's *wall motion* (how well the muscle relaxes and contracts) and *ejection fraction* (how much blood leaves a chamber of the heart when it contracts). Both tests give valuable information about the heart's health.

While X rays provide more detail, nuclear imaging can also be used to check *circulatory integrity,* or how open the veins and arteries are. Again, a radioactive isotope is injected into a vein near the target area and images are produced via a gamma-ray camera.

Evaluation of the ejection fraction, valve function, and pericardial fluid (found in the pericardial membrane that surrounds the heart) can also be done with ultrasound. In a process similar to that described earlier for the carotid arteries, *echocardiography* produces an image of the working heart.

The Digestive System, the Liver, and the Pancreas

The gastroenterologist specializes in disorders of the digestive system and the liver.

As in many other systems, X rays are the traditional diagnostic tool for gastrointestinal problems. Nuclear imaging, however, may be used for some specific complaints. For example, if you're having trouble with heartburn an *esophageal reflux* test may be done to determine whether or not you have a hiatus hernia. The patient eats nothing the night before the exam. A small balloon is placed over the stomach, held in place by a special inflatable belt. The patient then stands in front of a gamma-ray camera and drinks a glass of orange juice to which a radioactive isotope has been added. Pictures are taken as the fluid moves to the stomach. The patient then lies down on a table and the cuff is inflated, causing the balloon to apply pressure to the stomach. Pictures are taken to see if this pressure causes the liquid in the stomach to back up into the esophagus. If it does, a hiatus hernia is the diagnosis.

In a gastrointestinal examination, X rays are usually taken first, and an endoscopy is done if a tissue sample is needed for biopsy. Endoscopy gives the physician a direct view of the gastrointestinal tract. The endoscope is a flexible tube with a light source, a camera, and instruments for taking tissue samples. The patient eats nothing the night before the exam. After undressing and putting on a gown, the patient lies down and drinks a bitter-tasting local anesthetic to inhibit the gag reflex. A mild sedative is also administered.

The patient lies on his left side with the mouth open. The endoscope is then put in the mouth and advanced down toward the stomach. Photographs are commonly taken, and samples of tissue or gastric juice may also be taken. The exam takes about

The Digestive System

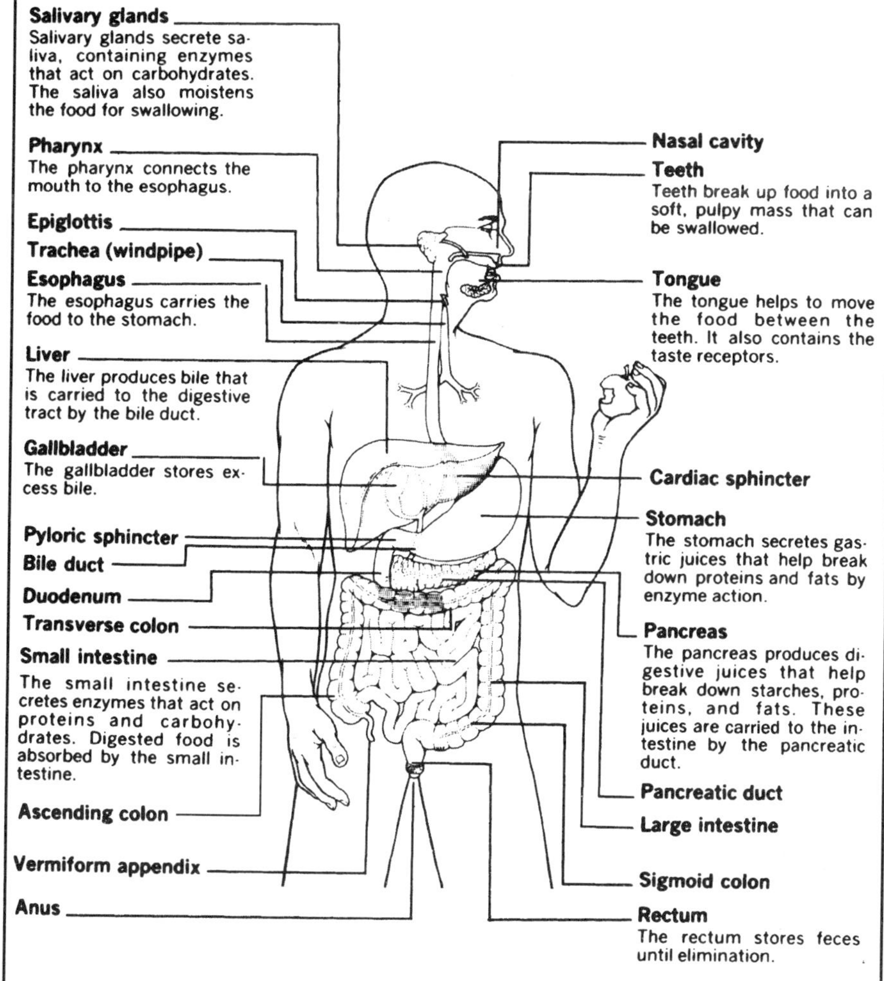

2 to 3 hours.

An *upper GI* may be in order if your doctor suspects an ulcer or tumor. No food is allowed for 8 hours before the test. An injection of glucagon (which may cause nausea or dizziness) is normally given to slow down the movements of the stomach. Next, the patient swallows a small cupful of granular material which produces gas and causes the stomach to distend. Finally, the patient is given a glass of barium and stands with his back to the X-ray table. A fluoroscopic screen is positioned in front of the patient, and the radiologist instructs him to take small swallows of the barium. A series of pictures are taken, with the patient changing position several times. If the entire small intestine is being studied, the patient is next taken to a waiting area and returns every 15 to 30 minutes for more pictures. A stomach—duodenum study takes about a half hour. The longer study takes from 1 to 3 hours.

A *lower GI,* often called simply a *barium enema,* is much more involved. It is used when there is a suspicion of diverticulitis, bowel obstruction, colon polyps, colitis, or other intestinal disorders. A strict diet is prescribed, along with laxatives, for several days before the test. Two enemas are given on the morning of the study. For this exam the patient lies down on the X-ray table. The doctor inserts a lubricated, gloved finger into the patient's rectum to make sure there are no obstructions and then inserts the enema tip. The tip has a built-in balloon that can be inflated if the patient feels unable to retain the enema. Like the upper GI, an injection of glucagon is often given to counteract the feeling of "fullness" experienced by most people. The fluoroscope is then positioned and the technologist begins the enema: a solution of barium is pumped into the rectum until it fills the large intestine. Air may then be pumped into the rectum for greater contrast. Both the enema and the air can cause a feeling of fullness and discomfort. The patient retains the enema and the air until all the pictures are taken.

There is a breath test used to detect the bacterium *Helicobacter pylori,* which is thought to be the cause of many ulcers. The patient simply blows into a small plastic bag, then drinks a glass of clear, tasteless liquid. The liquid consists of substances that will be broken down by any *H. pylori* in the stomach. Thirty minutes later, the patient exhales into another plastic bag. Both bags are sent to a laboratory to be tested for *H. pylori.* The breath test for *H. pylori* bacterium is about 95 percent accurate.

The gall bladder, an organ in the upper right abdomen responsible for storing the bile necessary for fat digestion, is a frequent site of infection and may also develop stones. Examination of the gall bladder can be done with X rays, ultrasound, or nuclear imaging. Most routine gall bladder studies are done with ultrasound. An 8-hour fast is required before the test. The patient is given a gown to wear, may be asked to drink a white liquid, and then lies down on the couch. The doctor applies a special lubricant to the abdominal area and moves the transducer over it. The patient can watch the results on a monitor.

If stones develop in the gall bladder and block the flow of bile, infection results—a condition called acute cholecystitis. Nuclear imaging is considered the most specific diagnostic tool for this disorder. The patient fasts for 4 hours before the exam. An isotope is injected and the patient lies down under a gamma-ray camera. Pictures are taken every 5 to 10 minutes for a half hour and then every 15 minutes for one and a half hours.

The liver makes the bile needed for fat digestion, and the pancreas makes the enzymes necessary for fat digestion. Neither the entire liver nor the entire pancreas can be seen with X rays. X rays of the blood supply and ductal structures, however, enable the skilled specialist to make accurate assumptions about the condition of either. CT imaging can give a full picture of both organs and is safer than X rays. Ultrasound is also useful.

If the results of lab tests suggest liver disease or if the organ is enlarged, a special *needle biopsy* may be done. The patient is normally asked to avoid eating the night before the test. Medication by mouth or injection may be given. The gastroenterologist feels the lower edge of the liver, selects a spot, and injects a small amount of local anesthetic under the skin. Next a larger needle with a syringe is inserted. There will be pressure and even a dull pain. The plunger of the syringe is pulled back, and liver cells are extracted. The needle is then removed and pressure is applied to the puncture site.

The Respiratory System

The respiratory system includes the pharynx, trachea, bronchi, and the lungs.

A chest X ray (described earlier) is usually the first test done when symptoms indicate a possible problem in the respiratory system. When the bronchi must be seen in more detail, a *bronchogram* may be done. This requires the suppression of the "coughing reflex" by spraying a local or topical anesthetic in the patient's mouth and back of the throat. Then a thin metal tube shaped like a candy cane (a cannula) will be placed in the mouth with the curved end over the back of the tongue. Anesthetic is injected into the cannula, which runs down the back of the throat into the bronchi. A rubber tube (catheter) is passed through the patient's nose, down the back of the throat, through the larynx, the trachea, and then into the bronchi of one or both lungs. A special dye is then instilled into the catheter, which runs down and fills the tubes. The dye highlights the bronchi, making it easier to see blockage and tight areas on the X ray.

A *bronchoscopy* may be in order if X rays or CT reveal potential problems and the physician needs a closer look or a tissue sample. The physician inspects the larynx, trachea and bronchi through a flexible fiber-optic tube called a bronchoscope. Miniature instruments are fed through the bronchoscope to collect tissue samples.

A group of tests called *pulmonary function tests* help the physician determine if certain symptoms may be due to either restrictive or obstructive lung disease. These tests measure how much air can be forcibly exhaled after inhaling as deeply as possible, how much air remains in the lungs after a forcible exhalation, and how much air is expired with each normal breath. They evaluate how well the lungs stretch with each breath inhaled and how well they collapse with each breath exhaled.

The Respiratory System

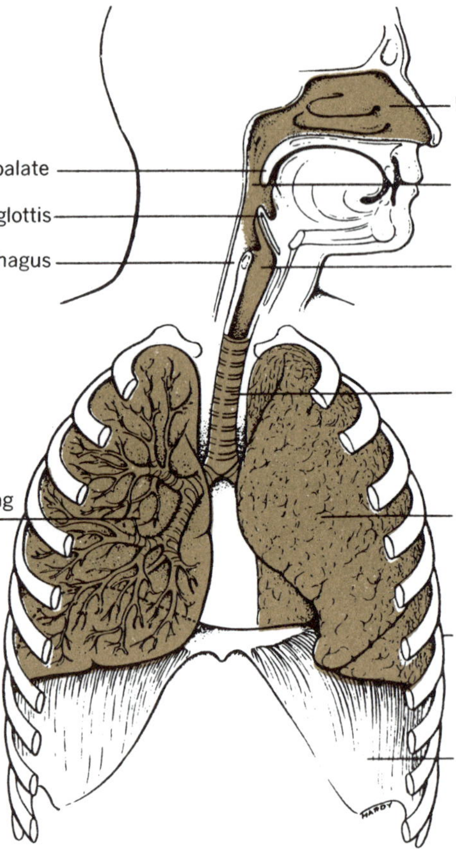

The patient is put in a pressurized plexiglass cabin called a body box, which looks like a large phone booth. The patient's nose is closed off with a nose clip and a special mouthpiece is inserted in the mouth. Then, the patient performs a series of breathing maneuvers by exhaling into the mouthpiece, which is attached to monitoring equipment. The tests take 15 to 45 minutes.

The Endocrine System

There are 7 endocrine glands that make up the endocrine system: pituitary, thyroid, parathyroids, adrenals, pancreas, ovaries (women), and testicles (men). The glands secrete hormones that produce a specific effect or regulate a certain action of other body organs. Laboratory tests of blood and urine are important diagnostic tools for the glands, and all can be visualized with X rays, CT, nuclear imaging, and ultrasound if lab tests indicate a potential problem. Some tests may necessitate the injection of a special dye to highlight the target area.

The Kidneys and the Urinary System

Laboratory tests of the urine are the most obvious way of beginning a diagnosis of kidney or urinary system problems. A resting EKG may also be done as well as nuclear imaging, ultrasound, and X rays. If a kidney biopsy is needed, the patient is normally given an anesthetic to induce drowsiness and is then instructed to lie face down on a table. The procedure is similar to that of the liver biopsy. First the anesthetic is injected, then the aspirating needle is inserted. This takes only a minute or so. An overnight stay is required for observation. Patients may experience a dull backache for several days after the biopsy.

An *intravenous urography* is a common test for urinary tract problems. Colon cleansing (strict diet, laxative, enemas) is often done before the test. Dye is injected into the patient's arm (or may drip in gradually from a diluted bottle of fluid). X rays are taken at timed intervals. A compression cuff (like a large blood pressure cuff) may be put around the abdomen to apply pressure just below each kidney, and more pictures are taken. The patient is then told to void his or her bladder; another X ray is taken, and the test is over.

Ears, Nose, and Throat

The otorhinolaryngologist specializes in treating problems of the ears, nose, and throat. Difficulty in hearing, faulty balance or vertigo, earache, and ringing in the ears (tinnitus) are common ear complaints. Congestion, discharge from the nose, postnasal drip, itching and sneezing, headaches over the eyes, pain over the upper teeth, and unexplained fever are complaints associated with the nose and sinuses. Laryngitis, sore throat, or difficulty in swallowing are common throat complaints.

An *audiogram* evaluates and measures hearing. The patient is seated in a booth and earphones are placed over the ears. A series of tones that vary in loudness are played through the earphones and the patient uses hand signals to indicate hearing a tone. Each ear is tested separately.

A *tympanogram* measures vibrations of the eardrum. A rubber plug is inserted in one ear and mild pressure is applied. The tympanogram reveals the type of hearing loss caused by a perforated eardrum, by an eardrum that has become thickened from an infection, or by an obstruction in the middle ear.

Patients who experience dizziness may be given an *electronystagmogram,* a series of neurological tests that rec-

A Guide to Some Home Medical Tests

Kind	Function	How It Works	Time Required
Blood glucose monitoring	Measures the level of glucose (a kind of sugar) in blood	Wash your hands thoroughly. Prick a finger or earlobe to obtain a drop of blood, then follow instructions.	1 to 2 minutes
Ovulation monitoring	Measures the quantity of luteinizing hormone (LH) in urine	A chemically treated strip is dipped in urine specimen and compared with a color guide.	20 minutes to 1 hour
Pregnancy	Detects human chorionic gonadotropin, produced by a developing placenta, in urine	Chemicals are mixed with a urine specimen in a small test tube. A ring formation or color change indicates pregnancy.	20 minutes to 2 hours
Urinary tract infections	Detects nitrite in urine	Chemically treated test strip is dipped in urine specimen on three consecutive mornings.	30 to 40 seconds
Occult fecal blood	Detects hidden blood in stools	A color change, appearing when stool specimen is brought into contact with peroxide and guaiac, indicates hidden blood.	30 seconds to 16 minutes
Gonorrhea	Detects the bacteria causing gonorrhea in the specimen of pus from the penis	Specimen, collected on a slide, is allowed to air-dry. Then follow directions.	Several days
Blood pressure	Measures the pressure of blood on the walls of the arteries	The center of a cuff is placed on the pulse point of the upper arm. With or without a microphone, the user listens for artery sounds.	2 to 5 minutes
Impotence	Detects, measures the rigidity of erections during sleep	Soft fabric band or stamps are placed around the penis before the subject goes to bed at night. The strips break at different degrees of pressure.	Overnight
Vision	Screens for visual acuity problems	Using three different tests, you read special eye charts.	2 to 3 minutes

ord eye movements. Abnormal movements of the eye can indicate a problem with the balance mechanism (vestibular system). The technician tapes a small metal disk under each eye and on the bridge of the nose. These sensors are attached by lead wires to a graph machine. The patient is then instructed to follow a slowly moving target with the eyes as eye movements are recorded. In the next test the patient, with eyes closed, lies down and turns to one side. Eye movements are recorded as water is placed into the external ear canal. This procedure often produces dizziness or nausea that persists for several hours.

Smears and cultures are the common lab tests for nose and throat complaints. X ray examinations may also be done. In some cases a biopsy may be necessary. For the nose, a needle aspiration is the common method, either through the nose or upper gum of the mouth. A local anesthetic is given first. An excisional biopsy may be necessary, in which case a small piece of tissue is removed. For the throat an excisional biopsy is commonly done, normally under general anesthesia, and an overnight stay in the hospital may be required. A laryngoscope is used to obtain the sample. The throat remains sore for several days afterwards.

The Eyes

Opthalmologists are certified doctors of medicine who specialize in medical and surgical care of the eye. As such, they have the greatest range of expertise among eye-care specialists. In addition to testing vision and prescribing corrective lenses, opththalmologists diagnose and treat all eye disorders, from minor infections to conditions such as glaucoma that can lead to blindness.

Optometrists diagnose vision problems and prescribe lenses, screen for glaucoma, and identify and treat other disorders. They are not physicians, but they have completed two years of study in an approved college followed by four years at a school of optometry.

Opticians fit and sell corrective lenses prescribed by an opthalmologist or optometrist.

The common eye exam includes tests for visual acuity, color blindness, and muscle integrity. Other tests are the slit-lamp exam, tonometry, and retinal exam.

The Snellen visual acuity chart is used to measure visual acuity. Letters, numbers, or symbols are arranged in rows, each row formed by characters of the same size. The top row contains large characters, with each succeeding row formed by smaller characters. The patient is asked to stand or sit 20 feet from the chart and identify the figures line by line from top to bottom until the figures are no longer recognizable. The doctor will check each eye individually while the patient covers the alternate eye; then both eyes are tested together. This test detects errors of vision such as nearsightedness, farsightedness, and astigmatism, which are the result of defects in the size and shape of the eye. Continuing the test, the opthalmologist fits the patient with a series of corrective lenses of different strengths. The patient looks through each sample lens and reads the Snellen chart again, identifying those lenses that help him see the letters or symbols most clearly.

Color blindness is the inability to recognize one or more colors. Various charts are used to detect color blindness. One commonly used chart contains patterns of colored dots. A color blind person will not be able to distinguish between dots of certain colors and therefore will not be able to discern a design defined by these dots.

The muscle integrity exam tests eye movement to determine if both eyes can focus together. The movement of the eye toward any desired direction is controlled through the coordinated action of six muscles at-

Focusing

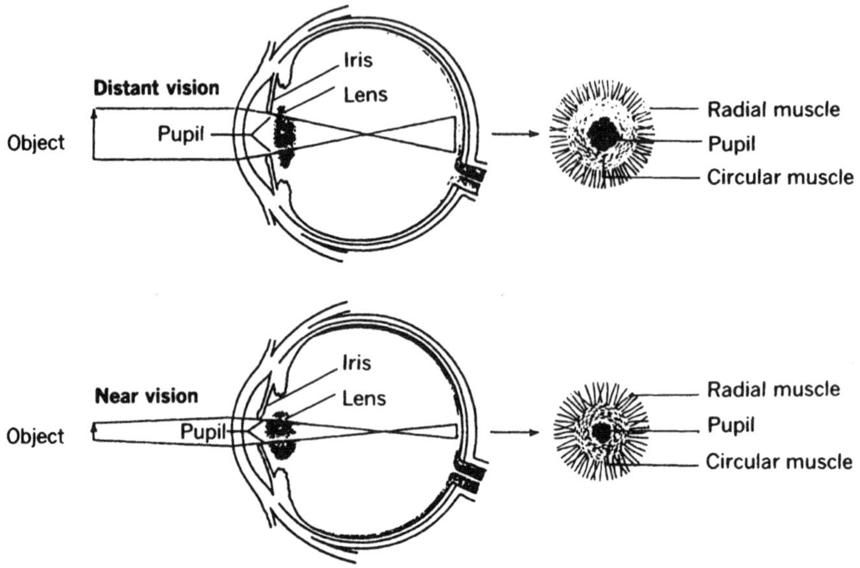

When viewing a distant object (more than 20 feet away), the lens flattens and the pupil dilates, allowing more light to enter the eye. The pupil is dilated by the action of the outer radial muscles of the iris, which contract and thus stretch the previously contracted circular muscles. When viewing a near object, the lens becomes more oval and the pupil contracts as more light enters the eye. This prevents overstimulation of the retina. The pupil is reduced in size by the contraction of the inner circular muscles, which serve to stretch the previously contracted radial muscles.

tached to the eyeball under the conjunctiva. For an object to be perceived properly, the eye muscles must work in unison to focus the image on the center of the retina at the back of the eye. In the muscle integrity exam, the patient is asked to look in various directions. Both eyes will move together if the muscles are working properly.

The slit-lamp microscope is used to obtain a magnified view of structures at the front of the eye—the sclera, iris, conjunctiva, cornea, and lens—which are carefully checked for signs of injury or disease. A common disorder detected by slit-lamp examination is the cataract, the clouding of the normally clear lens. The standard treatment for cataracts is surgical removal of the lens, which, in most cases, is then replaced with an artificial lens. Alternatives to an artificial lens include contact lenses or thick-lensed eyeglasses.

Glaucoma is a disease caused by inadequate drainage of the fluid within the eyeball. The resulting increase in the pressure of the fluid damages the optic nerve, leading to a gradual narrowing of the field of vision and, eventually, blindness. Glaucoma is the leading cause of blindness in the United States. An instrument called a tonometer is used to measure the pressure of fluid within the eyeball.

The tonometer is placed on the pupil after a drop of anesthetic has been applied to the eye, and a gauge records the resistance of the eye to the slight pressure applied. It is recommended that this painless procedure be done for those 40 and over every 2 to 3 years, or annually if there is a family history of glaucoma.

The final test in the general eye exam is the retinal exam. The room is darkened, and the doctor uses an ophthalmoscope to look through the pupil into the back of the eye.

A common disease of the retina is macular degeneration, an age-related disorder that causes increasingly blurred central vision in the elderly. A leading cause of blindness in the United States is diabetic retinopathy, a deterioration of the blood vessels of the retina brought on by diabetes.

Diagnostic Tests and the Patient's Rights

As medical costs continue to rise, questions about the necessity of various diagnostic tests will continue to be raised. For the healthy individual, it makes little sense to undergo more than the few routine screening tests necessary for his particular age group; there is always the chance of an error that may lead to additional tests at even greater expense, not to mention the emotional trauma that a false positive could cause.

For the patient experiencing particular symptoms, or those in high risk categories, the number and kind of diagnostic tests are a concern. Batteries, or sets, of tests are a particular cause for concern. The batteries can be complex, and the physician may not take the time to explain each one in detail so that the patient thoroughly understands what they mean in terms of discomfort, risk, and cost. The value of a particular test must also be weighed against its results. Expensive CT and MRI tests are the "study of choice" for many problems, but for others, the less expensive X ray might do just as well or better. When presented with the need for diagnostic tests, then, the patient should endeavor to become as informed as possible about what is necessary. As already mentioned, having a physician with whom you can converse easily and understand is an important factor in the quality of the medical care you receive.

27

Nutrition and Weight Control

Just as it was for our earliest ancestors, food is an integral part of our daily lives. Not only is food essential for survival, but oftentimes the way in which we structure our lives—our work habits, our recreational activities—revolves around how, when, and where we get food and eat it.

Ironically, however, because most of us live a much faster-paced lifestyle than we did even twenty years ago, we spend less time choosing, preparing, and eating food. We grab breakfast on the run (if we eat it at all), hurry through lunch, and rarely take time to plan and prepare a leisurely, well-balanced dinner. Often everyone in the family is on a different schedule, with the result that all too often we rely on prepackaged microwave dinners or take out fast food. Consequently, many of us are not eating properly, spending money on expensive vitamins to make up for poor nutrition, starving ourselves to lose weight, or gaining extra pounds by filling up on empty calories.

Practicing good eating habits may take a little more time and planning than we think we can afford, but its benefits will pay off in the long run in a healthier, happier way of life.

Basic Nutritional Requirements

The process by which food is converted into useful energy is called *metabolism*. It begins with chemical processes in the gastrointestinal tract that change plant and animal food into less complex components so that they can be absorbed to fulfill their various functions in the body—growth, repair, and fuel. Different foods have different energy values, measured in calories. An ideal diet for the average healthy individual provides the highest nutritional benefits from the fewest number of calories. Information on the protein, fat, and carbohydrate content in specific foods, as well as the number of calories, may be obtained by consulting the tables "Nutrients in Common Foods." The Metric Equivalents table converts spoon and cup measures into metric measures.

Protein

Of the several essential components of food, *protein* is, in many ways, the most important. This is so not only because it is one of the three principal sources of energy, but also because much of the body's structure is made up of proteins. For example, the typical 160-pound man is composed of about 100 pounds of water, 29 pounds of protein, 25 pounds of fat, 5 pounds of minerals, 1 pound of carbohydrate, and less than 1 ounce of vitamins. Because the muscles, heart, brain, lungs, and gastrointestinal organs are made up largely of protein, and because the protein in these organs is in constant need of replacement, its importance is obvious.

The recommended dietary allowance for protein is 0.8 g/Kg of body weight per day for persons aged 15 and up and 1 g/Kg of body weight for children under 15. (To convert your weight from pounds to kilograms, divide by 2.2. Thus a woman weighing 130 pounds weighs about 59 kilograms and needs about 47 grams of protein a day. A man weighing 175 pounds needs about 64 grams of protein a day.) Most Americans, however, eat about twice the amount of protein they need. Your body uses only what it needs. Some excess protein is excreted as urine; the rest is converted to fat.

Chemically, proteins are varying mixtures of amino acids that contain various elements, including nitrogen. There are 22 different amino acids that are essential for the body's protein needs. Nine of these must be provided in the diet and are thus called *essential* amino acids; the rest can be synthesized by the body itself.

Meat, fish, poultry, eggs, and milk or milk products are the primary protein foods and contain all of the essential amino acids; they are therefore called *complete* proteins. Grains, fruits, and vegetables are partly made up of protein, but more often than not, they do not provide all of the essential amino acids. When properly combined, however, these proteins, too, can be complete. For example, mixing rice and dried beans provides the same quality of protein as a steak (with a lot less fat).

One gram of protein provides four calories of energy.

Carbohydrates

Carbohydrates are another essential energy source. Called *starches* or *sugars,* they are present in large quantities in grains, fruits, and nuts. As *complex carbohydrates,* or *polysaccharides,* they are found in the foods named and particularly in breads, breakfast cereals, flours, pastas, barley, legumes, rice, and starchy vegetables. *Simple carbohydrates,* or mono- or disaccharides, are found in such foods as table sugars, candy, pastries, and soft drinks.

Complex carbohydrates are primary sources of calories, nutrients, and fiber—for such purposes as muscle contraction, weight reduction, and control of sodium and cholesterol. Simple carbohydrates, on the other hand, are pure sources of calories and contain little nutritional value. It is for this reason that they are often termed "empty" calories. Lack of adequate carbohydrates means the body will begin to convert body fat or protein into sugar.

Although there is no absolute dietary requirement for carbohydrates, it is generally recommended that more than half the energy requirement beyond infancy be provided by complex carbohydrates. One gram of carbohydrate provides four calories of energy. Thus the average man consuming about 2,900 calories per day should consume about 360 grams of carbohydrate. The average woman consuming about 2,200 calories per day should consume about 275 grams of carbohydrate.

Fats

Fats are a chemically complex food component composed of *glycerol* (a sweet, oily alcohol) and fatty acids. Fats exist in several forms and come from a variety of sources. One way to think of them is to group them as visible fats, such as butter, salad oil, or the fat seen in meat, and as invisible fats, which are mingled, blended, or absorbed into food, either naturally, as in nuts, meat, or fish, or during cooking. Another way is to think of them as solid at room temperature (fats), or as liquid at room temperature (oils).

Saturated and Unsaturated

Fats are also classified as *saturated* or *unsaturated.* This is a chemical distinction based on the differences in molecular structure of different kinds of fat. If the carbon atoms in a fat molecule are surrounded or boxed in by hydrogen atoms, they are said to be saturated. This type of fat tends to be solid at room temperature, and high consumption of it increases the cholesterol content of the blood, which can lead to heart disease. *Unsaturated* fats, such as those found in fish and vegetable oils, contain the least number of hydrogen atoms and do not add to the blood cholesterol content. They are either *monounsaturated* or *polyunsaturated.* In general, fats in foods of plant origin are more unsaturated than in those of animal origin (except for coconut and palm oils, which are highly saturated). It is recommended that you consume no more than 30 percent of your daily calories from fats, 10 percent of each of the three types.

Fats play several essential roles in the metabolic process. First, they provide more than twice the number of calories on a comparative weight basis than do proteins and carbohydrates (one gram of fat contains nine calories). They also can be stored in the body in large quantities (in adipose tissue) and used as a later energy source. They serve as carriers of the fat-soluble vitamins and—of no little importance—they add to the tastiness of food.

Vitamins

Vitamins, which are present in minute quantities in foods in their natural state, are necessary for normal metabolism and for the development and maintenance of the structure and function of the various tissues in the body. In the following sections, the amount of a nutrient that a person should consume daily is generally expressed as a Recommended Daily Allowance (RDA). An Adequate Intake (AI) is given in place of a RDA when the amount of the nutrient given is believed to meet a person's daily need, but does not qualify as a RDA.

Vitamin A

Vitamin A is essential for vision, growth, cell growth and development, reproduction, a strong immune system, and healthy hair, skin, and mucous membranes.

Vitamin A is fat soluble and is therefore stored by the body (in the liver). It comes in two forms: retinol, found only in animal foods (chiefly liver), and beta-carotene, found in fruits and vegetables (chiefly deep green or orange ones like spinach and sweet potatoes). Retinol is instantly available for bodily use, while beta-carotene must be converted by the body into retinol before it can be used. (Because the body will not convert excess beta-carotene into retinol, there is no danger of overdosing on this form of vitamin A. Retinol, however, can be extremely toxic at high levels.)

Symptoms of vitamin A deficiency include dry rough skin, slow growth, night blindness, thickening of bone, and increased susceptibility to infection. Vitamin A deficiency is rare in the United States.

Vitamin A content is expressed as retinal activity equivalents (RAE). The RDA for vitamin A for adult males is 900 RAE and for adult women, 700 RAE.

Modified Calorie/Weight Reduction Diet

Sample Menus

	1,500 Calories	1,800 Calories	2,000 Calories
Breakfast	1 serving fruit/juice 1 slice toast 1 serving egg or substitute 1 serving margarine 1 cup skim milk coffee/tea	1 serving fruit/juice 1 slice toast 1 serving egg or substitute 1 serving cereal 1 serving margarine 1 cup skim milk coffee/tea	1 serving fruit/juice 1 slice toast 1 serving egg or substitute 1 serving cereal 1 serving margarine 1 cup skim milk coffee/tea
Lunch	2-3 ounces meat 1 serving potato or substitute 1 serving bread vegetables salad/non-fat dressing 2 servings fruit 1 serving margarine coffee/tea	2-3 ounces meat 1 serving potato or substitute 1 serving bread vegetables salad/non-fat dressing 2 servings fruit/juice 1 serving margarine coffee/tea	2-3 ounces meat 1 serving potato or substitute 1 serving bread vegetables salad/non-fat dressing 2 servings fruit/juice 1 serving margarine 1 cup skim milk coffee/tea
Dinner	2-3 ounces meat 1 serving potato or substitute 1 serving bread vegetables salad/non-fat dressing 1 serving fruit 2 servings margarine coffee/tea	2-3 ounces meat 1 serving potato or substitute 1 serving bread vegetables salad/non-fat dressing 2 servings fruit/juice 2 servings margarine coffee/tea	2-3 ounces meat 2 servings potato or substitute 1 serving bread vegetables salad/non-fat dressing 1 serving fruit/juice 2 servings margarine coffee/tea
Snack	3 graham crackers 1 cup skim milk	1 ounce meat 1 slice bread 1 serving reduced-fat mayonnaise 1 cup skim milk	1 ounce meat 1 slice bread 1 serving reduced-fat mayonnaise non-alcoholic beverage

From the *Clinical Center Diet Manual*, Clinical Center Nutrition Department, National Institutes of Health, Department of Health and Human Services.

Vitamin D

Vitamin D is essential for proper metabolism of calcium, which is primarily responsible for the healthy growth of bones and teeth.

Vitamin D is fat soluble and therefore excessive intake can be toxic. It is consumed chiefly as an addition to milk and is also manufactured by the body by a reaction of sunlight on sterols present in the skin.

The major deficiency disease of vitamin D in children is rickets (deformation of the skeleton) and in adults, excessive bone loss and fractures. The Adequate Intake (AI) for children and adults under age 51 is 5 micrograms.

Vitamin E (tocopherol)

Vitamin E is essential for healthy nerve function and reproduction.

Vitamin E is found principally in plant oils, particularly wheat germ oil and nuts. It is fat soluble, but there is little danger of toxicity because absorption by the body is inefficient.

Vitamin E is measured in tocopherol equivalents (TE). The RDA for adults is 15 TE. Deficiencies in a normal diet are rare.

Vitamin K

Vitamin K is essential for proper clotting of the blood.

Vitamin K is fat soluble and is found primarily in green leafy vegetables. Another form of the compound is synthesized by intestinal bacteria. As with vitamin E, there is little danger from ingesting excessive vitamin K, and most diets provide an adequate supply.

The AI for adult males is 120 micrograms. The AI for adult women is 90 micrograms.

Vitamin C (ascorbic acid)

Vitamin C is essential for healthy skin, bones, teeth, and muscles, for producing and maintaining collagen, and for fighting infection.

Vitamin C is water soluble and therefore must be ingested every day. It is widely available in a variety of colorful fruits and vegetables, such as peppers, broccoli, cabbage, oranges, strawberries, and tomatoes. Unfortunately, vitamin C is also the most unstable of all vitamins and minerals: it is easily destroyed by heat and oxygen, so care should be taken in cooking and storing fruits and vegetables.

The classic vitamin C deficiency disease is scurvy, typified by the wasting away of muscles, wounds and bruises that don't heal, and bleeding, deteriorating gums. Milder forms of vitamin C deficiency produce milder versions of these symptoms. Vitamin C deficiency has also been linked to such health problems as the common cold, anemia, atherosclerosis, asthma, cancer of the stomach and esophagus, infertility in males, rheumatoid arthritis, and cataracts.

Vitamin C is measured in milli-

Average Daily Calorie Consumption

Men	Calories
Sedentary	2,500
Moderately active	3,000
Active	3,500
Very active	4,250
Women	**Calories**
Sedentary	2,100
Moderately active	2,500
Active	3,000
Very active	3,750

Guidelines for average daily calorie consumption by men and women. With increasing use of labor-saving devices, most Americans fall into the sedentary category.

Calorie Consumption for Some Activities

Type of Activity	Calories Per Hour
Sedentary: reading, sewing, typing, etc.	30–100
Light: cooking, slow walking, dressing, etc.	100–170
Moderate: sweeping, light gardening, making beds, etc.	170–250
Vigorous: fast walking, hanging out clothes, golfing, etc.	250–350
Strenuous: swimming, bicycling, dancing, etc.	350 and more

Table 1

Desirable Weights for Men and Women Aged 25 and Over[1]
(in pounds by height and frame, in indoor clothing)

MEN *(in shoes, 1-inch heels)*				WOMEN *(in shoes, 2-inch heels)*			
Height	Small Frame	Medium Frame	Large Frame	Height	Small Frame	Medium Frame	Large Frame
5′ 2″	112–120	118–129	126–141	4′ 10″	92– 98	96–107	104–119
5′ 3″	115–123	121–133	129–144	4′ 11″	94–101	98–110	106–122
5′ 4″	118–126	124–136	132–148	5′ 0″	96–104	101–113	109–125
5′ 5″	121–129	127–139	135–152	5′ 1″	99–107	104–116	112–128
5′ 6″	124–133	130–143	138–156	5′ 2″	102–110	107–119	115–131
5′ 7″	128–137	134–147	142–161	5′ 3″	105–113	110–122	118–134
5′ 8″	132–141	138–152	147–166	5′ 4″	108–116	113–126	121–138
5′ 9″	136–145	142–156	151–170	5′ 5″	111–119	116–130	125–142
5′ 10″	140–150	146–160	155–174	5′ 6″	114–123	120–135	129–146
5′ 11″	144–154	150–165	159–179	5′ 7″	118–127	124–139	133–150
6′ 0″	148–158	154–170	164–184	5′ 8″	122–131	128–143	137–154
6′ 1″	152–162	158–175	168–189	5′ 9″	126–135	132–147	141–158
6′ 2″	156–167	162–180	173–194	5′ 10″	130–140	136–151	145–163
6′ 3″	160–171	167–185	178–199	5′ 11″	134–144	140–155	149–168
6′ 4″	164–175	172–190	182–204	6′ 0″	138–148	144–159	153–173

[1]Adapted from Metropolitan Life Insurance Co., New York. New weight standards for men and women. *Statistical Bulletin* 40:3.

Table 2

Average Weights for Men and Women[1]
(in pounds by age and height, in paper gown and slippers)

Height	18–24 Years	25–34 Years	35–44 Years	45–54 Years	55–64 Years	65–74 Years	75–79 Years
MEN							
5′ 2"	137	141	149	148	148	144	133
5′ 3"	140	145	152	152	151	148	138
5′ 4"	144	150	156	156	155	151	143
5′ 5"	147	154	160	160	158	154	148
5′ 6"	151	159	164	164	162	158	154
5′ 7"	154	163	168	168	166	161	159
5′ 8"	158	168	171	173	169	165	164
5′ 9"	161	172	175	177	173	168	169
5′ 10"	165	177	179	181	176	171	174
5′ 11"	168	181	182	185	180	175	179
6′ 0"	172	186	186	189	184	178	184
6′ 1"	175	190	190	193	187	182	189
6′ 2"	179	194	194	197	191	185	194
WOMEN							
4′ 9"	116	112	131	129	138	132	125
4′ 10"	118	116	134	132	141	135	129
4′ 11"	120	120	136	136	144	138	132
5′ 0"	122	124	138	140	149	142	136
5′ 1"	125	128	140	143	150	145	139
5′ 2"	127	132	143	147	152	149	143
5′ 3"	129	136	145	150	155	152	146
5′ 4"	131	140	147	154	158	156	150
5′ 5"	134	144	149	158	161	159	153
5′ 6"	136	148	152	161	164	163	157
5′ 7"	138	152	154	165	167	166	160
5′ 8"	140	156	156	168	170	170	164

[1]Adapted from National Center for Health Statistics: Weight by Height and Age of Adults, United States. *Vital Health Statistics*. PHS Publication No. 1000—Series 11, No. 14.

grams (mg). The RDA for adult males is 90 mg. The RDA for adult females is 75 mg. Megadoses of vitamin C are often recommended to fight colds or as a general preventive measure against disease, although the body uses only as much as it needs; the rest is excreted in the urine. The risk of toxicity is rare.

Thiamin (vitamin B_1)

Thiamin is essential for the proper metabolism of carbohydrates and for a healthy nervous system.

Thiamin is water soluble and is

found primarily in cereals, wheat germ, pork, and nuts. It is strongly susceptible to destruction during cooking. Deficiency is not common among the general population, but studies have shown heavy drinkers, pregnant women, and the elderly to be more deficient. Severe thiamin deficiency results in beriberi, a disease that weakens the body, disables the mind, and permanently damages the heart. Symptoms of deficiency include loss of appetite, nausea, vomiting, constipation, depression, fatigue, poor eye-hand coordination, irritability, headaches, and anxiety.

Thiamin is measured in milligrams. The RDA for adult males is 1.2 mg and for adult women, 1.1 mg. Danger of toxicity is rare, because excess thiamin is excreted in urine.

Riboflavin (vitamin B_2)

Riboflavin is essential for growth and repair of tissues and aids in DNA synthesis. It helps metabolize proteins, fats, and carbohydrates.

Most Americans get plenty of this water-soluble vitamin, which is most readily found in liver, eggs, and milk products. Studies have found that children in low-income families, however, are less likely to get enough riboflavin. Signs of deficiency include a purplish-colored tongue; cracks at the corners of the mouth; sores and burning of the lips, mouth, and tongue; itchy inflamed eyelids; flaky skin around the nose, ears, eyebrows, or hairline; and light sensitivity of the eyes. Deficiency in riboflavin often means deficiency in other B vitamins as well. Cataracts, birth defects, and anemia have been linked to riboflavin deficiency.

Unlike vitamin C and thiamin, riboflavin is not easily destroyed by cooking. Risk of toxicity is very low; excess riboflavin is excreted in the urine.

Riboflavin is measured in milligrams. The RDA for adult males is 1.3 mg and for adult women, 1.1 mg.

Niacin (vitamin B_3)

Niacin is essential for the release of energy from carbohydrates, fats, and proteins and for the formation of DNA.

Most Americans get plenty of niacin from their diets. Severe deficiencies of niacin result in pellagra, a disease virtually wiped out in the United States since the 1930s with the advent of flour and cereals fortified with the vitamin.

Niacin is available in a variety of plant and animal foods, including fish, liver, turkey, cereals, and peanuts. The body is able to convert the amino acid tryptophan into niacin, and thus proteins high in tryptophan also provide plenty of niacin.

Niacin is measured in milligrams (60 mg of tryptophan equal 1 mg of niacin). The RDA for adult males is 16 mg and for women, 14 mg.

Recommended Dietary Allowances (RDAs)* for Fat-Soluble Vitamins

	Age	Vit. A (mcg RE)	Vit. D (mcg)	Vit. E (mgTE)	Vit.K (mcg)
Infants	0 to .5	400*	5*	4*	2.0*
	.5 to 1	500*	5*	5*	2.5*
Children	01 to 03	300	5*	6	30*
	04 to 08	400	5*	7	55*
Males	09 to 13	600	5*	11	60*
	14 to 18	900	5*	15	75*
	19 to 30	900	5*	15	120*
	31 to 50	900	5*	15	120*
	51 to 70	900	10*	15	120*
	71 +	900	15*	15	120*
Females	09 to 13	600	5*	11	60*
	14 to 18	700	5*	15	75*
	19 to 30	700	5*	15	90*
	31 to 50	700	5*	15	90*
	51 to 70	700	10*	15	90*
	71 +	700	15*	15	90*
Pregnant	19 to 50	770	5*	15	90*
Nursing	19 to 50	1,300	5*	19	90*

* Adequate Intakes (AIs) are given when RDAs are not available.

Vitamin B_6

Vitamin B_6 is essential for fat and carbohydrate metabolism and for the formation and breakdown of amino acids. It also helps regulate blood glucose levels and is needed to synthesize hemoglobin.

Vitamin B_6 occurs in three forms: pyridoxine, pyridoxal, and pyridoxamine, which are converted by the body into pyridoxal phosphate and pyridoxamine phosphate. It is most readily found in nuts, kidney, liver, eggs, pork, poultry, dried fruits, and fish.

Although few Americans get the full RDA of vitamin B_6, there is no evidence of corresponding overt deficiency symptoms. Aging and the following health problems, however, have been linked to B_6 deficiency: asthma, carpal tunnel syndrome, cancer (melanoma, breast, and bladder), diabetes, coronary heart disease, premenstrual syndrome, sickle-cell anemia, and dementia.

In moderate doses B_6 is not toxic. Although excessive amounts of this water-soluble vitamin are to a great extent flushed out of the body in the urine, high doses have produced neurological disturbances such as numbness in the hands, feet, and mouth.

Vitamin B_6 is measured in milligrams. The RDA for adults under age 51 is 1.3 mg.

Vitamin B_{12}

Vitamin B_{12} is important for normal growth, healthy nerve tissue, and normal blood formation.

Most Americans get plenty of B_{12}. It is found chiefly in animal foods: meat, fish, eggs, and milk products.

Recommended Dietary Allowances (RDAs)* for Water-Soluble Vitamins

	Age	Vit. C (mg)	Thiamin (mg)	Riboflav. (mg)	Niacin (mg)	Vit. B_6 (mg)	Folate (mcg)	Vit. B_{12} (mcg)
Infants	0 to .5	40*	0.2*	0.3*	2*	0.1*	65*	0.4*
	.5 to 1	50*	0.3*	0.4*	4*	0.3*	80*	0.5*
Children	01 to 03	15	0.5	0.5*	6	0.5	150	0.9
	04 to 08	25	0.6	0.6*	8	0.6	200	1.2
Males	09 to 13	45	0.9	0.9*	12	1.0	300	1.8
	14 to 18	75	1.2	1.3*	16	1.3	400	2.4
	19 to 30	90	1.2	1.3*	16	1.3	400	2.4
	31 to 50	90	1.2	1.3*	16	1.3	400	2.4
	51 to 70	90	1.2	1.3*	16	1.7	400	2.4
	71 +	90	1.2	1.3*	16	1.7	400	2.4
Females	09 to 13	45	0.9	0.9*	12	1.0	300	1.8
	14 to 18	65	1.0	1.0*	14	1.2	400	2.4
	19 to 30	75	1.1	1.1*	14	1.3	400	2.4
	31 to 50	75	1.1	1.1*	14	1.3	400	2.4
	51 to 70	75	1.1	1.1*	14	1.5	400	2.4
	71 +	75	1.1	1.1*	14	1.5	400	2.4
Parent	19 tp 50	85	1.4	1.4*	18	1.9	600	2.6
Nursing	19 to 50	120	1.4	1.6*	17	2.0	500	2.8

*Adequate Intakes (AIs) are given when RDAs are not available.

Only strict vegetarians (vegans), who eat none of these foods are in danger of vitamin deficiency. Problems arise with age for everyone, however; the stomach may become less able to absorb B_{12} and deficiency may result. Pernicious anemia is the classic B_{12} deficiency disease and may take years to appear. Other health problems that may be linked to B_{12} deficiency include infertility, nervous system disorders, and walking difficulties.

Cooking results in few losses of B_{12}, and toxicity is not a danger. The RDA for B_{12} for adults is 2.4 micrograms.

Folacin (folic acid, or folate)

Folacin is essential for many metabolic processes, especially cell growth and division.

Women, especially pregnant women, and alcoholics are most likely to be folacin deficient. Signs of deficiency include anemia, weakness, pallor, headaches, forgetfulness, sleeplessness, and irritability. Vitamin B_{12} deficiency can aggravate folacin deficiency because B_{12} is essential to release folacin from bodily storage. Other health problems that may be associated with folacin deficiency include depression, dementia, neuropsychological disorders, toxemia of pregnancy, infections, and fetal damage.

Folacin is widely distributed in fruits and vegetables, but it is easily

Copper

Copper is important as a cofactor in several enzyme systems and as a catalyst in the synthesis of hemoglobin. It also aids in collagen formation and is involved in the synthesis of phospholipids, which maintain healthy nerve fibers.

Copper deficiency is believed to be more common than once thought, and it has been linked to heart disease, central nervous system disorders, anemia, and bone disorders. Good sources of copper include shellfish, liver, nuts and seeds, meats, and green leafy vegetables. Copper supplements are not recommended because they can interfere with other minerals, and copper is toxic at more than trace amounts. The RDA for copper is 900 micrograms.

Manganese

Manganese has a variety of functions, some that other minerals can perform in its place. It is known to play a role in such processes as collagen formation, urea formation, synthesis of fatty acids and cholesterol, digestion of proteins, normal bone formation and development, and protein synthesis.

Manganese deficiency has not been observed in humans. Sources of manganese include liver, kidney, spinach, whole grain cereals and breads, dried peas and beans, and nuts. Excessive intake of manganese can interfere with iron absorption. More than trace amounts of manganese are not recommended. The AI for adult men is 2.3 mg. The AI for adult women is 1.8 mg.

Fluoride

Fluoride is essential for the development of healthy teeth and bones and the prevention of tooth decay.

Fluoride deficiency manifests in increased incidences of tooth decay. Fluoridated water is the most common source of fluoride for many people. For those without access to such water, fluoride tablets or toothpaste are helpful. Fish, tea, milk, and eggs are also sources of fluoride. The AI for adult men is 4 mg and for adult women, 3 mg.

Chromium

Chromium is important for maintaining normal glucose metabolism. It also acts as a cofactor for insulin.

Chromium deficiency can appear in the form of glucose intolerance in malnourished children and in some diabetics. Sources of chromium include whole grains, brewer's yeast, meats, and cheeses. Hard water also contains chromium. Chromium intake should not exceed trace amounts. The AI for adult men under age 51 is 35 micrograms. The AI for adult women under age 51 is 25 micrograms.

Recommended Dietary Allowanced (RDAs)* of Selected Vitamins and Minerals

		Biotin	Pant. acid	Copper	Manganese	Fluoride	Chromium	Molyb.
		(mcg)	(mg)	(mcg)	(mg)	(mg)	(mcg)	(mcg)
Infants	0 to .5	5*	1.7*	200*	0.003*	0.01*	0.2*	2*
	.5 to 1	6*	1.8*	220*	0.06*	0.5*	5.5*	3*
Children	01 to 03	8*	2*	340	1.2*	0.7*	11*	17
	04 to 08	12*	3*	440	1.5*	1*	15*	22
Males	09 to 13	20*	4*	700	1.9*	2*	25*	34
	14 to 18	25*	5*	890	2.2*	3*	35*	43
	19 to 50	30*	5*	900	2.3*	4*	35*	45
	51 +	30*	5*	900	2.3*	4*	30*	45
Females	09 to 13	20*	4*	700	1.6*	2*	21*	34
	14 to 18	25*	5*	890	1.6*	3*	24*	43
	19 to 50	30*	5*	900	1.8*	3*	25*	45
	51 +	30*	5*	900	1.8*	3*	20*	45
Pregnant	19 to 50	30*	6*	1,000	2.0*	3*	30*	50
Nursing	19 to 50	35*	7*	1,300	2.6*	3*	45*	50

* Adequate Intakes (AIs) are given when RDAs are not available.

Fiber

Fiber in the diet is important for proper elimination. Its use has been linked to the prevention of many health problems: constipation, colon cancer, diverticular disease, spastic colon, hiatal hernia, hemorrhoids, coronary heart disease, high blood pressure, gallstones, diabetes, obesity, ulcerative colitis, and Crohn's disease.

Fiber is found almost exclusively in plant foods and comes in two basic types: water soluble or water insoluble. Soluble fiber is found primarily in fruits and vegetables and in oat bran in the form of gums and pectin and affects the way the body metabolizes sugars and fats. Insoluble fiber is primarily associated with whole grains and with traditional "bran," such as wheat bran and rice bran. It is the fiber we think of when we think of laxatives.

Fiber in high doses can affect the absorption of other vitamins and minerals and can cause flatulence, bloating, nausea, diarrhea, and impaction or rupture of the bowel. Daily consumption of 20 to 35 grams of fiber is recommended for optimum health and safety.

Water

Water is not really a food in the fuel sense, but it is in many ways a crucial component of nutrition: the body's need for water is second only to its need for oxygen. It makes up from 55 to 65 percent of the body's weight, and it is constantly eliminated in the form of urine, perspiration, and expired breath. It must be replaced regularly, for although a person can live for weeks without food, he can live for only a few days without water.

Normally, the best guide to how much water a person needs is his sense of thirst. The regulating mechanism of excretion sees to it that an excessive intake of water will be eliminated as urine. The usual water requirement is on the order of two quarts a day in addition to whatever amount is contained in the solids which make up the daily diet.

Basic Daily Diets

Everyone should have the minimal amount of basic nutrients for resting metabolism. Each individual's needs are determined by whether he is still growing, and by his energy expenditure. All those who are still growing—and growth continues up to about 25 years of age—have relatively high food needs.

For Infants

That food needs of an infant are especially acute should surprise no one. The newborn baby normally triples his birth weight during his first year and is very active in terms of calorie expenditure.

For his first six months, breast milk or formula, or a combination of both, fills his nutritional needs. The amount of milk he should get each day is about two and a half ounces per pound of his body weight. This provides 50 calories per pound, and in the early months is usually given in six feedings a day at four-hour intervals.

If his weight gain is adequate and he appears healthy, and if his stomach is not distended by swallowed air, his appetite is normally a satisfactory guide to how much he needs. The formula-fed baby should get a supplement of 35 milligrams of ascorbic acid each day and 400 international units of vitamin D if the latter has not been added to the milk during its processing.

Solid Foods

Between two and six months of age, the baby should begin to eat solid foods such as cooked cereals, strained fruits and vegetables, egg yolk, and homogenized meat. With the introduction of these foods, it is not really necessary to calculate the baby's caloric intake. Satisfaction of appetite, proper weight gain, and a healthy appearance serve as the guides to a proper diet.

By one year of age, a baby should be getting three regular meals a day, and as his teeth appear, his food no longer needs to be strained. By 18 to 24 months, he should no longer need baby foods. For more information, see Ch. 2, *The First Dozen Years*.

Basic Food Groups

The recommended daily amounts of food for people over the age of two have been established with reasonable accuracy, but they always contain a fairly generous safety factor.

The Four Group Division

In general, foods are divided into four major groups:

- Meat, fish, eggs
- Dairy products
- Fruits and vegetables
- Breads and cereals

The Seven Group Division

For purposes of planning daily requirements, a more detailed way of considering food groupings is the following:

- Leafy green and yellow vegetables
- Citrus fruits, tomatoes, and raw cabbage

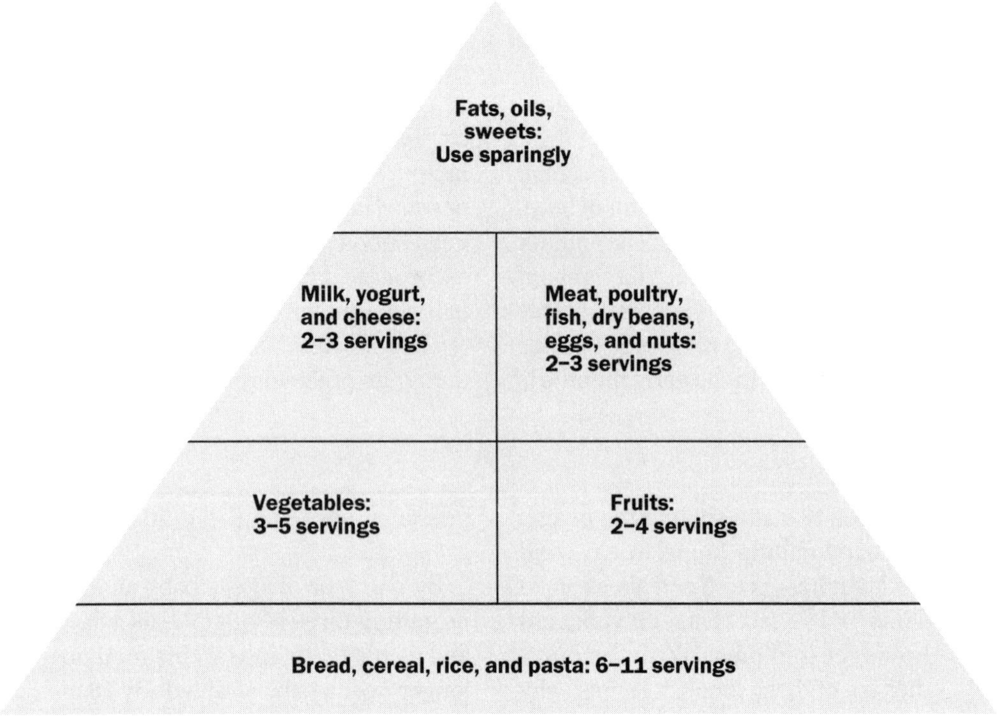

Derived from the U.S. Department of Agriculture's "Eating Right Pyramid."

- Potatoes and other vegetables and fruits
- Milk, cheese, and ice cream
- Meat, poultry, fish, eggs, dried peas, and beans
- Bread, flour, and cereals
- Butter and oils

The "Daily Food Guide" table can be used as a general guide to planning nutritionally balanced meals for preteens, teens, and adults of any age.

The Six Group Division (The Food Guide Pyramid)

Very similar to the seven group division, the six group division puts all vegetables into one group. The pyramid chart is meant to convey three key points: eat less fat, eat a variety of foods, and eat the recommended number of servings from each group.

The Years of Growth

A proper diet is crucial during the years from 2 to 18, since this is a period of tremendous growth.

Children should also learn about balanced diets, learn decent manners at the table, and develop a sense of timing about when to eat and when not to eat.

Creating a Pleasant Atmosphere at Mealtime

- Children should never be bribed with candy, money, or the promise of special surprises as a way of getting them to eat properly.
- They should not be given the idea that dessert is a reward for finishing the earlier part of the meal.
- Relatively small portions should be served and completely finished before anything else is offered.
- Between-meal snacks should be discouraged if they cut down on the appetite at mealtime.
- From time to time, childern should be allowed to choose the foods that they will eat at a meal.

Parents should keep in mind that the atmosphere in which childern eat and the attitudes instilled in them toward food can be altogether as basic as the nourishment for their bodies.

Teenage Diet

From the start of a child's growth spurt, which begins at age 10 or 11 for girls and between 13 and 15 for boys, and for several years thereafter, adolescent appetites are likely to be unbelievably large and somewhat outlandish. Parents should intervene with the youngster who is putting on too much weight, as well as with the one who is not eating enough and endangering their health. See "Diet" in Ch. 3 *The Teens.*

Adult Nutrition

The average American adult experiences slow, but steady, weight gain. For some, this can develop into an obesity problem. Because being even moderately overweight can pose health risks, weight gain as an adult should be viewed as a hazard that could jeopardize health. A sensible diet is recommended.

For Older People

People over 60 tend to have changes in their digestive system that are related to less efficient and slower absorption. Incomplete chewing of food because of carelessness or impaired teeth can intensify this problem. Avoiding haste at mealtimes ought to be the rule.

In cases where a dental disorder makes proper chewing impossible, food should be chopped or pureed.

Food for older people should be cooked simply; preferably baked, boiled, or broiled rather than fried, and foods high in fat should be avoided. A daily multivitamin capsule is strongly recommended.

Eating for Life

The U.S. Department of Agriculture and the U.S. Department of Health and Human Services recommend seven basic guidelines to avoid excess weight and maintain optimum health:

1. Eat a variety of foods.
2. Maintain a desirable weight.
3. Avoid too much fat, saturated fat, and cholesterol.
4. Eat foods with adequate starch and fiber.
5. Avoid too much sugar.
6. Avoid too much sodium.
7. If you drink alcoholic beverages, do so in moderation.

The guidelines are designed for healthy adult Americans, but are considered especially appropriate for people who may already have some of the risk factors for chronic diseases, including a family history of obesity, early heart disease, diabetes, high blood pressure, or high blood cholesterol levels.

The U.S.D.A. and the U.S.D. H.H.S. also recommend the "Choose More Often" approach to healthful eating.

Choose More Often:

Low-fat meat, poultry, fish
Lean cuts of meat trimmed of fat (round tip roast, pork tenderloin, loin of lamb chop), poultry without skin, and fish, cooked without breading or added fat.

Low-fat or Non-fat dairy products
1 percent or non-fat milk, buttermilk; non-fat or low-fat yogurt; lower fat cheeses (part-skim ricotta, fresh parmesan or feta); sherbet.

Dry beans and peas
All beans, peas, and lentils—the dry forms are higher in protein.

Whole grain products
Reduced-fat breads, bagels, and English muffins made from whole wheat, rye, bran, and corn flour or meal; whole grain or bran cereals; whole wheat pasta; brown rice; bulgur.

Fruits and vegetables
All fruits and vegetables: apples, pears, cantaloupe, oranges, grapefruit, pineapple, peaches, bananas, carrots, broccoli, Brussels sprouts, cabbage, kale, potatoes, tomatoes, sweet potatoes, spinach, cauliflower, turnips, etc.

Fats and oils high in unsaturates
Unsaturated vegetable oils, such as canola oil, corn oil, cottonseed oil, olive oil, and soybean oil, and margarine; reduced-fat and reduced-calorie mayonnaise and salad dressings.

Some tips for following the "choose more often" approach in grocery shopping, food preparation, and eating out:

When Grocery Shopping

Focus on variety. Using the above guidelines, choose a wide selection of low-fat foods rich in fiber. Although the goal is to reduce fat to 30 percent or less, when choosing foods that do contain fat, try to choose ones that contain primarily unsaturated fats.

Read food labels. Nutrition labels on most packaged foods give information on the nutrients in each serving: total calories and calories from fat; total and saturated fat; cholesterol; sodium; total carbohydrates, including dietary fiber, and sugars; protein; and certain vitamins and minerals. The label also calculates the percent daily value of each of these nutrients, meaning the percentage of the recommended amount of the nutrient that the food provides, based on a 2,000-calorie diet. Choose products that are low in fat—especially saturated fat—and high in fiber.

Beware of sodium. Many processed, canned, and frozen foods are high in sodium. Cured or processed meats, cheeses, soups and condiments (soy sauce, mustard, tartar sauce) are high in sodium. Check labels for salt, onion or garlic salt, and any ingredient with sodium in its name. Compare products and choose the ones with lower levels.

When Preparing Food

Use small amounts of fat and fatty foods when planning meals.
When you do use fat, use it sparingly and allow the full flavor of the foods to dominate, instead of a single element like cheese or butter. Try to use only ½ teaspoon of fat per serving. Gradually introduce nonfat or low-fat alternatives into your diet.

Use less saturated fat. While reducing your total fat intake, substitute unsaturated fat and oils for saturated. Instead of butter, try vegetable oil, margarine or a low-fat cooking spray. To substitute, use equal portions, or less.

Use low-fat alternatives. Substitute 1 percent, skim, or reconstituted nonfat dry milk for whole milk. Use buttermilk, nonfat or low-fat yogurt, or evaporated skim milk in place of cream and sour cream. Try reduced-fat or fat-free mayonnaise, sour cream and salad dressings. Also try using egg whites or egg substitutes in place of eggs, which are extremely high in fat and cholesterol.

Choose lean meat. Trim all visible fat from meat and poultry, including poultry skin. Canned, reduced fat and sodium stocks are now available for making soup.

Use low-fat cooking methods. Bake, steam, broil, microwave, or boil foods rather than frying. Avoid gravies and try vegetable-based instead of cream-based sauces.

Increase fiber. Substitute whole-grain flour for white flour. Have generous servings. Whenever possible, eat the edible fiber-rich skin as well as the rest of the vegetable or fruit.

Use herbs, spices, and other flavorings. For a different way to add flavor to meals, try lemon juice, basil, chives, curry powder, onion, cracked pepper, and garlic in place of fats and sodium. Try low-fat recipes and adjust old ones to reduce fat and sodium.

When Eating Out

Choose the restaurant carefully. Are low-fat, high-fiber items on the menu, like pasta? How are meat, chicken, and fish dishes cooked—broiled, baked, or fried? Avoid fast food places.

Try ethnic cuisines. Italian and Asian restaurants often feature low-fat dishes—though you must be selective and alert to portion size. Try a small serving of pasta or fish in a tomato sauce at an Italian restaurant. Many Chinese, Japanese, and Thai dishes include plenty of steamed vegetables and a high proportion of vegetables to meat. Steamed rice, steamed noodle dishes and vegetarian dishes are good choices, too. Ask for food without soy sauce or salt.

Make sure you get what you want. Be in control when you eat out. Ask how dishes are cooked. Don't hesitate to request that one food be substituted for another. Order a green salad or baked potato in place of french fries or order fruit or sherbet instead of ice cream. Request sauces and salad dressings on the side and use only a small amount. Ask that butter and rolls not be sent to the table. If you're not very hungry, order two low-fat appetizers rather than an entire meal, split a menu item with a friend, get a doggie-bag to take half of your meal home, or order a half-size portion. When you finish, let the waiter clear dishes to avoid post-meal nibbling.

Eat slowly. Don't eat to get your money's worth, eat to sate your hunger. Eating quickly can either leave you still feeling hungry or sick with indigestion. By deliberately slowing down your intake of food, you will more likely feel full earlier in the meal and your body will be able to properly digest your food.

Be reasonable. If you don't eat out very often, one meal won't ruin your health. If you feel like ordering a rich meal or having dessert, simply cut back on the extras; avoid the bread and butter, don't order an appetizer, have one glass of wine instead of two.

Raising Children with Healthy Eating Habits

Children who are raised with healthy eating habits are more likely to continue these habits in their adult life. For example, if dessert is more frequently fresh fruit than ice cream sundaes, a child will not grow up associating a special treat with only rich fatty sweets. The nectarine, pear or apple will seem just as special. Likewise, as an adult the same child will be less likely to overindulge with sweets or other fatty foods.

Malnutrition

The classic diseases of nutritional deficiency, or malnutrition, such as scurvy and pellagra, are now rare, at least in the United States. The chief reason for their disappearance is the application of scientific knowledge gained in this century of the importance of vitamins and minerals in the diet. Thus most bread is fortified with vitamins and minerals, and in ad dition, commercial food processing has made it possible for balanced diets of an appealing variety to be eaten all year round.

Many people do not have an adequate diet, either through ignorance or because they simply cannot afford it. A number of food programs have been created to assist them, but unfortunately, the programs don't reach everyone who needs help.

Metric Equivalents of Traditional Food Measures

1 teaspoon	=	5 milliliters
1 tablespoon	=	15 milliliters
1/4 cup	=	60 milliliters
1/3 cup	=	80 milliliters
1/2 cup	=	120 milliliters
2/3 cup	=	160 milliliters
3/4 cup	=	180 milliliters
1 cup	=	240 milliliters or 0.24 liter

Causes of Malnutrition

Some people, either because of ignorance or the influence of food fads, do not eat a balanced diet even though they can afford to. There are also large numbers of people with nutritional deficiency diseases whose eating habits are abnormal. Some are alcoholics; others are so depressed that they lack sufficient drive to feed themselves properly. A combination of any of these factors increases the likelihood of poor nutrition and often leads to health-damaging consequences.

Disease

People can also develop nutritional deficiencies because they have a disease that interferes with food absorption, storage, and utilization, or that causes increased excretion, usually in the urine, of substances needed for nutrition. These are generally chronic diseases, such as those of the gastrointestinal tract including the liver, or those involving the kidneys or the endocrine glands.

Medications

Nutritional deficiencies can also result from loss of appetite caused by medications, especially when a number of different medications are taken simultaneously. This adverse effect on the appetite is a strong reason for not taking medicines unless told to do so by a physician for a specific purpose.

Most people are not aware of inadequacies in their diet until there are

Nutrients in Common Foods

Food	Food energy	Protein	Fat	Carbohydrate
	Calories	Grams	Grams	Grams
Milk and Milk Products				
Milk; 1 cup:				
Fluid, whole	165	9	10	12
Fluid, nonfat (skim)	90	9	trace	13
Buttermilk, cultured (from skim milk)	90	9	trace	13
Evaporated (undiluted)	345	18	20	24
Dry, nonfat (regular)	435	43	1	63
Yogurt (from partially skimmed milk); 1 cup	120	8	4	13
Cheese; 1 ounce:				
Cheddar or American	115	7	9	1
Cottage:				
From skim milk	25	5	trace	1
Creamed	30	4	1	1
Cream cheese	105	2	11	1
Swiss	105	7	8	1
Desserts (largely milk):				
Custard, baked; 1 cup, 8 fluid ounces	305	14	15	29
Ice cream, plain, factory packed:				
1 slice or individual brick, ⅛ quart	130	3	7	14
1 container, 8 fluid ounces	255	6	14	28
Ice milk; 1 cup, 8 fluid ounces	200	6	7	29
Eggs				
Egg, raw, large:				
1 whole	80	6	6	trace
1 white	15	4	trace	trace
1 yolk	60	3	5	trace
Egg, cooked; 1 large:				
Boiled	80	6	6	trace
Scrambled (with milk and fat)	110	7	8	1
Meat, Poultry, Fish, Shellfish				
Bacon, broiled or fried, drained, 2 medium thick slices	85	4	8	trace
Beef, cooked without bone:				
Braised, simmered, or pot-roasted; 3 ounce portion:				
Entire portion, lean and fat	365	19	31	0
Lean only, approx. 2 ounces	140	17	4	0
Hamburger patties, made with				
Regular ground beef; 3-ounce patty	235	21	17	0
Lean ground round; 3-ounce patty	185	23	10	0
Roast; 3-ounce slice from cut having relatively small amount of fat:				
Entire portion, lean and fat	255	22	18	0
Lean only, approx. 2.3 ounces	115	19	4	0
Steak, broiled; 3-ounce portion:				
Entire portion, lean and fat	375	19	32	0
Lean only, approx. 1.8 ounces	105	17	4	0

Nutrients in Common Foods *(continued)*

Food	Food energy	Protein	Fat	Carbohydrate
	Calories	Grams	Grams	Grams
Beef, canned: corned beef hash; 3 ounces	155	8	10	9
Beef and vegetable stew; 1 cup	220	16	11	15
Chicken, without bone: broiled; 3 ounces	115	20	3	0
Lamb, cooked:				
Chops; 1 thick chop, with bone, 4.8 ounces:				
Lean and fat, approx. 3.4 ounces	340	21	28	0
Lean only, 2.3 ounces	120	18	5	0
Roast, without bone:				
Leg; 3-ounce slice:				
Entire slice, lean and fat	265	20	20	0
Lean only, approx. 2.3 ounces	120	19	5	0
Shoulder; 3-ounce portion, without bone:				
Entire portion, lean and fat	300	18	25	0
Lean only, approx. 2.2 ounces	125	16	6	0
Liver, beef, fried; 2 ounces	120	13	4	6
Pork, cured, cooked:				
Ham, smoked; 3-ounce portion, without bone	245	18	19	0
Luncheon meat:				
Boiled ham; 2 ounces	130	11	10	0
Canned, spiced; 2 ounces	165	8	14	1
Pork, fresh, cooked:				
Chops; 1 chop, with bone, 3.5 ounces:				
Lean and fat, approx. 2.4 ounces	295	15	25	0
Lean only, approx. 1.6 ounces	120	14	7	0
Roast; 3-ounce slice, without bone:				
Entire slice, lean and fat	340	19	29	0
Lean only, approx. 2.2 ounces	160	19	9	0
Sausage:				
Bologna; 8 slices (4.1 by 0.1 inches each), 8 ounces	690	27	62	2
Frankfurter; 1 cooked, 1.8 ounces	155	6	14	1
Tongue, beef, boiled; 3 ounces	205	18	14	trace
Veal, cutlet, broiled; 3-ounce portion, without bone	185	23	9	0
Fish and shellfish:				
Bluefish, baked or broiled; 3 ounces	135	22	4	0
Clams: raw, meat only; 3 ounces	70	11	1	3
Crabmeat, canned or cooked; 3 ounces	90	14	2	1
Fishsticks, breaded, cooked, frozen, 10 sticks (3.8 by 1.0 by 0.5 inches each), 8 ounces	400	38	20	15

Nutrients in Common Foods *(continued)*

Food	Food energy	Protein	Fat	Carbohydrate
	Calories	Grams	Grams	Grams
Haddock, fried; 3 ounces	135	16	5	6
Mackerel; broiled; 3 ounces	200	19	13	0
Oysters, raw, meat only; 1 cup (13-19 medium-size oysters, selects)	160	20	4	8
Oyster stew: 1 cup (6–8 oysters)	200	11	12	11
Salmon, canned (pink); 3 ounces	120	17	5	0
Sardines, canned in oil, drained solids; 3 ounces	180	22	9	1
Shrimp, canned, meat only; 3 ounces	110	23	1	—
Tuna, canned in oil, drained solids; 3 ounces	170	25	7	0
Mature Beans and Peas, Nuts				
Beans, dry seed:				
Common varieties, as Great Northern, navy, and others, canned; 1 cup:				
Red	230	15	1	42
White, with tomato or molassess:				
With pork	330	16	7	54
Without pork	315	16	1	60
Beans, dry seed:				
Lima, cooked; 1 cup	260	16	1	48
Cowpeas or black-eyed peas, dry, cooked; 1 cup	190	13	1	34
Peanuts, roasted, shelled; 1 cup	840	39	71	28
Peanut butter; 1 tablespoon	90	4	8	3
Peas, split, dry, cooked; 1 cup	290	20	1	52
Vegetables				
Asparagus:				
Cooked; 1 cup	35	4	trace	6
Canned, 6 medium-size spears	20	2	trace	3
Beans				
Lima, immature, cooked; 1 cup	150	8	1	29
Snap, green:				
Cooked; 1 cup	25	2	trace	6
Canned; solids and liquid; 1 cup	45	2	trace	10
Beets, cooked, diced; 1 cup	70	2	trace	16
Broccoli, cooked, flower stalks; 1 cup	45	5	trace	8
Brussels sprouts, cooked; 1 cup	60	6	1	12
Cabbage; 1 cup:				
Raw, coleslaw	100	2	7	9
Cooked	40	2	trace	9
Carrots:				
Raw: 1 carrot (5½ by 1 inch) or 25 thin strips	20	1	trace	5
Cooked, diced, 1 cup	45	1	1	9
Canned, strained or chopped; 1 ounce	5	trace	0	2
Cauliflower, cooked, flower buds; 1 cup	30	3	trace	6

some dramatic consequences. Nor is it easy to recognize the presence of a disorder that might be causing malnutrition. A physician should be consulted promptly when there is a persistent weight loss, especially when the diet is normal. He should also be informed of any changes in the skin, mucous membranes of the mouth or tongue, or nervous system function, because such symptoms can be a warning of dietary deficiency.

The family or friends of a person with a nutritional deficiency can often detect his condition because they become aware of changes in his eating patterns. They can also note early signs of a deficiency of some of the B vitamins, such as cracks in the mucous membranes at the corners of the mouth, or some slowing of intellectual function.

Correction of Nutritional Deficiencies

Nutritional deficiencies are among the most easily preventable causes of disease. It is important to realize that even mild deficiencies can cause irreparable damage, particularly protein deprivation in young children, which can result in some degree of mental retardation. Periodic medical checkups for everyone in the family are the best way to make sure that such deficiencies are corrected before they snowball into a chronic disease. In most cases, all that is required is a change of eating habits.

Weight

Probably the most important dietary problem in the United States today is obesity. It is certainly the most talked about and written about, not only in terms of self-esteem, but more importantly, in terms of good health.

Physicians, dieticians and other health experts use height and weight tables to calculate an average and these experts should be consulted to insure that the tables are being accurately applied and analyzed. While the notion of an "average" weight may be viewed by some with suspicion, the truth is that Americans are steadily gaining weight. Studies indicate that people who are obese have a higher rate of disease and a shorter life expectancy than those of average weight. Added weight places an added strain to the body, especially the heart. Obesity causes over 300,000 deaths a year and obese people need health care services more frequently than thinner people. Incredibly, thirty percent of the U.S. population is believed to be obese. Being too fat and being overweight are not necessarily the same, however. Heavy bones and muscles can increase a person's weight, but only an excess amount of fat tissue can make someone obese.

An individual is usually considered obese in the clinical sense if he weighs 20 percent more than the standard tables indicate for his size and age. Too much emphasis on the importance of the height and weight tables can be as harmful as too little emphasis. Increasingly, teenage girls and boys suffer from overly pessimistic assessments of their weights. Anxiety over acceptance by their peers and subtle pressure from advertising and media sources to be "model-thin," have pushed some teens into anorexia and bulimia.

The Pinch Test

Another method of determining obesity is to use the "pinch" test. In most adults under 50 years of age, about half of the body fat is located directly under the skin. There are various parts of the body, such as the side of the lower torso, the back of the upper arm, or directly under the shoulder blade, where the thumb and forefinger can pinch a fold of skin and fat away from the underlying bone structure.

If the fold between the fingers—which is, of course, double thickness when it is pinched—is thicker than one inch in any of these areas, the likelihood is that the person is obese.

The Problem of Overweight

The percentage of overweight people in this country has been increasing steadily, chiefly because people are eating more and using less physical energy than they used to. Americans do very little walking because of the availability of cars; they do very little manual labor because of the increasing use of machines. They may eat good wholesome meals, but they also snack at all hours, especially when sitting in front of the television screen.

These patterns usually begin in childhood. Youngsters rarely walk to school; they get there by bus or car. They often have extra money for snacks and soft drinks, and frequently parents encourage them to overeat without realizing that such habits do them more harm than good.

Most overweight children remain overweight as adults. They also have greater difficulty losing fat, and if they do lose it, they tend to regain it more easily than overweight adults who were thin as children. Many adults become overweight between the ages of 20 and 30. Thus, by age 30, about 12 percent of American men and women are 20 percent or more overweight. By age 60, about 30 percent of males and 50 percent of females are at least 20 percent overweight. As previously indicated, the phenomenon of weight gain while aging does not represent biological normalcy.

Why People Put on Weight

Why does weight gain happen? Excess weight is the result of the imbalance between caloric intake as food and caloric expenditure as energy, either in maintaining the basic metabolic processes necessary to sustain life or in performing physical activity. Calories not spent in either of these ways become converted to fat and accumulate in the body as fat, or *adipose* tissue.

A *calorie* is the unit of measurement that describes the amount of energy potentially available in a given food. It is also used to describe the amount of energy the body must use to perform a given function.

Counting Calories

If an adult gets the average 3,000 calories a day in his food from the age of 20 to 70, he will have consumed about 55 million calories. About 60 percent of these calories will have been used for his basic metabolic processes. The rest—22 million calories—might have resulted in a gain of about 6,000 pounds of fat, since each group of 3,500 extra calories could have produced one pound of fat.

In some ways, it seems like a miracle that people don't become more obese than they do. The reason, of course, is that most or all of these extra calories are normally used to provide energy for physical activity.

A reasonably good way for an adult to calculate his daily caloric needs for moderate activities is to multiply his desirable weight by 18 (for men) and 16 (for women). If one's typical day includes vigorous or strenuous activities, extra calories will, of course, be required.

Factors Affecting Obesity

Although there are exceptions, almost all overweight people consume more calories than they expend. The reasons for this imbalance are complex. Studies show that heredity is a factor. But heredity alone does not determine whether a person will become overweight. Environmental factors also play a role. Eating habits, lifestyle choices, and level of physical activity can affect weight. Psychological factors are also important. Some people may eat simply because they are bored. Others use food to comfort themselves when they are sad or angry, or to celebrate when they are happy. A habit of eating for reasons other than hunger often leads to weight gain.

Certain medications, such as steroids and antidepressants, may cause weight gain. Some illnesses may also lead to weight gain. Some obese people seem to have an impairment in the regulatory mechanism of the area of the central nervous system that governs food intake. Simply put, they do not know when to stop eating. Others may eat less than their nonobese counterparts, but they are considerably less active. In rare cases, some people appear to have an abnormality in the metabolic process that results in the accumulation of fat even when the balance between calories taken in and expended is negative and should lead to weight loss.

Nutrients in Common Foods *(continued)*

Food	Food energy	Protein	Fat	Carbohydrate
	Calories	Grams	Grams	Grams
Celery, raw: large stalk, 8 inches long	5	1	trace	1
Collards, cooked; 1 cup	75	7	1	14
Corn, sweet:				
Cooked; 1 ear 5 inches long	65	2	1	16
Canned, solids and liquid; 1 cup	170	5	1	41
Cucumbers, raw, pared; 6 slices (1/8-inch thick, center section)	5	trace	trace	1
Lettuce, head, raw:				
2 large or 4 small leaves	5	1	trace	1
1 compact head (4¾-inch diameter)	70	5	1	13
Mushrooms, canned, solids and liquid; 1 cup	30	3	trace	9
Okra, cooked; 8 pods (3 inches long, 5/8-inch diameter)	30	2	trace	6
Onions: mature raw; 1 onion (2½-inch diameter)	50	2	trace	11
Peas, green; 1 cup:				
Cooked	110	8	1	19
Canned, solids and liquid	170	8	1	32
Peppers, sweet:				
Green, raw; 1 medium	15	1	trace	3
Red, raw; 1 medium	20	1	trace	4
Potatoes:				
Baked or boiled; 1 medium, 2½-inch diameter (weight raw, about 5 ounce):				
Baked in jacket	90	3	trace	21
Boiled; peeled before boiling	90	3	trace	21
Chips; 10 medium (2-inch diameter)	110	1	7	10
French fried:				
Frozen, ready to be heated for serving; 10 pieces (2 by ½ by ½ inch)	95	2	4	15
Ready-to-eat, deep fat for entire process; 10 pieces (2 by ½ by ½ inch)	155	2	7	20
Mashed; 1 cup:				
Milk added	145	4	1	30
Milk and butter added	230	4	12	28
Radishes, raw; 4 small	10	trace	trace	2
Spinach:				
Cooked; 1 cup	45	6	1	6
Canned, creamed, strained; 1 ounce	10	1	trace	2
Squash:				
Cooked, 1 cup:				
Summer, diced	35	1	trace	8
Winter, baked, mashed	95	4	1	23
Canned, strained or chopped; 1 ounce	10	trace	trace	2

Nutrients in Common Foods *(continued)*

Food	Food energy	Protein	Fat	Carbohydrate
	Calories	Grams	Grams	Grams
Sweet potatoes:				
Baked or boiled; 1 medium, 5 by 2 inches (weight raw, about 6 ounces):				
Baked in jacket	155	2	1	36
Boiled in jacket	170	2	1	39
Candied, 1 small, 3½ by 2 inches	295	2	6	60
Canned, vacuum or solid pack; 1 cup	235	4	trace	54
Tomatoes:				
Raw; 1 medium (2 by 2½ inches), about ⅓ pound	30	2	trace	6
Canned or cooked; 1 cup	45	2	trace	9
Tomato juice, canned; 1 cup	50	2	trace	10
Tomato catsup; 1 tablespoon	15	trace	trace	4
Turnips, cooked, diced; 1 cup	40	1	trace	9
Turnip greens, cooked; 1 cup	45	4	1	8
Fruits				
Apples, raw; 1 medium (2½ inch diameter), about ⅓ pound	70	trace	trace	18
Apple juice, fresh or canned; 1 cup	125	trace	0	34
Apple sauce, canned:				
Sweetened; 1 cup	185	trace	trace	50
Unsweetened; 1 cup	100	trace	trace	26
Apricots, raw; 3 apricots (about ¼ pound)	55	1	trace	14
Apricots, canned in heavy syrup; 1 cup	200	1	trace	54
Apricots, dried; uncooked; 1 cup (40 halves, small)	390	8	1	100
Avocados, raw, California varieties: ½ of a 10-ounce avocado (3½ by 3¼ inches)	185	2	18	6
Avocados, raw, Florida varieties: ½ of a 13-ounce avocado (4 by 3 inches)	160	2	14	11
Bananas, raw; 1 medium (6 by 1½ inches), about ⅓ pound	85	1	trace	23
Blueberries, raw; 1 cup	85	1	1	21
Cantaloupes, raw, ½ melon (5-inch diameter)	40	1	trace	9
Cherries, sour, sweet, and hybrid, raw; 1 cup	65	1	1	15
Cranberry sauce, sweetened; 1 cup	550	trace	1	142
Dates, "fresh" and dried, pitted and cut; 1 cup	505	4	1	134
Figs:				
Raw; 3 small (1½-inch (diameter), about ¼ pound	90	2	trace	22
Dried; 1 large (2 by 1 inch)	60	1	trace	15
Fruit cocktail, canned in heavy syrup, solids and liquid; 1 cup	175	1	trace	47
Grapefruit:				
Raw; ½ medium (4¼-inch diameter, No. 64's)	50	1	trace	14
Canned in syrup; 1 cup	165	1	trace	44

Nutrients in Common Foods *(continued)*

Food	Food energy Calories	Protein Grams	Fat Grams	Carbohydrate Grams
Grapefruit juice:				
Raw; 1 cup	85	1	trace	23
Canned:				
Unsweetened; 1 cup	95	1	trace	24
Sweetened; 1 cup	120	1	trace	32
Frozen concentrate, unsweetened:				
Undiluted; 1 can (6 fluid ounces:	280	4	1	72
Diluted, ready-to-serve; 1 cup	95	1	trace	24
Frozen concentrate, sweetened:				
Undiluted; 1 can (6 fluid ounces)	320	3	1	85
Diluted, ready-to-serve; 1 cup	105	1	trace	28
Grapes, raw; 1 cup:				
American type (slip skin)	70	1	1	16
European type (adherent skin)	100	1	trace	26
Grape juice, bottled; 1 cup	165	1	1	42
Lemonade concentrate, frozen, sweetened:				
Undiluted; 1 can (6 fluid ounces)	305	1	trace	113
Diluted, ready-to-serve; 1 cup	75	trace	trace	28
Oranges, raw; 1 large orange (3-inch diameter)	70	1	trace	18
Orange juice:				
Raw; 1 cup:				
California (Valencias)	105	2	trace	26
Florida varieties:				
Early and midseason	90	1	trace	23
Late season (Valencias)	105	1	trace	26
Canned, unsweetened; 1 cup	110	2	trace	28
Frozen concentrate:				
Undiluted; 1 can 6 fluid ounces)	305	5	trace	80
Diluted, ready-to-serve; 1 cup	105	2	trace	27
Peaches:				
Raw:				
1 medium (2½-inch diameter), about ¼ pound	35	1	trace	10
1 cup, sliced	65	1	trace	16
Canned (yellow-fleshed) in heavy syrup; 1 cup	185	1	trace	49
Dried: uncooked; 1 cup	420	5	1	109
Pears:				
Raw; 1 pear (3 by 2½-inch diameter)	100	1	1	25
Canned in heavy syrup; 1 cup	175	1	trace	47
Pineapple juice; canned; 1 cup	120	1	trace	32
Plums				
Raw; 1 plum (2-inch diameter, about 2 ounces	30	trace	trace	7
Canned (Italian prunes, in syrup; 1 cup	185	1	trace	50

Nutrients in Common Foods *(continued)*

Food	Food energy	Protein	Fat	Carbohydrate
	Calories	Grams	Grams	Grams
Prunes, dried:				
Uncooked; 4 medium prunes	70	1	trace	19
Cooked, unsweetened; 1 cup (17–18 prunes and ⅓ cup liquid	295	3	1	78
Prune juice, canned; 1 cup	170	1	trace	45
Raisins, dried; 1 cup	460	4	trace	124
Raspberries, red:				
Raw; 1 cup	70	1	trace	17
Frozen; 10-ounce carton	280	2	1	70
Strawberries:				
Raw; 1 cup	55	1	1	12
Frozen; 10-ounce carton	300	2	1	75
Tangerines; 1 medium (2½-inch diameter), about ¼ pound	40	1	trace	10
Watermelon; 1 wedge (4 by 8 inches), about 2 pounds (weighed with rind	120	2	1	29
Grain Products				
Biscuits, baking powder, enriched flour; 1 biscuit (2½-inch diameter)	130	2	4	20
Bran flakes (40 percent bran) with added thiamine; 1 ounce	85	3	1	22
Breads:				
Cracked wheat:				
1 pound (20 slices)	1,190	39	10	236
1 slice (½-inch thick)	60	2	1	12
Italian; 1 pound	1,250	41	4	256
Rye:				
American (light):				
1 pound (20 slices)	1,100	41	5	236
1 slice (½-inch thick)	55	2	trace	12
Pumpernickel; 1 pound	1,115	41	5	241
White:				
1–2 percent nonfat dry milk:				
1 pound (20 slices)	1,225	39	15	229
1 slice (½-inch thick)	60	2	1	12
3–4 percent nonfat dry milk:				
1 pound (20 slices)	1,225	39	15	229
1 slice (½-inch thick)	60	2	1	12
5–6 percent nonfat dry milk:				
1 pound (20 slices)	1,245	41	17	228
1 slice (½-inch thick)	65	2	1	12
Whole wheat, graham, or entire wheat:				
1 pound (20 slices)	1,105	48	14	216
1 slice (½-inch thick)	55	2	1	11
Cakes:				
Angel food: 2-inch sector (1⁄12 of cake, 8-inch diameter)	160	4	trace	36
Butter cakes:				
Plain cake and cupcakes without icing:				
1 square (3 by 3 by 2 inches)	315	4	12	48

Nutrients in Common Foods *(continued)*

Food	Food energy	Protein	Fat	Carbohydrate
	Calories	Grams	Grams	Grams
1 cupcake (2¾-inch diameter)	120	2	5	18
Plain cake with icing:				
2-inch sector of iced layer cake (1⁄16 of cake, 10-inch diameter)	320	5	6	62
Rich cake:				
2-inch sector layer cake, iced (1⁄16 of cake, 10-inch diameter)	490	6	19	76
Fruit cake, dark; 1 piece (2 by 1½ by ¼ inches)	60	1	2	9
Sponge; 2-inch sector (1⁄12 of cake, 8-inch diameter	115	3	2	22
Cookies, plain and assorted; 1 cookie (3-inch diameter)	110	2	3	19
Cornbread or muffins made with enriched, degermed cornmeal; 1 muffin 2¾-inch diameter)	105	3	2	18
Cornflakes; 1 ounce	110	2	trace	24
Corn grits, degermed, cooked; 1 cup	120	3	trace	27
Crackers:				
Graham; 4 small or 2 medium	55	1	1	10
Saltines; 2 crackers (2-inch square	35	1	1	6
Soda, plain: 2 crackers (2½-inch square	45	1	1	8
Doughnuts, cake type; 1 doughnut	135	2	7	17
Farina, cooked; 1 cup	105	3	trace	22
Macaroni, cooked; 1 cup:				
Cooked 8–10 minutes (undergoes additional cooking as ingredient of a food mixture)	190	6	1	39
Cooked until tender	155	5	1	32
Noodles (egg noodles), cooked; 1 cup	200	7	2	37
Oat cereal (mixture, mainly oat flour), ready-to-eat; 1 ounce	115	4	2	21
Oatmeal or rolled oats, regular or quick cooking, cooked; 1 cup	150	5	3	26
Pancakes; baked; 1 cake (4-inch diameter):				
Wheat (home recipe)	60	2	2	7
Buckwheat (with buckwheat pancake mix)	45	2	2	6
Pies; 3½-inch sector (⅛ of 9-inch diameter pie):				
Apple	300	3	13	45
Cherry	310	3	13	45
Custard	250	7	13	27
Lemon meringue	270	4	11	40
Minced	320	3	14	49
Pumpkin	240	5	13	28
Pretzels; 5 small sticks	20	trace	trace	4

Nutrients in Common Foods *(continued)*

Food	Food energy	Protein	Fat	Carbohydrate
	Calories	Grams	Grams	Grams
Rice, cooked; 1 cup:				
Converted	205	4	trace	45
White	200	4	trace	44
Rice, puffed or flakes; 1 ounce	110	2	trace	25
Rolls:				
Plain, pan (16 ounces per dozen); 1 roll	115	3	2	20
Hard, round (22 ounces per dozen); 1 roll	160	5	2	31
Sweet, pan (18 ounces per dozen); 1 roll	135	4	4	21
Spaghetti, cooked until tender; 1 cup	155	5	1	32
Waffles, baked, with enriched flour: 1 waffle (4½ by 5½ by ½ inches)	215	7	8	28
Wheat, puffed; 1 ounce	100	4	trace	22
Wheat, rolled, cooked; 1 cup	175	5	1	40
Wheat flakes; 1 ounce	100	3	trace	23
Wheat flours:				
Whole wheat; 1 cup, sifted	400	16	2	85
All purpose or family flour: 1 cup, sifted	400	12	1	84
Wheat germ; 1 cup, stirred	245	17	7	34
Fats, Oils, Related Products				
Butter; 1 tablespoon	100	trace	11	trace
Fats, cooking:				
Vegetable fats:				
1 cup	1,770	0	200	0
1 tablespoon	110	0	12	0
Lard:				
1 cup	1,985	0	220	0
1 tablespoon	125	0	14	0
Margarine; 1 tablespoon	100	trace	11	trace
Oils, salad or cooking; 1 tablespoon	125	0	14	0
Salad dressings; 1 tablespoon:				
Blue cheese	90	1	10	1
Commercial, plain (mayonnaise type)	60	trace	6	2
French	60	trace	6	2
Mayonnaise	110	trace	12	trace
Thousand Island	75	trace	8	1
Sugars, Sweets				
Candy; 1 ounce:				
Caramels	120	1	3	22
Chocolate, sweetened, milk	145	2	9	16
Fudge, plain	115	trace	3	23
Hard	110	0	0	28
Marshmallow	90	1	0	23
Jams, marmalades, preserves; 1 tablespoon	55	trace	trace	14
Jellies; 1 tablespoon	50	0	0	13
Sugar; 1 tablespoon	50	0	0	12
Syrup, table blends; 1 tablespoon	55	0	0	15

Nutrients in Common Foods *(continued)*

Food	Food energy Calories	Protein Grams	Fat Grams	Carbohydrate Grams
Miscellaneous				
Beverages, carbonated, cola types; 1 cup	105	—	—	28
Bouillon cubes; 1 cube	2	trace	trace	0
Chocolate, unsweetened; 1 ounce	145	2	15	8
Gelatin dessert, plain, ready-to-serve; 1 cup	155	4	0	36
Sherbet, factory packed; 1 cup (8-fluid-ounce container)	235	3	trace	58
Soups, canned, prepared with equal amount of water; 1 cup:				
Bean with pork	168	8	6	22
Beef noodle	140	8	5	14
Bouillon, broth, and consomme	30	5	0	3
Chicken consomme	44	7	trace	4
Clam chowder, Manhattan style	80	2	3	12
Tomato	90	2	3	16
Vegetable beef	80	5	2	10
Vinegar; 1 tablespoon	2	0	—	1

Adapted from *Nutritive Value of American Foods* by Catherine F. Adams. Agriculture Handbook No. 456. U.S. Department of Agriculture, issued November 1975. The cup measure used in the following table refers to the standard 8-ounce measuring cup of 8 fluid ounces or one-half liquid pint. When a measure is indicated by ounce, it is understood to be by weight—1/16 of a pound avoirdupois—unless a fluid ounce is indicated. All weights and measures in the table are in U.S. System units.

Obesity and Health

There are many reasons why obesity is a health hazard. The annual death rate for obese people between the ages of 20 and 64 is half again as high as that for people whose weight is close to normal. This statistical difference is due primarily to the increased likelihood that the obese person will suffer from diabetes mellitus and from diseases of the digestive and circulatory systems, especially of the heart.

One possible reason for the increased possibility of heart disease is that there are about two-thirds of a mile of blood vessels in each pound of adipose tissue. Thus 20 or more pounds of excess weight are likely to impose a great additional work load on the heart.

Obese people are also poorer surgical risks than the nonobese, and it is often more difficult to diagnose and therefore to treat their illnesses correctly.

Permanent loss of excess weight makes the formerly obese person come closer to matching the life expectancy of the nonobese. However, losing and regaining weight as a repeated pattern is even more hazardous in terms of health than consistent obesity.

Psychological Consequences of Obesity

In ways that are both obvious and subtle, obesity often has damaging psychological consequences. This is particularly true for obese children, who tend to feel isolated and rejected by their peers. They may consider themselves victims of prejudice and blame their obesity for everything that goes wrong in their lives. In many cases, the destructive relationship between obesity and self-pity keeps perpetuating itself.

Obese adults are likely to experience the same feelings, but to a somewhat lesser degree. For some, obesity is an escape which consciously or unconsciously helps them to avoid situations in which they feel uncomfortable—those that involve active competition or relationships with the opposite sex.

Avoiding Excess Weight

Clearly, obesity is a condition that most people would like to avoid. Not putting on extra pounds does seem to be easier, in theory at least, than taking them off. One possible explanation for this is that additional adipose tissue consists of a proliferation of fat cells. Shrinking these cells is one thing, eliminating them is another. Our present lack of fundamental knowledge about the regulatory and metabolic mechanisms relating to obesity limits the technique of preventing overweight to recommending a balance between caloric intake and expenditure.

The real responsibility for preventing the onset of obesity in childhood rests with parents. It is important for the parents to set a good example and to instill early on all of the fundamentals of good nutrition and healthy eating habits; these are of the utmost importance in this connection. Caloric expenditure in the form of regular exercise is equally important.

Exercising by Habit

This does not necessarily mean that exercise should be encouraged for its own sake. What it does mean is making a habit of choosing an active way of approaching a situation rather than a lazy way: walking upstairs rather than taking the elevator; walking to school rather than riding; walking while playing golf rather than riding in a cart; running to get the ball that has rolled away rather than ambling toward it. These choices should be made consistently and not just occasionally if obesity is to be avoided. Those people who naturally enjoy the more active way of doing things are lucky. Those who don't should make an effort to develop new patterns, especially if obesity is a family problem.

Anyone with the type of physical handicap that makes a normal amount of exercise impossible should be especially careful about caloric intake.

Weight Reduction

The treatment of obesity is a complicated problem. In the first place, there is the question of who wants or needs to be treated and how much weight should be lost. Except in unusual situations, anyone who wants to lose weight should be encouraged to do so. Possible exceptions are teenagers who are not overweight but who want to be as thin as they can possibly be—the boy who is involved in an athletic event such as wrestling, or the girl who has decided she wants to look like a fashion model.

Crash dieting is usually unwise if the goal is to lose too much weight too rapidly and should be undertaken only after consulting a doctor about its advisability. As for adolescents who have become slightly overweight during puberty, they may be ill-advised to try to take off the extra pounds that probably relate to a temporary growth pattern.

Losing Weight Must Be Self-Motivated

Unless there are compelling medical reasons for not doing so, anyone weighing 20 percent or more over the normal limit for his age and body build should be helped to slim down. It is extremely important, however, for the motivation to come from the person himself rather than from outside pressure.

Unless an overweight person really wants to reduce, he will not succeed in doing so, certainly not permanently, even though he appears to be trying. He must have convinced himself—intellectually and emotionally—that the goal of weight loss is truly worth the effort.

It is very difficult not only for his friends and family but for the person himself to be absolutely sure about the depth of his motivation. A physician treating an overweight patient has to assume that the desire to reduce is genuine and will try to reinforce it whenever he can. However, if a patient has made a number of attempts to lose weight over a period of years and has either been unable to reduce to any significant degree, or has become overweight again after reducing, it is probably safe to assume that the emotional desire is absent, or that there are emotional conflicts that stand in the way.

It is very possible that such a person could be harmed psychologically by losing weight, since he might need to be overweight for some deep-seated reason. This can be true for both children and adults. Occasionally it is possible for a psychiatrist or psychologist to help the patient remove a psychological block against losing weight, after which weight reduction can occur if the caloric balance is straightened out.

Effective Planning for Weight Loss

The ultimate key to successful weight reduction is proper eating combined with proper physical activity. This balance is extremely difficult for many people to achieve because it involves a marked change in attitudes and be-

Effect of Fat Accumulation in Abdomen

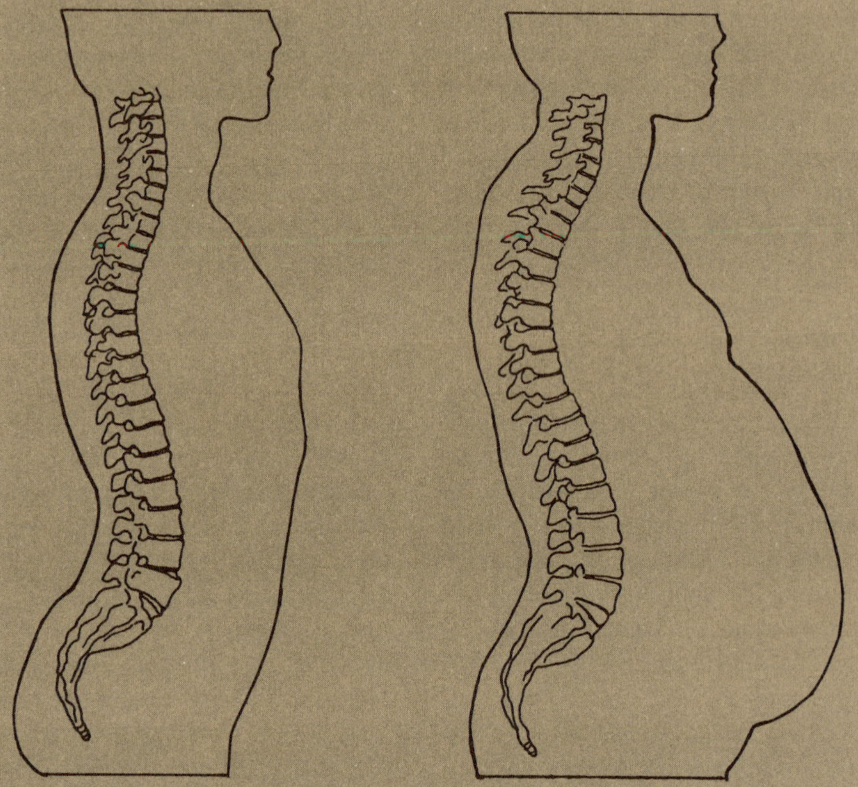

Fat accumulating in the abdomen puts severe stress on the lower vertebral column and can lead to many back problems.

havior patterns that are generally solidly established and of long duration. Furthermore, once the changes are made, they will have to endure for a lifetime if the weight that has been lost is not to be regained.

It is therefore important that the reducing diet should be somewhat similar to the person's usual eating pattern in terms of style and quality. Intake of fat and calories should be reduced and that of fiber increased, and probably the word "dieting" should not be used to describe the process, since most people don't find the idea of permanent dieting congenial.

Similarly, the increased physical activity that must accompany the new eating style should be of a type that the person enjoys. It is virtually impossible for an overeating person to reduce merely by restricting his caloric intake, or merely by increasing his caloric expenditure. The two must go together.

Cutting Down Step by Step

The first thing to determine when planning to lose weight is the number of pounds that have to go. A realistic goal to set is the loss of about one pound a week. This may seem too slow, but remember that at this rate, fifty pounds can be lost in a year.

Getting Started

Start by weighing yourself on arising, and then for two weeks try to eat in your customary manner, but keep a careful record of everything that you eat, the time it is eaten, and the number of calories it contains. During this period, continue to do your usual amount of physical activity.

When the two weeks are over, weigh yourself again at the same time of day as before. If you haven't gained any weight, you are in a basal caloric state. Then check over your food list to see what might be eliminated each day without causing discomfort.

Pay attention to portion size and try to think in terms of eliminating fats and simple carbohydrates first, because it is essential that you continue to get sufficient vitamins and minerals which are largely found in proteins, complex carbohydrates, fruits, and vegetables. The foods described in the "Food Guide Pyramid" should all continue to be included in your daily food consumption. If you are in the habit of having an occasional drink, remember that there are calories in alcohol but no nutrients, and that most alcoholic beverages stimulate the appetite.

Planning Meals

When you replan your meals, keep in mind that the items you cut down on must add up to between 300 and 400 calories a day if you are going to lose one pound a week.

Your total daily food intake should be divided among at least three meals a day—more, if you wish. If you need to eat more food or to eat more often, try snacking on low-calorie foods such as cabbage, carrots, celery, cucumber, and cauliflower. All of these can be eaten raw between meals.

There is definitely something to be said in favor of having breakfast every morning, or at least most mornings. This may be psychologically difficult, but try to do it, because it will be easier to control your urge to eat too much later in the day.

Increasing Exercise

At the same time that you begin to cut down on your food intake, start to increase your daily exercise in whatever way you find congenial so that the number of calories expended in increased exercise plus the number of calories eliminated from your diet comes to 500 or more. This is your daily caloric loss compared with your so-called basal caloric state.

Daily Food Guide

	Child	Preteen and Teen	Adult	Aging Adult
Milk or milk products *(cups)*	2–3	3–4 or more	2 or more	2 or more
Meat, fish, poultry, and eggs *(servings)*	1–2	3 or more	2 or more	2 or more
Green and yellow vegetables *(servings)*	1–2	2	2	at least 1
Citrus fruits and tomatoes *(servings)*	1	1–2	1	1–2
Potatoes, other fruits, vegetables *(servings)*	1	1	1	0–1
Bread, flour, and cereal *(servings)*	3–4	4 or more	3–4	2–3
Butter or margarine *(tablespoons)*	2	2–4	2–3	1–2

1. The need for the nutirents in 1 or 2 cups of milk daily can be satisfied by cheeses or ice cream. (1 cup of milk is approximately equivalent to 1½ cups of cottage cheese or 2–3 large scoops of ice cream.)
2. It is important to drink enough fluid. The equivalent of 3–5 cups daily is recommended.
3. The recommended daily serving of meat, fish, and poultry (3 oz.) may be alternated with eggs or cheese, dried peas, beans, or lentils.
4. Iron-rich foods should be selected as frequently as possible by teenage and adult females to help meet their high requirement for this mineral (liver, heart, lean meats, shellfish, egg yolks, legumes, green leafy vegetables, and whole grain and enriched cereal products).

From *Your Age and Your Diet* (1971), reprinted with permission from the American Medical Association.

Achieving Your Goal

You may wish to double your daily caloric loss so that you lose two pounds a week. Do not try to lose any more than that unless you are under close medical supervision.

If you gained weight during your two-week experimental period, you will have to increase your daily caloric loss by 500 for every pound gained per week. Thus, if you gained one pound during the two weeks, you will have to step up your daily caloric loss to 750 to lose a pound a week.

You'll have to keep plugging away to achieve your goal. It will be trying and difficult in many ways. You may get moody and discouraged and be tempted to quit. Don't. You'll probably go on periodic food binges. All this is natural and understandable, so try not to brood about it. Just do the best you can each day. Don't worry about yesterday, and let tomorrow take care of itself.

In many ways it can help, and in some cases it's essential, to have the support and encouragement of family and friends, particularly of those with whom you share meals. You may find it helpful to join a group that has been formed to help its members lose weight and maintain their weight loss. This is a good psychological support.

Maintaining Your Weight Loss

Once you have achieved your desired weight, you can test yourself to see what happens if you increase your caloric intake. Clearly, anyone who can lose weight in the manner described can't stay in a state of negative caloric imbalance indefinitely. But you will have to be careful, or you'll become overweight again. It's a challenge, but people who stick to a disciplined program can be rewarded by success.

Special Problems

If you do not succeed in losing weight in spite of carrying out the program described above, you may need professional help because of some special problem. A qualified physician may try some special diets, or he may even suggest putting you into a hospital so that he can see to it that you have no caloric food at all for as long as three weeks.

Perhaps the situation is complicated by a metabolic abnormality that can be corrected or helped by medication. Although such conditions are rare, they are not unheard of.

Obesity is almost never caused by a "glandular" problem—which usually means an underactive thyroid. Do not take thyroid pills to reduce unless your thyroid has been found to be underactive on the basis of a specific laboratory test.

The indiscriminate use of pills to reduce, even when prescribed, is never helpful in the long run, although it may appear to be at first. The unsupervised use of amphetamines, for example, can be extremely dangerous. See Ch. 29, *Substance Abuse,* for further information about the dangers of amphetamine abuse.

Because so many people are eager to reduce, and because losing weight isn't easy, there are many unethical professionals who specialize in the problem. Avoid them. All they are likely to do for you is take your money and make your situation no better—and often worse—than it was to begin with.

Underweight

Weighing too little is a problem that is considerably less common than weighing too much. In fact, in many cases, it isn't accurate to call it a problem at all, at least not a medical one.

There are some times, however, when underweight may indicate the presence of a disease, especially when a person rather suddenly begins and continues to lose weight, even though there has been no change in his eating habits. This is a situation that calls for prompt medical evaluation. Fortunately, such a person may already be under a physician's care at the time the weight loss is first noticed.

More often, however, underweight is a chronic condition that is of concern to the person who feels his looks would improve if he could only add some extra pounds. This is especially true in the case of adolescent girls and young women.

What To Do About Weighing Too Little

Chronic underweight is rarely a reflection of underlying disease. It is rather an expression of individual heredity or eating patterns, or a combination of both. Treatment for the condition is the opposite of the treatment for overweight. The achievement of a positive caloric balance comes first; more calories have to be consumed each day than are expended. An underweight person should record his food history over a two-week period in the manner described for an overweight one. Once this has been done, various adjustments can be made.

First of all, he should see that he eats at least three meals a day and that they are eaten in a leisurely way and in a relaxed frame of mind. All of the basic foods should be represented in the daily food intake, with special emphasis on protein and complex carbohydrates. The daily caloric intake should then be gradually increased at each meal and snacks added, so long as the snacks don't reduce the appetite at mealtimes.

Carbohydrate foods are the best ones to emphasize in adding calories. Since the extra food intake may cause a certain amount of discomfort, encouragement and support from family and friends can be extremely helpful. Just as there may be psychological blocks against losing weight, there may well be a complicated underlying resistance to adding it.

Anyone trying to gain weight should remain or become reasonably active physically. Adding a pound or two a month for an adult—and a little more than that for a growing youngster—is an achievable goal until the desired weight is reached. There will probably have to be some adjustments in eating and exercise patterns so that a state of caloric balance is achieved.

How Food Relates to Disease

Just as proper food is essential in the prevention of some diseases, it is helpful in the treatment of others. It also plays an important role in protecting and fortifying the general health of a patient while a specific illness is being treated.

The components of therapeutic diets are usually prescribed by the physician in charge, but some general principles will be presented here. Remember that diets designed to treat a given disease must supply the patient's basic nutritional requirements.

Ulcers

Special diet is a major treatment consideration in the case of peptic ulcer, whether located in the stomach (gastric) or in the small intestine (duodenal). A major aim of such a diet is the neutralizing of the acidity of gastric juices by the frequent intake of high protein foods such as milk and eggs. Foods which irritate an ulcer chemically, such as excessive sweets, spices, or salt, or mechanically, such as foods with sharp seeds or tough skins, and foods that are too hot or too cold, should be avoided. It is also advisable to eliminate gravies, coffee, strong tea, carbonated beverages, and alcohol, since all of these stimulate gastric secretion. Such a diet is called a *bland* diet. A soft diet is recommended for some forms of gastrointestinal distress and for those people who have difficulty chewing. It is often combined with the bland diet recommended for peptic ulcer patients to reduce the likelihood of irritation. See Ch. 11, *Diseases of the Digestive System,* for further information about ulcers.

Diabetes

As the section on diabetes mellitus indicates (see Ch. 15), the major objectives of the special diet are weight control, control of the abnormal carbohydrate metabolism, and as far as possible, psychological adjustment by the patient to his individual circumstances. To some extent, he must calculate his diet mathematically. First, his daily caloric needs have to be determined in terms of his activities.

If he is overweight or underweight, the total calories per pound of body weight will have to be adjusted downward or upward by about five calories per pound.

After his total daily caloric needs have been figured out, he can calculate the number of grams of carbohydrate, protein, and fat he should have each day: 58 percent of the calories should come from carbohydrates, 12 percent from protein, and 30 percent from fat. One-fifth of the total should be obtained at breakfast and the rest split between lunch and dinner. Snacks that are taken during the day should be subtracted equally from lunch and dinner.

It is important that meals and planned snacks be eaten regularly and that no food servings be added or omitted. Growing children from 1 to 20 years of age who have diabetes will require considerably more daily calories. A rough estimate is 1,000 calories for a one-year-old child and 100 additional calories for each year of age.

Salt-Free Diets

There are a number of chronic diseases which are treated in part by restricting the amount of sodium in the diet. These diseases, which are associated with fluid retention in the body, include congestive heart failure, certain types of kidney and liver diseases, and hypertension or high blood pressure.

The restriction of sodium intake helps to reduce or avoid the problem of fluid retention. The normal daily diet contains about seven or more grams of sodium, most of it in the form of sodium chloride or table salt. This amount is either inherent in the food or added during processing, cooking, or at mealtime. Half the weight of salt is sodium.

For people whose physical condition requires only a small restriction of the normal sodium intake, simply not salting food at the table is a sufficient reduction. They may decide to use a salt substitute, but before doing so should discuss the question with their physician.

A greater sodium restriction, for example, to no more than 5 grams a day, requires the avoidance of such high salt content foods as ham, bacon, crackers, catsup, and potato chips, as well as almost entirely eliminating salt in the preparation and serving of meals. Severe restriction—1 gram or less a day—involves special food selection and cooking procedures, as well as the use of distilled water if the local water has more than 20 milligrams of sodium per quart. In restricting sodium to this extent, it is important to make sure that protein and vitamins are not reduced below the minimum daily requirements. See "Sodium Restricted Diets."

Sodium Restricted Diets

Diets Moderately Restricted in Sodium

If only a moderate sodium restriction is necessary, a normal diet *without added salt* may be ordered. Such an order is interpreted to mean that the patient will be offered the regular salted food on the general selective menu with the following exceptions:

1. No salt will be served on the tray.
2. Soups that are salted will be omitted.
3. Cured meats (ham, bacon, sausage, corned beef) and all salted cheeses will be omitted.
4. Catsup, chili sauce, mustard, and other salted sauces will be omitted.
5. Salt-free gravies, sauces, and salad dressings will be substituted for the regular salted items.
6. Salted crackers, potato chips, nuts, pickles, olives, popcorn, and pretzels will be omitted.

This diet contains approximately 3 grams of sodium or 7.5 grams of sodium chloride, depending on the type and quantity of the food chosen.

Other Diseases Requiring Special Diets

There are several other disorders in which diet is an important consideration: all chronic gastrointestinal disorders, such as gallbladder stones, ulcerative colitis, enteritis, and diverticulitis; a variety of hereditary disorders such as phenylketonuria and galactosemia; atherosclerosis, especially when it is associated with elevated blood levels of cholesterol or triglycerides or both; liver disease such as cirrhosis; many of the endocrine diseases; kidney stones; and sometimes certain neurological diseases such as epilepsy. Diet also plays a special role in convalescence from most illnesses and in postsurgical care. A modified fat diet and low fat diet are recommended for some diseases of the liver and gallbladder. A minimal residue diet is recommended for some digestive troubles and before and after gastrointestinal surgery.

Diet and Individual Differences

Most discussions about food and eating tend to suggest that all normal people have identical gastrointestinal and metabolic systems. This is simply not true. There are many individual differences that explain why one man's meat is another man's poison. A person's intolerance for a given food may be caused by a disorder, such as an allergy or an ulcer, and it is possible that many of these intolerances will ultimately be related to enzyme deficiencies or some other biochemical factor.

More subtle are the negative physical reactions to particular foods as a result of psychological conditioning. In most such cases, the choice is between avoiding the food that causes the discomfort or eating it and suffering the consequences. Of course, compulsive overeating can also cause or contribute to discomfort. Practically no one can eat unlimited quantities of anything without having gastrointestinal discomfort or *dyspepsia.*

The establishment of so-called daily minimum food requirements suggests that every day's intake should be carefully balanced. Although this is beneficial, it is by no means necessary. Freedom from such regimentation can certainly be enjoyed during a holiday, or a trip to another country, or on a prolonged visit to relatives with casual food habits.

Sometimes a change in diet is dictated by a cold or an upset stomach or diarrhea. Liquids containing carbohydrates, such as tea with sugar and light soups, should be emphasized in treating a cold, while at the same time solid food intake should be somewhat reduced. In the case of an upset stomach or diarrhea, the discomfort may be eased by not eating or drinking anything at all for a whole day. This form of treatment may be helpful for an adult, but since children with diarrhea can become dehydrated in a day or so, professional advice is indicated when cutting down liquid intake.

Diet and Disease Prevention

More and more, medical specialists agree that diet can be helpful in preventing various diseases. Consensus has become general that a diet low in cholesterol and saturated fats can help prevent cardiovascular disease caused by atherosclerosis. Among the foods that reduce total cholesterol levels are rice bran and oat bran. Other sources of the soluble fiber that decreases blood cholesterol include peas, lentils, barley, and pectin fruits like apples, oranges, pears, and prunes. Also recommended are skinless poultry and fish, lean meat, and low-fat dairy products.

Food-Borne Diseases

There are several ways in which food can be the *cause* of disease, most commonly when it becomes contaminated with a sufficient amount of harmful bacteria, bacterial toxin, viruses, or other poisonous substances. The gastrointestinal diseases typically accompanied by nausea, vomiting, diarrhea, or stomach cramps that are produced in this way are not, strictly speaking, caused by the foods themselves, and are therefore called food-borne diseases.

Most food-borne illnesses are caused by a toxin in food contaminated by staphylococcal or salmonella bacteria. In general, milk, milk products, raw shellfish, and meats are the foods most apt to be contaminated. This is most likely to happen when such foods are left standing at room temperature for too long between the time they are prepared and the time they are eaten. However, food can also become contaminated at many different points in time and at various stages of processing. Standards enforced by federal and local government agencies provide protection for the consumer for foods bought for the home as well as for use in restaurants, although whether the protection is adequate is a matter of dispute.

Food Storage

Food is best protected from contamination when it is stored below 40 degrees Fahrenheit or heated to 145 degrees or more. Cold slows bacterial growth; cooking kills it. Bacteria present in food can double in number every 15 minutes at room temperature.

All food stored in the refrigerator should be covered except ripe fruits and vegetables. Leftover foods cannot be kept indefinitely, nor can frozen foods be stored beyond a certain length of time. Specific information about these time periods for individual items is available from the Agricultural Extension Service in each state.

Commercially processed foods sold in the United States are under government control and generally are safe. However, any food can spoil or become contaminated at any point in time, and the consumer should not buy or serve food whose container (package or can) has been broken, cracked, or appears unusual.

Food Additives

From time to time, concern is expressed about one or another food additive as a hazard to health. Most of these additives are put into foods during processing in order to increase their nutritional value, or to improve their chemical or physical characteristics, such as taste and color. Perhaps as many as 2,000 different substances are used in this way in the United States. Some are natural products such as vanilla, others are chemicals derived from other foods, and a few, like artificial sweeteners, are synthetic. Other additives are referred to as indirect, since they are residues in the food from some stage of growing, processing, or packaging. Although additives are controlled and approved by agencies such as the federal Food and Drug Administration, they continue to be a cause of concern to many people.

Pesticides

The pesticides and fertilizers used in growing fruits and vegetables and the additives given to livestock may pose additional health hazards to humans. The National Academy of Sciences, for example, in 1988 estimated the national risk of cancer from pesticide use alone at as many as 20,000 cases a year.

Although it is not known how much is too much, it only makes sense to try and eliminate as much of the risk as possible. This is fairly easy to do. First of all, eat a wide variety of foods to help minimize your exposure to any one pesticide. Eat what's in season and what's grown locally or domestically. (The right season and less transportation mean less chemicals to ripen and preserve food; food and animals from abroad are subject to different health standards that are hard to regulate and check.) Wash all meat and produce carefully; many toxins are easily removed with soap and water. Peel any fruit or vegetable with a wax coating. (Although it is generally advisable to retain as much of the skin of produce as possible for higher vitamin content, wax coatings hold in toxic residues.) Trim produce.

You may also want to go further in reducing your chances of consumption of added toxins by buying organically grown and raised produce and meat. These foods are not widely available in all areas of the country, and they often cost quite a bit more than foods raised with chemicals, but many people not only feel safer eating these foods, but find them tastier as well. Home gardening without the use of chemical fertilizers and pesticides is another healthful option. Be sure to wash and trim carefully all organic or home-grown vegetables, however, to guard against ingestion of naturally occurring toxins such as fungus.

Psychological Aspects of Food and Meals

Food and meals play an important role in emotional well-being and interpersonal relationships as well as in physical health and appearance.

During Infancy

The infant whose needs are attended to by a loving family develops a general sense of trust and security. The major contribution to his emotional contentment is probably made at mealtimes, and perhaps in a special way if he is breast-fed.

For most infants, food comes to be identified with love, pleasure, protection, and the satisfaction of basic needs. If there is an atmosphere of tension accompanying his feeding times, his digestion can be impaired in such a way as to cause vomiting, fretting, or signs of colic. If the tension and the baby's reaction to it—and inevitably the mother's increasing tension as a consequence—become a chronic condition, the result may be a failure to gain weight normally, and in extreme cases, some degree of mental retardation. Throughout life, good nutrition depends not only on eating properly balanced meals that satisfy the body's physiological requirements, but also on a reasonable degree of contentment and relaxation while eating.

Everybody develops individual emotional reactions and attitudes about food and its role as a result of conditioning during the years of infancy and childhood. These attitudes relate not only to food itself and to mealtimes in general, but also to other aspects of eating, including the muscle activities of sucking, chewing, and swallowing.

If food symbolized contentment during the early years, it probably will have the same role later on. If it was associated with conflict, then it may be associated throughout life with strife and neurotic eating patterns.

During Childhood

For the preschool child, mealtimes should provide the occasion for the development of interpersonal relationships, because they are a daily opportunity for both verbal and nonverbal self-expression. The child who eats with enthusiasm and obvious enjoyment is conveying one message; the one who dawdles, picks at food, and challenges his mother with every mouthful is conveying quite a different one.

Meals can become either positive or negative experiences depending in large part on how the adults in the family set the stage. Communication can be encouraged by relaxed conversation and a reasonably leisurely schedule. It can be discouraged by watching television or reading while eating, by not eating together, or by eating and running.

Reasonably firm attitudes about eating a variety of foods in proper quantities at proper times and avoiding excessive catering to individual whims can also help in the development of wholesome eating patterns.

Those who select and prepare the food can transmit special messages of love and affection by serving favorite dishes, by setting the table attractively, and by creating an atmosphere of grace and good humor. Or they can show displeasure and generate hostility by complaining about all the work involved in feeding everyone, or by constant criticism of table manners, or by bringing up touchy subjects likely to cause arguments at the table.

Diet Fads

There are many fads and fallacies about losing weight. Everyone wants an easy solution; cosmetic and food product manufacturers know this and develop products that play to this desire. Thus we have pills that are supposed to burn fat while we sleep; machines that are supposed to give us a "workout" while we're lying down by electrically stimulating our muscles; plastic suits that we wear while exercising that are supposed to produce dramatic weight loss; and special creams and body scrubbers that are supposed to take away unsightly cellulite.

The truth is that a pill will not burn calories for you, a machine will not do your exercise for you, a plastic suit will only make you lose water, not fat, and the idea that there is a special kind of fat called cellulite is a myth.

Cellulite, in fact, is fat, plain and simple; there are no special varieties. Much of the body's fat is stored directly beneath the skin where there is also a sheath of connective tissue, which tends to compartmentalize the fat cells. The more fat the more this tissue is stretched and the more the fat bulges around and through it, producing cellulite's characteristic dimpled effect. Women tend to have thinner skin and less flexible connective tissue, making them more "prone" to cellulite than men. There is no point in spending money on special creams or brushes; you cannot scrub away excess fat. You have to reduce your intake and burn it through exercise.

Similarly, most diet programs that consist of pills, powders, or foolish eating habits are ineffective and usually harmful. Many of them are addictive and those who benefit from the diet programs often gain back the weight lost once they return to their "normal" eating habits.

One drug often used in diet pills is phenylpropanolamine hydrochloride (PPA). PPA is a decongestant, but it also acts as a stimulant and an appetite suppressant. Its side effects include dry mouth, nausea, insomnia, increased heart rate, and increased blood pressure. When PPA is used at the same time as certain other drugs, the elevation of blood pressure can be dramatic, increasing the risk of stroke. PPA can also aggravate glaucoma and kidney disease.

Benzocaine, an ingredient in diet products such as gums and candies, is a local anesthetic that numbs taste receptors, which may briefly suppress the urge to eat. Benzocaine, however, can cause potentially fatal allergic reactions in some individuals.

Although there is no substitute for regular exercise and eating health-

Fat Content of Some Common Foods

Food	Percentage of calories from fat
Brazil nuts	92
Pecans	90
Avocado	83
Almonds	81
Peanuts	79
Pistachio nuts	77
Sunflower seed kernels, roasted	76
Cheese, American processed	76
Cheese, Cheddar	71
Salami, cooked	71
Mozzarella, whole-milk	68
Ricotta, whole-milk	67
Cheese, Swiss	67
Pork, ground, cooked	64
Mozzarella, part-skim	63
Ground beef, lean, broiled	62
Pot roast, braised	62
Egg	59
Ground beef, extra lean, broiled	58
Ricotta, part-skim	52
Granola	51
Cheese, Swiss, reduced-fat	51
Milk, whole, 3.3% fat	48
Croissant	47
Yogurt, plain, whole-milk	45
Sockeye salmon, baked or broiled	44
Chicken, roasted, dark meat, without skin	41
Milk, low-fat, 2% fat	37
Pork loin, tenderloin, roasted	31
Chicken drumstick, without skin	31
Chicken, roasted, light meat, without skin	28
Milk, low-fat, 1% fat	26
Yogurt, plain, low-fat	25
Halibut, baked or broiled	23
Turkey leg, without skin	20
Chicken breast, without skin	19
Oatmeal, instant	17
Hamburger or hot dog bun	15
Whole wheat bread	13
Cottage cheese, 1% fat	11
Shrimp, steamed, poached, or broiled	11
Corn	10
Milk, skim	<10
Egg noodles	8
Kidney beans, dry	8
Rice, brown	8
English muffin	7
Garbanzo beans (chickpeas), canned, solids and liquid	6
Bagel, plain	5
Spaghetti or macaroni	5
Rice, white	<4
Fruits	0
Green, leafy vegetables	0

Note: The U.S. Government recommends that no more than 30 percent of daily calories come from fat.

fully, obesity, which increases the risk of serious health problems, may be managed with the help of physician-prescribed appetite suppressants. These drugs, such as sibutramine (brand name Meridia), may be used for a short time to achieve a loss of ten percent of body weight, an amount thought to reduce health risks. They are not a substitute for long-term behavioral changes in diet and exercise.

Anybody interested in losing a substantial amount of weight should consult with his or her physician. The physician will know of a nutritionist who can provide a healthy program for weight reduction.

Weight loss involves a complete change in one's lifestyle. The solution includes eating balanced meals, reducing the intake of fat, increasing proportionately the consumption of carbohydrates, and exercising three or four times a week. It is a slow process that does not offer the quick yet temporary loss offered by over-the-counter diet programs. Rather, it is a permanent commitment to a healthy way of life. Only then, can a person maintain an optimal weight.

28

Mental and Emotional Disorders

The ability to adapt is central to being emotionally fit, healthy, and mature. An emotionally fit person is one who can adapt to changing circumstances with constructive reactions and who can enjoy living, loving others, and working productively. In everyone's life there are bound to be experiences that are anxious or deeply disturbing, such as the sadness of losing a loved one or the disappointment of failure. The emotionally fit person is stable enough not to be overwhelmed by the anxiety, grief, or guilt that such experiences frequently produce. His sense of his own worth is not lost easily by a setback in life; rather, he can learn from his own mistakes.

Communication and Tolerance

Even the most unpleasant experiences can add to one's understanding of life. Emerging from a crisis with new wisdom can give a sense of pride and mastery. The emotionally fit person can listen attentively to the opinions of others, yet if his decision differs from that being urged by friends and relatives, he will abide by it and can stand alone if necessary, without guilt and anger at those who disagree.

Communicating well with others is an important part of emotional fitness. Sharing experiences, both good and bad, is one of the joys of living. Although the capacity to enjoy is often increased by such sharing, independence is also essential, for one person's pleasure may leave others indifferent. It is just as important to appreciate and respect the individuality of others as it is to value our own individual preferences, as long as these are reasonable and do not give pain to others.

Ways of Expressing Disagreement

Communication should be kept open at all times. Anger toward those who disagree may be an immediate response, but it should not lead to cutting off communication, as it so frequently does, particularly between husbands and wives, parents and children.

Emotional maturity enables us to disagree with what another says, feels, or does, yet make the distinction between that person and how we feel about his thoughts and actions. To tell someone, "I don't like what you are doing," is more likely to keep the lines of communication open than telling him "I don't like you." This is particularly important between parents and children.

It is unfortunately common for parents to launch personal attacks when children do something that displeases them. The child, or any person to whom this is done, then feels unworthy or rejected, which often makes him angry and defiant. Revenge becomes uppermost, and communication is lost; each party feels misunderstood and lonely, perhaps even wounded, and is not likely to want to reopen communication. The joy in a human relationship is gone, and one's pleasure in living is by that much diminished.

Function of Guilt

The same principles used in dealing with others can be applied to ourselves. Everyone makes mistakes, has angry or even murderous thoughts that can produce excessive guilt. Sometimes there is a realistic reason for feeling guilty, which should be a spur to take corrective action. Differentiate clearly between thoughts, feelings, and actions. Only actions need cause guilt. In the privacy of one's own mind, anything may be thought as long as it is not acted out; an emotionally fit person can accept this difference.

Understanding Mental and Emotional Disorders

As recently as 200 years ago it was believed that the emotionally ill were evil, possessed by the devil. Their illness was punished rather than treated. The strange and sometimes bizarre actions of the mentally ill were feared and misunderstood.

Beginning in the late 1800's, Sigmund Freud made significant steps toward understanding mental functions. Since then, a number of physicians, psychologists, and scholars have made major contributions to the area of mental health.

Today, mental disorders are viewed and evaluated in the same way as physical diseases. Many are treatable using techniques similar to those used for physical diseases.

Mental Retardation

According to the American Association on Mental Retardation (AAMR) and the Diagnostic and Statistical Manual of Mental Disorders, 4th edition (DSM-IV), the diagnosis of mental retardation is appropriate when intellectual functioning is significantly below average, adaptive skills are limited, and the onset of the retardation occurs before the age of 18.

The term "mental retardation," while still valid diagnostically, is no longer the favored term in common usage. Instead the term "developmental disability" is widely used to refer to both mental retardation and to any other condition that results from a congenital abnormality, trauma, disease or deprivation that interrupts or delays normal growth and development.

The most common identifiable form of mental retardation is Down Syndrome. Physical characteristics include slanting eyes, slightly protruding lips and tongue, small hands and feet, and a short trunk. Compared to the general population, individuals with Down Syndrome are more likely to have congenital cardiac abnormalities, digestive tract problems, and cervical vertebrae problems. They are also more likely to develop upper respiratory infections, leukemia, or Alzheimer's Disease.

Other causes of mental retardation include hydrocephalus, an accumulation of fluid within the skull that destroys brain tissue; fragile X syndrome, a chromosomal abnormality resulting in moderate to severe retardation; phenylketonuria (PKU), the inability of a child's body to metabolize a certain kind of protein substance; Tay Sachs disease, an inherited disease that causes the progressive destruction of the central nervous system. Individuals with Tay Sachs disease appear to develop normally until about six months of age, when progressive deterioration of the infant's mental and motor skills begins. Most children who have the disease die from it before they are five years of age. Mental retardation from PKU can be prevented if the metabolic deficiency is detected within a few days after birth and treated with a special diet.

If a mother becomes infected with Rubella (German Measles) during her pregnancy, there is a chance her infant will be born with disabilities, including mental retardation. If a woman consumes alcohol during her pregnancy, there is a chance that her child will be born with Fetal Alcohol Syndrome (FAS). Characteristics of

FAS include mental and growth retardation, poor motor coordination, learning disabilities, and hyperactivity.

Early Intervention

An early intervention program is a very important part of the developmentally disabled child's life. It is an organized program of services necessary to prevent and/or minimize the effects of disability on young children with special needs. Programs are offered for children up to the age of 5 and may include speech, occupational and physical therapy, and medical care. Sometimes, eary intervention programming is all that a child needs, and thereafter they enter regular schooling with little or no need for further intervention.

Effects on the Family

When a member of a family is diagnosed with a developmental disability, the entire family is affected. Depending upon the extent of the disability, the family members usually must rearrange their lives based upon the needs of the developmentally disabled child. Families must choose between trying to care for the child at home, or finding suitable placement in the community. They must arrange for any medical care and therapy their child might need. They must also manage the financial obligations that result from their child's needs, which can be considerable.

There are many organizations devoted to providing services and support to individuals with developmental disablilites and their families. The Arc of the United States has many state and local chapters, and can provide families with information regarding the services available in their community. To find the Arc chapter nearest to you, contact the national Arc office.

The Arc of the United States
1010 Wayne Avenue, Suite 650
Silver Spring, MD 20910
(301) 565-3842

Mental Illness

Most people occasionally experience spells of anxiety, blue moods, or temper tantrums, but unless the psychological suffering they endure or inflict upon others begins to interfere with their job or marriage, they seldom seek professional guidance. There is no exacting scientific standard for determining when an eccentric pattern of behavior becomes a mental illness. Norms vary from culture to culture and within each culture. Norms also change from generation to generation.

Just how can a determination be made as to who is mentally ill? No temperature reading, no acute pain, no abnormal growth can be looked for as evidence of a serious problem. Yet there are warning signs, and among the common ones are these:

- Anxiety that is severe, prolonged, and unrelated to any identifiable reason or cause
- Depression, especially when it is followed by withdrawal from loved ones, from friends, or from the usual occupations or hobbies that ordinarily afford one pleasure
- Loss of confidence in oneself
- Undue pessimism
- A feeling of constant helplessness
- Uncalled for or unexplainable mood changes.
- Rudeness or aggression that is without apparent cause or which is occasioned by some trivial incident
- An unreasonable demand for perfectionism, not only in oneself but in one's loved ones, friends, business associates, and even from things or situations
- Habitual underachievement, especially if one is adequately equipped to do the work one is called upon to perform
- The inability to accept responsibility, often manifested by a recurrent loss of employment
- Phobias
- Unreasonable feelings of persecution
- Self-destructive acts
- Sexual deviation
- A sudden and dramatic change in sleeping habits
- Physical ailments and complaints for which there are no organic causes

If one or more of these warning signs occur frequently or in severe form, a mental illness may be present, and professional help should be sought to evaluate the underlying problem.

Types of Mental Illness

The following discussion of classifications and types of mental illnesses is based on criteria compiled by the American Psychiatric Association in the *Diagnostic and Statistical Manual of Mental Disorders.*

Anxiety Disorders

Anxiety disorders are the most common emotional disorders. They are characterized by chronic feelings of uneasiness. The symptoms of an anxiety disorder are more persistent and intense than the typical feelings of nervousness or anxiety everyone feels at various times. In addition, the symptoms typically occur for no clear reason and do not go away.

There are several types of anxiety orders. Symptoms of these disorders range from a mild, chronic sense of worry, to an overwhelming emotional condition, accompanied by such physical reactions as muscle tension, racing heart, nausea, and an increase in perspiration and blood pressure.

Panic Disorder

A person with *panic disorder* has recurrent attacks of intense apprehension, fear, or terror. Panic attacks may occur unexpectedly and seemingly without reason. This unpredictability tends to further intensify the feelings of fearfulness and terror.

Agoraphobia

A person with an anxiety of any place or situation from which a quick departure would be difficult or embarrassing may suffer from *agoraphobia*. The anxiety of agoraphobia is so severe that it can result in the outright avoidance of certain places or situations. Agoraphobia and panic disorder often occur together. People suffering from both have a fear of being in a place or situation in which they would not be able to get help if they had a panic attack.

Specific Phobias

A person with a *specific phobia* has an extreme or excessive fear of an object or situation that, under general conditions, is not harmful. The phobia often leads to avoidance of the object or situation altogether. People with specific phobias tend to realize that their reactions are irrational, but still are unable to overcome their fear without professional intervention. Common specific phobias include a fear of heights (acrophobia), a fear of flying (aerophobia), a fear of spiders (arachnophobia), a fear of confined spaces (claustrophobia), a fear of blood (hemophobia), and a fear of strangers (xenophobia).

Social Phobia

Also called *social anxiety disorder*, a *social phobia* is the fear of behaving in a way that could lead to public embarrassment or ridicule in specific social situations. A person with this phobia often avoids the problematic social situation altogether. Common social phobias include a fear of public speaking, a fear of using public restrooms, and a fear of meeting new people.

Obsessive-Compulsive Disorder

A person with *obsessive-compulsive disorder* experiences recurrent obsessions and recurrent compulsions. Obsessions are frequently occurring thoughts that usually reflect exaggerated anxiety or fears that have no foundation in reality. Although people with obsessions realize that their thoughts are irrational, this realization is not enough to alleviate their anxiety. Instead, they engage in repetitive rituals, or compulsions, to get rid of the obsessive thoughts and thereby reduce their anxiety. Compulsive behaviors can sometimes take up more than an hour a day, and can interfere with normal daily activities and social relationships.

Common obsessions, and the compulsions which result from them, include: a preoccupation with dirt or germs, resulting in repeated hand washing and the performing of excessive housekeeping chores; second-guessing previous actions, resulting in constant checking and rechecking to satisfy doubts; a need to have items in a very specific arrangement, resulting in strict regimens to ensure order and consistency.

Post-Traumatic Stress Disorder

Post-traumatic stress disorder is characterized by the repeated experiencing or "reliving" of a traumatic event, accompanied by extreme emotional, mental, and physical distress when exposed to situations reminiscent of the trauma. People with post-traumatic stress disorder repeatedly experience their ordeal through recurrent nightmares, memories of the event, and vivid flashbacks, which may make the person feel as if they were reliving the original event. Typical events which can result in post-traumatic stress disorder include: military combat, natural disasters, violent crime, and childhood abuse.

Acute Stress Disorder

Similar to post-traumatic stress disorder, *acute stress disorder* differs from it in duration. Whereas post-traumatic stress disorder lasts more than a month, acute stress disorder lasts a month or less; it occurs within a month after exposure to a traumatic event.

Generalized Anxiety Disorder

Generalized anxiety disorder is characterized by chronic and overwhelming anxiety that lasts for at least six months. People with this disorder experience such persistent worry and tension that it interferes with their daily lives. Symptoms of generalized anxiety disorder include: excessive concerns (about health, family, career, or finances) even when there is no apparent reason for such concern, inability to relax, tremors, insomnia, irritability, difficulty concentrating, fatigue, and headaches.

Substance-Induced Anxiety Disorder

In a *substance-induced anxiety disorder*, symptoms of anxiety are present because of drug abuse, the use of medication, or exposure to a toxin.

Mood Disorders

The predominant feature of these disorders is a serious disturbance in mood. Mood disorders can be caused by biological factors, drug abuse, use of medication, toxic substances, or various medical conditions—including thyroid disorders and Parkinson's disease. Some people have a genetic predisposition to developing mood disorders. The development and intensity of a mood disorder can also be affected by the personality of the individual. There are two types of mood disorders: ***depressive*** and ***bipolar.***

Depressive Disorders

In a ***major depressive disorder***, a person has strong feelings of depression for at least two weeks. The depression may have melancholic features—that is, there may be a loss of interest or pleasure in virtually all activities.

In a *dysthymic disorder*, a depressed mood exists for at least 2 years. This disorder is characterized by a moderate, lingering depression, in contrast to the more intense depression characteristic of a major depressive disorder.

Other symptoms of depressive disorders include periods of prolonged sadness, changes in appetite and sleep patterns, anger, anxiety, loss of energy, feelings of worthlessness, and recurring thoughts of death or suicide.

Bipolar Disorders

There are several variations of *bipolar disorders,* formerly known as *manic-depression.* These disorders are characterized by episodes of deep depression alternating with periods of extreme elation, or manic behavior. Examples of manic behavior include the need for less sleep without feeling tired, an increase in mental and physical activity, and exaggerated enthusiasm and feelings of self-worth. A person with a bipolar disorder might take unnecessary chances and engage in risky behavior.

Schizophrenia and Other Psychotic Disorders

The defining features of these disorders are psychotic symptoms, which include a loss of contact with reality, a disorganized thought process, hallucinations, and delusions.

A disorganized thought process is reflected by a person's actions and speech. The person may behave in a bizarre manner and not be able to give a coherent explanation for his or her actions. The person's speech will not make much sense to the average person.

Hallucinations are sensations that do not result from a "real" or external stimulus, although the person experiencing the hallucination might believe otherwise. They can occur with any of the five senses, but the most common are auditory hallucinations, particularly those of hearing voices.

Delusions are erroneous beliefs that usually involve a misinterpretation of experiences. One example of a delusion is the belief of being under surveillance by the police, although in actuality no surveillance is being made. A more extreme example of a delusion is the belief of certain people that their thoughts are under the control of or are being taken away by unknown entities. *Persecutory delusions*—delusions of being harassed, spied on, or tormented—are the most common type.

Schizophrenia

Schizophrenia is one of the most debilitating and puzzling mental illnesses. Symptoms may include not only psychotic symptoms—disorganized thought process, hallucinations, and delusions—but also withdrawal, social isolation, lack of emotional expression, and a decrease in normal thinking and speaking activity. Schizophrenia varies in severity from person to person, and, in a given individual, from one time to another.

Most mental health professionals agree that schizophrenia is a biological illness, and that it probably occurs in individuals with a genetic susceptibility to the illness who have been exposed to other factors. These factors include such prenatal problems as exposure to influenza or lack of nutrition while the individual was growing in the mother's womb. For someone with schizophrenia, stressful social and family interactions may affect the progression of the disease, but are they not the origin.

Contrary to popular belief, a schizophrenic does not have a "split personality." This notion probably developed from the fact that episodes of the illness may be separated by periods of normal behavior.

There are several types of schizophrenia, with behavior ranging from excitement and aggressiveness to withdrawal and immobility.

People with *paranoid schizophrenia* have strong feelings of persecution. They typically feel that someone (or a group of people) is plotting to harm or kill them.

People with *disorganized schizophrenia,* historically known as *hebephrenic schizophrenia,* experience such strong speech and behavior disorganization that their ability to perform daily activities is disrupted.

In *catatonic schizophrenia,* a person is usually in a state of extreme withdrawal and immobility. This may alternate with occasional periods of extreme agitation or excitement.

People with *residual schizophrenia* exhibit the absence of normal behaviors. For example, they may withdraw, lack emotional expression, isolate themselves from society, and experience a decrease in thinking and speaking activity.

In *undifferentiated schizophrenia,* a person exhibits a variety of schizophrenic symptoms, but none of them is dominant.

Psychotic Disorders

Other disorders included in the category of Schizophrenia and Psychotic Disorders follow, along with some defining features of each disorder.

Both *brief psychotic disorder* and *schizophreniform disorder* have the same symptoms as schizophrenia, but the symptoms do not last long enough to warrant a diagnosis of schizophrenia. In brief psychotic disorder, the symptoms last more than a day, but less than one month. In schizophreniform disorder, the symptoms last from one to six months.

In *schizoaffective disorder,* a person displays symptoms of a mood disorder—either bipolar or depressive—in addition to psychotic symptoms.

In a *delusional disorder,* a person experiences one or more delusions based on situations that could conceivably be happening to the person, but for which there is no evidence. The delusions must persist for at least one month in order to be classified as a delusional disorder.

In a *shared psychotic disorder,* a person is influenced by someone else who already has a similar delusion.

In a *substance-induced psychotic disorder,* the psychotic symptoms present are the result of drug abuse, the use of medication, or exposure to a toxin.

Personality Disorders

These disorders are characterized by a persistent pattern of noticeably unusual behavior and ways of thinking.

A *paranoid personality disorder* is characterized by a pattern of suspicion and distrust. A person with this disorder will misconstrue other people's intentions as being malicious.

A *schizoid personality disorder* is characterized by a pattern of disinterest in social relationships. A person with this disorder may be fearful of close interaction with others. They also have a limited range of emotional expression.

People with *schizotypal personality disorder* are socially and emotionally distant. Their thinking process is odd and distorted, and these oddities are evident through their speech and behavior.

An *antisocial personality disorder* is characterized by a pattern of disregarding and violating the rights of others. People with this disorder typically do not feel remorse or guilt after inflicting harm upon others. This disorder usually develops in adolescence and often continues into adulthood, although the severity of the disorder can diminish as a person ages.

A *borderline personality disorder* is characterized by a pattern of instability in relationships. A person with this disorder also displays symptoms of impulsiveness and irritability.

In *histrionic personalty disorder,* there is a pattern of attention-seeking behavior and excessive displays of emotion. A person with this disorder may easily fall under the influence of others in an effort to be the center of attention.

A *narcissistic personality disorder* is characterized by an exaggerated sense of self-importance. A person with this disorder requires excessive admiration and lacks empathy for others.

An *avoidant personality disorder* is characterized by feelings of inadequacy. A person with this disorder will avoid activities that require significant interpersonal interaction, and tends to be hypersensitive to negative evaluation.

A *dependent personality disorder* is characterized by an excessive need to be taken care of. A person with this disorder has a pattern of submissive and clinging behavior.

An *obsessive-compulsive personality disorder* is characterized by a preoccupation with orderliness, perfectionism, and control. A person with this disorder will appear inflexible and stubborn to others.

Dissociative Disorders

In these disorders, there is a disruption in consciousness, memory, identity, or perception. The disruption may occur suddenly, or it may gradually develop. It can also take the form of a brief affliction or a chronic condition.

A person with *dissociative amnesia* is unable to recall relevant personal information. The "forgotten" information is usually disturbing to the individual, and of a traumatic nature. For example, a person who attempts to commit suicide might not later remember anything at all regarding the incident.

A *dissociative fugue* is characterized by a sudden loss of personal identity and of the memory of one's past life. This is accompanied by the tendency to suddenly wander far from one's home or place of work. In some cases, the individual also assumes a new identity. The disorder can last from a couple of hours to several months. A dissociative fugue is usually brought on by traumatic events or an overwhelming accumulation of tension and stress. It is a rare disorder.

Dissociative identity disorder, formerly called *multiple personality disorder,* refers to the presence of two or more distinct personalities, each of which dominate an individual's behavior at different times. This disorder is also characterized by gaps in the individual's memory that vary, depending on which personality is currently dominant. For example, a weaker personality may not remember what happens during the times that a stronger personality is dominating the individual's behavior.

Depersonalization disorder is characterized by persistent feelings of detachment from one's own body or thoughts. The feelings of depersonalization can be severe and occur often enough that one's life is disrupted, and treatment is needed. In many cases, though, the sense of depersonalization is brief and minimal, and treatment is not needed.

Factitious Disorder

This disorder is characterized by physical or psychological symptoms that are deliberately produced or feigned in order to appear sick. People with this disorder might inflict harm upon themselves, exaggerate an existing medical complaint, or completely fabricate a new and false medical problem, for the sole purpose of appearing ill.

Somatoform Disorders

In these disorders, a person has physical symptoms of a physical disease, but does not have the disease. The physical symptoms are caused by psychological factors and are not intentionally produced by the individual. Examples of physical symptoms common in somatoform disorders include blindness, paralysis, respiratory distress, and heart problems.

A person with a *somatization disorder* has recurrent and multiple physical complaints and symptoms for which there is no known medical cause. There is evidence, or a strong presumption, that the symptoms are related to psychological reasons. Symptoms vary from person to person and also depend upon their underlying emotional conflict.

A person with a *conversion disorder* experiences emotional distress that is "converted" into physical symptoms. The physical symptoms have no biological cause, and are not a part of a somatization disorder. A person who witnesses a terrifying event and then develops blindness would be an extreme example of this disorder.

Hypochondriasis is the preoccupation with the fear of acquiring or the belief of having a serious disease. A person reaches this conclusion by overreacting to normal bodily functions and minor abnormalities. People with hypochondriasis will persist in their fears and beliefs despite medical tests and exams that prove that they do not have a serious disease.

A person with *body dysmorphic disorder* is preoccupied with an imagined or insignificant defect in one's own appearance.

Sexual and Gender Identity Disorders

These disorders involve sexual performance, sexual deviance, and concepts of appropriate gender roles. They include the categories of sexual dysfunctions, paraphilias, and gender identity disorders.

Sexual dysfunctions refer to changes in personal sexual desires and activities that the individual finds unfulfilling, or inadequate. Examples of sexual dysfuntions include pain during sexual activity and complications with sexual arousal and desire.

Persistent and intense sexual urges or behaviors that involve unusual objects or situations are called *paraphilias.* Examples of paraphilias include exhibitionism (exposing one's self), voyeurism (observing sexual activity), sadism (inflicting pain or humiliation), and masochism (receiving pain or humiliation).

A *gender identity disorder* is characterized by intense, persistent feelings of discomfort or inappropriateness with one's own gender, in addition to a strong identification with the opposite gender. People with gender identity disorders may engage in cross-dressing, hormone treatment, or surgery to acquire the physical appearance of the opposite sex.

Other Disorders

Several other types of disorders are discussed elsewhere in this encyclopedia. These disorders include:

Eating Disorders. See Chapter 3, *The Teens,* subtitles Anorexia Nervosa, and Bulimia.

Disorders Usually First Diagnosed in Infancy, Childhood, or Adolescence. See Chapter 2, *The First Dozen Years,* subtitles Autism, Brain Damage, Developmental Disability, Dyslexia, Hyperactivity, Learning Disability, Mental Illness, Mental Retardation, Pica, Speech Impediments, and Stuttering. Chapter 28, *Mental and Emotional Disorders,* subtitle Mental Retardation.

Sleep Disorders. See Chapter 2, *The First Dozen Years,* subtitles Dreams and Nightmares, Sleepwalking. Chapter 37, *Encyclopedic Guide to the Body, Health and Medicine,* subtitles Narcolepsy, Sleep, Sleep Apnea, Snoring. Chapter 5, *The Middle Years,* subtitle Rest and Sleep.

Treatment of Emotional Problems and Mental Disorders

When should help be sought for an emotional problem? Sometimes individuals themselves realize that they need help and seek it without urging. They may have symptoms such as anxiety, depression, or troublesome thoughts that they cannot put out of their mind. But many others who need help do not know it or do not want to know that they need it. They usually have symptoms that disturb others rather than themselves, such as irritability, impulsive behavior, or excessive use of drugs or alcohol that interferes with their family relationships and work responsibilities.

Other people in need of psychological guidance are those who have a physical disease that is based on psychological factors. They react to stress internally rather than externally. Instead of displaying anger, they feel it inside. We are all familiar with headaches or heartburn caused by tension.

The symptoms of many mental disorders seem only to be exaggerations of feelings and behavior found in "normal" people. At what point should help be sought for a problem? Generally, help should be sought when the problem begins to significantly and negatively impact the individual's life.

In all of the above situations, the individual's enjoyment of life is curtailed. He has no feeling of control over what he does and little or no tolerance for himself and others. Such an existence is completely unnecessary today, with the many agencies and specialists, capable of effectively treating these problems.

Mental Health Professionals

Who can help those with emotional problems? Confusion about the different professions in the mental health field is understandable. To add to the muddle, self-appointed counselors without professional training and experience have set themselves up in this field, so it is necessary to know whom to consult to obtain the best help possible. Every mental health professional you consult should be licensed, accredited, or associated with recognized groups of their peers.

Psychiatrists

Psychiatrists are medical doctors; that is, they have graduated from a medical school, served internships and afterwards residencies specializing in emotional disorders. They are specialists in the same way that a surgeon or an eye doctor is a specialist. Most are members of the American Psychiatric Association. They are experienced in treating medical illnesses, having done so for many years before being certified as specialists in emotional disorders.

The American Psychiatric Association, 1000 Wilson Blvd., Suite 1825, Arlington, VA 22209, can supply the names of members. The American Board of Psychiatry and Neurology, 500 Lake-Cook Road, Suite 335, Deerfield, IL 60015, examines and certifies psychiatrists who pass its tests. If a family physician is consulted about an emotional problem, he will often refer the patient to a psychiatrist, just as he would to any other specialist.

Psychologists

Psychologists have at least a master's degree in psychology; most psychologists have a doctoral degree. Like a psychiatrist, a psychologist can help you cope with many of life's problems. Unlike a psychiatrist, though, a psychologist is not a medical doctor and cannot prescribe medicine.

The American Psychological Association (APA), 750 First Street, NE, Washington, DC 20002, is the world's largest association of psychologists. They operate a telephone referral service. To find a psychologist in your area, call (800) 964-2000.

Pyschotherapists

Psychotherapy is the general term for any treatment that tries to effect a cure by psychological rather than physical means. A psychotherapist may be a psychiatrist, or he may be a psychologist, or may have no training at all. Anyone can set up an office and call himself a psychotherapist, psychoanalyst, marriage counselor, family therapist, or anything else he desires. It is up to the patient to check on the training and background of a therapist. Any reputable therapist should be pleased to tell patients his credentials and qualifications for helping them.

Social Workers

Social workers are another group of trained persons who may also counsel those with emotional problems. They may work either with individuals, families, or groups after meeting the educational requirements for the profession, which include a bachelor's degree and two years of professional training leading to a master's degree in social work.

Types of Therapy

Emotional problems and mental illnesses can be treated in a variety of ways, including psychotherapy, medication, or physical treatments. Psychotherapy, or "talking therapy," is an effective and commonly prescribed method of treatment for mild to moderate cases of emotional and mental disorders. In more severe cases, psychotherapy is used in combination with medication or physical treatments.

Psychotherapy

As noted above, psychotherapy applies to various forms of treatment that employ psychological methods designed to help people understand themselves. With this knowledge, or insight, a person learns how to handle life—with all its relationships and conflicts—in a happier and more socially responsible manner.

The best known form of psychotherapy is *psychoanalysis,* developed by Freud but modified by many others, which seeks to lift to the level of awareness the individual's repressed subconscious feelings. The information about subconscious conflicts is explored and interpreted to explain the causes of the individual's emotional upsets.

Another form of psychotherapy is *behavior therapy,* treatment based on the belief that many types of behavior are learned. Instead of probing an individual's unconscious, as in psychoanalysis, a behavior therapist focuses on the individual's observable behavior and tries to help the individual control it. In a method called *operant conditioning,* behavior is controlled using a *reinforcer,* anything that increases the likelihood that a particular behavior will be repeated. Praise or gifts given for good behavior are common examples of reinforcers.

Cognitive therapy is another form of psychotherapy. Unlike behavior therapy, cognitive therapy is based on changing thoughts. Cognitive therapy involves helping people change the patterns of thinking responsible for their emotional distress. The change is made by monitoring negative or distorted thoughts, then correcting or replacing them with positive thoughts.

Group therapy is a form of psychotherapy treatment in which a group of people, usually ten or fewer, discuss their mental and emotional problems. The group is under the guidance of a psychiatrist or clinical psychologist. By talking to one another about mutual problems and by interacting with one another emotionally under skillful guidance, people are often helped more quickly than when treated individually.

Psychodrama is a therapeutic technique in which an individual or members of a group create and act out situations based on their personal conflicts.

Play therapy is a type of treatment for young children who can more easily act out their problems through play activity, as opposed to discussing them. Play therapy may be a form of individual psychotherapy or group therapy. In both instances, the therapist observes the play activity.

Family problems can be treated with *family therapy.* Family members are sometimes able to discuss their problems of relating to each other within the context of a group better than they can on an individual basis with a therapist.

Medication

In the last half of the 20th century, the study of the relationship between biochemical processes of the brain and mental illness resulted in the development of psychiatric medication. Many people with mental illnesses have greatly benefitted from the use of these medications. However, many psychiatric drugs have side effects, some of which are severe, so close medical supervision is necessary while taking the drugs. With proper monitoring, psychiatric drugs can be a part of a safe, therapeutic approach to alleviating the negative effects of mental illness.

Depression is believed to be caused by low levels of *neurotransmitters,* chemicals of the nervous system. *Antidepressant drugs,* used to relieve the symptoms of depression, work by increasing the level of neurotransmitters present in the brain.

Antipsychotic drugs, sometimes called major tranquilizers, are used to relieve delusions, hallucinations and other psychotic symptoms. Antipsychotic drugs work by blocking the neurotransmitter *dopamine* from completing its function in the brain.

Antianxiety drugs, sometimes called sedatives or minor tranquilizers, are used to relieve anxiety or tension. By suppressing the brain chemistry responsible for anxiety, these drugs provide a sense of relaxation. They may also act as a muscle relaxant, and alleviate mild insomnia.

Mood stabilizers, like lithium, are used to treat bipolar depression. It is not known how lithium alleviates the symptoms of bipolar disorder, but it is effective. The blood level of lithium must be monitored carefully. If the level is too low, the medication will not be effective in stabilizing the person's mood, and if the level is too high, adverse side effects may result.

Physical Treatment

Electroconvulsive therapy (ECT) is a form of therapy in which regulated electric shocks are delivered to the brain to induce seizures. It is an effective treatment for severe depression, often providing relief much more quickly than psychiatric medication. Although psychiatric medication and psychotherapy are used much more frequently as treatments for depression, ECT is generally used in life-threatening situations or other circumstances where immediate relief from depression is needed.

Psychosurgery is another form of physical treatment. It involves physically altering the structure of the brain in an attempt to alleviate severe mental illness. Psychosurgery was widely used in 1950's. The use of psychosurgery has greatly diminished with increased knowledge of psychiatric illness and with the development of psychiatric drugs. Current pyschosurgery methods involve only microscopic alterations to the brain, and are only used in extreme cases of mental illness with a definite biological cause.

Options Available for the Mentally Ill

The last two decades have seen a number of changes in the facilities for treatment of mental disorders in the United States. The great majority of severely ill mental patients used to be cared for in county or state mental hospitals, many of which were crowded and able to offer custodial care but very little in the way of therapeutic programs. The picture has changed, however, and the extent and quality of care in these hospitals is expanding and improving. Also, other facilities now offer treatment for mental illnesses, including general hospitals, private psychiatric hospitals, mental heath clinics, and various social agencies.

Results of Treatment

There will always be things in life that are disappointing or otherwise upsetting. No treatment can eliminate such problems. After successful treatment, however, one should be better able to handle these stresses with flexible and constructive responses and to see individual difficulties in relation to the problems of others.

To feel emotionally fit is to have a capacity for enjoying life, working well, and loving others. Fear, shame, and guilt about undergoing needed treatment should not prevent anyone from reaching that potential.

29

Substance Abuse

Drug-Related Deaths up 59%." "Driving-and-Drinking Accident Claims 5 Lives." "Teen Drug Abuse—The News Is Bad."

The headlines tell a story with a moral, or lesson. The lesson is that the United States has a major health and social problem. Once called by a number of names, including *alcoholism, drug addiction,* and *drug abuse,* the problem today goes by the designation *substance abuse.* In this usage, the phrase applies to all forms of addiction or abuse, whether the substance is alcohol or such vegetation-derived drugs as marijuana, cocaine, and heroin.

In a broad sense, substances include any material aside from food that can be imbibed, injected, or taken into the body in any way and that changes or affects the body or mind. This definition covers aspirin, many medications, tobacco, and a broad range of other substances. But *substance abuse* refers to unhealthy or excessive use of any material, alcohol, or addictive drugs at an individual's discretion and not according to a physician's prescription.

The dimensions of the substance-abuse problem are almost incalculable. Americans in 1986 spent an estimated $110 billion on addictive drugs alone. At least 40 percent of all Americans between the ages of 18 and 25 had experimented with one or more illegal substances. As one authority wrote,

> Not only the poor, the uneducated, the deprived, or the shadow types are being destroyed. We're dealing with the privileged, the successful, the professional.

Alcohol Abuse

Alcohol abuse is not unique to the United States or to the twentieth century. Alcoholic beverages, and their use or abuse, have an ancient history. Long before humans began to keep records of any kind, these beverages were valued as food, medicine, and ceremonial drinks. When people today have a beer with dinner, or toast newlyweds with champagne, or share wine at a religious ritual or festival, they are continuing traditions that have deep roots in the past.

The consumption of alcoholic beverages has always been a fact of life. So, in a sense, has alcohol abuse. The immigrants who came to the United States brought their ethnic ceremonies and drinking habits with them. The frontiersmen who moved continually west found liquor to be a source of release and comfort. Inevitably, alcohol use and abuse occurred.

Most drinkers are able to control what they are doing when they drink and are none the worse for the habit. However, of the estimated 113 million drinkers in the United States, about 14 million have some kind of problem with alcohol: they are *alcohol abusers.* Drug and alcohol abuse is estimated to cost the economy some $240 billion annually. Drunken drivers are implicated in about 40 percent of the 40,000 traffic deaths occurring yearly.

Scientists have come to believe that habitual alcohol abuse is a disease and should be treated as such. In 1956, the American Medical Association officially termed alcoholism an illness and a medical concern.

Kinds of Alcohol

The alcohol in beverages is chemically known as *ethyl alcohol.* It is often called *grain alcohol.* Ethyl alcohol is produced by the natural process of *fermentation:* When certain foods such as honey, fruits, grains, or their juices remain in a warm place, airborne yeast organisms begin to change the sugars and starches in these foods into alcohol. Ethyl alcohol is in itself a food in the sense that its caloric content produces energy in the body, but it contains practically no essential nutriments.

Methyl alcohol, also called wood alcohol, because it is obtained by the dry distillation of maple, birch, and beech, is useful as a fuel and solvent. It is poisonous if ingested and can cause blindness and death. Other members of the same family of chemicals, such as *isopropyl alcohol,* are also used as rubbing alcohols—as cooling agents and skin disinfectants—and are also poisonous if ingested.

Present-Day Drinking Trends

On a per-capita basis, Americans drink twice as much wine and beer as they did a century ago, and half as much distilled spirits. Where drinking takes place has also changed. There is less hard drinking in bars and more social drinking at home and in clubs. The acceptance of drinking in mixed company has made it more a part of social situations than it was a century ago.

Here are some facts about the current consumption of alcoholic beverages in the United States:

- Drinking is more common among men than among women, but the gap is closing.
- It is more common among people who are under 40.
- It is more common among the affluent than among the poor.
- The number of drinkers over the age of 45 steadily declines.

Teenagers and Alcohol

One fact emerges clearly and consistently from all the surveys of teenage drinking in all parts of the country: The drinking behavior of parents is more related to what children do about drinking than any other factor. It is more influential than children's friends, neighborhoods, religions, social or economic status, or local laws.

Statistics on teenage (and adult) drinking vary from one ethnic group or one part of the country to another. But overall, the statistics show that about two-thirds of all Americans 18 and older consume alcoholic beverages. Some three-quarters of all students in the tenth-to-twelfth-grade-range also drink.

In general, for many youths drinking is an activity that is associated with growing up.

Kinds of Alcoholic Beverages

The way an alcoholic drink affects the body depends chiefly on how much alcohol it contains. The portion of alcohol can range from less than 1/20th of the total volume, as is the case with beer, to more than one-half, as is the case with rum. As a general rule, distilled drinks have a higher alcohol content than fermented ones.

The five basic types of alcoholic beverages are beers, table wines, dessert or cocktail wines, cordials and liqueurs, and distilled spirits such as brandy or whisky. The labels on beer and wine usually indicate the percentage of alcohol by volume. The labels on distilled spirits indicate the *proof.*

Proof

The proof number is twice the percentage of alcohol by volume. Thus a rye whisky that is 90-proof contains 45 percent alcohol, 80-proof bourbon is 40 percent alcohol, and so on. The word *proof* used in this way comes from an old English test to determine the strength of distilled spirits. If gunpowder soaked with whisky would still ignite when lighted, that fact was "proof" that the whisky contained the right amount of alcohol. The amount, approximately 57 percent, is still the standard in Canada and Great Britain.

How Alcohol Affects the Body

The overall effects of alcohol on the body and on behavior vary a great deal depending on many factors. One factor should be noted at once: if the blood reaching the brain contains a certain percentage of alcohol, there are marked changes in reaction. As the percentage increases, the functioning of the brain and central nervous system is increasingly affected. As the alcohol is gradually metabolized and eliminated, the process reverses itself.

If at any given time the blood contains a concentration of about 3/100 of one percent (0.03 percent), no effects are observable. This amount will make its way into the bloodstream after you have had a highball or cocktail made with one and one-half ounces of whisky, or two small glasses of table wine, or two bottles of beer. It takes about two hours for this amount of alcohol to leave the body completely.

Twice that number of drinks produces twice the concentration of alcohol in the bloodstream (0.06 percent) with an accompanying feeling of warmth and relaxation.

If the concentration of alcohol in the bloodstream reaches 0.1 percent—when one part of every thousand parts of blood is pure alcohol—the person is legally drunk in most states. The motor areas of the brain are affected; there is a noticeable lack of coordination in standing or walking. If the percentage goes up to 0.15 percent, the physical signs of intoxication are obvious, and they are accompanied by an impairment of mental faculties as well.

A concentration of as much as 0.4 percent can cause a coma. At the level of 0.5 to 0.7 percent there may be paralysis of the brain centers that control the activities of the lungs and heart, a condition that can be fatal.

Alcohol affects the brain and nervous system in this way because it is a depressant and an anesthetic.

How Alcohol Moves through the Body

Although it is negligible as nourishment, alcohol is an energy-producing food like sugar. Unlike most foods, however, it is quickly absorbed into the bloodstream through the stomach and small intestine without first having to undergo complicated digestive processes. It is then carried to the liver, where most of it is converted into heat and energy. From the liver, the remainder is carried by the bloodstream to the heart and pumped to the lungs. Some is expelled in the breath and some is eventually eliminated in sweat and urine. From the lungs, the alcohol is circulated to the brain.

People who use good judgment when drinking rarely, if ever, get drunk. The safe and pleasurable use of alcoholic beverages depends on the drinker's weight and his or her physical condition and emotional state. Other factors include the following:

1. *The Concentration of Alcohol in the Beverage* The higher the alcohol content in terms of total volume, the faster it is absorbed. Three ounces of straight whisky—two shot glasses—contain the same amount of alcohol as 48 ounces (or four cans) of beer.

2. *Sipping or Gulping* Two shots of straight whisky can be downed in seconds or, more normally, in a few minutes. The same amount diluted in two highballs can be sipped through an entire evening. In the latter case, the body has a chance to get rid of much of the alcohol.

3. *Additional Components of the Drink* The carbohydrates in beer and wine slow down the absorption of alcohol in the blood. Vodka mixed with orange juice travels much more slowly than a vodka martini.

4. *Food in the Stomach* The alcohol concentration in two cocktails consumed at the peak of the hunger before dinner can have a nasty effect. Several glasses of wine with a meal or a brandy sipped after dinner get to thebloodstream much more slowly and at a lower concentration. The sensible drinker doesn't drink on an empty stomach.

The Hangover

The discomfort that sometimes sets in the morning after excessive drinking is known as a hangover. It is caused by the disruptive effect of too much alcohol on the central nervous system. The symptoms of nausea, headache, dry mouth, diarrhea, fatigue, dizziness, heartburn, and a feeling of apprehension are usually most acute several hours after drinking and not while there is still any appreciable amount of alcohol in the system.

Although many people believe that "mixing" drinks, such as switching from whisky drinks to wine, is the main cause of hangovers, a hangover can just as easily be induced by too much of one type of drink or by pure alcohol. Nor is it always the result of drinking too much because emotional stress or allergy may well be contributing factors.

Some aspects of a hangover may be caused by substances called *congeners*. These are the natural products of fermentation found in small amounts in all alcoholic beverages, among them tannic acid and fusel oil. Some congeners have toxic properties that produce nausea by irritating certain nerve centers.

In spite of accumulated lore about hangover remedies, there is no certain cure for the symptoms. A throbbing head and aching joints can sometimes be relieved by aspirin and bed rest. Stomach irritation can be eased by bland foods such as skim milk, cooked cereal, or a poached egg. Persons seeking relief may also try analgesics such as aspirin or acetaminophen for the headache, antacids if the problem is upset stomach, or over-the-counter medications for the diarrhea.

Alcohol and General Health

It is known that alcohol has harmful effects when consumed in large quantities, but studies in the 1990s showed that alcohol may provide some health benefits. Moderate consumption—no more than one drink a day for women or two for men—has been associated with a lower risk of heart disease in some individuals. Some people, however, should not drink at all; for example, children and adolescents, people who cannot control their consumption, women who are pregnant or trying to become pregnant, and anyone taking medication. No one should drink before driving. The adverse effects of alcohol are detailed below.

Tissue Impairment

Habitual drinking of straight whisky can irritate the membranes that line the mouth and throat. The hoarse voice of some heavy drinkers is the result of a thickening of vocal cord tissue. As for the effect on the stomach, alcohol doesn't cause ulcers, but it does aggravate them.

There is no evidence to support the belief that port wine or any other alcoholic beverage taken in moderation will cause gout. Studies have shown that as many as 60 percent of all patients with this disease had never drunk any wine at all.

Brain Damage

Alcohol abuse continued over many years has been found to contribute to cognitive defects. These may, in turn, indicate brain impairment. Researchers do not know what the defects represent—whether greater susceptibility to the problems of aging or an actual, alcohol-caused "premature aging" effect. Whatever the case, long-term chronic alcohol abuse leads to more rapid aging of the brain. Neuropsychologically, the alcoholic's brain resembles that of an older nonalcoholic.

Long-term abuse can have many other effects. These include withdrawal symptoms beginning 12 to 48 hours after a person stops drinking, sometimes followed by *delirium tremens* (DTs), which brings hallucinations and can be fatal; the Werner-Korsakoff syndrome, a type of beriberi characterized by a lack of the B vitamins; alcoholic peripheral neuropathy, involving damage to the nerve tissue outside the brain and spinal cord; and liver damage, including alcoholic hepatitis and cirrhosis. In the latter the liver becomes hard and yellowed.

Alcohol and Immunity to Infection

Moderate drinkers who maintain proper health habits are no more likely to catch viral or bacterial diseases than nondrinkers. But heavy drinkers, who often suffer from malnutrition, have conspicuously lower resistance to infection. Even well-nourished heavy drinkers have a generally lower immunity to infection than normal. When the blood-alcohol level is 0.15 percent or higher, the alcohol appears to weaken the disease-fighting white blood cells.

Alcohol and Stroke

Studies have shown that heavy drinkers face nearly three times the teetotaler's risk of hemorrhagic stroke. Light drinkers face twice the risk. About one stroke in four occurring in the United States is hemorrhagic, but these strokes are more likely to be fatal than those caused by blood clots.

Alcohol and Life Expectancy

It is difficult to isolate drinking in itself as a factor in longevity. One study reported the shortest life span for heavy drinkers, a somewhat longer one for those who don't drink at all, and the longest for moderate drinkers. But other factors, such as general health and heredity, play important roles.

Alcohol and Sex Activity

Alcohol in sufficient quantity depresses the part of the brain that controls inhibitions. This liberating effect has led some people to believe that alcohol is an aphrodisiac, in men. This is a conclusion that is far from the truth. At the same time that alcohol increases the sexual appetite, it reduces the ability to perform.

Alcohol as an Irritant

Many otherwise healthy people cannot tolerate alcoholic beverages of any kind, or of a particular kind, without getting sick. In some cases, the negative reaction may be psychological in origin—connected with a disastrous experience with drunkenness in the early years or with an early hatred for a drinker in the family. Some people can drink one type of beverage but not another because of a particular congener, or because of an allergy to a specific grain or fruit. People suffering from such diseases as peptic ulcers, kidney and liver infections, and epilepsy should never drink any alcoholic beverages unless allowed to do so by a physician.

Uses and Hazards

At practically all times and in many parts of the world today, alcoholic beverages of various kinds have been and are still used for medicinal purposes. This should not be taken to mean that Aunt Sally is right about the curative powers of her elderberry wine, or that grandpa knows best when he says brandy is the best cure for hiccups. Today an American physician may recommend a particular alcoholic beverage as a tranquilizer, a sleep-inducer, or an appetite stimulant.

Use of Alcohol with Other Drugs

Alcoholic beverages should be avoided by anyone taking barbiturates or other sedatives. See "Drug Use and Abuse" later in this chapter for a discussion of barbiturates.

Alcohol and Driving

For many people, coordination, alertness, and general driving skills are impaired at blood-alcohol levels below the legal limit (0.1 percent). There are some people who become dangerous drivers after only one drink. Attempts are constantly being made, but so far with less than perfect success, to educate the public about the very real dangers of drunken driving.

Possible Causes of Alcohol Abuse

A popular myth holds that alcohol causes alcohol abuse. It doesn't—any more than sugar causes diabetes. Various theories have been evolved to explain what does cause alcohol abuse.

Physiological Causes

Although several physiological factors seem to be involved in the progression of alcohol abuse, no single one can be pinpointed as the cause of the disease. Among the theories that have come under investigation are the following: abnormal sugar metabolism, disorders of the endocrine glands, and dietary deficiencies.

Psychological Causes

Recent studies have pointed to a possible relationship between personality and alcohol abuse. Researchers indicate that one definable segment of the alcoholic population has the character disorder known as *antisocial personality.* Once called a *sociopath,* the person with an antisocial personality is usually charming in a social sense, manipulative, impulsive and rebellious, and egocentric. An estimated 25 percent of the alcoholic population falls in this category; in the general population the prevalence of antisocial personalities is about 3 percent.

Sociological Factors

Practically all studies of alcohol abuse in the United States indicate that ethnic groups vary dramatically in their rates of problem drinkers. A great deal of attention has therefore been focused on *learned attitudes* toward alcoholic beverages and how they are used or abused. Generally, in the low-incidence groups attitudes toward drinking are clearly defined and understood by all the members of the group. Drunkenness is consistently frowned upon. In the high-incidence groups, researchers have found extensive conflict over alcohol. The basic rules aren't clearly defined, and there are no clear-cut standards for acceptable and unacceptable drinking behavior.

Genetic Factors

Research into the genetics of alcohol abuse has led to a theory of "familial abuse." The theory holds that the person with a close relative who is alcoholic is at far greater risk of succumbing to the disease than are others without such connections. Familial abuse or "familial alcoholism" characterizes as many as three in four of all abusers. Therapy has thus begun to focus on the families of alcohol abusers—particularly young sons—as the ones most susceptible to the disease.

Recognizing the Danger Signals of Problem Drinking

The chronic alcohol abuser shows physical symptoms that a physician can recognize. Among them are hand tremors, deterioration of eye functions, reduced bladder control, liver disorders, anemia, memory lapses, and others. But there are many other symptoms that family members and friends can observe, among them these:

- Alcohol use as a way of handling problems or escaping from them
- Increased use of alcohol with repeated occasions of unintended intoxication
- Sneaking drinks or gulping them rapidly in quick succession
- Irritation, hostility, and lying when the subject of alcohol abuse is mentioned
- A noticeable deterioration in appearance, health, and social behavior
- Persistent drinking in spite of such symptoms as headaches, loss of appetite, sleeplessness, and stomach trouble

Treatment

Methods of treating alcohol abuse fall generally into three categories. Choice of any one form of treatment depends on the particular needs of a client, including the degree of dependency. The three categories include the hospital, the intermediate, and the outpatient settings. Other approaches to treatment may be geared to individual or group needs.

The family physician can in most cases provide guidance on what kind of treatment would most benefit a particular patient. The alcohol abuser may be referred first to a toxicologist for an interview and recommendations on treatment. A review of the patient's history is a typical first step in treatment. Family involvement during therapy may be critically important. More than 4,200 centers offer treatment programs; of these, many are nonprofit clinics while others are units owned by for-profit health care chains. Many centers and clinics specialize in team approaches to therapy.

The Hospital Setting

Whether undertaken voluntarily or involuntarily (for example, by court order) the treatment formats offered in a hospital can be individualized. Where some patients adjust best to inpatient care, others prefer partial hospitalization. In the latter case the patient is allowed to go home or to work at appropriate times, otherwise living in the hospital. In a hospital detoxification program, one designed to end physical addiction, the patient has a variable period, usually two weeks to a month, during which he or she undergoes a programmed regimen of activities. These may range from exercise classes to medications to bed rest and regulated diets.

The Intermediate Setting

The intermediate settings usually include at least halfway houses, quarterway houses, and residential care sites. The first of these offer not only living quarters but also job counseling, psychotherapy, and other services. In quarterway houses, the patient receives more attention in the form of counseling and psychotherapy. Residential care centers usually offer little beyond living quarters.

The Outpatient Setting

Again in the outpatient setting the patient has a range of treatment choices. Among them typically are individual counseling sessions held by a paraprofessional; individual therapy sessions with a professional who may have an advanced degree in social work, psychology, medicine, or a related specialty; and group therapy sessions supervised by either a paraprofessional or a professional.

Chemical Treatments

Some treatment programs utilize medications to help patients to "shake the habit." Tranquilizers may be used to reduce tensions and prepare the patient for a follow-up stage. In a program of *aversion therapy* a substance called emetine may be prescribed. Taken before an alcoholic drink, emetine causes nausea. The treatment should be undertaken only under medical supervision.

Where to Find Help

Volunteer organizations of various kinds offer the alcohol abuser and his or her family a wide range of services and programs. The best known is Alcoholics Anonymous (AA), which is supported by contributions from members. AA utilizes a group-support approach to treatment. Most larger communities have AA chapters as well as Al-Anon and Alateen units for family members, relatives, and friends of abusers. Alateen works with young people between 12 and 20 years of age. Counseling and referrals may be obtained from a local Alcoholic Treatment Center.

Information may also be obtained from the following national headquarters of organizations established to help alcohol abusers:

Alcoholics Anonymous
Grand Central Station
P.O. Box 459
New York, NY 10163
(212) 870-3400

National Association for Children of Alcoholics
11426 Rockville Pike, Suite 100
Rockville, MD 20852
(888) 554-2627

Al-Anon Family Group Hdqts
1600 Corporate Landing Parkway
Virginia Beach, VA 23454-5617
(888) 425-2666

National Council on Alcoholism and Drug Dependence
20 Exchange Place, Suite 2902
New York, NY 10005
(212) 269-7797

Drug Abuse

Like alcohol abuse, drug abuse can wreck lives and break up families. But to many experts the problem of drug abuse is far more serious than alcohol abuse. The trade in addictive, harmful drugs is not only unlawful; it has grown year by year, to the point where many believe it is out of control. Since the mid-1980's the U.S. government has spent approximately one and a half billion dollars a year to combat illegal drug importation, calling on units of the military to join the campaign. Nevertheless, the amount of illegal drugs seized and the amount estimated to elude detection increase each year.

The forms that drug abuse takes, and the numbers of drugs, are numerous and increasing. Many authorities believe we should examine our whole American society for the "pill-happy" context in which drug abuse occurs. Dr. Joel Fort, former consultant on drug abuse to the World Health Organization, called America

> "a drug-prone nation. . . . The average 'straight' adult consumes three to five mind-altering drugs a day, beginning with the stimulant caffeine in coffee, tea, and Coca Cola, going on to include alcohol and nicotine, often a tranquilizer, not uncommonly a sleeping pill at night and sometimes an amphetamine the next morning."

The social effects of drug abuse rank among the most alarming of all the symptoms of what has been called the drug crisis. By estimate, drugs are involved in one-third to one-half of all crimes committed in the United States in a typical year. In a single recent year, medical treatments for drug abusers cost the nation more than $2 billion. The costs of abuse to families, communities, and to abusers themselves cannot be calculated.

Making the problem of control of drug abuse unbelievably complex is the fact that literally thousands of drugs and drug combinations have basic roles in medical treatments. Legal and illicit uses may, because of the close connections, become confused. Physicians' instructions regarding use of such legal drugs as sleeping pills may be ignored or neglected. Legitimately prescribed drugs may, in some cases, unintentionally lead to abuse or dependency.

Other facts make it difficult to control drug abuse. More and more, for example, abusers are turning to multiple substance abuse. Cocaine "sniffers" may take alcohol in one form or another to soften the uncomfortable and even painful effects of cocaine withdrawal. Physicians report that "polydrug" abuse leads to progressive worsening of such medical symptoms as stomach ailments and liver problems.

Designer drugs add another complicating factor. Made in clandestine chemical laboratories, these drugs are created by altering the existing molecular structure of other drugs, such as cocaine, heroin, amphetamines, and many other controlled substances. The chemical composition of a designer drug is enough like that of the banned or controlled drug it imitates that it produces similar effects, but it is different enough to be a new drug. The federal Drug Enforcement Administration must then take steps to declare the new drug illegal. Far more powerful than the basic drugs they imitate, the designer forms have been implicated in hundreds of deaths.

A designer drug called Ecstasy is an imitation methamphetamine (speed). It contains the industrial chemical MPTP, a suspected causative element in cases of Parkinson's disease. A number of Ecstasy abusers also had classic Parkinson's symptoms: rigidity, tremors in the arms, legs, and even the head, and slow or difficult movement. Thus new research has focused on MPTP as a possible clue to the degenerative brain processes that lead to Parkinson's.

Over-the-Counter Drugs

Americans consume over-the-counter (OTC) drugs in enormous quantities. Purchasable without a physician's prescription, these drugs have limited but real potential for abuse. They range from headache remedies to cold nostrums and from acne ointments to vitamins. In general, good practice is to use OTC drugs as seldom as possible, for short-term, minor illnesses. Medicines of proven effectiveness should be used exclusively: taking an aspirin for a headache is a good example. The U.S. Public Health Service offers these guidelines:

- Self-prescribed drugs should never be used continuously for long periods of time. . . . A physician is required for abdominal pain that is severe or recurs periodically; pains anywhere, if severe, disabling, persistent, or recurring; headache, if unusually severe or prolonged more than one day; a prolonged cold with fever or cough; earache; unexplained loss of weight; unexplained and unusual symptoms; *malaise* lasting more than a week or two. . . .

The Food and Drug Administration (FDA), a branch of the U.S. Public Health Service, is responsible for establishing the safety and usefulness of all drugs marketed in the United States, both OTC and prescription. You can be assured that OTC drugs are safe provided you take them in strict accordance with the label instructions. These indicate the appropriate dosages, among other things, and carry warnings against prolonged or improper use, such as "discontinue if pain persists," or "do not take if abdominal pain is present." This labeling information is regulated by the FDA.

Drug Classifications

In addition to alcohol, the drugs of potential abuse fall into six categories: stimulants, depressants, and narcotic preparations, all of which can have legitimate medical uses; hallucinogens; cannabinoids such as marijuana; and inhalants (or volatile inhalants) such as aerosol sprays, glues, and fuels. See the accompanying table:

Major Drug Classification

Type	Examples
Stimulants	Amphetamines Cocaine derivatives
Depressants	Valium Seconal
Narcotics (opioids)	Morphine Codeine
Hallucinogens	LSD Mescaline Psilocybin

Drug abuse can lead to at least three kinds of addiction or dependency. *Physical addiction* results in unpleasant withdrawal symptoms, including, nausea, headache, or cold

Marijuana (cannabinoids)	Marijuana Hashish
Inhalants	Gasoline Amyl nitrate

sweats when the abuser does not take the drug. Sudden withdrawal from some physically addictive drugs can cause heart failure. *Psychological addiction,* more subtle, is a stage at which the abuser believes he or she cannot cope without the drug. In *functional addiction,* the abuser grows dependent on such drugs as decongestant nasal sprays to remain free of an uncomfortable physical condition.

Dependence and Addiction

Dependence and *addiction* are used to describe the compulsive and uncontrollable use of a substance. The use continues despite negative effects on health, lifestyle, work, or other aspects of one's life. Lack of the substance leads to physical or psychological discomfort and, at times, an overwhelming desire to obtain more of the substance to alleviate the negative sensations experienced from withdrawal.

Psychological dependence or *addiction* occurs when the user feels he or she cannot manage without the drug. This can occur for several reasons, with several types of drugs. The condition can be mild or can be extraordinarily severe.

Psychological addiction to painkillers—and this can include ibuprofen (Motrin), aspirin, and acetaminophen (Tylenol)—occurs when the user feels that pain may be too great without regular medication. As pain occurs without use, it fulfills the user's expectations. The pain may be real or may be psychosomatic (triggered by psychological expectations of pain), but it reassures the user that the drug is needed and does good. The problem is that with many types of drugs, the effectiveness decreases as use increases.

Psychological addiction can accompany physical addiction, and it is usually difficult to distinguish where psychological needs end and physical needs begin. Many addictions have both psychological and physical aspects.

Physical dependence or *addiction* occurs when the body has developed a physical need for the drug. Physical dependence is usually recognized when the user stops taking the drug. Withdrawal symptoms occur when the body is denied the chemicals to which it has become habituated. Withdrawal symptoms can include dizziness, anxiety, restless sleep, dull ache, acute pain, heart tremors, seizures and convulsions, and heart attack. Sudden withdrawal from some physically addictive drugs can kill the user. Many of the street drugs, such as cocaine and heroin, and many of the prescription drugs, such as Xanax and codeine, can produce severe symptoms if withdrawal is sudden from quantities that were abusive.

Tolerance is the term used for the effect that occurs when the quantity of drug is progressively increased to achieve the desired result. For some chemicals, the body becomes habituated to one quantity and the dosage must be increased to maintain the same level of relief or pleasure experienced from the drug. Increased tolerance for some drugs is what frequently leads to levels that are physically addictive.

Three Classes of Prescription Drugs

Among the drugs that may be prescribed for patients are some that have a tremendous potential for abuse. They include *stimulants,* such as amphetamines; *depressants,* such as sleeping pills; and *narcotic* painkillers, including morphine and codeine. When abused (that is, when taken in any way other than according to a physician's strict instructions), these drugs constitute a substantial part of America's burgeoning national drug problem.

Stimulant Drugs

The legitimate use of stimulant drugs and their great capacity for abuse stem from the same property: their ability to speed up the processes of the central nervous system. Physicians may prescribe amphetamines to counteract mild depression. More rarely, they use stimulant drugs to treat *narcolepsy,* a disease in which the patient is subject to irresistible bouts of sleep, and to counteract the drowsiness caused by sedatives. Amphetamines and an amphetamine-like drug (Ritalin) may be used to treat some hyperactive children who are extremely excitable and easily distracted. For reasons that are imperfectly understood, the drug calms these children instead of stimulating them. They are no longer recommended for weight loss or weight control.

Amphetamines

The major forms of the amphetamines are: amphetamine (Benzedrine), the more powerful dextroamphetamine (Dexedrine), and methamphetamine (Methedrine, Desoxyn). The street name for these drugs is "speed." The consumption of amphetamines is reportedly far greater than the prescription books indicate. Some 10 billion tablets are produced in the United States annually, enough for 50 doses for every man, woman, and child. Of this amount, probably half is diverted into illicit channels. Underground laboratories manufacture even more.

Amphetamines are a common "street" drug and are taken most often in powder form. Amphetamine abuse is most prevalent among younger age groups and at social events and gatherings. Amphetamines are usually used for their stimulant and euphoric effects, which last from 4 to 6 hours.

Used judiciously, amphetamines can improve performance, both mental and physical, over moderate periods of time. In effect, they delay the deterioration in performance that fatigue normally produces. Required to carry out routine duties under difficult circumstances and for extended periods, some astronauts have used amphetamines under long-range medical supervision.

Amphetamines give some persons feelings of self-confidence, well-being, alertness, and an increased ability to concentrate and perform. Others may experience an increase in tension ranging from the uncomfortable to an agonizing pitch of anxiety. High doses may produce dry mouth, sweating, palpitations, and raised blood pressure. Because amphetamines only defer the effects of fatigue, the letdown can be dangerous, especially for such users as long-distance truck drivers. In addition, the feelings of self-confidence about improved performance may be highly deceptive. Some college students who have crammed for exams while on speed have turned in blank examination books, or written a whole essay on one dense line.

Amphetamine abusers quickly develop a tolerance to the drug. They may have continually to increase dosages, and may undergo different kinds of drug experiences. Psychological dependence can build rapidly.

Amphetamine-like Stimulants

Several drugs that are chemically unrelated to the amphetamines produce very similar effects on the body. They are, also, equally amenable to abuse. Among them are methylphenidate (Ritalin) and phenmetrazine (Preludin). The latter has been commonly used as a diet pill.

Cocaine

Ranked as powerful stimulants to the central nervous system, cocaine and its derivatives were the trendy drugs of the late 20th century. An alkaloid found in the leaves of the coca bush, *Erythroxylon coca,* cocaine in its crystalline form is a white powder that looks like moth flakes. Cocaine can be sniffed, smoked, or taken intravenously. Abusers of cocaine may or may not develop a tolerance for the drug. But some evidence indicates that the same dose repeated frequently will not produce similar effects over a period of time.

Very little street-purchased cocaine is pure. Usually, the drug is mixed, or cut, with other drugs or with substances that resemble it, such as talcum powder or sugar.

Cocaine is a very addictive drug. When physical dependence develops, and the user does not consume more of the drug, the withdrawal symptoms may include hunger, irritability, extreme fatigue, depression, and restless sleep. With psychological dependence, abusers come to need the feeling of euphoria induced by cocaine. When a dose wears off, the abuser may go into a period of deep depression.

The use of cocaine as a legal anesthetic need not lead to addiction. It has been used particularly in surgical operations on the mouth, eyes, and throat because it can constrict blood vessels and because it is rapidly absorbed by the mucous membranes.

Cocaine's effects as a stimulant last only a short time. Generally, the effects depend on the size of the dose. A small dose may produce sensations of euphoria and illusions of increased strength and sensory awareness. A large dose may magnify these effects. The abuser may engage in irrational behavior, and may experience such physical side effects as sweating, dilation of the pupils, and rapid heartbeat.

In extreme cases abusers may have hallucinations and feelings of paranoia and depression. They may imagine that insects are crawling over their skins (formication) and may have chest pains. Injections by needle may produce skin abscesses. Both heavy and light users may develop runny noses, eczema around the nostrils, and deterioration of the nasal cartilage. The latter occurs because cocaine is usually "snorted" into the nostrils through a straw or a roll of paper, or from a spoon.

Death results, occasionally, from overdoses of cocaine, with respiratory arrest as a prime cause. The abuser may also have high fever, heart rhythm disturbances, or convulsions.

Crack Cocaine

Cocaine hydrochloride—cocaine in white powder form—can be converted into cocaine alkaloid, or *freebase,* by a simple procedure. The process involves mixing powdered cocaine with baking soda and water to form a paste. Once the concoction hardens, it looks like lumpy, off-white granulated sugar. Unlike powdered cocaine, the drug in this form, called *crack* or *rock,* can be smoked, eliminating the need for needles.

Crack is a purified cocaine base that is usually smoked in a special pipe with wire screens, or sprinkled on a tobacco or marijuana cigarette. The drug produces a high that may start in eight seconds and last five to ten minutes. By contrast, snorted cocaine takes effect after about five minutes and lasts for up to 30 minutes.

Crack produces a very intense euphoria along with other physical symptoms. Because the drug in this form is far more potent than powdered cocaine, the heartbeat speeds up and the abuser's blood pressure may rise. Heart-lung problems may follow, and seizures can occur. Death may ensue. Because of the variations in the strength and purity of crack, and because of the variability of a body's response, death can occur on the first use or the thousandth. Abuse of crack may lead to physical addiction in weeks, with the victim needing continually larger doses to achieve a high.

Depressant Drugs

Making up a second class of medically useful drugs that are also widely abused, the depressants act as sedatives on the central nervous system (CNS). They may also act as hypnotic, or sleep-inducing, agents.

The depressants include mainly barbiturates, which are both sedative and hypnotic, and tranquilizers, which can calm without producing sleep. Though they are available as main or secondary constituents of many brand name preparations, the barbiturates are readily abused.

Tranquilizers act selectively on the brain and the central nervous system. Divided into major and minor tranquilizers, these drugs are similar to barbiturates in many ways, including their sedative or calming effect. The major tranquilizers, called *neuroleptics* because they are useful in the treatment of mental disorders, are haloperidol and chlorpromazine. These drugs lead to virtually no addiction or dependence even in long-term therapy.

The minor tranquilizers, among them meprobamate (Miltown), chlordiazepoxide (Librium), and diazepam (Valium), are, by contrast, highly addictive. Abusers take such drugs to achieve euphoric states, as well as to offset the effects of alcohol, amphetamines, and other drugs.

Barbiturates

Barbiturates have many legitimate uses. For example, they may be prescribed to overcome insomnia, reduce high blood pressure, alleviate anxiety, treat mental disorders, and sedate patients both before and after surgery. Many doctors now prescribe benzodiazapines instead of barbiturates.

Barbiturates are metabolized, or broken down chemically, by the liver. They are then eliminated by the kidneys at different speeds depending on their types: ultra-short-, short-, intermediate-, and long-lasting. Long-lasting barbiturates, primarily phenobarbital and barbital, take effect on the brain in one to two hours and last for six to 24 hours. The intermediate- and short-acting barbiturates, including secobarbital and pentobarbital, take effect in 15 to 45 minutes and last five to six hours. The best known of the ultra-short-acting drugs, thiopental, can produce unconsciousness in a few minutes. Used mostly in hospitals as an anesthetic, thiopental is also injected by dentists to produce instant unconsciousness.

Abuse

Barbiturate abusers usually select the short-acting and intermediate-acting barbiturates. Abusers as a group generally fall into four categories, with some overlap.

The "silent abuser" takes sleeping pills at first to get some sleep, probably with a physician's prescription. Progressively, the drug helps the abuser to deal with tension and anxiety. Indulging at home, he or she finds the barbiturates producing an alcohol-like high, with slurred speech, confusion, poor judgment and coordination, and sometimes wild emotional swings. Eventually the abuser is obtaining the drug through illicit channels. Some may end up spending most of their time in bed.

A second group, taking barbiturates for stimulation, has already developed a high tolerance that makes drug stimulation possible. Some other abusers find that the drug releases inhibitions.

Made up mostly of young people who are experimenting with various drugs, a third group uses barbiturates to "come down" from an amphetamine high. Members of this group may find themselves in a vicious cycle of stimulation and sedation. To obtain both effects at once, some abusers take the barbiturate-amphetamine combination in the same swallow—a so-called "set-up."

A fourth group, abusers of heroin and other narcotics, uses barbiturates as a substitute when drugs of choice are not available. They may also combine barbiturates with heroin to prolong its effect. In one hospital surveyed, 23 percent of the narcotics users said they were also dependent on barbiturates.

Effects and Dangers

Barbiturate abuse is generally considered to be far more dangerous than narcotic abuse. Barbiturate overdose, accidental or intentional, is responsible for about one-third of all drug-related deaths that are reported. For such reasons many physicians believe barbiturates are the most dangerous of all drugs. Chronic abuse can lead to psychological dependence and increased tolerance, followed often by physical dependence of a particularly anguishing kind.

Abrupt withdrawal from barbiturates can be much more dangerous than withdrawal from heroin. Within a day the abuser withdrawing from barbiturates may experience headaches, muscle twitches, anxiety, weakness, nausea, and blood pressure drops. If the abuser stands up suddenly he or she may faint. Delirium and convulsions may come later. The latter can be fatal. Thus the withdrawal must always be undertaken under medical supervision. Even with supervision, a withdrawal from barbiturates may take two months.

Abuse of barbiturates presents other dangers. Unintentional overdosing frequently occurs when a person takes a regular dose to get to sleep and then remains awake or awakens soon afterward; tired and confused, the person may take another or repeated doses. Death may result. Mixing barbiturates and alcohol can produce the same outcome.

Other Barbiturate-Type Drugs

Some depressants are chemically unrelated to the barbiturates but have similar effects. These include *glutethimide* and *ethchlorvynol* (Placidyl). These too lead to tolerance when abused. For the most part, they have been replaced by the use of other medications.

Tranquilizers

The minor tranquilizers are manufactured as capsules and tablets in many sizes, shapes, and colors. They may also be purchased in liquid form for injection. Used legitimately to treat emotional tension and as muscle relaxants, these tranquilizers have high abuse potential because they produce both psychological and physical dependence. Tolerance develops with prolonged abuse.

Miltown, Librium, and Valium produce effects similar to those of barbiturates. But the minor tranquilizers act more slowly and have longer duration. Once considered completely harmless, these drugs came into such vogue that in the 1970s the federal government intervened. Both Valium and Librium as well as some other drugs were placed under federal control. From 1975 on anyone requiring a prescription for these drugs was limited to five prescription refills within a six-month period following the initial prescription. If more of the medication was required after that, a new prescription had to be written.

Withdrawal from the minor tranquilizers can be as dangerous and painful as withdrawal from barbiturates. Combining the tranquilizing drugs with others, including alcohol, is a highly dangerous form of abuse. Each drug reinforces the effects of the other. The result may be greater than the combined effects of the different drugs.

Narcotics (Opiates)

Narcotics are drugs that relieve pain and induce sleep by depressing the central nervous system. Under U.S. law, narcotics are addictive drugs that produce rapid and severe physical and psychological dependence; that category includes opium and such opium derivatives as heroin, morphine, and codeine. The narcotics, or *opioids,* also include the so-called synthetic opiates, among them *meperidine* and *methadone.*

Varieties of abused drugs

Name of Drug	Form	Classification
amphetamine methamphetamine	capsule, pill, liquid, powder, tablet, lozenge; swallowed	stimulant
barbiturate	sleeping pills, capsules, tablets; swallowed; injected	depressant, sedative
cocaine	white powder; sniffed, smoked, injected	stimulant, local anesthetic
hashish	resin; smoked	relaxant, euphoriant, hallucinogen (in large or strong doses)
heroin	powder; injected, or sniffed	narcotic
inhalants (for example, gasoline, paint, glue, aerosols, amyl nitrite)	aerosois, volatile substances, solvents; sniffed	
LSD (d-lysergic acid diethylamide)	tablet, capsule, liquid; swallowed	hallucinogen (psychedelic)
marijuana, marihuana	dried leaves; smoked	relaxant, euphoriant, hallucinogen (in large or strong doses)
mescaline	tablet, capsule; swallowed	hallucinogen
PCP	powder; smoked, swallowed	anesthetic (used only with animals)

Opium

The seedpods of the opium poppy, *Papaver somniferum,* produce a gummy resin that has narcotic effects when eaten or smoked. Opium has been used in many lands and many cultures since prehistoric times. It was used medicinally in ancient Egypt. But not until recently did its addictive properties become known. Of the more than two dozen active compounds, or *alkaloids,* that can be isolated from opium, the two most important are morphine and codeine.

Morphine

Morphine, named after Morpheus, the Roman god of dreams, is the chemical substance in opium that gives it sedative and analgesic properties. Isolated initially in the early 1800s, morphine was later synthesized in pure form. On the illicit drug market it appears usually as a white powder.

Morphine can relieve almost any kind of pain, particularly dull, continuous pain. It may also relieve the fear and anxiety that go with such suffering. In addition to drowsiness, euphoria, and impairment of mental and physical performance, morphine may have adverse effects including nausea, vomiting, and sweating. Intravenous injections of the drug may produce an orgasmic high sensation beginning in the upper abdomen and spreading throughout the body.

An overdose of morphine can lead to respiratory depression that is sometimes severe enough to cause coma or death. Morphine is highly addictive and is used only short-term in hospitals because prolonged use can easily lead to problems with addiction or withdrawal. Naloxone (Narcan) may be administered intravenously as an antidote for morphine overdose.

Codeine

Taking its name from the Greek word *kodeia,* meaning poppyhead, codeine is a mild pain reliever that can be produced from gum opium or through conversion from morphine. The effects of codeine peak in 30 to 60 minutes; they disappear in three to four hours. Codeine is milder than either morphine or heroin in its analgesic effect. All forms of codeine can induce addiction problems with prolonged use.

Heroin

Originally thought to be nonaddictive, heroin was, for a time, used as a cure for opium and morphine addiction. Later, it was found to be more addictive than either of those drugs. It was prohibited in the United States in 1924 and became a staple on the drug black market. Heroin is several times more powerful than morphine.

All of the opiates, including heroin, produce feelings of well-being or euphoria. They can also dull the senses and reduce or eliminate normal fear, tension, and anxiety. The drug also produces sleepiness and lethargy. Possible side effects include nausea, flushing, constipation, slowed respiration rates, retention of urine, and, eventually, malnutrition resulting from loss of appetite. When heroin is injected for the first time nausea and vomiting can occur almost immediately.

The heroin abuser rapidly develops tolerance to the drug. Progressively larger doses are then required to produce the same degree of euphoria. Used chronically, heroin leads to both psychological and physical dependence. The former is far more difficult to overcome.

Caught in a cycle involving desperate efforts to obtain the drug often by criminal means, and getting high, the heroin abuser is not necessarily driven by a search for escape. He or she may want, equally, to avoid withdrawal symptoms. For the chronic abuser such symptoms can be difficult and painful, and may include anxiety, sweating, muscle aches, vomiting, and diarrhea.

Heroin sold on the streets is cut with quinine, milk sugar, or baking soda. It may be cut several times before reaching the abuser. A bag may contain only 1 to 5 percent heroin. If the addict unknowingly buys a dose containing 30 percent or more pure heroin, the higher concentration can spell grave illness or death.

Because heroin can be taken in different ways, the drug's narcotic effects are variable. Sniffing is the mildest form of abuse, followed by skin-popping or subcutaneous injection anywhere on the body, and mainlining, injection directly into a vein, usually the large vein inside the elbow. Abscesses at the preferred site of injection are common, and the vein may become inflamed.

Heroin use does not necessarily lead to dependence. Many persons have experimented with the drug without becoming addicted. Others "joy-pop"—use the drug on weekends, usually for recreational purposes or "kicks."

Little agreement exists regarding treatments for heroin abuse. A promising yet controversial method is the substitution of controlled doses of *methadone* for heroin. Methadone is a synthetic opiate that does not produce the euphoria of heroin. The substitution can help the abuser to lead a normal life, but he or she may still be addicted—to methadone.

Other forms of treatment utilize group psychotherapy, often in live-in communities modeled after the West Coast's *Synanon.* Some experts believe that only multiple-approach treatment formats, combining chemical treatment, psychiatry, user communities, and rehabilitation, can be effective. But the five-year cure rate for heroin abusers is low—only about one-third of that for alcoholics.

Synthetic Opiates

Prescription pain-relievers such as Demerol, Dilaudid, Pantopon, and other synthetic opiates can become addicting if used indiscriminately. They occasionally appear on the illicit drug market. With the increased availability of methadone in treatment clinics, methadone itself is used illicitly, often in combination with alcohol or other drugs, and especially when heroin is in short supply.

The Hallucinogens: LSD and Others

LSD (lysergic acid diethylamide) is one of a class of drugs legally classed as *hallucinogens*—agents that cause the user to experience hallucinations, illusions, and distorted perceptions. Others include *mescaline, psilocybin* and *psilocin, PCP, DMT* (dimethyltryptamine), and *DOM* or *STP.*

A colorless, tasteless, odorless compound, LSD is a semisynthetic acid of immense potency. A single effective dose requires, on the average, only 100 millionths of a gram. A quantity of LSD equivalent to two aspirin tablets would furnish 6,500 such doses. When sold on the street, LSD is generally mixed with colored substances. It may be manufactured in capsule, tablet, or liquid form.

History of LSD

With names such as *California sunshine, acid, purple haze,* and others, LSD reached a peak of popularity in the 1960s. Today it cannot be made legally except for use in certain supervised experiments. Physicians may use it to treat alcoholism and some mental disease, but without uniformly convincing results. It may be sold illegally in sugar cubes, candy, cookies, on the surfaces of beads, even in the mucilage of stamps and envelopes. One dose may produce a 4- to 18-hour *trip,* a hallucinogenic experience.

In the 1960s this trip made LSD the drug of choice for many substance abusers. Among those who claimed that LSD and other psychedelic drugs were consciousness-expanding were well-known public figures. The drugs, in brief, were supposed to enhance the user's appreciation of everything in the environment, to increase creativity, open the gates of awareness to mind-bending mystical or religious experiences, and perhaps to bring about profound changes, hopefully for the better, in the user's personality.

While some users reported such results, various studies suggested that the improvements were illusory. Members of some groups nonetheless felt that it was "in" to be an *acidhead,* an LSD user. One authority estimates that less than 1 percent of the total population have experimented with LSD. Partly because knowledge of dangers in LSD use has become common, the drug has passed the peak of its popularity even though it can still be obtained illegally.

Addictive Aspects

Abuse of LSD is difficult; the drug produces such a spectacular high that daily ingestion is virtually out of the question. Thus LSD use does not lead to physical dependence. But the heavy user can develop a tolerance for the drug very quickly. The tolerance disappears after a few days of abstinence.

Effects

Taking LSD, the individual is usually prepared for minor physical discomforts: a rise in temperature, pulse, and blood pressure; the sensation of hair standing on end; and some nausea, dizziness, and headache. The trip begins about an hour after the drug is first taken. Vision is affected the most profoundly. Colors become more intense and more beautiful; those in a painting may seem to merge and stream. Flat objects become three-dimensional.

The LSD user's reactions are closely related to his or her expectations. Thus one trip may be mind-expanding, filled with brilliant sights and sensations as well as euphoric feelings of oneness with the universe. Another trip may bring anxiety, panic, fear, and depression verging on despair. The latter experience can be terrifying; some bad trips have ended in psychiatric wards, with the tripper suffering from a severe mental disorder, a *psychosis*. An individual's body image may be distorted; in the LSD-induced vision he or she may have no head, for example. Such psychotic episodes, or breaks, may clear up within a day or two. Others can last for months or years.

Some trips have ended in tragedy. Convinced that they could fly or float through the air, some trippers have walked through high windows to their deaths. Others have walked in front of trains or cars.

In effect, no one can predict what psychological changes LSD use will produce. One reason is that no one really knows how LSD works inside the body to affect the mind. What is known is that the drug moves quickly to the brain and throughout the body, acting on both the central and autonomic nervous systems. But all traces of the drug disappear from the brain in some 20 minutes. The effects, as noted, last many more hours.

As with all drugs, LSD should not be ingested by persons who have psychotic tendencies or who are unstable. A disquieting side effect, usually occurring after chronic or heavy use, appears in the flashback, a reexperiencing of the effects of the drug weeks or months after a trip. One theory holds that flashbacks are induced by stress or fatigue, or by resort to other drugs, but the theory remains a theory.

Studies have reported some statistical findings. One research project found that the children of LSD users are 18 times more likely to have birth defects than the children of nonusers. Some research also suggests that the drug may have toxic effects on some cells of the human body. An unproved, and possibly unprovable, theory indicates that there may be a link between LSD use and breaks in chromosomes that could conceivably lead to leukemia or to birth defects in users' children.

Other Hallucinogens

Many other substances, both natural and synthetic, are used as hallucinogens. Most of them produce effects similar to those of LSD, but are far less potent.

Mescaline

Mescaline is the active ingredient of *peyote,* a Mexican cactus that has been used by American Indians for centuries to achieve mystical states in religious ceremonies. Users consume cactus "buttons" either ground up or whole. Mescaline itself may be obtained as a powder or a liquid. It can also be synthesized in a laboratory.

Psilocybin and Psilocin

Psilocybin and psilocin are the active hallucinogenic ingredients in the Aztec mushroom *Psilocybe mexicana.* The mushroom grows in southern Mexico and has been eaten raw by the natives since about 1500 B.C. Both derivatives can be made in the laboratory.

PCP (Phencyclidine Hydrochloride)

First developed in 1959 as an anesthetic, PCP in its pure form is a white crystalline powder that is readily soluble in water or alcohol. It appears on the drug black market as tablets, capsules, and colored powders. Abusers snort, smoke, or eat PCP. They can also inject the drug, but do not usually do so. PCP appears as an adulterant in many drug mixtures—in mescaline, psilocybin, or LSD, for example. PCP reportedly has as many or more undesirable effects as positive ones, among them forgetfulness, loss of behavior control, feelings of depersonalization, paranoid episodes, hallucinations, and suicidal impulses.

DMT (Dimethyltryptamine)

Called the "businessman's high" because its effects may last only 40 to 50 minutes, DMT is similar in structure to psilocin. DMT can be smoked or injected; in either case the effect is a powerful wave of exhilaration. An ingredient of various plants native to South America, DMT has long been used by Indian tribes in the form of intoxicating drinks or snuff, often very dangerous. In the United States, DMT is synthesized from tryptamine in the laboratory.

DOM or STP

DOM or STP is a synthetic compound originally developed by the Dow Chemical Company for possible use in the treatment of mental disorders. The drug was never released. Manufactured illicitly, it was allegedly given the name STP for Serenity, Tranquillity, Peace. The drug is powerful, it produces vivid hallucinations, and it seems to last as long as LSD. It is also extremely poisonous, and can bring on fever, blurred vision, difficulty in swallowing, and occasionally death from convulsions. In some cases abusers suffer from manic psychoses lasting for days.

Marijuana (Cannabinoids)

Marijuana, or *marihuana,* is a Mexican-Spanish word originally used to refer to a poor grade of tobacco. Later it came to mean a smoking preparation made from the Indian hemp plant (*Cannabis sativa*). A tall, weedy plant related to the fig tree and the hop, cannabis grows freely in many parts of the world and in a variety of grades depending on climate and method of cultivation. The different grades produce drugs of varying strengths. Some 300 million people around the world obtain drug preparations of one kind or another from cannabis.

Drugs are obtained almost exclusively from the female hemp plants. The male plants produce the fiber for hemp. When the female plants are ripe, late in the summer, their top leaves and especially the clusters of flowers at their tops develop a minty, sticky, golden-yellow resin, which eventually blackens. This resin contains the highest concentrations of THC (tetrahydrocannabinol), the group of substances containing the active principles of the drug. The pure resin of carefully cultivated plants is the most potent form of cannabis. It is available in cakes, called *charas* in India, and as a brown powder called hashish in the Middle East.

An estimated 15,000 tons of marijuana are illegally smuggled into the United States annually. But cannabis cultivation has become a major underground business inside the United States. Most illegal shipments of the drug come from Colombia, Jamaica, and Mexico.

Abuse Potential

Marijuana has puzzling aspects. Scientists have not succeeded in establishing exactly what substances in the cannabis plant produce drug effects, or how. THC is, of course, believed to be the most important active element, but chemists believe it is not the only one.

Beyond that, marijuana seems to be in a special class as a drug. It is classed as a hallucinogen, but is less potent than the true hallucinogens. It is not a narcotic, and it resembles both stimulants and depressants in some of its effects. Its use does not lead to physical dependence, nor does the user or abuser develop tolerance. Some users, in fact, find that with regular use they need less marijuana to achieve the desired high.

Users do acquire a slight to moderate psychological dependence—less, in some experts' opinions, than do regular users of alcohol or tobacco. Thus much of the theorizing about marijuana is conjecture despite the fact that millions of persons use it regularly or occasionally.

Effects

Experimenters and newcomers to marijuana smoking may experience little at the beginning. A sense of panic may accompany early exposure to the drug. More serious reactions have been reported, however, including *toxic-psychosis* (psychosis caused by a toxic agent) with accompanying confusion and disorientation. But such reports are rare. Experimenters using large doses of marijuana, hashish, or THC have induced what they termed hallucinations and psychotic reactions.

The experienced smoker may feel halfway between elation and sleepiness. He or she may have some altered perceptions of sound or color, for example, and a greatly slowed-down sense of time. It is usually possible to control the extent of the high by stopping when a given point is reached. The smoker often experiences mild headache or nausea.

Medical Evidence

Some evidence indicates that marijuana may produce genetic damage. More definitely, marijuana has been found to be effective for reducing the pressure of fluids in the eyes of patients suffering from glaucoma. In a 1976 case, the Food and Drug Administration (FDA) approved the use of marijuana for such treatment.

In 1985 the FDA licensed a small drug firm to manufacture THC for use in combating the nausea associated with cancer chemotherapy. Other studies indicated that the drug may also be useful in the treatment of such other diseases as multiple sclerosis and AIDS.

Since 1996 a number of states have adopted initiatives to exempt patients using marijuana under a physician's supervision from state criminal penalties. Programs in some of these states use patient registries and limit the amount of marijuana a patient may cultivate and possess at once. However, federal law still maintains that it is illegal to grow or sell marijuana and does not make any exceptions for medical use of the drug.

Inhalants

The inhalants as a class include solvents used in cleaning compounds, aerosol sprays, fuels, and glues. Abusers of these substances sniff or inhale the fumes for recreational and mind-altering purposes. But the substances, primarily chemical compounds, were never meant for human consumption. With some exceptions, they are available commercially and thus have appeal for persons who cannot afford or cannot obtain the more conventional drugs.

Strictly speaking, tobacco, cocaine, and marijuana could be considered inhalants. But the term more commonly refers to three categories of products: solvents, aerosols, and anesthetics. Among the solvents are commercial items such as gasoline, transmission fluid, paint thinner, and airplane cement. The aerosol products include shoeshine compounds, insecticides, spray paints, and hair spray. The type of inhalant used appears to vary according to geographic location, the ethnic backgrounds of abusers, and availability.

Anesthetics comprise a special group of inhalants. Some of them, including nitrous oxide, ether, and chloroform, were used recreationally before medical applications were found for them. Because they are not widely available, they are not abused as much as solvents and aerosols.

Abuse Patterns

Young teenagers are the primary abusers of inhalants. But some groups or classes of adults, such as those in prison also use inhalants. Reasons for abuse vary; among teenagers, they range from hostility and lack of affection to peer pressure. Adults, say authorities, are attracted by the ready availability of many inhalants. Alcoholics may resort to inhalants to try to forestall the symptoms of withdrawal.

Effects

The active chemicals in many inhalants are toluene, naphtha, carbon tetrachloride, and acetone, among others. The fumes from these chemicals enter the bloodstream quickly. They are then distributed to the brain and liver. Entering the central nervous system, the fumes depress such body functions as respiration and heartbeat. It is possible for even first-time users to be killed by "huffing."

Classed as depressants, inhalants are sometimes referred to as "deliriants," because they can produce illusions, hallucinations, and mental disturbances. These effects are usually the result of overdose; in moderate doses, the abuser feels sedated, has altered perceptions and impaired judgment, and may experience fright or even panic. Depending on the dosage, the abuser may also feel intoxicated and may have lowered inhibitions, as well as feelings of restlessness, uncoordination, confusion, and disorientation.

Prolonged abuse can lead to nausea, muscular weakness, fatigue, and weight loss. Other effects of such abuse include extensive damage to the kidneys, bone marrow, liver, and brain. Inhalants have been implicated in some forms of cancer. A "high" can last from a few minutes to an hour or more. Repeated use can produce physical and psychological dependence.

In the 1960s, the many deaths resulting from glue-sniffing made inhalant abuse a matter of nationwide concern. Studies reported later that about two-thirds of these deaths came about because the abusers, usually children, put plastic bags over their heads to intensify the high and accidentally suffocated.

In recent years, inhalant abuse has become a serious problem. It is the fourth most commonly abused substance among eighth graders and is abused nearly as frequently as marijuana. Still, 9 out of 10 parents believe their children have never abused inhalants.

Where to Find Help

Substance abuse has many disturbing aspects aside from the physical, psychological, and social damage that it can cause. With addictive medicines, the progression from a *therapeutic* dose—the amount prescribed by a physician—to a *toxic* dose may seem, to some persons, natural and even inevitable. Ingestion or injection of a *lethal* dose may follow as an unintended consequence.

Other factors are causes for concern. The proliferation of illicit street drugs, the rapidity with which dependence or addiction can develop, and the costs and complexity of treatment or detoxification programs all add to the dangers inherent in abuse as a spreading phenomenon. Researchers are discovering weapons that may help in some cases to make treatment more effective: *naloxone* (Narcan), for example, can be given intravenously to reduce the toxic effects of narcotics. But too often a drug has done irreversible harm in a human system before help arrives.

American society has begun to mobilize resources to aid those who need information, assistance, or counsel, for themselves or others, in cases of substance abuse. A National Partnership to Prevent Drug and Alcohol Abuse has established a network of community groups to inform teenagers about narcotics and their potentially disastrous effects. Since 1997 it has been possible for parents to test their children's urine for traces of drugs with kits available over the counter at pharmacies.

Those seeking further information or help may call a toll-free number, 800-COCAINE, where counselors are linked to a network of treatment centers and hospitals throughout the country. The addresses and telephone numbers of four national groups are:

Cocaine Anonymous World Services (CAWS)
P.O. Box 2000
Los Angeles, CA 90049-8000
(310) 559-5833

National Family Partnership (NFP)
2490 Coral Way, Suite 501
Miami, Fl 33145
(800) 705-8997

Parent Resource Institute for Drug-Free Education (PRIDE)
4684 S. Evergreen
Newaygo, MI 49337
(800) 668-9277

Narcotics Anonymous
P.O. Box 9999
Van Nuys, CA 91409
(818) 773-9999

30

The Environment and Health

How pure is the soil in which our food grows? How clean is the air we breathe or the water we drink? How healthy are the animals that provide substantial portions of our diets?

The Environmental Protection Agency (EPA) monitors, among other things, the level of pollutants in drinking water, the disposal of toxic wastes, the threat of radiation from nuclear power plants and the seepage of poisonous chemicals.

Harmful ingredients in the environment may be the result of pollution, accidental or intentional. Some enter the environment as a result of deliberate planning. Asbestos, for example, a mineral fiber that will not burn, was used widely to insulate and fireproof buildings. The EPA banned the use of asbestos in construction in the 1970s, after researchers proved the fiber caused diseases and several forms of cancer.

Major health hazards fall in four categories: Air, water and noise pollution and food contamination. Other hazards include toxic wastes, nuclear radiation, and work-place dangers.

Air Pollution

Air pollutants can damage health in a number of ways. Even where little scientific proof links these pollutants to specific maladies, much statistical or circumstantial evidence suggests that air pollution can lead to various forms of respiratory disease. Some cases of air pollution outside the workplace and exclusive of nuclear radiation hazards have been documented.

Sulfur Dioxide

Sulfur dioxide enters the air from many sources. In the main, however, it is spewed into the atmosphere when heavy fuel oil and coal are burned to provide heat, generate electricity, and provide industrial power. Large cities are especially vulnerable because of their concentrations of heavy industry.

Sulfur dioxide apparently irritates the lungs and leads to a reduction of the lungs' oxygen-handling capacity. Persons who are particularly susceptible to carbon and sulfur dioxide-filled smogs are those suffering from bronchial asthma, chronic bronchitis, and emphysema. The respiratory systems of such persons are already defective. In emphysema, for example, the elasticity of the air sacs in the lungs has progressively broken down, usually after prolonged infection or repeated bronchial irritation. Cigarette smoking can produce such irritation; the sulfur dioxide only worsens the situation.

Lead

Substantial evidence indicates that lead in the air can cause neurological harm and impair body chemistry and bone growth. Most airborne lead comes from combustion of solid waste, coal, and oils; emissions from iron and steel production and lead smelters; and tobacco smoke. Children are most immediately affected because they have fewer natural defenses against toxic absorption than adults. But adults too may feel the effects of such absorption. They may, for example, feel tired, cramped, or confused.

Because their bodies absorb and metabolize substances rapidly, children may have rates of lead absorption four times as high as those of adults. Workers in some industries, including the ceramic, glass, and lead industries, are also at risk. One study showed that 44 percent of the lead workers in two U.S. smelters suffered from clinical poisoning.

Specific effects of lead poisoning range across a broad spectrum. The formation of red blood cells may be inhibited even by low-level exposure to lead in the air. At higher levels, lead may cause anemia. In children, bone cell growth may be stunted; in pregnant women, lead may prevent the normal development of the fetal skeleton. But lead affects the brain primarily, in some cases interfering with motor skills, auditory development, memory, and the nervous system. Children with higher levels of lead absorption have been found to have serious learning disabilities. Fortunately, lead levels may fluctuate, and the lead in blood and soft tissue may pass out of the human system four to six weeks after exposure ends. But lead remains in bone for periods lasting as long as three decades.

Other Fuel Contaminants

Auto exhausts are major sources of air pollutants. Exhaust emissions may include nitrogen oxides, carbon monoxide, hydrocarbons, and soot. The latter is made up of visible particles of carbon suspended in the air.

Nitrogen oxides irritate the eyes and the respiratory tract. When nitrogen oxide and hydrocarbons mix in sunlight, they form other noxious substances in the typical photochemical smog that has a yellowish cast. The new ingredients include *ozone,* a poisonous form of oxygen, and peroxyacetyl nitrate (PAN), which is intensely irritating to the eyes. Los Angeles was the first city to experience these smogs; they now occur in many other cities as well.

Worst of all, auto exhaust hydrocarbons include varieties that are possible *carcinogens,* causes of cancer in susceptible individuals.

Acid Rain

While so-called *acid rain* has not been found to harm humans directly, scientists say it has begun to damage the natural food chain in certain regions. As industrial smokestacks emit pollutants, including sulfur and nitrogen oxides, these rise into the upper atmosphere. Mixed with water vapor and other substances, the airborne chemicals are changed by sunlight, becoming tiny acid droplets. The droplets fall to earth as rain or snow, raising the acid content of freshwater lakes and damaging trees and other plants. Under conditions of extreme acidity, fish populations have disappeared. Where the food web is disrupted, aquatic animals, algae, and bacteria may dwindle in number. The effects of acid rain on crops and trees are less apparent but are thought to be harmful.

To some extent, acid rain is a geographic phenomenon in North America. Factories in the midwestern industrial belt throw off most of the pollutants, which are then carried east and north. Southeastern Canada and the northeastern and eastern regions of the United States are the areas primarily affected.

Indoor Air Pollution

Reports of illness associated with office and other nonresidential buildings have given rise to what has been termed the "sick building syndrome." The causes of this syndrome, or complex of symptoms, have not been completely and precisely explained. Among the possible explanations are the following:

- Building ventilation has been reduced to conserve energy, with the result that ventilation is simply inadequate

- Indoor air has become contaminated by emissions from the building fabric and associated systems, furnishings, office equipment, or maintenance materials

- Entrainment or cross contamination has taken place, with contaminants generated in a different part of the building or in a separate building drawn in by an air-handling system

- Bioeffluents, or volatile human substances, spread throughout a building, polluting the air with pyruvic acid, lactic acid, acetaldehyde, butyric acid, carbon dioxide, and other body effluents
- Combustion byproducts from smoking tobacco have produced substances, smoke included, that contaminate indoor air
- Microorganisms or airborne particles from molds, dust mites, and other sources cause such illnesses as Legionnaires Disease

A common tendency has been to identify a public building's heating, ventilating, and air conditioning (HVAC) system as the cause of indoor air pollution. But that conclusion may be premature and overly nonspecific. The symptoms described by persons affected by the sick building syndrome should be studied closely. At least four separate illnesses have been isolated according to their symptoms and causes. Hypersensitivity Pneumonitis and Humidifier Fever usually produce such symptoms as coughing, wheezing, chest tightness, muscular aches, chills, headache, fever, and fatigue. While these conditions are rarely fatal, Legionnaires Disease, produced by the bacterium *Legionella pneumonophilae,* is notable because of its 15 to 20 percent mortality rate. Both Legionnaires Disease and the relatively less serious Pontiac Fever are identified by their pneumonia-like symptoms.

Carbon Monoxide

Carbon monoxide poisoning is one of the most common dangers of modern living. A colorless, odorless and tasteless gas produced whenever organic, or carbon-containing, substances burn, carbon monoxide can be lethal in poorly-ventilated spaces. The gas rapidly combines with hemoglobin to replace oxygen in the blood. The heart and the brain are most vulnerable, since they rely heavily on oxygen to function properly, and symptoms generally mimic those associated with impaired heart or brain functions: shortness of breath, nausea, headache, fatigue, weakness, dizziness, irritability, and reduced ability to concentrate. During winter is when most deaths attributed to carbon-monoxide poisoning occur, primarily due to clogged furnace exhaust systems and doors and windows too tightly sealed against the cold. Other common sources are tobacco smoke, motor vehicle exhaust, house fires, wood-burning stoves and fireplaces, factory machines with gas-powered engines, charcoal-burning barbecues, kerosene heaters and water heaters that run on gas or oil. Improvements in ventilation systems and public warnings to consumers have lowered the number of carbon monoxide deaths in recent years. In addition, most hardware stores sell carbon monoxide detection devices that sound an alarm when unsafe levels of carbon monoxide are reached. Many cities now require all homeowners and landlords to install them.

Secondhand Smoke

While it has long been established that cigarettes are harmful to smokers, only in the last two decades has research begun to establish the risks of cigarette smoke to nonsmokers, those who passively inhale "secondhand" smoke. In 1986, the Surgeon General's Report examined the smoke inhaled directly by smokers and the smoke passively inhaled by nearby nonsmokers, concluding that the chemical composition of both types of smoke was similar enough to warrant further study and to issue a preliminary warning about the potential dangers. Since then, a heated debate has raged. While some research has linked passive smoking to an increased risk of diseases, including lung cancer, other research indicates a negligible effect. Despite the frequent contradictions in data, public opinion has sided with nonsmokers who fear potential harm from environmental tobacco smoke. Fewer and fewer public places even allow smoking and many places, including New York City, Boston, and the state of California, have legislatively declared most public spaces to be smoke-free environments.

The only exception to the debate on the risks of passive smoking are very young children exposed to passive smoke. Studies have proven that pregnant women who smoke not only increase their risk of miscarriage and stillbirth, but also risk delivering infants with low birthweight who, as a result, are highly susceptible to health and development problems. Infants and toddlers of smoking parents have an increased incidence of bronchitis and pneumonia and are much more likely to be hospitalized for respiratory infections than children of nonsmoking parents.

Household Chemicals

Depending on its location, structural characteristics, and other factors, the typical home may have as many as 350 or more organic chemical pollutants in its interior air. Household chemical products like spray paints, insecticides, and furniture polish disperse tiny (and toxic) droplets into the air, adding the propellant to the chemicals in the basic product. Among the hazard-producing chemicals, some solvents in particular are known or suspected carcinogens. One of the worst is methylene chloride, found in paint sprays and paint strippers and in some hair sprays and insecticides. Product labels may identify methylene chloride as a "chlorinated solution" or as "aromatic hydrocarbons."

Radon

After cigarette smoking, say scientists, the second leading cause of lung cancer may be radon gas. Considered by many to be the most dangerous of all indoor air pollutants, radon, a naturally occurring radioactive gas, diffuses out of the ground into houses that happen to be built above subsurface sources.

Invading homes, according to the U.S. Environmental Protection Agency, radon causes between 5,000 and 20,000 lung cancer deaths annually. The gas breaks down into unstable elements called "radon daughters"; these become attached to particles of dust or other matter floating in the air. If breathed in, the radon daughters lodge in the linings of the lungs. Radioactive decay takes place almost at once, with the daughters emitting alpha particles that damage the adjacent lung cells, sometimes causing cancer.

Private homes can be tested for radon and, if hazardous levels are found, can be equipped with ventilation or other equipment to remove the health threat. A charcoal-based detector is available. Finally, many firms can conduct home radon checks for a fee.

Water Pollution

To an increasing extent, water pollution has prevented or limited use of many once-valuable sources of water. This progressive deterioration of the nation's water supply has resulted from years of abuse in which natural lakes and waterways were inundated with quantities of raw sewage, waste products of industrial plants and slaughterhouses, petroleum residues, poisonous herbicides and insecticides, and so on. But the pollutants generally fall into two categories: materials that change with time and contact with water, and materials that remain unchanged in form. Organic materials in sewage and such industrial wastes as pulp and paper effluents belong in the first group; inorganic salts like sodium sulfate and such inert inorganic materials as pesticides represent the second.

Communities generate thousands of tons of municipal sewage daily. Industries, the greatest users of water, utilize more than half of all the water consumed in the United States for raw material, heating and cooling processes, and transporting, sorting, and washing operations. Agriculture, the second largest user, requires millions of gallons of water for irrigation and drainage; for spraying orchards and crops, often with insecticides, fungicides, or herbicides; for removal of animal and other organic wastes; and for manufacturing operations such as meat packing and canning.

Chemical Contamination

The continuing proliferation of chemicals, many of them toxic, suggests the dimensions of the problems relating to water pollution. One estimate by the EPA's Office of Toxic Substances indicated that more than

70,000 chemicals are manufactured or processed commercially in the United States. About 1,000 new chemical compounds are added annually. Literally hundreds of these compounds find their ways into the nation's water supply, some in potentially dangerous concentrations.

How directly and to what degree chemical contaminants contribute to America's health bill cannot be gauged with accuracy. But the roles of these contaminants as carcinogens is widely accepted. Federal health officials have estimated that environmental carcinogens, including those in water, account for 55 to 60 percent of all U.S. cancer cases annually. Some estimates run much higher.

Heavy Metals

A study by the U.S. Geological Survey reported that small amounts of seven toxic metals were present in many of the nation's lakes and streams, with dangerous concentrations occurring occasionally. The metals are mercury, arsenic, cadmium, chromium, cobalt, lead, and zinc. Aside from being generally poisonous, some of these metals are implicated in specific health problems. Cadmium, as one example, has been linked to hypertension caused by kidney malfunction. Some other substances represent special situations.

Mercury

Because mercury is heavier than water, experts thought for years that it could be dumped into lakes, the oceans, and waterways. In theory, the mercury would lie harmlessly on the bottom. In reality, bacteria can convert some of the metallic part of the element into water-soluble form. The new compound enters the food chain and ends up in fish. When dangerous levels of this form of mercury were found in some waters and in food fish, warnings were issued regarding canned tuna and swordfish. The government later announced that 97 percent of the tuna on the market was safe to eat. But lakes and rivers across the country were closed to commercial and sport fishing.

An extremely toxic substance, mercury can, even in small concentrations, produce blindness, paralysis, and brain damage. The U.S. Food and Drug Administration has established the safe limit of mercury in food at half a part per million—about the equivalent of a thimbleful in an Olympic-sized swimming pool.

PCBs

Among the chief water pollutants today are the *polychlorinated biphenyls* (PCBs), highly toxic chemicals used industrially in carbonless copying paper and as an additive in lubricants, paints, printing inks, coatings, waxes, and many other products. PCBs, which are *biodegradable* (capable of decomposing) only over a period of years, have been found in unusually large quantities in waterways downstream from manufacturing plants. The EPA banned the direct discharge of PCBs into any U.S. waterway in 1977 after tests showed that fish in some rivers, like the Hudson, had levels of PCBs far higher than the permissible levels.

No one knows what the long-term effects of ingesting small quantities of PCBs will be. But the chemical is a suspected carcinogen. PCB's have also caused severe skin and eye irritations and have been implicated in reproductive disorders, kidney damage, and liver ailments. Researchers believe that the millions of pounds of PCBs in the nation's water or in landfills will take many years to dissipate.

Sludge

Sewage treatment plants around the country also face the major health challenge of disposing of the sludge, or solid matter, that is removed from sewage in the treatment process. Sludge contains not only human wastes but the residues of petroleum products, detergents, toxic heavy metals such as cadmium, lead, and zinc, and many other contaminants. Disposal methods range from dumping on land to burning and to composting for use as fertilizer. But environmental experts maintain that the use of sludge as fertilizer constitutes a health hazard; and major food processors will not accept food grown with sludge as fertilizer. In refusing such food, the companies are following guidelines set by the National Food Processors Association, which has expressed concern for farm workers' health and for the health of the consumer.

The sludge comes from an estimated 6.8 billion gallons of sewage flushed daily into America's sewers. The sewage itself contains microorganisms that can endanger health. You may be risking gastrointestinal upsets if you swim at a beach that is posted with a sign proclaiming "polluted water." Scientists warn that the fish caught in sewage-polluted coastal waters and harbors may not only be cancerous, they may also be carcinogenic. A number of states including Michigan and New York have restricted or banned sales of tainted fish such as naturally grown carp, catfish, and striped bass.

Oil Spills

With the increasing reliance on supertankers to carry industrial and heating oil from abroad, the danger of major water-polluting oil spills in coastal areas has grown substantially. Several of these huge ships have gone aground and broken apart under heavy pounding by sea waves. Their cargoes have spilled into the oceans, where currents usually carry them many miles before they float ashore or sink to the ocean floor. The oil reaching land fouls beaches and kills water birds. Similar accidents on inland waterways have polluted rivers and lakes, killing fish and spoiling recreational areas.

Noise Pollution

"Pollution" refers generally to the various forms of physical pollution by liquids, gases, or solids. Few persons realize that we are all threatened by a pollutant so common that it tends to be overlooked: noise.

Noise assails us nearly everywhere. It fills homes with loud music or the dog's barking or the grinding of the washing machine and the workplace with the chatter of drill presses and the roar of huge engines. Neither city dwellers nor country people can live noise-free today; none of us can escape car and truck horns, motorcycles that belch sound, and the noisy throb of machinery.

Effects of Sound on the Eardrum

Noise is not just annoying; it is potentially dangerous, both physically and mentally. It has been described as "a slow agent of death." A form of energy, sound or noise is caused by anything that vibrates, that moves back and forth. Our ears receive the effects of this vibrating motion from a distance, great or small, via sound waves. These waves are successive series of regions of compressed air and partial vacuums, or areas of high and low air pressure. Sound can also travel through liquids and solids. We *hear* sound because our eardrums are moved back and forth by the changes in air pressure. The eardrum, or *tympanic membrane,* may perceive a sound that moves it only one billionth of a centimeter—the threshold of hearing. If the intensity of sound pressure becomes too great, we experience pain, and the eardrum or the delicate structures inside the ear may be damaged.

The intensity of sounds is often measured in units called *decibels,* or *db.* These units are logarithmic, that is, 10 db is ten times as powerful as 1 db, 20 db is 100 times as powerful, 30 db is 1,000 times as powerful, and so on. On this scale, 0 db is at the threshold of hearing; rustling leaves, 20 db; a quiet office, about 50 db; conversation, 60 db; heavy traffic, 90 db; a pneumatic jackhammer six feet away, 100 db; a jet aircraft 500 feet overhead, 115 db; a Saturn rocket's takeoff, 180 db.

For most people, the pain threshold is about 120 db; deafening ear damage can result at 150 db. But damage of various kinds can come from much lower exposures. Temporary hearing impairment can result from sounds over the 85 db now found in modern kitchens with all appliances going. If the ears do not get a chance to recover, the impairment will become permanent.

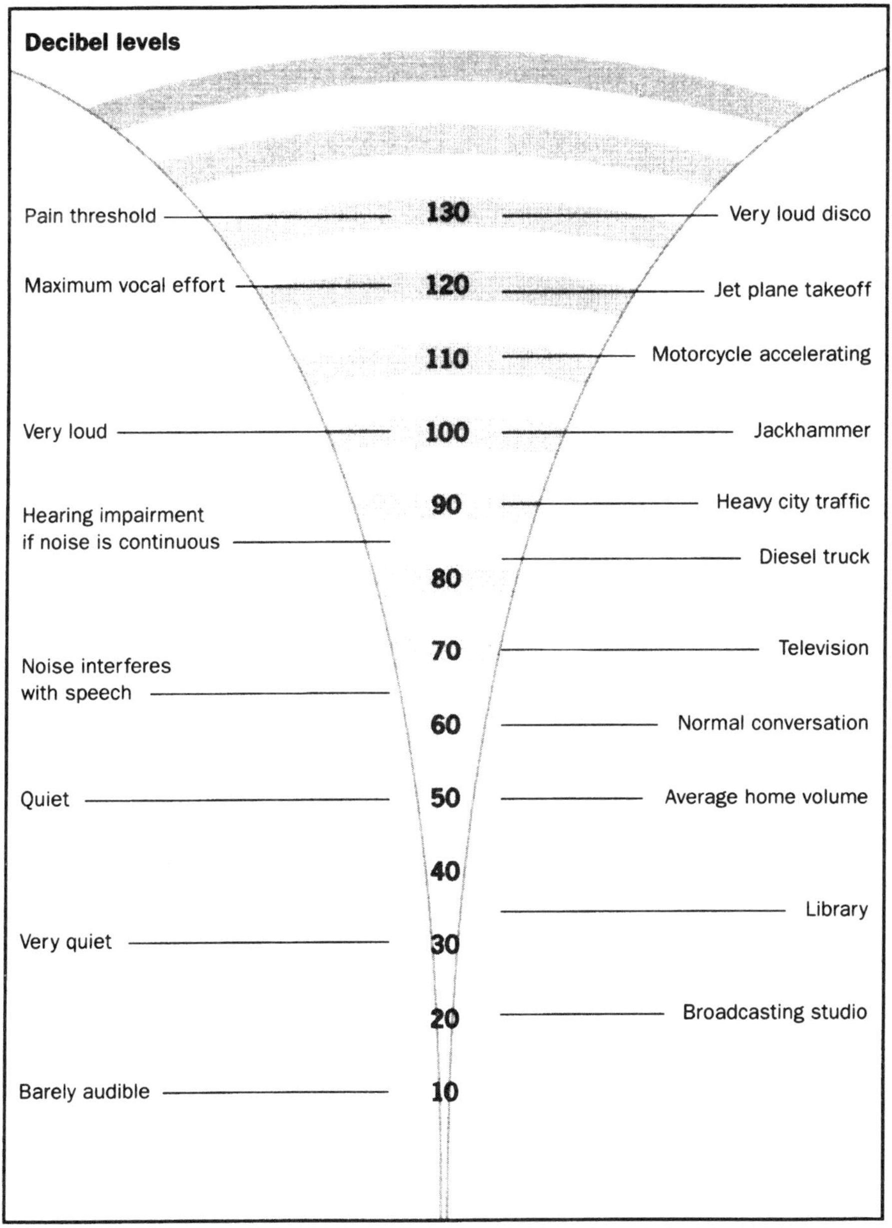

Damage to the Inner Ear

Although very loud noise can damage the eardrum, most physiological damage from noise occurs in the snail-shaped, liquid-filled *cochlea,* or inner ear. Sound transmitted to the cochlea produces waves in the liquid, which in turn move delicate and minute structures called hair cells or *cilia* in that part of the cochlea known as the organ of Corti. The motion of the cilia is transformed into electrical impulses that conduct the sensation of sound to the brain.

The cilia can easily be fatigued by noise, causing a temporary loss of hearing, or a shift in the threshold of hearing. If they are not given a chance to recuperate, they will be permanently damaged, and irreversible hearing loss will result. There are some 23,000 cilia in the average cochlea; different sets of cilia respond to different frequency bands. The cilia responding to sound frequencies of 4,000 to 6,000 cps (cycles per second) are especially vulnerable to damage. The region of 85 to 95 db is generally regarded as the beginning of dangerous sound intensities. In general, the louder the noise, the longer it lasts, the higher it is, and the purer in frequency, the more dangerous it is. Thus, jet engines and powerful sirens are particularly hazardous.

Noise and Stress

The EPA has estimated that some 20 million Americans live or work at noise levels that could cause hearing losses; about 18 million have experienced at least some hearing loss because of noise exposure. But sound, or noise, can lead to physical and psychological problems ranging from irritability to migraine headaches. Linked with many such problems is stress, which has been found to cause high blood pressure, insomnia, ulcers, digestive disorders, alcoholism, anxiety, and many other ills.

Excessive noise has been implicated in such problems as adrenaline flow, elevated heart rates, and blood pressure. All are associated with heart disease. Noise can also affect children in special ways. For example, researchers believe it can retard language development and impair reading ability. Pregnant women exposed to excessive noise may show symptoms of stress and may pass on the harmful effects to their unborn babies. Studies in several countries have shown that the newborns of women living near airport runways experience a higher than normal incidence of birth defects.

Noise-related stress has a definite effect on mental well-being. No one knows exactly how, but noise can produce irritability, tension, and nervous strain. More seriously, British medical authorities have reported a significantly higher incidence of mental illness among people exposed constantly to aircraft noise.

Workplace Noise

Workplace noise presents special problems. Persons working in such industries as construction, mining, steel, lumber, and textiles are almost universally exposed to loud noises. Certain operations in other industries expose workers to high decibel levels. Overexposure takes place when employees work eight hours a day at sites with noise levels exceeding 90 decibels. Such standards, established by the government's Occupational

Safety and Health Administration (OSHA), provide also that overexposure occurs where workers are subjected to higher decibel levels for shorter periods.

Workplace noise can lead to problems similar to those produced by overexposure elsewhere. But many workers have little choice as regards the places where they work. For their parts, companies may have limited options insofar as noise control or abatement is concerned. Changing the gears of a machine or building an enclosure around it may not always be feasible.

Some professional musicians find it difficult or impossible to avoid excessive noise on the job. Rock music artists, for example, spend hours at a stretch in enclosed places that magnify sound that is already greatly amplified. Such persons may be at serious risk of incurring hearing losses.

Food Hazards

Contaminants found in water often make their way into food products in the cooking and packaging processes, so that many of the comments on water pollution apply here. Some dilute water pollutants become highly concentrated as they pass up the food chain and end in fish or other foods for man. Mercury was cited earlier as one example. Contamination of food with harmful microorganisms is an everpresent concern wherever standards of cleanliness and sanitation are low.

Additives

Food entails a whole new set of problems because of the thousands of new ingredients that have been added to it, directly and indirectly, in recent years. These substances include many that have been deemed necessary because of the revolution in food technology: the rise of packaged convenience foods of all kinds. Labels on today's convenience foods list preservatives, nutrients, flavors, colors, and processing agents. The trouble with food additives is that we have had little time to learn about their long-term effects on the body. The Food and Drug Administration does set standards in this area; but in the opinion of many experts, these safeguards are inadequate.

What do the additives do and what are they? What kinds of health hazards do they present? The principal kinds are explained below.

Nutrients

Some additives are simply vitamins and minerals that increase the nutritional value of food. Iodine is added to salt as a goiter preventative; vitamins A and D go into fortified milk. The vitamin and mineral additives are generally beneficial.

Preservatives

Preservatives do what the name implies: they protect against spoilage from molds, yeasts, or bacteria, or prevent oxidation. In the first category are such substances as salt, sugar, vinegar, and—among the controversial additives—sodium nitrate, sodium nitrite, and the sulfiting agents. Where some of these substances guard against illnesses like salmonella and *Clostridium botulinum,* or botulism, a deadly form of food poisoning, the controversial types may cause serious illnesses and even cancers. For example, nitrates and nitrites can combine with the amines in protein to become nitrosamines, powerful carcinogens.

The antioxidants include lecithin from soybeans, ascorbic acid (vitamin C), and *butylated hydroxytoluene* (BHT) and *butylated hydroxyanisole* (BHA). The latter two have been studied because they appear to protect against stomach cancer and liver damage.

Flavors

Of the more than 1,500 different flavors used in food, some are natural and some synthetic. Among the natural flavors are cinnamon, vanilla, and citrus oils. The synthetics, some of which, like vanillin, have exactly the same chemical compositions as their originals, include monosodium glutamate (MSG), hydrolyzed vegetable protein, and maltol. MSG in particular has become controversial because it can cause "Chinese restaurant syndrome," with temporary headaches, dizziness, and other unpleasant symptoms.

Colors

As a group, the color additives are the most controversial. But they range from beta carotene, a yellow coloring that is used in carrots and sweet potatoes and is beneficial, to a number of coal tar dyes. The FDA has banned as unsafe more than a dozen of the latter in recent years. Others are readily available and are widely used in cereals, baked goods, ice cream, and beverages.

Processing Agents

Many useful processing agents, including yeast and baking soda, are standard kitchen items. They help to control stability, moisture, texture, and other food qualities and characteristics.

Chemical Residues

Some toxic substances found in food appear in the natural environment. An example: the trace amounts of arsenic in cow's milk. Other poisons are introduced into the environment by humans. These, including fungicides, herbicides, and pesticides, have aroused deep concern among environmentalists and a growing number of private physicians.

American farmers use more than 350 approved agricultural chemicals, including about one billion pounds of insecticides annually. Because of such heavy use, about 52 percent of the average American's diet contains one or more kinds of chemical residues. Measured often in parts-per-billion, these can collect in human bodies. Permanent damage can result, according to researchers. Among the compounds are not only weed- and bug-killers like parathion but also growth-enhancers like daminozide.

Researchers warn of other problems with contaminated food. The use of antibiotics in livestock feed, for example, promotes the development of bacteria that resist antibiotics. As one result, humans who eat beef or pork that is improperly cooked may acquire infections that resist penicillin or tetracycline.

Irradiated Foods

Consumer groups have urged further study and cautious use of irradiation as a means of preserving many foods. At least 30 countries have approved radiation exposure to retard spoilage and aging; but concerns remain. They focus particularly on the nutritional losses thay may occur if foods are exposed to more than one kind of preservative, on the effects of radiation exposure on workers handling irradiated foods, and on environmental hazards that could emerge in the transport, storage, and handling of radioactive food-processing wastes.

The possible long-term effects of irradiation have led to other concerns. Radiation kills the salmonella microorganism, but may not affect more virulent and dangerous bacteria such as those responsible for botulism and may, over time, strengthen those other organisms. Irradiation might even produce dangerous mutations of some bacteria. Researchers point out further that meat can become contaminated after irradiation, indicating that other preservatives might have to be used.

Other Hazards

Toxic Wastes

Various estimates place the number of toxic-waste disposal sites in the United States at 14,000 to 20,000. Poisonous substances left over from industrial processes are buried or simply dumped at these sites, many of which present serious health hazards. Primarily, according to scientists, the open dumps, landfills, bulk storage containers, and surface impoundments at the thousands of sites spill toxic chemicals into the surrounding soil and through it into groundwater systems. Noxious fumes and even flames burst from some sites at unpredictable moments. The wastes include a huge variety of substances, among them chlorinated solvents, aromatic hydrocarbons, pesticides, trace metals, and PCBs.

The locations of many waste disposal sites remain unknown, often, until a health or environmental problem is detected. Thus the health threats posed by waste dumps may lie dormant for years and may surface only after a container has rusted through or seepage has brought poisonous slush into contact with drinking-water sources.

Waste chemicals can enter the body through skin contact and inhalation as well as ingestion. But the latter is the most common method. Where dosage is substantial, ingestion usually leads to toxic effects on the liver and kidneys. Other parts of the body may be affected as well. Skin contact may produce lesions while inhalation can have direct respiratory effects.

Improved methods of disposing of toxic wastes have combined with public awareness and governmental action to build hopes of reduced waste problems in the future. In the meantime, as environmentalists contend, the thousands of existing toxic-waste sites pose continuing health hazards.

Nuclear Radiation

Among the most dangerous of all pollutants is nuclear or "ionizing" radiation. Made up of particles of energy, this radiation can attack the atoms that form the body's cells, causing both short- and long-term damage. Human tissues like skin, bone-marrow, and intestinal cells, all of which reproduce rapidly, feel the impact of radiation most intensely. But different isotopes in ionizing radiation concentrate in different body tissues, sometimes causing cancer or genetic mutations many years after exposure. Of the most common radioactive elements in radiation from a nuclear power plant, barium resembles calcium and therefore concentrates in the bones while iodine 131 concentrates in the thyroid.

Completely invisible, radiation reaches the earth from various natural and manmade sources. Some comes from the sun and outer space; larger amounts are given off by radioactive materials, including waste from nuclear power plants, the fallout from nuclear weapons explosions, and various electronic devices. The numbers of such devices are increasing steadily; among them are lasers, X-ray machines, TV sets, and microwave ovens.

The damage done to the human body as a result of exposure to radiation varies with the intensity of the "dose" and the isotopes involved. A dose of radiation above 1,000 rem, a unit of measurement, is always fatal. Smaller doses, with exposure over an extended period of time, may also be fatal. Victims can protect themselves to a limited degree if given time. For example, they can guard against thyroid cancer by taking potassium iodide. Ingested in pill form, the medication loads the thyroid gland with iodine, thus "blocking" the iodine 131 isotope and preventing its concentration in the thyroid.

In a simple operation physicians can transplant marrow into persons exposed to the barium isotope, and thus reduce the possibility of bone-marrow syndrome. This illness cripples the body's immune system. But donor marrow must match that of the victim, and the relatives of a victim are those most likely to supply marrow that is a genetic match. If the relatives have also been exposed to radiation, no donors may qualify.

Workplace Dangers

Air and noise pollution are, as noted, common in certain industries. The materials and machines used in manufacturing processes are the usual causes of such pollution. Many controls have been mandated by the federal Occupational Safety and Health Administration, but researchers have reported that some industries are experiencing increased health hazards, largely because of the materials they use.

High-tech microelectronics plants are especially threatened. According to scientists, many such plants use toxic chemicals that have been linked to reproductive disorders in both men and women. Among the high-tech hazards usually cited are glycol ethers, widely used as a solvent by manufacturers of printed circuit boards; arsenic, an element in the manufacture of some semiconductor chips; and lead, used in soldering and other operations. Some semiconductor plants are also employing radiofrequency radiation in potentially dangerous amounts to etch and clean silicon wafers.

Musculoskeletal Disorders

Carpal tunnel syndrome and other neurological and musculoskeletal disorders frequently occur in the workplace and are usually the result of a repetitive motion or series of movements which strain or damage nerves and muscles. Poor posture, uncomfortable or poorly-designed chairs and equipment, and lengthy periods of the same repetitive motion exposes the nerves and muscles of the body, often the hands and arms, to agonizing pain. In most cases, behavior modification, exercises, surgeries, and specially-designed furniture or equipment can completely eradicate pain and incidence of these disorders. A physician should be consulted for individualized diagnosis and treatment.

31

Health Insurance

The term "health insurance" refers to a broad range of insurance policies. To many people, health insurance means the kind of insurance offered by employers to employees. Health insurance has two basic purposes. It provides for reimbursement to families or individuals for health care costs. It may also guarantee replacement income when a person is unable to work because of sickness or injury. Reimbursement insurance can cover virtually all types of expenses connected with hospital care, medical treatment, and related services. Disability insurance usually involves periodic payments to make up for lost income.

From another perspective, health insurance offers protection to both groups and individuals. The groups may be company workforces that have *group insurance* as a benefit. Individuals can buy insurance from as many as 1,800 commercial insurance companies offering a huge variety of plans. Some insurers are general insurance companies. Others are hospital and medical service plans such as Blue Cross and Blue Shield, group medical prepayment plans such as health maintenance organizations (HMOs), and others.

What Health Insurance Is and Does

"Health insurance" means a number of things. It may be called "accident and health insurance" or "disability insurance." Various types of policies have other names. The different descriptions indicate that the policies vary regarding the types of expenses covered. While some policies cover only hospital expenses, others may cover virtually all kinds of medical expenses.

Two Types of Coverage

In general, private health insurance coverage is one of two kinds: *group* or *individual*. Employers, unions, and other kinds of organizations typically provide group insurance as an employee or membership benefit. An individual can buy individual insurance whether or not he or she is covered under a group policy. But a good group policy usually covers all the major health problems or contingencies that a person could face under normal circumstances.

Group insurance has a number of specific advantages over individual coverage, among them the following:

- Because a number of people can be included under a single contract, with consequent savings to the insurer in sales, administrative, and claims costs, the insurer can charge less per individual covered.
- In most cases the company, union, or organization holding the group contract pays part or all of the individual premiums.
- With group insurance, the health of the individual insured person is usually not a major factor in determining eligibility. The insurance company is more interested in the average age and overall health status of the group. The health of individuals may become a selection factor, however, when small groups of 10 or fewer persons are involved.
- Unless an individual leaves a job or gives up a membership, his or her group coverage cannot be canceled. Termination of the group plan itself would, of course, terminate coverage.

Despite the advantages of group insurance, individual and family policies fulfill at least two fundamental needs. First, they provide coverage for persons who are not members of an insured group. Such policies may also cover those who cannot, for whatever reason, obtain group coverage. Second, the individual or family policy can provide supplementary coverage when a group plan does not meet all basic health insurance needs.

Group and individual plans differ in basic ways. Whereas a group policy establishes the level of benefits for all group members, the individual policy can more easily be tailored to specific requirements. With the individual policy, too, each person or family is enrolled separately. The premiums of individual insurance are usually substantially higher because the insurer considers the age, health status of the insured, and other factors when setting premium rates.

Principles of Health Insurance

Private or commercial health insurance programs function according to certain key principles. Primarily, these programs are based on the theory that a relatively small, regular payment, the premium, can protect the insured against what might be a sizable loss.

A companion principle holds that the insured must pay the expenses of operating an insurance system. These expenses include the costs of maintaining offices, investigating claims, and otherwise administering the system as well as paying benefits.

Two other principles underlie the operation of most health insurance programs:

- The *large-loss principle,* which holds that the insured should try to obtain protection only against those costs or losses that he or she could not bear financially. Under the large-loss principle, the contract may exclude from reimbursement some specific kinds of costs. Most such policies contain a "deductible" clause specifying that the insured must pay a certain amount of initial costs.

  Major medical insurance plans probably exemplify best the large-loss, or large-risk, principle. These policies nearly always provide for a deductible. The higher the deductible, as a rule, the lower the premium.

- The *first-dollar principle,* under which the policy pays the full cost of all covered hospital and medical expenses. Policies of this kind have no deductible clauses or co-payments.

  Advocates of first-dollar policies stress the need for preventive health care. The policy in theory encourages the insured to see a physician and obtain treatment before a health problem becomes worse or even unmanageable.

Kinds of Insurance Plans

Private health insurance plans offer protection against abroad range of hospital and medical expenses. Some policies offer protection against a single illness such as cancer while others insure individuals, families, or groups against nearly all medical contingencies. Some of the many kinds of coverage are as follows:

Hospital

Blue Cross plans and most other commercial plans provide daily hospital room and board at a specified rate. Usually, they also cover miscellaneous hospital services, including drugs, operating room, and laboratory services up to a given cost level. Many commercial plans and most Blue Cross plans cover all costs in a semiprivate, or shared, room. Of all types of health insurance, hospital insurance is the most widely used.

Surgical

Typically, health insurance policies cover the costs of surgery according to a fee schedule that establishes specified amounts for listed procedures. The insurance contract sets a payment maximum for operations such as appendectomies or tonsillectomies, with that payment going toward coverage of the surgeon's bill. In the case of Blue Shield, certain surgeons perform surgical operations for low-income subscribers for no additional charge.

Regular Medical

This form of insurance, which is also referred to as general medical, provides coverage of physicians' fees in cases that do not involve surgery. The medical care may be provided in the home, in a hospital, or in a physician's office. A regular medical policy may also cover diagnostic X-ray and other laboratory expenses.

Major Medical

Major medical policies help cover the high costs of serious or catastrophic accidents or lengthy illnesses. As noted previously, such policies usually provide for deductibles. After an insured patient has reached a specified hospital-medical expense level, the insurer will pay, for example, 80 percent of all remaining expenses to a set maximum. The maximum may be $1 million or more. Some policies offer unlimited coverage. In some cases the policy sets a maximum, perhaps $5,000, $10,000, or $25,000, for a given illness in a one- or three-year period.

Comprehensive or Comprehensive Major Medical

This kind of health policy combines hospital, regular medical, major medical, and surgical coverage in one contract. Generally, little or no deductible applies to hospital and surgical charges. But the major medical coverage ordinarily comes with a deductible.

Dental

Dental insurance is usually available through group plans, and employers sometimes offer it as a fringe benefit. A basic dental plan may establish a set of allowances for each procedure to an annual maximum of, for example, $500 or $1,000. A comprehensive dental policy would cover, typically, 80 percent of all dental expenses above a specified minimum.

Special Perils

Although frowned upon by many insurance experts, "special perils" plans continue to appear. They cover such specific health hazards as cancer, polio, and vision problems. Under a special perils policy, the insurance company must provide coverage for the illness caused by the health hazard, unless it can prove that the specific health hazard is not excluded.

Auto and Travel

Many insurance companies offer auto and travel policies that cover insured persons in the event of an accident causing injury or death. Such policies may provide protection against almost any travel accident in various kinds of vehicles.

Loss of Income

Loss of income, or *disability insurance,* is the oldest kind of health insurance. It insures against loss of income and gives the insured person a flow of cash if, because of illness or disability, he or she cannot work. An individual commercial policy that limits coverage to accidental disability usually costs much less than broader coverage, or it provides for greater benefits. Accidental disability payments, usually monthly, may continue for life. Payments for disability resulting from illness are commonly limited to 6, 12, or more months, depending on the terms of the contract.

Many policies provide only for *hospital income insurance.* Such insurance pays a stipulated cash payment for every day of hospitalization. Insurance companies offer these policies to individuals only, not to groups.

Basic or Hospital-Surgical Protection

Of the various kinds of comprehensive health insurance, the so-called "basic protection" plan ranks among the most common. Basic protection covers the costs of hospital care and services and physicians' services.

Most basic protection policies specify that hospital room and board benefits will be paid in one of two ways. One kind of policy provides for reimbursement for a per-day dollar amount, which covers actual room and board charges up to a set daily maximum. Another kind offers a service type of benefit equaling the hospital's established semiprivate room and board daily rates. If the insured occupies a private room, he or she pays the additional room charge.

Surgical-Expense Insurance

Basic policies that provide hospital expense coverage generally offer surgical-expense benefits as well. That means coverage may extend to operations and postoperative, inpatient physicians' visits. The policy then becomes a "hospital-and-surgical-expense" or "hospital-surgical" plan.

Surgical-expense insurance normally pays benefits whether illness or accident makes the surgery necessary. Coverage may include benefits for anesthetics. A set schedule of surgical procedures and specified maximum benefits for each procedure is generally part of such a policy. Alternatively, physicians' fees may be covered to a "usual, customary, and ressonable (UCR)" level for the particular city or region. In this case, the policy would not contain a surgical schedule.

Physician's-Expense Insurance

The counterpart of the surgical-expense policy is the physician's-expense plan, sometimes called "regular medical expense insurance." This policy offers benefits to help cover the costs of nonsurgical physicians' services in a hospital, home, or office. The terms of the policy usually provide for maximum payments for specified services. The latter may include diagnostic X-ray and other laboratory expenses. It usually specifies a maximum benefit per visit (for example, $25 or $50) and a maximum number of visits per injury or illness.

Policy Provisions

Purchasing health insurance calls for close attention to the provisions of any given policy. Little standardization exists among the hundreds of types of policies, a factor that makes the buyer's task difficult. In four areas in particular the buyer should scrutinize closely the fine print in an individual policy.

Provisions Relating to Other Policies

Many policies include clauses that limit or prohibit payments when the policyholder has other insurance covering the same loss or expense. In this way insurers protect themselves against overpayments for specific losses. A typical clause of this kind reduces benefits payments to the policy's prorated share of the insured person's actual expenses.

Cancellation and Renewal

All health policies contain cancellation and renewal provisions. One type, the most favorable to the policyholder, specifies that the insurer cannot cancel or refuse to renew the policy before the insured turns 65. The same clause may state that the premium cannot be increased. Because it provides guaranteed coverage, this kind of policy is usually the most expensive.

Many policies contain a widely used modification of the no-cancel, guaranteed renewal clause. This alternative provides that the company must continue the coverage until the insured reaches 65, but that the premium can be increased for entire groups of insured persons. In a third variation, some policies permit the insurer to cancel or refuse to renew the coverage at anytime by giving written notice to the policyholder. This kind of policy is the least advantageous to the insured.

"Good-Health" Discounts

Increasingly, the disability, hospital, or medical policy provides for discounts for persons in good health. For example, the policy may specify that the applicant be a nonsmoker who exercises three to five times a week and does not have a high-risk job or hobby. Race-car driving would fall in the latter category.

Discounts of 5 to 15 percent have been available to nonsmokers since the 1960s. New discount arrangements broaden the range of qualifying factors and increase the discount levels. The new trend takes as a model the life insurance plan that may offer discounts of up to 50 percent if the applicant observes basic rules of health and safety. These include, in addition to those named, adhering to a nutritious diet, using seat belts while riding in a car, and avoiding excess salt in the diet.

Meeting Special Needs

Some health insurance policies are designed to meet special needs. They tend to provide coverage for individuals with long-term medical problems or chronic health conditions who represent above-average risks for insurers. Special policies may totally exclude coverage for the specified health problem while providing all other standard benefits, or they may impose a waiting period before beginning coverage of the problem. The section below provides more information regarding preexisting medical conditions.

Some insurance policies that were initially designed to meet special needs are now common to the point of being standard. For example, dental-expense coverage is now available through a majority of group and individual insurance plans. Many group policies also make provisions for the cost of vision care.

Making Insurance More Widely Available

Before 1997, the health insurance industry regularly imposed exclusions that prevented many people from obtaining adequate, uninterrupted coverage. Such coverage would be denied because of preexisting medical conditions, unemployment or a change in jobs, or a host of other reasons. As of July 1997, however, the Health Insurance Portability and Accountability Act, commonly known as the Kennedy-Kassebaum bill, changed the law and effectively ended most of these exclusions.

Preexisting Medical Conditions

Preexisting conditions are physical or mental problems that existed before an individual joined a new health plan. In the past, insurers would not provide any coverage for claims related to these conditions or would require a waiting period before coverage could begin. Now, provided a medical problem has existed for 12 months or more, coverage cannot be denied. It is, however, important to note that people with preexisting conditions may still have to pay higher rates for individual health insurance policies. This is because they are above-average risks, and insurers might stand to lose money by having to pay their claims.

Unemployment and Job Changes

Because most health insurance is a job-related benefit, many people used to find that their coverage terminated when they became unemployed. After passage of the Kennedy-Kassebaum bill, this can no longer happen, as long as individuals have had insurance for at least 12 months before losing their jobs. For those who become unemployed, their former employer's insurer must provide an individual health insurance policy. For those who change jobs, their new employer's insurer must accept them into the group health insurance policy. Individuals who previously did not have insurance, or who had it for fewer than 12 months before losing their jobs, can continue to receive health coverage for 18 months, at their own expense, under the provisions of COBRA (Consolidated Omnibus Budget Reconciliation Act).

Mental Health and Divorce

According to the Kennedy-Kassebaum bill, if an individual was already covered when he or she had a previous opportunity to join a health plan; has exhausted COBRA coverage; or lost coverage because of divorce, death, or a reduction in work hours, the individual must be allowed to join a group health plan, provided that he or she requests enrollment within 30 days of losing coverage. A 1998 amendment to the Kennedy-Kassebaum bill prohibits health plans from placing more restrictive limits on mental health coverage than on coverage for physical illness.

"Medigap Insurance"

Virtually all Americans over age 65 are insured by Medicare. Yet this federal health insurance program covers only a portion of all possible physician and health expenses. To help bridge the gap between Medicare and the 100 percent coverage that most people want, private insurance companies have developed "medigap" policies.

The terms of these policies vary, but most simply expand existing Medicare coverages. Few offer even partial protection against hospital and medical costs that Medicare does not cover, either fully or partially. Benefits not covered by medigap policies include hearing tests and hearing aids, dental care and vision care, and long-term care in-home or at a nursing facility. Clearly, policies with such exclusions leave people vulnerable. Those trying to supplement their Medicare coverage must search out more complete policies, such as Blue Cross/Blue Shield's.

When considering a medigap policy, consumers should research the reputation of the insurer by calling the Better Business Bureau. Understanding all the terms of coverage before buying the policy will prevent unpleasant surprises later. Basing decisions on premium levels is rarely wise: rates can and do increase at all companies. Finally, older people should make sure they have both parts of Medicare coverage (medical insurance *and* hospitalization) before purchasing additional policies.

Managed Care

Pressures to cut the costs of medical care have given rise to basic changes in the methods of delivering such care in the United States. Most people no longer call their family physicians and, if so advised, go to the nearest hospital. Insurance plans and programs now offer both more choices and more restrictions. Managed care in particular has changed the face of health insurance. Managed care includes many types of health insurance and health care plans. Five are discussed below.

Health Maintenance Organizations (HMOs)

HMOs are the oldest of the managed care plans. Operating clinic-style facilities, HMOs require that their subscribers pay a set monthly premium. In return, the HMO provides full medical care. However, members must select their primary care physicians from a list provided by the HMO.

Charging premiums that are lower than those for equivalent insurance coverage, HMOs provide incentives to avoid unnecessary expenses or treatments. They generally encourage subscribers to make use of preventive care to stay healthy. Thus, most HMOs offer vision and hearing check-ups, as well as podiatric and dental services, at little or no cost beyond the monthly fee.

There are drawbacks for HMO subscribers. An HMO member may go to a hospital only with the advance approval of their primary care physician, except in emergencies. In some cases, HMO physicians under great pressure to minimize costs have failed to recommend expensive treatments even when they were the most promising options.

HMOs account for a large share of the health care market. More than 50 million American are members of HMOs. As HMOs grow in number, new and better regulations will be developed to ensure a higher standard of care for subscribers. Many state and federal laws passed in recent years have already contributed to notable improvements in HMOs, and the future is similarly promising.

Preferred Provider Organizations (PPOs)

In this form of managed care, subscribers receive care at a reduced fee if they go to physicians and hospitals that are part of a preselected network. Generally, the insurance company underwriting the PPO allows employees in insured groups to go to a nonparticipating physician. In such a case, the PPO pays less of the costs.

Under the PPO arrangement, physicians, hospitals, and insurers work together to keep down overall costs. A PPO hospital provides care for insured persons at reduced rates. In exchange, the hospital enjoys increased utilization of its facilities.

Point-of-Service (POS) Plan

Point-of-service plans are becoming increasingly popular among patients and are a rapidly growing form of managed care. A POS is sometimes referred to an as "open-ended" HMO, although some PPOs also offer POS plans. In this plan, the primary care physician usualy makes referrals to other health care providers in the network, and the plan pays all or most of the expenses. However, members can refer themselves to providers outside the network if they wish and still receive some coverage. This is an important consideration for patients who want to see a specialist. The deductibles and copayments are higher in a POS plan than in an HMO or PPO, but the POS gives patients more freedom of choice.

Hospital Chains

Competition among health care providers has led to still another approach to both cost control and hospital utilization. Some for-profit hospital chains have bought insurance companies to obtain insurance licenses, then provided health insurance programs that required the insured to use the chain's facilities.

A variation on the HMO and PPO systems, the hospital chain approach makes possible insurance costs that are 10 to 15 percent lower than those of traditional plans. Chain officials contend that the lower charges are justified by more efficient hospital operation.

Insurance experts have noted characteristics of the hospital chains' programs that appear to justify caution on the part of the potential buyer. For example, the policies sold by the chains usually impose limits on lifetime benefits. Unlike the plans of such not-for-profit groups as Blue Cross/Blue Shield, the chains' policies provide for the termination of certain benefits at specified ages.

Long-Term Care

Increasingly, major insurance companies have begun to devise policies that cover the costs of long-term care for the elderly, in-home or at a nursing care facility. The terms of these policies vary, and some of them fall short of expectations. For example, rather than providing a live-in companion as soon as health begins to decline, many insurers will provide in-home care only after a stay in the hospital. Even individuals who have specific in-home care policies find that their insurers use their own stringent guidelines to determine if and when that care is needed.

Such specialized plans face a double financial difficulty. First, the insurance company needs to make a profit. Second, the costs of nursing home and in-home care that can cost several thousand dollars each month raises the possibility of enormous claims that could continue for many years. Some companies work through organizations like AARP. The memberships of such groups are usually large enough to reduce the premiums for the buyers and the risks of major claims for the insurers.

With long-term care policies in particular, it is important for people never to buy more insurance than they can afford, as they may never need to make a claim. They should also plan ahead as far as possible: purchasing coverage in advance of one's retirement years tends to secure lower premiums and better benefits. And, as with all policies, individuals should understand all the terms of coverage and the exclusions before making a purchase.

32

Home Care of the Sick

Patients suffering from serious illnesses or from certain communicable diseases should be hospitalized. Home care facilities do not normally include the expensive and delicate medical equipment required for the complete care of these diseases.

If, however, the physician in charge of a case decides that his patient does not need hospitalization and that adequate home nursing care can be provided, the well-being of the patient can be greatly enhanced by his being cared for in the comfortable and familiar surroundings of his own home.

When the decision to treat a patient at home is made, it must be understood that the physician's orders regarding rest, exercise, diet, and medications have to be rigorously adhered to. Nursing responsibilities assigned to the patient and whoever else is tending to the patient's recovery should be carried out as conscientiously as they would be if the patient's care were entrusted to a team of medical professionals in a hospital environment.

The physician in charge of a case should, of course, be notified of any significant changes in the condition of the patient. The physician should be contacted if, for example, the patient complains of severe pain, pain of long duration, or pain that apparently is not directly related to an injury or surgical procedure. The location and characteristics of the pain should be noted, and the physician will want to know whether the pain is affected by changing the position of the patient or if it seems to be related to the intake of food or fluids.

In addition to being informed of such potentially dangerous developments, the physician should get daily or frequent reports on the patient's progress. The easiest and best way to see that this is done is to keep a written record of the following functions, symptoms, and conditions of the patient:

- Morning and evening body temperature, pulse rate, and respiration rate
- Bowel movements—frequency, consistency of stools, presence of blood
- Urination—amount, frequency, presence of burning sensation, color
- Vomiting or nausea
- The amount and kind of solid foods and liquids taken by the patient
- Hours of sleep
- Medications given (should be administered only on the instructions of the physician)
- Patient's general appearance (includes any unusual swelling, skin rash, or skin discoloration)
- General mental and psychological condition of the patient, such as signs of irritability or despondency

Checking the Pulse and Respiration

The pulse and respiration are usually checked in the morning and again in the evening; the physician may recommend other times as well.

Pulse

The home nurse should learn how to measure the pulse rate in beats per minute. A watch with a second hand or a nearby electric clock will help count the passage of time while the pulse beat is counted. The pulse can be felt on the inner side of the wrist, above the thumb; the pulse also can be checked at the temple, the throat, or at the ankle if for some reason the wrist is not conveniently accessible.

The patient should be resting quietly when the pulse is counted; if the patient has been physically active the pulse count probably will be higher than normal, suggesting a possible disorder when none actually exists. Temperature extremes, emotional upsets, and the digesting of a meal also can produce misleading pulse rates.

What is a normal pulse rate? The answer is hard to define in standard or average terms. For an adult male, a pulse rate of about 72 per minute is considered normal. The pulse of an adult woman might range around 80 per minute and still be normal. For children, a normal pulse might be one that is regularly well above 100 per minute. Also, a normal pulse may vary by a few beats per minute in either direction from the average for the individual. The home nurse with a bit of practice can determine whether a patient's pulse is significantly fast or slow, strong or weak, and report any important changes to the physician.

Respiration

The patient's respiration can be checked while his pulse is taken. By observing the rising and falling of the patient's chest, a close estimate of the rate of respiration can be made. An average for adults would be close to 16 per minute, with a variation of a few inhalations and exhalations in either direction. The rate of respiration, like the pulse rate, is higher in children.

Sometimes the respiration rate can be noted without making it obvious to the patient that there is concern about the information; many persons alter their natural breathing rate unconsciously if they know that function is being watched.

Body Temperature

A fever thermometer, available at any drugstore, is specially shaped to help the home nurse read any tiny change in the patient's temperature, such changes being measured in tenths of a degree. Instead of being round in cross-section like an ordinary thermometer, a fever thermometer is flat on one side and ridge-shaped on the other. The inner surface of the flat side is coated with a reflective material and the ridge-shaped side actually is a magnifying lens. Thus, to read a fever thermometer quickly and properly, one looks at the lens (ridged) side.

How To Take the Temperature

The usual ways of taking temperature are by mouth (oral) or by the rectum (rectal), and fever thermometers are specialized for these uses. The rectal thermometer has a more rounded bulb to protect the sensitive tissues in the anus. Normal body temperature taken orally is 98.6° F. or 37° C. for most people, but slight variations do occur in the normal range. When the temperature is taken rectally, a normal reading is about 1° F. higher—99.6° F. or about 37.5° C.—because rectal veins in the area elevate the temperature slightly.

Before a patient's temperature is taken, the thermometer should be carefully cleaned with soap and water, then wiped dry, or sterilized in alcohol or similar disinfectant. The thermometer should then be grasped firmly at the shaft and shaken briskly, bulb end downward to force the mercury down to a level of 95° F. or lower—or 35°

C. or lower if the thermometer is calibrated according to the Celsius temperature scale. See the chart *Body Temperature in Degrees* for comparative values of the Fahrenheit and Celsius scales.

If the temperature is taken orally, the thermometer should be moistened in clean fresh water and placed well under the tongue on one side. If the temperature is taken rectally, the thermometer should be dipped first in petroleum jelly and then inserted about one inch into the opening of the rectum. If an oral thermometer is used in the rectum, special care should be taken to make sure that the lubrication is adequate and that it is inserted gently to avoid irritating rectal tissues. Whichever method is used, the thermometer should be left in place for at least three minutes in order to get an accurate reading.

Body Temperature in Degrees

Fahrenheit		Celsius
105.5		40.8
105		40.6
104.5		40.3
104		40
103.5		39.7
103		39.4
102.5		39.2
102		38.9
101.5		38.6
101		38.3
100.5		38.1
100		37.8
99.5		37.5
99		37.2
98.6	Normal	37.0
97.8	Range	36.6

If circumstances preclude an oral or rectal temperature check, the patient's temperature may be taken under the arm; a normal reading in that area is about 97.6° F. or 36.5° C.

Above-Normal Temperature

If the patient's temperature hovers around one degree above his normal reading, the home nurse should note the fact and watch for other signs of a fever that would indicate the presence of an infection or some other bodily disorder. A mild fever immediately after surgery or during the course of an infectious disease may not be cause for alarm. Also, the normal body temperature of a mature woman may vary with hormonal changes during her menstrual cycle. But when oral temperatures rise above 100° F. the change should be regarded as a warning signal. A rise of as much as three degrees above normal, Fahrenheit, for a period of several hours or more, could be critical, and a physician should be notified immediately.

Sleep

Another item to be checked each day for the at-home medical records is the patient's sleeping habits. While there is no standard number of hours of sleep per day preferred for healthy individuals, a regular pattern of sleep is very important during recovery from disease or injury, and an obvious change from such a pattern can suggest tension, discomfort, or other problems. Typical daily sleep periods for most adults range from 7 to 9 hours, while children and infants may sleep as much as 12 to 20 hours per day and be considered normal; sleep in the form of naps should be included in total amounts per day.

Making the Patient Comfortable

A good deal of the patient's time at home will be devoted to sleep or rest, most or all of it in bed. The bed should give firm support to the body; if the mattress does not offer such support, place a thick sheet of plywood between the springs and mattress. Pillows can be placed under the head and shoulders of the patient to raise those parts of the body from time to time. When the patient is lying on his back, a small pillow can be slipped under the knees to provide support and comfort. A small pillow can also be placed under the small of the back if necessary. Additional pillows may be placed as needed between the ankles or under one foot or both feet.

If the pressure of bed clothing on the feet causes discomfort, a bridge made from a grocery carton or similar box can be placed over the feet but beneath the blankets. To help maintain muscle tone and circulation in the feet and legs, a firm barrier can be placed as needed at the foot of the bed so the patient can stretch his legs and push against the barrier while lying on his back.

Changing Position

Helping the patient change position in bed is an important home-nursing technique. Unless a definite effort is made to help the patient change positions at regular intervals, the sick person may tend to curl up into a sort of fetal position, with the hips and knees flexed and the spine curved. While this position may be preferred by the patient in order to increase body warmth or to relieve pain, the practice of staying in one position for longer periods of time can lead to loss of muscle tone and even deformities.

Moving or positioning the patient in bed should, of course, be done according to directions outlined by the doctor for the specific medical problem involved. Body movements should not aggravate any injury or other disorder by placing undue strain or stress on a body part or organ system that is in the healing stage. At the same time, the patient should be stimulated and encouraged to change positions frequently and to use as much of his own strength as possible.

If the patient is likely to need a very long period of bed rest, and the family can afford the modest expense, it may be wise to purchase or rent a hospital-type bed. The basic hospital bed is higher from the floor than ordinary beds, making the tasks of changing bed linens, taking temperatures, etc., easier for the home nurse. More sophisticated hospital beds have manual or electrical controls to raise the head and foot of the bed.

Helping the Patient Sit Up

The patient can be helped to a sitting position in bed by placing one arm, palm upward, under the patient's shoulder while the patient extends an arm around the nurse's back or shoulders. The nurse also may slip both hands, palms facing upward, under the patient's pillow, raising it along with the patient's head and shoulders. The same procedures can be used to help move a patient from one side of the bed to the other if the patient is unable to move himself.

When the patient has been raised to a sitting position, he should try to brace his arms behind him on the bed surface with elbows straightened. If the patient feels dizzy or faint as a result of the effort, he can be lowered to the back rest position again by simply reversing the procedure.

When the patient is able to support himself in a sitting position, he should be encouraged to dangle his legs over the side of the bed, and—when his strength permits—to move to a chair beside the bed and rest for a while in a seated position.

Bathing the Patient

A patient who is unable to leave the bed will require special help in bathing. When bath time comes, the nurse will need a large basin of warm water, soap, a washcloth, and several towels, large and small. A cotton blanket also should be used to replace the regular blanket during bathing, and pillows should be removed from the bed unless they are necessary at the time.

One large towel should be placed under the patient's head and another should be placed on top of the bath blanket, with part of the towel folded under the bath blanket. This preliminary procedure should help protect the bed area from moisture that may be spilled during the bathing procedure.

The bath should begin at the area of the eyes, using only clear water and brushing outward from the eyes. Soapy water can be applied to the rest of the face, as needed, with rinsing afterward. After the face, bathing and rinsing are continued over the chest and abdomen, the arms and hands, the legs and feet, and the back of the body from the neck downward to the buttocks. The external genitalia are washed last.

During the washing procedure, the nurse uses firm strokes to aid circulation and checks for signs of pressure areas or bed sores. Skin lotions or body powders may be applied, and a back rub given, after washing. The teeth may be brushed and the patient may want to use a mouthwash. After the personal hygiene routine is completed, a fresh pair of pajamas can be put on. If bed linen needs to be changed, the bathing period provides a good opportunity for that chore.

Changing the Bed Linen

Changing the bed linen while the patient is in bed can be a challenge for any home nurse. However, there are a few shortcuts that make the task much easier. First, remove all pillows, or all but one, as well as the top spread if one is used. Loosen the rest of the bedding materials on all sides and begin removing the sheets from the head of the bed, top sheet first. By letting the patient hold the top edge of the blanket, or by tucking the top edges under his shoulder, the blanket can remain in place while the top sheet is pulled down, under the blanket, to the foot of the bed. If the top sheet is to be used as the next bottom sheet, it can be folded and placed on the side with the top spread.

Next, the patient must be moved to one side of the bed and the bottom sheet gathered in a flat roll close to the patient. Then the clean bottom sheet is unfolded on the mattress cover and the edges, top, and bottom,

Changing Patients' Bed

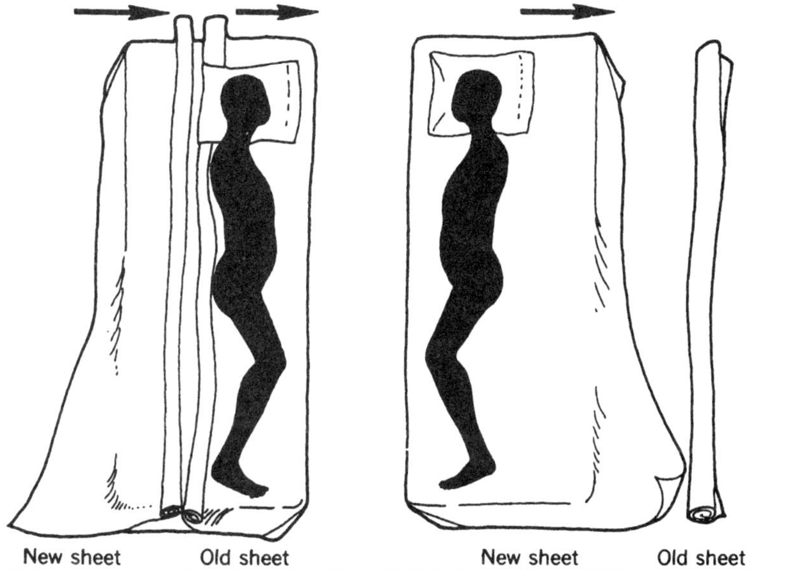

tucked under the mattress. The rest of the clean sheet is spread over the empty side of the bed and pushed in a flat roll under the soiled sheet next to the patient's back.

The next step is to roll the patient from one side of the bed onto the clean sheet that has been spread on the other side. The soiled bottom sheets can be pulled out easily and the new bottom sheet spread and tucked in on the other side.

The new top sheet can be pulled up under the blanket, which has been used to cover the patient throughout the change of bed linens. Finally, the top spread and pillows can be replaced, after the pillow cases have been changed. A special effort should be made, meanwhile, to keep the mattress cover and bottom sheet of the patient's bed as flat and smooth as possible and to allow room for the feet to move while the sheets are firmly tucked in at the foot of the bed.

The home nurse should handle the soiled linens carefully if the patient is being treated for an infectious disease; they should never be held close to the face.

Bowel Movements and Urination

If the patient is expected to remain bedridden for a long period of time, the home nurse should acquire a bedpan and perhaps a urinal from a drugstore. A sheet of oilcloth, rubber, or plastic material should also be provided to protect the bed during bowel movements and urination.

If the patient is unable to sit up on a bedpan because of weakness, his body can be propped up with pillows. If he is capable of getting out of bed but is unable to walk to the bathroom, a commode can be placed near the bed and the patient can be helped from the bed to the commode and back. Another alternative is to use a wheelchair or any chair with casters to move the patient between the bedroom and bathroom.

Administering an Enema

Occasionally, a physician may recommend an enema to help the patient empty his bowels or to stimulate the peristaltic action associated with normal functioning of the intestinal tract.

Since enemas are seldom an emergency aspect of home nursing, there usually is time to purchase disposable enema units from a drugstore. The disposable enema contains about four or five ounces of prepared solution packaged in a plastic bag with a lubricated nozzle for injecting the fluid into the patient's rectum. The entire package can be thrown away after it has been used, thus eliminating the need to clean and store equipment. The alternative is to use a traditional enema bag filled with plain warm water or a prescribed formulation.

An enema is best administered while the patient is lying on his side with his knees drawn up toward his chest. When using the disposable enema unit, the home nurse simply squeezes the solution through the lubricated nozzle that has been inserted into the rectum. When using an enema bag, the home nurse should lubricate the nozzle before insertion. After insertion of the nozzle, the enema bag should be held or suspended above the patient so that, upon the opening of the valve that controls the flow of the enema, the liquid will flow easily into the patient's rectum.

Feeding the Patient

It may be necessary at times for the home nurse to feed a patient unable to feed himself. An effort should be made to serve meals to the patient in an attractive and, when possible, colorful manner. The bedding should be protected with towels or plastic sheeting and the patient made as comfortable as possible with his head raised.

Liquids should be offered in a spoon filled about two-thirds full with any drops on the bottom of the spoon carefully wiped off. The spoon should be held so that the area between the tip and the side touch the patient's lower lip. Then the spoon is tilted toward the tip so the liquid will run into the patient's mouth. The process takes time, and much patience is required of the nurse. The patient may be slow to swallow and in no hurry to finish the meal.

If the patient can take liquids through a glass tube or plastic straw, the home nurse should see to it that the end of the tube inserted in the container of liquid is always below the surface of the fluid so that the patient will swallow as little air as possible.

A patient who can drink liquids from a spoon or tube may be able to drink from a cup. In making the step from tube or spoon to cup, the home nurse can help the patient by holding the cup by its handle and letting the patient guide the cup to his lips with his own hands.

The nurse should always make sure the patient is fully alert before trying to put food or liquid into his mouth; a semiconscious person may not be able to swallow. The nurse also should test the temperature of the food; cold foods should be served cold and warm foods should be served warm. But foods should never be too hot or too cold for the patient. Finally, the dishes, tubes, or other devices used to feed the patient should be carefully cleaned before storing them.

Ice Bags and Hot-Water Bottles

Ice bags and hot-water bottles frequently are used in home nursing to relieve pain and discomfort. The temperature of the water in a hot-water bottle or bag should be tested before it is placed near a patient's body. The maximum temperature of the water should be about 130° F., and preferably a few degrees cooler. The hot-water container should never be placed directly against the skin of a patient; it must be covered with soft material, such as a towel, to protect the patient against burns. A patient who is receiving pain-killing medications could suffer serious tissue damage from a hot-water bottle without feeling severe pain.

When ice is the preferred method of relieving pain, it can be applied in a rubber or plastic bag sealed to prevent leakage and covered with a soft cloth. Cold applications to very young and old persons should be handled cautiously and with medical consultation, particularly if ice packs are to be applied to large body areas for long periods of time; individuals at both age extremes can lack the normal physiological mechanisms for coping with the effects of cold temperatures.

Steam Inhalers

If the at-home patient suffers from a respiratory ailment that is relieved by steam inhalation, there are several devices to provide the relief he needs. One is the commercial electric inhaler that boils water to which a few drops of a volatile medication are added to provide a pleasantly moist and warm breathing environment. If a commercial inhaler is not available, a similar apparatus can be made by fashioning a cone from a sheet of newspaper and placing the wide end of the cone over the top and spout of a teapot containing freshly boiled water. The narrow end of the cone will direct the hot water vapor toward the face of the patient. If a medication is to be added, it can be applied to a ball of cotton placed in the cone; the steam or water vapor will pick up the medication as it passes through the cone.

If medicated vapor is intended for a small child or infant, the end of the cone can be directed into a canopy or tent made of blankets placed over a crib or the head of a bed. This arrangement should produce an effective respiratory environment for the child while keeping his body safely separated from the hot teakettle.

Still another method of providing steam inhalation for a patient requires only an old-fashioned washstand pitcher and bowl plus a grocery bag. An opening is cut in one corner of the bottom of the bag which is placed upside down over the pitcher filled with hot steaming water and, if needed, a medication. The patient simply breathes the hot moist air seeping through an opening in the bag. The pitcher of steaming water is placed in a bowl or basin as a safety precaution.

Improvising Sickroom Devices

With a bit of imagination, many sickroom devices can be contrived from items already around the house. A criblike bed railing can be arranged, for example, by lining up a series of ordinary kitchen chairs beside a bed; if necessary, they can be tied together to prevent a patient from falling out of bed. The bed itself can be raised to the level of a hospital bed by placing the bed legs on blocks built from scrap lumber. Cardboard boxes can be shaped with scissors and tape into bed rests, foot supports, bed tables, or other helpful bedside aids.

Plastic bags from the kitchen can be used to collect tissues and other materials that must be removed regularly from the sickroom. Smaller plastic bags may be attached to the side of the bed to hold comb, hairbrush, and other personal items.

Keeping Health Records

The family that keeps good records of past injuries and illnesses, as well as immunization information and notes on reactions to medications, has a head start in organizing the home care of a member who suddenly requires nursing. The file of family health records should include information about temperatures and pulse rates taken during periods of good health; such data can serve as benchmark readings for evaluating periods of illness. Also, if each member of the family can practice taking temperatures and counting pulse and respiration rates during periods of good health, the family will be better able to handle home nursing routines when the need arises.

Home Care Equipment Checklist

Following is a convenient checklist of basic supplies needed for home care of the sick:

1. Disinfectants for soaking clothing and utensils used by the sick. Not all disinfectants are equally effective for every purpose. For clothing and food utensils, corrosive or poisonous disinfectants are to be avoided. Antiseptics do not kill bacteria; they only retard their growth. Among the common disinfectants that can be used in the home are:

- Alcohol, 75 percent by weight, used for disinfecting instruments and cleaning the skin
- Lysol, for decontaminating clothing and utensils
- Soap with an antibacterial agent for scrubbing the hands
- Carbolic acid (phenol) for disinfecting instruments and utensils (it is corrosive, poisonous, and very effective if used in 5 percent solution)

- Cresol in 2.5 percent solution for disinfecting sputum and feces (less poisonous than phenol and can be obtained as an alkali solution in soap)
- Boric acid, a weak antiseptic eyewash
- Detergent creams, used to reduce skin bacteria

2. Disposable rubber gloves, to be used when handling patients with open wounds or contagious diseases, as well as for cleaning feces.

3. Paper napkins and tissues for cleaning nasal and oral discharges.

4. Rectal and oral thermometers. The former is used primarily for infants, while the latter is used for adults and older children. Thermometers should always be thoroughly disinfected after use by soaking in isopropyl alcohol, and they should be washed prior to reuse.

5. Eating and drinking utensils to be used only by the patient. Disposable utensils are preferable.

6. Urinal, bedpan, and sputum cup for patients who cannot go to the toilet. After use, they should be thoroughly disinfected with cresol and washed with liquid soap containing an antibacterial agent.

7. Personal toilet requisites: face cloths and towels, toilet soap, washbasin, toothbrush and toothpaste, comb, hairbrush, razor, and a water pitcher (if running water is not accessible to the patient).

8. Measuring glass graduated in teaspoon and tablespoon levels for liquid medication.

9. Plastic waste-disposal bags that can be closed and tied.

33

Health Care Delivery

A Changing Service

Unending change has characterized American health care in recent decades. The general practitioner in private practice, once the institutionalized symbol of medical care in the United States, has largely given way to specialists of many kinds. Whereas the general practitioner once sent a handwritten bill for services to the family home, he or she may now send a computerized invoice to an insurance company or a government agency. The "house call" has virtually disappeared.

Technology has taken over. Hospitals and other health care institutions may pay sums in seven figures for equipment that can save lives but that also demands to be used. A "technological imperative" requires that the new approach or instrument or drug at least be tried—experimented with, proven either useful or useless, and made available to those who need it. In diagnosis and therapy, physicians and other professionals are continually seeking the new and better.

In 2000, more than eleven million people were working in the American health care system. More than a half-million of those were physicians. The facilities in which the system's personnel work range from rural clinics to high-technology urban medical centers. On balance, the consumer dealing with this system has many choices. Understanding those choices may make the difference between a beneficial experience and a frustrating search for help.

Health care reaches the American public at three broadly defined levels. The three are primary, secondary, and tertiary care.

Primary Care

Essentially, *primary care* refers to "first contact" care as provided in physicians' offices or hospitals. Such care may also be provided in emergency rooms and outpatient clinics. The individual can obtain primary care without referral by a physician, but referrals from the primary care level are generally necessary to ensure that the patient will receive treatment at the next higher level. Among the types of services provided at the primary care level are health maintenance for infants and children, screening for infectious and communicable diseases, and treatment for minor injuries.

Secondary Care

At the *secondary care* level the patient usually comes under the care of a specialist or subspecialist, often in a community hospital or other, similar setting. Secondary level specialties include such well-known areas of medicine as obstetrics and gynecology, dermatology, otolaryngology, and cardiology. Although physicians often refer their patients for secondary level care, many other patients refer themselves.

Tertiary Care

At the tertiary care level, the patient receives highly specialized, high-technology care and treatment. Complex programs and unusual procedures, among them open heart surgery, organ transplantation, and neurological surgery, are provided by physicians with extensive training and the advantages of sophisticated equipment for diagnosis and treatment. Often, care at this level is obtainable only if the patient enters a hospital with specialized facilities. Of the various tertiary care institutions, three key ones are hospitals specializing in a certain disease or a group of diseases, hospitals associated with medical schools, and large regional referral centers. Many such institutions would be expected to have diagnostic equipment for such procedures as cardiac catheterization, nuclear magnetic resonance testing, and CT scanning.

Importantly, the three levels of care often overlap. The distinctions among them are not always clearly drawn or defined. For the patient, the most important factor may be the need for referrals at some levels and not at others.

Health Care Delivery Formats

The average American visits a physician three times a year. That statistic appears in a U.S. National Center for Health Statistics survey that also defines a visit as an encounter with a physician or other health professional under a physician's direction or supervision. The encounter can take place in the physician's office, in the patient's home, or in a hospital emergency department. The physician initiates about half of the encounters, usually as part of follow-up care.

Office and Clinic Care

In the main, the patient sees his or her physician in an office or at a site reserved for group practice; in a hospital outpatient department; in an ambulatory surgical center; or in a freestanding surgical center.

Office-Based Practice

Many physicians practice on their own; even so, the solo practice is declining as a way of medical life. The solo practitioner survives in isolated or rural areas, but hardly at all elsewhere. For the physician, solo practice is both simpler because of the independence and freedom it guarantees and more complex because the service responsibility may continue 24 hours a day, seven days a week. For the patient, the main advantage of solo practice is both the closer relationship that can develop and less fragmented care.

Partnerships

Very common today is the partnership, an agreement between two or more physicians under which the participants share office space, staff, and equipment. The physicians retain their independence in the sense that they have their own practices, but they usually share patient responsibilities under given circumstances. A physician who has to be out of contact with the office may, for example, give a patient another partner's number to ensure continuous backup. By spreading the care responsibilities and reducing the workload, each physician may also have more time for each patient.

The patient may find major advantages in the partnership. He or she can become acquainted with the physician's partner and in this way obtain personalized care at all times. Backup support may be especially important in obstetrics, where deliveries may occur without warning, and in cardiology, where emergencies are equally unscheduled.

Groups

When three or more physicians associate in an arrangement that is normally less formal than a partnership, they form a *group*. The physicians belonging to the group may practice in a single specialty or in diverse fields of medicine. An example of the latter is a group of three doctors offering internist, obstetrics-gynecological, and pediatric services. In other ways the group shares the advantages and disadvantages of the typical partnership. Like the partnership, the group has one particular advantage, however: other physicians are available for consultation and education. The group format may also make possible relatively sophisticated laboratory and other facilities.

Health Maintenance Organizations

The health maintenance organization (HMO) ranks as a special kind of group practice, one that involves a fixed monthly or annual fee system rather than a traditional fee-for-service arrangement. Usually, the HMO member is charged a small copayment for each doctor or emergency-room visit. The fixed fee ensures that the HMO member will receive all necessary health services, including hospitalization and the care of specialists. Preventive medicine at little or no extra cost to the member is a feature of the HMO that has ensured reduced usage of hospital facilities.

Preferred Provider Organizations

Like the HMO, the preferred provider organization (PPO) is at least partly a response to rising health-care costs. It is a combination of traditional fee-for-service and an HMO. In a PPO, a group of physicians contracts individually with an insurance company or employer to provide health services for fees that are usually lower than those prevailing in the community or area. Although the PPO charges on a fee-for-service basis, employees making use of the organization's medical services save money because they avoid the copayments of conventional insurance plans and the standard deductibles. Physicians belonging to the PPO have a stable pool of employed members whose health needs may be extremely diverse. For the employer or insurance company, a particular advantage is the ability to bargain for lower fees.

Three Alternative Systems

Office and clinic care take many forms. Three alternatives that provide relatively minor, low-level services are the hospital outpatient department, the ambulatory surgical center, and the freestanding emergency center. Each plays a particular role in the health care delivery network.

Hospital Outpatient Departments

Outpatient departments once offered free services as a means of training medical students and residents or because physicians volunteered their services for such departments. Today, outpatient departments charge for their services while delivering health care that varies broadly in quality. Patients leave the same day they come in and do not occupy a hospital bed overnight. Many operations that used to require a hospital stay, such as breast biopsy and hernia repair, can now be performed on an outpatient basis in most hospitals.

Ambulatory Surgical Centers

Sometimes called surgicenters, the ambulatory surgical center may be attached to a hospital or be completely independent. In either case, the surgicenter may be an effective alternative in the traditional situation when a patient needs an abortion, a dilatation and curettage (D & C), hernia repair, or tissue biopsy. Because they perform lower-risk procedures, ambulatory surgical centers can keep costs down. Local anesthesia is the norm, and usually the patient goes home on the day of the operation.

Freestanding Emergency Centers

Sometimes called *urgicenters* (because they treat urgent cases), freestanding emergency centers resemble hospital emergency departments. But private, for-profit groups usually run them. Open from 12 to 24 hours daily, they operate on a drop-in basis, meeting a definite need when a hospital emergency room is far away or when all physicians' offices have shut down for the day. Typically, emergency centers treat sprains and bruises, cuts that require stitches, and upper respiratory infections. Charges for such services are usually higher than visits to physicians' offices but lower than visits to hospital emergency rooms.

Community Health Care Facilities

Providing more evidence of the complexity of the United States' health care delivery complex, community health facilities fill a void in health services at a very basic level. At least six different modes of providing health care can to be considered community facilities.

School Health Programs

Once concerned primarily with the control of communicable diseases and screenings for dental, vision, and hearing problems, school health programs have taken on new functions. At the elementary and high-school levels, they may help with health and sex education programs, keep vaccination records, and consult with parents. Some colleges and universities provide inpatient care for acute illness. At larger schools, programs may deal with issues of contraception and pregnancy, as well as substance abuse and mental health problems.

Industrial Health Programs

Prevention and treatment of work-related injuries and minor illnesses are key functions of industrial health programs. The programs also give minor physical exams and provide general medical and dental care. But they have expanded their services in recognition of the value of preventive medicine. Newer or more modern programs offer comprehensive work-site education and screening programs, alcohol abuse counseling, smoking-cessation clinics, and exercise classes.

Health Screening

Provided by local health departments and voluntary health agencies (see Chapter 34), health screening varies from community to community regarding both availability and reliability. Depending on community funding, a local health department may or may not provide tests that screen for infectious or parasitic diseases, including sexually transmitted diseases (see Chapter 17), and chronic disorders such as high blood pressure, sickle cell anemia, or diabetes. Many health departments make referrals to follow-up medical care.

Neighborhood and Primary Health-Care Centers

Neighborhood and primary health-care centers were established in the 1960s to provide ambulatory care in underserved communities, both rural and urban. Often staffed by U.S. Public Health Service medical personnel or by nurse practitioners, the centers, for a time, had to limit their services according to income requirements or serve only specific communities. Because of cuts in federal spending, experts note, many such centers have been phased out.

Women, Infant, and Child Care

A federal agency, the Administration for Children and Families emphasizes provision of well-baby care, nutritious food, and nutrition education for pregnant women, infants, and children under three. Several other federal agencies have programs that promote the health and well-being of children and families.

Disease Prevention and Control

County or city health departments usually establish disease prevention and control programs to help control the spread of communicable diseases. Methods used include immunization, screening, and follow-up. Typical concerns include immunization for childhood diseases like diphtheria, measles, and polio; tuberculosis and sexually transmitted diseases; and influenza immunization for older persons.

Hospitals

Viewed a century ago as a deathhouse, the hospital has a new image. With an entirely revised role built on its ability to provide comforts and even amenities, some hospitals have added "hotel" functions to their fundamental "healing" function. But the hotel role does not affect the hospital's main medical purpose: to provide, within budgetary and other limits, sophisticated, technologically up-to-date care. The hospital has become the place to go for diagnostic and therapeutic care that a physician's office cannot provide.

A basic method of classifying hospitals is by length of the patient's stay. Viewed this way, hospitals fall into two groups, long-term or extended-care institutions and short-term hospitals. The former will be discussed later; the second group includes community, teaching, and public hospitals.

Community Hospitals

Most Americans receive medical care in community hospitals. Usually quite small, with 50 to 500 beds, this kind of hospital generally provides good to excellent secondary-level care. Traditionally, community hospitals were nonprofit corporations that depended heavily on community support. Today, the community hospital is increasingly likely to be proprietary. That means it is run for profit by investor-owned groups or corporations.

The costs of medical care at a proprietary community hospital may not be significantly different from those charged by a voluntary or nonprofit hospital.

Teaching Hospitals

Defined by the American Hospital Association as a type of community hospital, teaching hospitals range in size from a few hundred to a few thousand beds. They universally offer training for undergraduate medical students, postgraduate students, or fellows. Also, nearly all have ties to major medical schools. A state government may own a teaching hospital that is used by state medical schools; others are owned by the associated university or by a nonprofit corporation. Teaching hospitals provide care at all three levels: primary, secondary, and tertiary.

Public Hospitals

Public hospitals include not only county hospitals but others supported by public funds, among them public health service hospitals, Veterans Administration (VA) hospitals, and municipal short-term-stay hospitals. Many such institutions that are owned by federal, state, or city governments are teaching hospitals, and many also have associated rehabilitation units and nursing homes.

The Elderly: Home Care

According to the Administration on Aging (a program of the U.S. Department of Health and Human Services), one in four American families cares for an older relative, friend, or neighbor. Younger family members may need home care because of illness or injury, but typically the disabled or ill older person is the one receiving such care. A number of community resources are available to make home care—or self-care for those living alone—easier. These resources include home health workers, such services as Meals-on-Wheels, and various day-care programs.

Invaluable aids for those responsible for home care for an aging relative are unskilled companions and temporary help. With this kind of assistance, the elderly person may be able to enjoy continuity of care and independence while maintaining ties with family, home, and community.

Home Health Services

Some 2,500 home health agencies operate under the general direction of physicians to provide two kinds of services: skilled and supportive. Of the many types of home health service providers, the best known are private, either profit-making or nonprofit; public health agencies such as neighborhood health centers; hospital-based services; and local or county health department or community and church programs. The Visiting Nurse Associations of America is perhaps the most familiar.

Different communities and areas enjoy different levels and types of home health services. But most such agencies provide care to anyone who requests it. Fees vary, and may be paid by the individual or the family accepting the care. In other cases Medicare, Medicaid, or individual insurance plans may reimburse the family, partially or totally, for the fees charged. Hospital social workers or discharge-planners, the local Area Agency on Aging, the local office of the Social Security Administration, day-care centers, and churches and synagogues normally provide information on home health services.

Voluntary Health Agencies

Many voluntary health agencies provide aid and support to disabled or sick elderly persons (see Chapter 34). Such groups and organizations as the American Cancer Society and the Easter Seal Society may even offer "friendly visitor" services in specific communities. Most of the groups consider the education of the public as one of their most important functions. Thus they may provide films, lecturers, books and pamphlets, and other materials to groups and organizations of many kinds. Many such agencies have specialized equipment for those who need it as well as listings of community resources.

Drugstores and Medical Supply Houses

Two other basic sources of specialized equipment and sickroom supplies, the medically oriented drugstore and the medical supply house, play important roles. In many cases the family with home care responsibilities can obtain wheelchairs, walkers, portable oxygen equipment, and hospital beds from one source or the other. Often, the supplier will rent or sell the specialized equipment; the choice may be the family's to make.

Community Facilities for the Elderly

An entire new category of health care facilities has come into being in recent years in response to the needs of the elderly. These community facilities are designed specifically for elderly persons living at home who are not housebound.

Adult Day Care

A broad variety of community-based centers schedule adult day-care programs for the elderly. To some extent the programs provide an alternative to institutionalization. In each case the programs are tailored to meet specific needs. Each type has a basic therapeutic objective.

Medical Day Care

When chronically ill or disabled persons do not require frequent or intensive medical intervention, the medical day care service may be the solution. Located usually in a long-term care institution, nursing home, or freestanding community center, such a care service may include nursing and other supports. A physician's referral is required, and rehabilitation and maintenance are primary therapeutic goals. Reimbursement is by third-party (insurance company) payments on a sliding scale. Medicaid pays for medical day care in some states.

Mental Health Day Care

Offering a supervised environment along with mental health services to adults with various types of mental illness, the mental health day care service is usually located in a psychiatric institution or freestanding center. Referral by a psychiatrist is required. Three basic therapeutic goals are supervision, assistance with coping skills, and safety for the patient. Reimbursement is by third-party payment.

Social Adult Day Care

Title XX of the Social Security Act provides for funding of many social adult day care facilities, all of which are geared to the needs of adults who have difficulty functioning independently. Both families and health facilities can make referrals, but examination by a physician is normally required before admission. Third-party reimbursement is the norm. Program objectives and services vary widely, and are usually formulated by the funding source and the sponsoring organization. Program participants may attend part-days or full days five days a week; the facility may provide a midday meal and transportation within a specified area.

Nutrition Services

Nutrition ranks as a critical need for both homebound and more independent elderly persons. Meals-on-Wheels, a community service offered under voluntary auspices but funded partly by public funds, caters to the homebound. For a reasonable charge the service provides at least one hot meal daily for persons 60 and older. For the elderly attending senior centers, the local Area Agency on Aging provides both adequate nutrition and a chance to socialize. Agency personnel can keep in touch with clients' physical and social situations, giving the program an important outreach and prevention dimension.

Extended-Care, Long-Term Care, Nursing Homes

Closely related, the extended-care facility, long-term care facility, and nursing home nonetheless meet different needs. A relatively recent innovation, the extended-care facility provides a service that falls between that given in an acute-care hospital and that provided in a skilled nursing facility or nursing home.

Extended-Care Facility

Despite its name, the extended-care facility provides short-term inpatient care. This type of facility is designed mainly to aid patients who have been hospitalized but no longer need the full complement of hospital services. Such patients still require professional nursing and medical supervision. Typically attached to a hospital, the extended-care facility may also serve those who are not acutely ill but who require skilled care.

Because most extended-care facilities are physically attached to hospitals, patients often simply move from one hospital wing to another. Some nursing homes also meet the standards set for qualification as extended-care facilities by the Joint Commission on Accreditation of Healthcare Organizations (JCAHO). For the most part, extended-care facilities charge much less than the typical hospital.

Long- Term Care Facilities

Patients with chronic conditions that cannot be treated effectively in a general hospital generally qualify for care in a long-term care facility. Such conditions range from tuberculosis to mental retardation. The facilities also include chronic disease hospitals, rehabilitation hospitals, and psychiatric hospitals for both children and adults.

Nursing Homes

Also in the category of long-term care facilities, nursing homes comprise a special group of facilities of different kinds. They offer services ranging from sheltered living arrangements to around-the-clock nursing care. All nursing homes rank as residential facilities.

The approximately 18,000 nursing homes in the United States have between 1.3 and 1.5 million beds. Three-quarters of these nursing homes are proprietary, or for-profit, institutions that house about two-thirds of all the beds. Nonprofit organizations operate 15 percent of all the nation's nursing homes and make available about 20 percent of the beds. The government operates the remaining homes.

Nursing homes accommodate persons of all ages. A few younger residents have serious congenital illnesses or disorders, or have been recently discharged from a hospital. Others are recovering from recent surgery. But most patients are the chronically ill elderly. Typically, a nursing home resident is a woman in her 80s, single or widowed. Afflicted with three or more serious chronic illnesses, she has very likely exhausted all her assets except her monthly Social Security payments.

Residential-Care Facilities

Standing at the lowest level of nursing home care, the residential-care facility (RCF) or assisted-living residence is usually appropriate for the person who can no longer live alone and manage household chores. This type of resident does not need extensive medical attention but does require sheltered living, prepared meals, and some medical monitoring. The latter may include supervision of medications and tracking of signs and symptoms.

Intermediate-Care Facilities

The intermediate-care facility supplements typical RCF services with regular, but not round-the-clock, nursing care for residents who are unable to survive on their own. The intermediate-care facility may also provide social and recreational activities. Programs of physical therapy and rehabilitation, occupational therapy, speech therapy, and social work services may also be offered.

Skilled Nursing Facilities

With staffs of registered nurses, licensed practical nurses, physical and occupational therapists, speech-language pathologists, and audiologists, skilled nursing facilities can provide 24-hour care. They are, thus, appropriate for persons in need of intensive nursing care and rehabilitation. Like intermediate-care facilities, skilled nursing facilities are state-certified for the most part, a factor that makes them eligible for public funds as payment for services. Lack of certification may mean that an ICF or SNF has serious deficiencies.

Hospices

Described sometimes as more a philosophy than a type of physical facility, hospice is a form of care for the terminally ill. Whereas a normal medical setting concerns itself with healing a patient, the hospice environment concentrates on palliative treatment; in effect, treating and addressing pain and other symptoms of an incurable disease. Hospice programs emphasize quality, not length, of life. Hospice treats dying as a normal process and strives to help patients live comfortably and productively during their last days or months. Patients enter hospice programs at their own requests. A physician's referral, indicating that the prognosis is no more than six months, may also be required.

There are a variety of hospice settings. A hospice may be in a wing of a hospital or a separate building or institution. Many hospice programs are available to people in their homes. Families provide much of the care, although they are assisted by a team of hospice workers. At all times, the individual patient's comfort is of prime consideration.

For general information on hospice, contact the Hospice Association of America, 228 Seventh Street, SE, Washington, D.C. 20003-4306, (202) 546-4759.

34

Voluntary Health Agencies

Major Agencies

The establishment of more than 100 voluntary health agencies since the beginning of this century has been a major factor in the growth of health services to the American public. These agencies, whose activities are made possible by donations of time and money from the public, occasionally augmented by government grants for special projects, have the following objectives: spreading information about various diseases to the professional and lay public; sponsoring research; promoting legislation; and operating referral services on the community level to patients in need of diagnosis, treatment, and financial aid.

Some of these agencies, such as the American Diabetes Association, the Arthritis Foundation, the Cystic Fibrosis Foundation and United Cerebal Palsy, focus on a particular disease; others deal with problems arising from related disorders, such as the National Mental Health Association, the American Heart Association, the National Kidney Foundation, and the National Easter Seal Society.

To coordinate the activities of these many groups, to promote better health facilities, and to establish standards for the organization and conduct of these agencies, the National Health Council was founded in 1920. Its membership includes business and industrial, nonprofit, and professional organizations, as well as the 46 voluntary health agencies described below, which command a total budget of almost $4.3 billion and involve the services of almost 12 million volunteers.

All of these organizations function

on the national, state, and community level. Information and literature may be obtained through local chapters or by writing to the national office of the organization. Volunteers may offer their services in a variety of ways: as office workers, fund raisers, speakers, and community coordinators.

On the following pages, voluntary health agencies are discussed under the subjects with which they are concerned; the subjects are arranged alphabetically. Following these agencies is a brief discussion of other voluntary health agencies. Because of limitations of space, however, many worthwhile organizations have had to be omitted.

Accident Prevention

The National Safety Council, 1121 Spring Lake Drive, Itasca, Illinois 60143-3201; (630) 285-1121, was founded in 1913 to improve factory safety but soon broadened its activities to preventing every type of accident. The Council is now composed of groups and individuals from every part of the population: business, industry, government, education, religion, labor, and law. Its main efforts are devoted to building strong support for official safety programs at the national, state, and community levels in specific areas, such as traffic, labor, and home.

The Council believes that practically all accidents can be prevented with the application of the right safeguards. These safeguards include public education and awareness of danger, enforcement of safety laws and regulations, and improved design standards for machines, farm equipment, and motor vehicles.

It maintains one of the world's largest libraries of accident prevention materials, distributes a wide variety of safety literature, and issues awards for outstanding safety achievements. It also serves as a national and international clearing house of information about the causes of accidents and how they can be prevented.

In addition to campaigning for increased safety legislation on the national and state level, the Council's current programs include a defensive driving course, which provides effective adult driver training on a mass scale; a safety training institute; environmental and occupational health and "Right-to-Know" educational materials; and several approaches to the alcohol and driving problem.

Its publication, *Family Safety and Health,* is sold to companies who distribute it free to employees, and its manual called *Fundamentals of Industrial Hygiene* provides more than 1,000 pages of material essential to the safety of factory workers.

The Council in recent years has expanded its safety promotion work to include both on- and off-the-job safety for workers and their families, as well as 24-hour-a-day safety for all persons in all activities.

Alcoholism

The National Council on Alcoholism and Drug Dependence, 20 Exchange Place, Suite 2902, New York, New York 10005; (212) 269-7797, is the only national voluntary health agency founded to combat alcoholism as a disease by an extensive program on the professional and community level. The Council is completely independent of Alcoholics Anonymous, although the two organizations cooperate fully.

In more than 100 cities where the Council has affiliates, alcoholism information centers have been established that provide referral services for alcoholics and drug addicts and their families as well as educational materials for all segments of the community, including physicians and nurses, the clergy, the courts, social workers, and welfare agencies. Local affiliates also help to develop labor-management programs that provide help for employees who suffer from the disease.

The Council also sponsors research, professional training, and legislative action. Its publications department distributes a variety of fact sheets, pamphlets, posters, and videos. For a listing of publications or information on the Council's programs, write the national headquarters or contact the nearest local affiliate.

Arthritis

The Arthritis Foundation, P.O. Box 7669, Atlanta, Georgia 30357; (800) 283-7800, was established to help arthritis sufferers and their physicians through programs of research, patient services, public health information, and education on the professional and popular level. Its long-term goal is to find the cause, prevention, and cure for the nation's number one crippling disease.

The Foundation operates local chapters throughout the United States whose chief concern is the patient who has or might have arthritis. These chapters are centers for information about the disease itself and also serve as referral centers for treatment facilities. In addition, they distribute literature and sponsor forums on the latest developments in research and patient care.

Some chapters support arthritis clinics and home care programs; most conduct patient self-help programs such as discussion groups and exercise classes. Parent groups are often maintained for parents of children with arthritis.

Two special groups work within the Foundation: the Association of Rheumatology Health Professionals, which devotes itself to continuing education for health professionals caring for arthritis patients and the American Juvenile Arthritis Organization for those with a special interest in arthritis in children. A major part of the Foundation's work at the national level is providing funds for fellowships to young physicians and scientists so that they may continue their work in arthritis research and in funding through annual grants research at major institutions throughout the United States.

Cancer

The American Cancer Society, 1599 Clifton Rd. N.E., Atlanta, Georgia 30329; (800) 227-2345, was established in 1913 by a small group of physicians and volunteer workers to inform the public about the possibility of saving lives through the early diagnosis and treatment of cancer. The Society has 3,400 offices located in all 50 states plus Puerto Rico, devoted to the control and eradication of cancer. In addition to the physicians, research scientists, and other professional workers engaged in the Society's activities, more than two million volunteers are connected with its many programs.

The American Cancer Society conducts widespread campaigns to educate the public in the importance of annual medical checkups so that cancerous symptoms can be detected while they are still curable. Such checkups should include an examination of the rectum and colon and, for women, examination of the breasts and a Pap test for the detection of uterine cancer.

In another of its campaigns, the Society emphasizes the link between cigarette smoking and lung cancer. It also sponsors an extensive program to persuade teenagers not to start smoking. During its annual April Crusade against Cancer, the Society distributes approximately 40 million copies of a leaflet containing lifesaving information on early detection of cancer.

On the professional level, the major objective of the Society is to make every physician's office a cancer-detection center. To achieve this goal, it publishes a variety of literature, offers refresher courses, sponsors seminars, and cooperates closely with local and state medical societies and health departments on the diagnosis and treatment of cancer. It also arranges national and international conferences for the exchange of information on the newest cancer-fighting techniques, and finances a million-dollar-a-year clinical fellowship program for young physicians.

Among its special services to patients are sponsorship of the International Association of Laryngectomies, for people who have lost their voices to cancer; and Reach to Recovery, a program for women who have had treatment for breast cancer and who need support and guidance to return to normal living. On the community level, the American Cancer Society operates a counseling service for cancer patients and their families, referring them to the proper medical facilities and social agencies for treatment and care. Through its "loan closets," it provides sickroom necessities, hospital beds, medical dressings, and so on.

Some local divisions offer home

care programs through the services of the Visiting Nurse Association or a similar agency. Although the Society does not operate medical facilities, treat patients, or pay physicians' fees, some of the chapters support cancer detection programs and professionally supervised rehabilitation services.

Cerebral Palsy

The United Cerebral Palsy Associations, 1660 L Street, NW, Suite 700, Washington, DC 20036; (800) 872-5287, founded in 1948 by a small group of concerned parents, now has 203 affiliates across the country where those who have the condition may obtain treatment referral, therapy, and education. The Associations also play an important role in vocational training, job placement programs, housing, and recreational services.

The Research and Educational Foundation of this organization supports studies investigating possible causes of cerebral palsy. The Foundation also gives grants to universities and medical schools for research into the causes and prevention of cerebral palsy and new methods of therapy, for training medical and other professional personnel in the management of this condition.

Cystic Fibrosis

The Cystic Fibrosis Foundation, 6931 Arlington Road, No. 200, Bethesda, Maryland 20814; (800) 344-4823, was organized in 1955 by a group of concerned parents whose children were born with this lung disease. The Foundation now concerns itself with all serious lung ailments of children regardless of their medical names, and it engages in a broad program of research, medical education, public information, and the sponsorship of diagnostic and treatment centers.

The Foundation's 58 local chapters offer advice and information to parents of children with severe lung disease, and have direct connections with the more than 100 Cystic Fibrosis Centers throughout the country. They refer patients to sources of financial aid, make arrangements for the purchase of drugs at a discount, and lend home treatment equipment to families who cannot afford to buy it.

The national organization makes grants for research activities, conducts professional conferences, and publishes literature for physicians and the general public on various aspects of childhood lung diseases.

Diabetes

The American Diabetes Association, National Service Center, 1701 North Beauregard Street, Alexandria, Virginia 22311; (800) 342-2383, was established as a professional society in 1940. In recent years it has enlarged its scope so that it currently has 800 affiliated local chapters throughout the country that promote the creation of better understanding of diabetes among patients and their families; the exchange of knowledge among physicians and other scientists; the spreading of accurate information to the general public about early recognition and supervision of the disease; and the sponsorship of basic research.

Since 1948, the American Diabetes Association has conducted an annual Diabetes Detection Drive supported by widespread publicity in all news media. During this drive, approximately three million testing kits are provided to state and county medical societies to facilitate the early detection and prompt treatment of the disorder. This annual activity hopes to find the estimated millions of people who are unaware that they have diabetes.

Among the Association's publications of special interest to diabetics and their families are the *Diabetes Forecast,* a national magazine that presents news items on research and treatment; *Exchange Lists for Meal Planning,* prepared with the cooperation of the American Dietetic Association and the U.S. Public Health Services; and *The Complete Quick & Hearty Diabetic Cookbook,* which contains attractive recipes for meals that can be served to diabetics.

Other activities of the Association include encouraging the employment of diabetics and providing special groups such as teachers, police, and social agencies with information on the condition. It also established a classification of the disease according to its severity. Guidelines on emergency medical care and the scientific journal *Diabetes* are available to physicians.

Drug Abuse

Cocaine Anonymous World Services Office (CAWSO)
CAWSO, Inc.
P.O.Box 2000
Los Angeles, CA 90049-8000
(310) 559-5833

Parent Resource Institute for Drug-Free Education (PRIDE)
4684 Evergreen
Newaygo, Michigan 49337
(800) 668-9277

Eye Diseases

Prevent Blindness America, 500 E. Remington Rd., Schaumburg, Illinois 60173; (800) 321-2020, was founded in 1908 to reduce the number of cases of infants born with impaired sight. In subsequent years, it merged with the American Association for the Conservation of Vision and the Ophthalmological Foundation. The organization is now concerned with investigating all causes of blindness and supports measures and community services that will eliminate them. It also distributes information on the proper care and use of the eyes.

The organization's first and most significant victory was the adoption of laws by almost all states requiring that silver nitrate solution be routinely dropped into the eyes of all newborn babies to counteract the possibility of congenital blindness. This resulted in a dramatic drop in the number of children suffering from eye impairment dating from birth.

For almost half a century, Prevent Blindness America has actively campaigned to reduce the number of people suffering from glaucoma, one of the leading causes of blindness in the United States. It has also conducted a national program to educate the elderly in the ease, safety, and advantages of surgery for cataracts, the leading cause of blindness among the aged.

Since 1926, it has been conducting preschool vision screening programs administered by teams that travel from big cities to isolated rural communities. Current activities also include research into the cause, treatment, and prevention of eye diseases leading to blindness; assembling data and publishing reports; cooperating with community agencies to improve eye health; promoting conditions in schools and industry to safeguard vision; and advocating eye examinations in early childhood so that disorders can be properly and promptly corrected.

Family Planning

Planned Parenthood Federation of America, 810 Seventh Avenue, New York, New York 10019; (800) 669-0156, is the nation's oldest and largest voluntary family planning organization. Tracing its origins to 1916, when Margaret Sanger founded the first U.S. birth control clinic in Brooklyn, New York, Planned Parenthood maintains that every individual has the fundamental right to choose when or whether to have a child.

Planned Parenthood has five key goals:

- To increase the availability and accessibility of high-quality and affordable reproductive health care services and information, especially for underserved groups
- To reduce adolescent pregnancy and unwanted births to teens
- To meet the challenge of changes in health care delivery systems and maintain high-quality, efficiently run, and creative Planned Parenthood programs

- To further Planned Parenthood's role in the provision of education of human sexuality, reproduction, and population, and on the bioethical and legal implications of reproductive technology
- To increase access to safe and effective methods of voluntary fertility regulation for individuals in developing countries

Each year, more than three million individuals in 49 states and the District of Columbia obtain medical, educational, and counseling services through more than 900 clinics operated by Planned Parenthood's 171 affiliates. The organization is active in more than 100 developing countries throughout the world. In addition, Planned Parenthood conducts clinical research, provides professional training of health and education personnel, and serves as a resource to health agencies, government agencies at the state and federal levels, legislators and other policy makers, and the media.

Heart Disease

The American Heart Association, 7272 Greenville Avenue, Dallas, Texas 75231; (800) 242-8721, was founded in 1924 as a professional organization of cardiologists. It was reorganized in 1948 as a national voluntary health agency to promote a program of education, research, and community service in the interests of reducing premature death and disability caused by diseases of the heart and blood vessels. The complex of heart disorders, including atherosclerosis, stroke, high blood pressure, kidney diseases, rheumatic fever, and congenital heart disturbances, is by far the leading cause of death in the United States.

Since its first Annual Heart Fund Campaign in 1949, the Association has contributed more than $150 million to research and has been a major factor in the reduction of cardiovascular mortality statistics. It has spent more than $2 million since 1959 studying human heart transplantation procedures, and has contributed to the development of an artificial heart, plastic heart valves, and synthetic arteries.

Public and professional education programs designed to reduce the risk of heart attack through avoidance of cigarette smoking, obesity, and foods high in cholesterol are conducted on a nationwide and community level by the Association's affiliates throughout the country. The local chapters are also engaged in service programs for rheumatic fever prevention, stroke rehabilitation, school health, cardiopulmonary resuscitation, and industrial health. In addition, they conduct information and referral services for patients and their families.

The American Heart Association publishes many technical and professional journals as well as material designed for the general public.

Hemophilia

The National Hemophilia Foundation, 116 W. 32nd Street, 11th Floor, New York, New York 10001; (800) 424-2634, was established in 1948 to serve the needs of hemophiliacs and their families by ensuring the availability of treatment and rehabilitation facilities. It is estimated that there are as many as 100,000 males suffering from hemophilia, an inherited disease.

The long-term goal of the Foundation is to develop a national program of research and clinical study that will provide new information about early diagnosis and effective treatment of the disorder as well as trained professional personnel to administer patient care.

The development in recent years of blood-clotting concentrates is the most important advance to date in the treatment of the disease. This development, supported in part by the Foundation's 42 chapters, makes it possible for patients to have elective surgery and dental work, and to eliminate much of the pain, crippling, and hospitalization of those suffering from hemophilia.

The need for blood supplies from which to extract the clotting factor caused the Foundation to embark on an extensive campaign for blood donations. For this purpose, it has been working closely since 1968 with the American Red Cross and the American Association of Blood Banks. It also maintains close ties with various laboratories and research groups in the development of more powerful concentrates that can be manufactured and sold at the lowest possible cost.

The organization's activities include a national network of facilities with blood banks, clinics, and treatment centers as well as referral services. It has also established a Behavioral Science Department to explore the nonmedical aspects of hemophiliacs' problems, such as education, vocational guidance, and psychological needs.

Kidney Disease

The National Kidney Foundation, 30 E. 33rd Street, Suite 1100, New York, New York 10016; (800) 622-9010, formerly the National Kidney Disease Foundation, was founded in 1950 by a group of parents whose children had a disease with no cure—nephrosis. The ultimate goal was the total eradication of all diseases of the kidney and urinary tract. Today, although there remains no cure for nephrosis, the disease is almost totally treatable. The National Kidney Foundation and its 49 affiliates nationwide have funded millions of dollars in research to find cures for kidney and related diseases, including diabetes and high blood pressure.

The National Kidney Foundation and its affiliates sponsor a wide variety of programs in treatment, service, education, and prevention that are designed to aid the patient in the community. Examples of some affiliate programs include: information and referral programs for patients and their families, drug banks, support groups, summer camp programs for children on dialysis and transplantations, transportation services, counseling and screening, and direct financial assistance to needy patients.

The National Kidney Foundation seeks continually to increase the number of organs available for transplantation through its nationwide Organ Donor Program. To date, more than 50 million donor cards have been distributed by the Foundation and its affiliates. Distribution of public and professional educational materials continues to heighten public awareness of organ donation and the "Gift of Life" it can provide to thousands of people waiting for a kidney transplant.

Mental Health

The National Mental Health Association, 2001 North Beauregard Street, 12th Floor, Alexandria, Virginia 22311; (800) 969-6642, was founded in 1909 to work toward the improved care and treatment of people with mental illnesses, the promotion of mental health, and the prevention of mental disorders. The original National Committee for Mental Hygiene merged with the National Mental Health Foundation and the Psychiatric Foundation in 1950 to create the organization as it now stands.

The association implements its service programs through its 340 affiliates (local chapters and larger state divisions) across the country. These mental health associations tailor their efforts to the needs of their communities.

The National Mental Health Association is composed of one million volunteers and supporters who have a keen interest in mental health. They include family members whose loved ones have been affected by mental illnesses, current or former consumers, mental health professionals, and lay citizens.

Recent and ongoing activities include:

- Coordinated a national coalition to address the needs of people with mental illnesses who are homeless.
- Serves as a prime source of referral and educational information on mental illnesses and mental health issues through the NMHA Mental Health Information Center.
- Assists local and state MHA affiliates in serving communities through patient and family support groups, housing programs, suicide-prevention hotlines, and school mental health education programs.

- Helped extend the civil rights protection of the 8th and 14th Amendments to the U.S. Constitution to the mentally disabled by representing persons with severe mental illnesses before the Supreme Court.
- Specified a "state-of-the-art" program to prevent severe mental and emotional disabilities in a landmark 1986 report by its National Commission on the Prevention of Mental-Emotional Disabilities.
- Serves as the public-interest policy voice for mental health issues in the Congress and state legislatures.

Multiple Sclerosis

The National Multiple Sclerosis Society, 733 Third Avenue, New York, New York 10017; (800) 344-4867, was founded in 1946 with the primary goal of supporting research on this chronic neurological disease whose cause and cure are unknown. Some 250,000 Americans are estimated to have multiple sclerosis (MS).

Research aimed at finding the cause and methods of arresting MS is being conducted worldwide. From the beginning the Society has made every effort to increase professional and public awareness of the symptoms of MS and the best ways of treating them. This is done through a network of 143 chapters and branches and some 470,000 active members. The chapters, which are either affiliated with or support MS clinics around the country, provide home and hospital visits, recreational programs, referrals for medical care, job counseling, and other services. The chapters also arrange educational programs for physicians and social workers as well as for patients and their families. The society sponsors public education awards in magazine, radio, and television writing and conducts Project Rembrandt, a biennial competition for artists with MS.

The national office distributes publications for physicians and the interested public, including guides for the development of patient services and a quarterly magazine, *Inside MS.* Films, slide presentations, videocassettes and audiocassettes are available for purchase or loan.

Physical Disabilities

The Easter Seals national headquarters, 230 West Monroe, Suite 1800, Chicago, Illinois 60606; (800) 221-6827, has grown from its pioneering origins in 1919 to a national organization that serves more than one million disabled people of all ages. Among its network of facilities are comprehensive rehabilitation centers, treatment and diagnostic centers, and vocational training workshops, residential camps, special education programs, and transportation services in many different parts of the country.

Because many disabled children and adults in rural areas and small communities are unaware of the services available to them, the Society gives top priority to publicizing its information, referral, and follow-up activities. In recent years, it has also established mobile treatment units in hospitals and nursing homes in rural areas.

Other innovative activities include screening and testing programs to detect hearing loss in newborns and learning disabilities in preschool children, and providing treatment and referral for those who are disabled by respiratory diseases.

The Society collaborates with federal and professional agencies in all programs designed to eliminate architectural barriers to the disabled, and was instrumental in the enactment of legislation making it mandatory that all buildings constructed with government funds be fully and easily accessible to the disabled. It also initiates and supports significant studies in rehabilitation procedures as well as scientific research in bone transplant techniques.

Extensive literature is distributed to professionals, the public, parents, and employers. It also assembles special educational packets for parents of the disabled.

Sexually Transmitted Diseases

The American Social Health Association, P.O. Box 13827, Research Triangle Park, North Carolina 27709; (919) 361-8400, was organized in 1912 to promote the control of venereal disease and to combat prostitution. In the mid-1980s the Association faced new challenges in the field of sexually transmitted diseases (STDs) while also developing new strategies to augment and complement existing AIDS information programs, promote attention to chlamydia, the most widespread STD in the United States, exert influence in Congress for additional federal funding for STD prevention and control programs, and place STD information in the hands of high-school students.

The Association is in close touch with government agencies such as the Public Health Service, the National Institutes of Health, and the various branches of the armed forces. Through these channels, it promotes its program for STD education in the schools and for research toward the discovery of an immunizing vaccine against syphilis and gonorrhea.

It is the major national voluntary repository for information and consultation on STDs, and maintains the world's most comprehensive collection of source workshops, residential camps, special education programs, and materials on STDs. It constantly helps communities in diagnosing their problems and produces a number of publications for teachers, guidance counselors, and youth workers.

The Association stresses the importance of introducing family life education into the curriculum of elementary and secondary schools and of establishing training programs on this subject in teachers' colleges. These efforts have resulted in the inclusion of family life education in an increasing number of school systems throughout the United States.

Tuberculosis and Respiratory Diseases

The American Lung Association, 61 Broadway, 6th Floor, New York, New York 10006; (800) LUNG-USA, is the direct descendant of the first voluntary health organization to be formed in the United States. In 1904, when the National Association for the Study and Prevention of Tuberculosis was organized, this disease was the country's leading cause of death. Since 1973, with the sharp increase in the problems relating to smoking and air pollution, the association has been known by its present name, which was adopted to reflect the broader scope of its activities.

It now concerns itself not only with the elimination of tuberculosis but with chronic and disabling conditions, such as emphysema, and with acute diseases of the respiratory system, such as influenza. Through its affiliates and nationwide state organizations, it is actively engaged in campaigns against smoking and air pollution.

The early endeavor of the association to have tuberculosis included among the reportable diseases was accomplished state by state, and since the 1920s all states have required that every case in the country be brought to the attention of local health officials.

Public awareness of better care and the development of effective drugs have dramatically reduced the number of TB patients, but the association continues to concern itself with the fact that provisional data indicate that there are still about 22,000 new cases each year.

Through its local affiliates, the American Lung Association initiates special campaigns to combat smoking and air pollution, using radio and television announcements, car stickers, posters, and pamphlets, as well as films and exhibits. Educational materials on respiratory diseases are regularly distributed by the national office to local associations for physicians, patients, and the general public. Funds raised by the annual Christmas Seal drive also support research and medical education fellowships.

Other Voluntary Health Agencies

In addition to those voluntary health agencies that are members of the National Health Council, many other organizations function on a national scale and offer specialized services as well as literature and guidance to professionals, patients, parents, and concerned families. The following is a partial list.

Alcoholics Anonymous World Services, Grand Central Station, P.O. Box 459, New York, New York 10163; (212) 870-3400, is a fellowship of men and women who share their experiences and give each other support in overcoming the problem of alcoholism. Chapters exist throughout the country and offer referral services, literature, and information about special hospital programs.

Al-Anon Family Group Headquarters, Inc., 1600 Corporate Landing Parkway, Virginia Beach, Virginia 23454-5617; (888) 425-2666, is not affiliated with Alcoholics Anonymous, but cooperates closely with it. Al-Anon, which includes Alateen for younger members, is a primary community resource and self-help fellowship for the families and friends of alcoholics. Members share their experiences, strength, and hope at regularly held meetings, and learn to cope with the effects of being close to an alcoholic. Headquarters registers, services, and provides literature to 33,000 groups worldwide, of which 19,000 are in the United States.

Asthma and Allergy Foundation of America, 1233 20th Street, NW, Suite 402, Washington, DC 20036; (800) 727-8462, was established to help solve all health problems related to allergic diseases by sponsoring research and treatment facilities. It also grants scholarships to medical students specializing in the study of allergy.

Alzheimer's Association, 225 North Michigan Avenue, Suite 1700, Chicago, Illinois 60601; (800) 272-3900, was founded in 1980 to heighten public awareness of this degenerative brain disorder, provide support for patients and their families, aid research efforts, advocate for legislation that responds to the needs of Alzheimer's disease patients and their family members, and commemorate National Alzheimer's Disease Awareness Month each November. The network includes more than 200 chapters and affiliates across the country representing over 1,000 Family Support Groups. To obtain the most up-to-date information on Alzheimer's disease legislation and research, and for referral to local chapters, call or write the Association.

The American Foundation for AIDS Research (AmfAR), 120 Wall Street, 13th Floor, New York, New York 10005; (212) 806-1600, was created in the fall of 1985 as a result of the unification of two not-for-profit public foundations: the AIDS Medical Foundation (AMF), incorporated in the State of New York in April 1983; and the National AIDS Research Foundation (NARF), incorporated in the State of California in August 1985. AmfAR is an independent, national organization whose directors, committee members, and staff are professionals in the field of AIDS.

The Foundation has two main missions. First, it supports and facilitates laboratory and clinical research projects selected on the basis of scientific merit and relevance to achieve an understanding of the pathogenesis of AIDS, its prevention through the use of a vaccine, and its treatment. Second, the Foundation works to develop data and to serve as a source of accurate and up-to-date information about an epidemic that has profound repercussions in our society.

American Foundation for the Blind, 11 Penn Plaza, Suite 300, New York, New York 10001; (800) 232-5463, is a national nonprofit organization working with local and national services to improve the quality of life for all blind and visually impaired persons. It stocks many consumer products and publications and has recorded and produced millions of talking books for the Library of Congress.

Through its staff of national consultants and its regional offices, the Foundation maintains a direct liaison with state, regional, and local agencies.

Engender Health (formerly the Association for Voluntary Surgical Contraception), 440 Ninth Avenue, 3rd Floor, New York, New York 10001; (212) 561-8000, was founded in 1943 to promote the right of each individual to choose sterilization as a method of birth control. A nonprofit membership organization, Engender Health has increasingly collaborated with governmental and private sector providers to ensure effective access to sterilization facilities. The association also sponsors training, education, and program support for sterilization and family planning counselors and others; prepares annual estimates of male and female voluntary sterilizations in the United States; issues a variety of publications, and initiates and monitors research into medical, legal, psychological, ethical, and public health aspects of voluntary sterilization.

The C.D.C. National STD and AIDS Hotline, (800) 342-2437, is operated by the Federal Centers for Disease Control and provides confidential and anonymous information and referrals to local health organizations, counselors, and support groups. *The C.D.C. National Prevention Information Network,* P.O. Box 6003, Rockville, MD 20849, (800) 458-5231 provides free educational materials on the prevention of such diseases as tuberculosis and AIDS.

The Epilepsy Foundation of America, 4351 Garden City Drive, Landover, Maryland 20785; (800) 332-1000, is the result of a merger in 1967 of two similar organizations. At present, the Foundation has more than 60 local affiliates that provide information, referral services, and counseling. It conducts a research grant program for medical and psychosocial investigation and distributes a wide variety of literature on request to physicians, teachers, employers, and the interested public on such subjects as anticonvulsant drugs, insurance, driving laws, and emergency treatment. The national office also maintains an extensive research library.

The Leukemia & Lymphoma Society of America, 1311 Mamaroneck Avenue, White Plains, New York 10605; (800) 955-4572, was organized in 1949 and now has 57 chapters. It supports research in the causes, control, and eventual eradication of the disease that, though commonly thought of as a disorder of the blood, is in fact a disorder of the bone marrow, lymph nodes, and spleen, which manufacture blood. The society has a continuing program of education through special publications directed to physicians, nurses, and the public. Through its local affiliates, it conducts patient-aid services that provide counseling, transportation, and—to those who need financial assistance—drugs, blood transfusions, and laboratory facilities.

The Muscular Dystrophy Association, Inc., 3300 East Sunrise Drive, Tucson, Arizona 85718; (800) 572-1717, has as a primary goal the scientific conquest of muscular dystrophy and related neuromuscular diseases. The Association supports scientific investigators worldwide. In addition, through its 170 chapter affiliates nationwide, MDA provides a comprehensive patient and community services program to individuals diagnosed with any one of 40 neuromuscular disorders. The Association maintains a network of some 240 MDA clinics coast to coast to provide diagnostic services and therapeutic and rehabilitative follow-up care as well as genetic, vocational, and social service counseling to patients and their families. MDA also sponsors a summer camping program for youngsters aged 6 to 21 as well as adult outings, with activities geared to the special needs of those with neuromuscular diseases.

RESOLVE, (HelpLine: 888/623-0744) is a national non-profit consumer organization serving the unique needs of the infertile population and allied professionals with support, education and advocacy. RESOLVE, 1310 Broadway, Somerville, MA 02144-1779. Membership services include national newsletter, telephone helpline, physician referral service.

The Arc of the United States, 1010 Wayn Avenue, Suite 650, Silver Spring, MD 20910; (301) 565-3842, established in 1950, is the nation's largest voluntary organization specifically devoted to promoting the welfare of children and adults with mental retardation. It is estimated that there are six million such persons in the United States. Through its 1,500 affiliates the association conducts and supports research, sponsors employment programs, advocates for progressive public policy, and works for better community services. Counseling and referral services, as well as extensive literature for professionals and concerned families, are available on request.

The March of Dimes Birth Defects Foundation, 1275 Mamaroneck Avenue, White Plains, New York 10605; (888) 663-4637, was founded in 1938 to combat infantile paralysis (polio). In the 40 years since the conquest of polio, through the development of the Salk and Sabin polio vaccines, the March of Dimes has dedicated itself to the prevention of birth defects, the nation's number one child health problem. It does this through programs of birth defects research and medical service and education that provide new knowledge and understanding of birth defects and their prevention. More than a quarter-million babies are born with one or more of the 3,000 known birth defects each year. The Foundation also has established the Salk Institute in La Jolla, California, for the purpose of carrying on basic research in life processes to discover what causes birth defects and other diseases.

Special Health Services and Agencies

Many factors have contributed to the growth of the American system of health services. Specialists in various medical specialties have tried to meet needs for new types of health care. Medical care has become so effective that individual life expectancy has increased enormously; as one result, the number of Americans aged 65 and older tripled in the three-quarters of a century between 1900 and 1975. As the population of the United States has grown older, in percentage terms, the problems of the aged have received more attention. New methods and devices have been developed for the care and assistance of the ill or disabled of any age.

Special health services and agencies help to fill such needs. Many older persons have utilized the services of trained individuals who make survival possible—sometimes at home—or slow down the rate of deterioration. Other institutions and agencies perform simple maintenance tasks for the aged or the seriously ill or handicapped, or help with rehabilitation. Social service agencies and groups with health roles, for example, provide adult day care, homemaker assistance, and home health services that may include the following:

- Part-time or occasional nursing care, often under the supervision of a registered nurse
- Physical, occupational, or speech therapy
- Medical social services that help the patient and his or her family to adjust to the social and emotional conditions accompanying illness or disability of any kind
- Assistance from a home health aide, including help with such tasks as bathing and going to the bathroom, taking medications, exercising, and getting into and out of bed
- Under some circumstances, medical attention from interns or residents in training

The Complete Reference Guide to

MEDICINE AND HEALTH

The Complete Reference Guide to MEDICINE AND HEALTH

EDITED BY
Richard J. Wagman, M.D., F.A.C.P.
Assistant Clinical Professor of Medicine
Downstate Medical Center
New York, New York

Volume Four

FACTS ON FILE/NEW YORK

ISBN 0-8160-6144-0 (hardcover)

Printed in the United States of America

Editor
Richard J. Wagman, M.D., F.A.C.P.
Assistant Clinical Professor of Medicine
Downstate Medical Center
New York, New York

Contributors to The New Complete Medical and Health Encyclopedia

Consultant in Surgery

N. Henry Moss, M.D., F.A.C.S.
Associate Clinical Professor of Surgery
Temple University Health Sciences Center and Albert Einstein Medical Center;
Past President, American Medical Writers Association;
Past President, New York Academy of Sciences

Consultant in Gynecology

Douglass S. Thompson, M.D.
Clinical Professor of Obstetrics and Gynecology and Clinical Associate Professor of Community Medicine
University of Pittsburgh School of Medicine

Consultant in Pediatrics

Charles H. Bauer, M.D.
Clinical Associate Professor of Pediatrics and Chief of Pediatric Gastroenterology
The New York Hospital-Cornell Medical Center
New York, New York

Consultants in Psychiatry

Julian J. Clark, M.D.
Assistant Professor of Psychiatry
and
Rita W. Clark, M.D.
Clinical Assistant Professor of Psychiatry
Downstate Medical Center

Consulting Editor

Kenneth N. Anderson
Formerly Editor
Today's Health

Bruce O. Berg, M.D.
Associate Professor
Departments of Neurology and Pediatrics
Director, Child Neurology
University of California
San Francisco, California

D. Jeanne Collins
Assistant Professor
College of Allied Health Professions
University of Kentucky
Lexington, Kentucky

Anthony A. Davis
Vice President and Education Consultant
Metropolitan X-Ray and Medical Sales, Inc.
Olney, Maryland

Peter A. Dickinson
Editor Emeritus
Harvest Years/Retirement Living

Gordon K. Farley, M.D.
Associate Professor of Child Psychiatry
Director, Day Care Center
University of Colorado Medical Center

Arthur Fisher
Group Editor
Science and Engineering
Popular Science

Edmund H. Harvey, Jr.
Editor
Science World

Helene MacLean
Medical writer

Ben Patrusky
Science writer

Stanley E. Weiss, M.D.
Assistant Attending Physician, Renal Service
Beth Israel Hospital and Medical Center, New York

Jeffrey S. Willner, M.D.
Attending Radiologist
Southampton Hospital
Southampton, New York

Contents

Volume IV

35

Medical Emergencies

Anyone attempting to deal with a medical emergency will do so with considerably more confidence if he has a clear notion of the order of importance of various problems. Over and above all technical knowledge about such things as tourniquets or cardiac massage is the ability of the rescuer to keep a cool head so that he can make the right decisions and delegate tasks to others who wish to be helpful.

Cessation of Breathing

The medical emergency that requires prompt attention before any others is cessation of breathing. No matter what other injuries are involved, artificial respiration must be administered immediately to anyone suffering from respiratory arrest.

To determine whether a person is breathing naturally, place your cheek as near as possible to the victim's mouth and nose. While you are feeling and listening for evidence of respiration, watch the victim's chest and upper abdomen to see if they rise and fall. If respiratory arrest is indicated, begin artificial respiration immediately.

Time is critical; a human body has only about a four-minute reserve supply of oxygen in its tissues, although some persons have been revived after being submerged in water for ten minutes or more. Do not waste time moving the victim to a more comfortable location unless his position is life threatening.

If more than one person is available, the second person should summon a physician. A second rescuer can also assist in preparing the victim for artificial respiration by helping to loosen clothing around the neck, chest, and waist, and by inspecting the mouth for false teeth, chewing gum, or other objects that could block the flow of air. The victim's tongue must be pulled forward before artificial respiration begins.

Normal breathing should start after not more than 15 minutes of artificial respiration. If it doesn't, you should continue the procedure for at least two hours, alternating, if possible, with other persons to maintain maximum efficiency. Medical experts have defined normal breathing as eight or more breaths per minute; if breathing resumes but slackens to a rate of fewer than eight breaths per minute, or if breathing stops suddenly for more than 30 seconds, continue artificial respiration.

Artificial Respiration

Following is a description of the techniques used to provide mouth-to-mouth or mouth-to-nose artificial respiration. These are the preferred

Cardiopulminary Resuscitation (CPR)

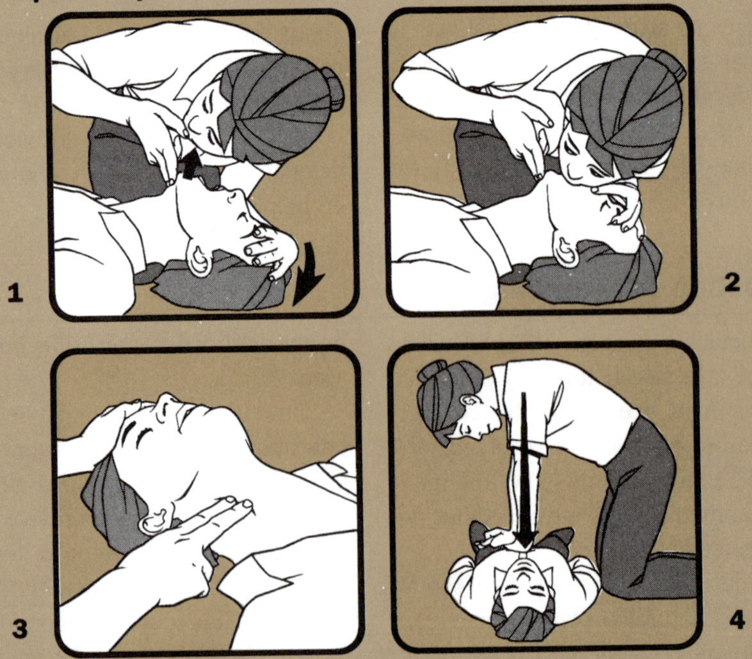

(1) Open airway: **tilt the head back** by the forehead and **lift the chin**. (2) If not breathing, begin rescue breathing. **Pinch nose, give 2 full breaths**, each of about five seconds in duration. If passage is blocked, reposition head and try again. If still no air enters the lungs, perform the Heimlich maneuver abdominal thrusts. (3) **Check pulse** at the carotid artery. (4) If heart is beating, continue mouth-to-mouth until breathing is started. **If no pulse, begin chest compressions**. Perform 15 compressions to every 2 full breaths. Check pulse after four cycles of compressions/breaths. **Warning:** Performing CPR is not recommended unless you have training. CPR incorrectly performed can cause physical injury and death. The American Red Cross and other organizations offer CPR certification.

methods of artificial respiration because they move a greater volume of air into a victim's lungs than any alternative method.

After quickly clearing the victim's mouth and throat of obstacles, tilt the victim's head back as far as possible, with the chin up and neck stretched to ensure an open passage of air to the lungs. If mouth-to-mouth breathing is employed, pull the lower jaw of the victim open with one hand, inserting your thumb between the victim's teeth, and pinch the nostrils with the other to prevent air leakage through the nose. If using the mouth-to-nose technique, hold one hand over the mouth to seal it against air leakage.

Next, open your own mouth and take a deep breath. Then blow forcefully into the victim's mouth (or nose) until you can see the chest rise. Quickly remove your mouth and listen for normal exhalation sounds from the victim. If you hear gurgling sounds, try to move the jaw higher because the throat may not be stretched open properly. Continue blowing forcefully into the victim's mouth (or nose) at a rate of once every three or four seconds. (For infants, do not blow forcefully; blow only small puffs of air from your cheeks.)

If the victim's stomach becomes distended, it may be a sign that air is being blown into the stomach; press firmly with one hand on the upper abdomen to push the air out of the stomach.

If you are hesitant about direct physical contact of the lips, make a ring with the index finger and thumb of the hand being used to hold the victim's chin in position. Place the ring of fingers firmly about the victim's mouth; the outside of the thumb may at the same time be positioned to seal the nose against air leakage. Then blow the air into the victim's mouth through the finger-thumb ring. Direct lip-to-lip contact can also be avoided by placing a piece of gauze or other clean porous cloth over the victim's mouth.

Severe Bleeding

If the victim is not suffering from respiration failure or if breathing has been restored, severe bleeding is the second most serious emergency to attend to. Such bleeding occurs when either an artery or a vein has been severed. Arterial blood is bright red and spurts rather than flows from the body, sometimes in very large amounts. It is also more difficult to control than blood from a vein, which can be recognized by its dark red color and steady flow.

Emergency Treatment

The quickest and most effective way to stop bleeding is by direct pressure on the wound. If heavy layers of sterile gauze are not available, use a clean

Pressure Points

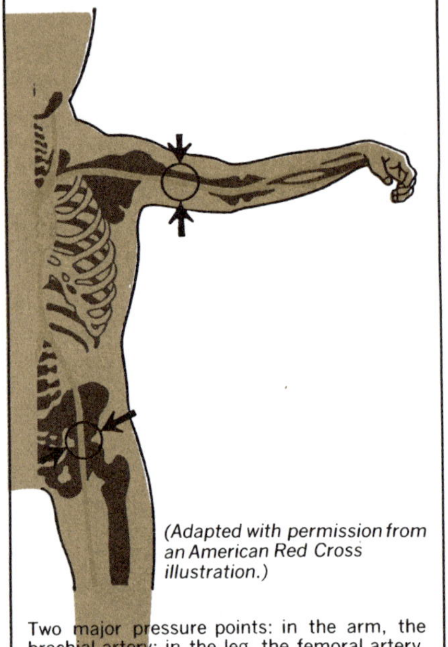

(Adapted with permission from an American Red Cross illustration.)

Two major pressure points: in the arm, the brachial artery; in the leg, the femoral artery. Continue to apply direct pressure and elevate the wounded part while utilizing pressure points to stop blood flow.

handkerchief, or a clean piece of material torn from a shirt, slip, or sheet to cover the wound. Then place the fingers or the palm of the hand directly over the bleeding area. The pressure must be *firm and constant* and should be interrupted only when the blood has soaked through the dressing. *Do not remove the soaked dressing.* Cover it as quickly as possible with additional new layers. When the blood stops seeping through to the surface of the dressing, secure it with strips of cloth until the victim can receive medical attention. This procedure is almost always successful in stopping blood flow from a vein.

If direct pressure doesn't stop arterial bleeding, two alternatives are possible: pressure by finger or hand on the pressure point nearest the wound, or the application of a tourniquet. No matter what the source of the bleeding, if the wound is on an arm or leg, elevation of the limb as high as is comfortable will reduce the blood flow.

Tourniquets

A tourniquet improperly applied can be an extremely dangerous device, and should only be considered for a hemorrhage that can't be controlled in any other way.

It must be remembered that arterial blood flows away from the heart and that venous blood flows toward the heart. Therefore, while a tourniquet placed on a limb between the site of a wound and the heart may slow or stop arterial bleeding, it may actually increase venous bleeding. By obstructing blood flow in the veins beyond the wound site, the venous blood flowing toward the heart will have to exit from the wound. Thus, the proper application of a tourniquet depends upon an understanding and differentiation of arterial from venous bleeding. Arterial bleeding can be recognized by the pumping action of the blood and by the bright red color of the blood.

Once a tourniquet is applied, it should not be left in place for an excessive period of time, since the tissues in the limb beyond the site of the wound need to be supplied with blood.

Shock

In any acute medical emergency, the

Pressure Points

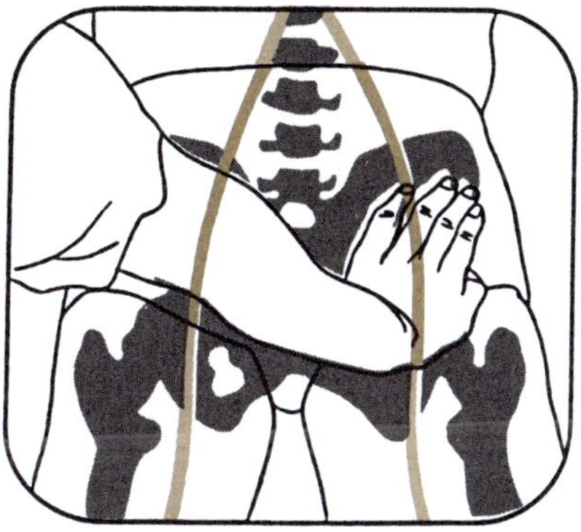

(Top) Use the femoral artery for control of severe bleeding from an open leg wound. Place the victim flat on his back, and put the heel of your hand directly over the pressure point. Apply pressure by forcing the artery against the pelvic bone. *(Bottom)* Use the brachial artery for control of severe bleeding from an open arm wound. Apply pressure by forcing the artery against the arm bone. Continue to apply direct pressure over the wound, and keep the wounded part elevated.

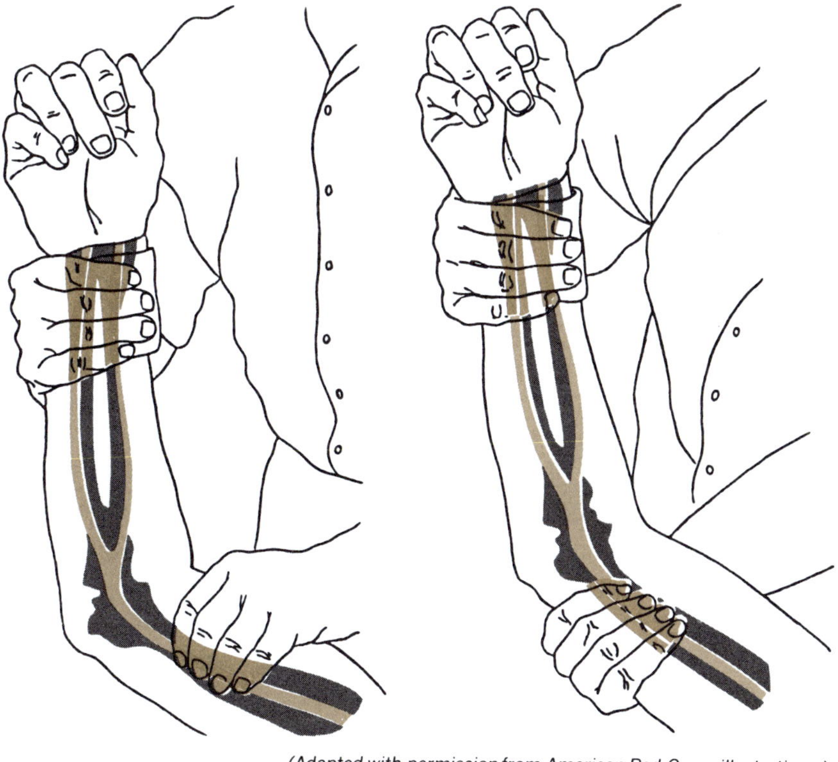

(Adapted with permission from American Red Cross illustrations.)

possibility of the onset of shock must always be taken into account, especially following the fracture of a large bone, extensive burns, or serious wounds. If untreated, or if treated too late, shock can be fatal.

Arterial Bleeding

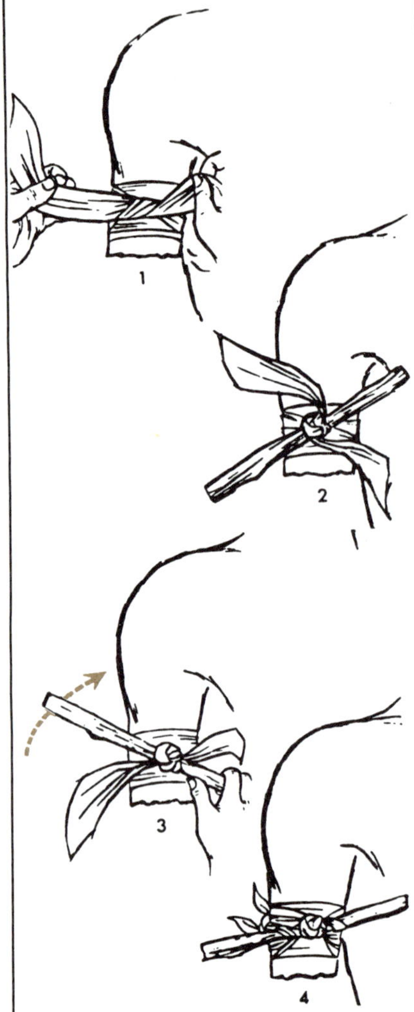

Severe arterial bleeding can be controlled by the correct application of a tourniquet. (1) A long strip of gauze or other material is wrapped twice around the arm or leg above the wound and tied in a half-knot. (2) A stick, called a windlass, is placed over the knot, and the knot is completed. (3) The windlass is turned to tighten the knot and finally, (4) the windlass is secured with the tails of the tourniquet. Improper use of a tourniquet can be very dangerous.

Shock is an emergency condition in which the circulation of the blood is so disrupted that all bodily functions are affected. It occurs when blood pressure is so low that insufficient blood supply reaches the vital tissues.

Types of Circulatory Shock and Their Causes

- *Low-volume shock* is a condition brought about by so great a loss of blood or blood plasma that the remaining blood is insufficient to fill the whole circulatory system. The blood loss may occur outside the body, as in a hemorrhage caused by injury to an artery or vein, or the loss may be internal because of the blood loss at the site of a major fracture, burn, or bleeding ulcer. Professional treatment involves replacement of blood loss by transfusion.
- *Neurogenic shock,* manifested by *fainting,* occurs when the regulating capacity of the nervous system is impaired by severe pain, profound fright, or other overwhelming stimulus. This type of shock is usually relieved by having the victim lie down with his head lower than the rest of his body.
- *Allergic shock,* also called *anaphylactic shock,* occurs when the functioning of the blood vessels is disturbed by a person's sensitivity to the injection of a particular foreign substance, as in the case of an insect sting or certain medicines.
- *Septic shock* is brought on by infection from certain bacteria that release a poison which affects the proper functioning of the blood vessels.

- *Cardiac shock* can be caused by any circumstance that affects the pumping action of the heart.

Symptoms

Shock caused by blood loss makes the victim feel restless, thirsty, and cold. He may perspire a great deal, and although his pulse is fast, it is also very weak. His breathing becomes labored and his lips turn blue.

Emergency Treatment

A physician should be called immediately if the onset of shock is suspected. Until medical help is obtained, the following procedures can alleviate some of the symptoms:

1. With a minimum amount of disturbance, arrange the victim so that he is lying on his back with his head somewhat lower than his feet. (*Exception:* If the victim's breathing is difficult, or if he has suffered a head injury or a stroke, keep his body flat.) Loosen any clothing that may cause constriction, such as a belt, tie, waistband, shoes. Cover him warmly against possible chill, but see that he isn't too hot.

2. If his breathing is weak and shallow, begin mouth-to-mouth respiration.

3. If he is hemorrhaging, try to control bleeding.

4. When appropriate help and transportation facilities are available, quickly move the victim to the nearest hospital or health facility in order to begin resuscitative measures.

5. *Do not* try to force any food or stimulant into the victim's mouth.

Cardiac Arrest

Cardiac arrest is a condition in which the heart has stopped beating altogether or is beating so weakly or so irregularly that it cannot maintain proper blood circulation.

Common causes of cardiac arrest are heart attack, electric shock, hemorrhage, suffocation, and other forms of respiratory arrest. Symptoms of cardiac arrest are unconsciousness, the absence of respiration and pulse, and the lack of a heartbeat or a heartbeat that is very weak or irregular.

Cardiopulmonary Resuscitation

If the victim of a medical emergency manifests signs of cardiac arrest, he or she should be given cardiopulmonary resuscitation (CPR), which is a combination of chest compressions and mouth-to-mouth resuscitation. Either one person or two can administer CPR. The procedure can be done in a moving vehicle en route to the hospital.

It is assumed that the victim is lying down with mouth clear and air passage unobstructed. The chest compressions are given in the following way:

1. The heel of one hand with the heel of the other crossed over it should be placed on the bottom third of the breastbone. The hands should be pressed firmly down with arms straight, using enough force so that the breastbone moves about two inches toward the spine, if the victim is an adult. Do not let the fingers press on the ribs.

2. The hands are then relaxed to allow the chest to expand.

3. If one person is doing both the chest compressions and the mouth-to-mouth respiration, he should interrupt the compressions after every 15 chest compressions and administer two very quick lung inflations to the victim.

4. The rescuer should try to make the rate of compression simulate restoration of the pulse rate. This is not always easily accomplished, but compression should reach 80 to 100 times per minute.

The technique for administering CPR to children is the same as that used for adults, except that much less pressure should be applied to a child's chest and, in the case of babies or young children, the rate of compression should be at least 100 times per minute and the pressure should be exerted with the tips of the fingers rather than the heel of the hand. Breaths should be administered after every fifth compression.

Caution

CPR can be damaging if applied improperly. Courses in emergency medical care offered by the American Red Cross and other groups are well worth taking. In an emergency in which CPR is called for, an untrained person should seek the immediate aid of someone trained in the technique before attempting it himself.

Choking or Obstructed Windpipe

Almost anyone can perform lifesaving measures quickly and easily and without special equipment. Choking usually occurs when a bite of food or an object becomes lodges at the back of the throat or at the opening of the trachea, or windpipe. Death can occur within four to five minutes, so quick action is crucial. The first step in helping a choking victim is to recognize the signs. Always call for help and the begin the rescue.

Signs of Choking

A choking victim cannot breathe, cough or speak. He may become pale and/or turn blue before collapsing. DO NOTHING if the person is coughing, breathing, or talking; he is getting air to his lungs and should be watched but have no rescue procedures performed on him. DO NOT slap the person on the back. The universal sign used to indicate choking is two hands placed on the throat, one hand on top of the other. Because people frequently grab or touch their throat when they are having difficulty swallowing or breathing, ask them if they are choking and need help.

Finger Probe

The finger probe should NEVER be performed on an infant or small child under the age of 8 years, except where indicated. If the object can be seen in an adult's mouth, a quick attempt to remove it can be made by probing with a finger. Use a hooking motion NOT a jabbing, poking motion to dislodge the object and extract it from the person's mouth. UNDER NO CIRCUMSTANCES should this method be pursued if it appears that the object is being pushed farther downward rather than being released and brought up. If no object can be seen or a finger probe fails to dislodge the object, the Heimlich maneuver should be given without delay.

The Heimlich Maneuver

This lifesaving technique works simply by squeezing the volume of air trapped in the victim's lungs. The object or piece of food literally pops out of the throat as if it were ejected from a squeezed balloon.

- for infants and small children (infant to 8 years) use the INFANT HEIMLICH MANEUVER
- for children and adults (8 years and older) use the ADULT HEIMLICH MANEUVER

Infant Back Blows and Heimlich Maneuver

This procedure should only be performed if you have seen or strongly suspect the baby is choking on an object and if breathing is becoming more difficult. Lips may appear to be blue. DO NOTHING if baby is coughing, breathing or talking. DO NOT probe throat with fingers. DO NOT hold baby upside down.

Using your lap, place baby face down on its stomach over your forearm, with its head resting on your hand. Keep the baby's head lower than its chest, but make certain your hand is fully supporting the baby's head. With the heel of your hand, give *five quick, firm* back blows between the shoulders. If water or vomit comes up, turn baby to the side and clear its mouth.

If this does not work, turn baby over onto its back, still holding head lower than chest, and place two to three fingers in center of baby's stomach about one to two finger widths below baby's nipples. Give five thrusts. Open baby's mouth, place thumb over tongue, and ONLY IF you see the object, remove it from the throat. DO NOT explore blindly. Repeat back blows and chest thrusts until obstruction is gone or infant becomes unconscious. If the infant becomes unconsious, begin emergency breathing.

The Heimlich Maneuver

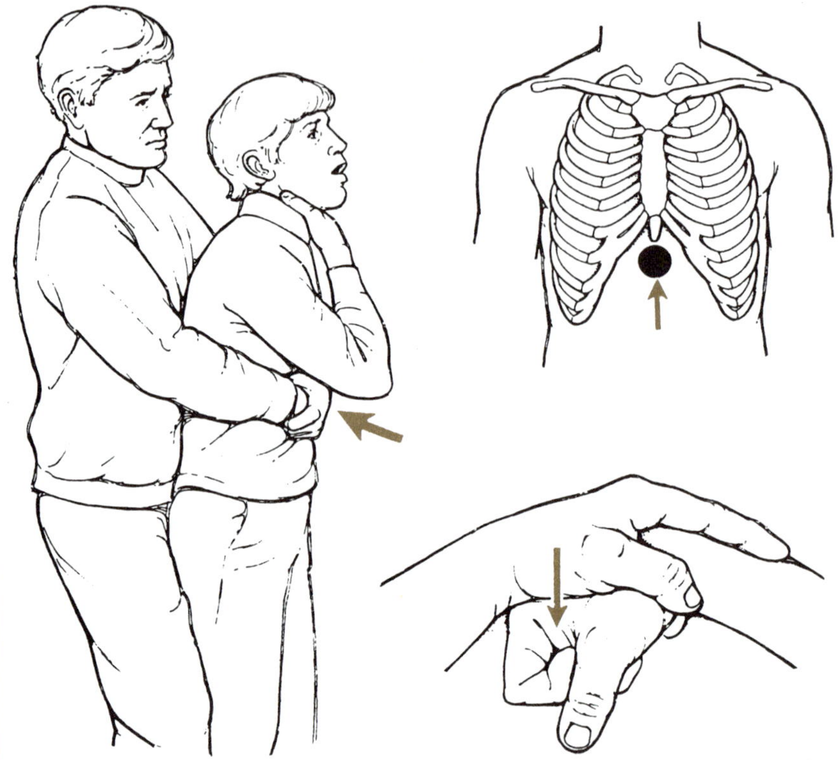

(Left) The rescuer stands behind the victim and grasps his hands firmly over the victim's abdomen just below the rib cage *(top right)*. The position of the rescuer's hands and the direction of thrust are shown at the bottom right.

Adult Heimlich Maneuver

To perform the technique on children and adults (8 years and older), hug the victim from behind and around the waist. Make a fist and place the thumb side against the stomach just above the naval but well below the lower tip of the breastbone. Grasp fist with your other hand. Pull your fist upward into victim's stomach with a quick upward thrust (see illustration). Repeat upward thrusts until obstruction is cleared or victim becomes unconsious. If victim becomes unconsious, begin emergency breathing. DO NOT administer back blows to children over age 8 or to adults.

If alone, you can perform the Heimlich maneuver on yourself, either by using your own fist or leaning into the back of a chair to simulate the thrust.

Poisoning

In all cases of poisoning, it is imperative to get professional assistance as soon as possible.

Listed below are telephone numbers for Poison Control Centers throughout the United States. These health service organizations are accessible 24 hours a day to provide information on how best to counteract the effects of toxic substances.

In the event of known or suspected poisoning, call the center nearest you immediately. Give the staff member to whom you speak as much information as possible: the name or nature of the poison ingested, if you know; if not, the symptoms manifested by the victim.

If for any reason it is impossible to telephone or get to a Poison Control Center (or a doctor or hospital), follow these two general rules:

1. If a strong acid or alkali or a petroleum product has been ingested, dilute the poison by administering large quantities of milk or water. Do not induce vomiting.

2. For methanol or related products such as window cleaners, antifreeze, paint removers, and shoe polish, induce vomiting—preferably with syrup of ipecac.

Calling for Help

Every household should have a card close by the telephone—if possible affixed to an adjacent wall—that contains the numbers of various emergency services. In most communities, it is possible to simply dial 911 or to dial the operator and ask for the police or fire department.

An ambulance can usually be summoned in one of the following ways: dialing 911; asking for a police ambulance; calling the nearest hospital; or calling whatever private ambulance service is available locally. Such services are listed in the classified pages of the telephone directory, and you should have their numbers on hand if an emergency service such as 911 is not available in your area.

Practically all hospitals have emergency rooms for the prompt treatment of accident cases. If the victim is in good enough physical condition, he can be placed lying down in a car for transportation to a hospital. However, under no circumstances should a person who has sustained major injuries or who has collapsed be made to sit upright in a car. First aid must be administered to him on the spot until a suitable conveyance arrives.

Every family should find out the telephone number of the nearest Poison Control Center (see section in this chapter) and note it on the emergency number card.

The Emergency-Free Home

Every year, hundreds of thousands of Americans go to hospital emergency rooms to obtain treatment for injuries or illnesses incurred in their homes. But many of these emergency health problems could have been prevented. In too many cases, no one took action to eliminate home hazards simply because they were easy to overlook or were not readily detectable.

Millions more Americans suffer less serious home injuries and do not go to hospitals. A cut finger, a stubbed toe, a fall that results in a bruise but no broken bones—all these minor accidents and many more occur daily.

With a little forethought, many of these home accidents can be prevented. This chapter provides basic guidelines for home safety.

First Aid Needs

The first step toward home safety is preparedness. This means ensuring that first aid equipment and medications are in the home, readily available.

Both materials and medicines should be chosen with care. Key considerations are the ages of those who live in the home, special requirements of particular family members, the seasons of the year, and other factors that may suggest a need for certain products or preparations.

First aid supplies should be kept in a medicine cabinet or in a larger storage place out of reach of children. Basic first aid items include:

- Soap
- Antiseptic wipes or solution
- Antiseptic/anesthetic ointment or spray
- Calamine/antihistamine lotion
- Sterile eye wash
- Activated charcoal for poison antidote (always call poison control center first)
- Blunt-tipped scissors
- Tweezers
- Bulb syringe
- Adhesive bandage strips
- Sterile cotton balls
- Sterile eye patches
- Sterile gauze pads, 4 by 4 inches
- Sterile nonstick pads
- Hypoallergenic adhesive tape
- Roller bandages
- Cotton swabs
- Triangular bandages
- Paper cups
- Butterfly bandages
- Cold packs, instant chemical-activated
- Elastic bandage, 3 inches wide
- Thermometer
- Eye wash cup

- Disposable latex gloves (for handling wounds)
- Flashlight
- Safety pin
- Candle and matches

Medicines and Medications

Don't overstock medications and, if possible, consult a physician or emergency hotline before attempting any emergency measures. Many medications only serve to delay proper medical attention. For example, syrup of ipecac, a preparation that induces vomiting in emergency situations, is a basic necessity in a household with children. However, if ipecac is used after the ingestion of certain liquids, the results can be very damaging and even fatal.

Leftover antibiotics should never be used a second time without consulting a physician. Because of their cost, many people are reluctant to dispose of leftover antibiotics, but severe allergic reactions could result or make it difficult for a physician to diagnose an illness if symptoms have been masked.

Antibiotics prescribed in series should be taken until the series is completed. Finally, no such medications should be passed on to friends or relatives for their use. Borrowed medications could harm, rather than help, the recipient.

What drugs or medications should be in your medicine cabinet? Some basic items are:

- Cold and allergy medications, including an antihistamine, a decongestant, a cough suppressant, an expectorant
- An antacid for indigestion
- Rubbing alcohol
- Antibiotic ointment
- Adhesive bandage strips
- An anti-diarrheal medicine
- A laxative
- Eyedrops
- Aspirin or an aspirin-free pain reliever
- Other items as required for chronic conditions.

Here are some additional safety rules regarding medicine cabinets:

- If possible, locate the medicine cabinet in a cool, dry, dark place, out of the reach of children.
- Check the contents periodically and throw away out-of-date or spoiled items (including aspirin that smells like vinegar).
- Remove the cotton from any medicine cabinet containers that may use cotton stoppers (because the cotton can absorb a medication's active ingredients).
- If even one pill in a bottle has deteriorated or spoiled, throw out the entire batch.
- Keep liquids in their amber containers to protect the contents from light.
- To discard medications, flush them down the toilet, then remove the labels on the containers to prevent

others from refilling the prescriptions.

- Keep emergency phone numbers (physician, pharmacist, fire, police, and so on; see the list of emergency phone numbers on the inside front cover of this volume) on the medicine cabinet or near it. When in doubt about which medication to use, call a doctor or pharmacist.

Reducing the Risk of Medicine Poisoning

Following certain safety rules can help ensure against the possibility of medicine poisoning. The rules are most important in homes where there are very young children or very old family members.

Medicines or preparations that are potentially harmful should be kept in a locked cabinet. If there are a number of such preparations in the home, they should probably be kept in a separate, locking storage place. If this is not possible, they should at least be stored out of the reach of young children.

Other safety rules are simply common sense. For example, one should never transfer a medicine into an unlabeled container. Special care should be taken with the dosages of both liquid and solid drugs. Sleeping tablets, tranquilizers, and even aspirin can, if taken in overdose, seriously harm the body.

If you plan to keep old medicine containers, wash them thoroughly and then store them carefully. Otherwise, they should be thrown away. If children resist taking their medicine, parents should never encourage them by pretending that the medicine is candy. Nor should parents rely too heavily on anti-tamper packaging. The shrink-wraps, push-and-turn bottle caps, foil inner seals, and other anti-tamper devices are valuable but not foolproof.

In any case of medicine poisoning, do not wait to seek help. Stay calm, call your physician or the nearest hospital or poison control center, and get instructions on correct procedures. If you take a poisoned family member to a hospital or elsewhere for help, you should bring with you the container(s) from which pills or liquid were taken. Do not administer salt and water to induce vomiting; the mixture is potentially fatal. With a child, a much more reliable method is to put a finger into the youngster's throat if the child is conscious.

Dangers of Alternative Medicines and Quack Remedies

Americans spend billions of dollars each year on "alternative" medicinal supplies and equipment. In too many cases the quack remedies not only do not help, they may do serious harm.

Examples of items that flood the marketplace but should not be found in your home are numerous. Among the many unproved procedures and preparations are hair analysis and cytotoxic tests for food allergies; oral chelation therapy, with vitamin and mineral capsules or tables for cardiovascular disease; and various "metabolic" programs, "non-toxic holistic medicines," radical dietary changes and regimens, and programs calling for massive doses of vitamins.

Still others include detoxification and drastic "cleansing" enemas, herbal mixtures to be applied to a sore or inflamed area, immune boosters that once were sold as cancer cures and now are promoted as treatments for AIDS, and laetrile, an unproven cancer treatment.

The following guidelines can help protect your family from such noneffective medications:

- Beware of testimonials in ads or on labels that purportedly come from satisfied users.
- Do not believe any promises of "money-back guarantees." They are rarely dependable.
- Be wary of advertising that claims a product is effective against numerous ailments.
- Be wary of promises of a "cure" or of "complete relief" from pain.
- Discount any "FDA-tested" or "FDA-recommended" testimonials. Federal law states that the Food and Drug Administration cannot be mentioned as giving marketing approvals.
- Beware of mentions of "natural" ingredients. The definition of natural is elusive, and the word is often abused.
- Think twice before buying *anything* that is advertised with such terms as these: "amazing," "vanish," "discovery," "breakthrough," "painless," "exclusive," or "instant."
- Finally,· warns the FDA, "If the product sounds too good to be true, it probably is."

Emergency-Proofing Your Home

The modern home is a marvel of timesaving, labor-saving, and comfort-producing devices and appliances. These include such products as space heaters, washers, dryers, refrigerators, gas and electric furnaces, and many others. To a great extent, the hazards that large or small appliances may introduce into your home are associated with fire. But householders should also take precautions against the dangers of electrocution, falls caused by poorly placed electrical cords, and other accident-producers.

Most emergencies arising from appliance use or misuse can be avoided by acting in advance to prevent possible hazards. Household items that are most likely to be hazardous are heating-cooling equipment, cooking equipment, heat tapes and humidifiers, and small electrical appliances.

Heating-Cooling Equipment

In the first category are furnaces, air conditioners, space heaters, and similar equipment. The primary safety rule with heating equipment is to make sure it is operating properly and efficiently. For furnaces of any kind, an annual checkup—usually in the summer or fall—is advisable. Many homeowners have maintenance policies that include such checkups.

All *space heaters* come with instructions for installation and operation. These instructions should be followed closely. Space heaters should be located so that they have plenty of room around them. They should be placed at a safe distance from all papers, clothing, draperies, furniture, and (if possible) children. Manufacturers' labels usually indicate what the proper clearance is for a particular model.

As with furnaces, space heaters should be kept in good working condition. Missing controls should be replaced; so should missing or defective guards or screens.

Electric space heaters should have tip-over shutoff switches that turn off the current if the unit is knocked over. These heaters should also have guards around their coils. The guard can be a wire grille or other protective "fence" that can keep fingers or fabrics away from the heating element.

If an extension cord is used with the space heater, the cord should have a power rating at least as high as the heater's rating. The cord should be in a safe place and out of the reach of children.

An important rule: Do not use a portable electric heater in a bathroom, near a sink, or close to water. This presents the risk of electrocution.

Gas space heaters may be vented or unvented. Both kinds need special care and attention.

If a gas space heater is vented, it should be vented correctly. That is, the vent pipe should be properly sized and free of cracks, leaks, and blockages, with tight joints and crack-free heat exchanger (to prevent leakage of carbon monoxide). If in doubt about the venting, call a servicer or your gas supplier.

When using an unvented gas space heater, you should always have a door or window slightly open in the room where the heater is located.

With either kind of gas heater, you should light the match *first* before you turn on the gas for the pilot light. This prevents flareups due to accumulated gas.

Woodburning, kerosene, or oil space heaters not only need to be installed properly; it would also be wise to have them inspected by a local fire safety official. Then you should use only the fuel, and in some cases the *grade* of fuel, for which the heater was designed.

The chimney of the heater or stove should be cleaned regularly, once every couple of months at least. In the case of a woodburning heater, it is best to use only paper or wood for kindling. *Never* use gasoline or another flammable or combustible fluid to start a woodburning stoves.

Cooking Equipment

The U.S. Consumer Product Safety Commission (CPSC) reports that more than 100,000 fires each year are associated with cooking equipment, especially stoves. These fires cause an estimated $300 million in property losses.

Some basic safety precautions can prevent most of these fires. For example, householders can avoid storing flammable or combustible items above the stove. The same applies to potholders, plastic utensils, towels, and other flammable items. Children's favorite foods, including cookies or candy, should never be kept above the range or in its immediate vicinity.

Clothing can be a trap for the unwary. Loose-fitting sleeves should not be worn while cooking. Also, you should never leave a stove unattended, especially when a burner is turned to a high setting.

Heat Tapes and Humidifiers

Heat tapes and ultrasonic humidifiers can pose home safety and health hazards. Heat tapes, used to keep exposed water pipes from freezing, present fire hazards. Ultrasonic humidifiers filled with tap water may discharge dangerous mineral particles into the air.

Electric heat tapes, or pipe heating cables, plug into wall or floor outlets. Once plugged in, they emit heat through their molded plastic insulation. Used in crawl spaces and in the substructures of homes and mobile homes, many tapes remain plugged in year-round. A thermostat in the power supply cord turns the tape on when the temperature falls below a certain level.

Improper installation of heat tapes has become a major cause of home fires in recent years. In many cases, lack of attention to the instructions that come with the product has resulted in faulty installation. Some homeowners lap the tape over itself when winding the tape around the pipe. Others ignore manufacturers' warnings that specific lengths of tape be used to protect pipes of given diameters and lengths.

If your home has heat tapes already installed you should (1) inspect all tapes, or have a licensed electrician inspect them, for proper installation or deteriorated installation; (2) check older tapes for cracks in the plastic insulation or bare wires, and replace worn tapes at once; (3) make certain, if you have plastic pipes, that the tapes you are using are recommended specifically for your kind of plastic piping; and (4) inspect all tapes to make sure none is wrapped over the thermal insulation on a pipe or near flammable objects.

Ultrasonic humidifiers using tap water have been found to spread such impurities as lead, aluminum, asbestos, or dissolved organic gases into the air. All these substances can be health hazards. To avoid such problems, use bottled, demineralized water or install demineralizing filters on your tap-water supply.

Other humidifiers pose no such mineral particle threat.

Home Electrical Safety

Have you conducted an audit of the connections, cords, gadgets (aside from major appliances), and other electrical equipment in your home? If not, such an audit is virtually a must.

You can start checking all lighting, including bulbs and sockets, all cords and extension cords, and all TV or audio equipment. Bulbs with wattages too high for the size of a fixture may overheat and cause a fire, so you should replace oversized bulbs with others of appropriate wattages. If the correct wattage is not indicated, use a bulb no larger than 60 watts.

Make sure all electrical cords are placed out of traffic areas so that people will not trip or fall over them. Stepping on cords can damage them, too, and produce fire hazards. Also check to make sure that cords do not have furniture resting on them. Cords should not be frayed, should not be wrapped around themselves or any object, and should *never* be attached to walls with nails or staples.

Extension cords should be equipped with safety covers and should never be expected to carry more than their proper loads. Both the cord and the electrical device will normally have electrical ratings.

Wall outlets and switches call for special attention. Whether they are in use of not, the same basic safety rules apply. All switches and wall outlets should be checked to make sure they are working properly and fixed if they are not. You can test them by touching: an unusually warm outlet or switch may indicate an unsafe wiring condition. Plugs should fit into outlets snugly, and all outlets should have face plates so that no wiring is exposed.

Kitchen countertop appliances, like TVs, radios, and other home entertainment equipment, should be placed so that they remain dry. If they give off heat, as does a toaster, they should have some space to "breathe." Countertop appliances should be unplugged when not in use.

Cords for countertop appliances are critically important. These should never be placed so that they can come into contact with hot surfaces; this applies especially to cords around toasters, ovens, and ranges. The same rule holds where water or wet surfaces are concerned.

Because ground fault circuit interrupters (GFCIs) can prevent many electrocutions, the Consumer Product Safety Commission recommends that all countertop outlets be equipped with them. They should also be used in bathrooms and other areas where there is a risk of electrical shock. Test your GFCIs regularly in accordance with the manufacturers' instructions.

Most current building codes require that bathrooms be equipped with GFCIs. Older homes may not have them.

Other electrical appliances and equipment require other kinds of safety care. These items can include hair dryers, curling irons, and electric blankets.

A universal rule is that such devices be unplugged when not in use. Plugged in and allowed to fall into water, they can cause an electrocution. They should also be in good operating condition, with no damaged wiring or other parts.

Do not use portable electric heaters in the bathroom or other rooms where they may come into contact with water. Keep *any* use of electrical devices or appliances in such rooms to a minimum.

Electric blankets also have to be used with care. They should be in good condition and have no charred spots on either the upper or the lower blanket surface. Before using them, look for cracks or breaks in wiring, connectors, and plugs.

To prevent overheating, do not cover electric blankets with other blankets, comforters, or other bedding. They should also be used flat, not folded back, and should not be tucked in except in accordance with the manufacturers' instructions.

Basement, garage, and workshop power tools and outlets constitute another extremely important area of safety concern. Power tools should have three-pronged plugs to indicate that they are double insulated. These plugs reduce the risk of electric shock.

Check your fuse box or circuit breaker. A fuse of the wrong size can present a fire hazard. If you do not know what sizes are correct, an electrician can tell you. Your circuit breakers should be "exercised" periodically if they are to remain in good working order. This procedure is simple:

1. Turn off your freezer, refrigerator, and air conditioner.

2. Flip each circuit breaker off and on three times.

3. Turn the appliances back on.

Repeat this routine at least once a year. Also check the GFCIs on your basement, garage, or workshop equipment to make sure they are working properly.

Receptacles located outdoors represent a final stage in your electrical audit.

These receptacles or outlets should have waterproof covers that keep water out and prevent malfunctions. The covers should be *closed* when not in use. If your home has no GFCIs on outside receptacles, you should have them installed.

As regards electric lawn movers and other electric garden tools and appliances, the basic rules of safety apply. But remember: extension cords used outside should be specifically designed for such use, or you may be risking a fire or a serious shock.

Home Fire Prevention and Protection

Many home fires have nothing to do with gadgets or appliances. Both the simplest and the most complex of our daily amenities can be fire hazards. Extremely flammable liquids provide power for our cars. Fabrics and upholstered furniture can ignite and burn. Some of us carry fire sources, matches or cigarette lighters, in our pockets.

In the sections that follow, effort will be made to call attention to the most important of these hazards.

Matches, Lighters, and Cigarettes

Some prohibitions that help to immunize your home against accidental fires are matters of common sense. Others have more technical origins.

Some 140 young children die each year in fires that they or their friends or siblings started. Children start thousands more home fires while playing with matches or lighters. Thus a basic rule is that children should not have access to either matches or cigarette lighters. Both should be kept out of sight and reach.

Adults should never use either matches or lighters as toys or sources of amusement. Cigarette butts should not be left burning in ashtrays that children can reach.

Ashtray and cigarette discipline is always appropriate. Lighted butts should not be thrown into the trash. A lighted butt can start a major fire. Ashtrays should not be placed on the arms of chairs, where they can be knocked off. As a precaution, check the furniture where smokers have been sitting to make sure that no lighted cigarettes have fallen unnoticed behind or between cushions or under furniture.

In a recent year, 46,700 mattress and bedding fires took some 700 lives. Thus, "No smoking in bed" represents a cardinal rule of home safety.

Furniture Precautions

Because many home fires start on pieces of furniture, you should take special care when selecting the items you need. In particular, you should look for furniture designed to reduce the likelihood of furniture fires that may be started by cigarettes.

This task has become simpler in recent years. Manufacturers are making upholstered furniture far more fire resistant than they have in the past. All furniture that meets the standards of the Upholstered Furniture Action Council (UFAC) carries a gold-colored tag with red letters that states, "Important Consumer Safety Information from UFAC."

The tag is a form of safety certification that the manufacturer attaches in compliance with UFAC's Voluntary Action Program. "The manufacturer of this furniture," states the tag, "certifies that it is made in accordance with the new, improved UFAC methods, designed to reduce the likelihood of furniture fires from cigarettes."

Other precautions help reduce the risks of injury or death from furniture fires. For example, look for upholstery fabrics made primarily from such thermoplastic fibers as nylon, polyester, acrylic, and olefin. These resist ignition by burning cigarettes better than do rayon or cotton, both cellulose fabrics.

Flammable Liquids

The federal Hazardous Substances Act establishes three labeling categories for liquid products:

1. *Extremely flammable liquids* include gasoline, the white gas commonly used in camping stoves, contact adhesives, and wood stains that produce ignitable vapors at room temperature. Once ignited, the vapors act as wicks to carry the fire to the container of the liquid.

2. *Flammable liquids* produce ignitable vapors at higher temperatures. In this group are such liquids as paint thinners, some paints, and automotive products such as brake fluids.

3. *Combustible liquids* can be ignited but are less likely to catch fire than the other kinds. This category includes furniture polishes, oil-based paints, fuel oil, diesel oil, and kerosene.

To some extent, you can shop wisely for flammable liquids. You can, for example, buy a product that is least likely to ignite but that still meets your needs. But remember: some products do not carry *flammable* labels because they will not catch fire in liquid form as they come from the container. Some paint strippers belong in this category. Once they are applied, however, they become quite flammable because their flame-suppressant chemicals evaporate.

Use solvent-based products with adequate moving air ventilation, and ventilate the work area. These precautions will keep fumes from building up and igniting. They will also protect you from the toxic effects of invisible and sometimes explosive vapors.

Wise Use of Flammable Liquids

At one time or another, nearly everyone has to use flammable liquids. Here are some fundamental rules for wise use:

- Never use such liquids near flames or a source of sparks, including pilot lights.
- Use gasoline only as a fuel, not as a cleaning fluid.
- Always shut off power mowers, chain saws, or other gas-powered equipment before refueling them. Refuel outdoors and wait for hot parts to cool before adding fuel.

- Use only liquids identified as *charcoal starters* to get charcoal fires going. Never pour on additional fluid after starting the fire.

Proper Storage

Gasoline and other extremely flammable liquids should be stored outside your house or apartment, but they should *not* be stored in the trunk of your car. Children should not be able to reach your safe-storage place. For added insurance, lock up all flammable liquids.

Never keep gasoline in glass bottles, plastic jugs, or other makeshift containers. If possible, invest in a gasoline container with such safety features as a pressure release valve or a flame arrester.

Flammable Fabrics

There are four basic safety principles regarding the flammability of fabrics:

1. All fibers used in ordinary clothing can burn. But some catch fire and burn less readily than others. The more-fire-resistant fabrics are fire-resistant cotton, wool, rayon, polyester, and modacrylic. Fabrics that burn most readily are acetate, untreated cotton and rayon, and linen.

2. The way in which a fabric is made determines the way it burns. As a rule, heavy, tightly constructed fabrics ignite with difficulty and burn more slowly than fabrics that are light, open, or fuzzy. Once ignited, however, the heavier fabrics burn longer than the lightweights and can cause very serious injuries.

3. "Flame resistant" does not mean "noncombustible." The phrase only indicates that a fabric is designed to resist ignition and burning. Under some conditions such fabrics will not only burn; they will be incapable of providing you with protection if you reach into a fireplace, a wood-burning stove, or an oven. To maintain a fabric's flame-resistant qualities, follow the manufacturer's instructions regarding care and cleaning.

4. A garment's style has much to do with safety. The safest clothes are those that fit closely, have large neck openings and quick release closures, and are wrap-style.

Remember the three rules for extinguishing a clothing fire:

1. Don't run.

2. Do try to remove the burning article of clothing.

3. If that fails, drop to the floor or ground and roll back and forth.

Smoke Detectors

There are two basic rules regarding smoke detectors. First, every home should have at least one smoke detector, approved by a recognized national testing laboratory. Second, at least one smoke detector should be

placed on each floor of your home.

These rules apply for both ionization and photoelectric detectors. Both types of detectors, if well designed and engineered, are effective. The particular layout of your home may determine whether you need plug-in or battery-powered devices. You may choose to have one or two of each type; both have advantages and disadvantages.

The battery-powered smoke detector can run out of power, usually after about a year. It then gives a warning sound, at which time you need to install new batteries.

The plug-in detector operates like a permanently burning lamp. However, it cannot operate if fire or some other interference breaks the electrical circuit that powers the detector. Other tips:

- Place detectors high up, on a ceiling or wall, close to where people sleep. Otherwise the alarm may not be heard.
- Never place a smoke detector in the kitchen or very near it. Airborne kitchen grease and cooking fumes can easily activate the device, touching off a false alarm.
- Even if a battery-powered detector does not give a signal that its batteries are running down, change the batteries at least once a year.
- With a photoelectric detector, the light source should be replaced as soon as it burns out.
- Test photoelectric detectors regularly with real smoke—from a just-extinguished candle, for example. Test ionization detectors using a *lighted* candle. Test detectors every two to four weeks.

Fire Extinguishers

Fire extinguishers complement your smoke alarms and should be part of your home "immunization" program. The extinguishers should be kept in areas where fires are most likely to occur: the kitchen, home workshop, or rooms where flammable materials are kept, where people may be smoking, or where there are hazard-producing activities or materials.

Fire extinguishers are rated according to size. A five-pound extinguisher rated ABC (meaning it can be used to fight fires of any kind) is considered minimal for home protection. Many homeowners, however, buy two-and-one-half-pound extinguishers specifically to fight small kitchen fires.

The best protection against home fires may be a common garden hose. Using extensions, it can be made long enough to reach every room in the house. You can also attach nozzles that make it possible to sprinkle, spray, or direct a solid stream. Keep the hose in one place so that it is always ready to use.

An Escape Plan

Fire causes most home emergencies, but other conditions can be just as disastrous. An accident outside the home may force immediate evacua-

tion; so may natural disasters such as storms or floods.

An escape plan should be part of your program for immunizing your home against emergencies. The plan, in a sense, is an admission that an emergency could occur, but it can save lives by preventing panic.

For Fires

Your escape plan has to take into consideration the possibility that you may have to evacuate for an hour or several days or longer. In cases of fire, you need to have two exits from each part of the house. You may want to consider installing rope or chain safety ladders outside windows that are too high above the ground for safe jumping. If you live in an apartment, you should obtain escape instructions from your building management or landlord or your local fire department.

Through informal fire drills, you can help to ensure that each member of your household understands the escape plan. You should include small children as part of your escape rehearsals, and the rehearsals should be repeated periodically. Everyone should know where they are to meet to be sure everyone got out safely.

Young children should understand clearly that they have to evacuate when everyone else does. They *must* escape; they cannot hide under a bed or in a closet.

Safe escape may require understanding of the tricks of self- preservation in case of fire. Three rules are critically important:

1. *Stay low.* Since most smoke rises, you need to keep low, crawling on hands and knees when necessary, to pass safely through a smoke-filled hallway or room.

2. *Feel doors before you open them.* If you find that the door panels, the knob, or the molding surrounding the door are hot to the touch, it may mean that the fire is just outside. Move toward another exit.

3. *Use wet cloths.* To avoid excessive smoke inhalation, a major cause of fire-related deaths, you can wet pillow cases, towels, or other fabrics and hold them over your face while you make your way to an exit.

For Natural Disasters

In case of natural disasters, you may need to obtain accurate, current information as well as warnings, advice, or instructions issued by various agencies. Disregarding such instructions or advice can endanger you and your family.

Your home should be equipped with a battery-powered portable radio. The radio could mean the difference between disaster and survival if your power is interrupted. You should have spare, sealed-in-the-package batteries for the radio. To prolong

their lives, you can keep them in a refrigerator freezer.

Other avenues of communication in an emergency are available in most communities in the United States. These include amateur radio, citizens' band (CB) radio, community disaster warnings, special signals and communications methods, and (of course) the telephone.

Amateur radio or "ham" operators have proven to be unusually helpful in emergencies. To locate such an operator in your community, you can inquire among your neighbors or write, enclosing a self-addressed, stamped envelope, to the Amateur Radio Relay League, 225 Main St., Newington, CT 06111.

Poisonous or Harmful Substances

Each year, more than 100,000 children under the age of five become victims of accidental ingestion of poisonous or harmful substances. These include medicines and such flammable liquids as gasoline, but they also include a vast range of liquids, solids, and gases that find their ways into the home.

Substances that require special precautions range from carbon monoxide to spoiled food, cleaning fluids, detergents, and pesticides. Some general guidelines are as follows:

- Bring such substances into your home only if necessary, and then in the smallest possible quantity.
- Keep all products in their original containers, never in containers customarily used for food or drinks.
- If a product comes in a child-resistant container, never transfer it to a container that has no such protection.
- Carefully separate foods from potentially harmful products.
- After using a product that comes in a child-resistant container, resecure the cap or other closure.
- Make sure that all products that entail any risk or hazard are properly labeled, and turn on lights before using such products.
- Store potentially hazardous products in a separate area from other household products, preferably in a locked cabinet.
- Because not all the harmful substances that enter your home have warnings on their containers, you should make it your business to learn whether hazards exist.

Lead Poisoning

Lead is a metallic element that has many uses in industry and manufacturing. In the latter half of the twentieth century, however, its use was

strictly curtailed because of the dangerous effects lead has on the human body. Nevertheless, significant amounts of lead still exist in the environment, both outdoors and in the home, and lead poisoning continues to be a public health concern.

Lead can be ingested, such as by consuming contaminated water, food, or paint chips, or by inhaling fumes that contain lead. It can also be absorbed through the skin. Although some lead is excreted, much of it remains in the body and accumulates, concentrating in the bone marrow, nerve tissue (including the brain), and the kidneys.

The symptoms of lead poisoning may be difficult to recognize or may not even be present. People with high levels of lead may be irritable and have diminished appetite and energy. Children may lose recently acquired developmental skills. There may be abdominal cramping.

The effects of long-term lead poisoning include anemia, high blood pressure, kidney damage, and damage to the reproductive organs in adults. Very high levels may cause diseases of the brain; symptoms of acute lead poisoning include vomiting, headache, staggering gait, seizures, and coma.

Children are particularly susceptible to the dangers of lead. They absorb a higher percentage of the lead to which they are exposed. It has been estimated that one in 11 children in the United States has dangerous levels of lead in the bloodstream. With prolonged or repeated exposure, the amount of lead in a child's body can accumulate and cause neurological damage. Lead poisoning has been associated, though not definitively, with mental retardation and lowered IQ in children.

Exposure to lead comes from various sources. Lead-based paint was often used in housing built before 1978, and this paint may still be on the walls. Small children become poisoned when they eat chips of the paint as it deteriorates. Old lead-based paint also disintegrates into dust that both children and adults can breathe in or consume accidentally. Older homes may have pipes that were soldered with lead, and such pipes can leach lead into drinking water. Lead can leach into food and drink from pewter dinnerware, from ceramic dinnerware coated with a lead-containing glaze, and from lead-crystal glasses and decanters. The inhalation of lead emissions is the major source of lead exposure for people working in factories and smelters that use lead. Such emissions also pose a threat to the general population, since airborne lead emissions not only pollute the air people breathe but also are eventually deposited in the soil.

A treatment called chelation therapy can remove lead from the body, but it cannot reverse any damage already done by exposure to lead. For this reason, the best treatment is considered to be prevention. Avoid storing acidic foods in ceramic containers. Do not store beverages in lead-crystal decanters. In homes that have pipes soldered with lead, only cold

water should be used for drinking and cooking (hot water absorbs more lead), and the water should be run for 30 to 60 seconds before use.

Test kits, available in hardware stores, can detect the presence of lead paint. In older housing having lead-based paint, the best prevention is to move out of the contaminated home. When moving out is not possible, regular, vigorous housecleaning can reduce lead-contaminated dust significantly. If there are certain rooms that have lead-based paint, children should be kept out of those rooms. Children who eat nutritious diets—low in fat and high in iron, calcium, and vitamin C—absorb less lead than those who do not eat well. Children's hands and their toys, pacifiers, and other objects should be washed frequently.

When doing major or minor renovations on a room or a house that has lead-based paint, take precautions to minimize the dangers. Protective equipment and clothing should be used. Lead paint should never be sanded off because it creates a large amount of small particles and dust that cannot be picked up by ordinary household vacuum cleaners. Similarly, using heat guns or torches to make lead paint easier to remove creates lead particles that can be inhaled. Painting over or paneling over lead paint is recommended instead of trying to take off the paint. If large-scale removal of lead contamination is necessary, it should be done by professionals.

The Allergen-Free Environment

Some 35 million Americans suffer from allergies. They may have hay fever, asthma, food intolerances or sensitivities, or adverse skin reactions to the stings of hornets, bees, or wasps. While medical scientists do not completely understand the causes and workings of allergies, great progress is being made in this area.

One result of allergy research is that most people with allergies are able to lead normal lives in spite of diverse symptoms and reactions. For hay fever sufferers, doctors can prescribe drugs to relieve irritating nasal inflammation, or allergic rhinitis. Cromolyn sodium may be prescribed to relieve the symptoms of asthma; the sodium can be inhaled through a spinhaler, nebulizer machine, or metered dose inhaler.

For most allergy victims, the best defense is to avoid the substances or circumstances that bring on attacks or symptoms. If there are allergy sufferers in your family, you may want to establish a home environment that is as allergen-free as possible. Furry pets are a major cause of allergic reactions. Carpeting, unless laid on a cement floor, serves as the perfect incubator for dust mites. Books can also harbor mites. Both feather and foam rubber pillows can be hazards. The best protection is cleanliness.

Radon, A Special Case

Radon is a colorless, odorless, radioactive gas that is almost impossible to detect without instruments. It seeps through the crevices or spaces in the soil or rock on which a home is built. It can enter your home through dirt floors, cracks in concrete floors and walls, joints, sumps, floor drains, and the tiny holes or pores in hollow-block walls.

Persons exposed to radon face serious health risks, specifically lung cancer. Also, continued exposure to radon increases the risk of illness. Many persons never realize that the gas is invading their homes.

Detection of radon requires special equipment but moderate cost. Two commercially available radon detectors are the charcoal canister and the alpha track detector. The former calls for a test period of three to seven days, and the latter requires two to four weeks. Trained personnel can provide other methods of detection. Reports on measurements of radon gas are made in terms of picocuries per liter (pCi/l).

If you obtain readings of above 1.0 WL (working level) or above 200 pCi/l, take follow-up measurements as quickly as possible.

Doing it yourself to close off the radon entry points in your basement begins with caulking. Using urethane or silicone caulk, seal up the gap (if any) between the basement floor and all walls; fill cracks in the mortar joints between concrete blocks; and lay a thick bead of caulk around the perimeter of sump openings. Treated plywood or a metal sheet can then be used to cover the sump, with more caulk used as a sealant.

Use ready-mix concrete to seal any large openings around pipes, pipe-chase openings, and spaces along the top rows of concrete-block walls. Inject insulation into the top rows of concrete-block walls before sealing them. Foam backing can be applied before the concrete sealing is applied to pipe-chase openings.

Ventilation supplements your efforts to close all gaps and holes in your basement's floors and walls. Without creating uncomfortable drafts, you can ventilate under your basement slab *if:* (1) you have a continuous slab with no large, unsealed openings to the earth beneath, and (2) there is a sufficiently porous bed under the slab to permit ventilating air to circulate through it. Given both conditions, you can create your own subslab vent system with pipes and a fan; the air intake and exhaust pipes should be located in opposite corners of the basement.

Other methods of ventilating your basement include forced-air systems using fans to maintain a balanced air exchange rate; heat-recovery ventilators that replace radon-tainted air with outside air; and use of a product called Enka-drain, which traps radon in a nylon mesh airspace that is then vented through an exhaust pipe.

Because it is a gas, radon always moves from a higher pressure area (the ground) to a lower-pressure one (your house). That means you have a final alternative to ventilation: pressurize your basement and home by providing outside air supplies for wood stoves, fireplaces, gas dryers, and furnaces.

The Food Department

Threats to your health can enter your home in a grocery bag. They can develop in your home in the forms of mold or bacteria on food. Poor food handling practices, either inside or outside the home, can contribute to these health hazards. The greatest threats are a lack of sanitation, insufficient cooking, and improper storage (see also "Food Hazards," pp. 967–970).

Bacteria cause about 95 percent of all cases of food poisoning. People can ingest illness-producing bacteria in contaminated foods; the bacteria can then multiply and spread infections in the digestive tract or the bloodstream. Such digestive problems occur most often in warm weather, when food may be taken to picnics or on cookout without proper refrigeration.

Contamination may also take place if parasitic animals such as the roundworm, found sometimes in pork, enter the body. The roundworm produces a disease called trichinosis.

There are four main kinds of bacteria that can contaminate foods and cause diseases: salmonella; "staph," or *staphylococcus aureus;* botulism; and *clostridium perfringens,* which causes diarrhea. However, you can avoid contamination if you take precautions. This is important because the four kinds of bacteria can produce symptoms as mild as an upset stomach or as severe as death, as in the case of botulism.

Food-Borne Poisons and Allergens

When shopping, you usually have to take on faith the food manufacturer's and the grocer's claims that their food is safe. But you can certainly be selective. You may want to avoid foods that touch off negative or allergic reactions. If certain foods have given you gastrointestinal or other problems in the past, it would be wise to avoid those foods when shopping.

Other factors may guide your shopping choices. You may be dieting; or, you may be trying to "beef up" your diet, for example, to provide more calcium or other minerals. You may have allergies—for example, to sulfites, the additives in many foods that can cause serious or even fatal reactions. Today, the labels on food packaging provide an abundance of dietary information to aid consumers in making choices.

Buying intelligently and carefully constitutes your first line of defense against food-borne illness and disease. Here are some guidelines for the conscientious shopper:

- Watch for possible spoilage in everything you buy, and *never* purchase food in a torn package or a dented or bulging can.
- Exercise your right to doubt: check display cases to make sure frozen foods are stored above the frost lines or load lines. Never buy frozen food that has softened.
- Always pick up meat, poultry, and dairy products last when making your grocery rounds.
- Never leave a sackful of groceries in the car on a hot day. Make the grocery store your last stop on the way home, and make sure perishable groceries are wrapped in an insulated bag for the trip home.
- Once home, put everything away quickly in the appropriate storage place, whether refrigerator, freezer, or storage cupboard.

Different foods require different storage methods. The labels on many packaged or canned foods provide instructions for storage procedures.

Food preparation under the wrong conditions creates many of the problems that Americans face when they sit down to eat. The wrong conditions range from unclean hands, hair, fingernails, and clothing to failure to wash one's hands thoroughly after using the toilet. You should wash your hands thoroughly after smoking or blowing your nose. You should also wash your hands after handling raw meat, poultry, or eggs and before working with other foods. Other precautions: Do not use your hands to mix foods; use clean utensils instead. Avoid using the same spoon more than once to taste food while preparing it. Never eat any food directly from the jar or can; this could contaminate the can's contents. Scrub potatoes and other raw foods before cooking them. Carefully clean all utensils, work surfaces, dishes, and kitchen equipment before using them. And drink only pasteurized milk.

It is best to serve foods soon after they are cooked; otherwise, refrigerate them. You can refrigerate hot or warm foods if you are sure they will not raise the refrigerator temperature above 45° F.

The temperatures at which you keep foods affect directly your home's level of food safety. Hot foods should be kept above 140 degrees for safety while cold foods should be stored at 40 degrees or lower. The danger zone in which foods can develop bacteria, sometimes in the space of two or three hours, lies between 60° and 125°. Keeping food warm for several hours in an oven can be hazardous if the oven's temperature is between 60° and 125°.

Some foods require special attention. Eggs, for example, should be used only if they are fresh, clean, uncracked, and odor-free. You may make exceptions if the eggs are unspoiled and if they are to be used in recipes that call for thorough cooking. When serving a dish that has eggs as a major ingredient, cool the dish quickly after it is cooked, preferably in cold water, if it is not to be served hot. Then refrigerate it.

Meat, poultry, and fish are also sensitive. If frozen, they should be thawed in the refrigerator. If you need to thaw these products more quickly, you can place them, sealed in watertight wrappers, in cold water. To cook frozen items of these types, allow about one-and-one-half times the ordinary cooking times for thawed products of the same weight and shape.

Meats, poultry, or fish should be stuffed just before they are cooked, not a day or two ahead of time. The stuffing should reach a temperature of at least 165° F. during cooking. Use reliable timetables or follow package directions when cooking these products, and take extra care with ground meat. Because it is handled several times in packaging, ground meat should be cooked thoroughly and never eaten raw. Some hams need to be cooked, and should be if you have any doubt.

Fish, meat, and poultry should be cooked entirely in a single process, not cooked partially one day and then finished on another. Poultry should always be cooked thoroughly. Ground poultry should be cooked to 165° F, and whole poultry should be cooked to 180° F in the thigh and 170° F in the breast. If you store poultry products before the day on which you plan to cook them, you should store the giblets and the rest of the bird separately in the refrigerator. Use hot dogs and cold meat within a few days after purchasing, and never more than a week later. Ground meats and all cuts of fresh pork should be cooked to 160° F. Beef, veal, lambsteaks, roasts, and chops may be cooked to 145° F.

Freezer practices should be grounded in common sense. A fundamental rule is that freezing does not kill the bacteria in food; it only keeps existing bacteria from multiplying. Thawing enables those bacteria to begin to proliferate again.

Do not refreeze food that has been frozen and thawed. To protect frozen foods, wrap or package each item carefully to keep air away from the product. Different items can be kept safely in a freezing compartment for different periods of time, depending on the product. Label each item with the date it went into the freezer and the type of food that it is.

Reaching a Physician

Emergencies are usually best handled in a hospital because they are likely to require oxygen, blood transfusions, or other services only a hospital can provide. There are many situations, however, in which a physician's guidance on the phone can be extremely helpful and reassuring.

Because there are times when the family physician may not be available by phone, it's a good idea to ask for the names and phone numbers of physicians who can be called when your own physician can't be reached. In many communities, it is also possible to get the services of a physician by calling the county medical society.

A family on vacation in a remote area or on a cross-country trip by car can be directed to the nearest medical services by calling the telephone operator or the nearest headquarters of the state police.

Emergency Transport

In the majority of situations, the transfer of an injured person should be handled only by experienced rescue personnel. If you yourself must move a victim to a physician's office or hospital emergency room, here are a few important rules to remember:

1. Give all necessary first aid before attempting to move the victim. Do everything to reduce pain and to make the patient comfortable.

2. If you improvise a stretcher, be sure it is strong enough to carry the victim and that you have enough people to carry it. Shutters, doors, boards, and even ladders may be used as stretchers. Just be sure that the stretcher is padded underneath to protect the victim and that a blanket or coat is available to cover him and protect him from exposure.

3. Bring the stretcher to the victim, not the victim to the stretcher. Slide him onto the stretcher by grasping his clothing or lift him—if enough bearers are available—as shown in the illustration.

4. Secure the victim to the stretcher so he won't fall off. You may want to tie his feet together to minimize his movements.

5. Unless specific injuries prevent it, the victim should be lying on his back while he is being moved. However, a person who is having difficulty breathing because of a chest injury might be more comfortable if his head and shoulders are raised slightly. A person with a severe injury to the back of his head should be kept lying on his side. In any case, place the patient in a comfortable position that will protect him from further injury.

6. Try to transport the patient feet first.

7. Unless absolutely necessary, don't try to put a stretcher into a passenger car. It's almost impossible to get the stretcher or injured person into a passenger car without further injuring him. If there is no ambulance,

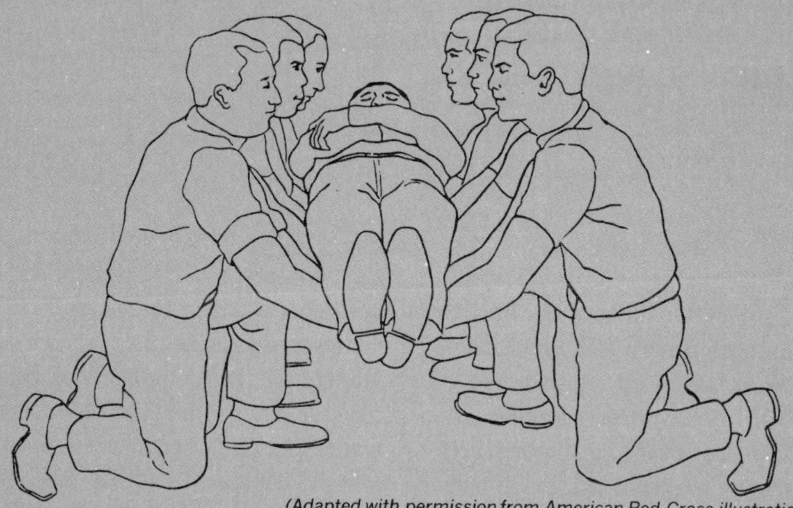

(Adapted with permission from American Red Cross illustrations.)

How to lift an injured or unconscious person to place him on a stretcher. Three bearers on each side of the victim kneel on the knee closer to the victim's feet. The bearers work their hands and forearms gently under the victim to about the midline of the back. On signal, they lift together as shown; on a following signal, they stand as a unit, if that is necessary. In lowering the victim to a stretcher or other litter, the procedure is reversed.

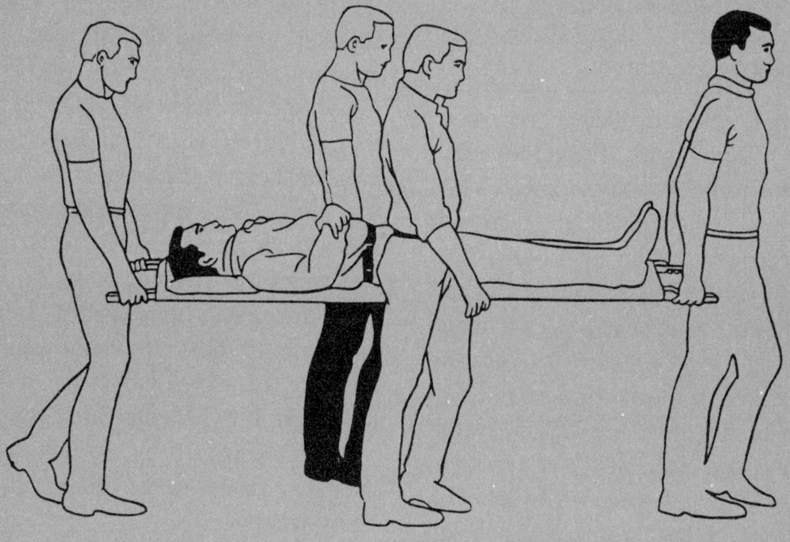

The proper way to carry a victim on a stretcher. One bearer is at the head, one at the foot, and one at either side of the stretcher. The victim should be carried feet first.

a station wagon or truck makes a good substitute.

8. When you turn the patient over to a doctor or take him to an emergency room of a hospital, give a complete account of the situation to the person taking charge. Tell the doctor what you've done for.

Alphabetic Guide to Medical Emergencies

Abdominal Wound

Abdominal wounds can result from gunshots during hunting or working with firearms, from falling on a knife or sharp object at home or work, or from a variety of other mishaps ranging from automobile accidents to a mugging attack. Such a wound can be a major emergency requiring surgery and other professional care. Call a physician or arrange for quick transportation to a hospital as quickly as possible.

Emergency Treatment

If there is severe bleeding, try to control it with pressure. Keep the victim lying on his back with the knees bent; place a pillow, coat, or a similar soft object under the knees to help hold them in the bent position. If abdominal organs are exposed, do not touch them for any reason. Cover the wound with a sterile dressing. Keep the dressing moistened with sterile water or the cleanest water available. Boiled water can be used to moisten the dressing, but be sure it has cooled before applying.

If the victim is to be moved to a hospital or physician's office, be sure the dressing over the wound is large enough and is held in place with a bandage. In addition to pain, you can expect the victim to experience nausea and vomiting, muscle spasms, and severe shock. Make the victim as comfortable as possible under the circumstances; if he complains of thirst, moisten his mouth with a few drops of water, but do not permit him to swallow the liquid.

Abrasions

Emergency Treatment

Wash the area in which the skin is scraped or rubbed off with soap and water, using clean gauze or cotton. Allow the abrasion to air-dry, and then cover it with a loose sterile dressing held in place with a bandage. If a sterile dressing is not available, use a clean handkerchief.

Change the dressing after the first 24 hours, using household hydrogen peroxide to ease its removal if it sticks to the abrasion because of clotted blood. If the skinned area appears to be accompanied by swelling, or is painful or tender to the touch, consult a physician.

Acid Burns

Among acids likely to be encountered at work and around the home are sulphuric, nitric, and hydrochloric acids. Wet-cell batteries, such as automobile batteries, contain acid powerful enough to cause chemical destruction of body tissues, and some metal cleaners contain powerful acids.

Emergency Treatment

Wash off the acid immediately, using large amounts of clean, fresh, cool water. Strip off or cut off any clothing that may have absorbed any of the acid. If possible, put the victim in a shower bath; if a shower is not available, flood the affected skin areas with as much water as possible. However, do not apply water forcefully since this could aggravate damage already done to skin or other tissues.

After as much of the acid as possible has been eliminated by flooding with water, apply a mild solution of sodium bicarbonate or another mild alkali such as lime water. Caution should be exercised, however, in neutralizing an acid burn because the chemical reaction between an acid and an alkali can produce intense heat that would aggravate the injury; also, not all acids are effectively neutralized by alkalis—carbolic acid burns, for example, should be neutralized with alcohol.

Wash the affected areas once more with fresh water, then dry gently with sterile gauze; be careful not to break the skin or to open blisters. Extensive acid burns will cause extreme pain and shock; have the victim lie down with the head and chest a little lower than the rest of the body. As soon as possible, summon a physician or rush the victim to the emergency room of a hospital.

Aerosol Sprays

Although aerosol sprays generally are regarded as safe when handled according to directions, they can be directed accidentally toward the face with resulting contamination of the eyes or inhalation of the fumes. The pressurized containers may also contain products or propellants that are highly flammable, producing burns when used near an open flame. When stored near heat, in direct sunlight, or in a closed auto, the containers may explode violently.

Emergency Treatment

If eyes are contaminated by spray particles, flush the eye surfaces with water to remove any particles of the powder mist. Then carefully examine eye surfaces to determine if chemicals appear to be imbedded in the surface of the cornea. If aerosol spray is inhaled, move the patient to a well-ventilated area; keep him lying down, warm, and quiet. If breathing fails, administer artificial respiration. Victims of exploding containers or burning contents of aerosol containers should be given appropriate emergency treatment for bleeding, burns, and shock.

The redness and irritation of eye injuries should subside within a short time. If they do not, or if particles of spray seem to be imbedded in the surface of the eyes, take the victim to an ophthalmologist. A physician should also be summoned if a victim fails to recover quickly from the effects of inhaling an aerosol spray, particularly if the victim suffers from asthma or a similar lung disorder or from an abnormal heart condition.

Alkali Burns

Alkalis are used in the manufacture of soap and cleaners and in certain household cleaning products. They combine with fats to form soaps and may produce a painful injury when in contact with body surfaces.

Emergency Treatment

Flood the burned area with copious amounts of clean, cool, fresh water. Put the victim under a shower if possible, or otherwise pour running water over the area for as long as is necessary to dilute and weaken the corrosive chemical. Do not apply the water with such force that skin or other tissues are damaged. Remove clothing contaminated by the chemical.

Neutralize the remaining alkali with diluted vinegar, lemon juice, or a similar mild acid. Then wash the affected areas again with fresh water. Dry carefully with sterile gauze, being careful not to open blisters or otherwise cause skin breaks that could result in infection. Summon professional medical care as soon as possible. Meanwhile, treat the victim for shock.

Angina Pectoris

Angina pectoris is a condition that causes acute chest pain because of interference with the supply of oxygen to the heart. Although the pain is sometimes confused with ulcer or acute indigestion symptoms, it has a distinct characteristic of its own, producing a feeling of heaviness, strangling, tightness, or suffocation. Angina is a symptom rather than a disease, and may be a chronic condition with those over 50. It is usually treated by placing a nitroglycerine tablet under the tongue.

An attack of acute angina can be brought on by emotional stress, overeating, strenuous exercise, or by any activity that makes excessive demands on heart function.

Emergency Treatment

An attack usually subsides in about ten minutes, during which the patient appears to be gasping for breath. He should be kept in a semireclining position rather than made to lie flat, and should be moved carefully only in order to place pillows under his head and chest so that he can breathe more easily. A physician should be called promptly after the onset of an attack.

Animal Bites/Rabies

Wild animals, particularly bats, serve as a natural reservoir of rabies, a disease that is almost always fatal unless promptly and properly treated. But the virus may be present in the saliva of any warm-blooded animal. Domestic animals should be immunized against rabies by vaccines injected by a veterinarian.

Rabies is transmitted to humans by an animal bite or through a cut or scratch already in the skin. The infected saliva may enter through any opening, including the membranes lining the nose or mouth. After an incubation period of about ten days, a person infected by a rabid animal experiences pain at the site of infection, extreme sensitivity of the skin to temperature changes, and painful spasms of the larynx that make it almost impossible to drink. Saliva thickens and the patient becomes restless and easily excitable. By the time symptoms develop, death may be imminent. Obviously, professional medical attention should begin promptly after having been exposed to the possibility of infection.

Emergency Treatment

The area around the wound should be washed thoroughly and repeatedly with soap and water, using a sterile gauze dressing to wipe fluid away from—not toward—the wound. Another sterile dressing is used to dry the wound and a third to cover it while the patient is taken to a hospital or physician's office. A tetanus injection is also indicated, and police and health authorities should be promptly notified of the biting incident.

If at all possible the biting animal should be identified—if a wild animal, captured alive—and held for observation for a period of 10 to 15 days. If it can be determined during that period that the animal is not rabid, further treatment may not be required. If the animal is rabid, however, or if it cannot be located and impounded, the patient may have to undergo a series of daily rabies vaccine injections lasting from 14 days for a case of mild exposure to 21 days for severe exposure (a bite near the head, for example), plus several booster shots. Because of the sensitivity of some individuals to the rabies vaccines used, the treatment itself can be quite dangerous.

Recent research, however, has established that a new vaccine called HDCV (human diploid cell vaccine), which requires only six or fewer injections, is immunologically effective and is not usually accompanied by any side effects. The new vaccine has been used successfully on people of all ages who had been bitten by animals known to be rabid.

Appendicitis

The common signal for approaching appendicitis is a period of several days of indigestion and constipation, culminating in pain and tenderness on the lower right side of the abdomen. Besides these symptoms, appendicitis may be accompanied by nausea and a slight fever. Call a physician immediately and describe the symptoms in detail; delay may result in a ruptured appendix.

Emergency Treatment

While awaiting medical care, the victim may find some relief from the pain and discomfort by having an ice bag placed over the abdomen. Do not apply heat and give nothing by mouth. A laxative should not be offered.

Asphyxiation

See GAS POISONING.

Asthma Attack

Emergency Treatment

Make the patient comfortable and offer reassurance. If he has been examined by a physician and properly diagnosed, the patient probably has an inhalant device or other forms of medication on his person or nearby.

The coughing and wheezing spell may have been triggered by the presence of an allergenic substance such as animal hair, feathers, or kapok in pillows or cushions. Such items should be removed from the presence of the patient. In addition, placing the patient in a room with high humidity, such as a bathroom with the shower turned on, may be helpful.

Asthma attacks are rarely fatal in young people, but elderly persons should be watched carefully because of possible heart strain. In a severe attack, professional medical care including oxygen equipment may be required.

Back Injuries

In the event of any serious back injury, call a physician or arrange for immediate professional transfer of the victim to a hospital.

Emergency Treatment

Until determined otherwise by a physician, treat the injured person as a victim of a fractured spine. If he complains that he cannot move his head, feet, or toes, the chances are that the back is fractured. But even if he can move his feet or legs, it does not necessarily mean that he can be moved safely, since the back can be fractured without immediate injury to the spinal cord.

If the victim shows symptoms of shock, do not attempt to lower his head or move his body into the usual position for shock control. If it is absolutely essential to move the victim because of immediate danger to his life, make a rigid stretcher from a wide piece of solid lumber such as a door and cover the stretcher with a blanket for padding. Then carefully slide or pull the victim onto the stretcher, using his clothing to hold him. Tie the body onto the stretcher with strips of cloth.

Back Pain

See SCIATICA.

Black Eye

Although a black eye is frequently regarded as a minor medical problem, it can result in serious visual problems, including cataract or glaucoma.

Emergency Treatment

Inspect the area about the eye for possible damage to the eye itself, such as hemorrhage, rupture of the eyeball, or dislocated lens. Check also for cuts around the eye that may require professional medical care. Then treat the bruised area by putting the victim to bed, covering the eye with a bandage, and applying an ice bag to the area.

If vision appears to be distorted or lacerations need stitching and antibiotic treatment, take the victim to a physician's office. A physician should also be consulted about continued pain and swelling about the eye.

Black Widow Spider Bites

Emergency Treatment

Make the victim lie still. If the bite is on the arm or leg, position the victim so that the bite is lower than the level of the heart. Apply a rubber band or similar tourniquet between the bite and the heart to retard venom flow toward the heart. The bite usually is marked by two puncture points. Apply ice packs to the bite. Summon a physician or carry the patient to the nearest hospital.

Loosen the tourniquet or constriction band for a few seconds every 15 minutes while awaiting help; you should be able to feel a pulse beyond the tourniquet if it is not too tight. Do not let the victim move about. Do not permit him to drink alcoholic beverages. He probably will feel weakness, tremor, and severe pain, but reassure him that he will recover. Medications, usually available only to a physician, should be administered promptly.

Bleeding, Internal

Internal bleeding is always a very serious condition; it requires immediate professional medical attention.

In cases of internal bleeding, blood is sometimes brought to the outside of the body by coughing from the lungs, by vomiting from the stomach, by trickling from the ear or nose, or by passing in the urine or bowel movement.

Often, however, internal bleeding is concealed, and the only symptom may be the swelling that appears around the site of broken bones. A person can lose three or four pints of blood inside the body without a trace of blood appearing outside the body.

Some Symptoms of Internal Bleeding

The victim will appear ill and pale. His skin will be colder than normal, especially the hands and feet; often the skin looks clammy because of sweating. The pulse usually will be rapid (over 90 beats a minute) and feeble.

Emergency Treatment

Serious internal bleeding is beyond the scope of first aid. If necessary treat the victim for respiratory and cardiac arrest and for shock while waiting for medical aid.

Bleeding, Minor

Bleeding from minor cuts, scrapes, and bruises usually stops by itself, but even small injuries of this kind should receive attention to prevent infection.

Emergency Treatment

The injured area should be washed thoroughly with soap and water, or if possible, held under running water. The surface should then be covered with a sterile bandage.

The type of wound known as a puncture wound may bleed very little, but is potentially extremely dangerous because of the possibility of tetanus infection. Anyone who steps on a rusty nail or thumbtack or has a similar accident involving a pointed object that penetrates deep under the skin surface should consult a physician about the need for antitetanus inoculation or a booster shot.

Blisters

Emergency Treatment

If the blister is on a hand or foot or other easily accessible part of the body, wash the area around the blister thoroughly with soap and water. After carefully drying the skin around the blister, apply an antiseptic to the same area. Then sterilize the point and a substantial part of a needle by heating it in an open flame. When the needle has been thoroughly sterilized, use the point to puncture the blister along the margin of the blister. Carefully squeeze the fluid from the blister by pressing it with a sterile gauze dressing; the dressing should soak up most of the fluid. Next, place a fresh sterile dressing over the blister and fasten it in place with a bandage. If a blister forms in a tender area or in a place that is not easily accessible, such as under the arm, do not open it yourself; consult your physician.

The danger from any break in the skin is that germs or dirt can slip through the natural barrier to produce an infection or inflammation. Continue to apply an antiseptic each day to the puncture area until it has healed. If it appears that an infection has developed or healing is unusually slow, consult a doctor. Persons with diabetes or circulatory problems may have to be more cautious about healing of skin breaks than other individuals.

Blood Blisters

Blood blisters, sometimes called hematomas, usually are caused by a sharp blow to the body surface such as hitting a finger with a hammer while pounding nails.

Emergency Treatment

Wash the area of the blood blister thoroughly with soap and water. Do not open it. If it is a small blood blister, cover it with a protective bandage; in many cases, the tiny pool of blood under the skin will be absorbed by the surrounding tissues if there is no further pressure at that point.

If the blood blister fails to heal quickly or becomes infected, consult a physician. Because the pool of blood has resulted from damage to a blood vessel, a blood blister usually is more vulnerable to infection or inflammation than an ordinary blister.

Boils

Boils frequently are an early sign of diabetes or another illness and should be watched carefully if they occur often. In general, they result from germs or dirt being rubbed into the skin by tight-fitting clothing, scratching, or through tiny cuts made during shaving.

Emergency Treatment

If the boil is above the lip, do not squeeze it or apply any pressure. The infection in that area of the face may drain into the brain because of the pattern of blood circulation on the face. Let a physician treat any boil on the face. If the boil is on the surface of another part of the body, apply moist hot packs, but do not squeeze or press on the boil because that action can force the infection into the circulatory system. A wet compress can be made by soaking a wash cloth or towel in warm water.

If the boil erupts, carefully wipe away the pus with a sterile dressing, and then cover it with another sterile dressing. If the boil is large or slow to erupt, or if it is slow to heal, consult a physician.

Bone Bruises

Emergency Treatment

Make sure the bone is not broken. If the injury is limited to the thin layer of tissue surrounding the bone, and the function of the limb is normal though painful, apply a compression dressing and an ice pack. Limit use of the injured limb for the next day or two.

As the pain and swelling recede, cover the injured area with a foam-rubber pad held in place with an elastic bandage. Because the part of the limb that is likely to receive a bone bruise lacks a layer of muscle and fat, it will be particularly sensitive to any pressure until recovery is complete.

Botulism

The bacteria that produce the lethal toxin of botulism are commonly present on unwashed farm vegetables and thrive in containers that are improperly sealed against the damaging effects of air. Home-canned vegetables, particularly string beans, are a likely source of botulism, but the toxin can be found in fruits, meats, and other foods. It can also appear in food that has been properly prepared but allowed to cool before being served. Examples are cold soups and marinated vegetables.

Emergency Treatment

As soon as acute symptoms—nausea, diarrhea, and abdominal distress—appear, try to induce vomiting. Vomiting usually can be started by touching the back of the victim's throat with a finger or the handle of a spoon, which should be smooth and blunt, or by offering him a glass of water in which two tablespoons of salt have been dissolved. Call a physician; describe all of the symptoms, which also may include, after several hours, double vision, muscular weakness, and difficulty in swallowing and breathing. Save samples of the food suspected of contamination for analysis.

Prompt hospitalization and injection of antitoxin are needed to save most cases of botulism poisoning. Additional emergency measures may include artificial respiration if regular breathing fails because of paralysis of respiratory muscles. Continue artificial respiration until professional medical care is provided. If other individuals have eaten the contaminated food, they should receive treatment for botulism even if they show no symptoms of the toxin's effects, since symptoms may be delayed by several days.

Brown House (or Recluse) Spider Bites

Emergency Treatment

Apply an ice bag or cold pack to the wound area. Aspirin and antihistamines may be offered to help relieve any pain or feeling of irritation. Keep the victim lying down and quiet. Call a physician as quickly as possible and describe the situation; the physician will advise what further action should be taken at this point.

The effects of a brown spider bite frequently last much longer than the pain of the bite, which may be comparatively mild for an insect bite or sting. But the poison from the bite can gradually destroy the surrounding tissues, leaving at first an ulcer and eventually a disfiguring scar. A physician's treatment is needed to control the loss of tissue; he probably will prescribe drugs and recommend continued use of cold compresses. The victim, meanwhile, will feel numbness and muscular weakness, requiring a prolonged period of bed rest in addition to the medical treatments.

Bruises/Contusions

Emergency Treatment

Bruises or contusions result usually from a blow to the body that is powerful enough to damage muscles, tendons, blood vessels, or other tissues without causing a break in the skin.

Because the bruised area will be tender, protect it from further injury. If possible, immobilize the injured body part with a sling, bandage, or other device that makes the victim feel more comfortable; pillows, folded blankets, or similar soft materials can be used to elevate an arm or leg. Apply an ice bag or cold water dressing to the injured area.

A simple bruise usually will heal without extensive treatment. The swelling and discoloration result from blood oozing from damaged tissues. Severe bruising can, however, be quite serious and requires medical attention. Keep the victim quiet and watch for symptoms of shock. Give aspirin for pain.

Bullet Wounds

Bullet wounds, whether accidental or purposely inflicted, can range from those that are superficial and external to those that involve internal bleeding and extensive tissue damage.

Emergency Treatment

A surface bullet wound accompanied by bleeding should be covered promptly with sterile gauze to prevent further infection. The flow of blood should be controlled as described under "Severe Bleeding" in this chapter. *Don't* try to clean the wound with soap or water.

If the wound is internal, keep the patient lying down and wrap him with coats or blankets placed over and under his body. If respiration has ceased or is impaired, give mouth-to-mouth respiration and treat him for shock. Get medical aid promptly.

Burns, Thermal

Burns are generally described according to the depth or area of skin damage involved. First-degree burns are the most superficial. They are marked by reddening of the skin and swelling, increased warmth, tenderness, and pain. Second-degree burns, deeper than first-degree, are in effect open wounds, characterized by blisters and severe pain in addition to redness. Third-degree burns are deep enough to involve damage to muscles and bones. The skin is charred and there may be no pain because nerve endings have been destroyed. However, the area of the burn generally is more important than the degree of burn; a first- or second-degree burn covering a large area of the body is more likely to be fatal than a small third-degree burn.

Emergency Treatment

If burns are minor, apply ice or ice water until pain subsides. Then wash the area with soap and water. Cover with a sterile dressing. Give the victim one or two aspirin tablets or acetaminophen to help relieve discomfort. A sterile gauze pad soaked in a solution of two tablespoons of baking soda (sodium bicarbonate) per quart of lukewarm water may be applied.

For more extensive or severe burns, immediately seek professional treatment. While help is being obtained, there are a few things you can do. Get the victim away from the fire or heat. Monitor the victim's breathing and stop any bleeding. Cool the burn with cool water. Cut—never pull—clothing from burned areas. If fabric is stuck to the burn, cut around it and leave it in place. Cover the burn with a cool, moist sterile pad or clean sheet. Do not apply oils, sprays, or ointments. If fingers or toes are burned, gently separate them with dry, sterile, non-adhesive dressings.

To prevent shock, make sure the victim's head is lower than his feet. Be sure that the victim is covered sufficiently to keep him warm, but not enough to make him overheated; exposure to cold can make the effects of shock more severe. Provide the victim with plenty of nonalcoholic liquids such as sweetened water, tea, or fruit juices, so long as he is conscious and able to swallow.

To prevent infection, do not permit absorbent cotton or adhesive tape to touch the wound caused by a burn. Do not apply iodine or any other antiseptic to the burn. Do not open any blisters. Do not permit any unsterile matter to touch the burn area. Do not cough, sneeze, or even breathe toward the wound resulting from a burn. Serious infections frequently develop in burn victims from contamination by microorganisms of the mouth and nose.

Skin Grafts

In serious burn cases, it is very important to get the wounds closed as quickly as possible to protect against infection. Left to itself, the skin will contract over the wound, resulting in scarring that is disfiguring and often disabling. A graft of the patient's own healthy skin (autograft) is the best covering for a burn wound, but patients with extensive burns often do not have enough healthy skin for autografting. It is possible to grow, over the course of several weeks, grafts of skin from small samples of uninjured skin taken from the patient's body. Grafts of cadaver skin or pig skin may be used—especially as a temporary covering—but they are often rejected by patients' immune systems.

Artificial skins can take the place of cadaver and pig skin grafts. One type of artificial skin, called INTEGRA, has an inner layer made from collagen fibers from animal tissues and an outer, protective layer of silicone. It can be left in place for up to two months and encourages the growth of the patient's own skin underneath it. TransCyte artificial skin combines a bioengineered human dermal layer with a synthetic covering.

See also CHEMICAL BURNS OF THE EYE.

Carbuncles

Carbuncles are quite similar to boils except that they usually develop around multiple hair follicles and commonly appear on the neck or face. Personal hygiene is one factor involved in the development of carbuncles; persons apparently susceptible to the pustular inflammations must exercise special care in cleansing areas in which carbuncles occur, particularly if they suffer from diabetes or circulatory ailments.

Emergency Treatment

Apply moist hot packs to the boil-like swelling. Change the moist hot packs frequently, or place a hot-water bottle on the moist dressing to maintain the moist heat application. Do not handle the carbuncle beyond whatever contact is necessary to apply or maintain the moist heat. The carbuncle should eventually rupture or reach a point where it can be opened with a sterile sharp instrument. After the carbuncle has ruptured and drained, and the fluid from the growth has been carefully cleaned away, apply a sterile dressing.

Frequently, carbuncles must be opened and drained by a physician.

Cat Scratch Fever

Although the scratch or bite of a house cat or alley cat may appear at first to be only a mild injury, the wound can become the site of entry for a disease virus transmitted by apparently healthy cats. The inflammation, accompanied by fever, generally affects the lymph nodes and produces some aches and pains as well as fatigue. Although the disease is seldom fatal, an untreated case can spread to brain tissues and lead to other complications.

Emergency Treatment

Wash the scratch thoroughly with water and either soap or a mild detergent. Cover with a sterile dressing.

Watch the area of the scratch carefully for the next week or two. If redness or swelling develop, even after the scratch appears healed, consult your physician. The inflammation of the scratch area may be accompanied by mild fever and symptoms similar to those of influenza; in small children, the symptoms may be quite serious. Bed rest and antibiotics usually are prescribed.

Charley Horse

A charley horse occurs because a small number of muscle fibers have been torn or ruptured by overstraining the muscle, or by the force of a blow to the muscle.

Emergency Treatment

Rest the injured muscle and apply an ice pack if there is swelling. A compression dressing can be applied to support the muscle. Avoid movement that stretches the muscle, and restrict other movements that make the victim uncomfortable. If pain and swelling persist, call a physician.

During the recovery period, which may not begin for a day or two, apply local heat with a hot water bottle or an electric heating pad, being careful not to burn the victim. A return to active use of the muscle can begin gradually as pain permits.

Chemical Burns of the Eye

Emergency Treatment

Flush the victim's eye immediately with large quantities of fresh, clean water; a drinking fountain can be used to provide a steady stream of water. If a drinking fountain is not available, lay the victim on the floor or ground with his head turned slightly to one side and pour water into the eye from a cup or glass. Always direct the stream of water so that it enters the eye surface at the inside corner and flows across the eye to the outside corner. If the victim is unable, because of intense pain, to open his eyes, it may be necessary to hold the lids apart while water pours across the eye. Continue flushing the eye for at least 15 minutes. (An alternate method is to immerse the victim's face in a pan or basin or bucket of water while he opens and closes his eyes repeatedly; continue the process for at least 15 minutes.)

When the chemical has been flushed from the victim's eye, the eye should be covered with a small, thick compress held in place with a bandage that covers both eyes, if possible; the bandage can be tied around the victim's head. *Note:* Apply nothing but water to the eye; do not attempt to neutralize a chemical burn of the eye and do not apply oil, ointment, salve, or other medications. Rush the victim to a physician as soon as possible, preferably to an ophthalmologist.

Chemicals on Skin

Many household and industrial chemicals, such as ammonia, lye, iodine, creosote, and a wide range of insecticides can cause serious injury if accidentally spilled on the skin.

Emergency Treatment

Wash the body surface that has been affected by the chemical with large amounts of water. Do not try to neutralize the chemical with another substance; the reaction may aggravate the injury. If blisters appear, apply a sterile dressing. If the chemical is a refrigerant, such as Freon, or carbon dioxide under pressure, treat for frostbite.

If the chemical has splashed into the eyes or produces serious injury to the affected body surface, call a physician. The victim should be watched closely for possible poisoning effects if the chemical is a pesticide, since such substances may be absorbed through the skin to produce internal toxic reactions. If there is any question about the toxicity of a chemical, ask your doctor or call the nearest poison control center.

Chigger Bites

Emergency Treatment

Apply ice water or rub ice over the area afflicted by bites of the tiny red insects. Bathing the area with alcohol, ammonia water or a solution of baking soda also will provide some relief from the itching.

Wash thoroughly with soap, using a scrub brush to prevent further infestation by the chiggers in other areas of the body. Apply sulfur ointment as protection against mites that may not have attached themselves to the skin. Continue applications of ice water or alcohol to skin areas invaded by the insects. Clothing that was worn should be laundered immediately.

Chilblains

Emergency Treatment

Move the victim to a moderately warm place and remove wet or tight clothing. Soak the affected body area in warm—but not hot—water for about ten minutes. Then carefully blot the skin dry, but do not rub the skin. Replace the clothing with garments that are warm, soft, and dry.

Give the victim a stimulant such as tea or coffee, or an alcoholic beverage, and put him to bed with only light blankets; avoid the pressure of heavy blankets or heavy, tight garments on the sensitive skin areas. The victim should move the affected body areas gently to help restore normal circulation. If complications develop, such as marked discoloration of the skin, pain, or blistering and splitting of the skin, call a physician.

Cold Sores/Fever Blisters

Emergency Treatment

Apply a soothing ointment or a medication such as camphor ice. Avoid squeezing or otherwise handling the blisters; moisture can aggravate the sores and hinder their healing. Repeated appearances of cold sores or fever blisters, which are caused by the herpes simplex virus, may require treatment by a physician.

Concussion

See HEAD INJURIES.

Contusions

See BRUISES.

Convulsions

Emergency Treatment

Protect the victim from injury by moving him to a safe place; loosen any constricting clothing such as a tie or belt; put a pillow or coat under his head; if his mouth is open, place a folded cloth between his teeth to keep him from biting his tongue. Do not force anything into his mouth. Keep the patient warm but do not disturb him; do not try to restrain his convulsive movements.

Send for a physician as quickly as possible. Watch the patient's breathing and begin artificial respiration if breathing stops for more than one minute. Be sure that breathing actually has stopped; the patient may be sleeping or unconscious after an attack but breathing normally.

Convulsions in a small child may signal the onset of an infectious disease and may be accompanied by a high fever. The same general precautions should be taken to prevent self-injury on the part of the child. If placed in a bed, the child should be protected against falling onto the floor. Place him on his side—not on his back or stomach—if he vomits. Cold compresses or ice packs on the back of the neck and the head may help relieve symptoms. Immediate professional medical care is vital because brain damage can result if treatment is delayed.

See also EPILEPTIC SEIZURES.

Cramps

See MUSCLE CRAMPS.

Croup

Croup is a breathing disorder usually caused by a virus infection and less often by bacteria or allergy. It is a common condition during childhood, and in some cases, may require brief hospitalization for proper treatment.

The onset of a croup attack is likely to occur during the night with a sudden hoarse or barking cough accompanied by difficulty in breathing. The coughing is usually followed by choking spasms that sound as though the child is strangling. There may also be a mild fever. A physician should be called immediately when these symptoms appear.

Emergency Treatment

The most effective treatment for croup is cool moist air. Cool water vaporizers are available as well as warm steam vaporizers. Another alternative is to take the child into the bathroom, close the door and windows, and let the hot water run from the shower and sink taps until the room is filled with steam.

It is also possible to improvise a croup tent by boiling water in a kettle on a portable hot plate and arranging a blanket over the back of a chair so that it encloses the child and an adult as well as the steaming kettle. A child should never be left alone even for an instant in such a makeshift arrangement.

If the symptoms do not subside in about 20 minutes with any of the above procedures, or if there is mounting fever, and if the physician is not on his way, the child should be rushed to the closest hospital. Cold moist night air, rather than being a danger, may actually make the symptoms subside temporarily.

Diabetic Coma and Insulin Shock

Diabetics should always carry an identification tag or card to alert others of their condition in the event of a diabetic coma—which is due to a lack of insulin. They also should advise friends or family members of their diabetic condition and the proper emergency measures that can be taken in the event of an onset of diabetic coma. A bottle of rapid-acting insulin should be kept on hand for such an emergency.

Emergency Treatment

If the victim is being treated for diabetes, he probably will have nearby a supply of insulin and a hypodermic apparatus for injecting it. Find the insulin, hypodermic syringe, and needle; clean a spot on the upper arm or thigh, and inject about 50 units of insulin. Call a physician without delay, and describe the patient's symptoms and your treatment. The patient usually will respond without ill effects, but may be quite thirsty. Give him plenty of fluids, as needed.

If the victim does not respond to the insulin, or if you cannot find the insulin and hypodermic syringe, rush the victim to the nearest physician's office.

Insulin shock—which is due to a reaction to too much insulin and not enough sugar in the blood—can be treated in an emergency by offering a sugar-rich fluid such as a cola beverage or orange juice. Diabetics frequently carry a lump of sugar or candy that can be placed in their mouth in case of an insulin shock reaction. It should be tucked between the teeth and cheek so the victim will not choke on it.

If you find a diabetic in a coma and do not know the cause, assume the cause is an insulin reaction and treat him with sugar. This will give immediate relief to an insulin reaction but will not affect diabetic coma.

Diarrhea

Emergency Treatment

Give the victim an antidiarrheal agent; all drugstores carry medications composed of kaolin and pectin that are useful for this purpose. Certain bismuth compounds also are recommended for diarrhea control.

Put the victim in bed for a period of at least 12 hours. Do not let the victim become dehydrated; if he is thirsty, let him suck on pieces of ice. If the diarrhea appears to be subsiding, let him sip a mild beverage like tea or ginger ale; cola syrup is also recommended.

Later on the patient can try eating bland foods such as dry toast, crackers, gelatin desserts, or jellied consomme. Avoid feeding the patient rich, fatty, or spicy foods. If the diarrhea fails to subside or is complicated by colic or vomiting, call a physician.

Dizziness/Vertigo

Emotional upsets, allergies, and improper eating and drinking habits—too much food, too little food, or foods that are too rich—can precipitate symptoms of dizziness. The cause also can be a physical disorder such as abnormal functioning of the inner ear or a circulatory problem. Smoking tobacco, certain drugs such as quinine, and fumes of some chemicals also can produce dizziness.

Emergency Treatment

Have the victim lie down with the eyes closed. In many cases, a period of simple bed rest will alleviate the symptoms. Keep the victim quiet and comfortable. If the feeling of dizziness continues, becomes worse, or is accompanied by nausea and vomiting, call a physician.

Severe or persistent dizziness or vertigo requires a longer period of bed rest and the use of medicines prescribed by a physician. While recovering, the victim should avoid sudden changes in body position or turning the head rapidly. In some types of vertigo, surgery is required to cure the disorder.

Drowning

Victims of drowning seldom die because of water in the lungs or stomach. They die because of lack of air.

Emergency Treatment

If the victim's breathing has been impaired, start artificial respiration immediately. If there is evidence of cardiac arrest, administer cardiac massage. When the victim is able to breathe for himself, treat him for shock and get medical help.

Drug Overdose (Barbiturates)

Barbiturates are used in a number of drugs prescribed as sedatives, although many are also available through illegal channels. Because the drugs can affect the judgment of the user, he may not remember having taken a dose and so may take additional pills, thus producing overdose effects.

Emergency Treatment

If the drug was taken orally, try to induce vomiting in the victim. Have him drink a glass of water containing two tablespoons of salt. Or touch the back of his throat gently with a finger or a smooth blunt object like the handle of a spoon. Then give the victim plenty of warm water to drink. It is important to rid the stomach of as much of the drug as possible and to dilute the substance remaining in the gastrointestinal tract.

As soon as possible, call a physician or get the victim to the nearest hospital or physician's office. If breathing fails, administer artificial respiration.

Drug Overdose (Stimulants)

Although most of the powerful stimulant drugs, or pep pills, are available only through a physician's prescription, the same medications are available through illicit sources. When taken without direction of a supervising physician, the stimulants can produce a variety of adverse side effects, and when used frequently over a period of time can result in physical and psychological problems that require hospital treatment.

Emergency Treatment

Give the victim a solution of one tablespoon of activated charcoal mixed with a small amount of water, or give him a glass of milk, to dilute the effects of the medication in the stomach. Then induce vomiting by pressing gently on the back of the throat with a finger or the smooth blunt edge of a spoon handle. Vomiting also may be induced with a solution made of one teaspoonful of mustard in a half glass of water. Do not give syrup of ipecac to a victim who has been taking stimulants.

As soon as possible call a physician or get the victim to the nearest hospital or physician's office. If breathing fails, administer artificial respiration.

Earaches

An earache may be associated with a wide variety of ailments ranging from the common cold or influenza to impacted molars or tonsillitis. An earache also may be involved in certain infectious diseases such as measles or scarlet fever. Because of the relationship of ear structures to other parts of the head and throat, an infection involving the symptoms of earache can easily spread to the brain tissues or the spongy mastoid bone behind the ear. Call a physician and describe all of the symptoms, including temperature, any discharge, pain, ringing in the ear, or deafness. Delay in reporting an earache to a doctor can result in complications that require hospital treatment.

Emergency Treatment

This may include a few drops of warm olive oil or sweet oil held in the ear by a small wad of cotton. Aspirin can be given to adults help relieve pain. Professional medical treatment may include the use of antibiotics.

Ear, Foreign Body in

Emergency Treatment

Do not insert a hairpin, stick, or other object in the ear in an effort to remove a foreign object; you are likely to force the object farther into the ear canal. Instead, have the victim tilt his head to one side, with the ear containing the foreign object facing upward. While pulling gently on the lobe of the ear to straighten the canal, pour a little warmed olive oil or mineral oil into the ear. Then have the victim tilt that ear downward so the oil will run out quickly; it should dislodge the foreign object.

Wipe the ear canal gently with a cotton-tipped matchstick, or a similar device that will not irritate the lining of the ear canal, after the foreign body has been removed. If the emergency treatment is not successful, call a physician.

Electric Shocks

An electric shock from the usual 110-volt current in most homes can be a serious emergency, especially if the person's skin or clothing is wet. Under these circumstances, the shock may paralyze the part of the brain that controls breathing and stop the heart completely or disorder its pumping action.

Emergency Treatment

It is of the utmost importance to break the electrical contact *immediately* by unplugging the wire of the appliance involved or by shutting off the house current switch. **Do not touch the victim of the shock while he is still acting as an electrical conductor.**

If the shock has come from a faulty wire out of doors and the source of the electrical current can't be reached easily, make a lasso of dry rope on a long sturdy dry stick. Catch the victim's hand or foot in the loop and drag him away from the wire. Another way to break the contact is to cut the wire with a dry axe.

If the victim of the shock is unconscious, or if his pulse is very weak, administer mouth-to-mouth respiration and cardiac massage until he can get to a hospital.

Epileptic Seizures

Epilepsy is a disorder of the nervous system that produces convulsive seizures. In a major seizure or *grand mal,* the epileptic usually falls to the ground. Indeed, falling is in most cases one of the principal dangers of the disease. Then the epileptic's body begins to twitch or jerk spasmodically. His breathing may be labored, and saliva may appear on his lips. His face may become pale or bluish. Although the scene can be frightening, it may not truly be a medical emergency; but may become so if prolonged.

Emergency Treatment

Make the person suffering the seizure as comfortable as possible. If he is on a hard surface, put something soft under his head, and move any hard or dangerous objects away from him. **Make no attempt to restrain his movements, and do not force anything into his mouth.** Just leave him alone until the attack is over, as it should be in a few minutes. If his mouth is already open, you might put something soft, such as a folded handkerchief, between his side teeth. This will help to prevent him from biting his tongue or lips. If possible, turn the person's head so if he vomits, the matter will be expelled, and he won't choke. If another seizure begins, or if the seizure lasts more than ten minutes, call a physician. If his lower jaw sags and begins to obstruct his breathing, support of the lower jaw may be helpful in improving his breathing. After a seizure has stopped, turn the person's head to the side so he can breather normally.

When the seizure is over, the patient should be allowed to rest quietly. Some people sleep heavily after a seizure. Others awake at once but are disoriented or confused for a while. If it is the first seizure the person is aware of having had, or if it does not resolve, see a physician promptly.

Eye, Foreign Body in

Emergency Treatment

Do not rub the eye or touch it with unwashed hands. The foreign body usually becomes lodged on the inner surface of the upper eyelid. Pull the upper eyelid down over the lower lid to help work the object loose. Tears or clean water can help wash out the dirt or other object. If the bit of irritating material can be seen on the surface of the eyeball, try very carefully to flick it out with the tip of a clean, moistened handkerchief or a piece of moistened cotton. Never touch the surface of the eye with dry materials. Sometimes a foreign body can be removed by carefully rolling the upper lid over a pencil or wooden matchstick to expose the object.

After the foreign object has been removed, the eye should be washed with clean water or with a solution made from one teaspoon of salt dissolved in a pint of water. This will help remove any remaining particles of the foreign body as well as any traces of irritating chemicals that might have been a part of it. Iron particles, for example, may leave traces of rust on the eye's surface unless washed away.

If the object cannot be located and removed without difficulty, a small patch of gauze or a folded handkerchief should be taped over the eye and the victim taken to a physician's office—preferably the office of an ophthalmologist. A physician also should be consulted if a feeling of irritation in the eye continues after the foreign body has been removed.

Fever

Emergency Treatment

If the fever is mild, around 100°F. by mouth, have the victim rest in bed and provide him with a light diet. Watch closely for other symptoms, such as a rash, and any further increase in body temperature. Aspirin usually can be given in adults.

If the temperature rises to 101°F. or higher, is accompanied by pain, headache, delirium, confused behavior, coughing, vomiting, or other indications of a severe illness, call a physician. Describe all of the symptoms in detail, including the appearance of any rash and when it began.

Fever blisters

See COLD SORES.

Finger Dislocation

Emergency Treatment

Call a physician and arrange for inspection and treatment of the injury. If a physician is not immediately available, the finger dislocation may be reduced (put back in proper alignment) by grasping it firmly and carefully pulling it into normal position. Pull very slowly and avoid rough handling that might complicate the injury by damaging a tendon. If the dislocation cannot be reduced after the first try, go through the procedure once more. But do not try it more than twice.

Whether or not you are successful in reducing the finger dislocation, the finger should be immobilized after your efforts until a physician can examine it. A clean flat wooden stick can be strapped along the palm side of the finger with adhesive tape or strips of bandage to hold it in place.

Fingernail Injuries

Emergency Treatment

Wash the injured nail area thoroughly with warm water and soap. Trim off any torn bits of nail. Cover with a small adhesive dressing or bandage.

Apply petroleum jelly or cold cream to the injured nail area twice a day, morning and night, until it is healed. If redness or irritation develops in the adjoining skin area, indicating an infection, consult a physician.

Fish Poisoning

Emergency Treatment

Induce vomiting in the victim to remove the bits of poisonous fish from the stomach. Vomiting usually can be started by pressing on the back of the throat with a finger or a spoon handle that is blunt and smooth, or by having the victim drink a solution of two tablespoons of salt in a glass of water.

Call a physician as soon as possible. Describe the type of fish eaten and the symptoms, which may include nausea, diarrhea, abdominal pain, muscular weakness, and a numbness or tingling sensation that begins about the face and spreads to the extremities.

If breathing fails, administer mouth-to-mouth artificial respiration; a substance commonly found in poisonous fish causes respiratory failure. Also, be prepared to provide emergency treatment for convulsions.

Food Poisoning

Emergency Treatment

If the victim is not already vomiting, try to induce it to clear the stomach. Vomiting can be started in most cases by pressing gently on the back of the throat with a finger or a blunt smooth spoon handle, or by having the patient drink a glass of water containing two tablespoons of salt. If the victim has vomited, put him to bed.

Call a physician and describe the food ingested and the symptoms that developed. If symptoms are severe, professional medical treatment with antibiotics and medications for cramps may be required. Special medications also may be needed for diarrhea caused by bacterial food poisoning.

Fractures

Any break in a bone is called a fracture. The break is called an *open* or *compound fracture* if one or both ends of the broken bone pierce the skin. A *closed* or *simple fracture* is one in which the broken bone doesn't come through the skin.

It is sometimes difficult to distinguish a strained muscle or a sprained ligament from a broken bone, since sprains and strains can be extremely painful even though they are less serious than breaks. However, when there is any doubt, the injury should be treated as though it were a simple fracture.

Emergency Treatment

Don't try to help the injured person move around or get up unless he has slowly tested out the injured part of his body and is sure that nothing has been broken. If he is in extreme pain, or if the injured part has begun to swell, or if by running the finger lightly along the affected bone a break can be felt, *do not* move him. Under no circumstances should he be crowded into a car if his legs, hip, ribs, or back are involved in the accident. Call for an ambulance immediately, and until it arrives, treat the person for shock.

Splinting

In a situation where it is imperative to move someone who may have a fracture, the first step is to apply a splint so that the broken bone ends are immobilized.

Splints can be improvised from anything rigid enough and of the right length to support the fractured part of the body: a metal rod, board, long cardboard tube, tightly rolled newspaper or blanket. If the object being used has to be padded for softness, use a small blanket or any other soft material, such as a jacket.

The splint should be long enough so that it can be tied with a bandage, torn sheet, or neckties beyond the joint above and below the fracture as well as at the site of the break. If a leg is involved, it should be elevated with pillows or any other firm support after the splint has been applied. If the victim has to wait a considerable length of time before receiving professional attention, the splint bandaging should be checked from time to time to make sure it isn't too tight.

In the case of an open or compound fracture, additional steps must be taken. Remove that part of the victim's clothing that is covering the wound. Do not wash or probe into the wound, but control bleeding by applying pressure over the wound through a sterile or clean dressing.

Frostbite

Emergency Treatment

Begin rapid rewarming of the affected tissues as soon as possible. If possible, immerse the victim in a warm bath, but avoid scalding. (The temperature should be between 102°F. and 105°F.) Warm wet towels also will help if changed frequently and applied gently. Do not massage, rub, or even touch the frostbitten flesh. If warm water or a warming fire is not available, place the patient in a sleeping bag or cover him with coats and blankets. Hot liquids can be offered if available to help raise the body temperature.

For any true frostbite case, prompt medical attention is important. The depth and degree of the frozen tissue cannot be determined without a careful examination by a physician.

Gallbladder Attacks

Although gallstones can affect a wide variety of individuals, the most common victims are overweight persons who enjoy rich foods. The actual attack of spasms caused by gallstones passing through the duct leading from the gallbladder to the digestive tract usually is preceded by periods of stomach distress including belching. X rays usually will reveal the presence of gallstones when the early warning signs are noted, and measures can be taken to reduce the threat of a gallbladder attack.

Emergency Treatment

Call a physician and describe in detail the symptoms, which may include colic high in the abdomen and pain extending to the right shoulder; the pain may be accompanied by nausea, vomiting, and sweating. Hot water bottles may be applied to the abdomen to help relieve distress while waiting for professional medical care. If the physician permits, the victim may be allowed to sip certain fluids such as fruit juices, but do not offer him solid food.

Gas Poisoning

Before attempting to revive someone overcome by toxic gas poisoning, the most important thing to do is to remove him to the fresh air. If this isn't feasible, all windows and doors should be opened to let in as much fresh air as possible.

Any interior with a dangerous concentration of carbon monoxide or other toxic gases is apt to be highly explosive. Therefore, gas and electricity should be shut off as quickly as possible. **Under no circumstances should any matches be lighted in an interior where there are noxious fumes.**

The rescuer needn't waste time

covering his face with a handkerchief or other cloth. He should hold his breath instead, or take only a few quick, shallow breaths while bringing the victim to the out-of-doors or to an open window.

Emergency Treatment

Administer artificial respiration if the victim is suffering respiratory arrest. Arrange for medical help as soon as possible, requesting that oxygen be brought to the scene.

Head Injuries

Accidents involving the head can result in concussion, skull fracture, or brain injury. Symptoms of head injury include loss of consciousness, discharge of a watery or blood-tinged fluid from the ears, nose, or mouth, and a difference in size of the pupils of the eyes. Head injuries must be thought of as serious; they demand immediate medical assistance.

Emergency Treatment

Place the victim in a supine position, and, if there is no evidence of injury to his neck, arrange for a slight elevation of his head *and* shoulders. Make certain that he has a clear airway and administer artificial respiration if necessary. If vomitus, blood, or other fluids appear to flow from the victim's mouth, turn his head gently to one side. Control bleeding and treat for shock. Do not administer stimulants or fluids of any kind.

Heart Attack

A heart attack is caused by interference with the blood supply to the heart muscle. When the attack is brought on because of a blood clot in the coronary artery, it is known as *coronary occlusion* or *coronary thrombosis*.

The most dramatic symptom of a serious heart attack is a crushing chest pain that usually travels down the left arm into the hand or into the neck and back. The pain may bring on dizziness, cold sweat, complete collapse, and loss of consciousness. The face has an ashen pallor, and there may be vomiting.

Emergency Treatment

The victim ***must not be moved*** unless he has fallen in a dangerous place. If no physician is immediately available, an ambulance should be called at once. No attempt should be made to get the victim of a heart attack into an automobile.

Until help arrives, give the victim every reassurance that he will get prompt treatment, and keep him as calm and quiet as possible. Don't give him any medicine or stimulants. If oxygen is available, start administering it to the victim immediately, either by mask or nasal catheter, depending on which is available.

If the victim is suffering from respiratory arrest, begin artificial respiration. If he is suffering from cardiac arrest, begin cardiac massage.

Heat Exhaustion

Heat exhaustion occurs when the

Toxic Mushrooms

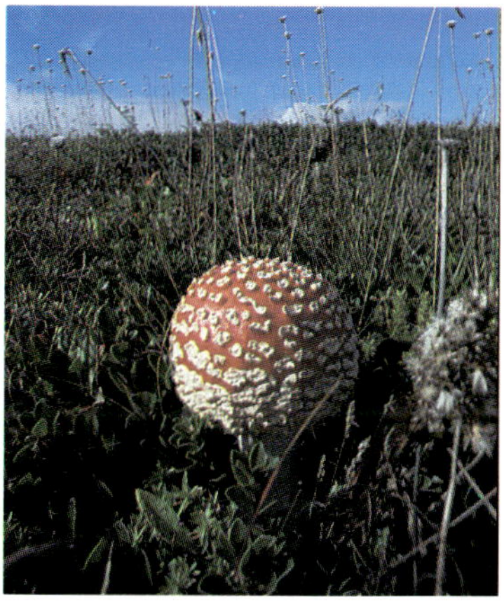

Tom Stack and Associates

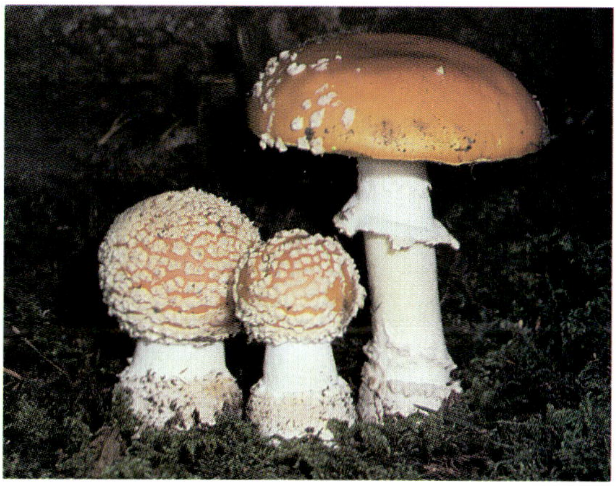

Tom Stack and Associates

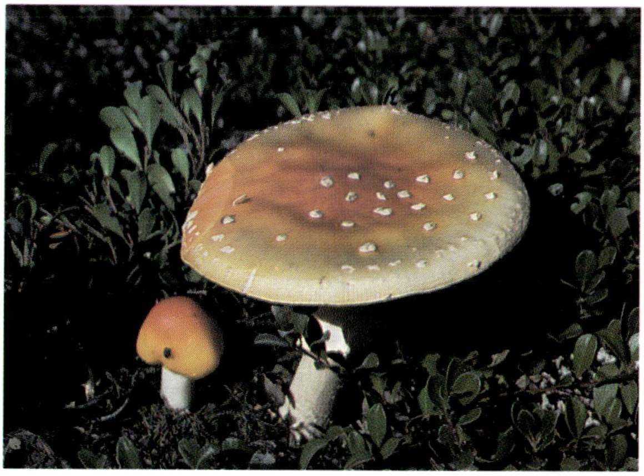

Tom Stack and Associates

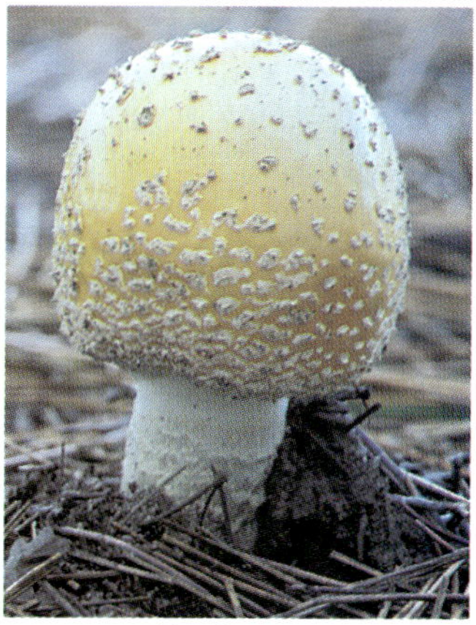

Tom Stack and Associates

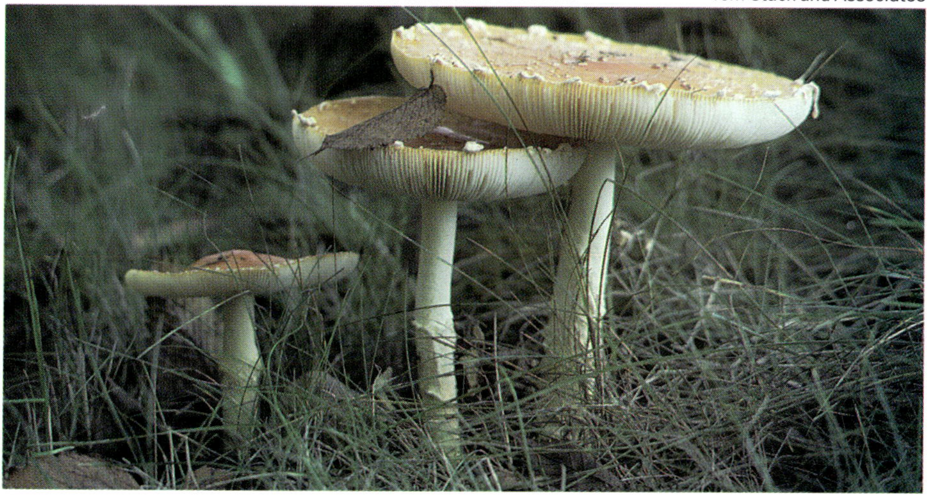

James P. Rowan (Shedd Aquarium)

The poisonous mushroom Amanita Muscaria shows many different shapes, forms, and colors and grows in many parts of the United States.

Common Poisonous Plants

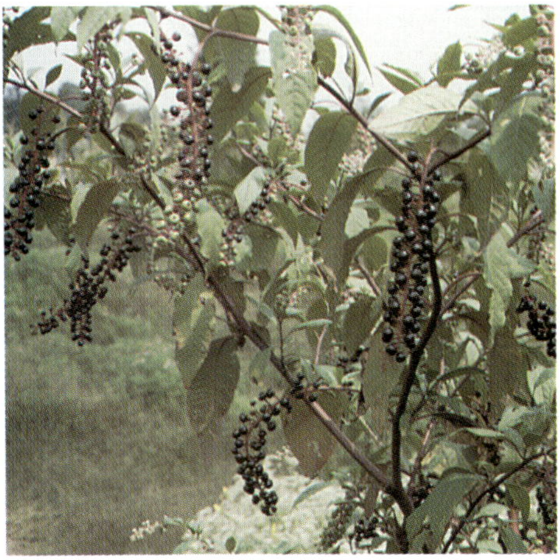

Pokeweed. Poke or Pokeweed is a bush of the eastern United States. Eating uncooked leaves, the roots, or using the cooking water in a soup, causes abdominal cramps and vomiting.

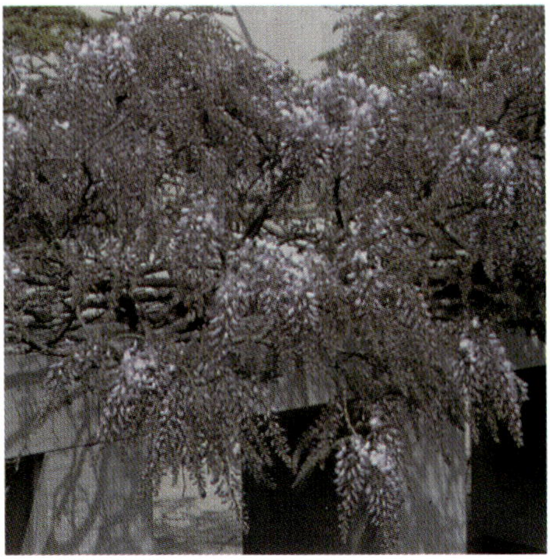

Wisteria. All parts of the vine—leaves, flowers, or the seeds in the pod—may cause a prolonged nausea, abdominal pain, and vomiting.

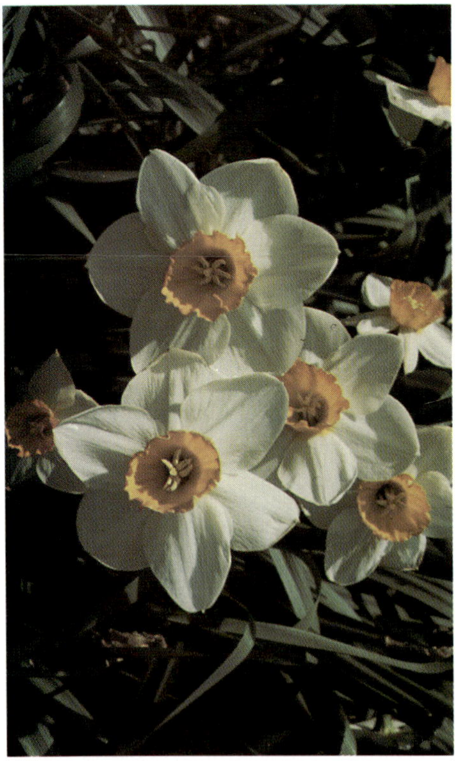

Daffodil or Narcissus. Mistaking the bulb of this plant for an onion is the cause of most poisonings.

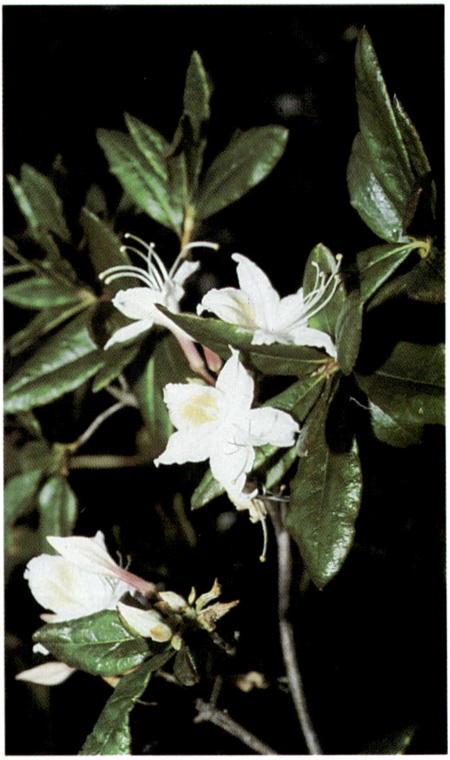

Rhododendron and Azalea. Some, but not all, of these bushes are poisonous. The one pictured from the state flower of California is toxic.

Common Poisonous Plants

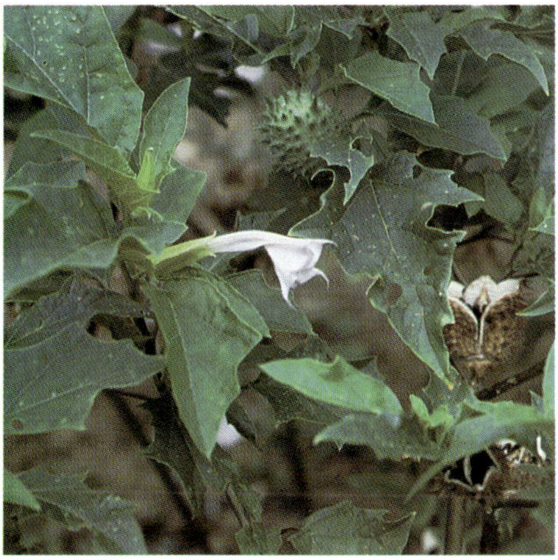

Jimson Weed. This weed is the cause of the first recorded plant poisoning in the United States, in the Jamestown Settlement. The seeds and leaves are toxic.

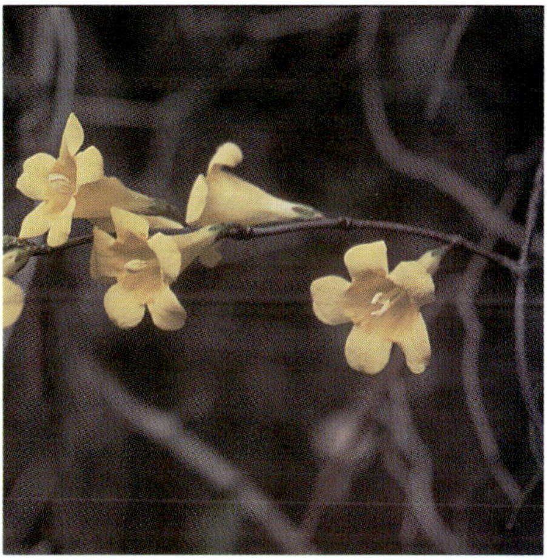

Yellow Jessamine or Carolina Yellow Jasmine. Children have been poisoned sucking the nectar from the trumpet shaped flowers. The muscles become weak.

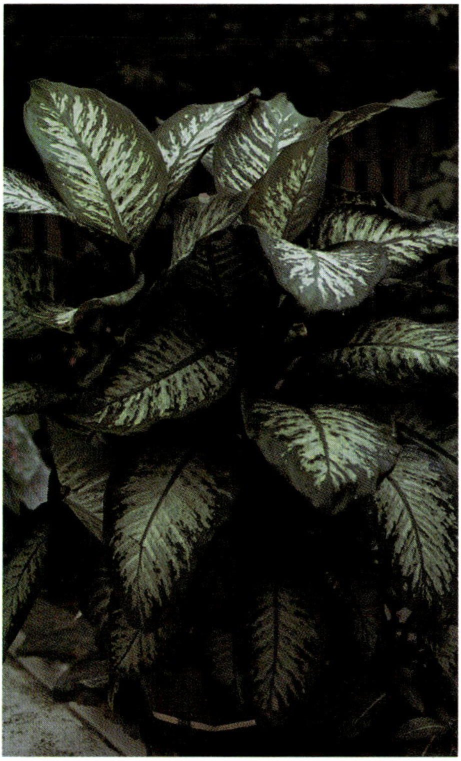

Dieffenbachia or Dumbcane. Biting into the leaf causes an immediate intense, painful burning in the mouth. This houseplant is the one most frequently involved in injury to young children.

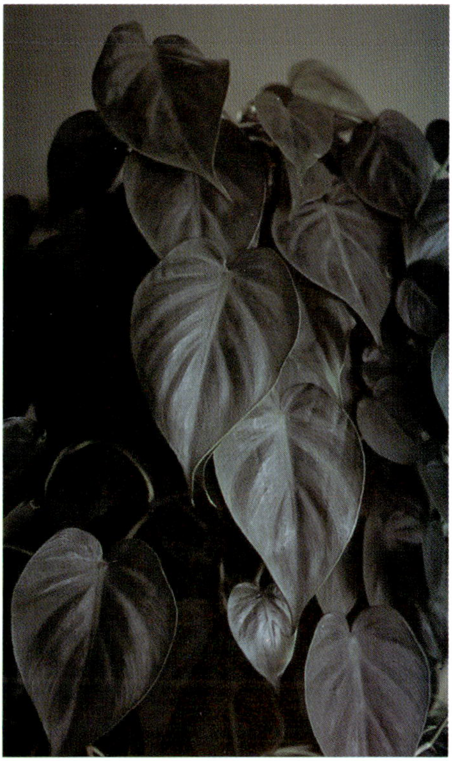

Philodendron or Heart-Leaf Ivy. This produces a response similar to Dieffenbachia, but not usually as intense.

Common Poisonous Plants

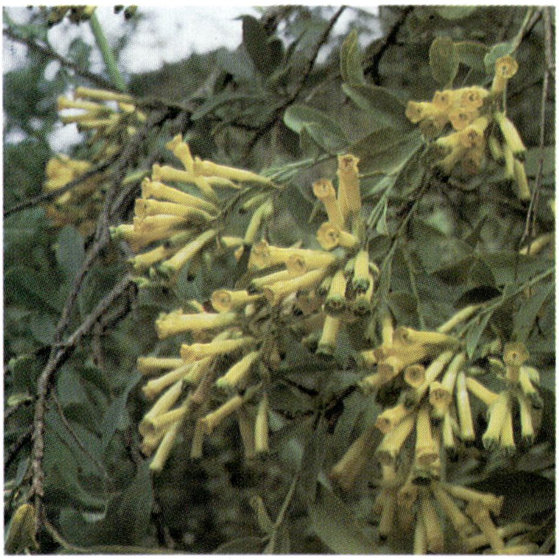

Tree Tobacco. Primarily a plant of the southwest, it has been responsible for a number of deaths, usually from eating the leaves prepared in a salad.

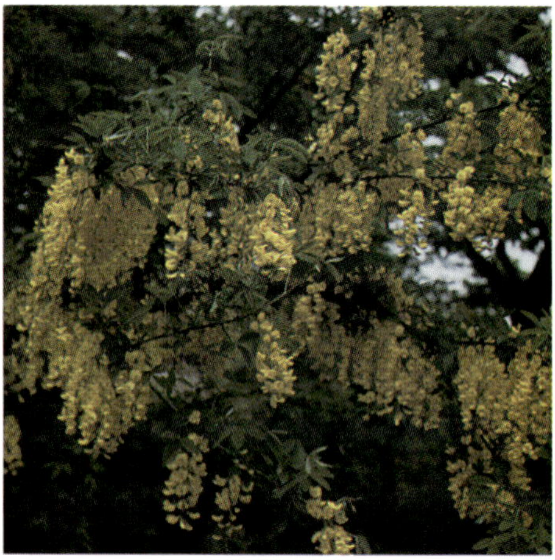

Golden Chain or Laburnum. All parts of the plant, but particularly the seeds in the flat pods, are poisonous. Intoxications rarely are serious.

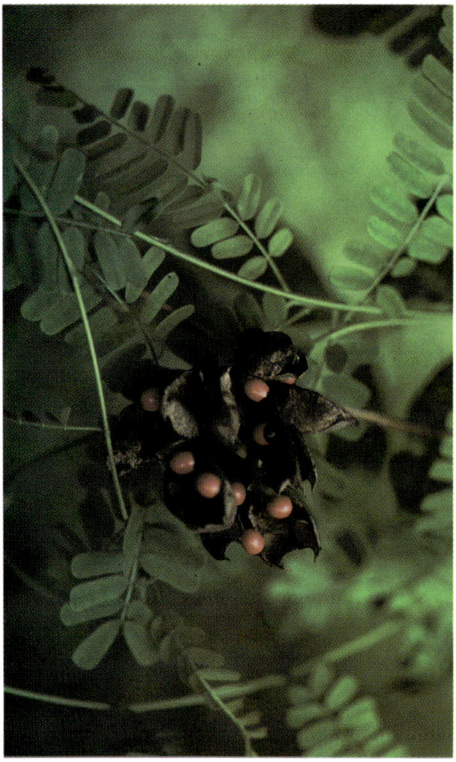

Rosary Pea. This vine grows as a weed in Florida, the Virgin Islands and Puerto Rico, Mexico, and Hawaii. The toxic seeds are strung as jewelry and rosaries, and, may be found throughout the United States.

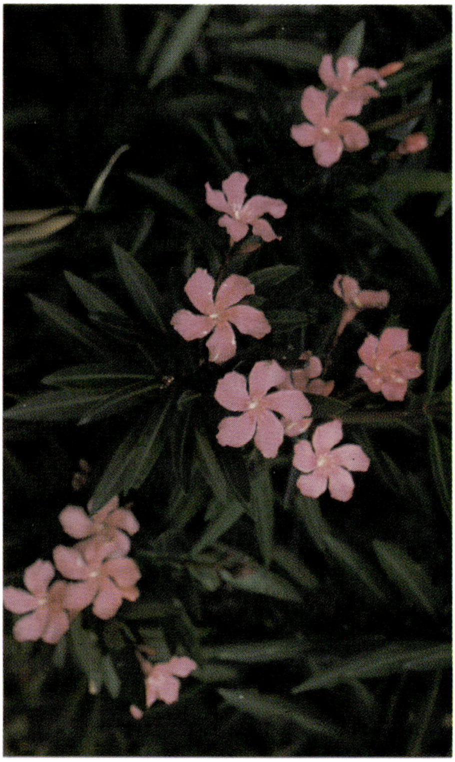

Oleander. All parts of this attractive bush contain a toxin similar to digitalis. Most poisonings have involved ingestion of the leaves.

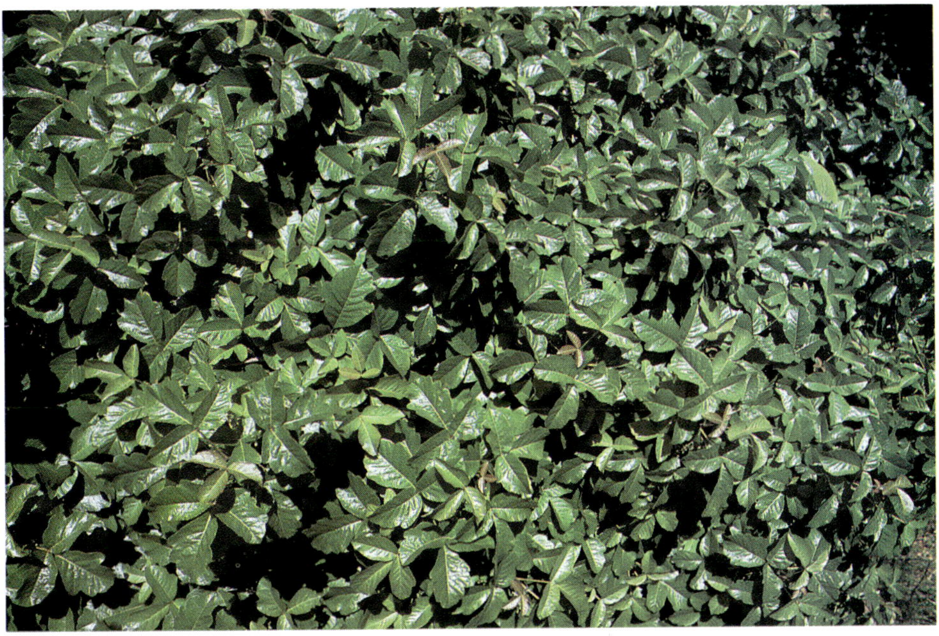

Poison Oak
Tom Stack and Associates

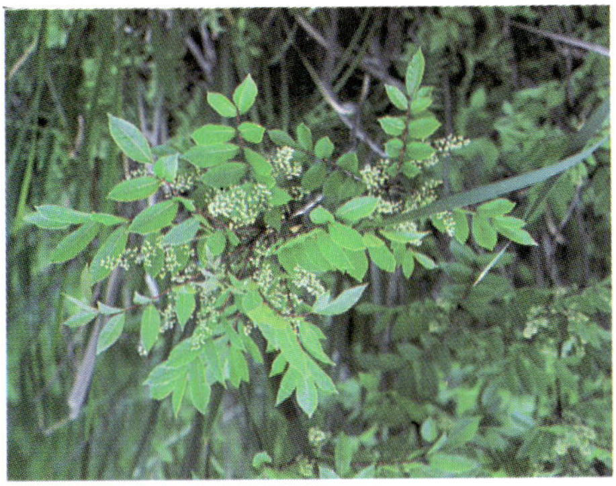

Poison Sumac
James P. Rowan

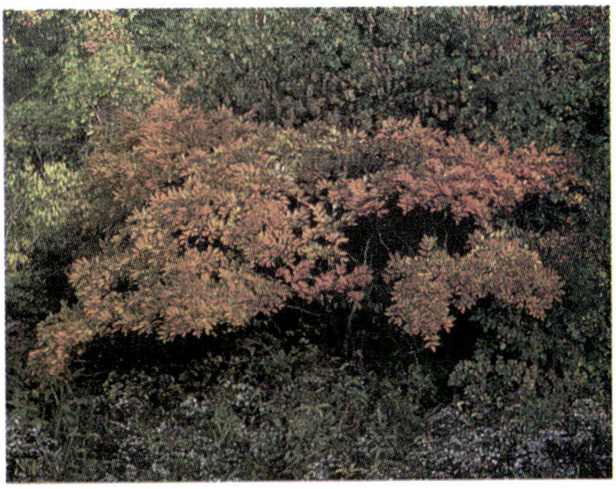

Poison Sumac in Autumn
Tom Stack and Associates

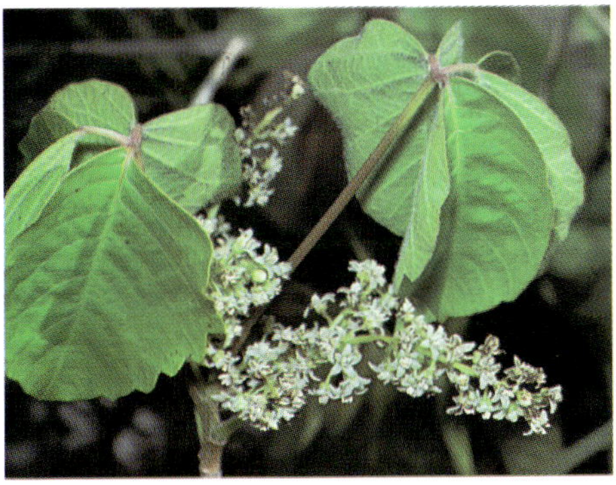

Poison Ivy
Tom Stack and Associates

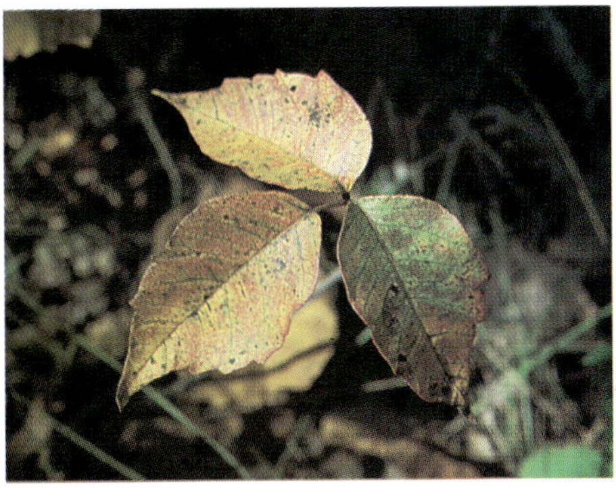

Poison Ivy in Autumn
James P. Rowan

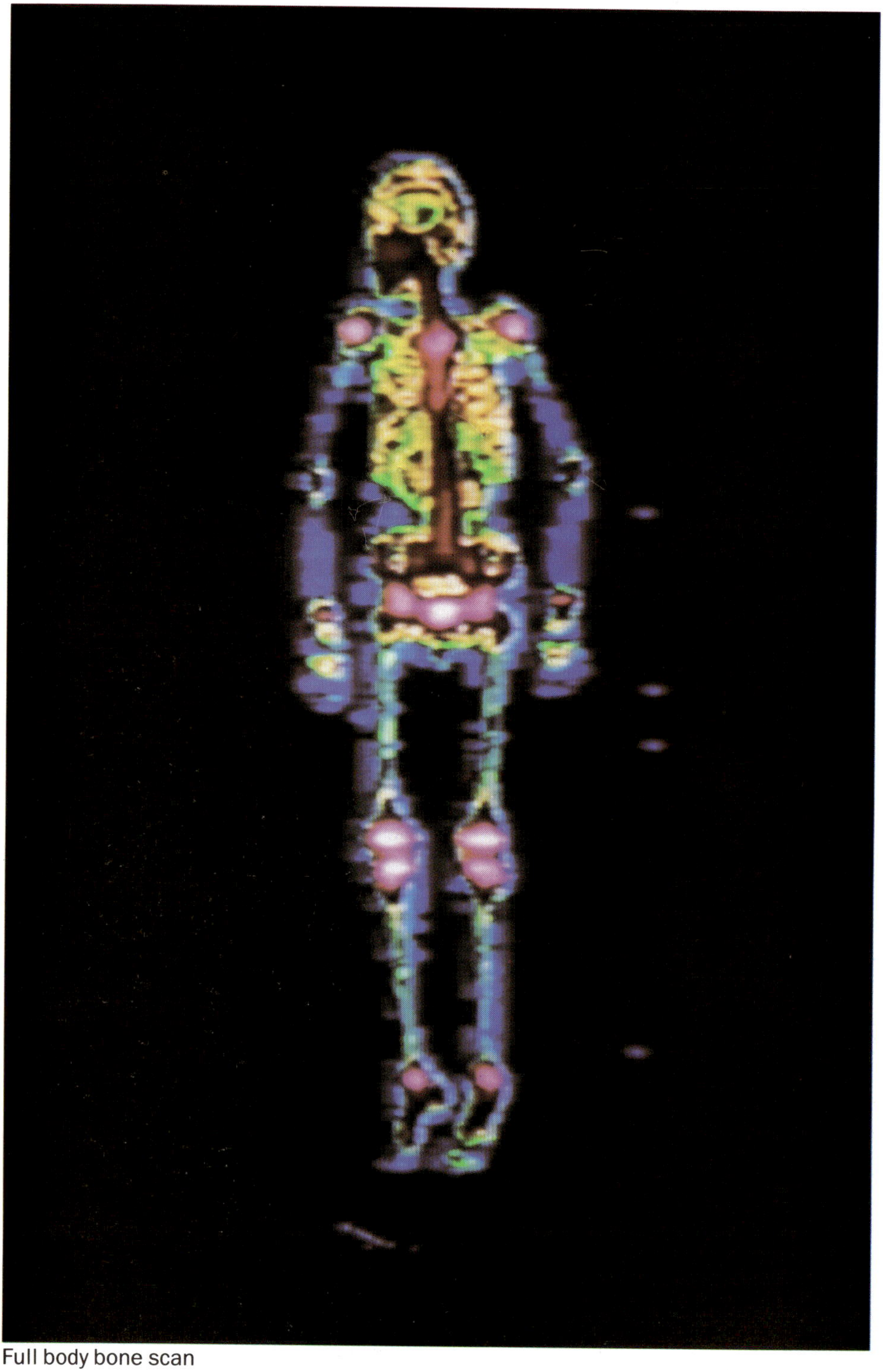
Full body bone scan

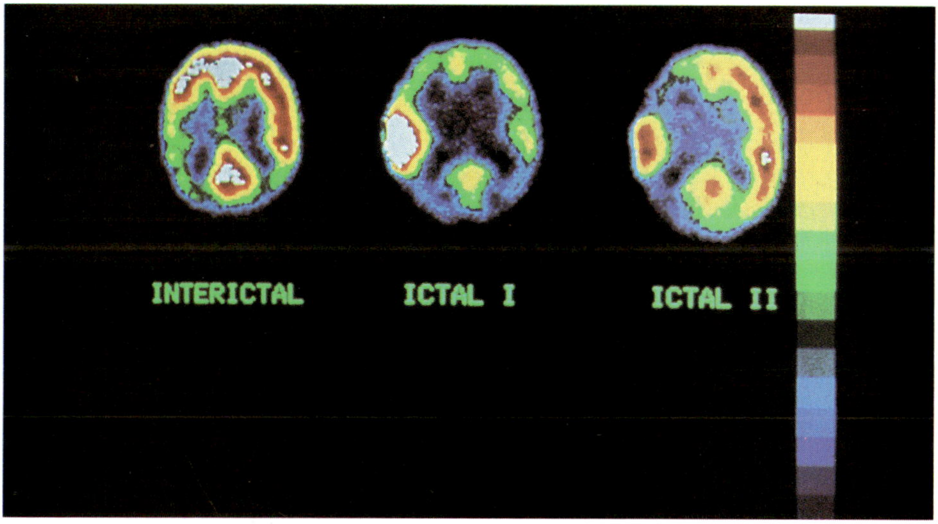

PET scan of human brain in stages of epileptic seizure

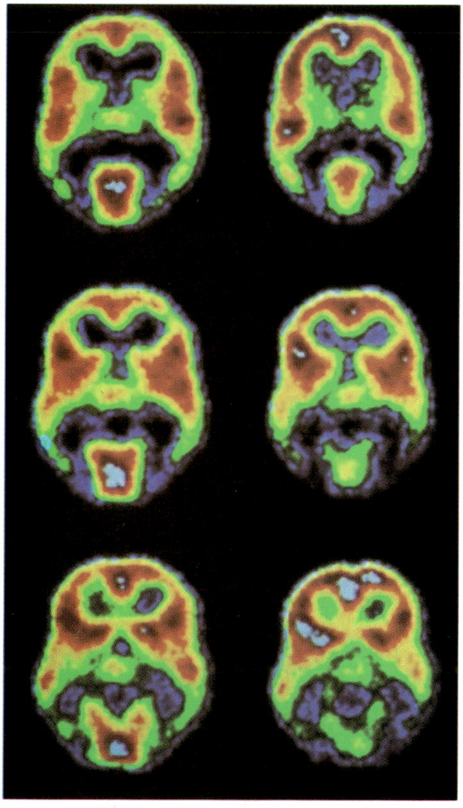

ECAT scans of normal brain

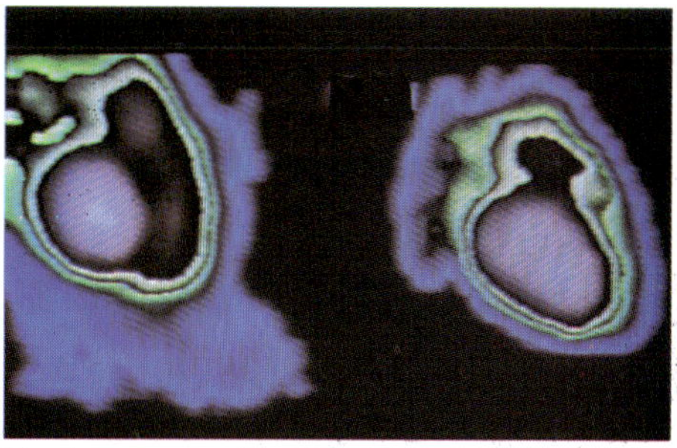

Nuclear scan showing heart volume

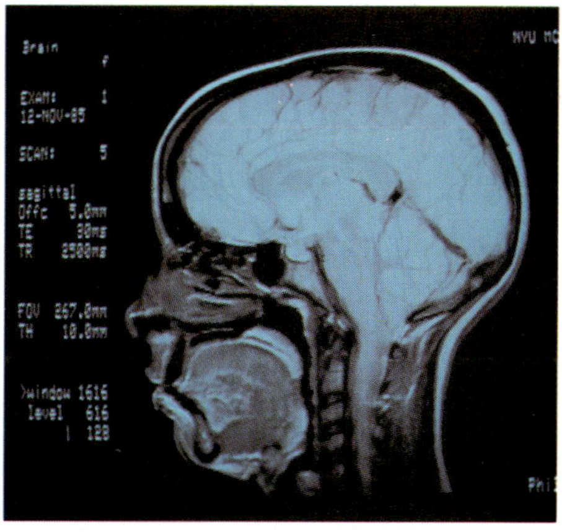

MRI scan of human brain to diagnose blood supply

(All photographs © Photo Researchers, Inc.)

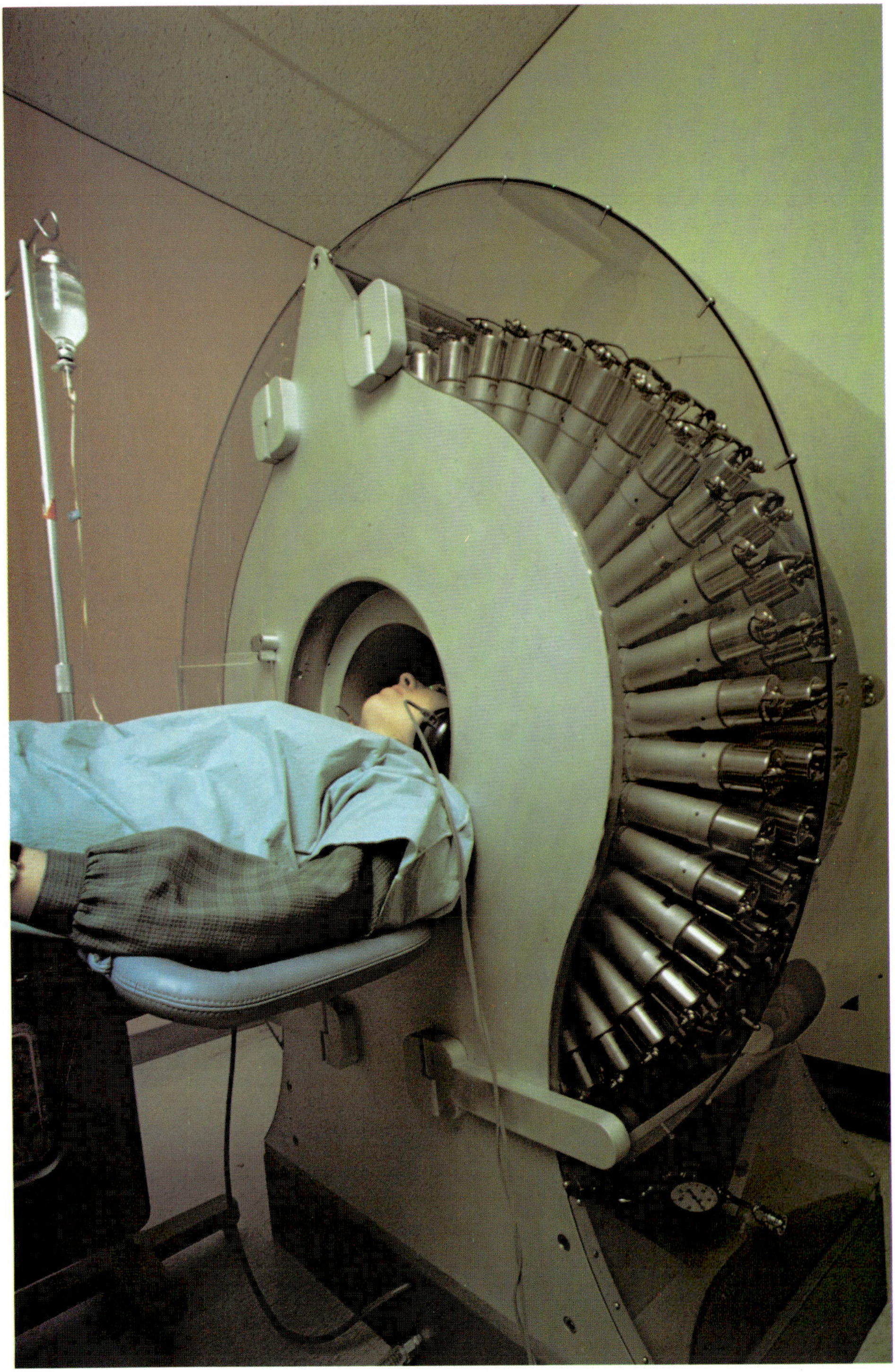

Positron emission tomography

(PET scan
© Dan McCoy—Rainbow)

body is exposed to high temperatures and large amounts of blood accumulate in the skin as a way of cooling it. As a result, there is a marked decrease in the amount of blood that circulates through the heart and to the brain. The victim becomes markedly pale and is covered with cold perspiration. Breathing is increasingly shallow and the pulse weakens. In acute cases, fainting occurs. Medical aid should be summoned for anyone suffering from heat exhaustion.

Emergency Treatment

Place the victim in a reclining position with his feet raised about ten inches above his body. Loosen or remove his clothing, and apply cold, wet cloths to his wrists and forehead. If he has fainted and doesn't recover promptly, smelling salts or spirits of ammonia should be placed under his nose. When the victim is conscious, give him sips of salt water (approximately one teaspoon of salt per glass of water), the total intake to be about two glasses in an hour's time. If the victim vomits, discontinue the salt solution.

Heatstroke/Sunstroke

Heatstroke is characterized by an acutely high body temperature caused by the cessation of perspiration. The victim's skin becomes hot, dry, and flushed, and he may suffer collapse. Should the skin turn ashen gray, a physician must be called immediately. Prompt hospital treatment is recommended for anyone showing signs of sunstroke who has previously had any kind of heart damage.

Emergency Treatment

The following measures are designed to reduce the victim's body temperature as quickly as possible and prevent damage to the internal organs:

Place him in a tub of very cold water, or, if this is not possible, spray or sponge his body repeatedly with cold water or rubbing alcohol. Take his temperature by mouth, and when it has dropped to about 100°F., remove him to a bed and wrap him in cold, wet sheets. If possible, expose him to an electric fan or an air conditioner. Then call for medical aid.

Hiccups

Emergency Treatment

Have the victim slowly drink a large glass of water. If cold water is not effective, have him drink warm water containing a teaspoonful of baking soda. Milk also can be employed. For babies and small children, offer sips of warm water. Do not offer carbonated beverages.

Another helpful measure is breathing into a large paper bag a number of times to raise the carbon dioxide level in the lungs. Rest and relaxation are recommended; have the victim lie down to read or watch television.

If the hiccups fail to go away, and continued spastic contractions of the diaphragm interfere with eating and sleeping, call a physician.

Insect Stings

Honeybees, wasps, hornets, and yellow jackets are the most common stinging insects and most likely to attack on a hot summer day. Strongly scented perfumes or cosmetics and brightly colored, rough-finished clothing attract bees and should be avoided by persons working or playing in garden areas. It should also be noted that many commercial repellents do not protect against stinging insects.

Emergency Treatment

If one is stung, the insect's stinger should be tweezed or scraped gently from the skin as soon as possible; don't squeeze it. Apply Epsom salt solution to the sting area. Antihistamines are often helpful in reducing the patient's discomfort. If a severe reaction develops, call a physician.

There are a few people who are critically allergic to the sting of wasps, bees, yellow jackets, or fire ants. This sensitivity causes the vocal cord tissue to swell to the point where breathing may become impossible. A single sting to a sensitive person may result in a dangerous drop in blood pressure, thus producing shock. Anyone with such a severe allergy who is stung should be rushed to a hospital immediately.

Allergic persons should always have on hand an insect-sting emergency kit, which can be obtained through a prescription.

Insulin Shock

See DIABETIC COMA AND INSULIN SHOCK.

Jaw Dislocation

The jaw can be dislocated during a physical attack or fight; from a blow on the jaw during sports activities; or from overextension of the joint during yawning, laughing, or attempting to eat a large mouthful of food. The jaw becomes literally locked open so the victim cannot explain his predicament.

Emergency Treatment

Reducing a dislocated jaw will require that you insert your thumbs between the teeth of the victim. The jaw can be expected to snap into place quickly, and there is a danger that the teeth will clamp down on the thumbs when this happens, so the thumbs should be adequately padded with handkerchiefs or bandages. Once the thumbs are protected, insert them in the mouth and over the lower molars, as far back on the lower jaw as possible. While pressing down with the thumbs, lift the chin with the fingers outside the mouth. As the jaw begins to slip into normal position when it is pushed downward and backward with the chin lifted upward, quickly remove the thumbs from between the jaws.

Once the jaw is back in normal position, the mouth should remain closed for several hours while the ligaments recover from their displaced condition. If necessary, put a cravat bandage over the head to hold the mouth closed. If difficulty is experienced in reducing a jaw dislocation, the victim should be taken to a hospital where an anesthetic can be applied.

Jellyfish Stings

Emergency Treatment

Wash the area of the sting thoroughly with alcohol or fresh water. Be sure that any pieces of jellyfish tentacles have been removed from the skin. Aspirin or antihistamines can be administered to relieve pain and itching, but curtail the use of antihistamines if the victim has consumed alcoholic beverages. The leg or arm that received the sting can be soaked in hot water if the pain continues. Otherwise, apply calamine lotion.

If the victim appears to suffer a severe reaction from the sting, summon a doctor. The victim may experience shock, muscle cramps, convulsions, or loss of consciousness. Artificial respiration may be required while awaiting arrival of a doctor. The physician can administer drugs to relieve muscle cramps and provide sedatives or analgesics.

Kidney Stones

Emergency Treatment

Call a physician if the victim experiences the agonizing cramps or colic associated with kidney stones. Discuss the symptoms in detail with the doctor to make sure the pain is caused by kidney stones rather than appendicitis.

Comforting heat may be applied to the back and the abdomen of the side affected by the spasms. Paregoric can be administered, if available, while waiting for medical care; about two teaspoonsful of paregoric in a half glass of water may help relieve symptoms.

Knee Injuries

Emergency Treatment

If the injury appears to be severe, including possible fracture of the kneecap, immobilize the knee. To immobilize the knee, place the injured leg on a board that is about four inches wide and three to four feet in length. Place padding between the board and the knee and between the board and the back of the ankle. Then use four strips of bandage to fasten the leg to the padded board—one at the ankle, one at the thigh, and one each above and below the knee.

Summon a physician or move the patient to a physician's office. Keep the knee protected against cold or exposure to the elements, but otherwise do not apply a bandage or any type of pressure to the knee itself; any rapid swelling would be aggravated by unnecessary pressure in that area. Be prepared to treat the patient for shock.

Laryngitis

Laryngitis is associated with colds and influenza and may be accompanied by a fever. The ailment can be aggravated by smoking, and it is possible that the vocal cords can be damaged if the victim tries to force the use of his voice while the larynx is swollen by the infection.

Emergency Treatment

Have the victim inhale the warm

moist air of a steam kettle or vaporizer. A vaporizer can be improvised in an emergency by pouring boiling water into a bowl and forming a "tent" over the steaming bowl with a large towel or sheet, or by placing a large paper bag over the bowl and cutting an opening at the closed end of the bag so the face can be exposed to the steam. The hot water can contain a bit of camphor or menthol, if available, to make the warm moist air more soothing to the throat, but this is not necessary.

Continue the use of the vaporizer for several days, as needed. The victim should not use the vocal cords any more than absolutely necessary. If the infection does not subside within the first few days, a physician should be consulted.

Leeches

Emergency Treatment

Do not try to pull leeches off the skin. They will usually drop away from the skin if a heated object such as a lighted cigarette is held close to them. Leeches also are likely to let go if iodine is applied to their bodies. The wound caused by a leech should be washed carefully with soap and water and an antiseptic applied.

Lightning Shock

Emergency Treatment

If the victim is not breathing, apply artificial respiration. If a second person is available to help, have him summon a physician while artificial respiration is administered. Continue artificial respiration until breathing resumes or the physician arrives.

When the victim is breathing regularly, treat him for shock. Keep him lying down with his feet higher than his head, his clothing loosened around the neck, and his body covered with a blanket or coat for warmth. If the victim shows signs of vomiting, turn his head to one side so he will not swallow the vomitus.

If the victim is breathing regularly and does not show signs of shock, he may be given a few sips of a stimulating beverage such as coffee, tea, or brandy.

Motion Sickness

Emergency Treatment

Have the victim lie down in a position that is most comfortable to him. The head should be fixed so that any view of motion is avoided. Reading or other use of the eyes should be prohibited. Food or fluids should be restricted to very small amounts. If traveling by car, stop at a rest area; in an airplane or ship, place the victim in an area where motion is least noticeable.

Drugs, such as Dramamine, are helpful for control of the symptoms of motion sickness; they are most effective when started about 90 minutes before travel begins and repeated at regular intervals thereafter.

Muscle Cramps

Emergency Treatment

Gently massage the affected muscle, sometimes stretching it to help relieve the painful contraction. Then relax the muscle by using a hot water bottle or an electric heating pad, or by soaking the affected area in a warm bath.

A repetition of cramps may require medical attention.

Nosebleeds

Emergency Treatment

Have the victim sit erect but with the head tilted slightly forward to prevent blood from running down the throat. Apply pressure by pinching the nostrils; if bleeding is from just one nostril, use pressure on that side. A small wedge of absorbent cotton or gauze can be inserted into the bleeding nostril. Make sure that the cotton or gauze extends out of the nostril to aid in its removal when the bleeding has stopped. Encourage the victim to breathe through the mouth while the nose is bleeding. After five minutes, release pressure on the nose to see if the bleeding has stopped. If the bleeding continues, repeat pressure on the nostril for an additional five minutes. Cold compresses applied to the nose can help stop the bleeding.

If bleeding continues after the second five-minute period of pressure treatment, get the victim to a physician's office or a hospital emergency room.

Poison Ivy/Poison Oak/Poison Sumac

Emergency Treatment

The poison of these three plants is the same and the treatment is identical. Bathe the skin area exposed to poison ivy, poison oak, or poison sumac with soap and water within 15 minutes after first contact. If exposure is not discovered until a rash appears, apply cool wet dressings. Dressings can be made of old bed sheets or soft linens soaked in a solution of one teaspoon of salt per pint of water. Dressings should be applied four times a day for periods of 15 to 60 minutes each time; during these periods, dressings can be removed and reapplied every few minutes. The itching that often accompanies the rash can be relieved by taking antihistamine tablets.

Creams or lotions may be prescribed by a physician or supplied by a pharmacist. Do not use such folk remedies as ammonia or turpentine; do not use skin lotions not approved by a physician or druggist. Haphazard application of medications on poison ivy blisters and rashes can result in complications including skin irritation, infection, or pigmented lesions of the skin.

Rabies

See ANIMAL BITES.

Rape

Rape has been defined as any unlawful

sexual intercourse or sexual contact by force or threat. Most commonly, men commit rape against women; but homosexual rape involving men only may occur, for example, in a prison.

Of the million or more Americans who are raped each year, one in five is under the age of 12. Boys are the victims of sexual assault as often as girls. In seven to ten percent of all reported adult cases, men are the victims.

Emergency Response

The victim of rape may not always be able to help him- or herself. Because violence may accompany the rape, the victim may find it impossible to seek help at once. But where possible, the recommended course of action is to go to a hospital for physical examination. Reporting to a hospital in itself may reduce the feelings of shock, depression, anxiety, and revulsion that generally follow a sexual assault. The physical examination that takes place at the hospital may produce evidence that could be important in a court trial if the rapist is later apprehended. Victims are also advised to report the rape to the police as soon as possible.

For additional information on ways to avoid rape and what to do if it occurs, see "The Rape Victim" in Ch. 25, *Women's Health.*

Sciatica/Lower Back Pain

Although lower back pain is frequently triggered by fatigue, anxiety, or by strained muscles or tendons, it may be a symptom of a slipped or ruptured disk between the vertebrae or of a similar disorder requiring extensive medical attention.

Emergency Treatment

Reduce the pressure on the lower back by having the victim lie down on a hard flat surface; if a bed is used there should be a board or sheet of plywood between the springs and mattress. Pillows should be placed under the knees instead of under the head, to help keep the back flat. Give aspirin to relieve the pain, and apply heat to the back. Call a physician if the symptoms do not subside overnight.

Scorpion Stings

Emergency Treatment

Apply ice to the region of the sting, except in the case of an arm or leg, in which event the limb may be immersed in ice water. Continue the ice or ice-water treatment for at least one hour. Try to keep the area of the sting at a position lower than the heart. No tourniquet is required. Should the breathing of a scorpion sting victim become depressed, administer artificial respiration. If symptoms fail to subside within a couple of hours, notify a physician, or transfer the victim to a doctor's office or hospital.

For children under six, call a physician in the event of any scorpion sting. Children stung by scorpions may become convulsive, and this condition can result in fatal exhaustion unless it receives prompt medical treatment.

Snakebites

Of the many varieties of snakes found in the United States, only four kinds are poisonous: copperheads, rattlesnakes, moccasins, and coral snakes. The first three belong to the category of pit vipers and are known as *hemotoxic* because their poison enters the bloodstream. The coral snake, which is comparatively rare, is related to the cobra and is the most dangerous of all because its venom is *neurotoxic.* This means that the poison transmitted by its bite goes directly to the nervous system and the brain.

How to Differentiate among Snakebites

Snakes of the pit viper family have a fang on each side of the head. These fangs leave characteristic puncture wounds on the skin in addition to two rows of tiny bites or scratches left by the teeth. A bite from a nonpoisonous snake leaves six rows—four upper and two lower—of very small bite marks or scratches and no puncture wounds.

The marks left by the bite of a coral snake do not leave any puncture wounds either, but this snake bites with a chewing motion, hanging on to the victim rather than attacking quickly. The coral snake is very easy to recognize because of its distinctive markings: wide horizontal bands of red and black separated by narrow bands of yellow.

Symptoms

A bite from any of the pit vipers produces immediate and severe pain and darkening of the skin, followed by weakness, blurred vision, quickened pulse, nausea, and vomiting. The bite of a coral snake produces somewhat the same symptoms, although there is less local pain and considerable drowsiness leading to unconsciousness.

If a physician or a hospital is a short distance away, the patient should receive professional help *immediately.* He should be transported lying down, either on an improvised stretcher or carried by his companions—with the wounded part lower than his heart. He should be advised to move as little as possible.

Emergency Treatment

If several hours must elapse before a physician or a hospital can be reached, the following procedures should be applied promptly:

1. Keep the victim lying down and as still as possible.

2. Tie a constricting band *above* the wound between it and the heart and tight enough to slow but not stop blood circulation. A handkerchief, necktie, sock, or piece of torn shirt will serve.

3. If a snakebite kit is available, use the knife it contains; otherwise, sterilize a knife or razor blade in a flame. Carefully make small cuts in the skin where the swelling has developed. Make the cuts along the length of the limb, not across or at right angles to it. The incisions should be shallow because of the danger of severing nerves, blood vessels, or muscles.

4. Use the suction cups in the snakebite kit, if available, to draw out as much of the venom as possible. If suction cups are not available, the venom can be removed by sucking it out with the mouth. Although snake venom is not a stomach poison, it should not be swallowed but should be rinsed from the mouth.

5. This procedure should be continued for from 30 to 60 minutes or until the swelling subsides and the other symptoms decrease.

6. You may apply cold compresses to the bite area while waiting for professional assistance.

7. Treat the victim for shock.

8. Give artificial respiration if necessary.

Splinters

Emergency Treatment

Clean the area about the splinter with soap and water or an antiseptic. Next, sterilize a needle by holding it over an open flame. After it cools, insert the needle above the splinter so it will tear a line in the skin, making the splinter lie loose in the wound. Then, gently lift the splinter out, using a pair of tweezers or the point of the needle. If tweezers are used, they should be sterilized first.

Wash the wound area again with soap and water, or apply an antiseptic. It is best to cover the wound with an adhesive bandage. If redness or irritation develops around the splinter wound, consult a physician.

Sprains

A sprain occurs when a joint is wrenched or twisted in such a way that the ligaments holding it in position are ruptured, possibly damaging the surrounding blood vessels, tendons, nerves, and muscles. This type of injury is more serious than a strain and is usually accompanied by pain, sometimes severe, soreness, swelling, and discoloration of the affected area. Most sprains occur as a result of falls, athletic accidents, or improper handling of heavy weights.

Emergency Treatment

This consists of prompt rest, the application of cold compresses to relieve swelling and any internal bleeding in the joint, and elevation of the affected area. Aspirin is recommended to reduce discomfort in adults. If the swelling and soreness increase after such treatment, a physician should be consulted to make sure that there is not a fracture or a bone dislocation.

Sting Ray

Emergency Treatment

If an arm or leg is the target of a sting ray, wash the area thoroughly with salt water. Quickly remove any pieces of the stinger imbedded in the skin or flesh; poison can still be discharged into the victim from the sting-ray sheath. After initial cleansing of an arm or leg sting, soak the wound with hot water for up to an hour. Apply antiseptic or a sterile dressing after the soak.

Consult a physician after a sting-ray attack. The physician will make a thorough examination of the wound to determine whether stitches or antibiotics are required. Fever, vomiting, or muscular twitching also may result from an apparently simple leg or arm wound by a sting ray.

If the sting occurs in the chest or abdomen, the victim should be rushed to a hospital as soon as possible because such a wound can produce convulsions or loss of consciousness.

Strains

When a muscle is stretched because of misuse or overuse, the interior bundles of tissue may tear, or the tendon that connects it to the bone may be stretched. This condition is known as strain. It occurs most commonly to the muscles of the lower back when heavy weights are improperly lifted, or in the area of the calf or ankle as the result of a sudden, violent twist or undue pressure.

Emergency Treatment

Bed rest, the application of heat, and gentle massage are recommended for back strain. If the strain is in the leg, elevate the limb to help reduce pain and swelling, and apply cold compresses or an ice bag to the area. Aspirin may be taken to reduce discomfort.

In severe cases of strained back muscles, a physician may have to be consulted for strapping. For a strained ankle, a flexible elastic bandage can be helpful in providing the necessary support until the injured muscle heals.

Stroke

Stroke, or apoplexy, is caused by a disruption of normal blood flow to the brain, either by rupture of a blood vessel within the brain or by blockage of an artery supplying the brain. The condition is enhanced by hardening of the arteries and high blood pressure, and is most likely to occur in older persons. A stroke usually occurs with little or no warning and the onset may be marked by a variety of manifestations ranging from headache, slurred speech, or blurred vision, to sudden collapse and unconsciousness.

Emergency Treatment

Try to place the victim in a semireclining position, or, if he is lying down, be sure there is a pillow under his head. Avoid conditions that might increase the flow of blood toward the head. Summon a physician immediately. Loosen any clothing that may be tight. If the patient wears dentures, remove them.

Before professional medical assistance is available, the victim may vomit or go into shock or convulsions. If he vomits, try to prevent a backflow of vomitus into the breathing passages. If shock occurs, do not place the victim in the shock position but do keep him warm and comfortable. If convulsions develop, place a handkerchief or similar soft object between the jaws to prevent tongue biting.

Sty on Eyelid

Sties usually develop around hair follicles because of a bacterial infection. They are most likely to develop in association with poor health and lowered resistance to infection.

Emergency Treatment

Apply warm, moist packs or compresses to the sty for periods of 15 to 20 minutes at intervals of three or four hours. Moist heat generally is more penetrating than dry heat.

The sty should eventually rupture and the pus should then be washed carefully away from the eye area. If the sty does not rupture or is very painful, consult a physician. Do not squeeze or otherwise handle the sty except to apply the warm moist compresses.

Sunburn

Emergency Treatment

Apply cold wet compresses to help relieve the pain. Compresses can be soaked in whole milk, salt water, or a solution of cornstarch mixed with water. The victim also may get some relief by soaking in a bathtub filled with plain water. Soothing lotions, such as baby oil or a bland cold cream, can be applied after carefully drying the skin. Don't rub the burn area while drying. Avoid the use of "shake" lotions, like calamine, which may aggravate the burn by a drying action. The victim should, of course, avoid further exposure to sunlight.

If pain is excessive, or extensive blistering is present, consult a physician.

A severe or extensive sunburn is comparable to a second-degree thermal burn and may be accompanied by symptoms of shock; if such symptoms are present the victim should be treated for shock. See also BURNS, THERMAL.

Sunstroke

See HEATSTROKE.

Tick Bites

The most common tick-borne illness is Lyme disease which is carried by a bacterium that infects mice, ticks, deer and humans. It is distinguished by a red bull's eye rash, fatigue, chills headaches and fever within three to 30 days after infection and has been fatal in some rare cases. Lyme disease can be treated with antibiotics which should be administered in the condition's early stages.

Emergency Treatment

To make the tick drop away from the skin, cover it with a heavy oil, such as salad, mineral, or lubricating oil. Oil usually will block the insect's breathing pores, suffocating it. If oil is not readily available, carefully place a heated object against the tick's body; a lighted cigarette or a match that has been ignited and snuffed out can serve as a hot object.

Carefully inspect the bite area to be sure that all parts of the tick have been removed. Use a pair of tweezers to remove any tick parts found. Then carefully wash the bite and surrounding area with soap and water and apply an antiseptic. Also, wash your hands and any equipment that may have come in contact with the tick. Consult a physician if symptoms of tick fever or tularemia, such as unexplained muscular weakness, occur following a bite.

Toothaches

Emergency Treatment

Rinse the mouth with warm water. Give an adult one or two aspirin tablets. The aspirin should be swallowed with plenty of water. Do not let it dissolve in the mouth or be held near the aching tooth. Aspirin becomes effective as a painkiller only after it has gone through the digestive tract and into the bloodstream; if aspirin is held in the mouth, it may irritate the gums. A young child may be given acetaminophen during this time.

Gently use dental floss to make sure that there is no food or other material lodged around the tooth. If the jaw is swollen, apply an ice bag for periods of 15 minutes at a time, at intermittent intervals. Never apply heat to a swollen jaw when treating a toothache. Arrange to see your dentist as soon as possible.

Tooth, Broken

Emergency Treatment

If a tooth is broken, the mouth should be rinsed with warm water, and cold compresses should be applied to the area to keep the swelling down. Get to a dentist as soon as possible.

If the tooth has been knocked out of its socket, time is critical. It is important to retrieve it and get to a dentist as soon as possible—within 30 minutes is best—because it may be possible to save the tooth. Hold the tooth by the crown and rinse off the root if it is dirty, but do not scrub or otherwise clean the root. If possible, place the tooth gently back in its socket; otherwise, put it in milk or water and take it to the dentist immediately.

Unconsciousness

Unconsciousness is the condition that has the appearance of sleep, but is usually the result of injury, shock, or serious physical disturbance. A brief loss of consciousness followed by spontaneous recovery is called *fainting.* A prolonged episode of unconsciousness is a *coma.*

Emergency Treatment

Call a physician at once. If none is available, get the victim to the nearest hospital. If the loss of consciousness is accompanied by loss of breathing, begin mouth-to-mouth respiration. If the victim is suffering cardiac arrest, administer cardiopulmonary resuscitation (CPR). Don't try to revive the victim with any kind of stimulant unless told to do so by a physician.

36

Commonly Prescribed Drugs

Disclaimer: This is only a generalized classification based on the Food & Drug Administration (FDA) indications for pharmaceutical usage. Physicians reserve the right to prescribe medications as they see fit within their field of practice. The FDA approves a drug for safety and efficacy of a particular indication of use. Therefore, a physician may properly prescribe a medication for a use other than that described in its classification in this chapter.

The products listed in this chapter are just some of the commonly prescribed drugs available to the consumer. The listings do not imply equivalency of brand names or that they are substitutable or interchangeable. The products listed may come in different dosage forms, tablets, capsules, extended release, sustained release, etc. Your doctor will select the appropriate dosage and form of a product that best suits your therapeutic needs. Drugs shown below list first the generic name followed by trade name in parentheses.

The Action, Use, Possible Side Effects and Precautions of the eleven classifications are very general and not specific to each drug. These classifications should increase your knowledge and involvement in your own or your loved one's therapy. Use other resources including your family doctor and pharmacist to learn more information regarding usage, precautions, and possible side effects for the medication that is prescribed to you.

I. ANTI-INFECTIVES

ACTION: Inhibit nutrition, growth, or reproductive growth of infective agents.

USE: Follow your doctor's directions for use of these medications. Do not miss any doses. Take your medication for the full course of treatment even if you feel better after a few days of use. Some of these medications must be taken with regard to food or other medications.

POSSIBLE SIDE EFFECTS AND PRECAUTIONS: Common side effects include nausea, vomiting, mild diarrhea, or irritation of mouth or throat. Contact your doctor if they continue or become bothersome. Contact your doctor immediately if you have a severe reaction to any of these medications. A severe reaction can include a severe rash or hives, difficulty in breathing, fever, dizziness, tightness in the chest, or swelling of the eyelids, face, or lips. If you experience any other side effects not listed above, contact your doctor.

A. Antibiotics

Penicillins

Amoxicillin (Amoxil, Biomox, Polymox, Trimox, Wymox)
Amoxicillin/clavulanate (Augmentin)
Ampicillin (Omnipen, Polycillin, Principen)
Cloxacillin (Cloxapen, Tegopen)
Dicloxacillin (Dynapen, Dycill, Pathocil)
Penicillin V (Veetids, Pen-Vee-K)

Cephalosporins

Cefaclor (Ceclor)
Cefadroxil (Duricef)
Cefixime (Suprax)
Cefpodoxime (Vantin)
Cefprozil (Cefzil)
Ceftibuten (Cedax)
Ceforoxime (Ceftin)
Cephalexin (Biocef, Keflex, Keftab)
Loracarbef (Lorabid)

Fluroquinolones

Ciprofloxacin (Cipro)
Lomefloxacin (Maxaquin)
Norfloxacin (Noroxin)
Ofloxacin (Floxin)

Macrolides

Azithromycin (Zithromax)
Clarithromycin (Biaxin)
Dirithromycin (Dynabac)
Erythromycin (E.E.S., E-Mycin, Ery-Tabs, EryPed, Erythrocin, Erythromycin Stearate, Ilosone, PCE)
Troleandomycin (TAO)

Tetracyclines

Doxycycline (Doryx, Doxy Caps, Monodox, Vibramycin, Vibra-Tabs)
Minocycline (Dynacin, Minocin)
Tetracycline (Achromycin V, Panmycin, Sumycin)

Other Miscellaneous Antibiotics

Metronidazole (Flagyl, Metric 21, Protostat)
Sulfamethoxazole and Trimethropin (Bactrim, Cotrim, Septra, Sulfatrim)

B. Antifungals

Butoconazole (Femstat)
Fluconazole (Diflucan)
Itraconazole (Sporanox)
Ketoconazole (Nizoral)
Miconazole (Micatin, Monistat)
Nystatin (Mycostatin, Nilstat, Nystex)

C. Antivirals

Acyclovir (Zovirax)
Amantadine (Symadine, Symmetrel)
Didanosine (Videx)
Famciclovir (Famvir)
Lamivudine (Epivir)
Rimantadine (Flumadine)
Valacyclovir (Valtrex)
Zidovudine (Retrovir)

D. Antituberculous

Ethambutol (Myambutol)
Isoniazid (Laniazid, Nydrazid)
Pyrazinamide (various manufacturers)
Pyrimethamine (Daraprim)
Rifabutin (Mycobutin)
Rifampin (Rifadin, Rimactane)

II. ANALGESICS

ACTION: Act upon several (known and some unknown) processes to alleviate pain. Some known processes include the reduction of inflammation and action upon the transmission of pain.

USE: Follow your physician's directions in using these medications. Many analgesics can be upsetting to the stomach. Take analgesics with food if using them as directed upsets the stomach.

POSSIBLE SIDE EFFECTS AND PRECAUTIONS: Common side effects include dizziness, drowsiness, nausea, vomiting, and constipation. If these symptoms continue or become bothersome, contact your doctor. If you have a severe reaction to any of these medications, contact your physician immediately. A severe reaction can include a serious rash, hives, difficulty in breathing, fever, dizziness, tightness in the chest, or swelling of the eyelids, face, or lips. CAUTION: THESE MEDICATIONS MAY CAUSE DROWSINESS. Use of these medications alone, or with alcohol or other medications may reduce your ability to use machinery or drive a motor vehicle. Some of these medications, specifically the narcotics, can be addictive. If you experience any other side effects not listed above, contact your doctor.

A. Narcotics

Codeine (various manufacturers)
Hydromorphone (Dilaudid)
Methadone (Dolophine)
Morphine Sulfate (MS Contin)
Propoxyphene (Darvon)

B. Acetaminophen (Tylenol, various other manufacturers)

C. Aspirin (Bayer, Ecotrin, Empirin)

D. Nonsteroidal Anti-Inflammatory Drugs (NSAIDs)

Diclofenac (Voltaren)
Etodolac (Lodine, Lodine XL)
Flurbiprofen (Ansaid)
Ibuprofen (Advil, Medipren, Motrin, Nuprin, Rufen)
Indomethacin (Indocin, Indocin SR)
Ketoprofen (Orudis, Oruvail)
Meclofenamate (Meclomen)
Nabumetone (Relafen)
Naproxen (Aleve, Anaprox, Anaprox DS, Naprosyn)
Piroxicam (Feldene)
Sulindac (Clinoril)
Tolmetin (Tolectin, Tolectin DS)

III. BLOOD PRESSURE AND HEART

ACTION: Work in a variety of ways to lower blood pressure and relieve stress on the heart. Some medications may act specifically on the rhythm of the heart.

USE: Follow your doctor's directions for use of these medications. The use of some of these medications must be evaluated with regard to mealtimes or other medications.

POSSIBLE SIDE EFFECTS AND PRECAUTIONS: Drowsiness, dizziness, or weakness may occur temporarily but diminish during treatment. If side effects continue or become bothersome, contact your physician. If you experience irregular heartbeat or fainting, contact your physician immediately. Do not stop taking these medications without the consent of your doctor. Drowsiness or dizziness may occur in some cases. Do not drive or use machinery until you are familiar with the effects of these medications. If you experience any other side effects not listed above, contact your doctor.

A. Antihypertensives

Diuretics

Amiloride (Midamor)
Chlorothiazide (Diuril)
Furosemide (Lasix)
Hydrochlorothiazide (Esidrix, Hydrodiuril)

Indapamide (Lozol)
Methyclothiazide (Aquatensen, Enduron)
Metolazone (Diulo, Zaroxolyn)
Spironolactone (Aldactone)
Spironolactone w/Hydrochlorothiazide (Alazide, Alactazide)
Triamterene (Dyrenium)
Triamterene w/Hydrochlorothiazide (Dyazide, Maxzide)

Beta-Blockers

Atenolol (Tenormin)
Metoprolol (Lopressor)
Nadolol (Corgard)
Pindolol (Visken)
Propranolol (Inderal)

Calcium Channel Blockers

Amplodipine (Norvasc)
Diltiazem (Cardizem, Dilacor, Tiazac)
Nifedipine (Adalat, Procardia)
Verapamil (Calan, Isoptin, Verelan)

Angiotensin Acting Drugs

Captopril (Capoten)
Enalapril (Vasotec)
Lisinopril (Prinivil, Zestril)
Losartan (Cozaar)
Ramipril (Altace)
Trandolapril (Mavik)
Valsartan (Diovan)

B. Antiarrhythmic Drugs

Amiodarone (Cordarone)
Disopyramide (Norpace)
Mexiletine (Mexitil)
Procainamide (Procanbid, Procan SR, Pronestyl)
Quinidine (Quinidex Extentabs, various manufacturers)
Tocainide (Tonocard)

C. Antianginal

Nitrates

Isosorbide (Imdur, Ismo, Isordil, Monoket)

Nitroglycerin

Nitrostat (sublingual)
Minitran, Nitro-Dur (transdermal)

D. Others

Clonidine (Catapres)—antihypertensive
Digoxin (Lanoxin)—antiarrhythmic
Methyldopa (Aldomet)—antihypertensive
Prazosin (Minipress)—antihypertensive

IV. BLOOD MODIFIERS

ACTION: Enhance or inhibit the process of clotting or thinning of the blood.

USE: Follow your doctor's directions for use of these medications. DO NOT TAKE ASPIRIN OR ASPIRIN PRODUCTS WITH THESE MEDICATIONS WITHOUT THE CONSENT OF YOUR DOCTOR. Always consult with your doctor or pharmacist if you are taking one of these medications with another type of drug. Your doctor may require frequent testing of blood while these medications are being used.

POSSIBLE SIDE EFFECTS AND PRECAUTIONS: Contact your doctor if you experience any signs or symptoms of bleeding. Bleeding may include unusual bruising, pain, swelling, nosebleeds, bleeding from the gums, unexplained vaginal bleeding; discoloration of urine or stool; black, tarry stools; or any signs of illness. If you experience any other side effects not listed above, contact your doctor. DO NOT STOP TAKING THESE MEDICATIONS WITHOUT THE CONSENT OF YOUR DOCTOR. Before having emergency treatment or surgery, tell health care workers you are using this type of medication.

A. Antiplatelet Agents

Dipyridamole (Persantine)
Ticlopidine (Ticlid)

B. Anticoagulants

Heparin Sodium (Calciparine, Liquaemin)
Warfarin (Coumadin)

V. HORMONES

ACTION: Replace, stimulate, or inhibit normal hormonal activity.

USE: Follow your doctor's directions for use of these medications. Do not stop taking these medications without the consent of your doctor. The use of most of these medications must be evaluated with regard to mealtimes. Regular checkups and blood testing may be required.

POSSIBLE SIDE EFFECTS AND PRECAUTIONS: Some common side effects include nausea, vomiting, increase or loss of appetite, and change in body weight. If these continue or become bothersome, contact your doctor. Contact your doctor immediately if you experience unusual weight gain, black, tarry stools, severe nausea or vomiting, changes in or irregular menstrual periods, cold symptoms, or fever or sore throat. If you experience any other side effects not listed above, contact your doctor.

A. Sex Hormones

Female

Estrogen (Estraderm, Premarin, Ogen)
Oral Contraceptives (Demulen 1/35, Ortho-Novum 7/7/7, Ortho-Novum 1/35, Tri-Levlen)
Progestin (Medroxyprogesterone, Provera)

Male

Fluoxymesterone (Halotestin)
Methyltestosterone (Android, Metandren)

B. Thyroid Drugs

Levothyroxine (Levoxine, Levoxyl, Synthroid)
Methimazole (Tapazole, Thiamazole)
Propylthiouracil (various manufacturers)

C. Antidiabetic Agents

Insulin

Regular
- Humulin R
- Novolin R
- Regular Iletin II

NPH
- Humulin N
- Novolin N
- NPH Iletin II

Lente
- Humulin L
- Lente Iletin II
- Novolin L

Ultralente
- Humulin U
- Ultralente U

Premixed
- Humulin 70/30
- Novolin 70/30

Oral Antidiabetic Agents

Acarbose (Prandase, Precose)
Chlorpropamide (Diabinese)
Glipizide (Glucotrol, Glucotrol XL)
Glyburide (DiaBeta, Glynase Prestab, Micronase)
Metformin (Glucophage, Glucophage XR)
Tolazamide (Tolinase)

D. Adrenal Cortical Steroids

Cortisone Acetate (Cortone)
Dexamethasone (Decadron, Dexone)
Hydrocortisone (Cortef, Hydrocortone)
Methylprednisolone (Medrol)
Prednisolone (Delta-Cortef, Prelone)
Prednisone (Deltasone, Liquid Pred, Orasone)
Triamcinolone (Aristocort, Kenacort)

VI. MENTAL AND EMOTIONAL

ACTION: These medications work in a variety of ways to increase, decrease, or eliminate selective nerve transmissions.

USE: Follow your doctor's directions for use of these medications. DO NOT STOP taking these medications without the consent of your doctor. Some of these medications may require several days or weeks of use before a desired effect may be achieved.

POSSIBLE SIDE EFFECTS AND PRECAUTIONS: CAUTION: THESE MEDICATIONS MAY CAUSE DROWSINESS. Use of these medications with alcohol, other medications, or alone may reduce your ability to use machinery or operate a motor vehicle. Some of these medications may be habit forming if you exceed the recommended dosage or take them longer than they are prescribed for. Some common side effects are dizziness, drowsiness, weakness, blurred vision, dry mouth, and constipation. Contact your doctor immediately if you experience muscle spasms or severe agitation, tremors, slurred speech, or confusion. If you experience any other side effects not listed above, contact your doctor.

A. Sedatives, Tranquilizers, and Sleeping Pills

Alprazolam (Xanax)
Buspirone (BuSpar)
Chlordiazepoxide (Librium)
Clonazepam (Klonopin)
Diazepam (Valium)
Flurazepam (Dalmane)
Lorazepam (Ativan)
Temazepan (Restoril)
Triazolam (Halcion)

B. Antidepressants

Amitriptyline (Elavil, Endep)
Bupropion (Wellbutrin, Zyban)
Desipramine (Norpramin, Pertofrane)
Fluoxetine (Prozac)
Fluvoxamine (Luvox)
Imipramine (Tofranil)
Nefazodone (Serzone)
Nortriptyline (Aventyl, Pamelor)
Paroxetine (Paxil)
Phenelzine (Nardil)
Sertraline (Zoloft)
Venlafaxine (Effexor)

C. Antipsychotics

Chlorpromazine (Thorazine)
Clozapine (Clozaril)
Fluphenazine (Permitil, Prolixin)
Haloperidol (Haldol)
Risperidone (Risperdal)
Thioridazine (Mellaril)
Thiothixene (Navane)
Trifluoperazine (Stelazine)

D. Anticonvulsants

Carbamazepine (Tegretol)
Clonazepam (Klonopin)
Clorazepate Dipotassium (Tranxene)
Diazepam (Valium)
Phenobarbital (Solfoton)
Phenytoin (Dilantin)
Primidone (Mysoline)
Valproic Acid (Depakene, Depakote)

VII. RESPIRATORY

ACTION: Dilatation, constriction, or inhibition of the respiratory cells.

USE: Follow your doctor's directions for use of these medications. The use of some of these oral medications must be evaluated with regard to mealtimes. Do not exceed the recommended dosage of these medications.

POSSIBLE SIDE EFFECTS AND PRECAUTIONS: Some common side effects include nausea, vomiting, dizziness, drowsiness, irritability, and insomnia. If these symptoms continue or become bothersome, contact your doctor. CAUTION: THESE MEDICATIONS MAY CAUSE DROWSINESS. Use of these medications—especially antihistamines—with alcohol or other medications may reduce your ability to operate machinery or drive a motor vehicle. If you experience any other side effects not listed above, contact your doctor.

A. Bronchodilators

Albuterol (Proventil, Ventolin)
Metaproterenol (Alupent, Metaprel)
Pirbuterol (Maxair)
Terbutaline (Brethine)
Theophylline (Theo-24, Theo-Dur, Slo-bid Gyrocaps)

B. Respiratory Inhalants

Albuterol (Proventil, Ventolin)
Beclomethasone Dipropionate (Beclovent, Vanceril)
Cromolyn Sodium (Intal, Nasalcrom)
Flunisolide (AeroBid)
Fluticasone Propionate (Flovent)
Ipratropium Bromide (Atrovent)
Pirbuterol (Maxair)
Salmeterol (Serevent)
Triamcinolone Acetonide (Azmacort)

C. Intranasal

Beclomethasone (Beconase, Vancenase)
Budesonide (Rhinocort)
Fluticasone (Flonase)
Triamcinolone Acetonide (Nasacort)

D. Nasal Decongestants

Levmetamfetamine (Vicks Inhaler)
Oxymetazoline (Afrin, Duration, 4-Way 12-Hour Nasal, Neo-Synephrine 12 Hour Spray)
Phenylephrine (Neo-Synephrine)
Pseudoephedrine (Sudafed)

E. Antihistamines

Brompheniramine Maleate (Dimetane)
Cetirizine (Zyrtec)
Chlorpheniramine Maleate (Chlor-Trimeton)
Clemastine Fumarate (Tavist, Tavist-1)
Cyproheptadine HCL (Periactin)
Diphenhydramine (Benadryl, Benylin)
Promethazine (Phenergan)
Terfenadine (Seldane)

F. Cough and Cold Combinations

Syrups & Elixirs

Dimetapp
Hycodan
Phenergan
Phenergan VC
Phenergan w/codeine
Robitussin AC
Robitussin DAC
Rondec
Rondec DM
Tussionex
Tussi-organidin

Tablets & Caplets

Actifed
Benadryl
Claritin-D
Coricidin
Dallergy
Rynatan
Sudafed
Tavist
Tavist-D

VIII. STOMACH AND DIGESTION

ACTION: Increase or decrease the motility of the gastrointestinal tract and reduce or neutralize acidity of the stomach. Most cholesterol lowering drugs work with the digestive process to decrease the absorption or formation of cholesterol.

USE: Follow your doctor's directions for use of these medications. Do not use for prolonged periods of time without the consent of your doctor. The use of some of these medications must be evaluated with regard to mealtimes.

POSSIBLE SIDE EFFECTS AND PRECAUTIONS: Some common side effects include dizziness, drowsiness, nausea, vomiting, flatulence, and diarrhea or constipation. If these side effects continue or become bothersome, contact your doctor. Contact your doctor immediately if you experience severe cramping, weakness, fever, severe headache, rash, yellow skin or eyes, or severe vomiting. If you experience any other side effects not listed above, contact your doctor.

A. Antacids

Aluminum Hydroxide (Gaviscon)
Calcium Carbonate (Alka-Mints, Tums)
Calcium Carbonate & Magnesium (Rolaids)
Magnesium Hydroxide & Aluminum Hydroxide (Maalox, Mylanta)
Magnesium Hydroxide (Phillips' Milk of Magnesia)

B. Anti-Gas

Simethicone (Mylanta Gas, Phazyme)

C. Acid Blockers

Cimetidine (Tagamet)
Famotidine (Pepcid)
Lansoprazole (Prevacid)
Nizatidine (Axid)
Omeprazole (Prilosec)
Ranitidine (Zantac)

D. Antispasmodics

Dicyclomine (Bentyl)
L-Hyoscyamine (Anaspaz, Cystospaz, Levsin)

Combinations

Barbidonna
Bellergal-S
Donnatal
Librax

E. Laxatives

Citrate of Magnesia
Colace
Dulcolax
Ex-Lax
Feen-a-mint
Fleet Phospho-soda
Metamucil
Milk of Magnesia
Peri-Colace
Senokot

F. Antidiarrheals

Bismuth Subsalicylate (Pepto-Bismol)
Diphenoxylate & Atropine Sulfate (Lomotil, Lonox)
Loperamide (Imodium)

G. Cholesterol Lowering Drugs

Atorvastatin (Lipitor)
Cholestyramine (Prevalite, Questran)
Fluvastatin (Pravachol)

Gemfibrozil (Lopid)
Lovastatin (Mevacor)
Pravastatin (Pravachol)
Simvastatin (Zocor)

IX. OPHTHALMICS

ACTION: Reduce inflammation, treat infection, reduce intraocular pressure. Some ophthalmic products provide lubrication of the eyes.

USE: Follow your doctor's directions for use of these medications. Always wash your hands before and after the use of any eye medication. To use eye drops, tilt your head back and with your index finger, pull the lower lid away from the eye to form a pouch. Drop the medicine into the pouch and gently apply pressure to the inside corner of the eyes for 1 to 2 minutes. Do not blink and keep your eyes closed during this time. Do not touch the applicator tip to any surface, including your eye. If using more than one eye drop medicine, use them at least ten minutes apart.

POSSIBLE SIDE EFFECTS AND PRECAUTIONS: Some common side effects include temporary blurring of vision, headaches, sensitivity to bright light, itching, and dryness or bitter taste in the mouth. If these side effects continue or become bothersome, contact your doctor. Contact your doctor immediately if you experience a rash or irritated eyelids. If you experience any other side effects not listed above, contact your physician.

A. Glaucoma

Betaxolol (Betoptic, Betoptic S)
Brimonidine (Alphagan)
Dipivefrin HCL (Propine)
Dorzolamide (Trusopt)
Latanoprost (Xalatan)
Levobunolol (Betagan)
Pilocarpine HCL (Isopto Carpine, Pilocar)
Timolol Maleate (Timoptic)

B. Anti-Inflammatory

Nonsteroidal

Diclofenac (Voltaren)
Flurbiprofen (Ocufen)
Ketorolac (Acular)

Steroidal

Dexamethasone (Decadron, Maxidex)
Fluorometholone (Flarex, FML Forte)
Prednisolone (Inflamase Forte, Pred Forte)

C. Anti-infectives

Ciprofloxacin (Ciloxan)
Erythromycin (Ilotycin)
Gentamicin (Garamycin)
Norfloxacin (Chibroxin)
Sodium Sulfacetamide (Bleph-10, Sodium Sulamyd)
Tobramycin (Tobrex)

D. Artificial Tears

Hypotears
Isopto Tears
Liquifilm Tears
Moisture Drops
Refresh
Tears Naturale

X. VITAMINS AND MINERAL SUPPLEMENTS

Organic substances found in most foods that are essential, in small amounts, for the regulation of the metabolism and normal growth and functioning of the body. Recommended Dietary Allowances (RDA) are published and revised periodically by the Food and Nutrition Board of the National Research Council—National Academy of Sciences. These are guidelines for nutritional problems and for providing standards of good nutrition for different age groups.

XI. HERBAL REMEDIES

For thousands of years herbs have been used for flavoring in the preparation of food and for their medicinal and healing properties. In the United States, there is no comprehensive system in place for the approval of traditional herbal claims. Nutritional supplements are given legal definition and legitimacy under the Dietary Supplement Health and Education Act (DSHEA). Under DSHEA, herbal products will be standardized and regulated for product labeling.

The United States Pharmacopeia (USP) is a non-profit organization that uses subcommittees and advisory panels to set drug, nutritional supplement, and herbal standards. These standards are subject to public review and are continuously updated and published. The USP Subcommittee on Natural Products is developing public standards for certain botanicals and their dosage forms.

Until herbal products are standardized and regulated, there is no way to determine standards for safe dosing and effectiveness. Currently, we can not judge their potential for dangerous interactions with other herbal products or with legitimate pharmaceutical products.

37

Physical Fitness

The Target: Total Fitness

Total fitness has been described in many ways. Most aptly, perhaps, it involves looking your best, feeling your best, and performing to the best of your ability. In the totally fit body stamina, strength, and flexibility have been brought to peak levels of development.

Total fitness may mean different things to different people. The level of fitness that a person can achieve varies with his or her physical or medical history. The level also depends on the person's height, weight, age, musculature, body type, and other characteristics. Thus, total fitness for any individual is the highest level of fitness to which that person can go, given the limitations imposed by the various factors.

Physicians and fitness experts agree that movement of some kind is mandatory for anyone who wants to achieve total fitness. Movement in the form of a planned, timed, repetitive program of exercise brings the human body to the goal of fitness in the shortest possible time.

Total physical fitness has many aspects. It calls for adequate rest and relaxation and it requires proper nutrition. The totally fit person has to follow sound health practices and have good dental and health care. Otherwise, fitness may prove difficult or impossible to achieve.

In broader terms, fitness brings many advantages and benefits to various aspects of a person's life. Fitness enhances an individual's ability to work with endurance and vigor and to enjoy work and leisure activities. A person who achieves total fitness can usually avoid undue fatigue, so that he or she has energy left for hobbies, recreation, and for meeting unforeseen emergencies.

Getting Started

Starting your fitness program may call for resolution of some final questions. Got a place in which to work out? Know what you're going to wear? Need any special equipment?

Think of a few other things. The process of warming up and cooling down. The problems of pain and strain, especially at the beginning—problems such as shin splints, which you may remember from college or high school.

You'll want to have these and other items clear in your mind. The questions of where to exercise, when during the day and week, what to wear, and how vigorously to exercise trouble many persons starting out on their self-tailored fitness programs. This is natural; the questions are important. The program has to fit into your life. It has to be practical.

The Where

We are talking, obviously, of the person who has decided on a personalized program that can be carried out alone. However, the person may not have decided on a place to do his or her exercises. One useful guideline to follow is to choose a space, or develop one, that ensures that the program can be "lived with." Designers of fitness programs suggest that the following three basic provisions should be made if you plan to work out at home.

Find Enough Space

Floor exercises and weight lifting take a floor area measuring approximately 7.5 by 10.5 feet. A larger area would, of course, be welcome. But to avoid bouncing off the walls you should have the space indicated. The height of the ceiling does not matter unless a trapeze or rings are to be installed. In either case the exercise area would require an 11-foot ceiling. For all other purposes, a ceiling clearance of eight feet is adequate.

Set Up a Mirror

A mirror set up close to the exercise area expands the space in a visual sense. More importantly, the mirror makes it possible for the person to check the accuracy of his or her exercise positions and routines when working out alone. If possible, the mirror should be six feet high by three feet wide so that it provides a full-length view.

Creating Your Own Exercise Equipment

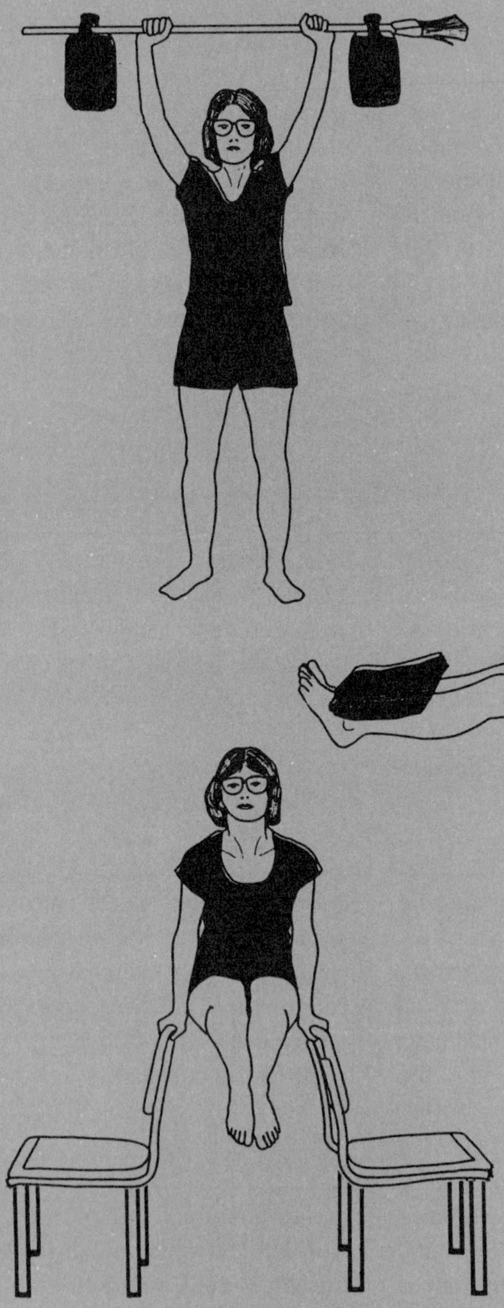

Ensure Safety Underfoot

Because slippery floors can present major safety hazards, the footing should be tested and retested for safety. Carpeting helps unless the exercise program includes dance routines. In general, a tightly woven, looped-pile, industrial-grade carpeting is recommended. This kind of carpeting has one major advantage over cut-pile—shag or velvet surface—carpeting: the looped-pile type is more durable. Just incidentally, the looped-pile type is cheaper.

Special Equipment

Keeping a program simple ordinarily rules out expensive equipment. But some equipment will make it possible to add the spice of variety to the program. For example, barbells may help to make flexibility an easily achieved goal.

One or two exercise mats provide the base for many lying-down exercises. Mats can be purchased from sporting goods stores, ordered from mail-order houses, or made at home out of 1.5-inch foam rubber. If made at home, the mats can be covered with a fabric that goes with the room. The material may be terry cloth, vinyl-coated fabric, canvas, or some other type that is soft, easily washed or wiped off, and durable.

If the mat has a line running down its center lengthwise, it will make body alignment a simple task. The line can be made out of a similar fabric of a different color from the mat covering proper.

The mat or mats should be sized to fit the individual's body. The perfect mat is somewhat longer than the user is tall, and wide enough to provide protection against bumps and bruises. That means it should be wider than a line drawn from heel to heel when the person lies flat and stretches both legs as far apart as possible. Another way to measure the ideal mat width is to lie flat and extend the elbows as far as possible straight out from the shoulders. The points reached by the elbows indicate a good width. The good mat has plenty of "give." It also springs back into position when pressure is removed.

Choosing and arranging permanent equipment may take a little thought. With care and planning, the room's appearance need not really suffer. Equipment may come in chrome, steel, or natural wood.

Handling Space Problems

Got a space problem? No room at all for privacy while charging through a workout? No place to install and use an exercycle or treadmill? Think a minute.

Can space be created? If the exercise equipment had to be stored, where would it go? Can that storage space be turned into an exercise area? A separate room isn't necessarily the only solution. Closets may be useful in solving the no-space problem. A walk-in closet may serve as a special niche for some types of equipment. A two-foot-deep enclosure can be created along a wall by installing folding doors; some equipment can then be hidden behind the barrier. When the doors are opened, presto! The area becomes a miniature gym.

Because exercise equipment has to be ready for use without much advance preparation, it may be desirable to feature it as part of the overall layout. An exercycle may be placed in a corner in a cleared space. A set of barbells may rest on a simple bench that holds them in notches for safety. Ballet bars may double as towel bars when not serving their fitness functions. For real permanence and solidity, exercise benches might be recessed into the walls. They could be covered with throws when not in use.

Homemade Equipment

If, on the other hand, Spartan simplicity is preferable, formal equipment may be dispensed with totally. Many exercises can be performed without any equipment at all. For example, various sets of exercises have been designed for practice in the shower, sitting down at the work desk, or standing up in an ordinary room. More on that later.

Many household items can be converted to exercise props. Weights can be made out of plastic dish detergent or bleach containers. The containers need only be filled with sand or water. If desired, the weights can be attached to the ends of a bar made of a broom or mop handle. Numerous heavy objects such as ski boots, telephone books, or bricks wrapped in towels can also be incorporated into exercise routines.

A little creativity can turn other everyday items into perfectly adequate fitness equipment. A length of clothesline makes an admirable jump rope. Two solid chairs of the same size can be placed back to back a couple of feet apart to form parallel bars. A heavy towel, held with arms spread an appropriate distance, can be used to provide both variable resistance and a massaging effect. Different exercises to increase endurance, equilibrium, speed, suppleness, strength, and coordination have been devised utilizing lengths of cloth.

Time Out for Exercise

Some trial and error may be necessary in determining the amount of time needed for exercising. At first, repetitions should be in short series, after which the principle of overload dictates a gradual step-up. Particularly at the beginning, those who have not exercised much for years should consider cowardice the better part of fitness valor. Instead of starting with 45-minute sessions that include a mile run, a 30-minute session including a run of a block or two may be adequate. Once it has been established that such minimal achievement levels do not cause overstrain, the program's general shape should be maintained until the specific short-term goals have been reached.

For those in better condition, a faster start is more appropriate. Again, the rule requiring regularity in all the basic phases of the program should be observed.

Some Important Factors

Mealtimes should be carefully considered in scheduling the daily exercise round. Most authorities believe that engaging in vigorous exercise within an hour before or after a meal may interfere with the digestive processes. That suggests that the exercise time should start at least an hour to an hour and one-half after eating. Conversely, one should allow at least an hour between an exercise session and the next meal.

Some other factors are important. Exercise taken immediately before bedtime may interfere with relaxation, and sleep, through stimulation of the adrenalin flow. Late-evening exercise should, in fact, be followed by an hour or so period of winding down. At other times of the day the wind-down period may be somewhat shortened, and may often be dispensed with altogether.

A psychological element appears to enter into the choice of time during the day. Many persons feel that by scheduling the fitness session in the early morning, they can "get it over with" and thus avoid having other responsibilities of the day interfere with exercising. Others prefer the noon hour. Some like the later afternoon, when the exercise round provides a break in the day's routine. The late-day session acts as a kind of after-work, before-dinner tonic for many persons.

The Systematic Approach

An orderly, systematic approach to exercising calls for establishing a special time during the day for working on fitness. The principle of repetitiveness and its corollary—overload—are also founded on the idea of system and regularity.

Most fitness authorities even suggest that system ought to govern the order in which exercises are taken. One version of an exercise circuit for ten different parts of the body is illustrated here. Each person has options here: depending on personal fitness goals, other exercises may be more appropriate for the same circuit.

The systematic approach should also govern decisions on the numbers of repetitions for each exercise. Exercise patterns to be presented later will be accompanied by specification of typical repetition cycles for each exercise.

The Sweater Myth

For decades people have been donning sweaters after heavy exercise. The name sweater, in fact, has obvious origins. The sweater began as a means of keeping the body warm and covered once it had become hot and sweaty.

Unless exposure to inclement weather is a problem, or the individual has particular reasons for putting on a sweater at the end of a hot workout, the sweater myth is just that. Under normal temperature, weather, and other conditions, the sweater simply prolongs the body's hot state. That helps not at all.

Some stiffness can, of course, result from exercise. But wearing a sweater is not the way to prevent that. Stiffness usually has its sources in the body's condition—or lack of it.

Physical Activity and Fatigue

The advice that counsels moderation in launching a fitness program or in starting new phases of it has a sound basis in physiology. The purpose is to avoid excessive fatigue. Muscular fatigue is defined as stimulation of a muscle or group of muscles beyond their ability to recover. A second type of fatigue affects the entire body. Known as physical fatigue, this form can be regarded as normal after physical exercise if it does not suggest undue stress.

Planning a Level of Intensity

Keep in mind that a flexible plan may call for different adjustments under different circumstances. It may indicate sometimes that it is best to terminate the day's activities. On other occasions it may require elimination of some exercises and continuation with others.

- Your knee begins to bother you. You drop the exercises calling for knee exertion and retain those that don't.
- You get a "stitch" in your side. Because it hurts continually, you decide to downplay those exercises—for that day—that produce or exacerbate the discomfort.
- While running in place, you find yourself troubled by shin splints, those pains along the sides of the

shin bones. You stop running and turn to something else.

Flexibility can exist alongside dedication to a program. As common sense dictates, the individual should sometimes slow down or blow the whistle completely on some exercises. Even Napoleon retreated now and then.

Another important principle should be noted: the individual will build and take to a fitness program most readily if he believes it will do him some good. And if he has faith and confidence in it, he is likely to stay with the program over the long haul.

Climbing the Fitness Ladder

Three stages of fitness have been identified. The individual who stays with an intelligently devised program moves through beginning, intermediate, and advanced stages. These have been termed by some authorities the low, medium, and excellent stages or phases. Some experts add a fourth level: the elite stage at which a person finds himself able to take part in highly competitive and demanding athletic activities.

The Exercise Tolerance Factor

Fatigue places basic strictures on the human body. Exercise tolerance refers to an individual's ability to take part in a demanding sport or game, jog, do a series of exercises, or engage in some other activity without reaching the undue fatigue stage.

At the start-up stage of a fitness program, the beginner should make certain that all the exercises selected are adjusted to his or her own exercise tolerance level. That adjustment has both positive and negative sides: the exercises should not be too difficult, nor should any be chosen that do not make the body work sufficiently hard. Exercises that are too easy will not produce fitness and should be eliminated or made more difficult. Pulse rate provides a good indication of whether the body is being asked to do an appropriate amount of work.

Decreased heart rate usually comes with advancing age. At the same time the older person has decreased work capacity or exercise tolerance. But age is only one villain producing the decreased work capacity. Reduced elasticity in the blood vessels also affects physical performance.

Warm-up and Cool-down

The rules for warm-up and cool-down are simple. A gradual progression in intensity of exertion should introduce the fitness session. At the end of the session there should be a tapering-off period, during which the body returns to normal. Actually, authorities disagree to some extent on the need for a warm-up and cool-down. But most feel that a preexercise warm-up should be mandatory for everyone taking part in demanding exercises. For those who have not exercised seriously for a long time and who are restarting, the warm-up should last 10 to 15 minutes. For those in better condition, the warm-up can be shorter, even as little as four or five minutes.

An effective warm-up period has several physiological effects. For one thing, it stretches ligaments. The warm-up also raises body temperature and increases cardiovascular activity. In all such ways the warm-up prepares the body for exercise.

Warm-up: What and How?

The warm-up begins, for best results, with light, rhythmical exercises performed at a slow pace. Stretching and deep breathing both loosen the muscles and increase the body's oxygen supply. Stretching also makes deeper breathing possible.

Most sets of warm-up exercises include about four or five very simple movements. The body should be sweating lightly when the set is done. A typical group of four exercises is shown.

1. The *deep-breathing* exercise requires that you rise on your toes, inhaling deeply at the same time. First extend your arms straight out to the side. While breathing in and rising on your toes, raise your arms from shoulder level until your hands come together over your head. That position should be held for a moment or two. Then lower your arms to your sides and exhale while returning to the flat-footed standing position. Six to a dozen repetitions will suffice.

2. The *arm rotation* exercise calls again for extension of your arms straight out to the sides from your shoulders. The hands are then rotated in circles about a foot in diameter. Your hands should describe 20 circles while rotating forward and 20 more while rotating in the other direction.

3. In the *body rotation* exercise, after placing your feet wide apart and bending forward at the waist, rotate your body from the belt up in slow circles. The upper body should describe circles large enough to stretch all the affected muscles. You can rotate five times in one direction, five more in the other.

4. In the *bend and bounce*, bend far over with your legs spread apart. Try to touch your fingers to the ground three times in front of your right foot, then three times in front of the left. The touching should be done with downward bouncing motions of the body. The beginner may want to

Warm-up Exercises

Arm rotation

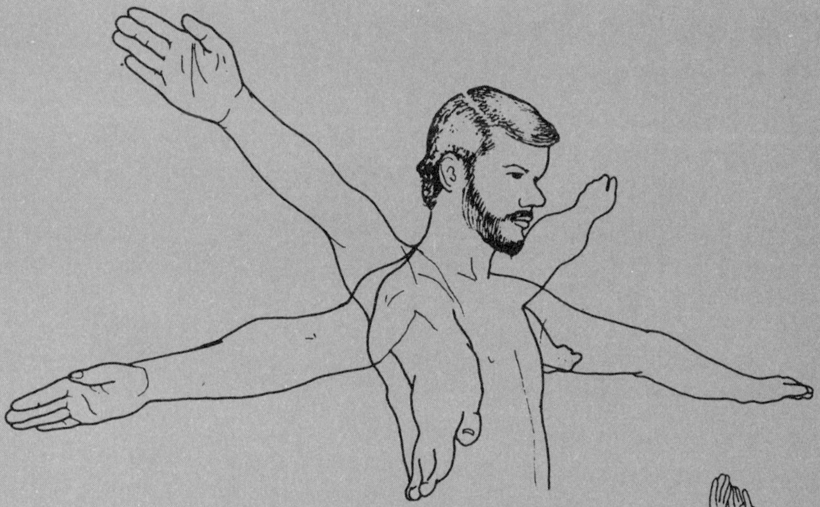

Deep breathing

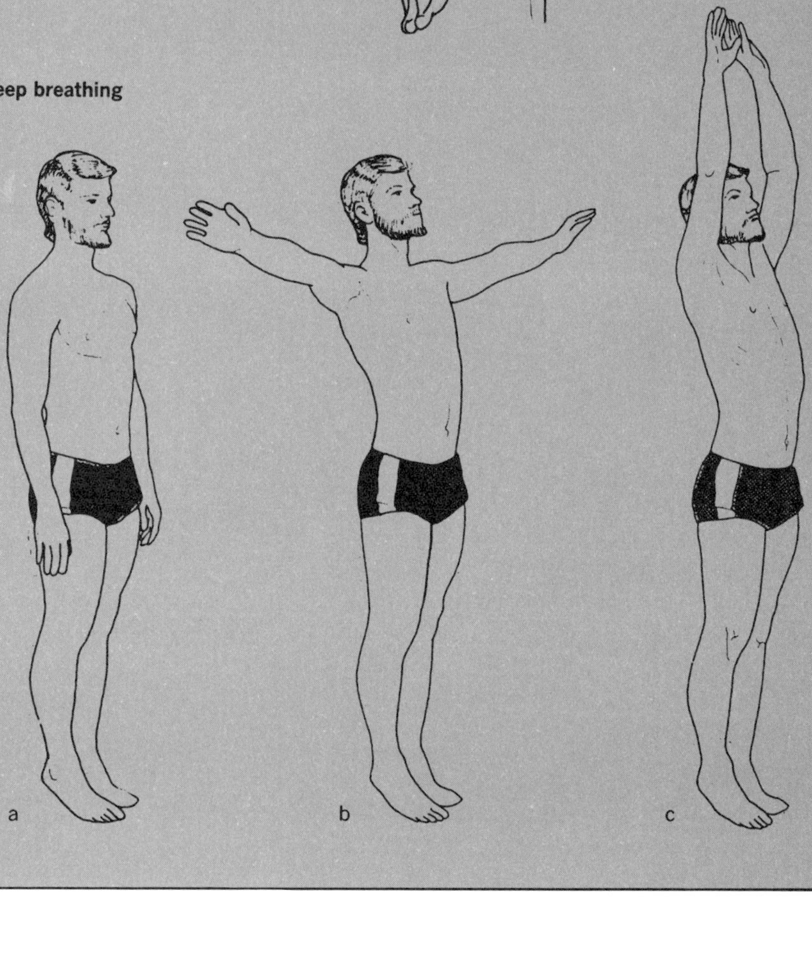

Warm-up Exercises

Body rotation

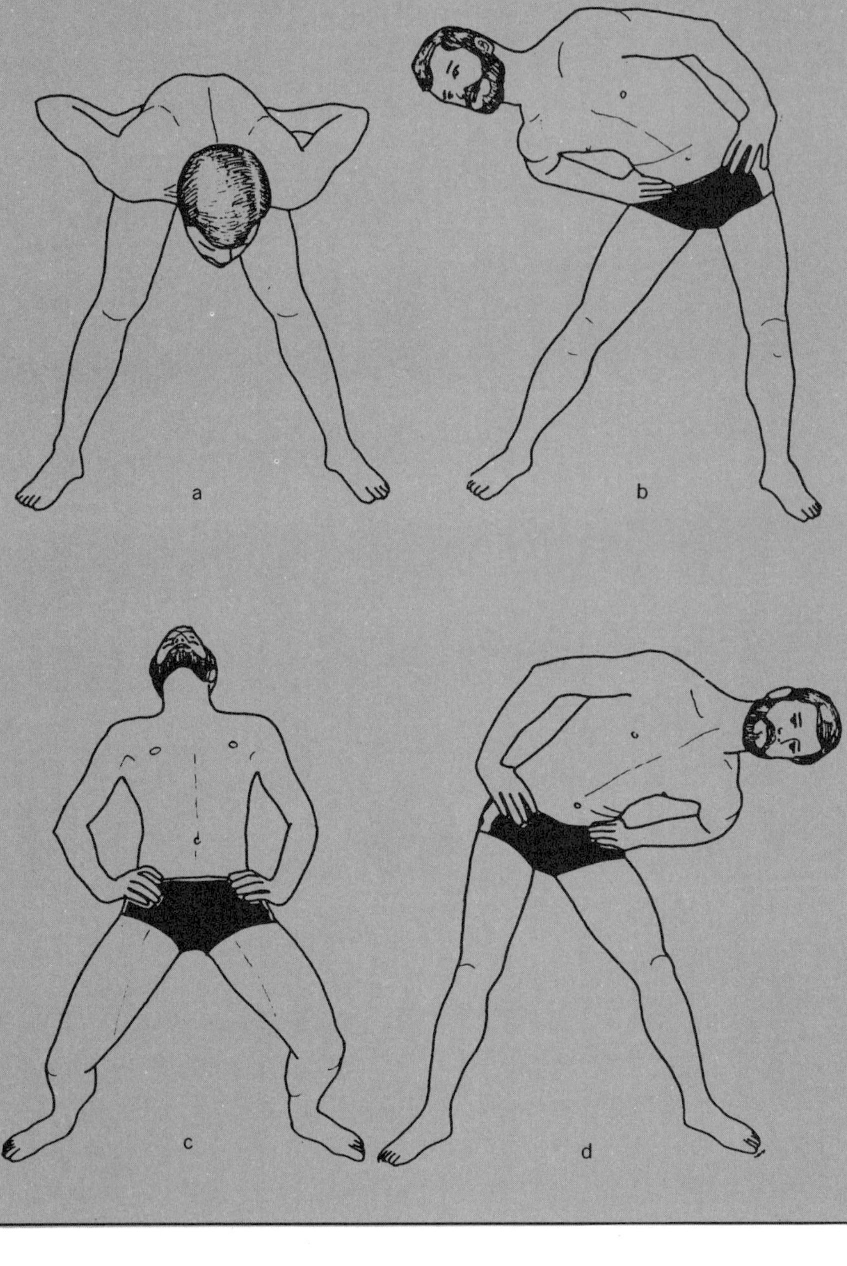

Warm-up Exercises

Bend and bounce

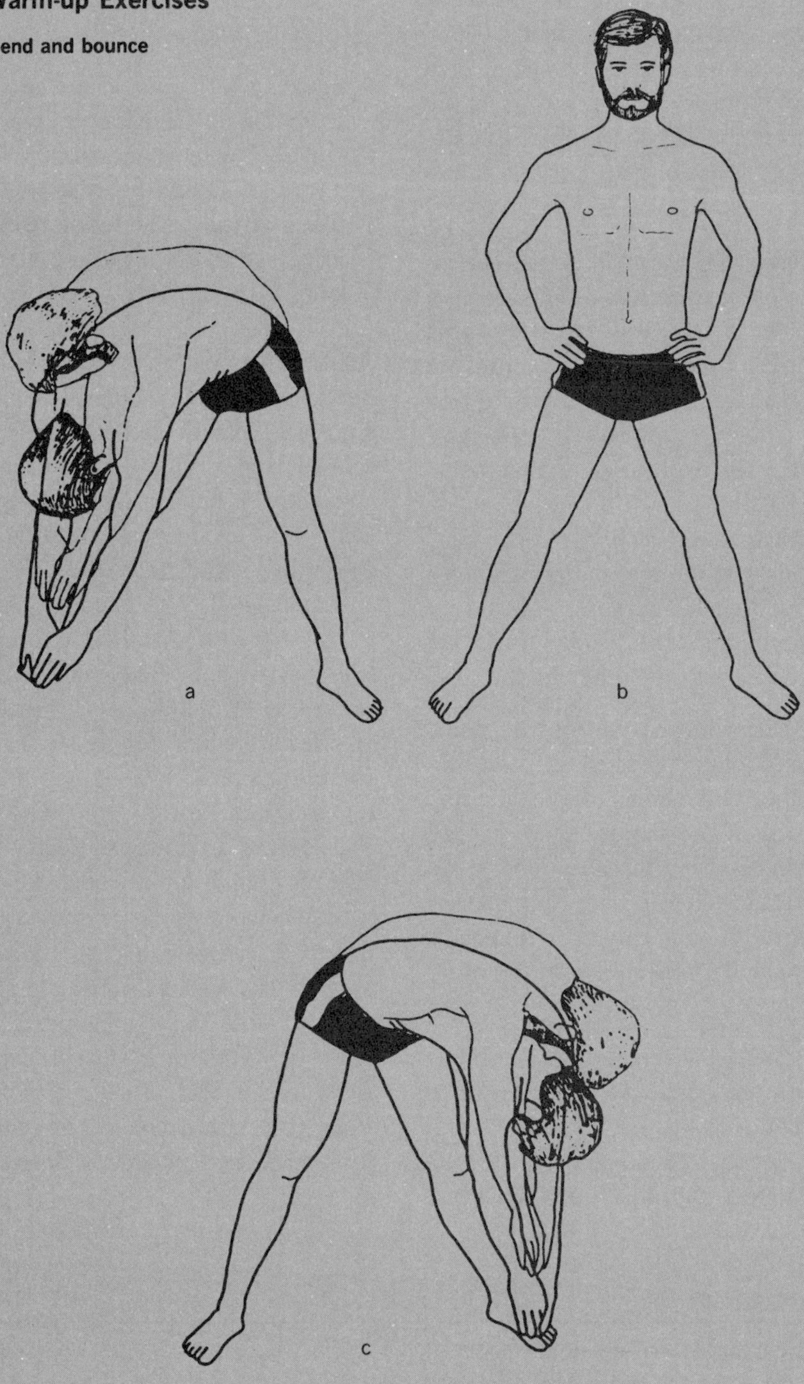

bend without touching the ground at all—just bouncing and bending low. The bend and bounce should stretch the back muscles. The tension on the muscles should be increased daily until flexibility returns.

The same warm-up series can include other exercises designed to get the feet in tune with the body. This final set of movements helps prevent the damage that can be inflicted on the feet by neglect or a premature start on the exercise program proper.

- While sitting, pick up a dozen marbles with the toes of the right foot. Drop each marble in turn into a container. The procedure is repeated with the other foot.
- Again while sitting on the floor, with one leg crossed over the other at the knee, take hold of the toes of the upper leg with both hands. Using that pressure as resistance, try to curl your toes as hard as you can. The exercise should be repeated with the other foot.
- Again while seated on the floor, flex one leg at the knee and place that foot on the floor. Hold the other leg straight out with the toes pointed, and describe a full circle with the foot. Repeat this exercise 10 times with each foot.
- Standing with your hands on your hips, rise up on tiptoe, then lower yourself to the floor quickly. The exercise should be repeated 10 times in the early sessions, then increased to 20 or more times for later warm-ups.

Note that you can invent your own warm-up exercise routine. It should, if possible, parallel the exercises that you will be performing in the main fitness activity. Indeed, warm-up movements may be identical to those later exercises, particularly where sports are concerned. The handball player warms up with throwing exercises and special shots. The tennis player warms up by rallying easily until his muscles are completely ready for the sometimes violent demands of the regular game.

Those who decide to create their own warm-up routines should keep in mind the basic characteristics of any satisfying set of exercises. Whole-body activity such as running in place or jumping is usually included in a warm-up. The warm-up set should also exercise each of the major body areas: trunk and hips; arms and shoulders; neck; legs and knees; and ankle and foot.

The Cool-off

If a careful warm-up helps prevent muscle soreness, what does the cool-off period do? Can't you just lie down and let the sweat dry until you go to the shower?

In answer to the first question, the

cool-down period allows the blood to be gradually redistributed in the normal resting pattern. The body temperature returns to normal. Your heart rate goes back to normal.

The answer to the second question is No. The best procedure is to keep moving for at least several minutes after vigorous exercise. You are trying to get your breathing and heart rate back to normal. You want your body literally to cool down.

Why not just lie down—or sit down—to cool off? An abrupt and complete cessation of the exercise reduces the flow of venous blood to the heart. A complete stop may also decrease the heart stroke volume. The heart may have to work much harder to maintain an adequate blood flow. Thus abruptly terminating exercise may lead to dizziness, fainting, shock, or other strain on the heart. Most heart attacks that afflict older persons in exercise situations take place during the postexercise period.

The ideal cool-down exercise is slow jogging or walking. At the same time the subject should swing his or her arms. Once the pulse rate has reached about 120—a ten-second count of 20—the readjustment has been largely accomplished.

Showers, Saunas, and Steam Baths

Hot showers, saunas, and steam baths also are not recommended for the immediate postexercise period. The hot shower, sauna, or steam bath merely adds strain. While they can be enjoyable and relaxing, be sure to wait until body temperature and heart rate has returned to normal before indulging in them.

Ice-cold showers present their own dangers. Ice-cold water flowing over the chest increases the blood pressure. It also raises the heart rate and cardiac output. While a healthy individual can tolerate the additional load, a person with cardiovascular problems could experience difficulties. Such a person may or may not know of his condition; the ice-cold shower would take its toll in either case.

The need to shower after heavy exercise cannot, of course, be minimized. A noted educator once stated that a social gap exists between those who bathe daily and those who do not. The gap would widen if the shower were not a postexercise priority. But the shower water should have a moderate temperature—about 70 degrees. At that temperature the shower tones the skin while also cleaning.

Some experts recommend a warm shower followed by a cool one. The warm shower opens the skin pores; the cool one closes them. Medical authorities agree generally that the practice has merit for persons in good health.

Living with Stress

Ten Ways to Get a Handle on Stress

Exercise is a key method of working off stress and tension. But there are many other useful approaches to managing these problems. Ten ways to cope are:

1. *"Blow off steam!"* When angry or upset, or when feeling any kind of stress or tension, it's wise to engage in some kind of physical activity. You can garden, jog, play tennis, lift weights, or walk. Virtually any kind of physical activity provides an outlet for the "fight" impulse—as contrasted with a "flight" urge—thus relieving mental or emotional stress.

2. *Talk it out:* Is there someone in your life whom you trust and respect? That person may be the one to sit down and "talk it out" with. The person need not be close; it could be a clergyman, a physician, a teacher, a counselor. Professional listeners like psychologists and guidance counselors may be the answer.

3. *Accept what you cannot change:* Many problems lie beyond our powers of control. These the individual has to accept—at least until they can be changed. Why spin your wheels? Why beat your head against a brick wall? Even a padded brick wall?

4. *Avoid self-medication:* The person who treats himself or herself with medications in hopes of relieving the distress of stress may have a fool for a patient. Many agents and chemicals, including alcohol, may seem to alleviate stress, but they do not help you to adjust to the stress itself. Also, many such substances are habit-forming and should not be taken without a doctor's prescription or approval.

5. *Get enough sleep and rest:* Lack of sleep and rest can reduce your ability to deal with the stress that invades every life at one time or another. Most people need seven to eight hours of sleep in every 24-hour day. If stress interferes with sleep, a physician should be consulted.

6. *Balance work and recreation:* "All work and no play can make you the richest man in the graveyard." On the way there, you may become a nervous wreck. Because the mind needs recreation just as the body does, you should include some time off in your schedule. Loafing may do it if no other kind of recreation is possible.

7. *Help someone:* Doing things for others provides a genuine stress reducer. In many cases stress involves overconcentration on oneself and one's problems. Doing something for someone else helps you to get your mind off your problems as it gets your mind off yourself—and you may win a new friend.

8. *Take one thing at a time:* Tackling a dozen tasks at once usually means that none of them will get done right. If you can, line them up either in writing or in your mind and take one at a time.

9. *Give in now and then:* A common source of the stress experienced by many people is other people. One possible solution is to give in now and then; try to relax and enjoy your own defeat or change of mind. Stress may fly out the window.

10. *Make yourself available:* Does stress hit you when you are feeling bored, left out of life, mired in the slow track? The answer may be to go where the action is. Make yourself available to those who may be able to involve you in an interesting way—in life, in activities, in cultural programs, in whatever you find exciting or important. To withdraw with your stress and feel sorry for yourself is the worst response.

Stress and tension are normal parts of life. But many persons can combat and even eliminate them through regular exercise. Although the program that the fitness novice draws up will generally be geared to the achievement of other goals, elimination of stress should be a by-product of the exercises.

The Physiological Effect

Stress and tension in the human body encourage the production of adrenaline. Exercise counteracts stress and tension in at least three ways:

- It helps the body to distribute the stress effects over a wider area. That in turn removes the danger that the stress may have a disproportionately damaging effect on one body part, such as the heart. Approached sensibly, exercise thus lessens the danger that a heart attack may follow a stressful situation.
- Exercise also strengthens the body as a whole and its vital organs in particular. The organs can then better withstand the effects of stress.
- Exercise literally "works off" the stress by attacking the physiological and emotional symptoms. Vigorous exercise can often reduce stress to pleasant, normal, physical fatigue.

Sleep

Sleep is the body's key mechanism for combating fatigue. Like exercise, sleep helps to reduce or eliminate tension. But healthy, sound sleep may elude persons suffering from prolonged stress. In a state of moderate fatigue resulting from exercise, by contrast, the body normally finds sleep a welcome refreshment.

The consensus among physicians today is that vitamins and tranquilizers are almost never the right answers to severe fatigue, nor are alcohol and sleeping pills. Caffeine can be counterproductive to the point where the body cannot really relax. Too much caffeine may even cause anxiety symptoms and an increase in stress and tension.

Curiously, most persons require less—not more—sleep once they have begun an exercise program. The reasons may be psychological or physical or both; physicians are not certain. Those who find it difficult to fall asleep while pursuing an exercise program should examine their schedules. Strenuous exercises shortly before bedtime can interfere with sleep more than help it.

Muscle-Relaxing Techniques

Muscular tension accompanies psychological stress. The causes of the stress may differ, ranging from fear to worry to anger and frustration, but the muscular tension is always there. The muscle tone or tonus increases beyond the normally low level of contraction.

Exercises designed to reduce muscular tension can have a therapeutic effect on one's emotional state. The basic concept in all the various techniques for reducing stress through exercise is to reduce tension by depressing muscular activity and by degrees induce a state of relaxation. The exercises incidentally contribute to total fitness, but generally to a minor degree.

Rhythmic exercises for the trunk help to reduce tension and build muscles. These exercises also contribute to improved circulation. Other types of muscle-relaxing exercises help to improve breathing.

Regional Relaxation

Muscle-relaxing exercises are effective in reducing tension because the mind can affect or control groups of muscles even though the causes of stress may not be reachable—or even recognizable. Learning to relax controllable muscles, the individual can attack first the muscular tension, then the psychological stress that undergirds it. "Uncontrollable tensions" thus come under the influence of the mind. The source of the stress may or may not be still at work; the exercise nonetheless relieves the symptoms that it has caused.

For the purpose of relieving muscular tension, the person first concentrates on muscle regions or groups. Effort is then exerted to recognize voluntary muscle contractions. In one muscle group after another, the levels of voluntary contraction are progressively lowered. With practice, the subject's perceptions of his own muscular state improves. Eventually he can identify and eliminate any slightest degree of in voluntary muscle tension of any kind in any part of the body.

Often, a kind of meditational relaxation takes place. The subject gradually and for short periods achieves a state of high concentration. Nagging life-problems are—briefly—forgotten.

Tension-reducing exercises fall into a basic pattern. To a large extent, they take their cues from the model developed in 1929 by Dr. Edmund Jacobson. In this model, a formal training method for teaching a person to relax groups of muscles at will, the subject consciously alternates contracting with relaxing various muscle groups at maximum, half-strength, and very slight levels of intensity.

Patterned methods of relaxing muscles should be practiced five or ten minutes a day. They can become part of an exercise program, or they can be completely separate. They do, after all, have their own rationale.

One set of exercises for relaxation of muscle groups follows:

Relaxation Breathing

Lying on your back on the floor, bend your knees so that your feet can rest flat. While taking a deep breath, let both the chest and the abdominal wall rise and expand. The breath should be held for a few seconds. Then expel it through your mouth with a rush. Repeat the exercise four or five times at regularly spaced intervals.

Arm Tension

Standing erect, swing both arms forward and back, then side to side. At the same time the arms should be allowed to drop during the swings; the hands should brush your thighs at each pass. Keeping the shoulders low and as relaxed as possible, repeat several times.

Next, sit on the edge of a chair and clench one hand tightly. The hand is kept clenched while the arm is swung vigorously in wide circles. Repeat the movement with the other arm.

Leg Tension

While sitting on the edge of a table, swing your legs freely backward and forward, bending at the knee. Try to keep your legs moving in rhythm.

Stomach Tension

In a kneeling position, lower your body so that your feet are under your hips. Extend your arms over your head and clasp your hands. Then swing your trunk down to one side and around. At the same time swing your arms in a wide circle over your head until you come up on the other side.

For an alternative stomach relaxer, stand with your buttocks against a wall. With feet spread apart and a few inches from the wall, bend your body forward and let it sway from side to side. Keep arms and head loose.

Relaxation for the Neck Muscles

With your head forward and lowered, back straight, and shoulders loose, turn your head first to one side and then the other. Your chin should touch first one collarbone and then the other. Movements should be slow and rhythmic.

Stretching and Pulling

The personal war against stress, tension, and fatigue ought to take posture and working positions into account. For example, the secretary who has to sit for long periods while working may want special exercises to counter back fatigue, aching muscles, and even headaches. The train conductor who has to stand for long periods may utilize similarly patterned exercises.

One six-part set of simple tension and fatigue-combating exercises calls for stretching and pulling motions:

1. *Shoulder/head pull:* In a sitting or standing position, place your arms behind your back. The left hand grasps the back of the right. The hands are pressed against the buttocks. Push your hands downward slowly, at the same time pulling the shoulders back and the shoulder blades down. The head should be tilted as far back as possible. Next, pull your shoulders forward and your shoulder blades up. Bring the head forward as far as possible. Repeat the exercise two or three times.

2. *Shoulder shrug:* In a sitting or standing position, hold your arms at your sides. Slowly pull your shoulders up and back as far as possible while holding the head upright. Finally, let the shoulders drop into a normal, completely relaxed position.

3. *Shoulder roll:* Again while sitting or standing with your arms at your sides and your head upright, pull your shoulders forward and down. Then push them back as far as you can. Finally let them drop into the normal, relaxed position.

4. *Back fold and unfold:* Sitting or standing, hold your arms relaxed at your sides. Go through two or three twisting, bending movements. Then bend far forward and gradually compress your body into a ball shape. The head should be dropped and the back rounded, with the arms hanging loosely. Straighten the spine slowly and by degrees—the lower back first, then the upper back. Try to be aware of each vertebra as you work your way upwards. The shoulders, chest, and head follow into the starting position. Repeat two or three times. If done in a standing position, this exercise can pay an added dividend. Simply stand with the knees bent slightly to relieve tension in the backs of the legs.

5. *Foot stretch and pull:* Sitting on the floor or on the edge of a chair, with your legs extended straight out, curl your toes under slowly. Straighten the feet as far as they will go. Then turn your toes back toward your face as far as possible while spreading your toes at the same time. Release and let your feet relax. Repeat two or three times.

6. *Foot roll:* Rotate the feet at the ankle while sitting as in step 5. Rotate slowly, first clockwise, then counterclockwise. Stretch the feet as far as possible. Repeat two or three times.

The stretching and pulling exercises, or variations on them, can be used during the warm-up part of an exercise session. The stretchers and pullers promote flexibility while preparing the muscles, joints, and ligaments for the more strenuous exercise which follows.

Body Problems

If you encounter physical problems at any time during your workout, it may be desirable to modify what you are doing. Dr. Lenore Zohman, a prominent exercise cardiologist, and her associates have summarized some possible body problems into two categories:

The Stop Exercising Group

(See a physician before resuming):

- Abnormal heart activity, including such signs and symptoms as irregular pulse (missed beats or extra beats), fluttering, jumping or palpitations in the throat, a sudden burst of rapid heartbeats, or a sudden slowdown in a rapid pulse rate.
- Pain or pressure in the center of the chest, arm, or throat during or immediately after exercise.
- Dizziness, light-headedness, a sudden lack of coordination, confusion, cold sweating, glassy stare, pallor, "blueness," or fainting.
- Illness, in particular a viral infection, which can lead to myocarditis, a viral infection of the heart muscle. Exercise should, in fact, be avoided during and immediately following an illness.

The Attempt Self-Correction Group

- Persistent rapid pulse for five to ten minutes or more. Self-correction technique: reduce the intensity of the activity, raising heart rate to a lower level, then move on to higher levels of activity at a slower rate. Consult a physician if the problem persists.
- Nausea or vomiting after exercise. Self-correction technique: reduce the intensity of the endurance exercise and lengthen the cool-down period. Avoid eating for at least two hours before the exercise period.
- Extreme breathlessness after exercise. Self-correction technique: reduce the intensity of the exercise. If the condition persists, consult a doctor.
- Prolonged fatigue for up to 24 hours following exercise. Self-correction technique: if the condition persists, reduce the intensity of the exercise and of the total workout session. If those corrective methods fail, see a physician.

Local Complaints

Many local complaints can afflict the person starting out on a full-scale program. By being careful and taking precautions, you can minimize adverse effects. In many cases they can be eliminated entirely.

Some of the best measures for combating local body problems resulting from exercise or participation in sports have already been described. They include provision of sensible clothing and shoes and the warm-up and cool-down periods. Specific problems such as the following may call for other corrective or curative measures.

Achilles Tendon Pains or Injuries

This runner's problem, like so many others having to do with the lower extremities, is usually caused by improper footwear. Shoes that lack heel wedges or that rub against the Achilles tendon may be the culprits. The only remedy is total rest and applications of ice (and the purchase of good shoes). Preventive methods include adequate warm-up, part of which should be a heel-stretching exercise.

Ankle Problems

Ankle problems, afflicting primarily those who take part in sports that require quick changes of direction, should receive immediate attention if they are at all serious. An ankle sprain should be placed in ice at once. A physician should examine a serious sprain. Prevention should begin with protecting the ankle and the surrounding muscles by wearing high-top gym or basketball shoes or by taping. Both methods may be used together.

Athlete's Foot

Clean socks and shoes do the most to prevent athlete's foot, which is caused by a fungus that develops between the toes. Symptoms are itching, burning, and scaling skin; the problem may lead to serious infections. Preventive methods include careful drying between the toes after showering and airing both the shoes and feet. Sprinkling powder between the toes will also help.

Blisters

Prevention should start with the proper footwear and socks. Socks should be snug enough to remain in place and not "bunch up." If blisters appear anyway, they should be cleaned with an antiseptic solution and covered with light gauze. Growth of an incipient blister may be halted if gauze is taped over the irritated spot.

Bone Bruises

Where handball players may acquire bone bruises on their hands, participants in other sports activities may experience them on the bottoms of their feet. The cause is usually a single blow or other severe trauma to the flesh and bone. Applying ice and providing padding over the bruised area should help. Appropriate footwear, including protective inner soles, serves to prevent foot bruises. Handball players who continue to play after incurring bone bruises may find that the condition persists long after it should have disappeared. The cause in such cases is repeated blows to the bruised area.

Knee Problems

Because the knee performs such a crucial role in so many different types of exercise and sports activities, it sees extensive use. Joggers and runners in particular develop knee complaints. Most of them can avoid difficulties by wearing the proper footwear and running on soft, level surfaces. Grass or a cinder track is usually the most comfortable. Staying away from sharp turns should also help. A physician should be consulted if knee problems persist.

Muscle Cramps

While the specific causes of muscle cramps have proved difficult to pinpoint, they appear to result usually from salt and potassium imbalances in muscles. The cramps are involuntary muscle spasms, or contractions. Stretching and massage usually relieve the problem. Preventive measures include adequate warm-up, replacement of the potassium and salt lost in sweating, and stretching during the cool-down period.

Muscle Soreness

Sore muscles, usually encountered at the start of a fitness program, virtually dictate that the beginner go slowly. Progressing slowly and steadily from a very moderate start through the upper level of a program should reduce or eliminate soreness. Thorough warm-ups and cool-downs are mandatory. Massage and warm baths should help to relieve soreness when it appears.

Shin Splints

Shin splints are pains that appear along the sides of the shinbone, or tibia. The causes vary and include lowered arches, tearing in a muscle where it attaches to the bone, irritated membranes, hairline fractures of the bone, and others. Running or jogging on hard surfaces, such as streets, and improper running techniques may bring on shin splints. Rest represents the only real cure, but the pains can be alleviated by wrapping or taping the leg.

What do you do when a jogging or running program has to be suspended because of problems in or injuries to a lower extremity? One possibility is to continue the program by cycling, using a regular bicycle or an exercycle. The program can then be continued and fitness maintained.

Starting With Some Easy Exercises

Feel like starting slowly? A lot of people don't launch a full-scale program all at once. Rather, they test themselves, try out some simple exercises, stay with those on some kind of schedule for two to six weeks or longer, depending on how they take to their newly exercise-oriented lifestyle, and make sure they are enjoying the whole thing. Others integrate the simple exercises into full-scale programs from the beginning.

A simple preliminary program can introduce the neophyte to the world of exercise. A couple of simple rules will be useful. First, the exercise should feel good while you are doing it. The feeling should persist after the exercise is over.

Starting slowly ensures that the Great Resolution that has brought you to a total fitness program will not die a horrible death. If the road to perdition is paved with good intentions, the road to fitness is flooded with them.

Five-Minute Routines

Five-minute routines can be devised that give a person a wide-awake start to the day or help fill in the waiting period just before Aunt Sally arrives for lunch; they can utilize the desk in the study as a prop, or be performed propless in a standing, sitting, or prone position. A four- or five- or six-minute routine can be performed in an odd moment during a busy workday—at home, at the office—wherever the time and privacy are available.

Five-minute routines may look like warm-up exercises, but they are simpler. They stretch muscles and tendons without preparing the body to spring into the high gear of strenuous activity. They bring major muscle groups into action, but in a relaxed way, thereby inducing a general feeling of relaxation. By calling on different parts of the body for gentle exertion, short routines may warm the body, but they should not work up a heavy sweat.

In brief, instituting a short, standardized routine lays the groundwork for the more formal exercise in a total fitness program that will follow. Once that program starts, five-minute routines can still be part of your day, testimony to the fact that exercise has indeed become part of your lifestyle.

"Quick-time" Wake-up and Relaxer Routines

The "quick-time" routines are designed for use in the morning and evening. The morning set stretches the muscles that may have become cramped during sleep, placing major emphasis on the legs, hips, and balance. The evening set is intended to help the body to unwind gently and prepare for sleep.

The Wake-up Routine

The morning routine awakens the body and readies it for the day's mental and physical challenges through seven separate exercises—or several of the seven, according to choice.

1. *Side stretch:* Lying flat on your back with arms stretched out above the head, slide the right knee up and at the same time extend the left arm as far as possible. The whole left side of the body should be stretched. Reverse, using the left knee and the right arm. Repeat eight to ten times with both sides.

2. *Heel haul:* Sitting up, stretch the legs out in front of the body. Leaning forward, grasp the heels, or the legs as close as possible to the heels, and pull the torso toward the knees. Bend the knees slightly if necessary. The back should be rounded, the toes pointed up and, if you are bending your knees, slightly to the side. Let go and sit up, straightening the spine, then repeat, grasping the heels and pulling forward again. Repeat eight to ten times.

3. *Knee bounce:* Sitting up straight, spread your legs and place the soles of the feet together. They need not fit flat against each other. Now gently bounce the knees toward the floor 16 times. Lower the torso over the still-joined feet, then straighten. Repeat five to ten times.

4. *Sky reach:* Sit on the floor with your feet apart as far as they will go. Reach for the sky with first the right arm, then the left. You should feel the pull on the muscles of the back and sides down to your hips. Repeat 16 times on each side.

5. *Forward reach:* In the seated, legs-spread position, slowly lower the chest toward the floor. At the same time place the hands on the floor directly in front of you and push them out ahead of the lowering upper body. Try to achieve a good stretch. In that position, bounce the torso very gently eight to ten times.

6. *Torso bend:* From the same beginning position on the floor, bend the torso gently to the right, at the same time reaching over the head with the left arm. The right arm moves toward the left knee. Gently straighten and bend eight to ten times. Reverse side and repeat.

7. *Knee tug:* Lying on your back with your toes pointing up, pull the left knee up toward the chest. Hold that position, gently tugging at the knee with both hands four times in a bouncing motion. Grasping your leg at the ankle or calf, pull it out straight so that your foot is over your head, keeping the other leg straight. Gently pull for eight counts. Next grasp the ankle of the upward-stretched leg and bend it gently out to the side. Hold for eight counts. Repeat with the other leg.

The Relaxer Routine

The evening routine includes six exercises. You should maintain breathing at a regular, relaxed pace, and exhale through the mouth.

1. *Sky reach #2:* While sitting on a chair with the ankles crossed, stretch arms overhead. Reach first with one arm, repeating 16 times, then with the other for another 16 repetitions.

2. *Rollover:* Lying flat on your back with your arms at your sides, raise both legs straight up, pointing your toes. Bring the legs back over your head with your knees straight, then—if you can—press your toes to the floor and support your back with your hands. Hold until you have counted to 16. Collapse your legs around your ears and hold for another 16-count. Roll back to the supine position.

3. *Modified push-up:* Lie facedown on the floor, then place your hands on the floor and support your upper body on hands and knees. Keeping your back and elbows straight, tilt your chin up and your head back gently. Bend the knees and bounce the toes upward toward your head eight times.

4. *Slow knee pull:* While sitting on a chair, cross the right leg over the left and gently pull the right knee toward the chest. Hold for a 16-count. Reverse and repeat with the left leg.

5. *Leg extensor:* Lying on your back with your knees drawn up, bounce your right leg up toward your chest four times. Then extend the leg upward, grasping the ankle or calf, and bounce the leg toward your head eight times. Repeat with the left leg.

6. *Crouch-and-breathe:* Starting from a kneeling position, crouch down in a ball on the floor, right ear to the floor and knees drawn up under you. Breathe in deeply through your nose. Exhale slowly through your mouth. Repeat three times. Turn the head to the other side and repeat.

Muscle Locators

If you find it difficult to come up with enough valuable exercises to fill a half-hour to 45 minutes three times a week, why not select some "muscle locators" for the central part (between warm-up and cool-down) of the session? In this section, we will offer two approaches to a set of basic exercises. You may wish to choose some favorites to program into your fitness schedule. By making the selection yourself, you ensure that the program's personalized character will be maintained.

Use caution when performing some of the muscle locators on the Phillips-Hatch list, particularly half situps and squats.

Simplicity characterizes the 11 basic muscle locators. They are:

1. *Side bends:* Standing with your feet wide apart, knees slightly bent, lean first to the right, then to the left. Keep your hips as stationary as possible. Starting with ten bends to each side in the first week, increase the number as directed until you are doing 30 in the fifth week.

Basic Muscle Locators

Sidebends

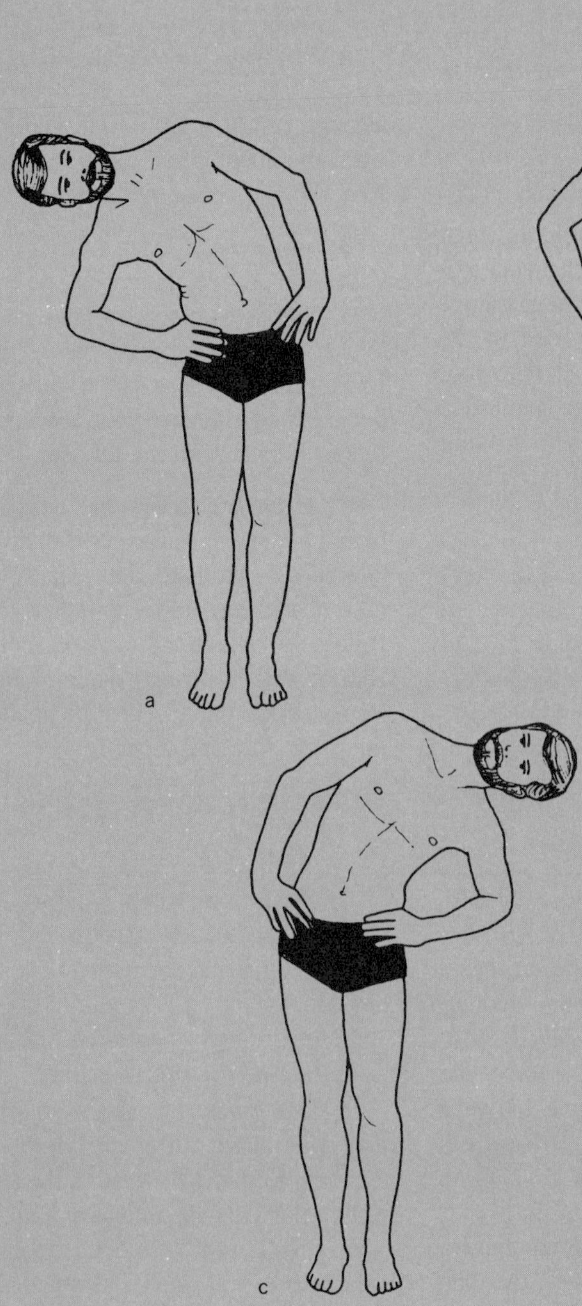

Basic Muscle Locators

Good mornings

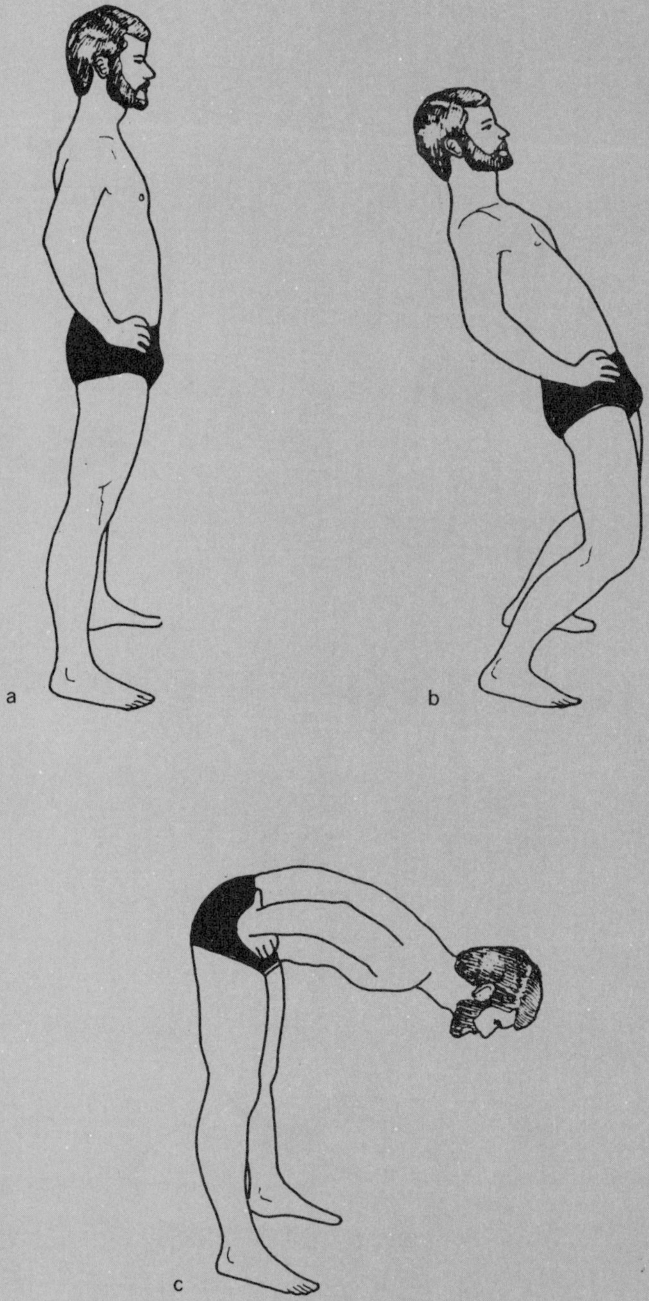

Basic Muscle Locators

Squats

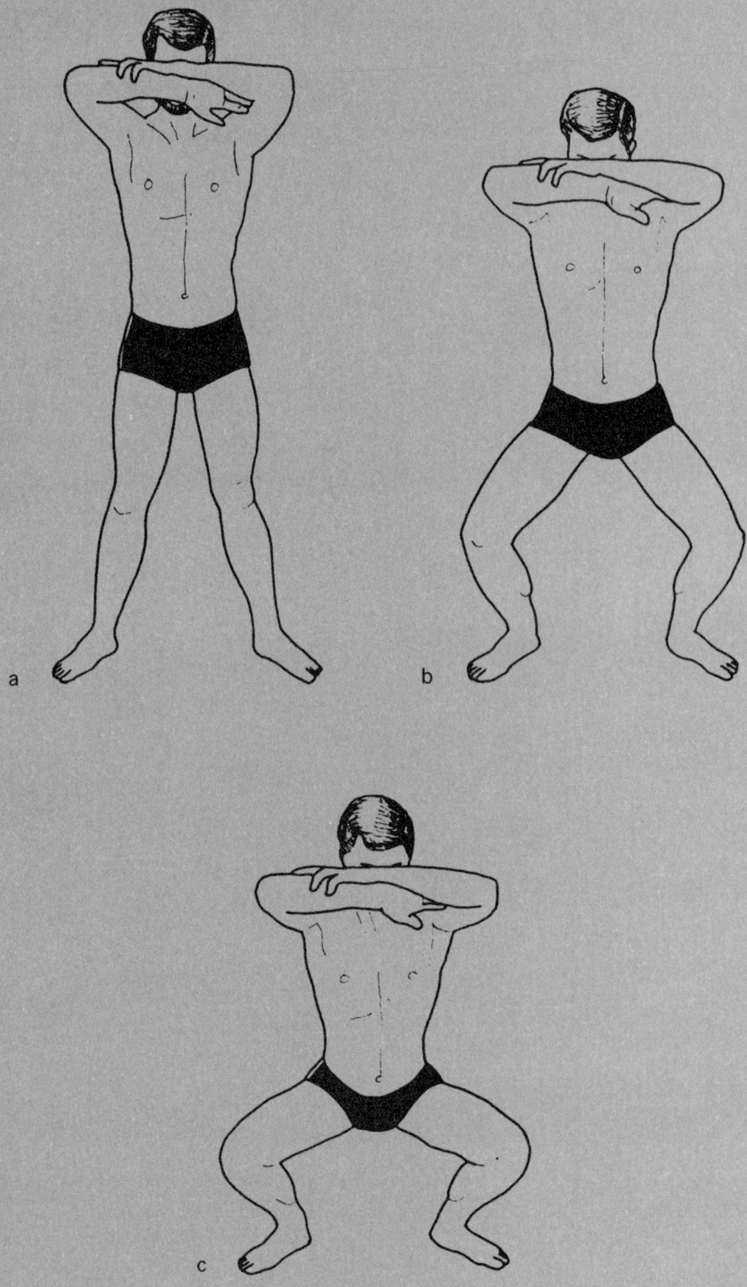

Basic Muscle Locators

Seated stretch

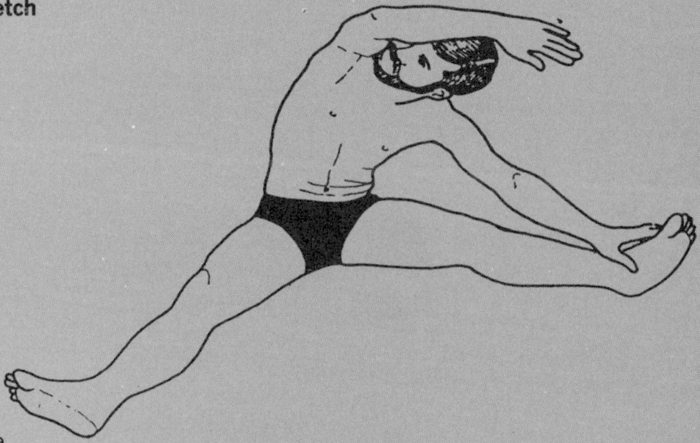

a

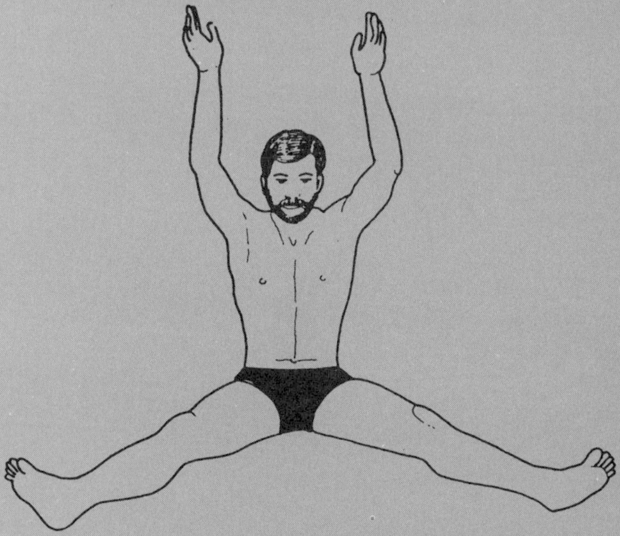

b

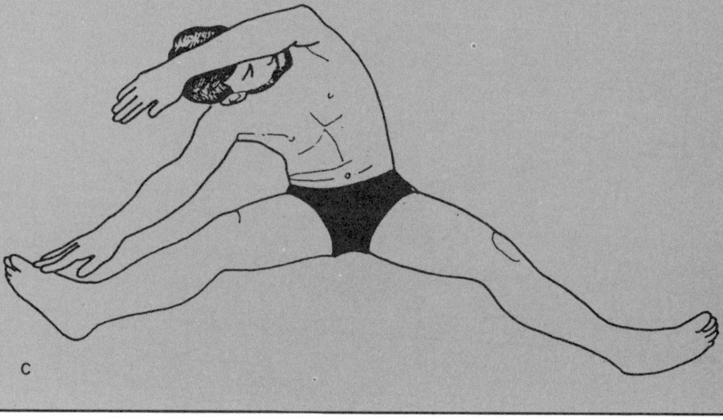

c

Basic Muscle Locators

Curl-ups

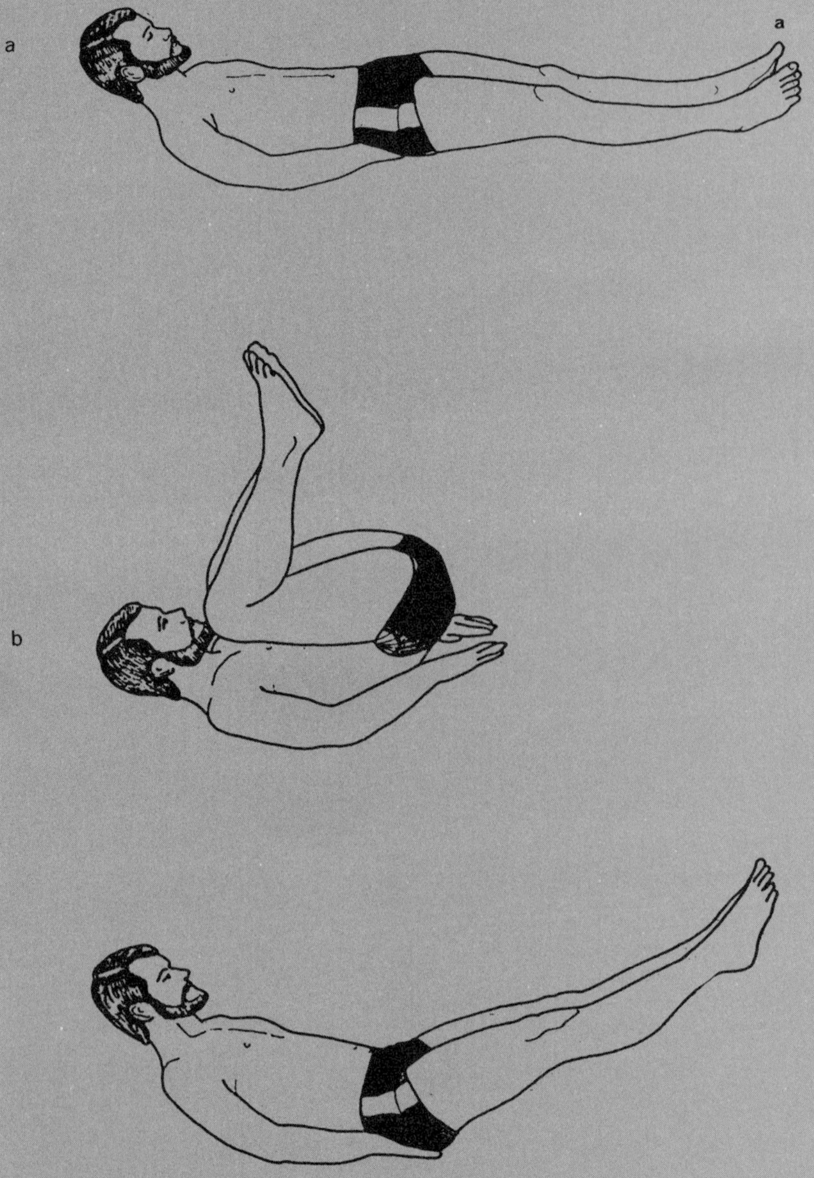

Basic Muscle Locators

Scissors

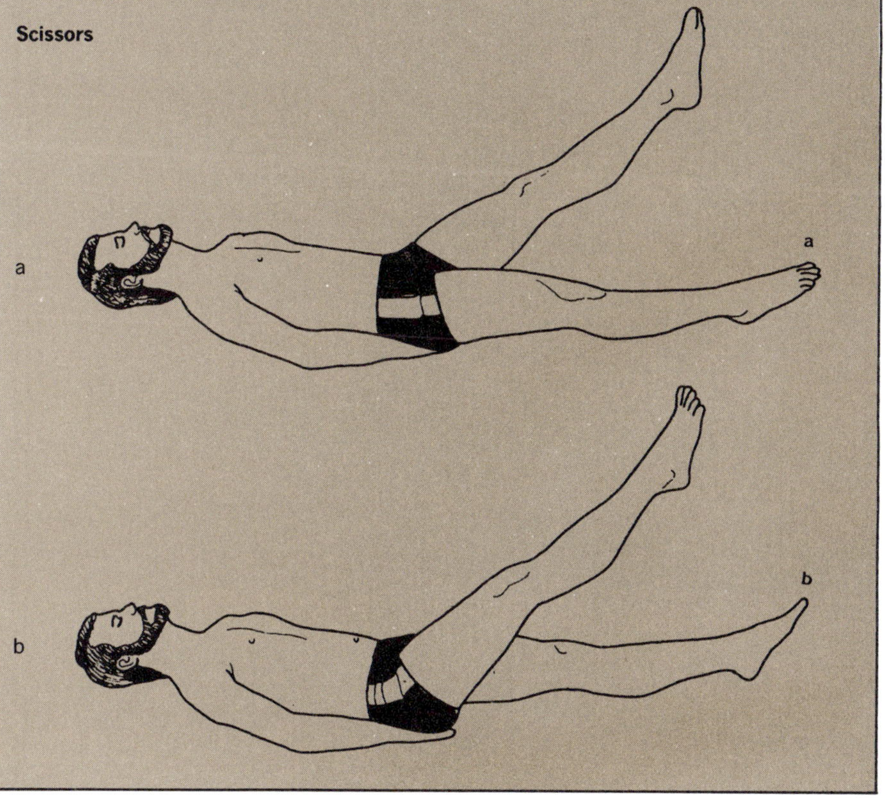

2. *Good mornings:* Starting again with feet wide apart, knees bent slightly, lean forward. Keep your hips as stationary as possible. Straighten up and then arch gently backward. Repeat as directed.

3. *Seated stretch:* Seated on the floor, spread your legs as far apart as possible. With your right hand on your left knee, try to touch your left toes with your left hand. At the same time, bring your nose close to your knee. In the first week repeat five times, then reverse for five on the right side.

4. *Feet raisers:* Lying on the floor with your hands under your buttocks, palms down, lift your head off the floor. With your legs straight and toes pointed, lift your legs off the floor to an angle of about 45 degrees. Lower your legs.

5. *Curl-ups:* Lying on your back with your hands under your buttocks and head slightly raised off the floor, bring your knees up under your chin. Straighten your legs out until they are hovering at a 45-degree angle from your body. Lower your legs and repeat as directed.

6. *Scissors:* Again lying on your back, hold up your legs at an angle of 20 to 30 degrees from your body.

Basic Muscle Locators

Side leg raisers

a

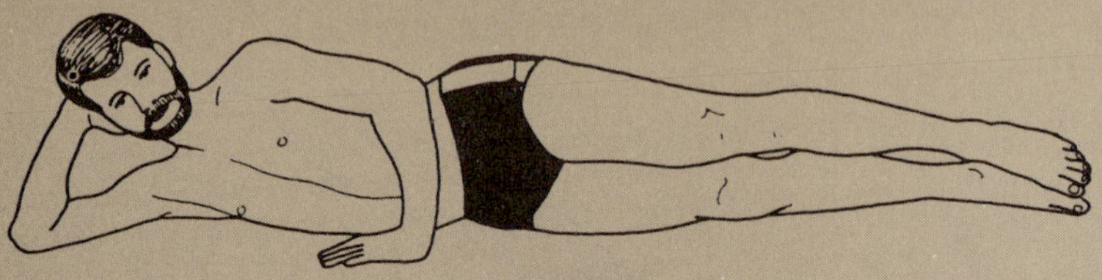

b

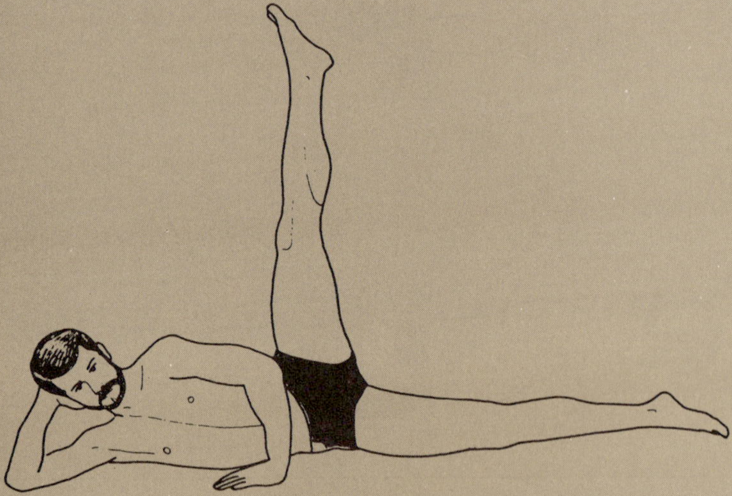

Keep your hands under your bottom. Work your legs like a pair of scissors, crisscrossing them repeatedly.

7. *Half sit-ups:* The half sit-up is the same as the whole, but it is not completed. Lie on the floor, knees up, with your hands on your thighs, then sit up to an angle of 45 degrees. Try not to move your legs or hips. As you sit up, bring your head down toward your chest.

8. *Side leg raisers:* Lying on your side and balancing yourself by holding one hand on the floor, prop your head up on your other hand. Lift your top leg as high as possible for the specified number of times, then lie on your opposite side and lift the other leg the same number.

9. *Simple press-ups:* standing with your back straight and your bottom tucked in, lean forward, placing your hands on a table edge. Still keeping your back straight, lower yourself down to the table. If the "simple" press-up is too simple, try a regular push-up.

10. *Squats:* Standing with your

Basic Muscle Locators

Hip kicks

a

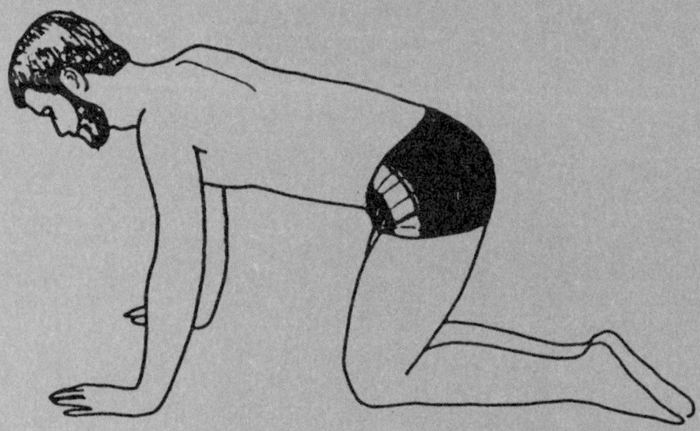

b

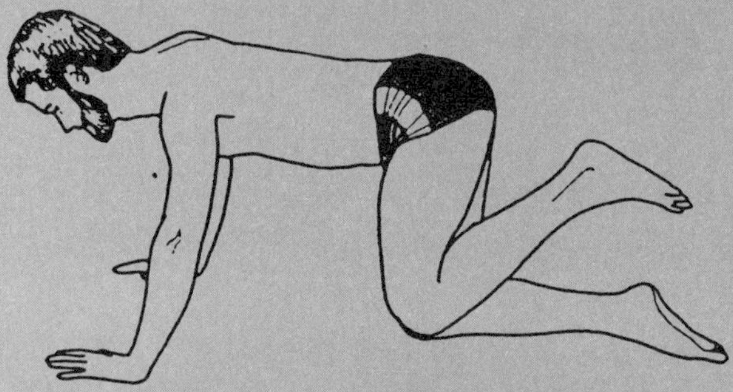

c

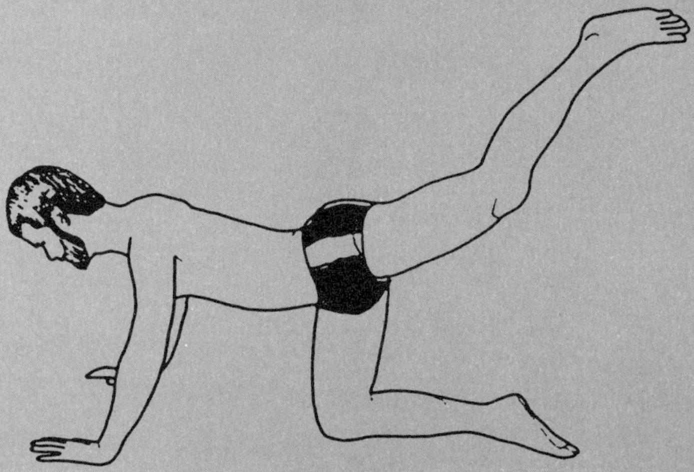

Basic Muscle Locators

Simple press-ups

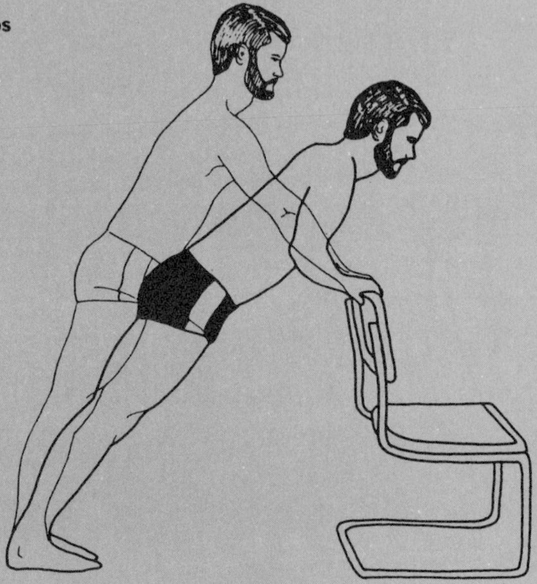

Half sit-ups

a

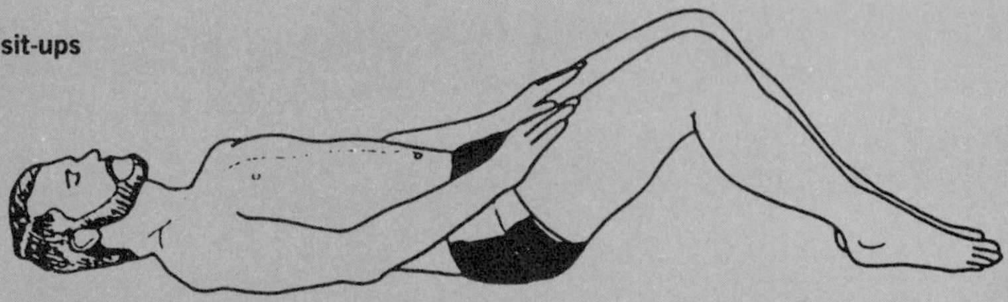

b

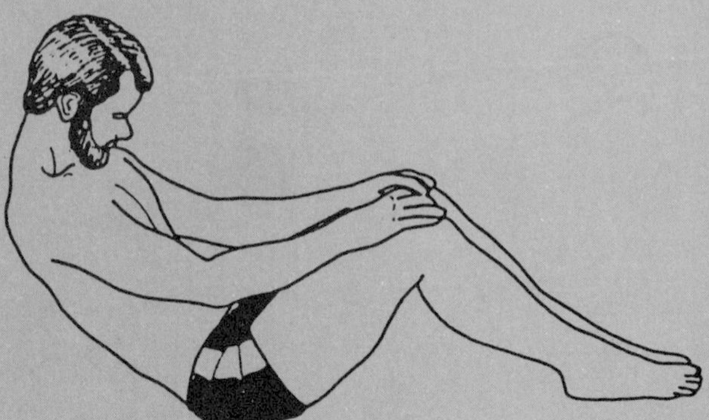

Special pelvic strengthener

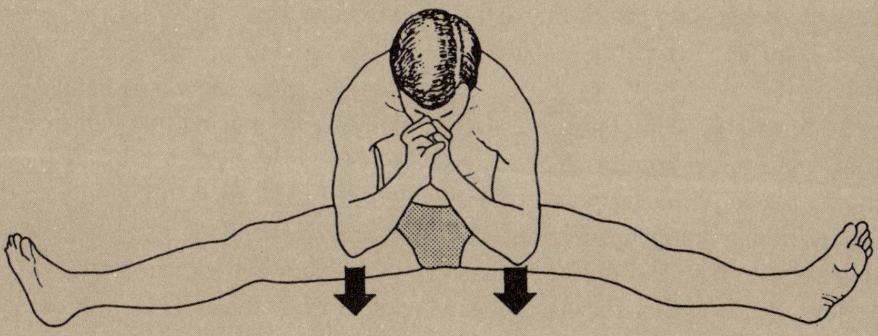

feet 15 to 20 inches apart, and with a one- or two-inch block under each heel, bend your knees to a full squatting position. Keep your back as straight as possible at all times and hold your arms folded at shoulder level. Remember the caveat about deep knee bends that involve bringing your buttocks all the way down to your heels.

11. *Hip kicks:* Kneeling on all fours, bring one knee forward off the floor and toward your face. Now push that leg straight back and upward as high as you can. Repeat with the other leg.

Sitting, Towel, and Other Exercise Routines

As emphasized earlier, a basic exercise program can include a variety of supplementary movements and exercises that add zest. Additional exercises can also be practiced separately from regular exercise sessions and under the most informal of circumstances: when taking a shower, toweling off after the shower, sweeping the floor with a broom, and in other situations. Any of these can be programmed into the basic fitness schedule without difficulty.

Sitting-down Exercises

With no more special equipment than a sturdy, dependable chair, you can do at least ten different exercises. For some of the exercises you will need a chair with arms. Each of these movements contributes in its own way to your basic program.

Cardiorespiratory Endurance Exercises

Two of the special chairborne exercises contribute to cardiorespiratory endurance.

1. Sitting in your chair, stretch your arms out straight in front at shoulder level. Holding your arms in that position, stand up. Do not use your arms. While standing, inhale deeply. Sit down, then exhale. Repeat the exercise 20 to 30 times at a moderate pace.

2. Sitting on the chair, breathe deeply, at the same time bending your knees and hugging them so that your feet leave the floor. Exhale, then let go of your knees, bringing your feet down to the floor and pushing your bent elbows back. Gently arch your spine while inhaling. Repeat 20 to 30 times.

Flexibility and Balance Exercises

Six other exercises utilizing a chair contribute to flexibility and balance.

1. Sitting on the chair, inhale deeply and bend forward to touch the floor. Let your breath out as you bend. Straighten up. Bring one arm up and back and let the other swing down and back, gently stretching your shoulders and spine as you inhale. Repeat 15 to 20 times.

2. Start by kneeling sideways on the chair seat on your left knee, with the right hand holding the back of the chair and the left arm dangling down. Raise and extend your right leg and left arm, arch your back, and inhale. Exhale as you return to your original position. Repeat several times, then change position and do the same exercise while kneeling on the other knee.

3. Sitting in the chair, bend one knee and lift it toward your shoulder. Touch your raised foot with the opposite hand when your knee has come up to shoulder level. Repeat with the other leg and hand. Keep up a moderate pace while repeating 20 or more times for each side. Breathe regularly at a slow tempo. If possible, accelerate the pace as you go.

4. Standing behind a chair that has arms, bend your body forward. Place your hands on its arms, then with your midriff resting on the chairback, carefully raise and extend one leg, then the other. If possible, raise both and balance on the chair. With one or both legs in the air, arch your body gently. Lower your legs and repeat slowly, exhaling when bringing your legs up, inhaling when arching your body. Caution: make sure of your chair before starting. It should be well balanced and solid.

5. Sitting on the edge of the chair with your body straight and your arms hanging over the side of the chair, try to raise one leg slowly, keeping it straight, while at the same time trying to reach the upraised foot with the opposite hand. Alternate sides. Exhale when you touch; inhale while you change legs and hands.

6. Sitting deep in the chair and grasping the sides of the seat tightly, hold your legs together and swing them from side to side. Accelerate the tempo while continuing the swinging motion 20 to 30 times.

Muscular Strength Exercises

Two final exercises with a chair help build muscular strength.

1. Sit straddling an armless chair, facing its back. Place both hands on the chair back and raise both knees while bending forward and exhaling. Slowly extend your legs out and slightly to the sides. Lean back cautiously and inhale. Repeat 10 to 30 times.

2. Sitting on the floor in front of the chair, raise your feet and place them on the chair seat. Try to reach up and touch your toes with your fingertips. As a somewhat more difficult alternative, sit in the chair with your hands on the chair arms. Bend and lift your knees, at the same time trying to lift yourself up with your arms. Exhale when you bend and inhale when you relax. Repeat 10 to 30 times.

Towel Exercises

In six other exercises a towel can, in effect, be a portable gym. The towel serves as a means of providing resistance and also has a massaging effect.

1. To build cardiorespiratory endurance, hold a bath towel by the ends behind you and stretch it taut horizontally at hand level. Inhale deeply, then pull the towel ends forward, crossing your arms in front. Push your crossed arms so as to stretch the towel as far as possible. Exhale while pushing. Uncross your arms, go back to the starting position with your hands stretched out from your sides, and inhale. Repeat 15 to 30 times.

2. For flexibility and balance, while in a standing position hold the towel taut in front of you at waist level. Your hands should be held apart about the width of your shoulders. Try to pass one leg over the towel and then bring it back. Repeat with the other leg. Exhale when your knee is highest and inhale when your knee is down. Repeat 10 to 20 times with each leg.

3. For muscular strength, hold the towel taut behind your head. Bend one arm, then the other, as you maintain tension in the towel and slowly move it back and forth behind your neck. Inhale when both your arms are extended upward; exhale when one arm is down. Overload gradually by increasing the tension. Repeat 20 to 30 times.

4. Again for flexibility and balance, hold the towel stretched across the back of your neck. Take a deep breath and swing your right arm downward

Towel Exercises

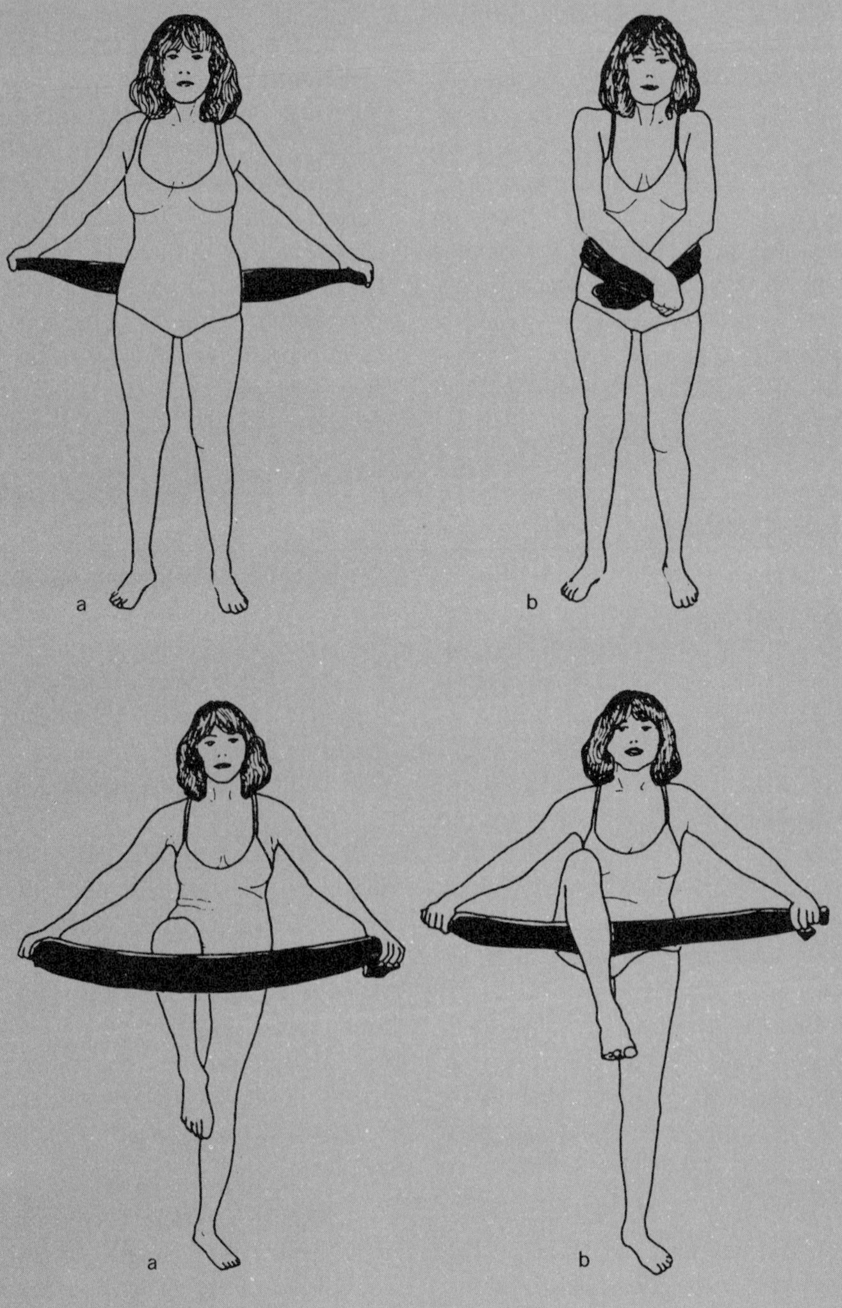

Towel Exercises

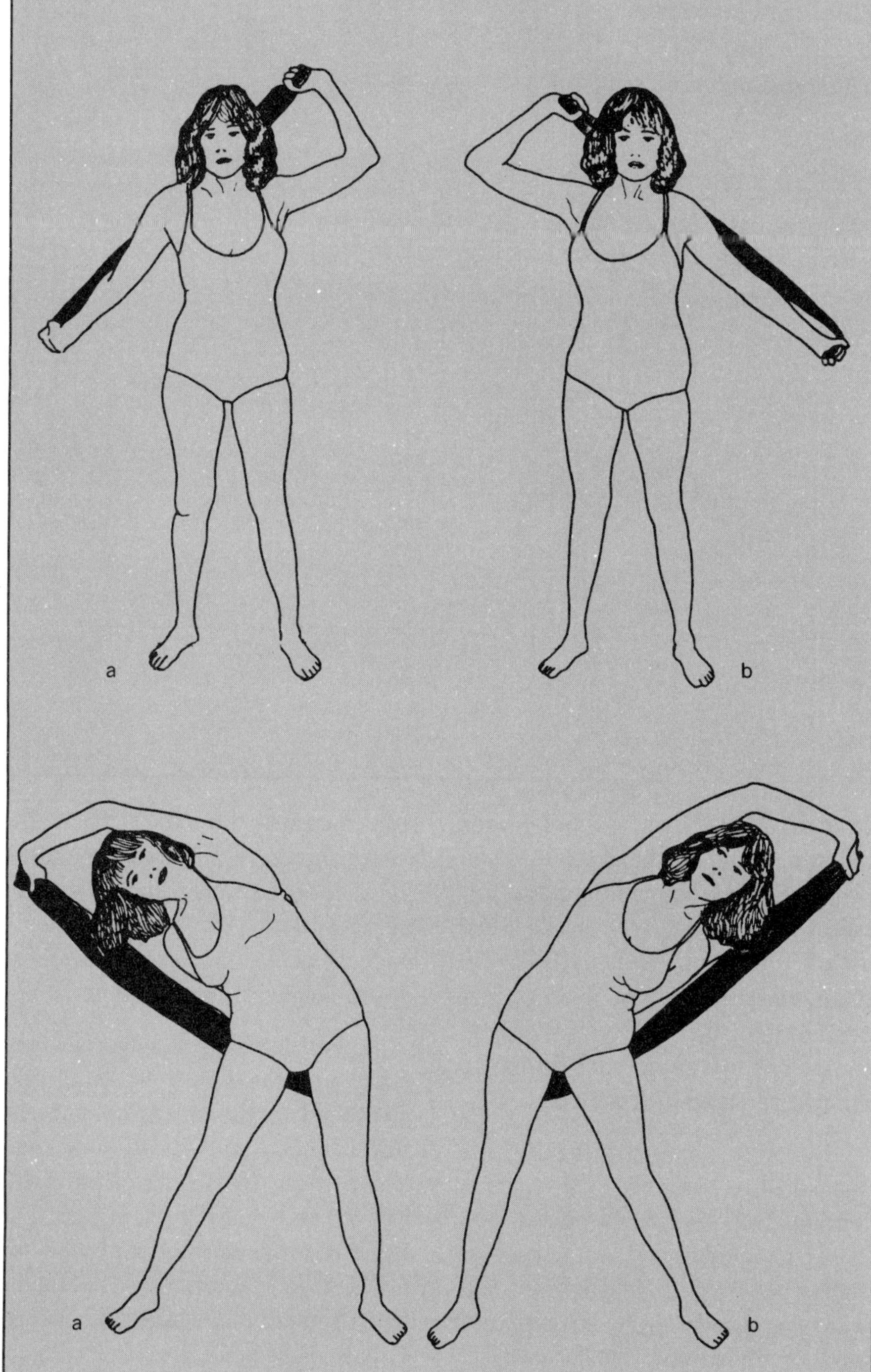

Towel Exercises

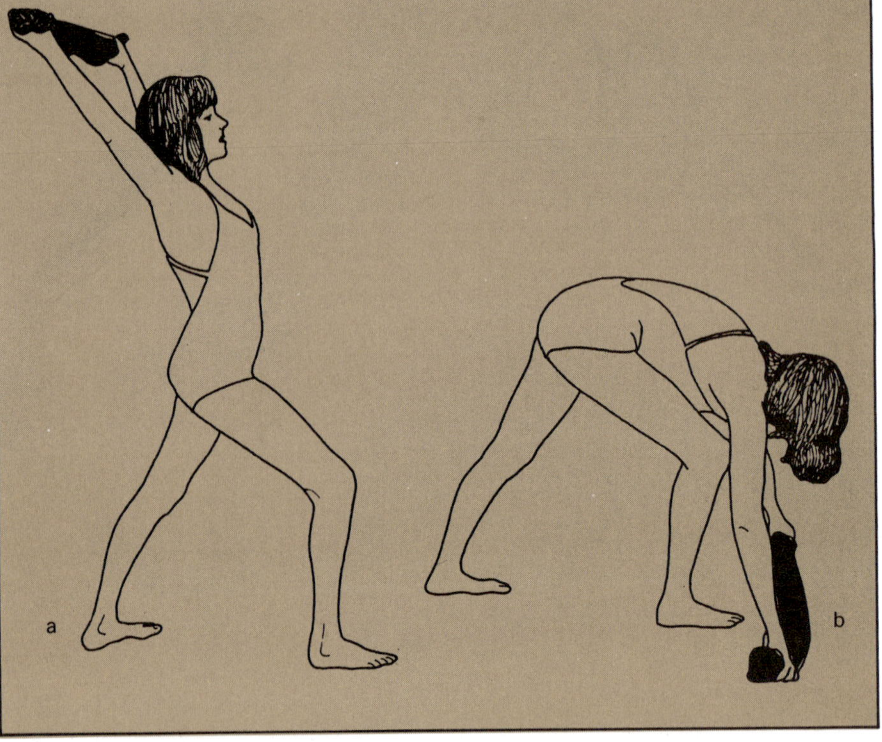

behind your back as you bring your left arm up and overhead as far as you can. Bend your body to the right. Exhale while bending over, inhale while straightening up. Repeat 10 to 30 times, then change arm positions and bend to the left, exhaling at the same time. Try to keep your arms as straight as possible at all times.

5. For flexibility and agility, assume a lunge position as you would in fencing. One leg should be set well ahead of the other and bent; the other should be straight. Holding the towel with your hands apart, stretch your arms up above your head and back, arching the body slightly. Bring your arms forcefully down to the floor. The towel should, if possible, touch the floor. The exercise should be repeated 10 to 15 times at a steady pace. Exhale as your arms come down, inhale as they come up.

6. For flexibility and coordination, stand upright with your arms outstretched to the sides, holding the towel behind you. Raise your right leg, twisting your trunk to the right. Try to reach your right foot with your left hand while still holding both ends of the towel. Alternate legs. Inhale when you are in the straight position. Exhale at the end of the twist. Repeat 15 to 20 times.

Shower Routines

Shower shape-ups have two advantages. First, they are simple. Second, they provide the mild movement that in the morning in particular can increase circulation and help the body to wake up.

The shower shape-ups can, of course, be done other places than in a shower. But if you perform them in the shower, be sure the surface on which you are standing and exercising is covered with a nonslip mat—for safety. If you do these exercises while the shower is running, breathe through the mouth, not the nose. Pretend you are swimming.

1. For cardiorespiratory endurance, take a deep breath while standing, then slowly bring your arms and shoulders forward. Cross your arms in front of you to squeeze your chest, exhaling at the same time. Slowly move your arms and shoulders back while inhaling. Repeat 10 to 20 or more times.

2. For flexibility, while in a standing position take a deep breath and slowly bend your body forward. Move your arms back and up as far as possible while exhaling. Straighten up slowly, inhaling, and repeat 10 to 20 or more times.

3. For flexibility and balance, again standing, place your hands on your hips and bend your right knee. Holding your right foot up, try to remain balanced on your left foot for ten seconds. See if you can retain your balance with your eyes closed. Do the same with the other foot. Breathe slowly and deeply. Repeat 10 to 20 or more times with each foot.

4. For muscular strength, stand in a slightly crouched position, hands on knees, and slowly bend your knees while keeping your head forward. Press gently on your knees with your hands. Breathe regularly. Exhale when your knees are bent and inhale when they are straight. Repeat 15 to 30 times.

5. For flexibility and agility, while standing bend up one arm after the other at the elbow, accelerating gradually. Breathe with every two to six motions of the arms. Repeat as desired.

6. For flexibility and coordination, place your left hand behind your neck, inhale deeply, then bend your left knee slowly. Raise your left foot off the floor slowly, bringing it as high as possible. Try to reach your toes with your right hand as you twist your body gently. Exhale as you straighten up. Change arms and do the exercise with the other leg. Repeat with each leg 10 to 30 times.

The Broom Way

Like the chair and shower routines, the broom exercises are a simple set of movements intended as enjoyable adjuncts to a fitness program. The broom is the only required piece of equipment. But the broom wielder will need a rather large space in which to work out. Otherwise, he or she might find the broom banging on walls, furniture, pictures, and so on.

The half-dozen broom exercises are designed to increase cardiorespiratory endurance (No. 1), build flexibility and agility (Nos. 2, 3, 5, and 6), and develop muscular strength (No. 4).

1. Stand with your body bent forward, arms out to the sides, and hands holding the broomstick across the back of your shoulders. Slowly, without touching the broom handle to your head, bring the handle over your head and extend your arms all the way forward. Inhale while your arms are extended in front and exhale as they are bent.

2. In a sitting position, with your legs wide apart and arms outstretched to the sides, holding the broom across the back of your shoulders, twist your torso while continuing to hold the broom, trying to reach your right foot with your left hand and then your left foot with your right hand. Maintain a steady pace, exhaling when you reach down and inhaling when you straighten up. Repeat 15 to 20 or more times.

3. Again standing, with your arms forward and holding the broomstick horizontal with both hands in front of you, extend one leg behind you as far as it will go. Move that leg forward and up, raising it as high as you can while maintaining your balance on the other foot. Repeat with the other leg. Inhale while you are bringing your raised leg down; exhale while raising it. Repeat 15 to 25 times.

4. In a standing position, with your legs wide apart, hold the broomstick vertically in front of you with both hands. The handle end should rest on the floor. Slowly bend one knee after the other, using the broomstick as support, so that the body shifts from side to side. While bending a knee, exhale. Inhale while straightening up. Repeat 15 to 30 times.

5. Standing with your legs wide apart, bend your body forward. The broomstick should be held across the back of your shoulders, hands on either end. Slowly twist your torso until the broom has gone from the horizontal position to a vertical. Accelerate gradually as you repeat the exercise on alternate sides. Breathe in rhythm and repeat 15 to 25 times.

6. Kneeling on your left knee, with your right leg extended behind you, hold the broomstick across the back of your shoulders with your outstretched arms. First turn your torso to the left, then slowly twist to the right. Move your right leg sideways and forward and try to reach your right foot with your left hand. Return to the original position and reverse the movement while kneeling on your right knee. Exhale when you are reaching toward your foot, inhale when your body is vertical. Repeat 15 to 25 times.

Some Movements to Beware of

For varying reasons, controversy surrounds the use of some exercises. Whatever your program, you will want to cast a wary eye on these movements for the reasons indicated:

1. *Deep knee bends:* Particularly for the beginner, the deep knee bend, lowering the buttocks until they touch the heels, poses hazards. The deep knee bend stretches the knee's lateral

Movements to Beware of

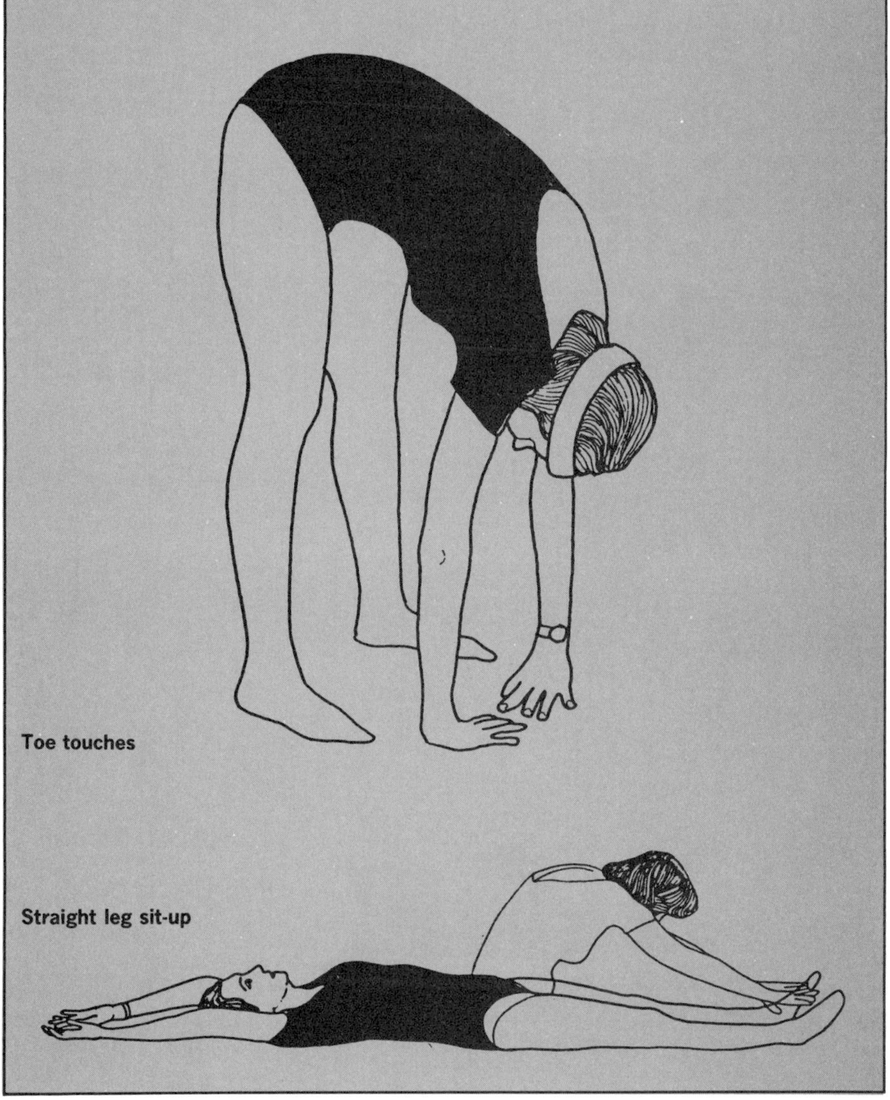

Movements to Beware of

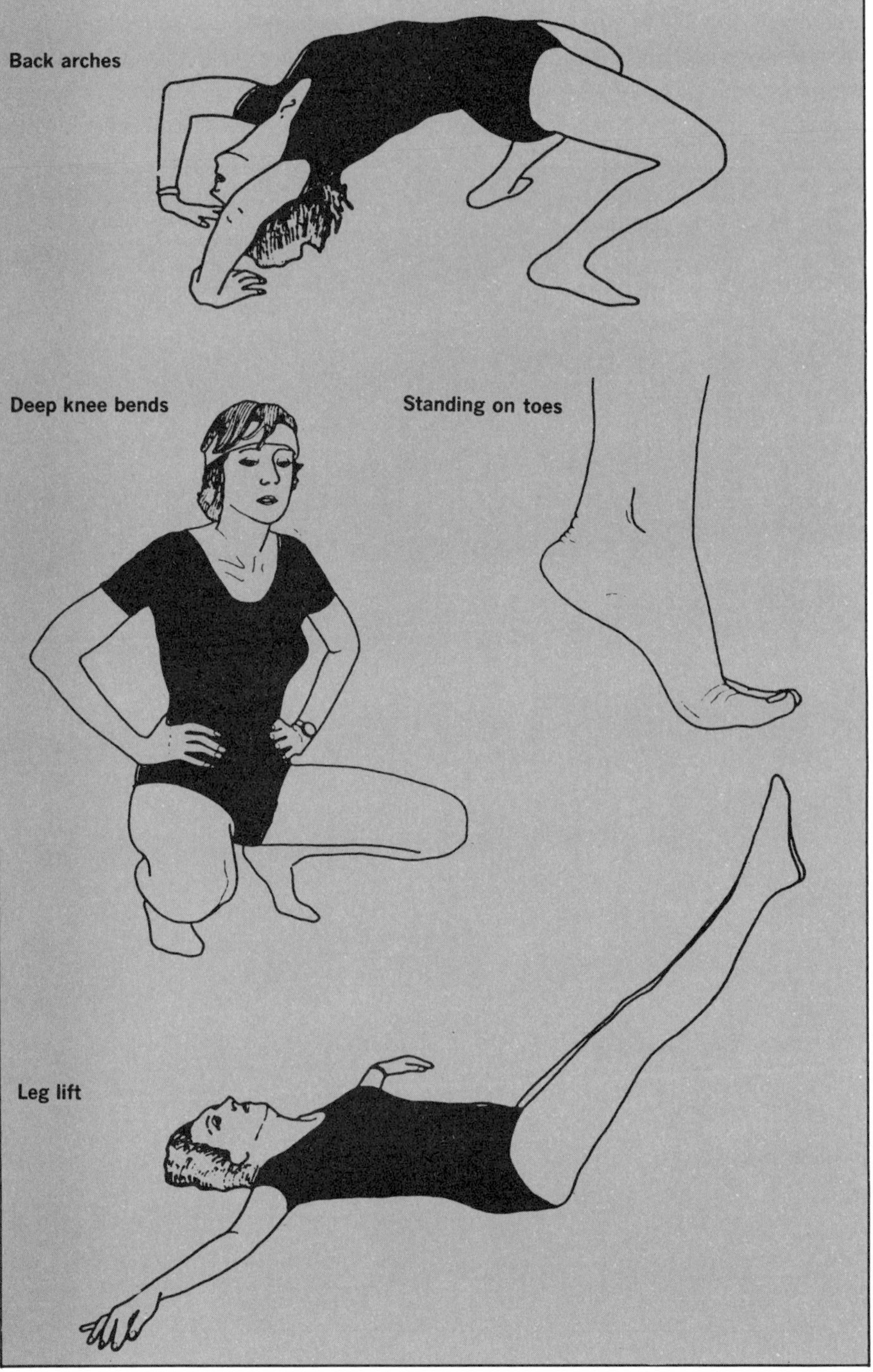

ligaments. Stretched too far, the ligaments cease to protect the knee. If the ligaments become overextended, cartilage problems can result.

2. *Back arches:* The danger in back arches is that hyperextension may occur. Persons with difficulties such as weak abdominal muscles may find that their conditions become worse if they do this exercise. Physicians maintain that a fitness program should, in the beginning at least, stress abdominal exercises rather than low-back work.

3. *Leg lifts:* Performed while the exerciser is lying on his back, leg lifts have been found to help trim the waistline. But they can also lead to problems in persons with a tendency to the low-back ailment called lordosis. The reason is that leg lifts are accomplished through the use of the iliacus and psoas muscles, a set of muscles that can be easily strained when they are not in good condition.

4. *Standing on toes:* Recommended in many exercise programs, the repetitive toe stand allegedly strengthens the longitudinal arch. But in reality high toe stands may produce stresses that weaken the arch. Substitutes for high toe stands include heel cord stretches or walking on the heels.

5. *Straight-leg sit-ups:* The straight-leg sit-up also requires the use of the iliacus and psoas muscles. But in sitting up the exerciser can hyperextend and strain the back. The effort in sitting up with legs extended in effect tugs at the muscles along the spinal column. Low-back problems in particular can be aggravated.

6. *Toe touches:* Toe touching not only forces the knees to overextend; it also exerts heavy pressure on the lower spine. Since the exercise doesn't help to trim the waistline, as it has been alleged to do, toe touching both fails to provide the exercise value claimed for it and presents the risk of back problems.

Low-Back Pain

Health authorities have estimated that nearly one in every six Americans suffers from low-back pain. Drugs and medications for the relief of such pain earn their manufacturers millions of dollars a year. But low-back pains may often be most effectively attacked with carefully planned and regularly pursued exercise routines.

The causes of low-back pains can vary. Tension can be to blame. A similar result occurs when the lower vertebrae have been compressed or crowded together. In other instances body positions of movements cause direct muscle or ligament strain.

Where such body mechanics have led to low-back pain, the fault usually lies with posture. If the pelvis slants downward, the lower back develops an abnormal curve and presses on the nerves of the spinal column. The pressure becomes so severe sometimes that the disks of cartilage that protect the nerves cannot do their job.

Muscle Weakness and Tension

Some medical authorities hold that vertebral compression produces only about one-fifth of all the cases of low-back pain that afflict Americans. The other 80 per cent result from simple weakness of the muscles of the back, the abdomen, the hips (the psoas group), the hip extensors (gluteals), and the hamstrings.

Tension also plays a major role. The muscle groups that support and control the movements of the torso tighten up, often because they lack strength and flexibility. And lack of strength and flexibility results from inadequate exercise.

Relief of Low-Back Syndrome

Is it any wonder that medications that promise to reduce low-back pain sell so well? The search for relief from such pain may occupy many of the waking hours of the sufferer—and cost a substantial amount of money. Yet the best way to relieve low-back syndrome is to avoid it. That means the individual must keep the important muscles involved in trunk support and movement strong and flexible. Such flexibility, once achieved, not only reduces the chances of low-back pain, but also provides the body with greater agility and mobility.

If low-back syndrome cannot be avoided in the first place, it can be relieved through exercise. Physical activities, sports, and games of nearly all kinds that involve movement of the body help eliminate muscle tension. The activities also provide a safe outlet for nervousness and tension which can, as noted, make their own contribution to low-back syndrome.

The Exercises

Many movements, exercises, and activities that help the fitness beginner to rid himself of low-back pain can be included in a fitness program. They should generally be performed on a firm, flat surface. They require repetition, but the number of repetitions can often be a judgment matter. Each person should gauge his tolerance for such exercises by the ways in which his or her body reacts to them.

The exercises described below are particularly adapted to alleviating the specific conditions for which they are prescribed. But many others to be mentioned later will also help to improve these conditions, if less directly, while also serving one or more

Good-bye Backache Exercises

Alternate hamstring stretch

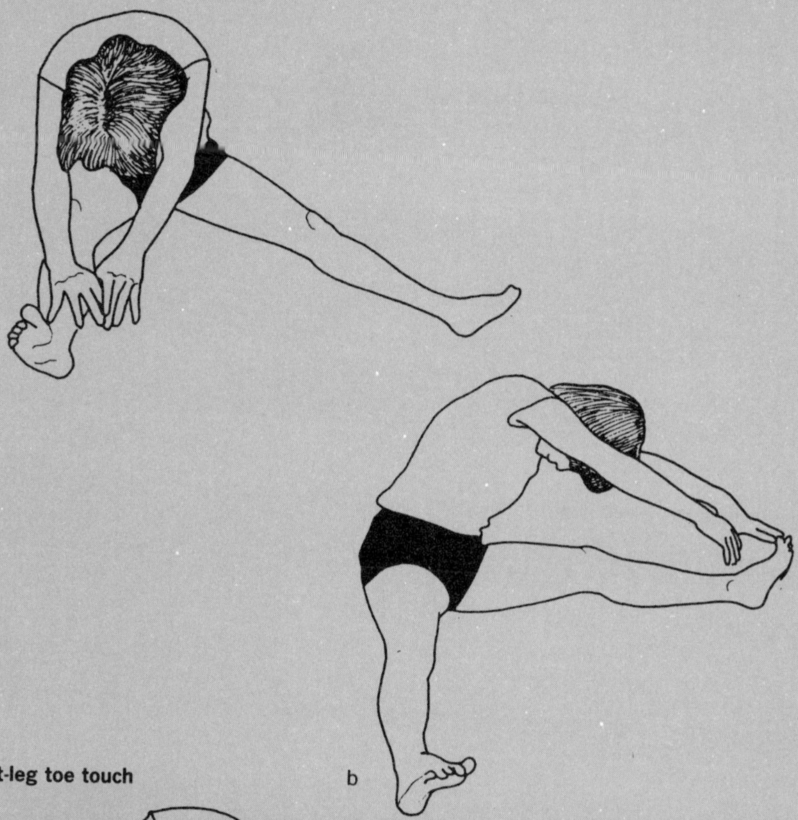

a b

Bent-leg toe touch

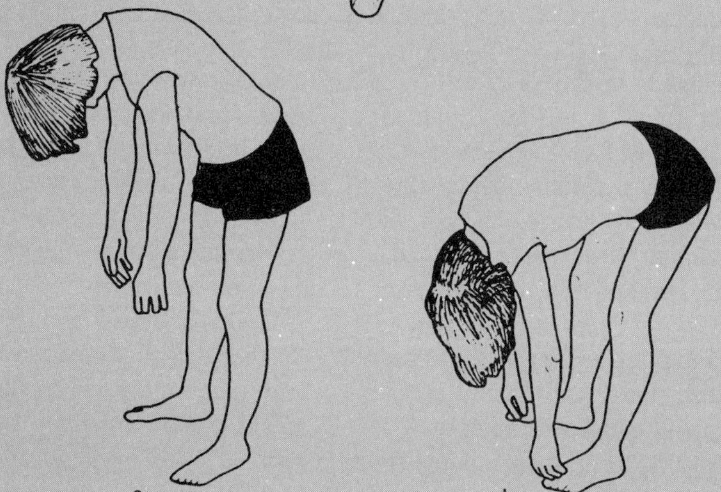

a b

Good-bye Backache Exercises

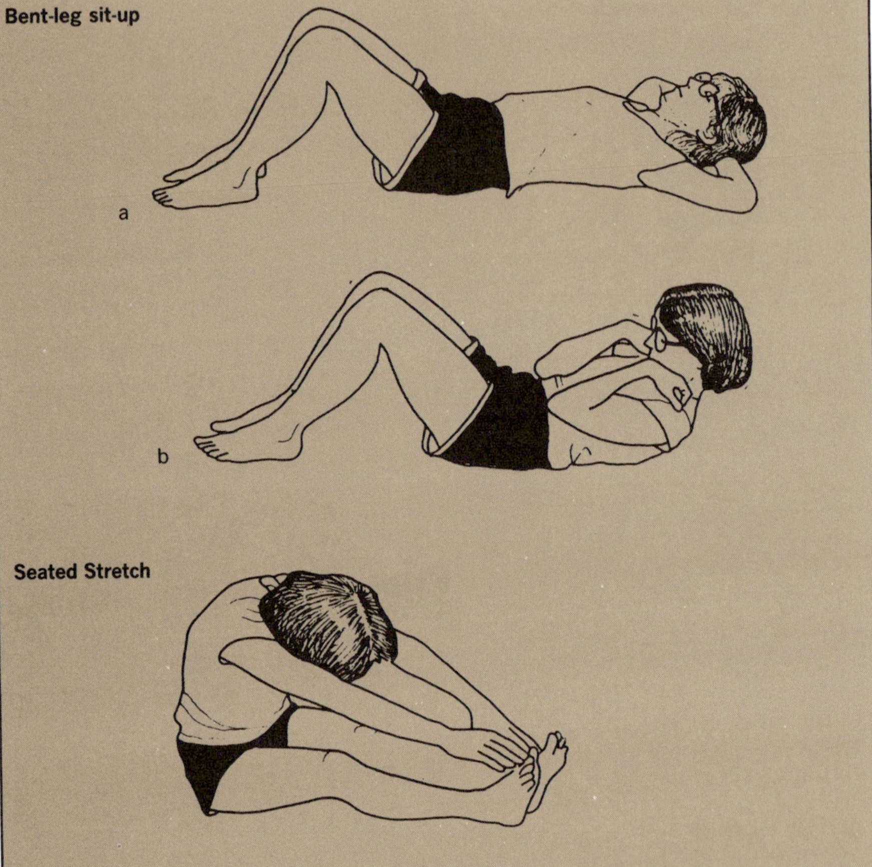

of the five basic fitness goals.

Like those in the preceding set, these exercises should be performed slowly and carefully. The subject should begin by lying on his back with his arms at his sides, palms facing down. The knees should be flexed, either by resting them on a pillow or by placing the feet flat on the ground. Breathe slowly and deeply at least five times, inhaling through the nose and exhaling through the mouth. Thus relaxed, you are ready to proceed with these exercises:

1. Contract your abdominal and gluteal muscles at the same time so as to bring your back flat against the floor. After holding that position for six seconds, relax. Repeat the process ten to 20 times. You can perform the same movements with your legs straight. You may want to try contracting the abdominals and gluteals from time to time during the day as a means of strengthening these muscles.

2. To stretch your back, starting from the same position and with your

Good-bye Backache Exercises

Alternate knee pull

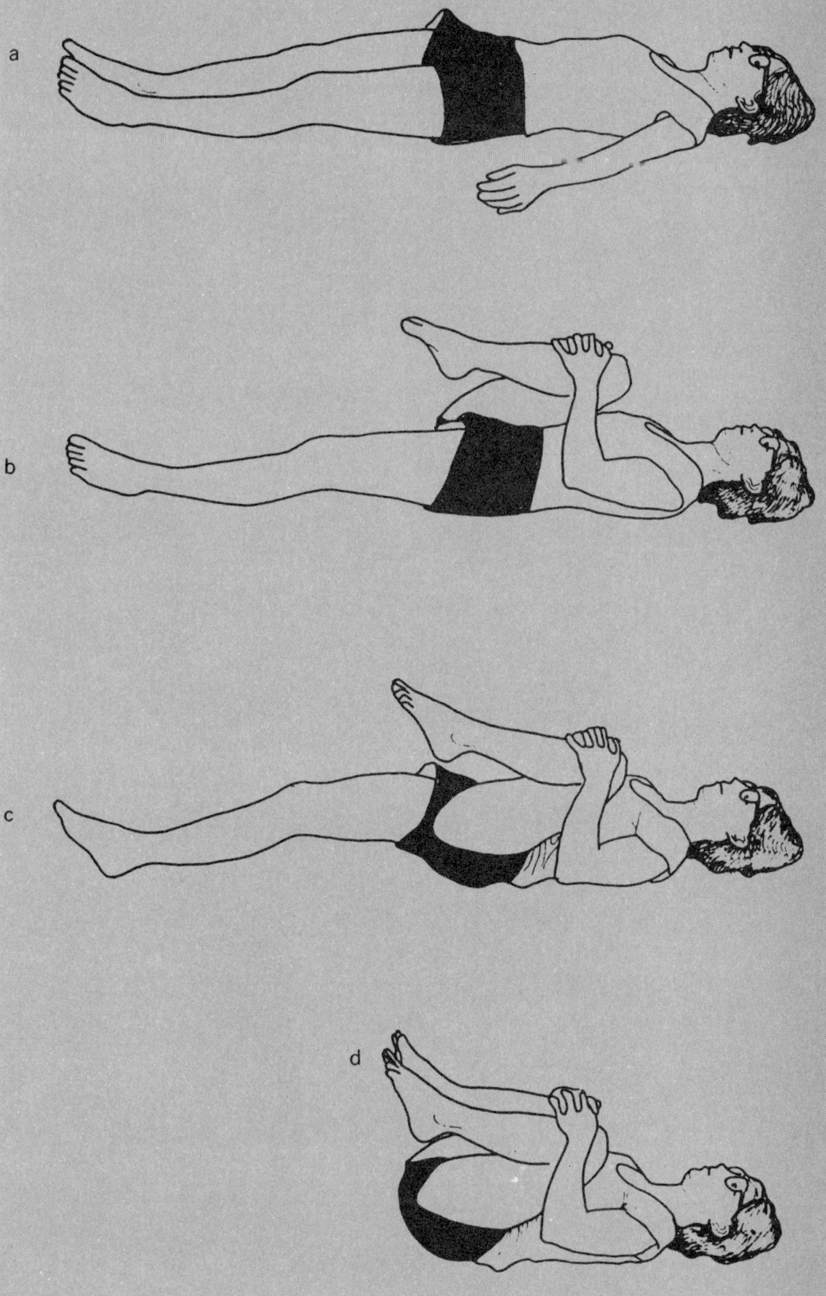

Good-bye Backache Exercises

Stand and stretch

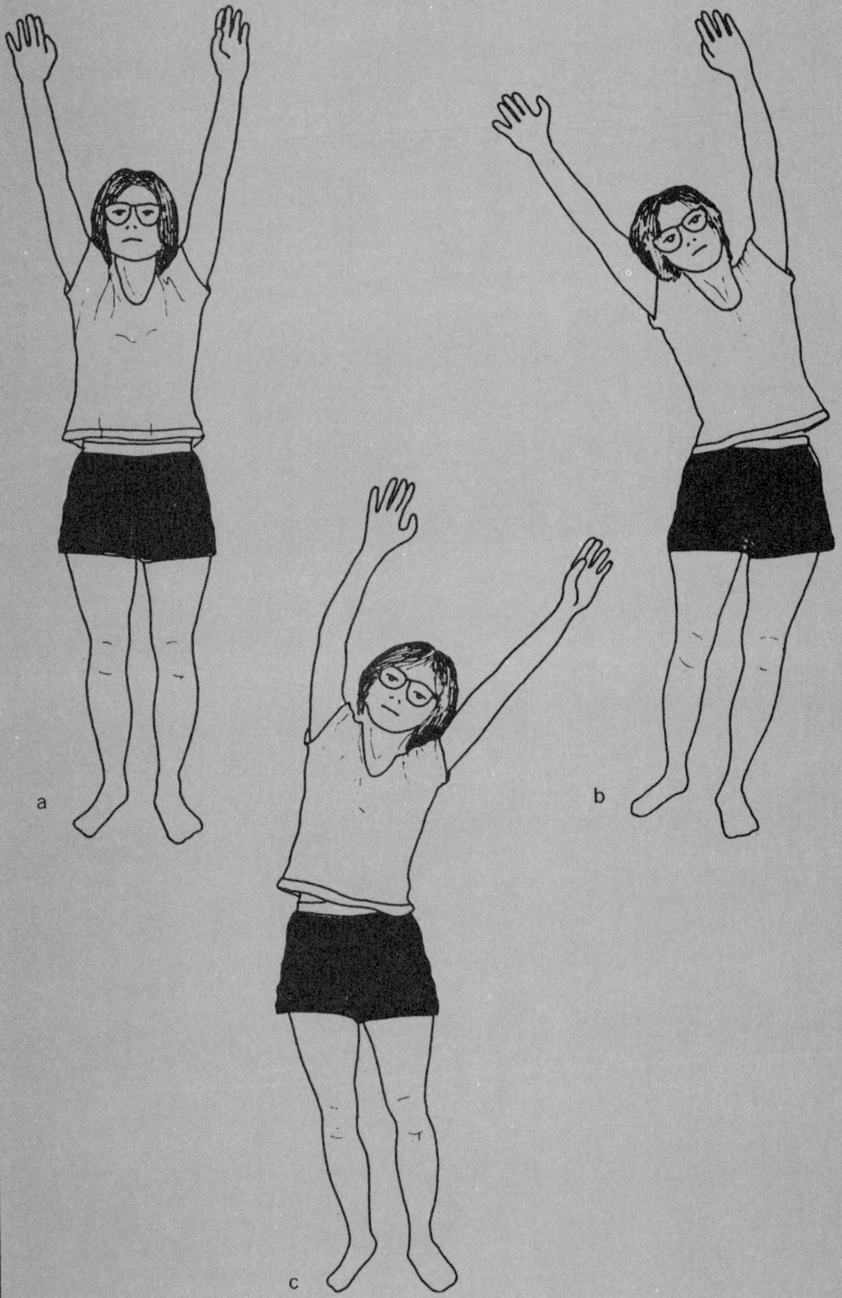

back flat against the floor as above, raise your head. At the same time bring both knees up as far as your chest while clasping your hands around your knees. Exert pulling pressure with your hands for six seconds, then relax and resume your original position. Repeat 10 to 20 times.

3. To strengthen the muscles of the hip joint start in the same position, with your arms at your sides. Your knees should be relaxed, your legs stretched out. Simultaneously contract your stomach muscles and flatten your back. Raising your head, bring one knee up to your chest. The other knee should remain relaxed. Repeat 10 to 20 times, alternating legs.

4. Beginning on your hands and knees and keeping your head, neck, and back straight, raise one knee up and back as far as possible. Keep your upraised leg flexed and your back straight. Return to your starting position on hands and knees and repeat 10 to 20 times, alternating legs.

5. Stand with your feet together and your hands at your sides. To strengthen your low-back muscles and at the same time stretch your hamstrings, bend over slowly from the hips. Bring your arms back as far as possible. Return slowly to the starting position. Repeat 10 to 20 times.

Supplementary Back-pain Relievers

Two other exercises help relieve the low-back pains that make life miserable for so many persons. Both exercises contribute to flexibility; both are simple and easy to master.

1. In the *head pull-back,* drop your head until your chin touches your chest. Clasp your hands behind your head. Moving your head upward slowly and then backward as far as possible, keep pressure on the back of your head with your hands. In this isometric movement your head should go back as far as you can move it. Once back, count slowly to five while maintaining the hand pressure. Relax and repeat half a dozen times. Rest for about five seconds between repetitions.

2. In the *monkey slump,* stand with your feet spread apart and your knees slightly bent. With your hands on your knees, and while breathing in deeply, tense all your body muscles to a moderate degree. Then exhale slowly and let your hands slip from your knees. Your body should slump forward until your hands touch—or almost touch—the floor. Your chin should be level with your thighs. Maintain the slump for three to five seconds. Repeat half a dozen times.

Yoga

An introduction to yoga can do little more than sketch some of the main features of this Eastern system of body control and movement. An estimated 300 or more books of relatively recent vintage deal with the subject in greater or less detail. More than 60 authors have written on hatha (physical, or force) yoga alone.

The claims made for yoga cover a broad range. Where one exponent may proclaim yoga's reducing or weight-control merits, another may stress its capacity to restore youth and vitality. A third may emphasize that yoga relieves stress and tension as no other discipline can. A fourth may swear that yoga eliminates low-back pain, straightens shoulders, and cures a multitude of other disorders.

Unquestionably, yoga can do much for the faithful practitioner. But the question for the person seeking total fitness is simple: can yoga help me?

With some qualifications, the answer is Yes.

Some Background

Yoga began in India some 5,000 years ago. It represents much more than a system of body control. Yoga promises the faithful student that he can, in time, achieve union with the source of all knowledge. The student will thus be awakened to the farthest reaches of his intellectual and spiritual potential.

Yoga means union. It has been described as one of the six main schools of Hindu philosophy. At least 16 systems of yoga have come into currency in Western countries. The 16 promote different paths to similar goals. But of them all, hatha yoga stands out as the form most concerned with revitalizing the body, improving physical health, and providing relaxation. Hatha yoga promises to do these things by teaching a variety of asanas, or postures. The student also learns breathing control. He achieves mental control as well by concentrating on the postures and on their effects.

A brief listing of some of the purposes of yogic postures suggest how broad is the possible range of objectives. Included are postures especially for weight control, sagging abdominal muscles, or back trouble, exercises for women, for relaxation, and for general self-help. Persons over 60 can benefit from specially adapted routines.

Yoga Can Help

The logic of many asanas is readily apparent. They call, for example, for progressive flexing of the curving segments of the spine from the neck on down through the upper back, lower back, and spinal base. Flexing is accompanied by strengthening. Every joint and ligament undergoes the systematic stretching process. Pressure may also be applied to specific areas of the body to promote improved circulation of the blood. By degrees, the body becomes conditioned to increased demands.

While in various postures, the yoga student learns to practice deep breathing. Deep breathing, properly done from the diaphragm, can encourage relaxation. If it is correctly performed, both the stomach and the chest expand during inhalation and recede during exhalation. A session may close with a final extended relaxation period. Meditation makes it possible to replenish inner resources while absorbing the full benefit of the asanas.

The asanas promote correct deep breathing and thus provide a means of relaxing that can be important to a fitness program. For the fitness worker who wants to learn deep breathing as a road to relaxation, here are two multistep exercises derived from yoga.

The First Breathing Exercise

1. While lying on your back, draw up your knees. Your feet should be placed slightly apart. Inhaling deeply, allow the stomach to relax, then expand. Exhale, at the same time pulling the stomach in so that the diaphragm rises to the point where it presses against the rib cage.

2. Continue to breathe diaphragmatically. First slowly fill the lower portions of the lungs, then try to fill the middle and upper parts.

3. Exhale. Try to picture the air slowly leaving the upper, then the lower, parts of the chest cavity.

4. Continue to breathe in this fashion. Breathe slowly and deeply. Let your breathing become very slow. Your body should relax completely.

The Second Breathing Exercise

1. Start by sitting on a chair with your hands on your thighs and your elbows at your sides. Straighten your spine. Do not lean back against the back of your chair—or touch the back at all.

2. Breathe in and out rapidly through your nose. Repeat about 12 times, keeping a wood-sawing rhythm.

3. Exhale slowly through your nose until you have emptied your lungs.

4. Inhale to the count of seven. Pause for one second, then exhale. Pause again for a second. Repeat until you have completed seven breathing cycles.

An Overall Assessment

Yoga has been found to be useful in a total fitness program, but it can effect only a limited range of improvements. While it cannot substantially benefit muscular endurance, it does build flexibility and grace. The postures and breathing exercises help to induce relaxation, and may in that process reduce high blood pressure. But evidence indicating that it helps to improve blood circulation is minimal. Yoga does not build muscular strength, but it can help to firm up specific muscle groups. It does not produce a smooth, taut skin despite claims to that effect. Finally, its value in weight control has been questioned. The beginner should take those factors into consideration when deciding whether to schedule yoga sessions into the basic fitness program.

Calisthenics

Calisthenics have gone out of style to a degree because of the limited effect that they have on circulorespiratory fitness. But they still have many valuable uses. For example, many older people can take part in calisthenic exercises without danger.

Calisthenics have other advantages. They are easy to perform. They require little or no special equipment. They can be used in a fitness program to enhance circulorespiratory benefits. Contrary to the traditional approach, which calls for constantly starting and stopping activity, some calisthenics programs require continuous performance. In these programs the cardiorespiratory benefits can be considerable.

Calisthenics programs for individuals alone or for groups can include vigorous workout patterns that begin producing positive effects, such as increased strength or greater flexibility, in a very short time in nearly all the body's muscle groups. However, calisthenics programs have been found to be of limited value for "spot reducing." In fact, the spot-reducing concept has been attacked as deceptive. Different parts of the body that are burdened with excess fat can be strengthened through exercise: the protruding abdomen will benefit, for example, from sit-ups, V-seats, and curl-ups. But the benefit comes from stronger muscles. The stomach may also become flatter, but the exercise will not remove the fat.

To remove abdominal—or other—fat, the individual should probably choose some other program format, not calisthenics. These persons should, rather, take part in activities that require large-muscle motion, such as walking, swimming, cycling, and jogging.

Adult Physical Fitness

The Adult Physical Fitness program developed by the President's Council on Physical Fitness is generally acknowledged to be very good. Essentially a calisthenics program, it includes a jog-walk sequence that is

Calisthenics (Men)

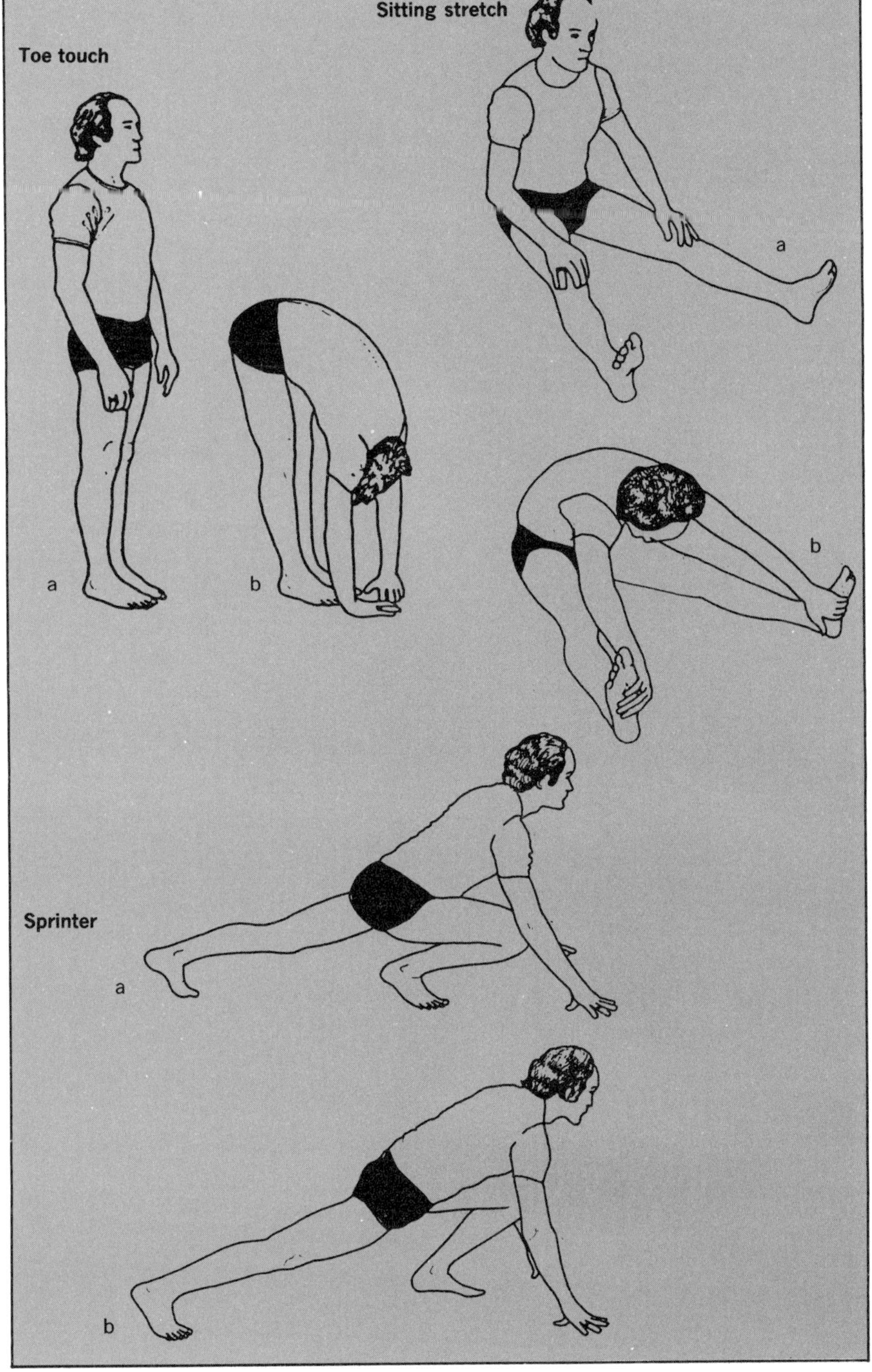

Calisthenics (Men)

Sit-up

a

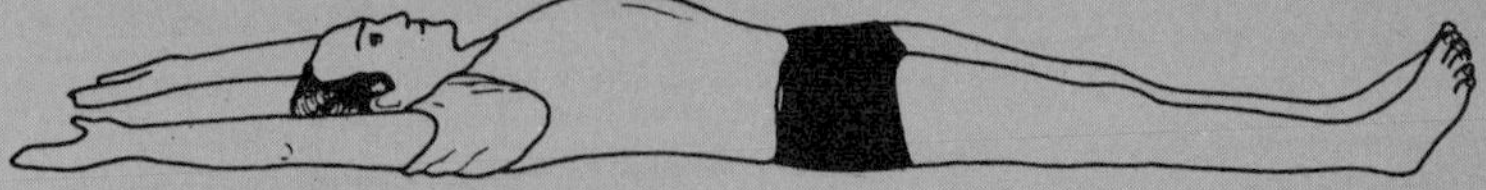

b

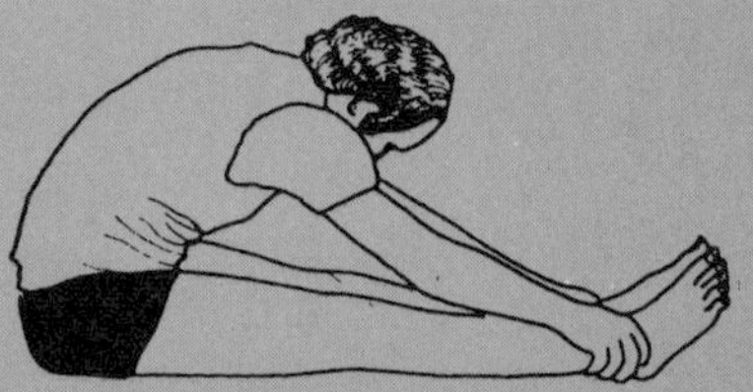

Leg raiser

a

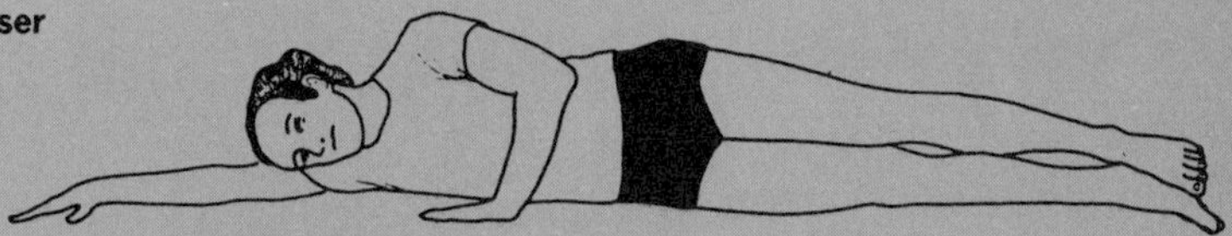

b

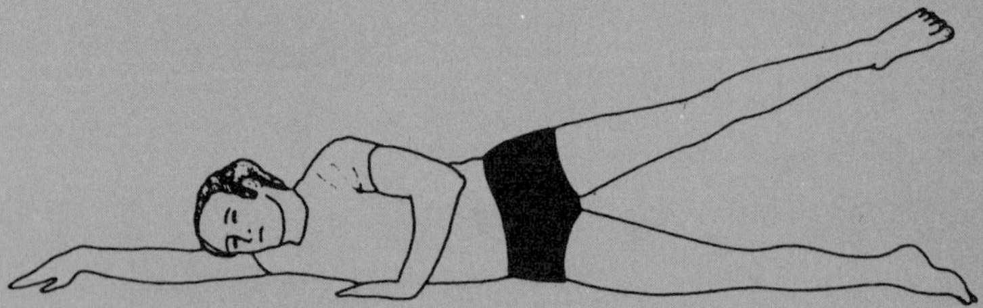

Calisthenics (Men)

Push-up

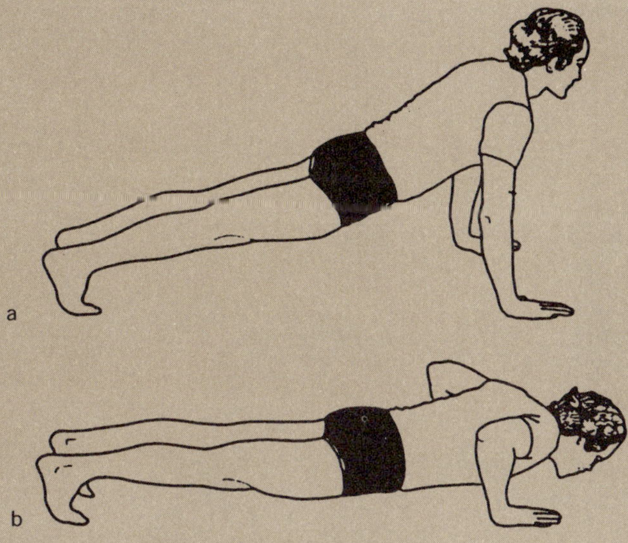

vital to the program's effectiveness. If that sequence is omitted the program fails to measure up to the standards set for basic fitness programs that seek to produce the five basic body improvements.

The program contains separate exercise regimens for men and women. The exercises are basically sound, and participants are led through progressively more difficult levels of activity. In all, five levels are included following an orientation program that introduces the regimen to the beginner. Exercises are described and illustrated for clarity, and charts are provided for those who want to keep records.

Calisthenics Programs

Calisthenics programs, like most others, fall into discernible patterns. They stress different types of exercise depending on how they were originally conceptualized and drawn up. They can be completely adequate as individualized fitness programs for home use if the exerciser pays attention to certain basics.

Before adapting a calisthenics program to his or her own needs, the individual should make sure that the program has the following characteristics:

The program should include exercises that develop circulorespiratory fitness. These can be added to the basic calisthenics program if they are not integral parts of it from the beginning. For example, a walking or walk-

Calisthenics (Women)

Bend and stretch

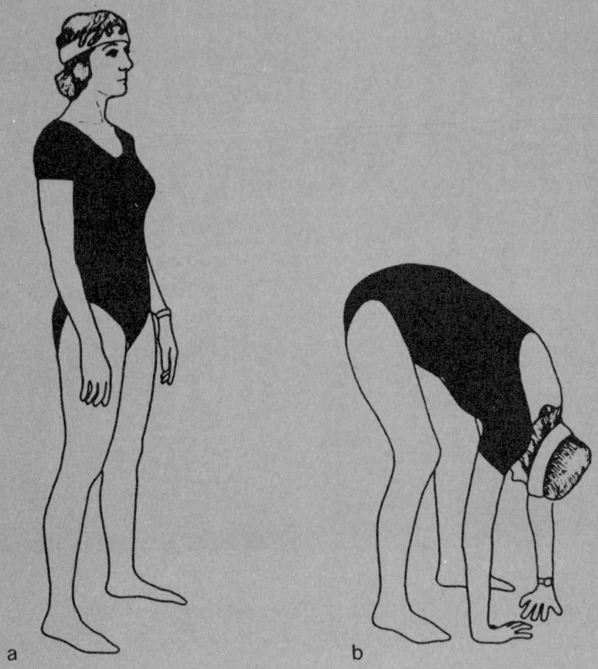

Knee lift

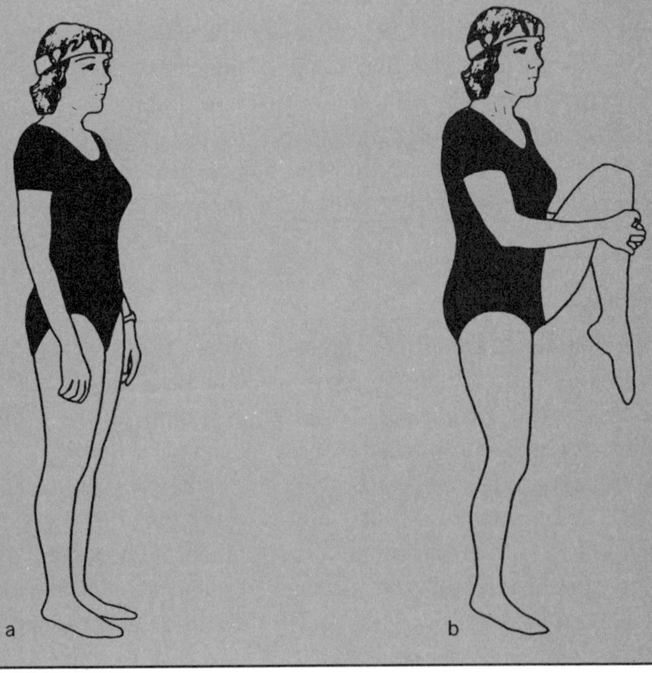

Calisthenics (Women)

Wing stretcher

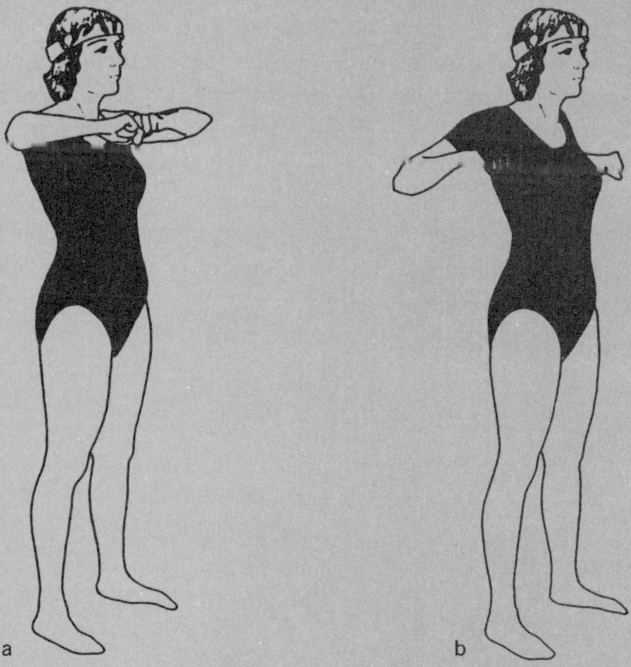

a b

Half knee-bend

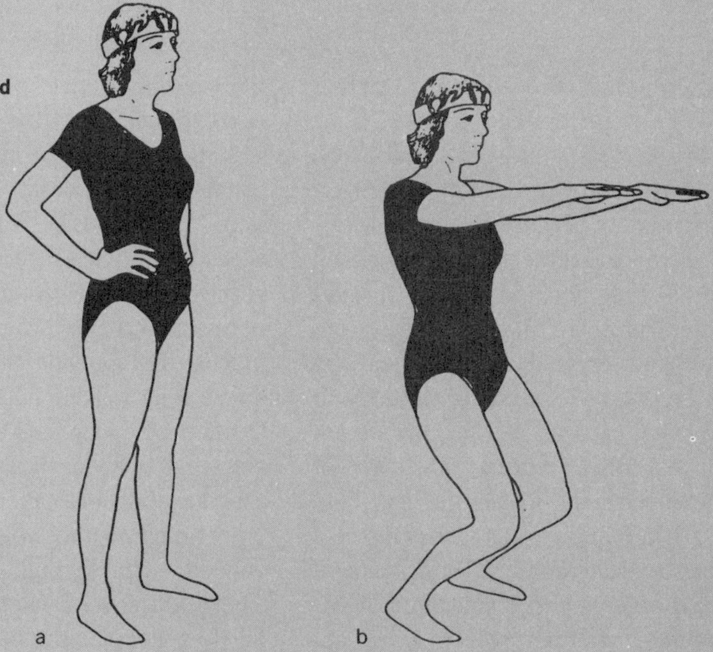

a b

jog section can be added to the basic program. Running in place between calisthenics routines is sometimes a desirable approach.

The program should include exercises that provide work for all the body's major muscle systems.

The program should allow for challenging rates of progression for the out-of-shape beginner as well as the person in very good condition. Progress in the areas of muscular strength and endurance and cardiorespiratory efficiency are particularly important.

Each session should include a warm-up and a cool-down.

As with other fitness programs, the calisthenics program should include at least three sessions weekly, and each session should last at least 30 minutes.

Questionable exercises should be approached with caution or eliminated.

Other Fun Exercises

In a period of weeks after starting a fitness program—usually 12 to 24—the dedicated person will probably be ready to branch out into a wide variety of more strenuous activities. More diverse types of exercises are likely to seem attractive. A good fitness program should be preparing the beginner for locomotor sports—those that require the whole body to be in motion—and for brachiation activities, which require movement of the upper body, mainly the arms.

The program, after all, has the goal of maximizing body peformance in all areas of life. In branching out, consideration should be given to those activities that provide enjoyment and at the same time meet physical, social, recreational, and other needs. The activities should not be purely seasonal or participation will be part-time. It may be necessary to mix types of activities so as to ensure year-round participation.

Special training programs in calisthenics may provide the answer, as may a daily walking hour, or dancing. Other people may want to keep it simple—and turn to ancillary exercises that can be performed alone. Still others might opt for yoga or some advanced strength builder exercises. There are several factors to bear in mind as you plan the best way to expand your fitness horizons:

Model Exercise Circuit Chart

Station 1: Neck

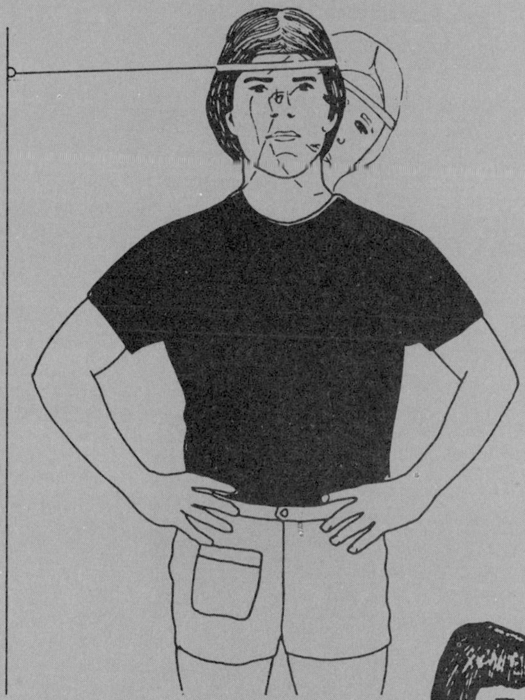

Station 2: Arms

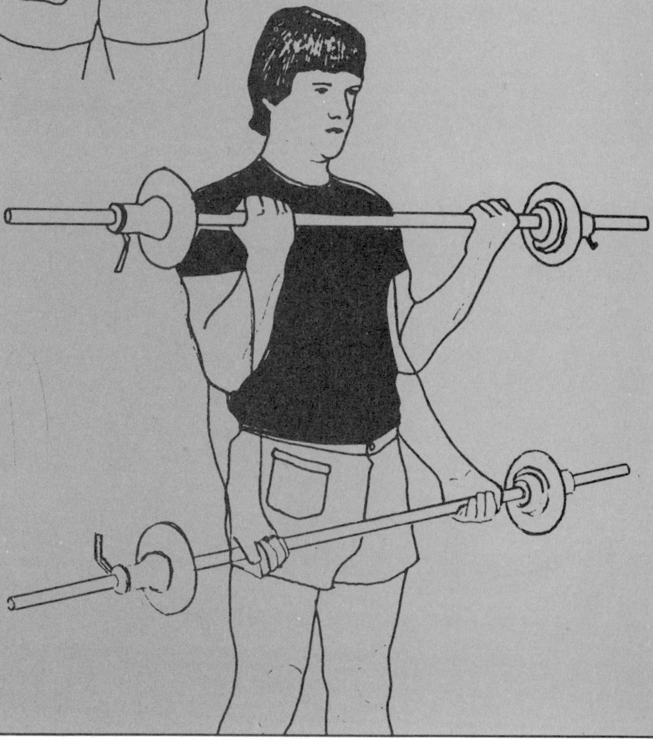

Model Exercise Circuit Chart

Station 3: Hands

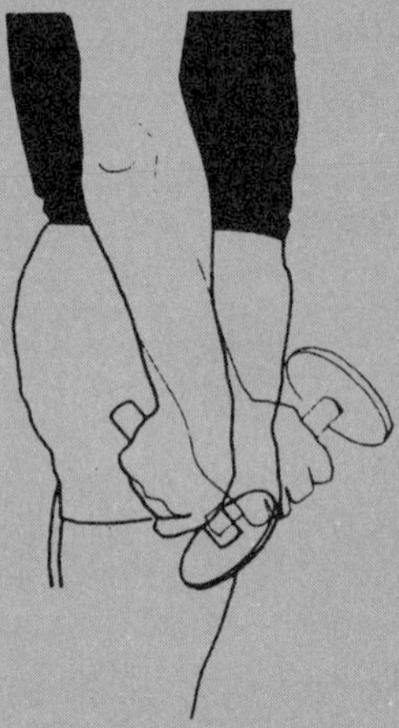

Station 4: Shoulders

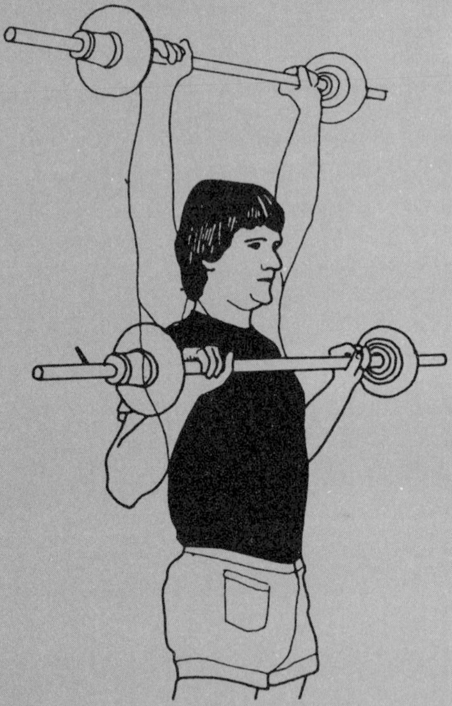

Station 5: Abdomen

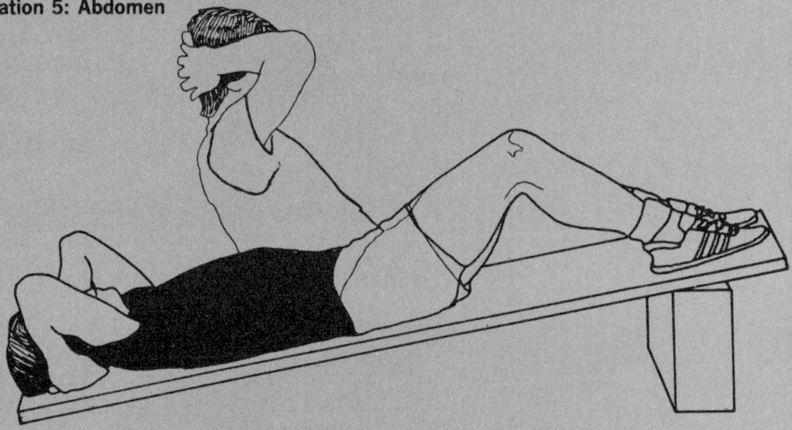

Model Exercise Circuit Chart

Station 6: Back

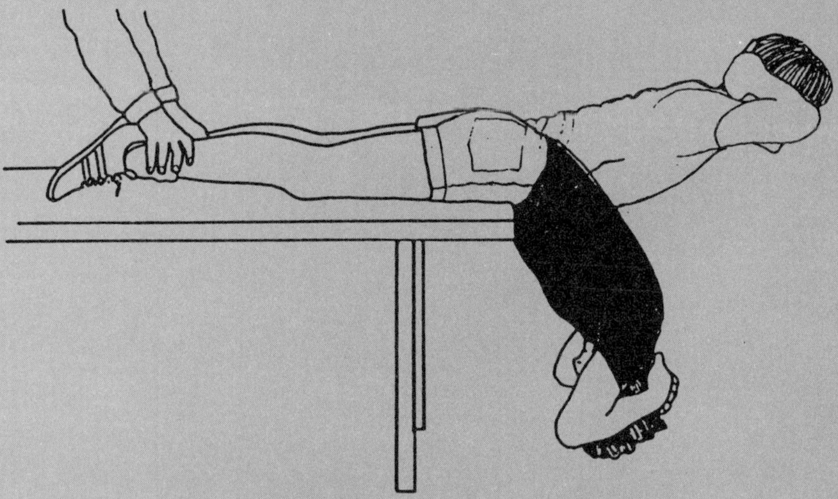

Station 7: Chest

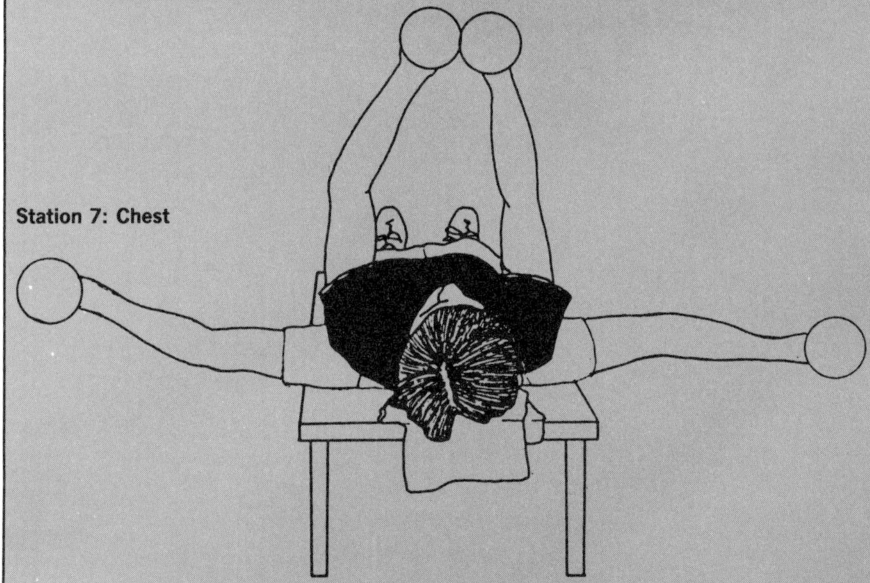

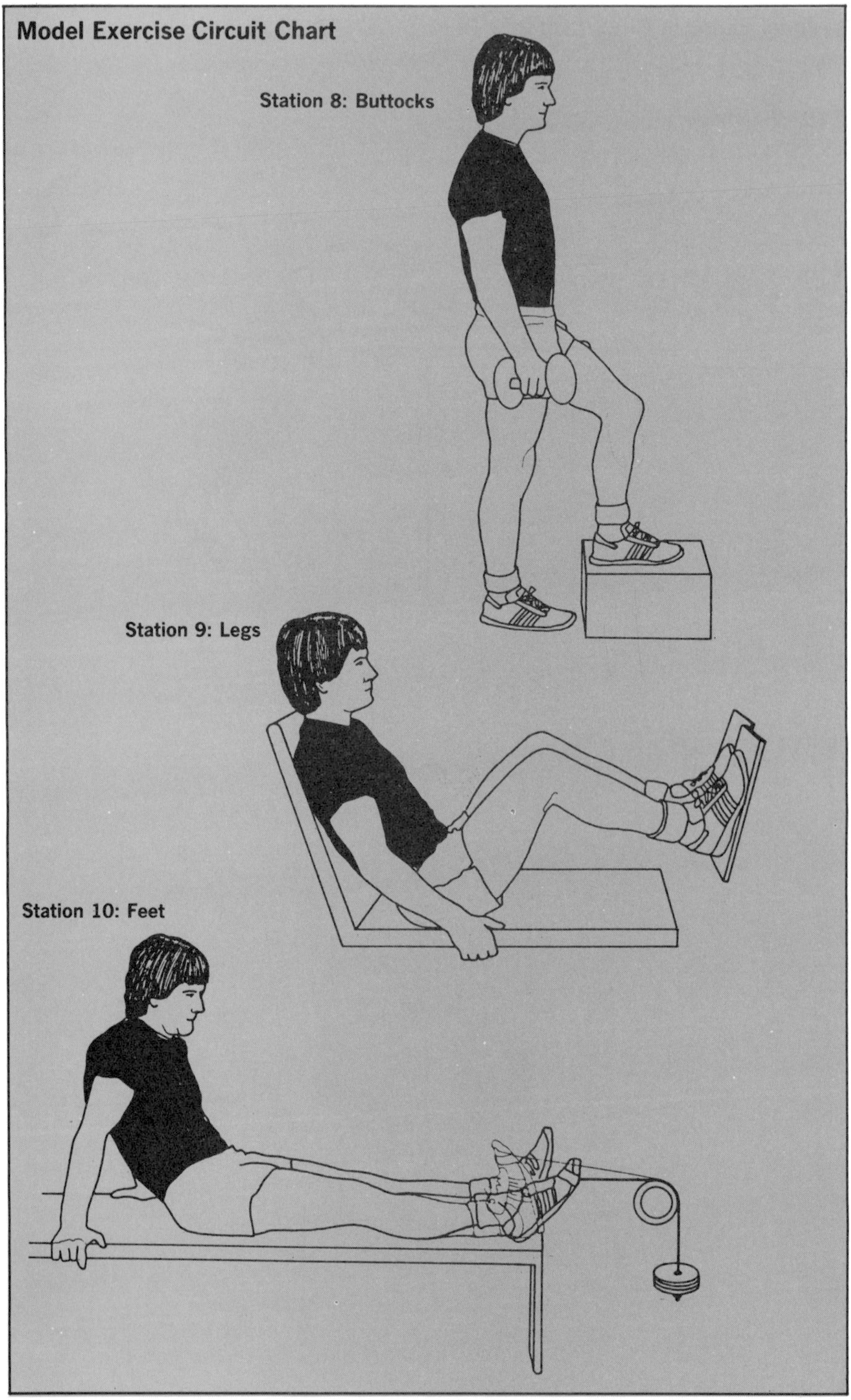
Model Exercise Circuit Chart
Station 8: Buttocks
Station 9: Legs
Station 10: Feet

Group One: Muscle Builders

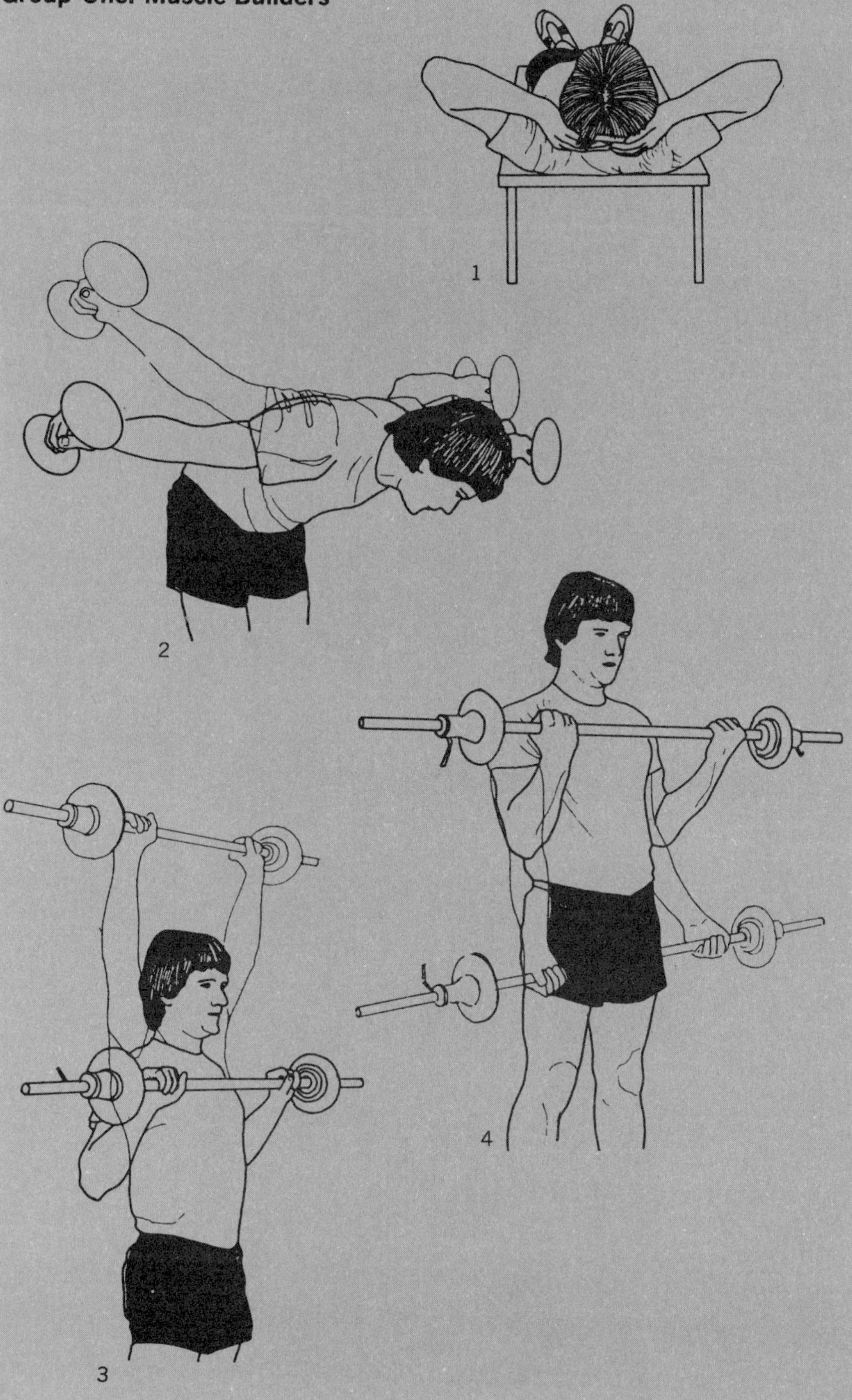

Group One: Muscle Builders

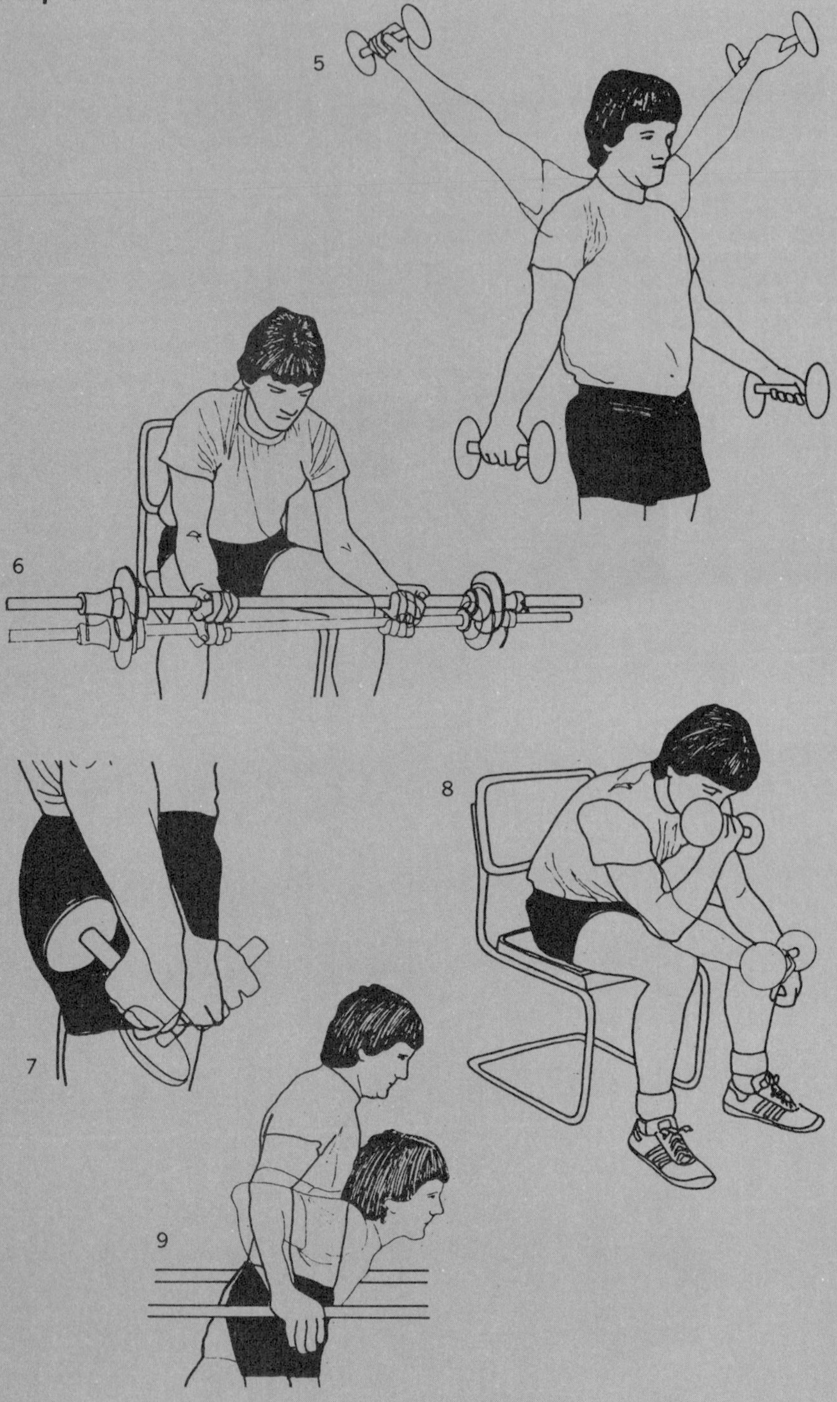

Group Two: Muscle Builders

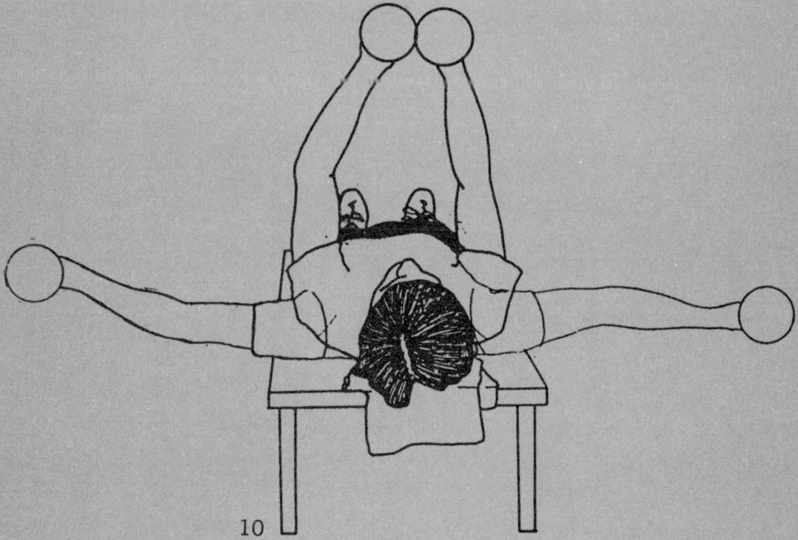

10

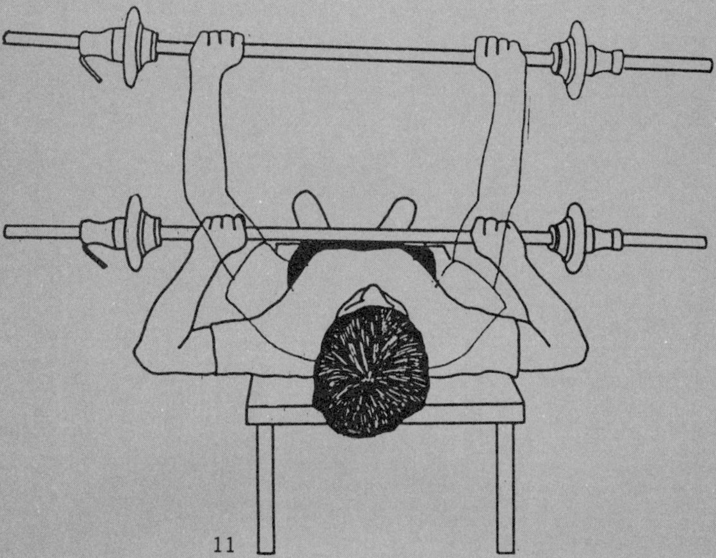

11

Group Two: Muscle Builders

12

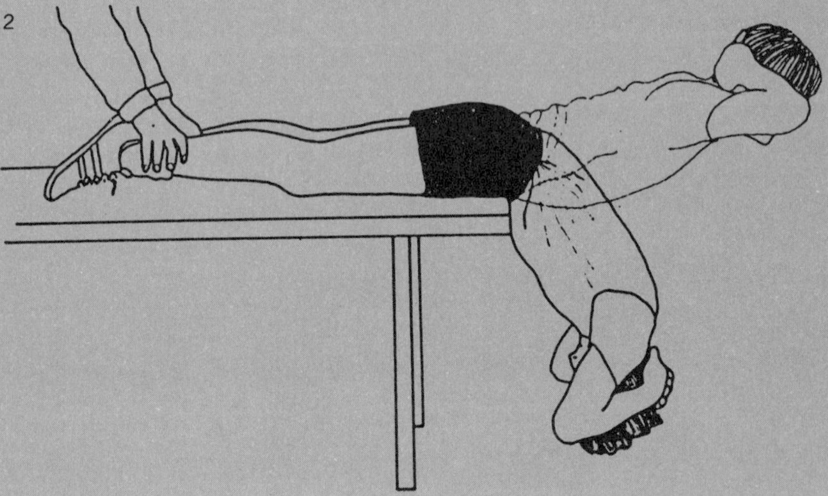

13

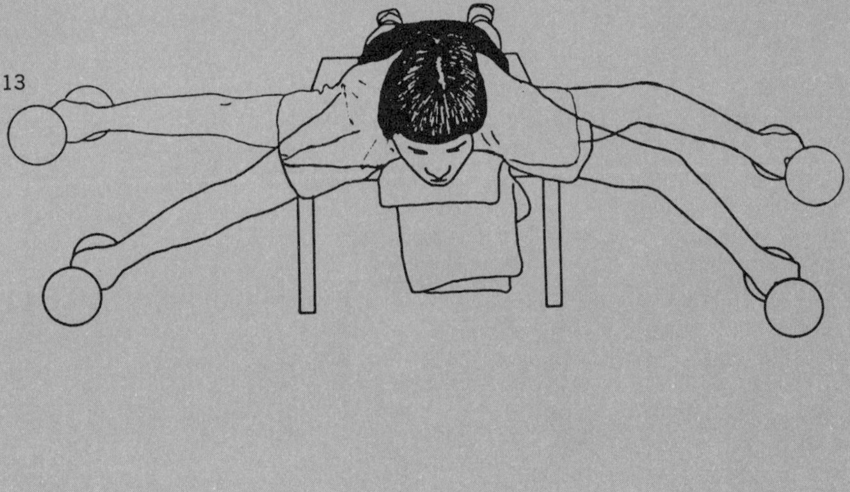

Group Two: Muscle Builders

14

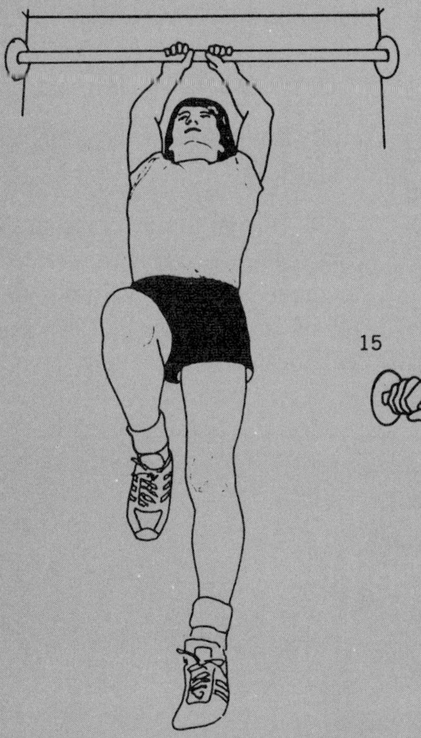

15

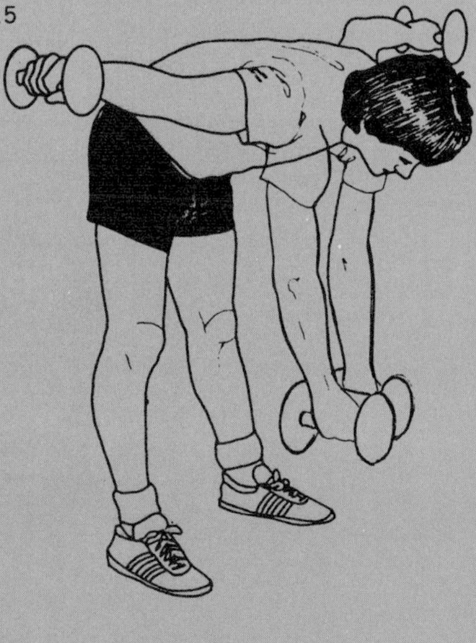

16

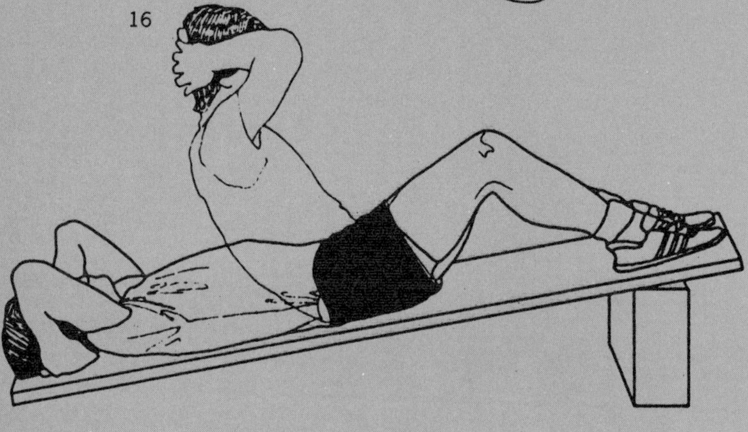

Walking

Americans love to walk, fitness experts say. But many people don't get the most from the walking they do because they don't approach it as exercise.

Walking does qualify as exercise, however—one of the best. To ensure that you get the benefits that walking can bring, a seven-part procedure is suggested.

1. Picture walking as a separate fitness activity. Learn to take your own pulse. Then calculate what your target pulse rate per minute should be for your age. That usually means 70 to 85 percent of your maximum rate (220 minus your age in years).

2. Buy a pair of comfortable running shoes.

3. Design a starter program for your own use. Promise yourself, for example, that you will walk 20 minutes four days a week. Raise that target to 25 minutes a day, four days,

Warm-up Exercises for Joggers

Adductor stretch

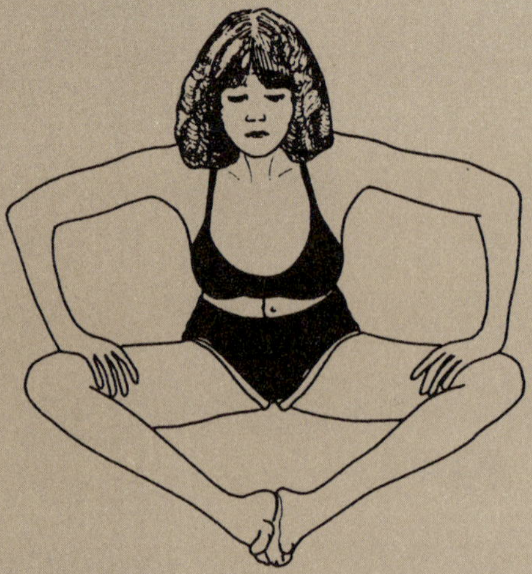

Back stretch

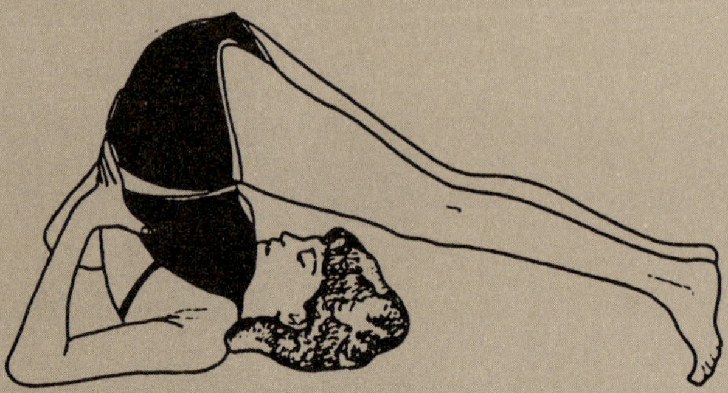

Warm-up Exercises for Joggers

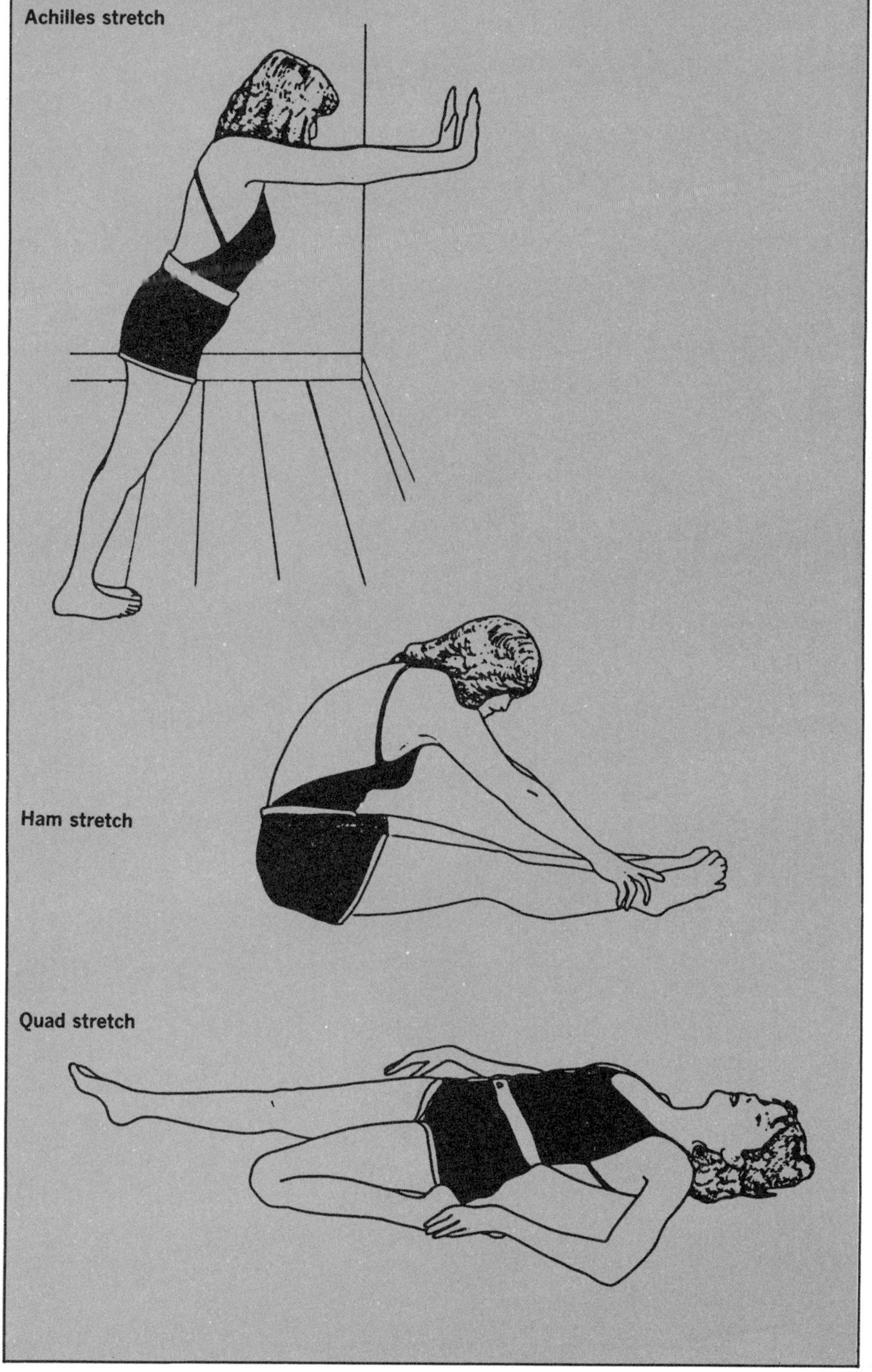

Aerobic Dance Step

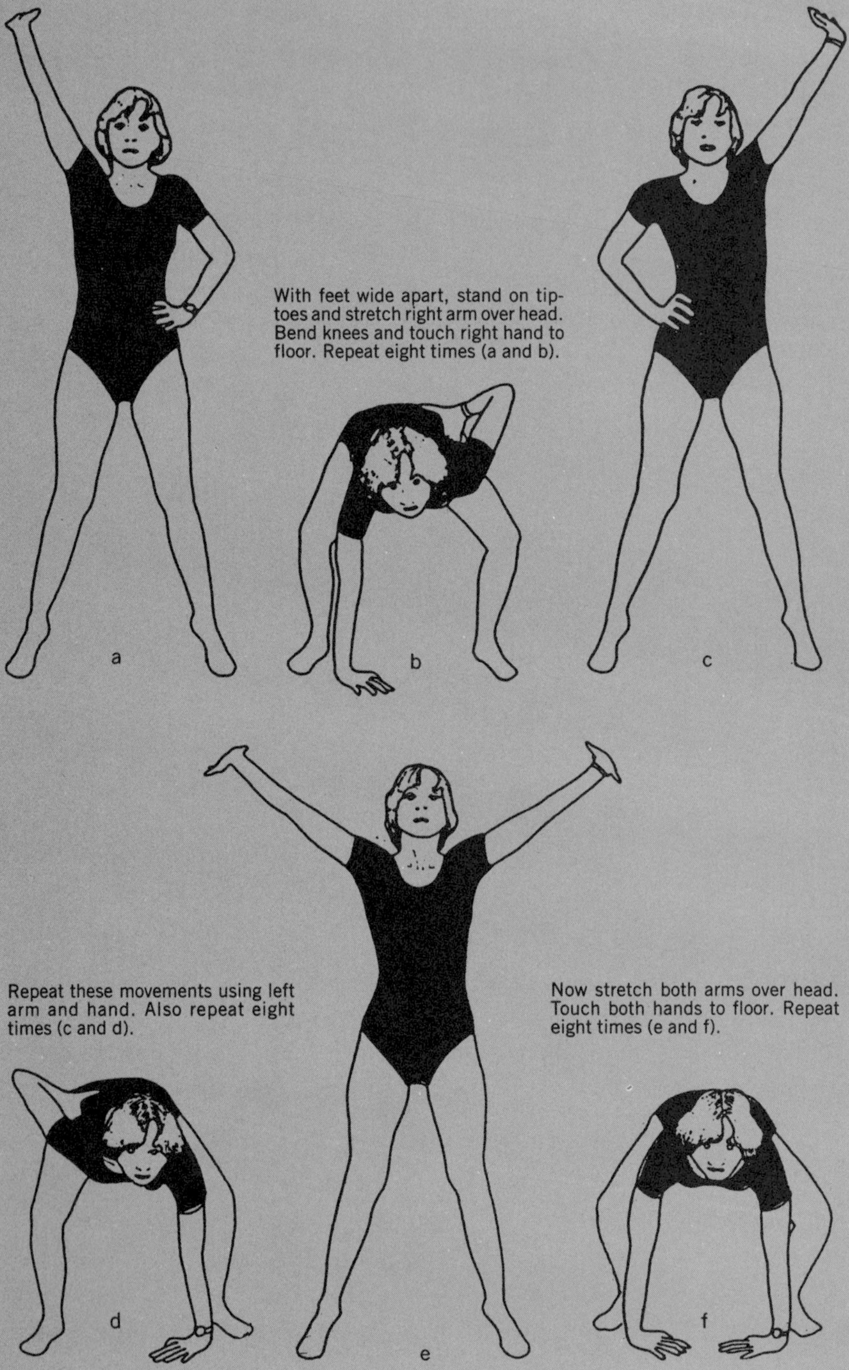

With feet wide apart, stand on tiptoes and stretch right arm over head. Bend knees and touch right hand to floor. Repeat eight times (a and b).

Repeat these movements using left arm and hand. Also repeat eight times (c and d).

Now stretch both arms over head. Touch both hands to floor. Repeat eight times (e and f).

and then increase the level by increments of five minutes. A good final target might be 45 minutes four days a week.

4. Take your own pulse every day and keep a record of your findings. Watch your pulse rate decline as your body becomes more efficient.

5. In walking, breathe rhythmically. Let your arms swing by your sides.

6. Use your walk as recreation even though you've planned it as a kind of independent fitness program. As you walk, notice colors, trees, buildings, people. Try not to think of work.

7. Schedule mini-walks in the midafternoon, when your body may be starting to drag. Walk, if possible, instead of taking the usual coffee break. You should obtain a fresh charge of energy and a clearer head.

Everybody walks, it seems. Why regard walking as exercise, then? Because walking can do almost as much for individual fitness as jogging.

There are other reasons for making walking a part of a fitness program, or for walking at every opportunity apart from the program. Walking burns up calories. Walking does not strain joints and muscles as some other exercises do. Walking can be enjoyable, as dedicated walkers have testified down through history.

Conceivably, the typical modern American could go through an entire day without taking more than 15, 20, or 50 long strides. To do so, it would only be necessary to utilize the elevators, autos, escalators, and other devices that make walking unnecessary. But for those who consider walking both fun and a learnable art, walking as exercise puts those devices into the shade.

Let's consider some of the types of walking that the individual can incorporate into his or her life.

Speedwalking

A technique of walking as fast as possible while swinging the arms back and forth, speedwalking or racewalking is rapidly gaining in popularity. The arms are used to provide rhythm and momentum. The elbows remain bent at 90-degree angles. The speedwalker, like other walkers, needs only comfortable exercise clothes and shoes. Many speedwalkers wear runners' shoes.

Speedwalking burns up 620 to 870 calories an hour. As an exercise, it puts every muscle to work in an aerobic and circulorespiratory way. The exaggerated hip movements help firm up buttocks, thighs, and hips. The beginner should aim for three half-hour speedwalking tours a week, over that period maintaining a rate of three or four miles per hour. Leg-stretching warm-ups before starting and cooldowns at the end of the walk will help in the same ways as warm-ups and cool-downs before and after other exercise sessions.

As the speedwalker progresses, he or she can step up the walking pace to five or more miles per hour. If possible, keep records of the date, the distance walked, and the time consumed.

Interval Walking

Other approaches to walking are less strenuous, but they offer many of the advantages of speedwalking if performed regularly. Interval walking, for example, involves walking briskly for 30 seconds, then slowly for 30 more seconds. That process is continued until the walker is reasonably tired. Ideally, again, records are kept in interval and other approaches to walking.

Continuous Walking

In continuous walking the exerciser sets himself an objective and walks until he achieves it. The first time out, wisdom dictates an easy pace. On subsequent walks, perhaps every two or three days, the pace is stepped up.

Tempo Walking

In the walking format known as tempo walking, the walker moves easily for five minutes. Then he walks at top speed for one minute. The relaxed-then-rapid repetitions are continued over a set distance. Every few workouts, the rapid phase of the tempo walk should be lengthened by five seconds. The cool-down is accomplished by walking easily for five final minutes.

Long-Stride Walk

A variation on tempo, continuous, and interval walking, the long-stride walk involves what the name indicates: a period of long-stride walking that is inserted into the basic continuous, interval, or tempo walk. Walking with the longest possible strides helps in particular to condition the hips and buttocks. As a variation on the variation, the walker can insert into his walk periods of walking with short strides while the body inclines well forward.

Hill Walking

After a warm-up of five minutes of easy walking in a flat area, the hill walker sets off to mount a low hill. For best body conditioning, the uphill pace is rapid, the downhill pace moderate. Hill walking calls for discretion; the walker should not attempt too much too soon—as in every other area of fitness conditioning. Steep hills may have to be avoided at first.

Stationary Walking

Walking in place, or stationary walking, involves little more than simulated walking in which the exerciser lifts his knees as high as possible. Starting at an easy pace, he gradually "walks" faster. Stationary walking can be done according to the continuous, interval, or tempo methods.

Variety Walking

Excepting the speedwalk, the several approaches to walking can be combined and recombined to taste. One approach can be used one day, another approach the next. In this way, the exerciser injects variety into the walking phase of his fitness program.

Hopping, Jumping, and Stepping

Various hopping, jumping, and stepping activities can add spice and enjoyment to the fitness program and can prepare the individual for sports and games involving similar movements. All three exercises should be approached with the same respect that is paid to other parts of the fitness program. That means heart rates should be monitored as necessary, the exercises should become regular features of the fitness program, and, if possible, records of performance should be kept.

Jumping

In the jump, or side-to-side jump, the legs remain relatively straight and are flexed only slightly while the body is in the air.

A small object may be placed on the floor to serve as a guide in side-to-side jumping. A stripe on the floor or carpeting will accomplish the same purpose. Make sure that you clear the stripe or object in a lateral direction. In jumping again, clear it in the other direction. You should maintain a continuous side-to-side motion, with both feet leaving the floor and touching down again at the same time. Jumping, like hopping, should be continued for a minute or more.

Hopping

If done properly, the kangaroo hop, or plain hop, can build agility as well as circulorespiratory capacity. To hop, place both feet together, bend over with hands reaching backward, crouch slightly, and jump upward. Your knees should be brought up toward your chest while your body is in the air.

Hopping should be continued for one minute or more. Persons in good physical condition, can, of course, continue the exercise for longer periods. It then becomes a genuine aerobic activity.

Stepping

An exercise routine including hopping and jumping may also include the step exercise. The step involves stepping up onto a bench or other raised, firm object in repetitive movements that are continued for a minute or more.

The jump, hop, and step have been combined in a training circuit that was specifically designed as preparation for participating in high-movement sports. The circuit includes six stations or stages covering up to six minutes each:

1. Side-to-side jumping
2. Quad sitting, in which the seated exerciser tightens his quadriceps or front thigh muscles for 40 to 50 seconds
3. The kangaroo hop
4. Heel and toe raises, in which the exerciser stands with feet apart, rises on his toes, returns to the floor, turns his toes outward, straight ahead, and inward, then rolls back on his heels
5. The bench step
6. Half squats

Exercise for the Heart Patient, for Postop Patients, and for the Hospitalized

Exercise has been portrayed as a means by which the healthy person can build more health, strength, and fitness. The weight of medical opinion today holds that exercise can and should have an important place in the life of the sick, disabled, or seriously handicapped person.

In each individual case the exercise has not only to be approved and recommended by a physician; the exercises or sports should also be specifically designed to correct problems or help the person regain physical health. At the least, exercises should make it possible for the ailing person to maintain some level of fitness.

Each exercise should be geared to fulfilling a particular purpose. Following breast surgery, a doctor may prescribe arm and shoulder exercises designed to restore strength in the woman's upper body. Following a coronary attack, a graduated program of walking or swimming may be prescribed. Before a heart attack, a person showing signs of severe tension may be told that he should engage in any of dozens of kinds of relaxing activities. These can range from yoga to golf to simple stretching exercises. Or they can include many other activities discussed in this chapter. In each instance, the exercises are chosen with the patient's problems and condition in mind.

After the Heart Attack

Through regular exercise the heart attack victim earns a second chance in life. But he faces a difficult challenge. He has to devote constant effort to his exercise regimen. If he backslides, or drops out of the program, he usually finds that deterioration sets in within days or weeks.

The training program that the heart attack victim undertakes should be geared to his personal physical situation. He should start it only with the approval of his physician, and should progress at the prescribed rate. In most cases the post-heart attack exerciser will be asked to keep track of his rate of progression. In all cases he will be asked to see his physician at prescribed intervals.

Postcoronary exercise has, like all exercise, specific goals. It can be very effective in increasing cardiac efficiency by decreasing the heart rate and the consumption of oxygen at a given workload. The training, taken initially in small doses, makes it possible for the muscles to extract more oxygen from the blood. The heart can then pump less blood for a given task. In time, the heart becomes less susceptible to the ill effects of stress hormones, or catecholamines, that circulate in the blood. The patient usually learns to respond better to stress-filled situations. He can control his weight more easily.

With improved physical condition may come other benefits. The patient may experience little or none of the depression that is so common following a heart attack. Chest pains may dwindle or disappear entirely. Many patients experience relief from angina—a cramp-like chest pain—as their fitness levels improve.

Problems and Preparations

The postcoronary exercise regimen calls for advance consideration of a number of problems. A practical problem is that the patient may find that the program cuts into his work, family, and social life. If he lives in a large city, he may have difficulty commuting to and from the clinic, YMCA, or other institution offering the program.

In consultation with his physician, the patient can in most cases develop an exercise program that eliminates many such problems. In so doing, he increases the likelihood that he can continue to exercise consistently. Typically, he reduces the number of medically supervised sessions to a minimal weekly number compatible with training effectiveness and safety. The "minimal number" may be once or twice weekly. Some physicians give their patients specific instructions and then trust the individual to continue on his own.

Authorities believe that a heart attack victim's assumption of responsibility for all or part of his own fitness program teaches the patient to cope with the stresses, strains, and difficulties that he inevitably faces as he moves toward complete rehabilitation. Also, he grows accustomed to normal living more quickly. In a sense, he becomes by degrees independent of physician, clinic, or other medical advisor without neglecting basic precautions or the prescribed periodic checkups.

A stress test should precede the start of the fitness program. The patient can determine his own sustained maximum heart rate by subtracting his age from the figure 220. Thus a man of 40 would have a maximum sustained rate of 180.

In later stress retesting, usually carried out at four to eight week intervals, the patient may be asked to exercise until his heart rate approaches the maximum. Initially, in each of the four to six exercise sessions each week, he works his heart for half an hour at a rate equal to about 70 or 75 percent of the maximum. The man of 40, mentioned earlier, is thus able to bring his exercising heart rate to about 126.

In a second phase, again undertaken with his physician's approval, the patient may be allowed to bring his exercising heart rate as high as 85 per cent of the maximum. A third and even a fourth phase might follow if necessary.

The stress test may be administered with a bicycle ergometer or a treadmill. During the test, the electrocardiogram is monitored continuously. Breath analyses may be taken as a means of estimating the patient's actual maximum oxygen consumption. Afterward, depending on the program, the patient may be placed in a "complicated" or "uncomplicated" category. In the uncomplicated group are those who have worked their hearts to 70 to 75 percent of the maximum heart rate without developing abnormalities in the electrocardiogram. In the complicated group are those who cannot finish the tests because evidence of cardiac ischemia, or lack of oxygen for the heart muscle, has appeared.

As a final preparatory step, the patient may receive a personal exercise prescription. After later stress tests, he learns, he will receive new prescriptions as he progresses. He may, if needed, receive instructions in the methods of taking a pulse count.

Exercises of Choice

Recommended exercises of postcoronary patients include walking, jogging, swimming, and others. But the exercises cannot be taken randomly. The patient should walk or jog a specific distance, or swim a specified number of laps, while timing himself with a stopwatch. He will probably be told that he cannot use a regular watch in timing his sessions because such a method of measurement lacks accuracy.

A typical clinic session for a postcoronary group might start with a talk or discussion. Patients learn that they can discuss problems relating to their physical situation or their home exercise prescriptions. They also find out about the "do's" and "don't's" that apply to them, about medications and their uses, and about the meanings of various cardiac signs. Sexual problems may come up for discussion; so may fad diets and the values of "cures" for heart disease that have been reported in the media.

The beginner's session may continue with a 10- to 20-minute warm-up. While music provides a rhythmic accompaniment, the patient may go through simple flexibility exercises interspersed with light walking and jogging. In a class session, the group may halt all activity at specified intervals to take a pulse count. If any individual indicates that he is having chest pains or other problems, he may be asked to stop and undergo a further medical assessment, including electrocardiograms. Instruction for all participants will usually cover proper jogging techniques. Following the warm-up, participants go into their prescribed exercise series. They conclude with a cool-down period lasting 10 to 15 minutes.

As postcoronary exercise sessions continue, the patient may be asked to keep a detailed log. Entries cover current prescriptions, the time and distance data on each workout, and pre- and postworkout heart rates. Periodically—usually once a month—the patient takes his resting heart rate, preferably before he gets out of bed in the morning. He may be asked to ascertain the average of three consecutive morning heart counts. In all cases, the distance, speeds, and heart rates are carefully charted for each patient.

Using such information, a physician can easily gauge a patient's progress. In most cases a patient will show improvement within weeks. But doctors believe that an exercise regimen should be continued for at least a year if substantial benefits are to be achieved. Two years may be necessary in many cases.

When Not to Exercise

Many heart attack patients cannot wait to get started on an exercise program. They may not understand that when a physician advises against exercise of any kind, or prescribes very light exercise at the beginning of a program, he usually has reasons that relate to the condition of the patient's heart.

In myocardial infarction, for instance, a scar forms on the heart. The scar may take as long as six weeks to heal. Exercise taken before the healing process has been completed may cause the heart wall to bulge, forming an aneurysm. The bulging can occur with each heartbeat and can lead to additional serious heart problems.

If a patient has experienced an acute myocardial infarction, a relatively rare occurrence, either the right or the left sides of the heart may be seriously affected. Exercise may not become permissible until complete recovery of pump efficiency has taken place. The period may last for two or three months or more.

An aneurysm in one of the large blood vessels, such as the aorta, may preclude vigorous training for a period of weeks or months.

A patient who senses rapidly progressing anginal pain while exercising may be receiving warnings of another heart attack. Normally, he should stop exercising at once and not resume until he has medical clearance.

A generalized infection of the heart area can accompany such major diseases as rheumatic fever or diphtheria. Infection may also occur with viral problems such as poliomyelitis, influenza, or infectious mononucleosis. The heart involvement, known as myocarditis, makes exercise hazardous, especially where the patient is feverish. A doctor may suggest that the patient wait a week after his temperature returns to normal before resuming his exercise regimen.

Irregular heart action may lead to serious and even fatal ventricular fibrillation, or rapid, irregular contractions of the heart muscle. Fibrillation always precludes additional exercising until the normal heart action can be restored through use of medication. Mild rhythm irregularities may not, however, be considered serious enough to terminate a training program.

Other types of heart problems that may necessitate cessation or modification of an exercise program include some types of valvular heart disease, blood clots in the lungs or peripheral arteries, repetitive heart failure that leads to enlarged heart, and complete heart block. Hypertension that cannot be controlled by medication may indicate that exercise will drive the blood pressure up higher, possibly to dangerous levels. Some forms of congenital heart disease make exercise inadvisable.

In still other cases a physician who recommends that a patient avoid exercise may be basing his judgment on noncardiac conditions. Heavy exercise may, for example, be contraindicated where the patient has severe uncontrolled diabetes. The same may be true of patients with epilepsy or narcolepsy, a tendency to experience sudden, uncontrollable attacks of sleepiness. Because exercise increases the demands made on the lungs, kidneys, and liver, exercise may be ruled out if the patient has kidney or lung diseases, tuberculosis, or other conditions affecting these vital organs.

Inappropriate exercise can aggravate other diseases and physical problems. Those falling in this category include some types of arthritis; chronic low-back trouble, a complaint that may be exacerbated by jogging; anemia; and some relatively rare kinds of neurological, muscular, or glandular diseases.

Basic Program

While every postcoronary exercise program must be tailored to the needs and capabilities of the individual patient, some generalizations can be made. An outline of a typical walking-jogging program includes, for example, four basic phases. In each, the regimen includes five weekly sessions, with two days of rest taken at any time during the week.

1. *Adjustment phase:* In this phase, the patient works into the program by gradual stages. For two weeks he may be asked to walk a mile in 30 minutes. In each of three follow-up two-week periods, he walks 1.5 miles in 42 minutes, 2 miles in 50 minutes, and 2.5 miles in 57.5 minutes.

2. *Action phase 1:* In action phase 1, beginning with the conclusion of the adjustment phase, the patient walks a mile in 20 minutes, continuing that routine for two weeks. For two additional weeks he walks two miles in 40 minutes; then for a final two weeks he covers a three-mile course five times weekly in 60 minutes. The time allotted for each walk is slightly higher for the patient who is over 45 years of age.

It should be noted that patients with higher levels of maximum oxygen consumption may be allowed to pass through the three stages with shorter time prescriptions. The patient with a very good level of consumption would probably be allowed to complete the three-mile course in as little as 42 minutes. In approaching the target, he would be moving through a walking-jogging phase of training. The point at which full-time jogging becomes part of the regimen is usually reached where the patient faces the task of covering a mile in 14 or 15 minutes.

3. *Action phase 2:* In this phase, the patient graduates to jogging exclusively. The transition may take many months. The exercising patient should always watch for adverse heart symptoms. He may have to make adjustments in his program on the basis of what he observes.

In action phase 2, the patient again

increases the intensity of the workout while simultaneously decreasing the distance covered. Starting out, for example, the patient might walk-jog over a one-mile course in 18 minutes. After two weeks he might allow himself 16 minutes to walk-jog a mile, then continue that program for two weeks. By such easy stages he increases the pace to one mile in ten minutes. He then goes back to the 18-minute mile, but covers a two-mile course. In the end, having gradually reduced the number of minutes per mile, he is covering a three-mile course in 30 minutes, jogging all the way.

4. *Action phase 3:* Using the same gradual approach, the patient progresses to the point where he is jogging five miles in 50 or 60 minutes. The process requires, normally, one year. The ability to undertake such long-distance jogging represents a major accomplishment. In most cases it pays off in terms of high levels of cardiorespiratory fitness. Some heart attack patients have progressed to the point where they have entered marathons.

Caveats

Even after he has reached a satisfactory fitness level the heart attack victim may have to be careful. He may, for example, avoid exercising at higher altitudes. At elevations over 4,000 or 5,000 feet, the oxygen pressure in the air sacs of the lungs decreases. The oxygen content in the circulating blood is correspondingly reduced.

The postcoronary patient should also watch for signs of overtraining, or staleness. This condition is characterized by chronic fatigue, irritability, susceptibility to minor infections including colds, insomnia, loss of appetite, and loss of concentration. The answer in such cases is to rest for a week or two. The body can then recuperate and adjust.

In many other situations the postcoronary program may have to be modified or suspended temporarily. Exercise types, times, and places may have to be chosen carefully. No recuperating patient should exercise heavily after a heavy meal; a wait of two hours is usually suggested. Outdoor exercise in very cold weather may have to be ruled out. The cold air may act as an irritant on the large air passages in the lungs—or exposure to cold may cause a sharp rise in blood pressure. Many physicians believe that a heart attack victim should never do isometric exercises.

Finally, patients on medication should consider the effects of exercise-plus-medicine on their heart rates. Small doses of some medications may not affect the heart rate, but larger doses may do so. Medication may also affect the individual's endurance levels; fatigue may set in more quickly where a patient is taking medication.

All Men (and Women) Were Created Equal

If men and women are essentially equal, can they take up the same sports? Can they participate in the same exercise regimens? Can they fill in their leisure hours with the same recreational activities?

They can, and they should. Women are taking up weight training, to name one example. Women are learning that bodily strength need not necessarily mean bulging biceps and triceps, and that they can be strong and healthy as a result of exercise and athletic endeavor—while also looking—and feeling—more graceful and attractive.

Increasingly, women are taking up exercise programs; indeed, many more women than men of comparable ages are going into sports activities. And, they are developing the exercise and sports-recreation programs that best suit their temperament and tastes. Jogging is only one of many possible answers.

There are some physiological differences between men and women that are of special relevance in a recreational or fitness program. For example, women are more flexible than men at all ages. Also, women normally carry a somewhat greater percentage of fat than men. For that reason, among others, women do not so readily develop the muscle bulges that male weight lifters have.

Women have heart rates that are five to ten beats per minute faster than those for men. This finding is interesting in view of the fact that before puberty girls and boys do not differ substantially in terms of maximum oxygen consumption. It prompts the question of whether or not women's heart rates are culturally conditioned. Are they more rapid than those of men because of the traditions that have long forced different patterns of exercise and other behavior for girls and women? That question has not yet been answered.

Some other differences may be mentioned. The working capacity of the average woman in the postpuberty years has been found to be about 85 percent of that of the average man of comparable age. That effect comes about because of the woman's smaller heart muscle size and strength capacity. Thus women generally find that while exercising their pulse rates rise more rapidly and to higher levels than those of men.

Some Misconceptions about Competition

It follows that if men and women can take part in the same exercises and sports, they can also take part in the same competitive activities, whether athletic or of some other kind. However, consideration should be given to the physiological differences between the sexes, including the different heart rates. Testing conducted in a physician's office, laboratory, or clinic should follow the same procedures as for men. Training effects should be sought by the same means. And the same precompetition protocols that apply to men apply to women.

Some authorities maintain that women are assuming unnecessary and perhaps serious risks when they take part in competitive activities or sports that involve heavy body contact. The risks center in the breast area, where bruises and contusions can do permanent, painful damage.

But physicians see little difference between the sexes with respect to the desirability of engaging in noncontact activities. Girls and boys, men and women, have nearly equal capacity for competitive sports and games—aside from the limitations noted—and can enjoy such activities equally.

Some Gynecological Facts

On the basis of extensive evidence, gynecologists agree that:

- Neither premenstrual changes in the body nor menstruation itself need interfere with a fitness program or ancillary activities. A woman should not assume that menstruation and its accompanying inconvenience need necessarily determine her participation or nonparticipation at any given time. That decision should, rather, be made with overall considerations of health and attitude in mind. Bear in mind that female Olympic athletes compete without regard to whether they are menstruating or not.

- Physically fit women appear to avoid many of the leg, back, hormonal, and other problems that seem to afflict women in general more than they do men. The problems thus need not be considered inevitable. They may be outgrowths of the state of "unfitness."

- Menopause need not involve a decrease in fitness activities. On the contrary, keeping fit means keeping normal, "doing your thing," and living and enjoying life. If menopause interferes seriously with the effort to keep fit, something may be complicating the situation, and a doctor should be consulted.

Exercise during Pregnancy and Postpartum

A fitness program can be continued with modifications during pregnancy. After pregnancy, the new mother can gradually resume—or start—a fitness program. In both cases the physician's advice should control both the

Expecting the Yoga Way

The cat/bidalasana

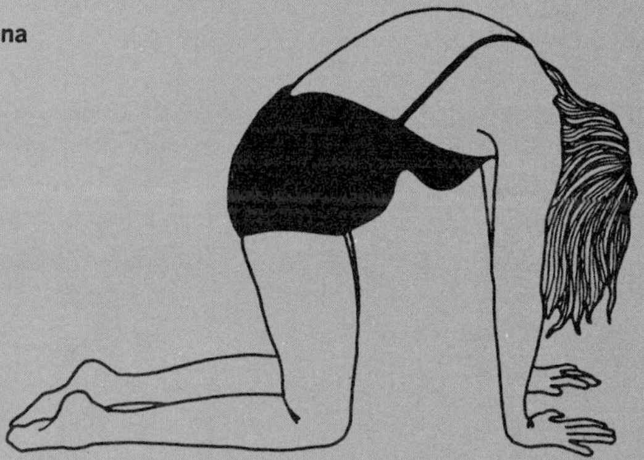

a

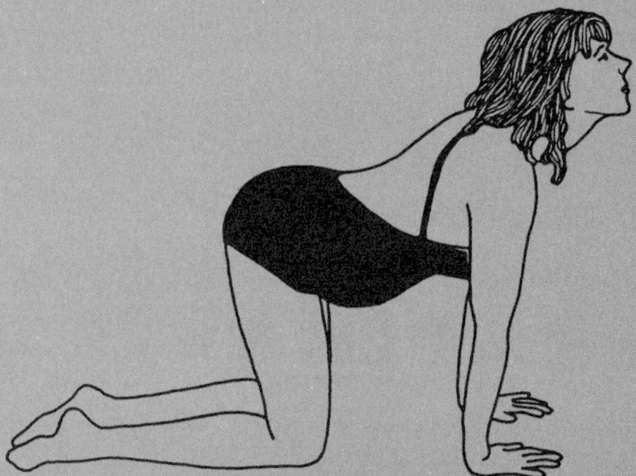

b

Variation for aswini-mudra

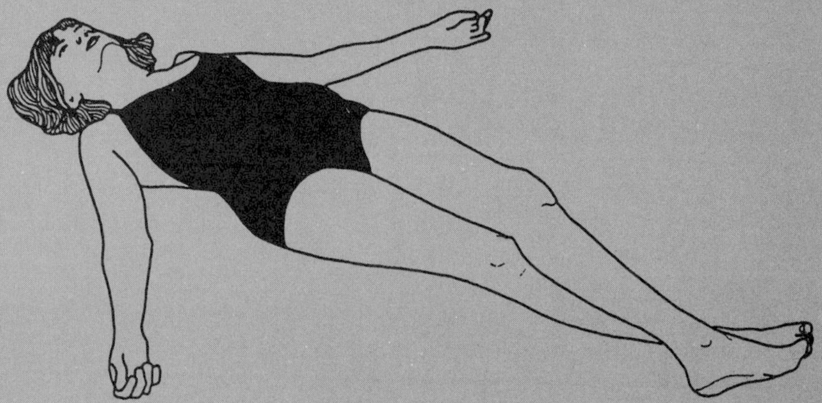

Expecting the Yoga Way

Deep breathing asana

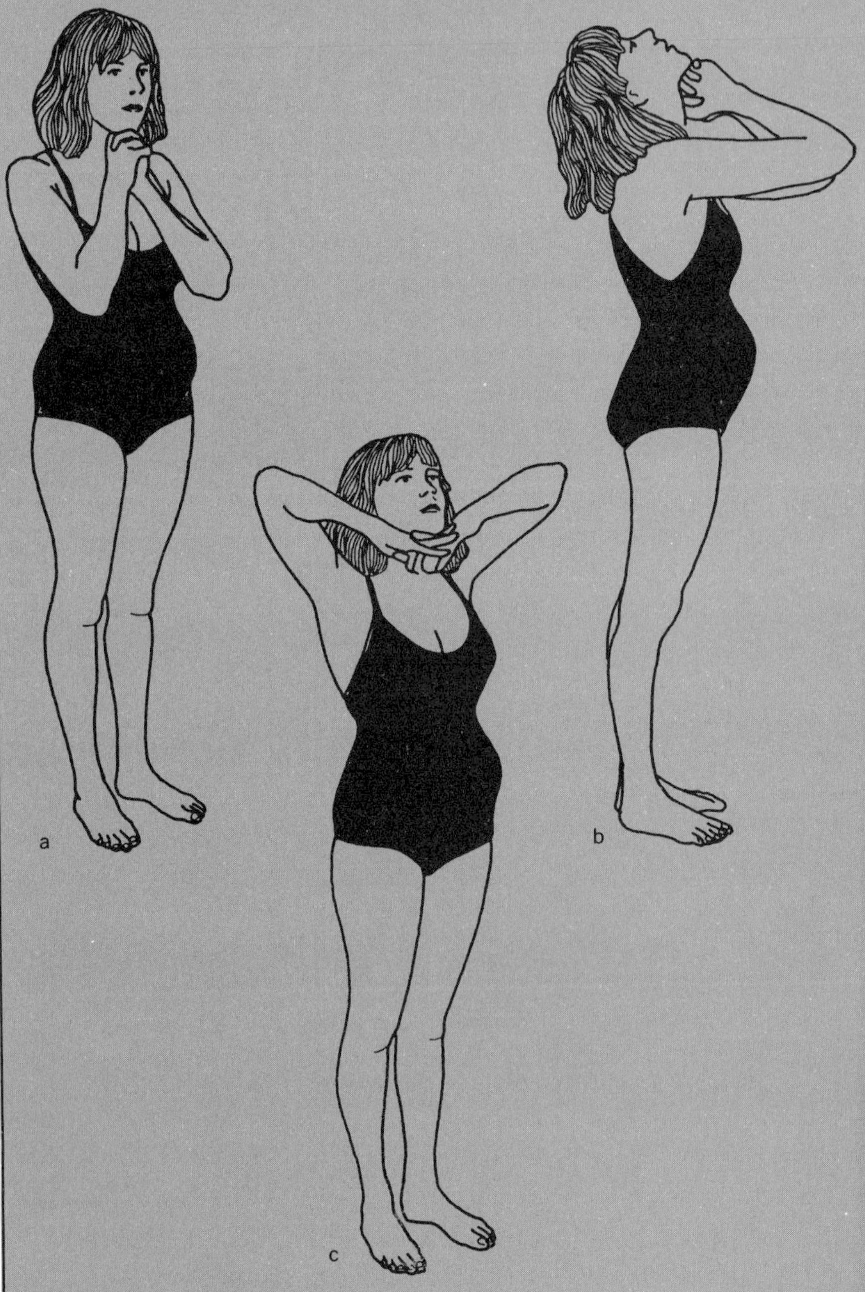

intensity of participation and the types of activities.

Clearly, the growing fetus interferes increasingly with strenuous activity. Activity of any kind may become difficult and tiring. After delivery, the problem may become one of "getting your figure back." *The Complete Book of Good Health,* by Phoebe Phillips and Pamela Hatch, contains exercises that your physician may approve for pregnancy and postpartum.

During Pregnancy

1. Start by sitting on the floor with legs spread wide. Placing your hands on your knees, lean forward gently. Let your head sink forward as far as you comfortably can. Let your hands slide toward your toes, stretching down; then bounce two or three times, gently.

2. While lying flat on your back with your feet anchored under a bed or chair, extend your arms straight up. Then pull yourself up to a sitting position, moving slowly.

3. This one is designed to relieve the backaches commonly encountered in pregnancy. Lying on your back with your knees bent, your soles flat on the floor, arms resting on the floor, press the small of your back against the floor. Hold that position for a slow four-count and release. Breathe deeply. Repeat four or five times.

Postpartum Exercises

The postpartum exercises can start the day after you deliver if your physician approves. Care should be taken to avoid overexertion or strain, but on the other hand, delaying too long can make it more difficult to get back in shape.

As a separate relaxer, try the back bend. Standing erect, feet slightly apart, let your head fall forward, dragging your upper body with it. Let your hands hang free. Take a deep breath and hold it while straightening up slowly. Once back in the erect position, exhale slowly. Breathe normally. Remember that as you straighten up your lower back muscles should do the work.

After-the-Baby

Here are eleven more after-the-baby exercises for slimming. The first four can start almost immediately after delivery. Three or four days later, try Nos. 5, 6, and 7. Leave the remaining exercises until about two weeks after delivery.

1. Lie on your back, knees bent and feet flat, and breathe in as deeply

Sexercises

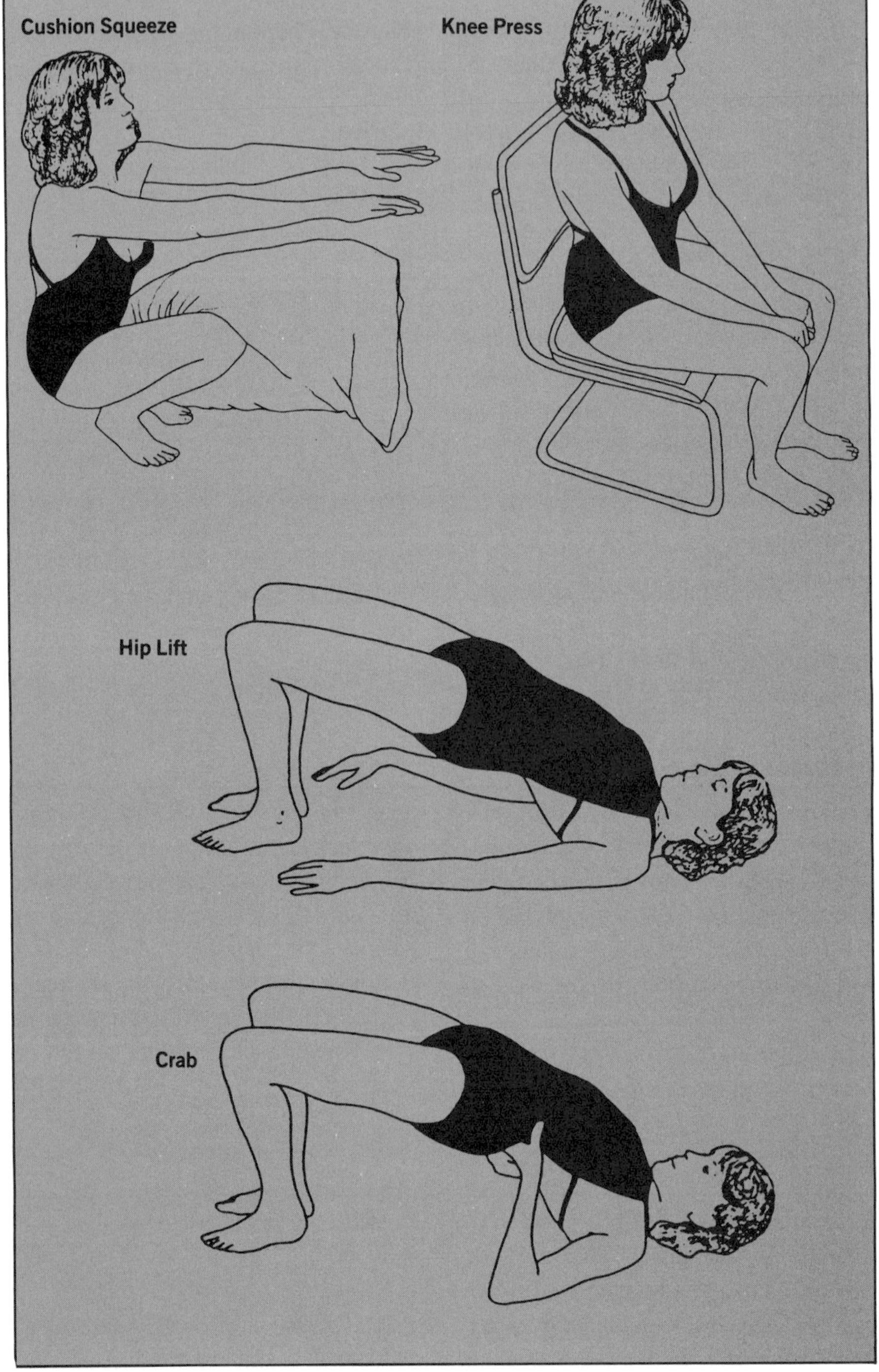

as you can. Let your stomach inflate. As you breathe out, draw your stomach in as far as possible. Repeat four times, three times a day.

2. Lying on your back still, with legs straight out, bend and stretch your ankles. Point your feet upward. Keeping your ankles as still as possible, wiggle your toes, then rotate your feet at the ankles. Repeat as in No. 1 above.

3. Again lying down with your legs straight, press your knees and thighs down as hard as you can. Relax between presses. Repeat as above.

4. To strengthen the pelvic muscles, lie on your back with your knees bent and slightly apart. Tighten the pelvic muscles slowly, with the pressure centering at mid-pelvis. Relax, then repeat as before.

5. While lying on your back with one leg bent, keep that leg still while trying to shorten the other leg. To "shorten," draw that straight leg up at the hips and waist. Then stretch it down in the same way. Repeat four times once a day.

6. While lying on your back with knees bent and feet flat, tighten your stomach muscles and draw them in. Press your waist down with your hands. While keeping your lower back flat, lift your hips slightly. Repeat four times, relaxing between exercises.

7. Again lying on your back with your knees bent and arms stretched out at your sides, twist from the waist only. Swing both knees over to the left, then repeat toward the right. Your feet and shoulders should remain in position. Repeat four times, once a day.

8. Lie on your back with your arms at your sides and lift your head slightly. Let your shoulders follow your head up. While raised, bend over to one side and reach down with your arm. Repeat on the other side.

9. Lying on your back, place your hands on the top part of your chest. Keeping your waist and back on the floor, raise your head and shoulders. Keep your eyes on your knees. Lower and relax.

10. Start as you do No. 9, but your hands should be at your sides. Lift your head and shoulders slightly. Bring your right arm up and over and touch the floor on the left side. All movement should come from the upper body.

11. In a final exercise, fold your arms under your head. Relax your neck muscles. Lift the right leg and bring it down. Relax and repeat with the left leg.

Exercises for Early Ages

The wise parent finds out about his child's physical needs and capabilities and tries to provide activity opportunities that match them. The unwise parent tries to force the child into an activity mold in which the child feels uncomfortable or downright embarrassed.

The wise parent understands that maturation refers to both physical and mental aspects of the child's makeup. Maturation in both areas may determine the child's ability to perform well in sports or games that demand a high level of coordination or skill. Maturation may in fact be more important than experience.

Do's and Don'ts

In regard to this maturation process here are a few "do's" and "don't's" for the parent:

- DO encourage your child to develop good activity habits.
- DO encourage your child to develop good posture habits as a way to be kind to his body.
- DO instruct your child in the rules of safety, good sportsmanship, and other aspects of exercise, sports, and athletic activity.
- DO make sure that your child has adequate medical and dental care.
- DON'T compare your child's performance unfavorably with the performances of others.
- DON'T force your child to take part in any game, exercise, or sport against his will or at too rapid a pace.
- DO take part in exercises or other activities with your child to teach techniques and attitudes in the most personal of all ways—by sharing time.
- Without forcing it, DO encourage your child to become fitness conscious.

Warning Signs

Children become sick just as adults do. As with adults, a sickness can be primarily physical or primarily emotional. In either case the sensation of weakness or incapacity will be completely real.

A physician should be consulted when a child, during play or exercise, displays any of the following symptoms:

- Blue lips or nails. Blueness should not occur unless the child is playing in cold, damp air—and that in itself might be unhealthful.

- Unusual fatigue. Excessive fatigue does not mean the child is reacting with laziness; it can mean that he needs rest, or a respite from the game.

- Excessive loss of breath. Breathlessness is normal after vigorous activity, but where it persists more than three to five minutes after termination of the activity, a medical examination may be in order.

- Shakiness. Shakiness that lasts more than ten minutes after strenuous activity may be abnormal.

- Cold sweat. The young person who breaks out in a cold sweat is rarely showing a normal reaction.

- Muscle twitching. Muscle twitches may or may not be normal, and should be watched.

In addition, children may exhibit other symptoms after taking part in exercise, games, or sports. These may require a physician's attention, especially if they continue. Among such symptoms are digestive upsets, fainting, headache, dizziness, pain not associated with an injury, disorientation, personality changes, uneven heartbeat, and interrupted sleep.

Fun Exercises for Preteens

The following exercises, adapted from Pat Stewart's *U.S. Fitness Book,* comprise a simple, easy-to-learn method of introducing a preteen child to a fitness program. The exercises have been designed for children six years old and older. Adult participation or supervision is appropriate if the young exercisers are six to ten years old. For those older than ten, supervision should not be necessary.

1. *The wheelbarrow:* Performed with two children, develops arm, shoulder, and abdominal strength. One participant kneels on the floor and places his hands down flat, directly under the shoulders. The fingers should point forward. The other child grasps the kneeling child's ankles and raises the legs. The first child "walks" forward on his hands while the partner keeps his feet suspended in the air at waist height. The walker should travel only three or four feet at the beginning.

2. *The tortoise and hare:* An aerobic exercise, the participants stand at attention. On the count of 1, the youngsters start to jog slowly in place. On the count of 2, the command "Hare" is given and the children double the tempo, lifting their knees high while their arms pump vigorously. On the count of 3, the command "Tortoise" brings the tempo back to an easy jog. The commands can be repeated every minute for four minutes.

3. *Trees in the wind:* Helps to develop trunk flexibility. The children

Exercises for Preteens

Trees-in-the Wind

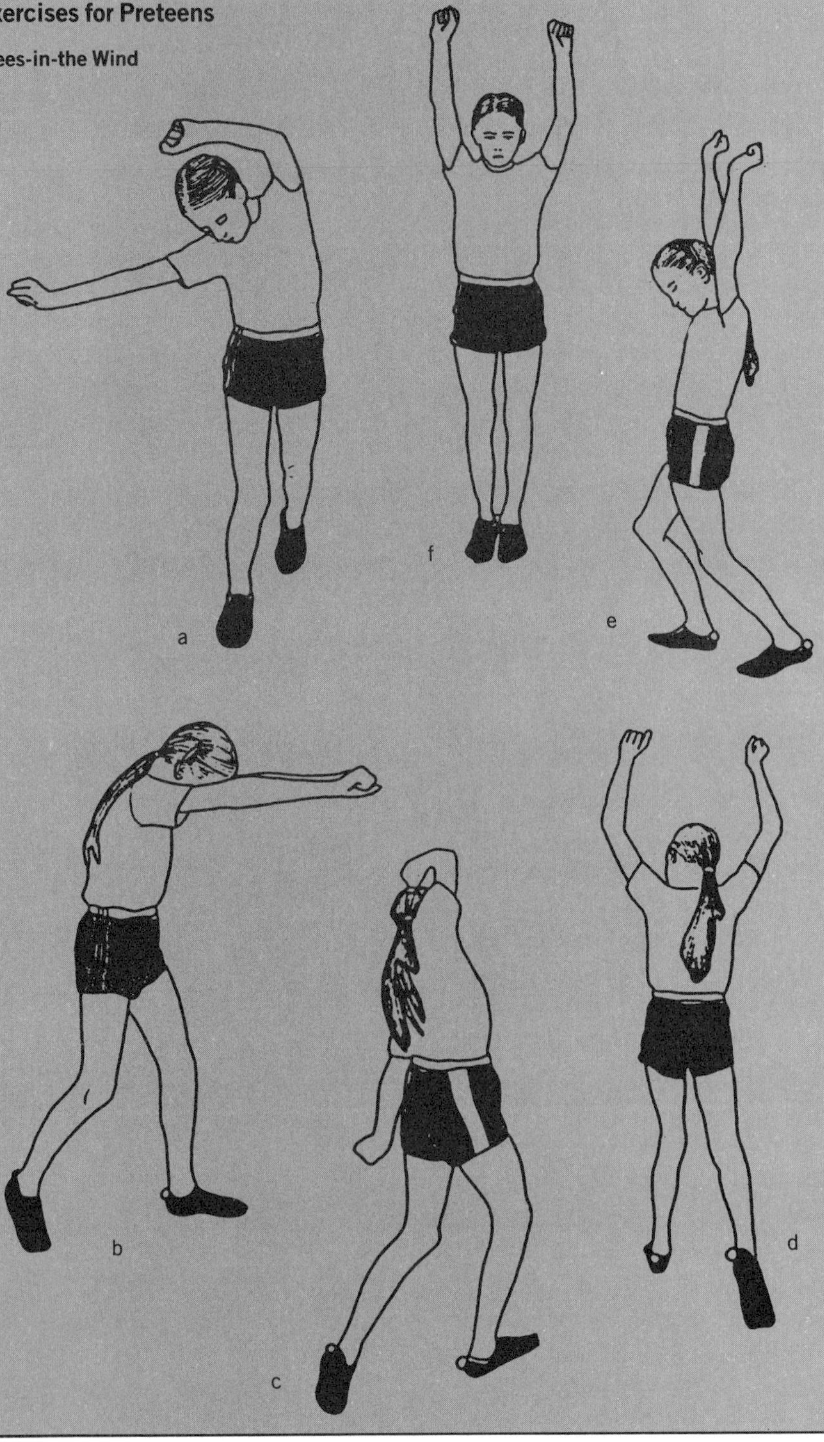

Exercises for Preteens

Bear Walk

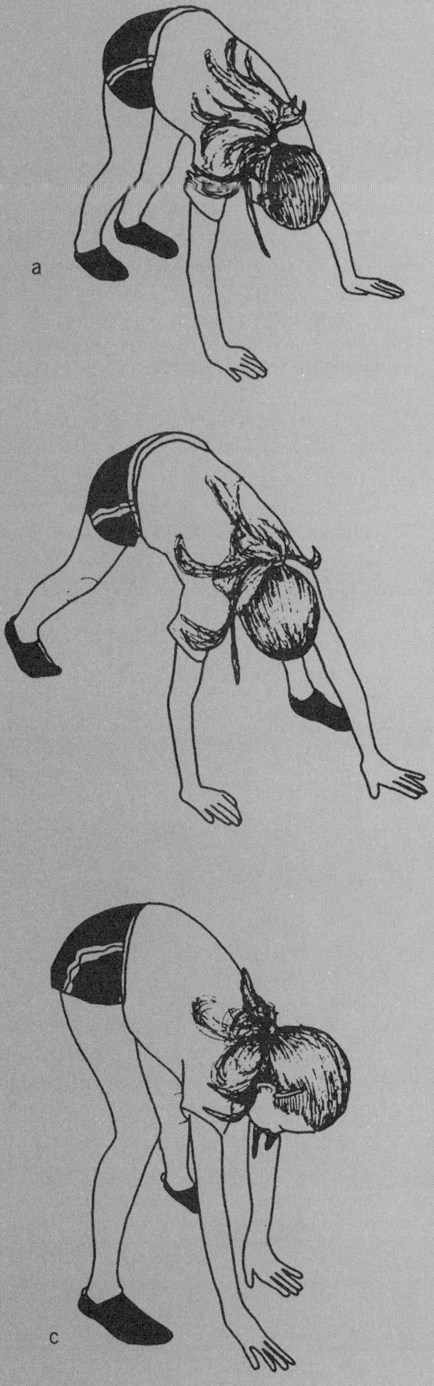

Exercises for Preteens

Measuring Worm

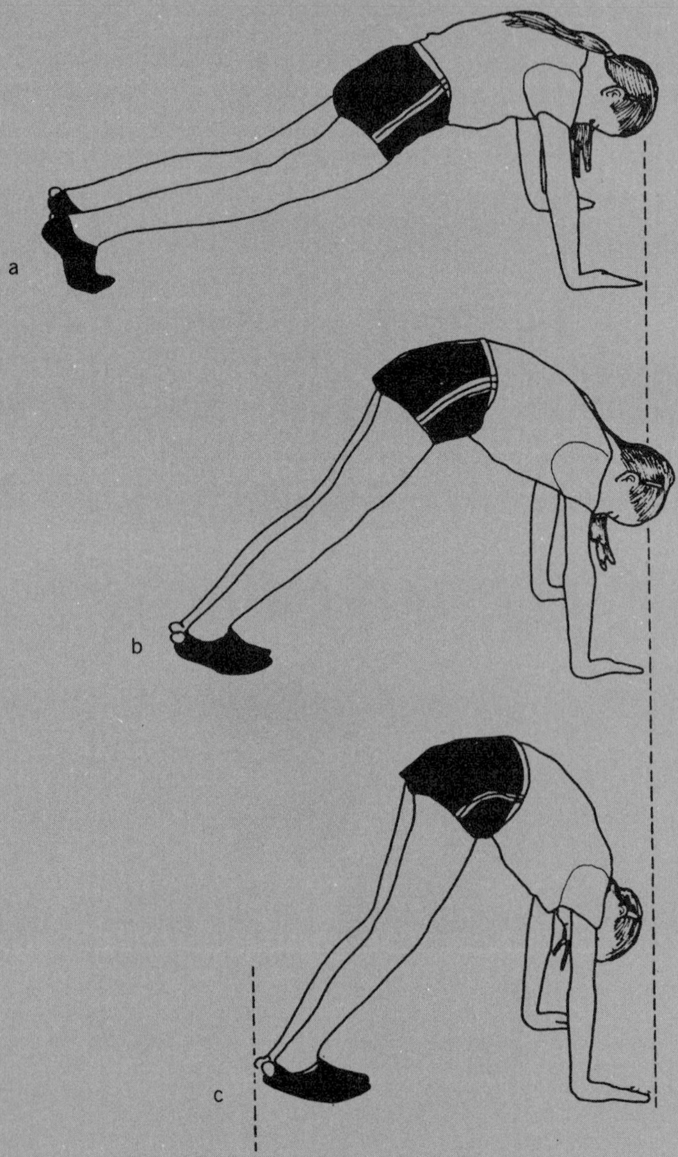

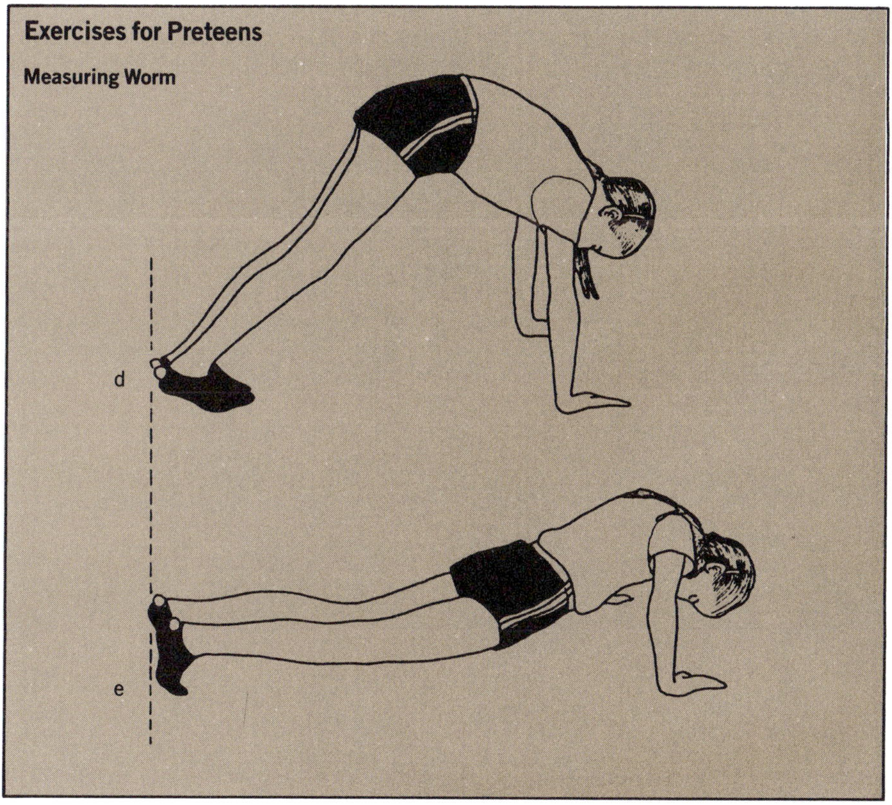

stand in a circle, arms extended overhead. As the children run slowly in a circle, they bend left, forward, and right, then forward and back like trees swaying in a wind. The exercise can be continued for three or four minutes.

4. *The gorilla walk:* For flexibility and coordination, begins with the children standing and spreading their feet to shoulder width. They then bend at the waist and grasp their ankles. The knees should be kept straight. The participants walk forward while holding their ankles. A walk of three or four feet should be a good starting distance.

5. *The hop:* A leg-muscle builder, starts with the child standing straight. The child hops forward on the left foot only, taking long steps. Then he repeats on the right foot. A forward trip of three or four feet on each foot is enough.

6. *The bear walk:* For leg flexibility requires that the child bend forward from the waist. He places his hands on the floor. Moving around in a circle, the child moves his right arm and right leg at the same time as one step. Then he moves the left arm and left leg. Four circles will do.

7. *The rabbit race:* Another exer-

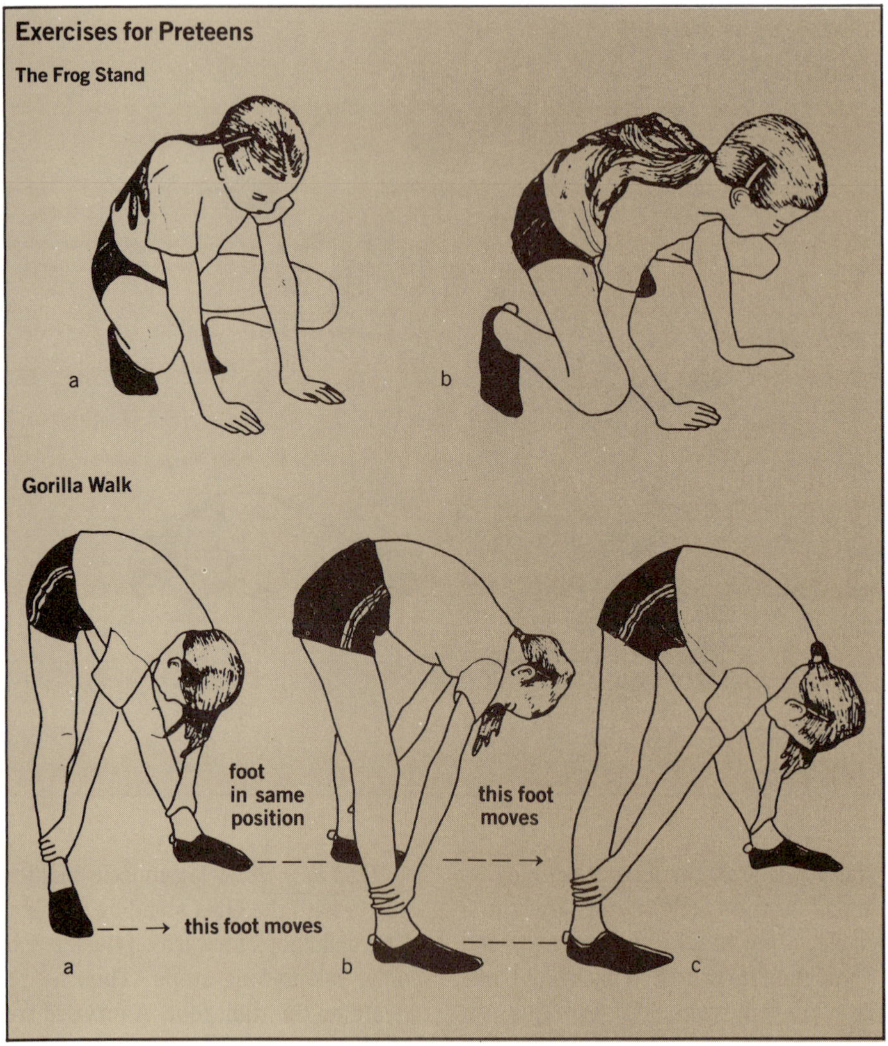

cise for two or more children, the rabbit race promotes circulorespiratory fitness. The participants line up exactly as if they were taking part in a foot race; but they stand three feet apart, side by side, facing a marked finish line 60 feet away. The children race by hopping. They hold their feet together over the entire course, hopping with their toes pointed first toward the left, then toward the right, then straight ahead. They repeat these movements until they reach the finish line. Variations may be introduced. The children may hop on one leg, for example.

8. *The frog stand:* Strengthens the arms and enhances balance. The participant squats and places his hands on the floor. The fingers point forward

Exercises for Preteens

The Wheel Barrel

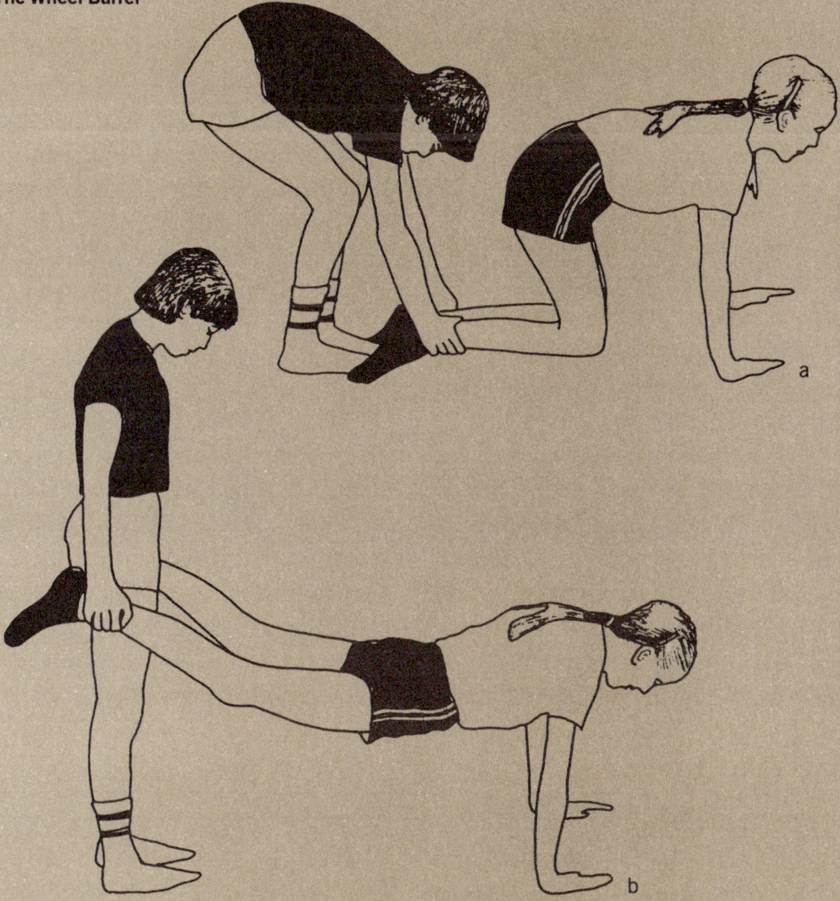

and the elbows press against the inside of the knees. Leaning forward slowly, the child transfers his weight to his hands, going up on his toes and, if possible, raising his toes off the floor. He balances on his hands, keeping his head up. After several seconds in that position, he returns to the starting position. In repetitions the child tries to maintain his balance for increasingly longer periods.

9. *The coffee grinder:* An upper-body strength builder, the coffee grinder requires that the child support his extended body on the right hand and his feet. The body is kept straight. The right arm and both legs are fully extended. The feet are slightly apart. In that position, the child "walks" his feet in a circle around the right arm, which serves as a pivot. The exercise should be repeated with the left arm supporting the body weight.

10. *The measuring worm:* Has been found effective in the development of strength in the lower back and hamstrings. The child assumes the push-up position with both hands on the floor and arms straight. Holding his hands in one place, the child "walks" his feet toward his hands. His back arches up. When he has walked his feet forward as far as possible, the child walks his hands forward by slow stages until he has assumed the original push-up position. Both walking actions should be repeated five times.

Two other exercises for children may be used or omitted depending on the child's strength, coordination, and flexibility. Both present a significant hazard of overextension of the knee muscles. Also, in the second exercise, a soft mat may have to be used for the child to kneel on to prevent bruises.

11. *The bunny hop:* Requires that the child assume a full squat position. His hands are placed alongside his head behind his ears, palms forward, to represent rabbit ears. The child hops in a circle with both feet together. Completing each hop, he lands again in the squat position. The hopping continues for two minutes.

12. *The knee down:* In the knee down, the child stands with the toes of both feet on a line. The child drops to both knees without taking his hands from his sides or moving his toes from the line. Then he returns to the standing position, again without using his hands or other aids. Five repetitions are prescribed.

The Teen Years

The teenager is approaching maturity in both the physical and the emotional senses. During these years between the ages of 13 and 19, most teens develop an interest in team sports and games. Growth may continue throughout the entire period. Activities requiring stamina become part of the teen's life. If no total or maintenance fitness program has been introduced into the young person's schedule in the earlier years, the time for such a program may have arrived.

Various factors suggest that conclusion. Many teens reduce the range of their physical activities to make time for school work, social activities, television, and other interests. Many walk less as they learn to drive the family car. As the teen years move on, bicycling comes to be regarded as demeaning or "too much work."

It may help for the parents to take part in fitness activities with their teenagers. But many teens have the maturity to start and continue a total fitness program on their own.

The Goals

The overall goal remains fitness—fitness for school; for homework; for the part-time job, if any; for dancing; for anything else requiring alertness, bodily movement, and endurance. But more limited goals may be set if the teen does not appear to be ready for an ambitious, graduated program.

Parental eagerness may have to be tempered with moderation in this regard. Remember, if the program seems overly ambitious, the young person will be less likely to stick with it. And if the teen does not stay with the program, the overall goals will never be met.

Goals of a more specific nature range across the basic spectrum established for this book. The teen should work—as the adult does—toward circulorespiratory endurance, good body composition, muscular strength and endurance, and flexibility. Training for specific sports and games can be included if that is desired. A 30-minute exercise session three times a week should constitute minimal exposure.

The teen's needs and preferences should always be respected. Few persons, teen or adult, can continue a fitness program if they feel no personal involvement or interest.

Caveats

The precautions already noted with reference to preteens apply equally to teens. Where a teen has encountered special problems in earlier years, a doctor should be consulted before a program is launched.

Just as adults should be tested, so should teens. The stress test may be accompanied by physical strength and endurance tests similar to those prescribed for adults.

Some teens will want to practice exercises before starting a total program or when adding new movements to an initially limited program. If so, they should be allowed to take as much time as necessary to learn the various movements. A week or two usually suffices.

The Exercises

The exercises that are adapted particularly to teen use echo some of those that have already been introduced. But many of them add or subtract an element to ensure that they are actually suited to the teenage group. The first three of the teen exercises described below may be regarded as warm-ups.

1. *The deep breather:* To perform this circulorespiratory warm-up, you simply stand at attention. On the count of 1, moving slowly and rhythmically, rise on your toes and simultaneously circle your arms inward and upward so that they cross in front of you. Move slowly. Inhale deeply. Completing the 1-count, raise your arms overhead. On the count of 2, circle your arms backward and downward. Lower your heels to the floor and exhale. Repeat for one to two minutes.

2. *The wing stretcher:* To increase your flexibility, try the wing stretcher. Standing straight with your elbows at shoulder height, fists clenched, hold your palms in front of your chest. Throw your elbows back vigorously. Then bring them back forward just as vigorously. Keep your head erect. Your elbows should remain at shoulder height. Repeat for one to two minutes.

3. *The one-foot balance:* In this balancing exercise, first stand at attention. On count 1, stretch your left leg backward. Bend your trunk forward, extending your arms sideward until you are "flying." Your head is up, your upper body parallel to the floor, and your left leg is extended back and up, toes pointed. Try to hold this position for five to ten seconds, then return. On count 2, switch to the other leg and repeat. Continue the repetitions for one to two minutes.

4. *The jumping jack:* In this coordination exercise, first stand at attention. On the count of 1, swing your arms sideward and up. Touch your hands above your head with your arms straight. At the same time move your feet apart toward the sides in a single jumping motion. On count 2, bring your feet back together and your hands to your sides. Repeat for two minutes.

5. *The body bender:* This flexibility exercise has four counts or separate movements. To prepare, simply stand erect with your hands against the back of your head. On count 1, bend sideways to the left as far as you can, moving only from the hips. While keeping your feet stationary and your toes pointed forward, return to the starting position on count 2. On count 3, repeat, but bend to the right. At count 4, return to the starting position. Continue for 15 to 30 repetitions.

6. *The windmill:* Another four-count exercise, the windmill promotes flexibility in the middle body. Stand with your knees flexed and apart and your feet spread to shoulder width. Your arms should be extended outward to the sides at shoulder level. On count 1, twist and bend your trunk while bringing your right hand to the left toe. Keep your arms straight and your knees flexed. The other three counts bring you (2) back to the starting position, (3) twisting and bending while bringing your left hand to your right toe, and (4) returning to the starting position. Repeat 10 to 20 times.

7. *Back stretcher:* In this exercise for the lower back and thighs, while standing with your feet apart extend your arms overhead. On the count of 1, bend forward from your hips, bending your knees, and touch the floor by extending your arms between your legs and behind them. On count 2, return to the starting position.

8. *The jump and touch:* In this leg exercise, go into a half crouch. Pretend you are going to start a broad jump. Your arms should be extended backward. Springing upward, bring your knees toward your chest and your heels toward your buttocks. While in the air swing your arms down and around your legs and attempt to bring your hands together. Come down in the starting position and repeat 5 to 15 times.

9. *The squat thrust:* A circulorespiratory exercise, the *squat thrust* was described earlier. The teen version exactly parallels the adult version. Repeat 10 to 20 times.

10. *The bear hug:* In the bear hug, a thigh thinner, stand with your feet spread comfortably and your hands on your hips. On the count of 1, step out diagonally to the right. Keep your left foot anchored. Circle your arms around your right thigh, "tackling" your right leg. On count 2, return to the starting position. On counts 3 and 4, perform the exercise on the left side. Repeat 15 to 30 times.

11. *The Coordinator:* Stand at attention to start this cardiorespiratory conditioner. On count 1, hop on your left foot. Swing your right leg forward and touch your right toe to the floor in front of your left foot. At the same time raise both arms in front of your body until they reach shoulder level. On count 2, hop again on the left foot. Swing your right foot out to the right and touch the toe to the floor. At the same time bring your arms sideward at shoulder level.

12. *Squat jump:* A leg strengthener, the *squat jump* begins as you assume a semisquat position. Clasp your hands on top of your head with feet apart and the heel of your left foot on a line with the toes of the right foot. On count 1, spring upward in a ballet-like movement, reversing the positions of your feet while in the air. Come down to the semisquat position with your hands still on your head. The same movement is repeated on count 2, but the feet are reversed. Continue, reversing your feet on each jump, until you have jumped 10 to 20 times.

13. *Knee raise (single and double):* This hip and abdominal-muscle flexor requires that you first lie on your back. Your knees should be slightly bent, with your feet flat on the floor and your arms at your sides. On count 1, raise one knee as high as possible, bringing it close to your chest. On count 2, extend the leg fully so that it is perpendicular to the floor. Count 3: bend your knee and return it to your chest area. Count 4: straighten the leg and return to the starting position.

During this exercise, you should alternate legs. Repeat 15 to 30 times. For variety and even better exercise, move both of your legs simultaneously.

14. *Head and shoulder curl:* The curl has also been described earlier. The head should be held up for a 4-count, then returned to the starting position. Repeat 15 to 30 times.

15. *Leg extension:* To start this hip and abdominal flexor, you should sit on the edge of a table and extend your legs. Keep your body erect and your hands on your hips. On count 1, flex your knees quickly and swing your feet backward toward your buttocks. Your toes should drag on the floor. With count 2, extend your legs back to the starting position. Keep your head and shoulders high throughout the exercise. Repeat 15 to 30 times.

16. *The up oars:* Begin this exercise, another hip and abdominal exercise, by lying on your back. Extend your arms above your head. On the count of 1, sit up and reach forward with the extended arms. Pull your knees up against your chest. Your arms should remain outside your knees. On count 2, return to the starting position. Remember that you are simulating rowing, and keep your movements rhythmic. Repeat 10 to 20 times.

17. *Snap and twist:* Still another exercise that helps the muscles of the hips and abdomen, the snap and twist has a count of 4. Lie on your back with your arms stretched out above your head. On the count of 1, sit up quickly and bring the left knee up to your chest. At the same time extend your right arm forward and your left elbow backward. The movements should be vigorous.

On count 2, return to the starting position. Repeat on the opposite side on count 3, and on count 4 return to the starting position. Keep it as rhythmic as possible. Repeat 10 to 20 times.

18. *The back twist:* One more for the hip and abdominal muscles, this exercise requires that you lie on your back with your arms extended to the sides and your palms on the floor. Your legs should be pointed straight up. On count 1, keeping your feet together, swing your legs slowly to the left. They should almost touch the floor. Your arms, shoulders, and head should remain on the floor. On the count of 2 return to the starting position; on count 3, repeat to the right, and on count 4 return again to the starting position. Repeat 10 to 20 times.

19. *Side leg raise:* Designed to strengthen the lateral muscles of the leg, the side leg raise has a two-count. Lie on your side with your arms extended overhead. Rest your head on your lower arm. Your legs should be extended fully, one on top of the other. On the count of 1, raise your upper leg vertically. On count 2, bring the leg back down. Repeat 10 to 20 times and then turn to the other side and repeat an identical number of times.

20. *The sprinter:* In this circulorespiratory exercise, assume the sprinter's squatting position. Your hands are on the floor, your fingers pointed forward, your left leg extended far back. On the count of 1, reverse the positions of your feet. Bring the left foot forward to your hands and move the right leg back in a single motion. On count 2, reverse again and return. Repeat 15 to 30 times.

21. *Push-ups:* The push-up strengthens the arm, shoulder, and chest muscles. For boys, the standard push-up is recommended—with the entire body straight and supported on hands and toes. For girls the modified push-up is often preferable. The body is kept straight, but the knees rest on the floor. With practice, both boys and girls should be able to repeat the push-up 10 or 20 times.

22. *Bouncing ball:* Another arm-shoulder-chest exercise, the bouncing ball challenges the physically very fit person. From the regular push-up position, push yourself off the floor with your hands. Your hands should actually leave the floor. With practice, you may be able to clap your hands while you are in the air. Repeat as possible.

Alternatives

Other exercises, or variations of those already described, may tempt the teen fitness enthusiast. At the least, these alternatives inject some variety into the program. The following exercises, as well as those already described, can be overloaded in the three standard ways: by working out with weights, by speeding up the tempo, or by increasing the number of repetitions. (Note: these exercises require somewhat more space than the earlier ones.)

1. *All fours:* Get down on your hands and feet (note feet, not knees). "Walk" for two to four minutes.

2. *Bear walk:* From the same position, "walk" forward by moving the right arm and right leg simultaneously. Then take another step by moving the left arm and left leg in unison. Continue for two to four minutes.

3. *Leap frog:* This old familiar game requires at least two persons, but it can be done with virtually any number. Participants should count off by twos and, on command, the "evens" leap over the "odds." Then the odds leap over the evens. Repeat for two to four minutes.

4. *Indian walk:* With your knees bent slightly and your trunk bent far forward, let your arms hang down until the backs of your hands touch the floor. Holding this position, walk forward. Continue for two to four minutes.

5. *Crouch run:* Leaning forward at the waist, and keeping your upper body parallel to the ground, run slowly. Continue for two to four minutes.

6. *Straddle run:* While running forward, leap off to the right at an angle as you put down your right foot. Leap to the left as your left foot advances. Continue for two to four minutes.

7. *Knee-raised run:* Run with your knees moving up as high as possible on each step. At the same time pump your arms vigorously. Continue for two to four minutes.

8. *One-leg hop:* Hop forward on your left foot, then on your right. Take five to ten hops on each foot in succession and continue for two to four minutes.

Some Beginner's Weight-Training Exercises for Teenage Girls

Muscle-building exercises for teenage girls should differ from those prescribed for teen boys in at least two ways. First, the girls' exercises should involve more repetitions and less weight—usually no more than two to 12 pounds. Second, the exercises for girls should be designed to lengthen or stretch muscles—not to build bulging biceps.

Depending on their conditioning levels, some adult women may want to follow the girls' somewhat lighter weight-training regimen. Here are four basic routines recommended for teens:

1. *The pullover:* To firm up and tone the chest muscles, and thus build a more attractive bust, lie down on a bench with a two-pound dumbbell or other weight in each hand. Extend your arms straight up and hold for a count of four to six. Lowering the weights to your bent knees, raise them until your arms are extended straight up again. Repeat 10 to 15 times.

2. *Thigh high:* For the muscles in the front of your thighs, sit on the floor with your legs straight out and your hands on the floor behind you for support. With a 2½ pound leg weight strapped to each ankle, raise your right leg slowly. Hold for a count of four to six. Lower to the floor and repeat 10 to 15 times. Go through the same routine with the other leg.

3. *A leg up:* To give shape to the backs of your legs, try the leg up. Lying on your stomach on the floor with a weight strapped to each ankle, bend your right knee. Your right foot should point up straight. Raise and lower that leg five times, flexing the foot each time, then push your right leg up so that it comes entirely off the floor. Straighten that leg. Repeat 10 to 15 times with that leg, then do the routine with the other leg the same number of times.

4. *Leg lifts:* A stomach strengthener, the leg lift requires that you strap one five-pound weight to both feet. Sitting on a chair or bench, hold your feet about two inches off the floor, then raise your legs, keeping them straight, until they are level with your hips. Slowly lower your legs to the two-inches-off-the-floor position. Repeat 10 to 15 times.

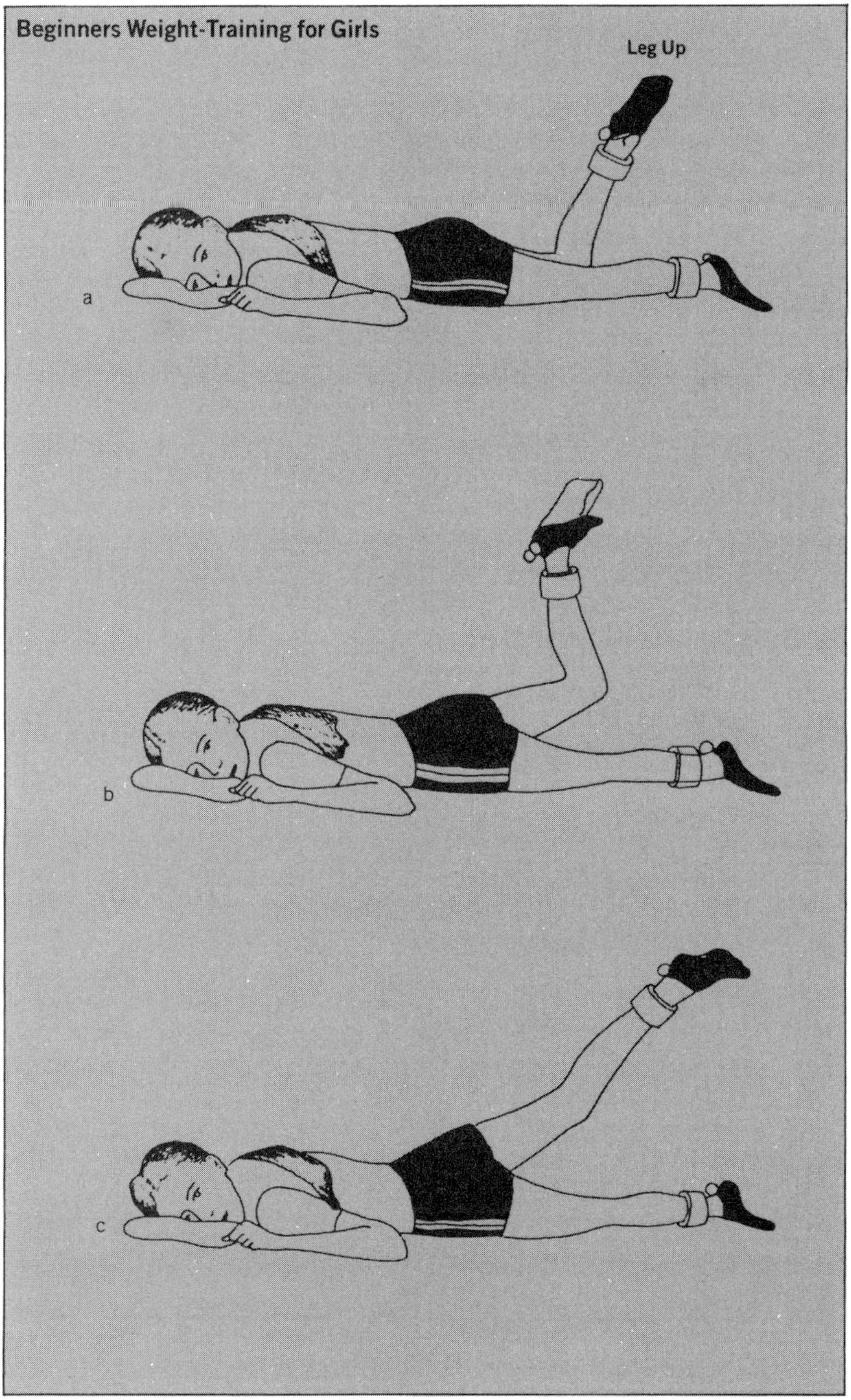
Beginners Weight-Training for Girls
Leg Up
a
b
c

Beginners Weight-Training for Girls

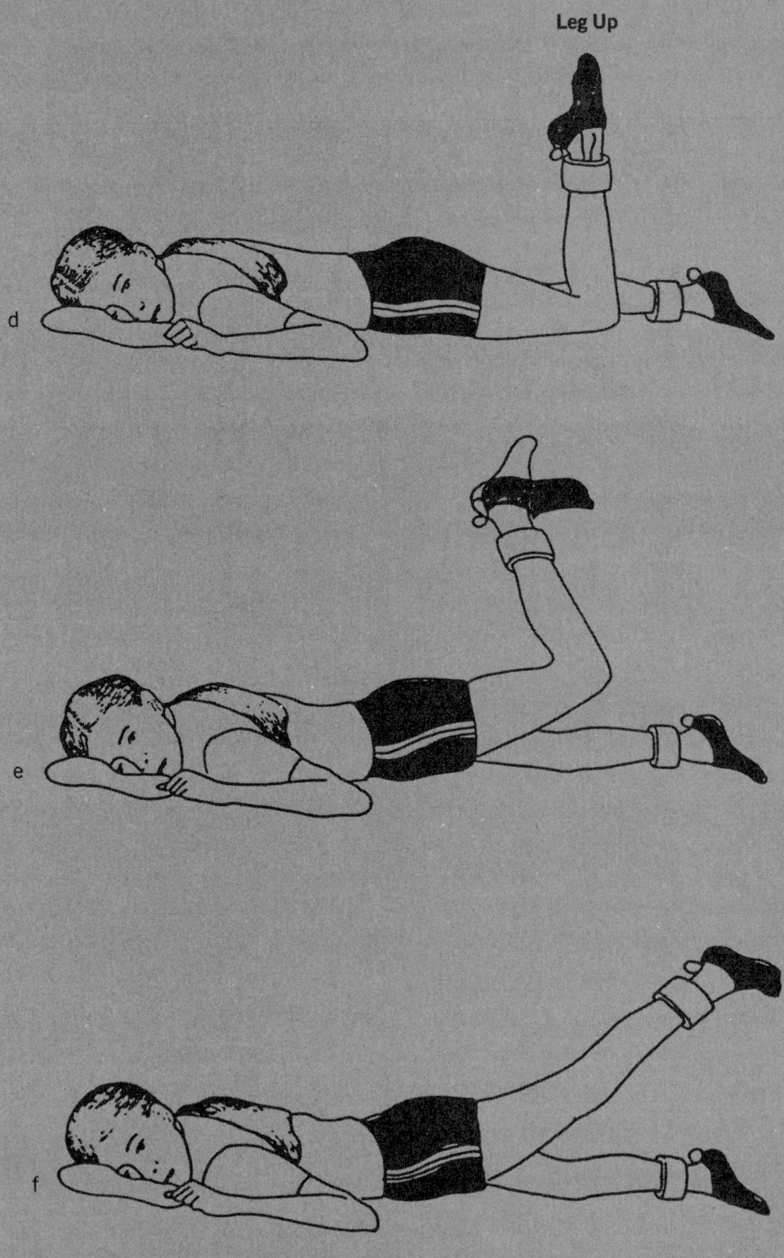

Beginners Weight-Training for Girls

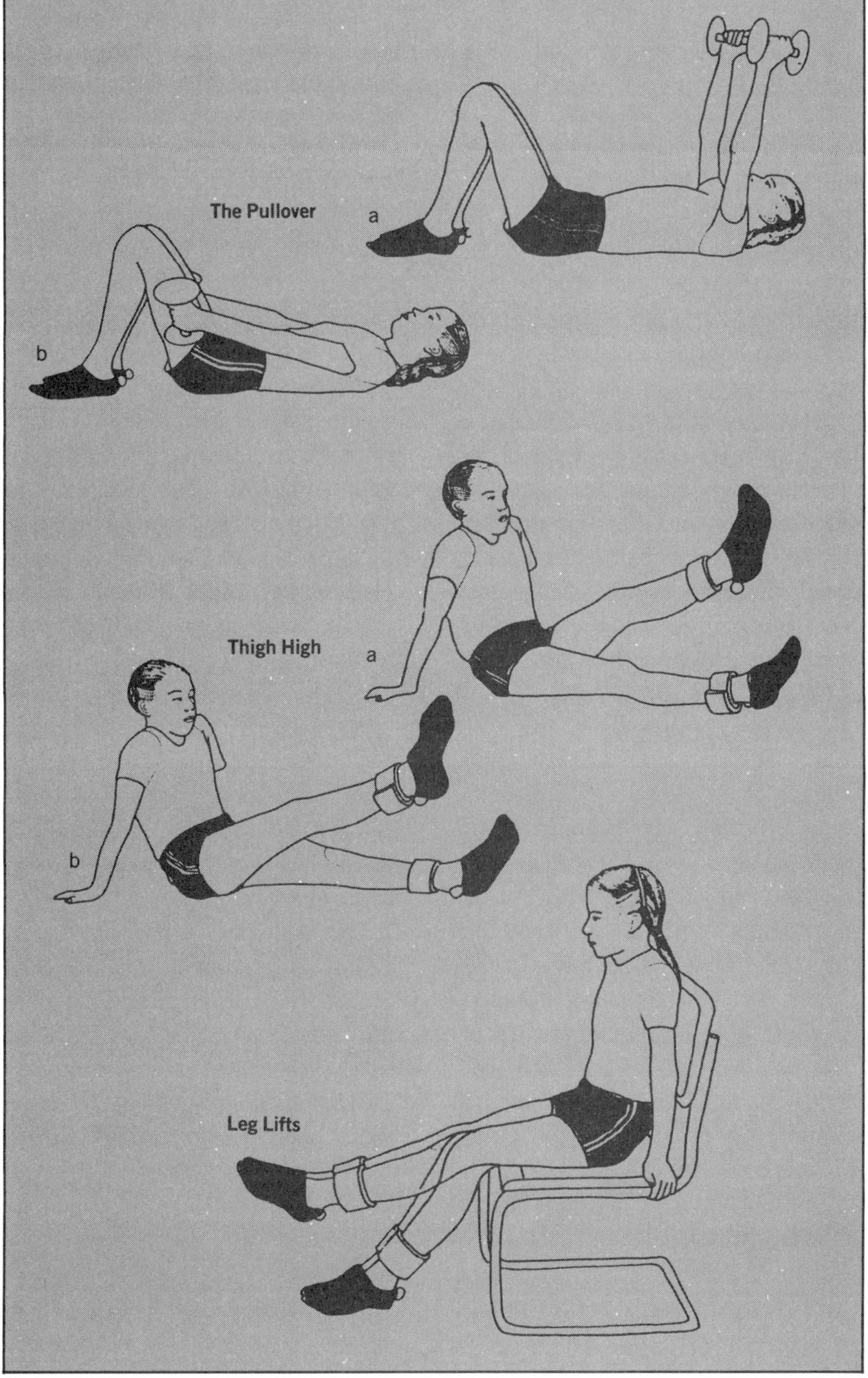

Exercises for Later Life

Young muscles that are not used come to resemble the muscles of the aged. To a very considerable extent, the reverse of that statement is also true: symptoms of aging may in fact be symptoms of disuse. Many senior citizens who exercise can hold off these symptoms and succeed in preserving a youthful appearance, psyche, and level of fitness.

The mention of "psyche" is important. Upon entering his 60s, or the retirement period, or any significant stage of later life, a person may feel that he is dying a small death. He may find it difficult to face the changes that later life brings: reduced involvement, more time to think about himself, a sense of diminishment and decreased importance, and so on.

He may find it less difficult if he has remained physically active, or if he can become physically active. By retaining some vigor, he may also retain a positive feeling about himself. He may have greater courage, and thus be able to try out new and stimulating experiences. He may move with greater ease and grace, presenting a trim and attractive figure. And the fit older person has a degree of independence that his less fit neighbor does not have. He need not call on friends, relatives, or others for help. He retains a large measure of personal freedom.

Basic Principles

The principles behind a golden-age fitness program are essentially the same as those already specified for younger and mature adults. But the older person, perhaps even more than the younger one, has to move in easy stages. Even after testing and medical clearance, he should not undertake too much too fast. He will probably want to increase repetitions as his program progresses, and gradually add more difficult exercises. The main alternative, to overload by increasing intensity, might cause undue strain.

Physiologically, the older person faces a slightly different problem from the younger. He cannot reach the same high heart rates that the younger one achieves. Thus the older person has a correspondingly lower target heart rate.

The older person may be exercising just as hard as his younger counterpart. But the older person's pulse rate response will be lower. He will have reached the same percentage of his maximum as the younger person, only sooner. Those realities apply to women as well as to men. Women can achieve approximately the same maximum heart rates as men of comparable ages.

Warm-up and cool-down are as important or more so for older people as for younger. Running in place warms up the body effectively; so do easy stretching, pulling, and rotating exercises. In the main part of the workout, vigorous exercise should be alternated with periods of less strenuous activity.

A Warm-up Routine

The older person planning his or her own fitness program may want to invent a warm-up series of exercises. Alternatively, he may want to try the plan devised as part of the Senior Citizen's Exercise Program. Sponsored

Walking Warm-Ups for the Senior Citizen

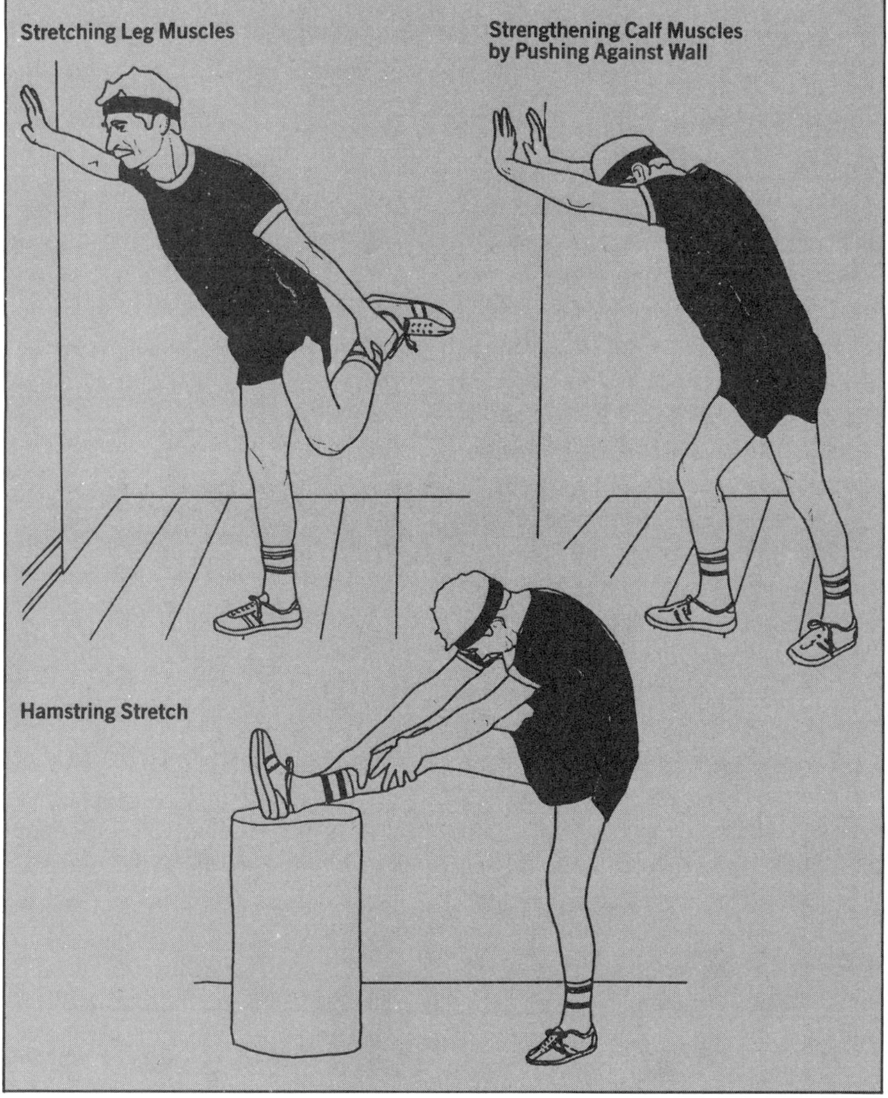

by the Travelers PEP (Physical Exercise Pays) program, the senior citizen's routine has been recognized by the President's Council on Physical Fitness and Sports. The routine is performed over a five- or six-minute period:

1. Take a deep breath while rising on your toes with arms extended over your head. Exhale slowly. Repeat three times, then lift your left and right knees in succession. Repeat the knee lifts ten times.

2. Start walking. You will want to increase the amount of walking you do by small increments. Walk erect, keeping your head up and remaining comfortable. Concentrate on walking heel to toe. That means that as you put your foot down, rock forward to your toes, thus strengthening your leg muscles. Gradually pick up the pace of your stride.

A Ten-part Set for Seniors

The normally mobile older person has many options. He or she can, obviously, create a routine for thrice-weekly or more frequent use. A ready-made program, such as the following program presented by Linda Webb in the Good Housekeeping Institute Exercise and Diet Program, may also do the trick.

The first three movements in the ten-part program can be used by nearly anyone, including persons who are confined to wheelchairs. But such persons are advised to keep the number of repetitions to three in all cases.

1. *Arm swing:* One of the simplest of all exercises, the arm swing involves rotating the right arm forward five times, then reversing the motion and rotating backward an equal number of times. Repeat with the left arm. Place both arms together, windmill fashion, and swing five times.

2. *Finger squeeze:* Extending your arms forward at shoulder height, with palms down, squeeze the fingers together slowly into a fist, then release. After repeating five times, turn your palms up and squeeze again five times. With your arms extended toward the front, shake your fingers five times.

3. *Arm turn:* Extend your arms straight out to the sides. With palms up, cup your hands and rotate your arms so the palms face down. Return to the starting position. Repeat five times. Starting with your palms down, cup hands, and move your arms in the opposite direction. Repeat five more times.

4. *Shoulder roll:* Beginning with arms at your sides, roll your shoulders forward slowly. Your shoulders should describe a full circle. After five repetitions, reverse the direction of the roll and repeat five more times. End with a shrug.

5. *Body stretch:* Keeping your left foot firmly planted, extend your right

Ten Exercises for the Senior Citizen

Arm Swings

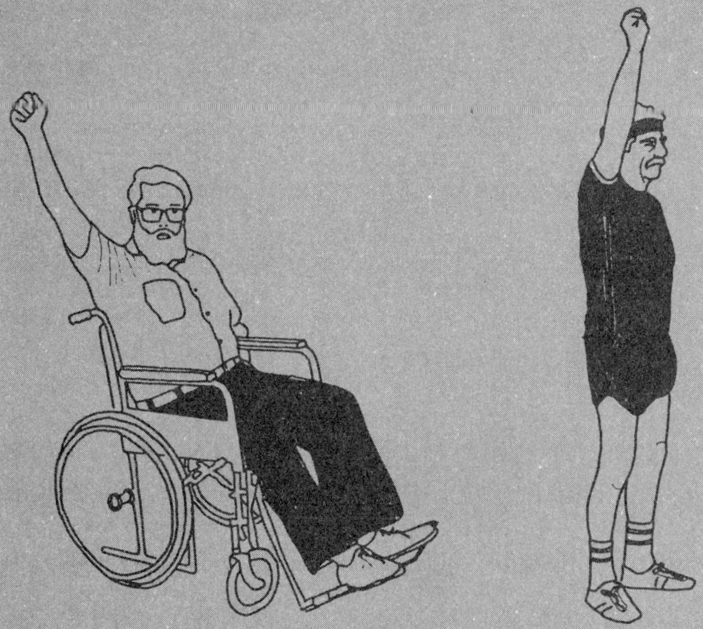

Finger Squeeze

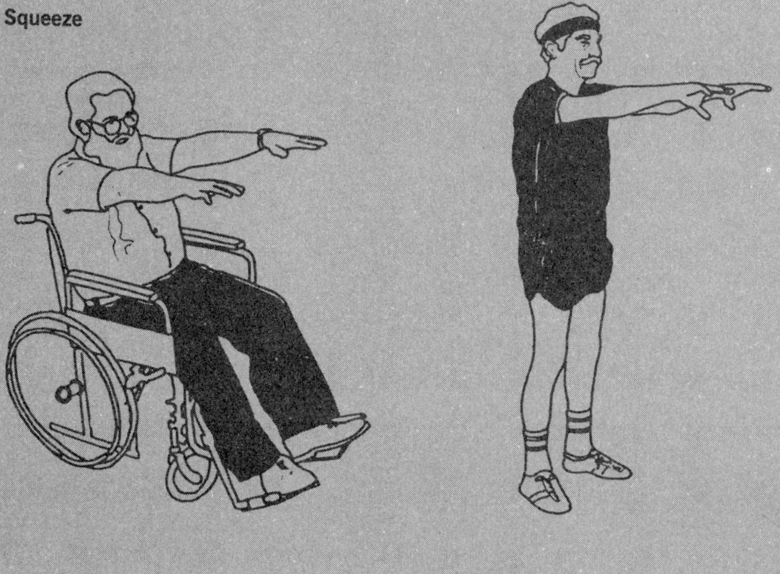

Ten Exercises for the Senior Citizen

Arm Turns

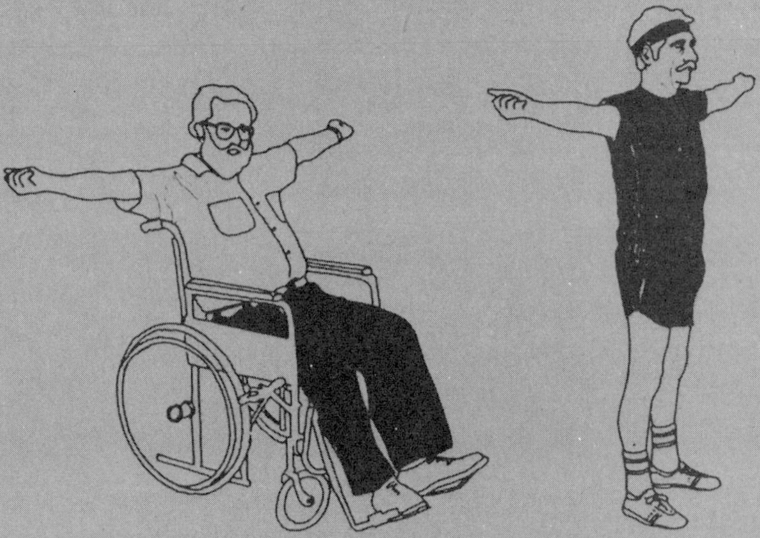

Shoulder Rolls

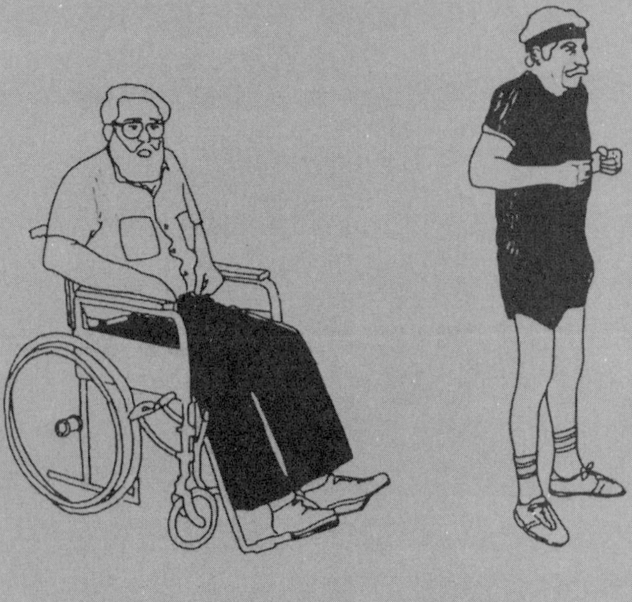

Ten Exercises for the Senior Citizen

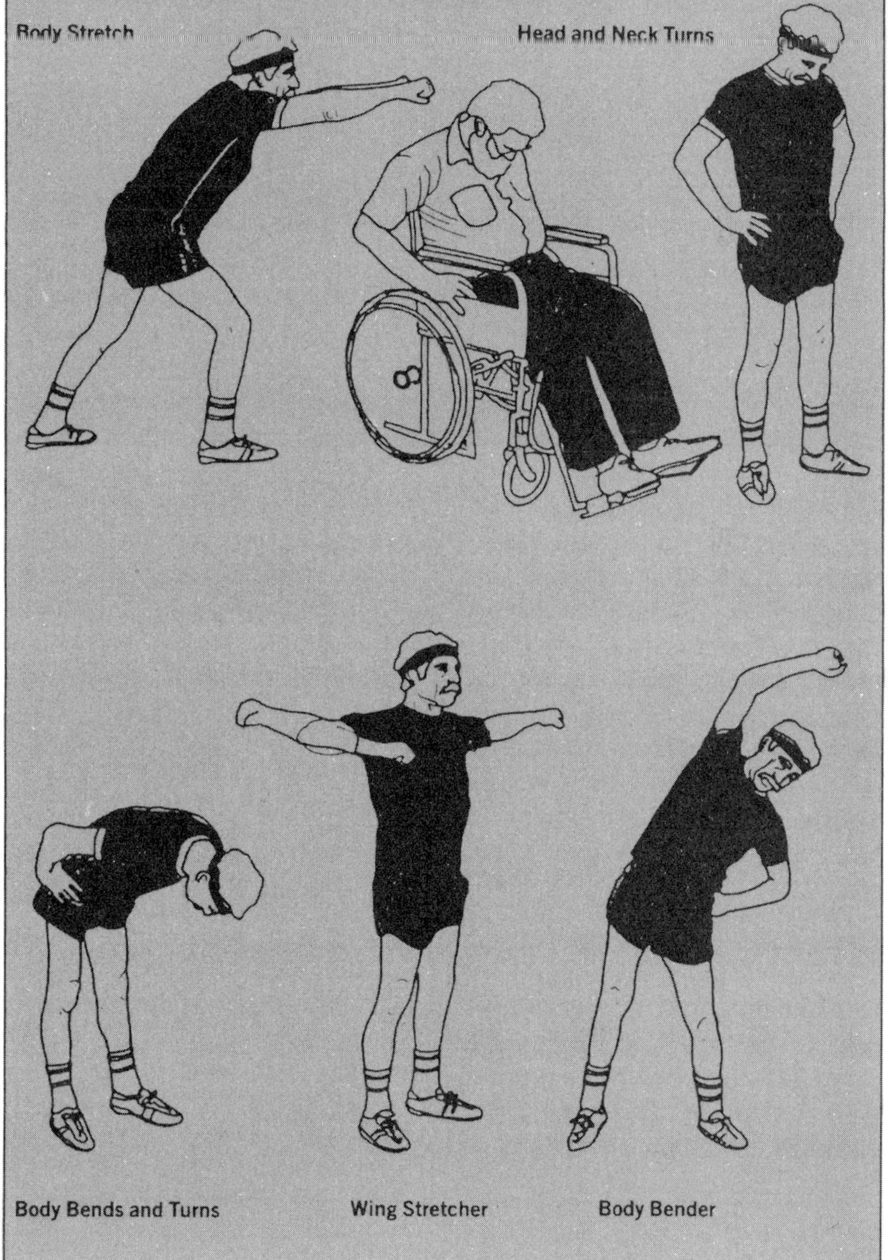

Ten Exercises for the Senior Citizen

Arm Thrusts

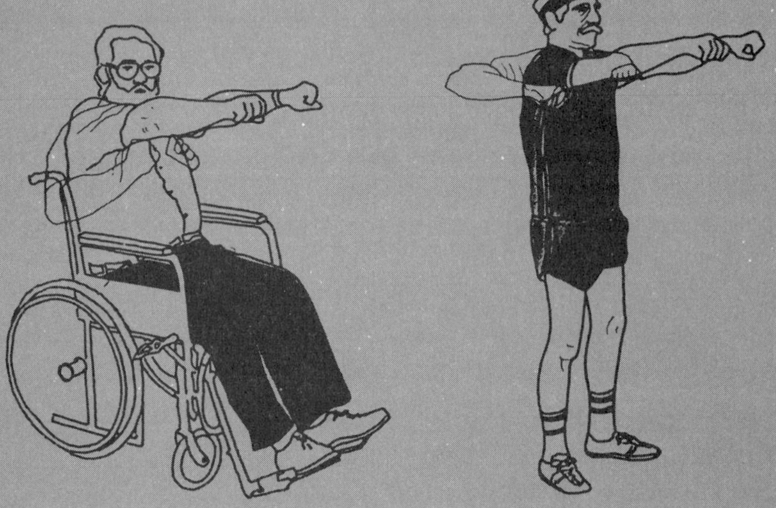

foot forward as far as possible. Bend your body forward at the same time, arms extended out in front, in a kind of lunge. Count to five, stretching a little more on each count. Switch, extending the left foot and keeping the right planted. With each stretch, while holding for the five-count, lift up on the toes of your back foot. Repeat five times with each foot.

6. *Head and neck exercise:* Hands on hips, bring your head down and forward so that your chin touches your chest. Then bend your head backward as far as you comfortably can. Bring your head back to the starting position, erect, then turn it slowly to the left, then to the right. Repeat the entire cycle five times.

7. *Body bend and turn:* Again with your hands on your hips, bend slowly forward from the waist until you can bend no farther. Stand straight and lean back from the hips. Return to the starting position, bend slowly to the left, then to the right, and come back to the erect position. Repeat five times.

8. *Body bender:* Place your left hand on your left hip. Raise your right hand straight overhead. To a count of two, bend toward the left. Returning to the starting position, change hands, raising the left and putting the right on your right hip. Bend toward the right. Each bend should be done to a count of two. Repeat five times on both sides.

9. *Wing stretcher:* Standing with your feet about six inches apart, tighten your leg muscles and draw in your stomach while extending your chest. Bring your arms up, fists clenched, so that both elbows and

fists are at shoulder level and your fists are in front of your chest. In this position, with muscles taut, take a deep breath and release it slowly. Vibrate your arms toward the back for a count of three. Repeat three times and work up to five.

10. *Arm thrust:* From the same starting position, clenched fists again in front of your chest, thrust your arms forward at shoulder height. Bring your fist back toward your chest and swing your arms out to the sides. Bring your arms back to the chest and thrust them vigorously up and down. Repeat three times.

Progressing through Fitness Levels

The exercises described above take the fitness-aware senior citizen into a program in the simplest possible way. They should cause little pain or strain. But for optimal results, any program for any participant at any age should provide for progression.

A three-level program may be the perfect answer. The program is self-contained: it offers the older person a long-term alternative that need never be abandoned because it can be overloaded almost limitlessly. On the other hand, the man or woman who wants to utilize the program as a springboard to a more ambitious schedule of physical activities can use it in that way too.

The three-level program that follows is adapted from Pat Stewart's *U.S. Fitness Book.* It has a relatively simple level 1, a more difficult level 2, and a most challenging level 3. At each level the exerciser achieves a balanced workout, using all the muscle groups and giving primary emphasis to circulorespiratory fitness. Before starting, the older person should make sure that he or she is entering the program at the proper level. Standard walking or walk-jog tests along with others noted earlier can provide guidance in determining where to begin.

The Who and the How

Both men and women can take part in the exercises recommended below. Couples may find mutual encouragement if they can take part together—and may be more inclined to continue the program for that reason. But in the experience of fitness authorities, men usually start at a somewhat higher level than women of comparable ages.

For both men and women, the watchword should be, "Take it easy!" The tempo of the exercise session and the numbers of repetitions should be increased very gradually. In this way, stiffness and soreness can be minimized. But some stiffness and soreness may be expected. If that occurs, it means only that the exerciser needed the workouts.

To encourage consistency and to provide a means of checking

progress, records should be kept—as always. The records should include the date, the exercises performed, the number of repetitions, and so on. Without such records, it may prove difficult to overload sensibly, with an eye to past accomplishments. Without gradual overloading, much of the potential benefit of the program may be lost.

Music that suits the tempo of the various exercises may make the exercise session more enjoyable. Comfortable clothing such as slacks or shorts, plus short-sleeved blouses or T-shirts, makes free, rhythmic movement easier. Wear comfortable, properly fitted shoes with nonskid soles and low or no heels.

The Exercises

The older person should follow the instructions given with each exercise. If two repetitions are called for, the exerciser should repeat only twice. The reason is that the exercises have been arranged in such a way that a warm-up, or preparation for a succeeding exercise, is built into each set or station. Thus the exercises should be performed as prescribed if they are to give optimal results.

Level 1

As much as possible, the exercises at level 1 should be performed in a continuous sequence, with only brief rests between sets. But a rest is always called for if the exerciser feels that he is straining or pushing himself too hard.

It is important to remember that the ability to go through the level 1 exercise routines in continually shorter spans of time indicates progress. But no one should overdo it, or try to set any records. The person should maintain an even pace, avoiding jerkiness. If, after a week of performing the exercises as prescribed, he or she feels that the pace is too strenuous, the pace should be slowed, or some exercises should be eliminated for the time being. Wherever possible the exerciser ought to stick with the set routines for another week, making such adjustments as are necessary.

Where a range of repetitions is indicated, gradual overloading calls for the addition of one repetition in the second week. But the senior exerciser should proceed with overloading only if he feels ready for it. After the second week, two or more repetitions can be added where allowed—again depending on the way in which he is taking to the program. Many persons will reach the highest number of repetitions on level 1 in three or four weeks.

Once at the level 1 maximum, the exerciser should continue at the same level until he or she can complete the entire series without resting between exercises. Having done that for three successive days, he can move on to level 2.

Level 2

At level 2, the person follows generally the same procedure as at level 1. Initially, he performs the minimum number of suggested repetitions. In three to five weeks he should have completed the level 2 conditioning phases and be prepared for level 3.

As at the preceding level, the exerciser should move on to level 3 only when, in three consecutive sessions, he is able to perform all the repetitions of the level 2 exercises without stopping to rest between sets.

Level 3

The same general approach should govern at level 3 as at levels 1 and 2. The exerciser starts slowly and progresses gradually. When the exerciser is able to perform without strain all the prescribed repetitions of the level 3 exercises in three consecutive sessions, he is ready to face the maintenance phase. At this point, several alternatives lie open:

- Go back to the exercise routines indicated earlier for mature adults and devise a completely new program.
- Get into walking and jogging on a more advanced or demanding level.
- Consider a program of relatively easy sports, to be dealt with in the next three chapters, and recreational activities, already covered.
- Take up yoga or calisthenics.
- Construct an augmented program out of the activities in levels 1, 2, and 3.

Whatever the choice, remember that muscles that aren't used deteriorate.

Beyond the Daily Schedule

Whatever the older exerciser does to extend or supplement the daily schedule, he should keep in mind that he can retain the high level of fitness already achieved only on one condition. The new activities have to include the same basic tasks, and give the same benefits, as those already mastered.

Many persons turn to group activities. YMCAs across the country offer exercise classes for senior citizens, as do local recreation centers. Where a senior exerciser joins a group, he can usually skip his regular level 3 exercises on the days on which classes or meetings are held.

For other persons, sports beckon irresistibly. Swimming is excellent because the exerciser can proceed at his own pace while deriving outstanding physical—in particular circulorespiratory—benefits. But bicycling, tennis, and many other sports are also possibilities. In each of these alternatives, the objective is more movement, and more beneficial movement.

A-Z Index Reference Guide

A Note on Using the Index

The pages that follow contain a reference tool that should be very useful for the layman. In using this glossary-index combination the reader will be able to find brief definitions for medical terminology and locate the pages where each major topic is discussed. Where appropriate, cross references to similar or related topics are given. Illustrations and photos are indicated by the page numbers which are in italics.

Index

Medical Glossary

a- (*prefix*): not, as in afebrile, not feverish
abdomen: in human beings, the cavity between the diaphragm and the floor of the pelvis, in which the stomach, intestines, liver, and other organs are located
abortion: the expulsion of a nonviable fetus prior to term, either induced or involuntary (miscarriage or spontaneous abortion)
abrasion: scraped place on the skin, as from a fall
abscess(es): collection of pus in a body cavity formed by tissue disintegration, and often accompanied by painful inflammation
absorption: assimilation by means of the digestive process
accommodation: the thinning or thickening of the lens of the eye in order to adjust the focus of vision at different distances
acetabulum: the hip socket
achalasia: failure of a sphincter muscle to relax, causing, in the case of the cardiac sphincter, abnormal dilation of the esophagus
Achilles tendon: the thick tendon that connects the muscles at the back of the calf of the leg to the bone of the heel
acid: any of various chemical compounds that in water solution are sour in taste, turn blue litmus paper red, and are capable of reacting with another compound (a base) to form a salt
acidosis: chemical imbalance in the blood marked by an excess of acid, sometimes affecting diabetics and leading possibly to diabetic coma
acidotic: having or marked by acidosis
acinous cell: cell in the pancreas that secretes digestive juice, as distinguished from the cells of the islets of Langerhans
acne: common eruptive skin disorder resulting from the clogging or inflammation of the sebaceous glands
acoustic nerve: auditory nerve
acromegaly: disorder of the pituitary gland characterized by enlarged head, hands, feet, and most body organs
acrophobia: fear of heights
acupuncture: the Oriental art of traditional medicine in which needles are inserted at specific points through the skin to treat disease and induce anesthesia
acupuncturist: one skilled in acupuncture
acute: sudden and severe, as a disease
Adams-Stokes disease: temporary loss of consciousness caused by the heart's missing a beat, i.e., its failure to contract and pump blood on schedule
addiction: the compulsive habitual use of a drug for other than medical reasons
Addison's anemia: anemia, pernicious
Addison's disease: chronic hypofunction (underfunctioning) of the adrenal cortex, characterized by weakness, loss of body hair, and increased skin pigmentation
adenocarcinoma: carcinoma involving epithelial tissue of a gland
adenoid(s): enlarged lymphoid growth behind the pharynx
adenoidectomy: surgical removal of the adenoids

adenoma: benign tumor which can cause hyperfunction of the parathyroid glands
adenopathy: any glandular disease characterized by swelling of the lymph nodes
adenotonsillectomy: T and A operation
adipose: of or pertaining to fat; fatty
adolescents: age groups, teenagers
adrenal cortex: the outer part of the adrenal gland, which produces several hormones that affect metabolism of foods, secondary sex characteristics, skin pigmentation, and resistance to infection
adrenalectomy: surgical removal of an adrenal gland
adrenal gland: either of two small ductless glands situated above each kidney
adrenaline/epinephrine: adrenal hormone that acts to stimulate the heart, dilate the blood vessels, and relax bronchial smooth muscles
adrenal medulla: inner part of the adrenal gland
adrenocorticotrophic hormone/ACTH: hormone secreted by the anterior lobe of the pituitary gland which stimulates the growth and function of the adrenal cortex
aerobic: capable of living only in air or free oxygen, as certain bacteria
aerobics: exercises that involve a workout for the lungs and heart as well as the muscles
affect: emotion, as distinguished from thought or perception
afferent: applied to nerves receiving sensations; sensory
afferent nerves: nerves, sensory
aflatoxin: toxic substance produced by a fungus that develops typically in stored grains or legumes such as peanuts and that is associated with cancer of the liver
African trypanosomiasis: *see* sleeping sickness
afterbirth/the placenta: so called when expelled from the uterus after the birth of a baby
agoraphobia: fear of open spaces
agranulocytosis: acute disease characterized by almost total disappearance of neutrophils from the blood, and often following the use of certain drugs
AHF: antihemophilic factor
AIDS (acquired immune deficiency syndrome)**:** a serious condition whose main characteristic is a deficiency in the body's natural immunity against various diseases
ailurophobia: fear of cats
airway: 1. passageway for air 2. plastic breathing tube for administering artificial respiration from rescuer's mouth to victim's mouth
albino: organism with deficient pigmentation. In human beings, skin is usually milky or translucent, hair is white, and eyes appear pink
albumin: any of a class of protein substances found in the blood
albuminuria: the presence of protein in the urine
alcohol: colorless, flammable liquid distilled from fermented grains, fruit juices, and starches
alcoholic: one suffering from alcoholism
alcoholism: disease characterized by excessive and compulsive use of alcoholic beverages
aldose: a kind of sugar
algophobia: fear of pain
alimentary tract or **canal/gastrointestinal tract** or **canal:** passageway for food utilized in the digestive process, extending from the mouth to the anus, and including the esophagus, stomach, intestines, and rectum
alkali: any of various chemical compounds that neutralize acids and turn litmus paper blue
alkaloid: organic substance containing nitrogen and having a powerful toxic effect on animals and man, as morphine or strychnine
alkalosis: chemical imbalance in the blood marked by an excessive alkali content
allergen: substance or material capable of causing an allergic reaction
allergenic: having the properties of an allergen
allergic: pertaining to or caused by allergy
allergic rhinitis/hay fever: annually recurring inflammation of the mucous membranes of the nose and eyes caused chiefly by the pollen of certain plants
allergic shock/anaphylactic shock: violent shock reaction, often accompanied by a rash, resulting from an oversensitized reaction to a foreign substance such as medication or the substance transmitted by an insect bite
allergist/allergologist: physician specializing in the diagnosis and treatment of allergies
allergology: the branch of medical science dealing with the diagnosis and treatment of allergies
allergy(ies): condition of heightened susceptibility to a substance that in similar amounts is innocuous to others
allograft: *see* homograft
alopecia: baldness
alopecia areata: baldness, patchy
alveolar bone: either of the bones of the upper and lower jaws that include sockets for the teeth
alveoli (*sing., alveolus*)**:** air sacs situated in the lungs
Alzheimer's disease: presenile dementia
amalgam: mercury and silver compound, often used to fill teeth
amblyopia: dimness of sight not resulting from refractive error or disease
ambulation: act of walking or moving about, postoperative
ambulatory: able to walk

amenorrhea: absence or cessation of menstruation
amenorrhea, acquired: *see* amenorrhea, secondary
amenorrhea, primary: failure of menarche (the onset of menstruation) to occur
amenorrhea, secondary/acquired amenorrhea: cessation or interruption in the occurrence of menstruation
American trypanosomiasis: *see* Chagas' disease
amino acid: any of a group of compounds that form an essential part of the protein molecule
amnesia: loss or impairment of memory, sometimes temporary
amniocentesis/prenatal diagnosis: procedure for determining whether a fetus is afflicted with an inherited disorder by sampling the amniotic fluid of a pregnant woman
amnion/amniotic sac: membranous sac enclosing the embryo in mammals, birds, and reptiles
amniotic fluidbag of waters: the fluid within a membrane surrounding an embryo in the uterus of a pregnant woman
amoebic dysentery: form of dysentery caused by an amoeba
amphetamine/Benzedrine: any of a class of drugs that stimulate the central nervous system, used medically to treat depressive mental disorders and sometimes to retard appetite, and used illicitly to induce a state of abnormal alertness and excitement
Amphotericin B: antibiotic substance used to treat histoplasmosis and other deepseated fungus infections
ampulla (*pl., ampullae*)**:** any dilated part or sac, as the base of each of the semicircular canals of the inner ear
amputate: to remove surgically by cutting, as a gangrenous limb
anabolism: the process by which nutrients are built up into the living organism; constructive metabolism
anaerobic: capable of living without air or free oxygen, as certain bacteria
anal fissure: crack, split, or ulceration in the area of the two anal sphincters that control the release of feces
analgesia: incapacity to feel pain
analgesic: drug that lessens or eliminates the capacity to feel pain
anal sphincter: the ring of muscle fibers surrounding the anus and controlling the passage of wastes from the body
anaphylactic shock: allergic shock
androgen: any of various hormones found in males that control the appearance and development of masculine characteristics, also present although in smaller amounts in females
androsterone: an androgen secreted in the urine
anemia: deficiency in the amount or quality of red blood corpuscles or of hemoglobin in the blood
anesthesia: loss of sensation
anesthesiologist: physician specializing in the study and administration of anesthetics
anesthesiology: the branch of medical science that deals with the study and administration of anesthetics
anesthetic: drug, gas, or other substance or procedure that produces anesthesia
anesthetist: person trained to administer anesthetics
aneurysm: localized dilation of the wall of an artery, forming a pulsating sac and usually accompanied by pain resulting from abnormal pressure
angina pectoris: condition causing acute chest pain because of interference with the supply of oxygen to the heart
angiocardiography: visualization by X ray of the heart and its major blood vessels after injection of an opaque fluid
angioedema: swelling of the subcutaneous tissues
angiogram: X ray of a blood vessel obtained by the injection of an opaque liquid material into the blood vessels that supply the brain
angiography: visualization of the blood vessels
angiology: the branch of medical science dealing with the blood vessels and lymph vessels
ankylosing spondylitis: spondylitis, rheumatoid
ankylosis: the stiffening or fixation of a joint, as by disease or surgery
annular: having the shape of a ring
anorexia: loss of appetite
anorexia nervosa: emotional disturbance, especially of young women, characterized by aversion to food and resulting emaciation
anovulatory: without ovulation
anoxemia: deficiency of oxygen in the blood
anoxia: oxygen deficiency of the body tissues
antacid: any alkaline substance that can neutralize stomach acidity caused by gastric juices, often prescribed in ulcer diets
anterior: toward the front
anterior lobe hypophysis: the anterior part of the pituitary gland that produces growth hormones and hormones that stimulate other glands
anterior urethra: the meatus, or external opening, of the urethra in the penis
anthrax: malignant, infectious disease of sheep, cattle, and other animals, caused by a bacillus and sometimes transmitted to humans
anti- (*prefix*)**:** against; opposed to; opposite to

antibiotic(s): any of a large class of substances, such as penicillin and streptomycin, produced by various microorganisms and fungi that have the power to destroy or arrest the growth of other microorganisms, including many that cause infectious diseases
antibody: substance produced by the body to counteract infection and in response to specific antigens
anticlotting compounds: anticoagulant
anticoagulant: substance that retards clotting of the blood
anticonvulsant: medicine used to control epileptic seizures
antidepressant: drug that stimulates physiological activity, thereby tending to alleviate depression
antidiuretic hormone: vasopressin
antidote: anything that neutralizes or counteracts the effects of a poison
antigen: any of several substances, including toxins, enzymes, and proteins, that cause the development of antibodies when introduced into an organism
antihelminthic: drug or remedy used to destroy intestinal worms, or helminths
antihemophilic factor/AHF: substance that causes clotting and stops bleeding in hemophiliacs
antihistamine: any of a number of drugs that counteract the nasal engorgement and vasoconstrictor action of histamine in the body, often used in the treatment of hay fever
antimetabolite: chemical that interferes with cell metabolism
antiperspirant: astringent preparation that acts to diminish or prevent perspiration
antitoxin: antibody produced in response to the presence of a specific toxin, which it neutralizes
antivenin: antitoxin to venom or serum prepared to counteract the effects of venom
anuria: inability to urinate
anus: the opening at the lower extremity of the alimentary canal
anvilincus: the middle of the three ossicles of the middle ear, the bone between the hammer and the stirrup
anxiety reaction: neurosis characterized chiefly by anxiety unrelated to any apparent cause
aorta: the large artery originating from the left ventricle of the heart that forms the main arterial trunk from which blood is distributed to all of the body except the lungs
aortic valve: the membranous valve between the left ventricle of the heart and the aorta
Apgar system: system of rating the health of newborn babies
aphasia: partial or total loss of the power of articulate speech resulting from a disorder in the cerebrum of the brain
aplasia: arrested development or congenital absence of a part or organ of the body
aplastic: marked by aplasia; underdeveloped
apnea: cessation or interruption of breathing
apoplexy: stroke
appendectomy: surgical removal of the vermiform appendix
appendicitis: inflammation of the vermiform appendix characterized by pain in the right lower abdomen, nausea, and vomiting
appendicular skeleton: skeleton
appendix vermiformis: vermiform appendix
aqueous humor: the clear, limpid alkaline fluid that fills the anterior chamber of the eye from the cornea to the lens
arachnoid: the middle of the three membranes that envelop the brain and spinal cord
areola: the dark circular area around the nipple of a breast or around a pustule
arrest: slow or stop the progress of, as a disease
arrhythmia: variation from the normal heartbeat
arterial: having to do with or carried by the arteries
arteriogram: X-ray picture of an artery
arteriography: technique of injecting an opaque substance into the coronary arteries and observing the material by X ray as it runs its course through the heart muscle
arteriole: small artery, especially the one that leads to a capillary
arteriosclerosis: thickening and hardening of the walls of an artery, with impairment of blood circulation
arteritis: inflammation of an artery
artery: any of a large number of muscular, tubular vessels conveying blood away from the heart to all parts of the body
arthritis: inflammation of a joint, characterized by pain, swelling, and tenderness
arthropathy: any disease of the joints
articulate: form a joint, as one bone with another
artificial respiration: artificial maintenance of respiration in someone who has ceased to breathe, especially mouth-to-mouth resuscitation
ascaris: roundworms
ascorbic acid/vitamin C: white, odorless, crystalline compound found in citrus and other fresh fruits and green leafy vegetables, and also made synthetically, that prevents scurvy
asepsis: prevention of infection by the maintenance of sterile conditions
aseptic: free from disease-causing microorganisms
aseptic meningitis: *see* meningitis, aseptic

asphyxiation: loss of consciousness caused by too little oxygen in the blood, generally as a result of suffocation by drowning or the breathing in of noxious gases
aspirate: withdraw by suction
aspiration: act or process of aspirating
aspiration, vacuum: *see* vacuum aspiration
aspirin (acetylsalicylic acid): analgesic drug that has fever-reducing properties, widely used to treat symptoms of the common cold, rheumatoid arthritis, and many other conditions
assimilation: the process by which digested food is made an integral part of the solid or fluids of an organism
asthenia: lack or loss of strength; weakness
asthma: chronic respiratory disorder characterized by recurrent paroxysmal coughing caused by spasms of the bronchi or diaphragm, and resulting in many cases from an allergic reaction
astigmatism: distorted vision caused by an uneven curvature of the cornea
asymptomatic: condition in which antibodies for a disease are present in the blood but no symptoms of the disease can be observed
ataxia: absence or failure of muscular coordination
atherosclerosis: hardening of the inner walls of the arteries, resulting in a loss of elasticity, and accompanied by the deposit of fat and degenerative tissue changes
athetosis: derangement of the nervous system in which the hands and feet, especially the fingers and toes, keep moving or twitching
athlete's foot: ringworm of the foot, caused by a parasitic fungus
atrioventricular block: disruption of normal transmission of signals between the upper and lower chambers of the heart, as from scar tissue, that may affect blood flow to the brain and cause blackouts or convulsions
atrium (*pl., atria*)/**auricle:** one of the two upper chambers of the heart, which receive blood from the veins and transmit it to the ventricles
atrophy: the wasting or withering away of the body or any of its parts, as from disease or lack of use
attenuated: weakened in strength, as a microorganism for use in a vaccine
audiologist: one who specializes in the treatment of those with hearing problems
audiometer: device that measures hearing
auditory canal/auditory meatus: either of two passageways, the *external auditory canal* leading from the outer ear to the tympanic membrane or eardrum, and the *internal auditory canal* passing through the temporal bone to the brain
auditory nerve/acoustic nerve: nerve consisting of the cochlear nerve and the vestibular nerve and connecting the inner ear with the brain, conveying the sense of hearing and of equilibrium
aura: subjective, momentary sensory perception of an unusual nature that occurs just before the onset of an epileptic convulsion
Aureomycin: trade name for the antibiotic tetracycline
auricle: atrium
auscultation: diagnostic procedure of listening, as to sounds in the chest with a stethoscope
autism: mental disorder of children, marked by lack of response to external activities
autistic: suffering from or pertaining to autism
autograft: tissue graft taken from one part of a patient's body for transplanting in another part
autonomic nervous system: network of nerves originating in the spinal column, and including the sympathetic and parasympathetic nervous systems, that controls and stimulates the functions of body tissues and organs not subject to voluntary control, such as the heart or stomach
autopsy: postmortem examination of a body, as to determine the cause of death
avulsion: a tearing or wrenching away, as a structure or part of the body, as a result of an accident or by surgery
axillar: underarm
axillary: pertaining to or in the region of the armpit
axon: cylindrical fiber in neurons carrying impulses away from the cells

Babinski reflex: reflex of the toes, normal in infants, in which the large toe is extended upward and the other toes splayed when the underside of the foot is stroked, an indication in adults of neurological disease
baby: *see* infant; newborn
baby teeth/deciduous teeth/milk teeth: the first temporary set of human teeth, 20 in all, which begin to appear about the age of six months and are usually complete by the end of the second year
bacillary dysentery: a usually acute form of dysentery caused by bacilli
bacillus (*pl., bacilli*): any of a class of straight, rod-shaped bacteria having both beneficial and disease-causing effects
backbone: *see* spinal column
bacteria (*sing., bacterium*): one-celled microorganisms that come in three varieties —bacillus, coccus, and spirillum—and that range from the harmless and beneficial to the virulent and lethal
bacteriophobia: fear of germs
bag of waters: amniotic fluid

baldness/alopecia: common hereditary condition of males marked by a gradual loss of hair on the crown of the head until only a fringe remains around the sides and in the back, often called *male pattern baldness*
barber's itch: sycosis
barbiturates: any of a class of drugs derived from barbituric acid that depress the central nervous system, used medically as sedatives and sleeping pills and in the treatment of epilepsy and high blood pressure, and illicitly to counteract the effects of stimulant drugs
barium: metallic element used in compounds, especially barium sulfate, in radiography of the gastrointestinal tract because it is radiopaque—impervious to X rays
barium enema: enema in which a barium mixture is used to visualize the inner walls of the large intestine by X ray; used to detect cancer and other diseases
barium meal: liquid containing barium taken orally for the visualization of the upper gastrointestinal tract by X ray
barium sulfate: an insoluble barium compound used to facilitate X-ray pictures of the stomach and intestines
barium swallow: X-ray examination of the esophagus as the patient swallows a liquid containing barium
baroreceptors/barostats: sensitive nerve cells that respond to changes in blood pressure and may help to regulate it
Basal Body Temperature/BBT: accurate measure of body temperature taken under uniform conditions, used to determine a woman's day of ovulation
basal ganglia: group of nerve cells embedded in the cerebral hemisphere, the largest part of the human brain
basal metabolism: the minimum energy, measured in calories, that the body needs to maintain essential vital activities when it is at rest
basal thermometer: thermometer scaled in tenths of degrees instead of fifths, used by women to determine the time of ovulation
BBT: *see* Basal Body Temperature
bed-wetting: enuresis
belladonna: plant with purple-red flowers whose leaves and roots yield a number of poisonous alkaloids used in medicine
Bell's palsy: facial paralysis resulting from a lesion of the facial nerve
bends: *see* decompression sickness
benign: mild or nonmalignant, and responding to treatment
Benzedrine: amphetamine
beriberi: disease of the peripheral nerves characterized by partial paralysis and swelling of the legs, caused by the absence of B complex vitamins
bicuspid/premolar: one of the four upper or four lower cusped teeth located between the cuspids (or canine teeth) and the molars
bile: bitter, viscid alkaline fluid used in digestion, especially of fats, that is secreted by the liver and stored in the gallbladder
bilharziasis: *see* schistosomiasis
biliary tract: duct that conveys bile
bilirubin: pigment found in bile
biodegradable: capable of being broken down, as a chemical compound, by microorganisms
biodegrade: break down (a substance) chemically by the action of microorganisms
biological death: death of the brain, following clinical death
biomicroscope: slit lamp microscope
biopsy: excision of tissue or other material from a living subject for clinical and diagnostic examination
birth abnormalities: birth defects
birth canal: passageway formed by the cervix and vagina through which a fetus passes in the birth process
birth control: the regulation of conception by employing preventive methods or devices
birthmark: mark or stain existing on the body from birth
bite, improper: *see* malocclusion
black cancer: *see* melanoma
black fever: *see* kala-azar
black lung disease: form of pneumoconiosis common in coal miners and caused by constant exposure to coal dust
bladder: elastic membranous sac near the front of the pelvic cavity, used to store urine temporarily
bleb: blister formed in the epidermis
bleeder: *see* hemophiliac
blepharoplasty: surgical technique to correct congenital defects in the eyelids or to alter their size or shape
blister: small rounded sac, especially on the skin containing fluid matter, often resulting from injury, friction, or scalding
blood blister: blister containing blood from broken capillaries, often resulting from a pinch or other injury
blood count: examination of blood components, used in diagnosis. A *complete blood count* reveals the size, shape, and number of white and red cells and platelets in a cubic millimeter of blood. A *differential blood count* determines the percentage of leukocytes and other cells
blood groupblood type: classification of the blood, commonly designated AB, A, B, and O, based on the specific generic differences in the composition and chemical properties of the blood
bloodletting: *see* phlebotomy

blood poisoning/septicemia: introduction of virulent bacteria into the bloodstream, usually from a local infection such as a boil or wound and marked by chills, fever, and fatigue
blood pressure: diagnostic procedure of measuring the pressure of the blood on the walls of the arteries, varying with the resilience of the blood vessels and with the heart's contraction (*systole*) or relaxation (*diastole*), usually represented by two numbers, the systolic pressure followed by the diastolic pressure
blood serum: the watery, clear portion (*serum*) of blood
blue baby: infant born with cyanosis (imperfect oxygenation of the blood) resulting from a congenital heart defect
body scanner: *see* CT scanner
body scanning: *see* CT scanning
Boeck's sarcoid: *see* sarcoidosis
boil: abscess of the skin caused by bacterial infection of a hair follicle or sebaceous gland
bolus: lump or mass of food that has been chewed and softened with saliva
bone(s): hard tissue of which the skeleton of a vertebrate animal is largely composed
bone atrophy: decalcification
botulism: poisoning caused by eating spoiled or improperly prepared or canned food and characterized by acute gastrointestinal and nervous disorders
bowel, large: *see* intestine, large
Bowman's capsule: dilated structure surrounding a glomerulus as part of the nephron of a kidney
boy (*slang*): heroin
brain cage: cranium
brain damage: tissue destruction of the brain caused by an injury before, at, or after birth
brain death: biological death
brain scan: procedure of injecting a radioactive substance into the brain tissue or fluid and recording its movement by X rays
brain scanning: *CT scanning* of the brain
brain stem: all of the brain except the cerebellum, cerebrum, and cerebral cortex; the midbrain
brain surgeon: neurosurgeon
breastbone: *see* sternum
breathalyser: device for measuring the concentration of alcohol in the bloodstream of drivers of motor vehicles
breech presentation: birth with the baby positioned to present the buttocks first instead of the head first
bridge: a mounting for holding false teeth, attached to adjoining teeth on each side
Bright's disease: *see* nephritis
bromidrosis: perspiration odor
bronchi (*sing., bronchus*): the two forked branches of the trachea
bronchial asthma: *see* asthma
bronchial tree: the bronchi and bronchial tubes
bronchial tubes: the subdivisions of the trachea conveying air into the lungs
bronchiole: minute subdivision in a bronchial tube
bronchitis: inflammation of the bronchial tubes, characterized by coughing, chest pain, and fever
brucellosis/Malta fever/undulant fever: persistent infectious disease caused by a bacterium (*Brucella*) transmitted to humans from infected animals, as goats, cattle, or swine, and marked by recurrent fever, sweating, weakness, and generalized aches and pains
bruxism: habit of grinding the teeth during sleep or when otherwise under strain
bubo: inflammatory swelling of a lymph gland, especially in the groin or armpit
bubonic plague: form of plague characterized by buboes
buccal: pertaining to the cheek or mouth cavity
Buerger's disease: circulatory disorder associated with cigarette smoking
bulbar: pertaining to a bulb, especially the bulb of the medulla oblongata of the brain
bulimia: disorder involving overeating followed by self-induced vomiting
bunion: painful swelling of the foot, usually at the outer side of the base of the big toe
Burkitt's lymphoma: malignant lymphoma affecting the jaw, found especially among children in Africa
bursa: any of the fluid-filled sacs within the body that tend to lessen friction between movable parts
bursitis: inflammation of a bursa
byssinosis/white lung disease: lung disorder caused by inhaling cotton dust

cadaver: dead human body, especially one intended for dissection
Caesarian section: surgical delivery of a baby by cutting through the abdominal wall into the uterus
caffeine: chemical found in the leaves and berries of coffee, used as a stimulant and diuretic
caisson disease: *see* decompression sickness
calcification: the degenerative hardening of tissue because of the deposit of calcium salts
calcinosis: interstitial calcinosis
calcitonin: hormone secreted by the parathyroid glands, important in regulating the amount of calcium in the body
calculus: collection of hard material, as a deposit on the teeth
calorie(s): unit of heat used especially to express the heat- or energy-producing content of foods
calyx (*pl., calyces*): cup-shaped recess in the kidney pelvis that serves as a collecting point for urine

canalization: formation of new channels or ducts within tissues
canals of Schlemm: ringlike vein in the sclera of the eye that helps maintain a proper balance of aqueous humor
cancer: any of various diseases that probably have different causes and originate in different tissues, but which all involve neoplasms that spread by metastasis, resulting in progressive tissue degeneration
cancer-producing agents: carcinogens
candidiasis: *see* moniliasis
canine teeth: the sharp, pointed teeth, two in the upper jaw (called *eye teeth*), and two in the lower jaw, located between the incisors and the molars
canker sore: small ulcerous lesion in the mouth near the molar teeth, inside the lips or in the lining of the mouth
cannabis: hashish or marihuana
Cannabis sativa: the Indian hemp plant, from whose flowering tops are derived marihuana and hashish
cannula: narrow tube inserted into a body cavity or vessel, as to extract a substance or introduce a medication
capillary(ies): minute blood vessel
caput succedaneum: swelling under a newborn baby's scalp soon after birth, that usually dissolves in a few days
carbohydrate(s): any of a group of compounds, including sugars, starches, and cellulose, that contain carbon combined with hydrogen and oxygen, essential in the metabolism of plants and animals
carbolic acid/phenol: powerful caustic poison distilled from coal tar oil and used as a disinfectant
carbon monoxide: colorless, odorless gas that is highly poisonous when inhaled because it combines with the hemoglobin in the blood and thus excludes oxygen
carbon tetrachloride: colorless liquid that can be poisonous if inhaled over a long period, and often used as a fire extinguisher or cleaning fluid
carbuncle: painful, extensive inflammation of the skin, marked by hardness and the discharge of pus
carcinogen: cancer-producing agent
carcinogenic: causing cancer or increasing the incidence of cancer in a population
carcinoma: malignant tumor that arises in the tissue that lines body cavities and ducts (epithelial tissue)
cardia: the opening between the esophagus and the stomach
cardiac: of or relating to the heart
cardiac arrest: a stopping of the heartbeat
cardiac catheterization: the advancing of a catheter, or thin tube, through the veins to the heart chamber, in order to detect abnormalities and obtain blood samples
cardiac massage/cardiovascular pulmonary resuscitation/CPR: emergency procedure consisting of the application of rhythmic pressure on the chest in order to compress the heart and start it beating again
cardiac muscle: the striated but involuntary muscle of which the heart is composed
cardiac sphincter: ring of muscle at the entrance of the stomach, or cardia, that opens to allow food to enter from the esophagus
cardiac X-ray series: chest X rays taken after the patient has swallowed an opaque liquid such as barium sulfate
cardiogram: 1. record produced by a cardiograph 2. electrocardiogram
cardiograph: 1. instrument for recording the force of the movements of the heart 2. electrocardiograph
cardiologist: physician specializing in the diagnosis and treatment of heart disease
cardiology: the branch of medical science dealing with the heart, its physiology, and its pathology
cardiovascular: pertaining to the heart and blood vessels
cardiovascular disease/heart disease: disorders affecting the heart and blood vessels
cardiovascular pulmonary resuscitation: *see* cardiac massage
cardiovascular specialist: physician specializing in the diagnosis and the treatment of diseases of the heart and blood vessels
caries: decay of a bone or tooth (dental caries); see tooth decay
cariogenic: causing caries, or tooth decay
carotene: orange or red crystalline pigment converted to vitamin A in animal metabolism
carotid artery: either of two major arteries of the neck supplying blood to the head
carpal(s): pertaining to the bones of the carpus, or wrist
carpus: the wrist
carrier: person who is immune from infection of specific disease-causing bacteria that his body carries and that can be transmitted to others who are not immune
cartilage: tough, elastic supporting tissue
cartilage plate/epiphysis: extremity of a long bone, originally separated from it by cartilage but later consolidated with it by ossification
cast(s): bit of tissue, often microscopic, having taken the shape of a vessel or cavity in which it was formed, that is found in excretions and may indicate the presence of disease
catabolism: the destructive aspect of metabolism, in which living matter breaks down nutrients into simpler substances

catalepsy: abnormal condition characterized by lack of response to stimuli and by muscular rigidity, often associated with a psychological disorder
catalyst: substance or agent that causes a chemical reaction while remaining stable, such as an enzyme or hormone in the human body
cataract: the gradual clouding and opacity of the lens of the eye, leading to impaired passage of light and loss of vision
catatonic schizophrenia: *see* schizophrenia, catatonic
cathartic: medicine for purging the bowels
catheter: slender tube for drawing off fluid from a body cavity, especially urine from the bladder
catheterization: the introduction of a catheter into the body
caudal: situated at the tail end or bottom; posterior
caudal anesthesia/caudal/caudal block: form of anesthesia in which the patient is injected in the region of the lower spinal cord (sacral canal) to block pain in the pelvic area
caul: membrane (*amnion*) surrounding the fetus if it is unruptured and intact about the baby's head at delivery
cautery, chemical: chemosurgery
cavities: dental caries; *see* tooth decay
CBC: complete blood count; *see* blood count
cc: cubic centimeter
cecum: blind pouch or cavity open at one end, especially the cavity below the ileocecal valve that forms the first section of the large intestine
celiac: pertaining to the abdomen
celiac disease: *see* malabsorption syndrome
cellular therapy: treatment for the process of aging in which a person is injected with cells from healthy embryonic animal organs with the idea that the animal cells from the particular organ injected will then migrate to the same organ in the aging body and reactivate it
cementum: the layer of body tissue developed over the roots of the teeth
central nervous system: the portion of the nervous system that contains the brain and spinal cord and controls voluntary action and movement
centrifuge: 1. (*n.*) rotary machine employing centrifugal force to separate substances having different densities, as the constituents of blood 2. (*v.*) subject to a whirling motion to separate component parts, as of blood, that have different densities
cephalhematoma: swelling under a newborn baby's scalp, that usually dissolves within a few weeks
cerebellum: large section of the brain located below and behind the cerebrum, consisting of a central lobe and two lateral lobes, and which coordinates voluntary muscle movements, posture, and equilibrium
cerebral arteriogram: an X-ray picture of the brain used to investigate brain damage, especially after a hemorrhage or stroke, and made by injecting opaque dye into the blood vessels serving the brain and X raying them
cerebral arteriosclerosis: degenerative changes in the arteries of the brain
cerebral cortex: the cells and fibers that look like a convoluted layer of gray matter and that cover the cerebral hemisphere of the brain
cerebral hemisphere: one of the two halves into which the brain is divided
cerebral hemorrhage: hemorrhage into the cerebrum of the brain or within the cranium
cerebral palsy: inability to control movement caused by nonprogressive brain damage resulting from a prenatal defect or birth injury
cerebrospinal fluid/CSF: the clear, colorless fluid that surrounds the brain and spinal cord
cerebrospinal meningitis: inflammation of the membranes that cover the brain and spinal cord
cerebrovascular: of or relating to the vessels supplying blood to the brain
cerebrum: the upper anterior part of the brain, consisting of two hemispherical masses that constitute the chief bulk of the brain in man and is assumed to be the seat of thought and will
cervical: 1. pertaining to the cervix of the uterus 2. pertaining to the neck or any necklike part
cervical cap: contraceptive device made usually of soft plastic that fits over the cervix
cervical spine: cervical vertebrae
cervical vertebrae/cervical spine: the top seven vertebrae of the backbone, which are located in the neck and support the head
cervicitis: inflammation of the cervix of the uterus
cervix: neck of the uterus
cestode: tapeworm
chafing: inflammation of two opposing skin surfaces, caused by warmth, moisture, or friction
Chagas' disease/American trypanosomiasis: disease of Central and South America, a form of trypanosomiasis, caused by certain protozoa and spread by the bite of the assassin bug, characterized by fever, edema, and chronic heart disease
chancre: primary syphilitic lesion resembling a sore with a hard base
chancroid/soft chancre: venereal disease that produces a soft chancre
change of life: menopause

chapping: condition where skin is irritated, cracked, or roughened, more common in wintry weather
character disorder: *see* personality disorder
charas: resin obtained from the Cannabis sativa (marihuana) plant
chemical diabetes: *see* diabetes, chemical
chemosurgery: medical technique that utilizes chemistry, surgery, and microscopic analysis, especially used in the treatment of skin cancers
chemotherapy: medical technique used in the prevention or treatment of disease by chemical disinfection of affected organs and tissues, especially through the use of synthetic drugs whose action is specific against certain pathogenic microorganisms but nontoxic to the patient
chest cavity/thoracic cavity: body cavity corresponding to the chest, enclosed by the ribs
chest/thorax: part of body enclosed by ribs
chest X ray: X-ray photograph of the chest cavity that may reveal various abnormalities of the heart, blood vessels, or lungs
chicken pox: contagious viral disease, especially of children, marked by a rash
chilblains: localized inflammation of the skin, usually on the extremities or face, causing itching, swelling, and redness
chin, plastic surgery on: mentoplasty
chiropodist: podiatrist
chiropody: podiatry
chiropractic: method of therapy based on the theory that disease is mainly a result of nerve malfunction, which may be corrected by manipulation
chloasma: liver spots
Chloromycetin: brand name of an antibiotic used to treat typhoid
chloroquine: drug used in the treatment of gout and other conditions
cholecyst: *see* gallbladder
cholecystectomy: *see* gallbladder, removal of
cholecystitis: inflammation of the gallbladder
cholecystogram: visualization of the gallbladder by X ray
cholera: acute, infectious, chiefly epidemic bacterial disease characterized by diarrhea, vomiting, prostration, and dehydration
cholesterol: fatty crystalline alcohol derived principally from the bile and present in gallstones, the blood, and in brain and nerve tissues
chondromalacia: the softening of a cartilage, as under the kneecap
chondrosarcoma: form of cancer originating in the cartilage at the end of a bone
chorea/St. Vitus dance: disease of the nervous system characterized by involuntary muscular twitching
choroid: the middle, vascular coat of the eyeball
chromosome: one of the rod- or loop-shaped bodies, usually paired, found in the nucleus of every cell and containing genes
chronic: occurring gradually over an extended period of time, as a disease
chyme: partly digested food, in semiliquid form, as it passes from the stomach to the small intestine
cilia (*sing., cilium*)**:** tiny hairs in the nose and breathing passages that help filter out foreign particles that enter the body
ciliary muscles: the set of muscle fibers, attached to ligaments, that support the lens of the eye
cirrhosis: condition associated with excessive drinking in which there is an abnormal formation of connective tissue and a wasting of the tissue of the liver
clap: *see* gonorrhea
claustrophobia: fear of being in an enclosed place
clavicle: the bone connecting the shoulder blade and breastbone; the collarbone
cleft lip/harelip: genetic defect in which the upper lip is not completely joined
cleft palate: genetic defect in which the hard palate is not completely joined
climacteric, female: *see* menopause
climacteric, male: in men, the psychological equivalent of the menopause, characterized by forgetfulness, depression, and declining sexual interest
clinical: pertaining to or based on the actual process or symptoms of a disease as observed, as distinguished from those described as typical from a statistical or theoretical point of view
clinical death: cessation of respiration and heartbeat
Clinoril: sulindac
clitoris: small, erectile organ of the female in the front part of the vulva
clonic: of or characteristic of clonus
clonic phase: the period during a grand mal epileptic convulsion when spasms of rigidity and relaxation (or jerking) occur in rapid succession
clonus: muscular spasm characterized by rapid alternation of contraction and relaxation
closed bite: form of malocclusion, a severe overbite in which upper teeth extend far over lower teeth when the jaws are together
closed-chest massage: *see* external cardiopulmonary resuscitation
closed fracture/simple fracture/complete fracture: fracture in which bone is completely broken, but without accompanying break in the skin
clotting-deficiency diseases: hemorrhagic diseases
coagulation: clotting, as of blood

coarctation: stricture or contraction, as of a cavity or blood vessel
coated tongue: condition in which the tongue is coated with a whitish substance, consisting of food particles and bacteria, which can indicate fever, illness, or a temporary lack of saliva
cocaine: white, bitter, crystalline alkaloid used as a local anesthetic and a narcotic
cocarcinogen: substance that is not cancer-producing but reacts with other substances to produce cancers
coccidioides fungus: fungus, the spores of which can cause coccidioidomycosis
coccidioidomycosis/desert rheumatism/valley fever: infectious disease caused by fungus spores and characterized by symptoms resembling pneumonia and tuberculosis and the formation of reddened bumps
coccyx: the tail end of the spinal cord
cochlea: spiral-shaped structure of the inner ear containing the essential organs of hearing, including the organ of Corti
cochlear nerve: the part of the auditory nerve leading from the cochlea of the inner ear to the brain, conveying the sense of hearing
codeine: white, crystalline alkaloid, derived from morphine and used in medicine as an analgesic and to suppress coughing
coitus: sexual intercourse
coitus interruptus: contraceptive method whereby the male withdraws before he ejaculates
cold, common: viral infection of the respiratory tract
cold sores: herpes simplex
colitis: inflammation of the colon
collagen: fibrous protein that forms the chief constituent of the connective tissues of the body, such as cartilage, skin, bone, and hair
collapsed lung: pneumothorax
collarbone: clavicle
colon: the part of the large intestine extending from the cecum to the rectum and divided into the ascending colon, transverse colon, descending colon, and the sigmoid
colonoscope: speculum used to examine the colon
color blindness: inherited vision defect consisting of the total or partial inability to discriminate between certain colors, usually red, green, and blue
colostomy: the formation of an artificial opening in the colon through which solid wastes can pass
colostrum: the creamy, yellowish, milklike substance rich in proteins, that is produced by a mother's breasts the first few days after having given birth
colposcopy: microscopic technique for visual examination of the cervix and vagina
coma: prolonged loss of consciousness
comminuted fracture: fracture in which bone is splintered or crushed
common bile duct: duct formed by the juncture of the hepatic and cystic ducts, and carrying digestive enzymes from the liver, pancreas, and gallbladder to the duodenum
complete fracture: *see* closed fracture
compound fracture/open fracture: fracture accompanied by an open wound, often exposing bone that is completely broken
compulsion: urgent need to perform certain ritualistic acts, often irrational, a symptom of certain neuroses
computed tomography: *see* CT scanning
conception: union of spermatozoon and ovum, first step in the birth process; fertilization
concussion: violent shock to the brain, typically caused by a blow to the head, as in a fall, that impairs the functioning of the brain, usually temporarily
condom: membranous sheath for the penis that serves as a contraceptive device
condyloma acuminatum: *see* venereal wart
cone: one of many photosensitive cone-shaped bodies in the retina of the eye, sensitive to color and daylight vision
congener: natural product of fermentation found in small amounts in all alcoholic beverages
congenital: acquired prior to or at birth, or during development as a fetus, as fetal abnormality because of the mother's contraction of rubella
congenital defects: *see* birth defects
congenital heart disease: deformity of the heart or of major blood vessels existing from birth
congestion: excessive accumulation of blood or fluid in an organ or tissues
conjunctiva: mucous membrane on the inner part of the eyelid and extending over the front of the eyeball
conjunctival sac: the small sac at the inner corner of the eye between the eyeball and the lower lid that serves as a collecting pool for tears
conjunctivitis: inflammation of the conjunctiva (pinkeye)
connective tissue: the fibrous tissue that binds together or supports the parts of the body, as cartilage, tendons, and ligaments
conscience: superego
conservative: of or involving procedures or treatment intended to preserve function of diseased or injured parts, utilizing established therapeutic methods
constipation: inactivity of the bowels resulting in difficult, infrequent, or incomplete evacuation
constrict: to become narrower, as a blood vessel
contact dermatitis: *see* dermatitis, contact

contact lens: one of a pair of glass or plastic lenses fitted directly over the cornea of each eye to correct vision defects
contagion: communication of disease by contact, direct or indirect
contagious: (of a disease) transmitted by direct or indirect contact
continuous positive airway pressure: procedure in which high-oxygen is forced into the lungs of newborns suffering from respiratory difficulty
contraception: the prevention of conception
contraceptive: device or substance designed to prevent conception
contraindication: symptom or sign that makes a particular course of treatment inadvisable
conversion hysteria: *see* conversion reaction
conversion reaction/conversion hysteria: neurosis characterized by manifestation of physical symptoms, such as blindness or deafness, without organic cause, as an expression of psychic conflict
convulsion/seizure: spontaneous violent and abnormal muscular contraction or spasm of the body
Cooley's anemia: *see* thalassemia
corium: dermis
corn(s): horny thickening of the cuticle common on the feet
cornea: the transparent lens surface of the eye
coronary: encircling or crowning, such as the two arteries branching from the aorta and encircling the heart
coronary arteries and veins: the network of arteries and veins that nourishes the muscle and tissue of the heart
coronary artery disease: fatty obstructions in the coronary vessels that nourish the heart, thus impairing adequate delivery of oxygen to the heart
coronary attacks: heart attacks
coronary insufficiency: insufficient blood circulation through the coronary arteries
coronary occlusion: closure of the coronary artery resulting from buildup of fatty deposits or coronary thrombosis
coronary thrombosis: interference with the blood supply to the heart muscle because of a blood clot in the coronary artery
corpus callosum: fibrous tissue connecting the two hemispheres of the cerebrum of the brain
corpuscle: one of the cells that make up blood, either a red corpuscle (*erythrocyte*) or a white corpuscle (*leukocyte*)
corpus luteum: mass in the ovary formed by the rupture of a Graafian follicle that releases an ovum during each menstrual cycle
cortex: the outer layer or covering of an organ or part, as of the cerebrum or cerebellum of the brain (called *gray matter*), of the adrenal glands, or of the kidneys
corticoids: any of the hormones manufactured in the adrenal cortex
corticosteroid: 1. any of the steroids secreted by the cortex of the adrenal gland 2. any steroid hormone resembling in its effects the steroids secreted by the adrenal gland
corticosterone: steroid hormone of the adrenal cortex associated with blood sugar levels and other metabolic functions
Corti, organ of: *see* organ of Corti
cortisone: powerful hormone extracted from the adrenal cortex and also made synthetically
coryza: inflamed mucous membranes in the nose, with discharge of mucus characteristic of a head cold
cosmetic surgeon: physician specializing in cosmetic surgery
cosmetic surgery: plastic surgery concerned with improving the appearance of parts of the body
costal: pertaining to or near a rib or ribs
cough: to expel air or phlegm from the lungs in a noisy or spasmodic manner
cowpox: live calf lymph virus, used in smallpox vaccinations
coxa: the hip or hip joint
coxa vara: deformity of the hip joint caused by curvature of the femur toward the joint, thus shortening the affected leg and causing a limp
Coxsackie virus: any of a group of viruses causing various diseases in humans, including a form of meningitis
cradle cap: disease of the scalp, especially in babies, marked by yellowish crusts
cranial nerves: the twelve pairs of nerves that originate within the brain
cranioplasty: surgical correction of the skull, as to repair a congenital defect
craniotomy: any surgery involving an opening in the skull
cranium: the part of the human skull that encloses and protects the brain
crash: (*slang*) amphetamine
cresol: compound obtained by destructive distillation of coal, beechwood, or pinewood, used as an antiseptic and disinfectant
cretinism: stunted or impaired physical and mental development because of deficiency of thyroxin, a secretion of the thyroid gland, in infancy or during the fetal period
crib death: *see* sudden infant death syndrome
crossed eyes/crosseye: strabismus characterized by a tendency of the eyes to turn inward toward the nose
cross-match: to intermix constituents of the blood of a prospective donor with that of a prospective recipient to check blood compatibility
croup: spasm of the trachea, especially the larynx, occurring in children and marked by difficulty in breathing and a barking cough

crown: the part of a tooth exposed beyond the gum and covered with enamel
cryosurgery: type of surgery in which extremely low temperatures are employed either locally or generally to destroy tissue, as in malignant skin lesions
cryotherapy: inducement of peeling by freezing the skin with carbon dioxide to improve appearance of flat acne scars and shallow wrinkles
cryptorchidism/cryptorchism: failure of the testicles to descend normally
CSF: *see* cerebrospinal fluid
CT scanner/body scanner: computerized X-ray machine used in CT scanning
CT (computed tomography) scanning/body scanning: procedure for producing a cross-sectional, computer-generated, composite X-ray picture of the body or an organ, as the brain, by rotating about a site and taking a series of radiographs directed to it
culdoscopy: technique for examining the female reproductive organs within the abdominal cavity
culture: the development of microorganisms or living cells in a special medium, as gelatin, often as a means of analyzing a body fluid or tissue for the presence of disease
Cuprimine: penicillamine
cupula: structure within each of the semicircular canals of the inner ear, communicating changes in motion
curettage: the scraping of a cavity with a curette, as to remove morbid matter or obtain tissue for diagnosis
curette: small instrument, usually resembling a spoon or scoop with sharpened edges, used in curettage
Cushing's syndrome: excess of hormones secreted by the adrenal cortex, characterized by weakness, purple streaks in the skin, and a moon face
cusp: 1. one of the projections or points on the crown of a tooth 2. one of the triangular flaps of a heart valve
cuspid/canine tooth/eye tooth: one of the two upper or two lower sharp, pointed teeth located between the incisors and the bicuspids
cutaneous: pertaining to, affecting, or on the skin
cuticle: 1. epidermis 2. crescent of toughened skin around the base of the nail
cyanosis: disordered circulatory condition resulting from inadequate oxygen supply in the blood and causing a livid bluish color of the skin
cyanotic: bluish in color because of cyanosis
cyclamates: sodium cyclamate
cycloid: *see* cyclothymic
cyclothymic/cycloid: describing a personality disorder in which the individual is subject to sharply defined moods of elation or depression
cynophobia: fear of dogs
cyst: saclike mass containing liquid or semisolid material
cystectomy: 1. surgical removal of the gallbladder or of the urinary bladder 2. surgical removal of a cyst
cystic duct: duct that carries bile from the gallbladder to the juncture with the hepatic duct, where the common bile duct is formed
cystic fibrosis: hereditary disease of infants and young children marked by cysts, excessive fibrous tissue, and mucous secretion
cystitis: inflammation of the bladder, characterized by a burning sensation when voiding, frequent need to urinate, and sometimes blood in the urine
cystocele: hernia in which part of the bladder protrudes through the wall of the vagina
cystoscope: device used to view the interior of the bladder after being inserted in the urethra
cystoscopy: the technique of viewing the interior of the bladder by means of a cystoscope
cystostomy: the making of an artificial outlet from the urinary bladder

D and C: *see* dilation and curettage
dandruff: condition marked by itching and flaking of the skin, especially of the scalp
db: decibel
DBI/phenformin: drug that stimulates the production of insulin in the pancreas
D.D.S.: Doctor of Dental Surgery
decalcification/bone atrophy: the loss of lime or calcium salts from the bones or teeth
decibel/db: unit for measuring the intensity of sound
deciduous teeth: baby teeth
decision-maker: ego
decompression sickness/caisson disease/the bends: painful, sometimes fatal condition that results from bubbles of nitrogen formed in the blood when a rapid reduction in pressure occurs, as when a diver returns directly to the surface after a period deep under water
decongestant: agent designed to relieve congestion
defecation: the discharge of feces
defibrillation: act or process of stopping fibrillation of the heart muscle and restoring normal rhythm, as by jolting it with an electric current
defibrillator: device that sends a jolt of electricity into the heart muscle in order to stop fibrillation and get the heart back to normal rhythm
degenerative: characterized by deterioration or change from a normally active state to a lower or less active form, especially of body tissue, as in a disease process
degenerative joint disease: *see* osteoarthritis
deglutition: act of swallowing

dehydration: loss or removal of water, as from body tissues
déjà vu: distortion of memory in which a new situation or experience is regarded as having happened before
delirium tremens/DTs: violent form of delirium characterized by nausea, confusion, crawling sensation on the skin, and hallucinations caused especially by rapid lowering of blood alcohol levels in very heavy drinkers
dementia: mental deterioration resulting from an organic or functional disorder
Demerol: meperidine
demyelination: gradual loss of myelin, resulting in paralysis, numbness, or other loss of nerve function
dendrites: short, gray filaments in neurons that conduct impulses toward the cell body
dental calculus/tartar: hard deposit of minerals and other substances that collects on teeth
dental caries/cavities: ulceration and decay of teeth; *see* tooth decay
dental floss: strong, silky filament for cleaning between the teeth
dental surgeon: *see* oral surgeon
dentin: the hard calcified substance that forms the body of a tooth
dentist: one who specializes in the diagnosis, prevention, and treatment of disease affecting the teeth and their associated structures
dentistry: the branch of medical science that concerns the study, diagnosis, prevention, and treatment of diseases of the teeth, gums, and associated structures
dentition: the kind, number, and arrangement of the teeth in the mouth
denture(s): frame of plastic or other material adapted to fit the mouth and containing one, several, or a complete set of artificial teeth to replace natural teeth that have been lost
depilatory: chemical product capable of removing or loosening hair
depressant: drug or other substance that reduces or calms the physiological processes of body or mind
depression: 1. mental state marked by melancholy, pessimism, or dejection 2. psychotic condition characterized by stuporous withdrawal from reality and intense guilt feelings
depressive reaction: 1. neurosis characterized by persistent feelings of depression and pessimism unrelated to any apparent cause 2. (involutional melancholia) psychosis usually occurring in women around the time of menopause, and in men during their 50s, characterized by hopeless melancholy, anxiety, weeping, and often delusions
dermabrasion: the removal of layers of skin by planing with an abrasive tool to dispose of wrinkles or skin blemishes
dermal: of or relating to the skin
dermatitis: inflammation of the skin
dermatologist: physician specializing in the diagnosis and treatment of disorders of the skin
dermatology: the branch of medical science dealing with disorders of the skin
dermis/corium/true skin: the inner layer of the skin, which contains blood vessels, nerves, connective tissue, sweat glands, and sebaceous glands
DES: *see* diethylstilbestrol
desert rheumatism: coccidioidomycosis
Desoxyn: methamphetamine
detached retina/separated retina: eye disorder in which the membrane at the back of the eye (retina) is separated from its bed, as by being torn, thus impairing vision
developmental disability: any condition which interferes with a child's development, especially one which will constitute a handicap throughout the individual's life, such as mental retardation or cerebral palsy
Dexedrine: dextroamphetamine
dextroamphetamine (d-amphetamine)/Dexedrine: isomer of the amphetamine compound, considered to have a more stimulating effect on the central nervous system than amphetamine
dextrose: form of glucose (a sugar) found normally in animals, used in intravenous feeding because it is readily assimilated by the blood
diabetes, chemical/prediabetic condition: condition indicating predisposition to development of diabetes, when blood sugar level remains abnormally high for too long after taking a glucose tolerance test
diabetes insipidus: production of excessive amount of urine because of deficiency of antidiuretic hormone
diabetes mellitus: disease associated with inadequate production of insulin and characterized by excessive urinary secretion containing abnormal amounts of sugar, accompanied by emaciation, excessive hunger, and thirst
diabetic: one who has diabetes
diabetic acidosis: advanced stage of diabetes treated with insufficient insulin, characterized by increasing buildup of ketone bodies, drowsiness, and, if untreated, coma
diabetic coma: state of unconsciousness in a diabetic resulting from insufficient insulin, characterized by deep, labored breathing and a fruity odor to the breath
diabetic ketosis: early stage of diabetes treated with insufficient insulin, characterized by excessive urination, thirst, and hot, dry skin
diabetic retinopathy: disease of the eye associated with diabetes in which new, abnormal blood vessels form on the surface of the retina, sometimes marked by bleeding
diacetylmorphine: heroin

diagnosis: identification of a disease or disorder by its characteristic symptoms, or the conclusions reached in a particular instance
dialysis: the separating of mixed substances by means of wet membranes, as the action of the kidneys, especially applied to an artificial process to remove waste products and excess fluid from the bloodstream of a patient with defective kidneys
diaper rash: rash caused by the ammonia produced by the urine in diapers
diaphragm: 1. dome-shaped layer of muscle between the chest and abdomen whose contraction enlarges the rib cage for inflation of the lungs in breathing 2. contraceptive device of molded rubber or soft plastic material used to cover the cervix and prevent entry of spermatozoa
diaphragmatic hernia: hernia, hiatus
diarrhea: frequent and fluid evacuation of feces
diastole: the instant when the heart is relaxed as the ventricles fill with blood prior to contraction and pumping (systole)
diastolic pressure: measure of blood pressure taken when the heart is resting, the lower of the two figures in a reading
diathermy: treatment by means of heat generated within the body of high-frequency radiation
diethylstilbestrol/DES/stilbestrol: synthetic hormone resembling estrogen implicated in the formation of vaginal and cervical cancers in the daughters of women who had taken the hormone during pregnancy
differential blood count: *see* blood count
digestion: process of dissolving and chemically changing food in the alimentary tract so that it can be assimilated by the blood and its nutrients can be absorbed by the body
digestive tract: *see* gastrointestinal tract
digitalis: the dried leaves of foxglove, containing several glycosides, often used as a heart tonic
dilate: to become larger, as the pupil of the eye in diminished light
dilation and curettage/D and C: enlarging the opening into the uterus and the scraping of the uterus with a curette
dimethyltryptamine: *see* DMT
diphenylhydantoin: phenytoin
diphtheria: respiratory, bacterial disease marked by the formation of a false membrane that obstructs breathing
diplopia: *see* double vision
disclosing tablets: tablets which, after being chewed, leave a temporary stain on plaque remaining on teeth after brushing
disinfectants: germicides
dislocation(s): the partial or completed displacement of one or more of the bones at a joint
displacement: transference of intense anxiety unconsciously felt about a particular conflict to a substitute, which is regarded consciously with the same intensity of anxiety, a manifestation of the phobic reaction
dissociative reaction: neurosis characterized by escape from a part of the personality by means of dream states, amnesia, forgetfulness, etc.
distal: relatively remote from the center of the body, or from a point considered as central
distal muscles: the muscles of the extremities (the hands and the feet)
distillation: separation of the more volatile parts of a substance from the less volatile by boiling and condensing the vapors into separate liquids
diuresis: excessive excretion of urine
diuretic(s): substance stimulating the secretion of urine
diverticula (*sing., diverticulum*)**:** pouches or sacs opening off the large intestine
diverticulitis: inflammation of diverticula in the digestive tract, especially in the colon
diverticulosis: the presence of diverticula in the digestive tract
diverticulum (*pl. diverticula*)**:** abnormal pouch or bulge protruding from an organ or part, as from the colon or the intestines
DNT/dimethyltryptamine: synthetic hallucinogen
DNA (deoxyribonucleic acid): chemical in the human cell that controls body development
Dolly (*slang*)**:** methadone
DOM/STP: synthetic hallucinogen
dopamine: chemical compound found in the brain, needed in the synthesis of norepinephrine and epinephrine
Doriden: glutethimide
dorsal: toward, near, or in the back
double vision/diplopia: condition in which a single object is perceived as two images because of an inability to coordinate focusing of the eyes
douching: flushing of a body part or cavity, especially the vagina, with water as a means of cleansing
Down's syndrome/Mongolism: congenital mental and physical retardation resulting from a chromosomal anomaly, accompanied by variable signs, including a flat face and pronounced epicanthic folds
downs/downers/goof balls (*slang*)**:** barbiturates or other drugs that depress the central nervous system
DPT injection: injection to provide immunity against diphtheria, pertussis (whooping cough), and tetanus
Dramamine: proprietary drug used to counteract motion sickness
dreamer (*slang*)**:** morphine

dropsy: former term for edema, especially when caused by cardiac insufficiency
drug(s): 1. any substance other than food that changes or has an effect on the body or mind 2. narcotic drug
dry socket: painful complication of a tooth extraction in which underlying tissue of the alveolar bone is exposed to infection
DTs: delirium tremens
Duchenne's muscular dystrophy: pseudohypertrophic muscular dystrophy
duct/hepatic: either of two ducts of the liver that join to form the common hepatic duct and that carry bile
ductless glands: *see* endocrine glands
dumdum fever: *see* kala-azar
duodenal ulcer: ulcer of the duodenum of the small intestine
duodenum: the first section of the small intestine, leading from the stomach to the jejunum
dura mater: the tough, fibrous, outermost membrane of the three membranes covering the brain and spinal cord
dwarfism: disorder characterized by stunted growth
dysentery: severe inflammation of the mucous membrane of the large intestine, characterized by bloody stools, pain, cramps, and fever
dysfunction: impairment or abnormal functioning, as of an organ
dyslexia: 1. impairment or loss of the ability to read, as from a stroke 2. in children, impairment of ability to acquire language skills because of motor or perceptual disabilities
dysmenorrhea: painful menstruation
dyspareunia: painful sexual intercourse
dyspepsia: indigestion, characterized by heartburn, nausea, pain in the upper abdomen, and belching
dysphagia: difficulty in swallowing
dysphasia: disorder of the cerebral centers characterized by difficulty in understanding or using speech
dyspnea: labored, difficult breathing
dystrophy: 1. defective or faulty nutrition 2. any of various neurological or muscular disorders, as muscular dystrophy
dysuria: difficult, painful, or incomplete urination

eardrum/tympanic membrane/tympanum: drumhead membrane separating the middle ear from the external ear
earwax: waxy substance secreted by the glands lining the passages of the external ear
ECG: electrocardiogram
echocardiogram: graph recording the pattern of deflection of sound waves by the heart, used in diagnosing heart abnormalities
eclampsia: toxemia of pregnancy involving convulsions
E. coli/Escherichia coli: common bacillus found normally in the human intestines, usually harmless but having certain strains that cause urinary tract and other infections
ECPR/external cardiopulmonary resuscitation: closed-chest massage, used for those suffering cardiac arrest
ectoderm: outermost layer of tissue
ectopic/atopic: out of normal place or position
ectopic pregnancy: abortive pregnancy outside the uterus, as in the Fallopian tubes or abdominal cavity
eczema: noncontagious skin condition characterized by itching and scaling of the skin
edema: swelling of tissues because of abnormal fluid accumulation
edentulous: toothless
EEG: *see* electroencephalogram
efferent: applied to nerves, communicating impulses so that directive action can be taken
egg cell: ovum
ego: the self, considered as the seat of consciousness
ejaculation: expulsion of semen during orgasm
EKG: *see* electrocardiogram
elective surgery: surgery that is not essential for the maintenance of physical health, as cosmetic surgery
Electra complex: repressed sexual attachment of daughter to father, analogous to the Oedipal complex involving the son and mother
electric shock: the body's reactions to the passage through it of an electric current, as involuntary muscular contractions
electrocardiogram/ECG/EKG: graph recording the pattern of electric impulses produced by the heart, used in the diagnosis of heart disease
electrocardiograph: machine used to record the electric current produced by the heart muscle
electrocardiography: technique of producing electrocardiograms and interpreting them
electroencephalogram/EEG: graph recording the pattern of electric impulses produced by the brain, used in the diagnosis of neurological disorders
electroencephalograph: machine used to record the electric current produced by the brain
electroencephalography: technique of producing electroencephalograms and interpreting them
electrolysis: technique for removing unwanted hair by destroying the hair root with an electric current
electromyogram/EMG: graph recording the electrical activity of a muscle
electromyography: technique of producing electromyograms and interpreting them

electroshock: describing a form of treatment for psychological disorders in which a controlled electric current is passed through the patient's head, producing convulsions and unconsciousness, usually given in series
electrosurgery/surgical diathermy: surgical procedure utilizing electricity to destroy tissue
elephantiasis: lymphatic edema, especially of the legs and scrotum, a symptom of filariasis
embolism: the stopping up of a vein or artery, as by a blood clot, that has been brought to the point of obstruction by the bloodstream
embolus: object moving within the bloodstream, as a blood clot or air bubble, that is capable of causing an obstruction (embolism) in a smaller vessel
embryo: the rudimentary form of an organism in its development before birth, usually considered in the human species to be the first two months in utero
emetic: medicine or substance used to induce vomiting
emphysema: puffed condition of the alveoli or air sacs of the lung (or other tissues or organs) because of infiltration of air and consequent loss of tissue elasticity
enamel: the layer of hard, glossy material forming the exposed outer covering of the teeth
encephalitis: inflammation of the brain
encephalogram: X-ray picture of the brain made by encephalography
encephalography: X-ray visualization of the brain following the removal of cerebrospinal fluid and its replacement with air or other gases
endarterectomy: surgical procedure in which carbon dioxide is forced through hardened arteries to ream out fatty blockages
endemic: confined to or characteristic of a given locality, as a disease
endocarditis: inflammation of the membrane (endocardium) lining the chambers of the heart, sometimes caused by bacteria
endocardium: the delicate membrane that lines the chambers of the heart
endocrine gland: one of several ductless glands that release secretions (hormones) directly into the blood or lymph and that exert powerful influences on growth, sexual development, metabolism, and other vital body processes
endocrinologist: physician specializing in endocrinology
endocrinology: the branch of medical science dealing with the structure and function of the endocrine glands and their hormones
endoderm: innermost layer of tissue
endodontics: branch of dentistry dealing with root canal work and the dental pulp
endodontist: dentist specializing in root canal work
endogenous insulin: self-produced insulin
endolymph: fluid within the semicircular canals of the inner ear
endometrial: of or pertaining to the endometrium
endometrioma: mass of tumorlike endometrial cells as a result of endometriosis
endometriosis: condition in which tissue that lines the uterus (endometrium) grows outside the uterus in the pelvic cavity
endometrium: the lining of the uterus
endoscope: instrument for examining a hollow organ or an internal cavity, as the urinary bladder or the urethra
endoscopy: examination with an endoscope
enema: liquid injected into the rectum as a purgative or for diagnostic purposes
ENT: otolaryngology (ear, nose, and throat doctor)
enteric: pertaining to the intestines
enteric fever: *see* typhoid
enteritis: inflammation of the intestines, especially of the small intestine
enterocele: hernia in which part of the small intestine protrudes through the wall of the vagina
enuresis/bed-wetting: involuntary urination during sleep at night
enzyme(s): organic substance, usually a protein, produced by cells and having the power to initiate or accelerate specific chemical reactions in metabolism, such as digestion
eosinophil: any of a type of white blood cell that stains easily when a particular red dye (eosin) is applied
ephedrine: drug that dilates the bronchi, used to reduce nasal congestion and relieve asthma
epicanthic fold/epicanthus: vertical fold of skin at the inner corner of the eyelid, found chiefly in certain Asian peoples
epicanthus: *see* epicanthic fold
epidemic: 1. (*adj.*) affecting many in a community at once, as a disease 2. (*n.*) the temporary prevalence of a disease in a community or throughout a large area
epidemiologist: physician specializing in epidemiology
epidemiology: the branch of medical science concerned with the study and prevention of epidemic diseases
epidermis/cuticle: the outer, nonvascular layer of the skin, overlying the dermis
epididymis: portion of the seminal ducts just above the testis
epigastric: pertaining to the upper middle part of the abdomen
epigastrium: the upper middle (epigastric) part of the abdomen
epiglottis: the leaf-shaped plate of cartilage at the base of the tongue that covers the trachea during the act of swallowing

epilepsy: chronic nervous disorder characterized by sudden loss of consciousness and sometimes by convulsions
epileptic: 1. (*adj.*) pertaining to epilepsy 2. (*n.*) person who has epilepsy
epinephrine: *see* adrenaline
epiphysis: cartilage plate on the extremity of a long bone
episiotomy: incision made during labor to enlarge the vaginal area enough to permit passage of the baby
epistaxis: nosebleed
epithelial: pertaining to the epithelium
epithelium: membranous tissue that lines the canals, cavities, and ducts of the body, as well as all free surfaces exposed to the air
erection: enlarged and firm state of the penis when sexually stimulated
eruption: 1. emergence of a tooth through the gums 2. a breaking out of a rash on the skin
erysipelas: acute bacterial skin infection characterized by bright red patches
erythema: redness of the skin, a symptom occurring in various forms in different conditions having various causes, as from infection or a burn
erythremia: polycythemia vera
erythrocyte/red blood cell/red corpuscle: cell found in the bloodstream, often lacking a nucleus, the carrier of hemoglobin
erythrophobia: fear of blushing
eschar: dry crust or scab left by a burn caused by heat or corrosive chemical action
Escherichia coli: *see* E. coli
esophagoscope: device inserted into the esophagus to permit its inspection
esophagus (gullet): the tube through which food passes from the mouth to the stomach
essential: of unknown cause, as a disease or condition
essential hypertension: *see* hypertension, essential
estrogen: any of several hormones found in the ovarian fluids of the female which promote growth of secondary sex characteristics and influence cyclical changes in the female reproductive system
ethanol: ethyl alcohol
ether: colorless, volatile, flammable chemical compound used as an anesthetic
ethmoid bone: sievelike bone at the base of the skull behind the nose
ethyl alcohol/grain alcohol/ethanol: product of the distillation of fermented grains, fruit juices, and starches, used in beverages, and having intoxicating properties
etiologist: physician specializing in studying the causes of disease
etiology: 1. the cause or causes of a disease 2. the branch of medical science dealing with the causes of disease
eunuch: in males, the failure at puberty to develop secondary sex characteristics because of removal or disorder of the testicles
Eustachian tube: passage connecting the middle ear to the upper throat which equalizes air pressure on both sides of the eardrum
Ewing's sarcoma: malignant tumor of the shafts of the long bones in children
excise: cut out or remove by surgery
excision: act or procedure of cutting out or removing surgically
excrete: to eliminate, as waste matter, by normal discharge from the body
excretion: 1. the act of excreting 2. the body's waste matter, as sweat, urine, and feces
exocrine gland: any of various glands, such as mammary or sebaceous glands, having ducts that carry their secretions to specific locations
exophthalmic goiter: hyperthyroidism
expectorant: medicine that promotes the discharge of mucus from the respiratory tract
expectorate: discharge from the mouth, as saliva or phlegm
exploratory: performed for the purpose of making a diagnosis: said of a surgical operation
extension: state of being extended or straightened
extensor: muscle whose function is to extend or straighten a part of the body
external cardiac massage: cardiac massage
extraction: surgical removal of a tooth
extrinsic: originating or situated outside an organ or part
exudate: substance filtered through the walls of living cellular tissue, sometimes as a result of disease or injury, as in the case of inflammation
eyeground: the inner side of the back of the eyeball
eyestrain: disorder caused by excessive or improper use of the eyes and characterized by fatigue, tearing, redness, and a scratchy feeling in the eyelids
eye teeth: the upper canine teeth

face lift: rhytidoplasty
facial canal: Fallopian canal
facial neuralgia: *see* trigeminal neuralgia
facial plasty: rhytidoplasty
fainting: brief loss of consciousness
Fallopian canal/facial canal: bony canal in the skull
Fallopian tubes: the pair of tubes connecting the ovaries and the uterus, through which the egg must pass at the time of ovulation
family therapy: form of group therapy in which the patient group are members of the same family
farsightedness/hypermetropia/hyperopia: inability to see nearby objects clearly

fascia: fibrous tissue in the form of sheets that connect, surround, and support muscles and organs of the body
fascitis: inflammation of the fascia
fat: chemical compound forming an important food reserve and a source of hormones, vitamins, and other products essential in metabolism
fat pad: mass of fatty tissue
FDA: Food and Drug Administration
febrile: feverish
feces/stool: animal waste discharged following a bowel movement, usually containing indigestible foods, bacteria, bile, and mucus
femur: the long bone that supports the thigh; the thigh bone
fermentation: the conversion of glucose into ethyl alcohol, especially through the action of an enzyme (zymase) found in yeast
fetus: organism developing in the uterus before birth, sometimes considered in the human species to begin with the third month in utero, prior to which is called an embryo
fever/pyrexia: body temperature above the normal
fever blisters: *see* cold sores
fiberoptic: consisting of or making use of fibers of glass or plastic, as in optical instruments designed for viewing the intestines or stomach
fibrillation: irregular, uncoordinated contraction (arrhythmia) of muscle fibers of the heart
fibrin: insoluble protein that forms an interlacing network of fibers in clotting blood
fibrinogen: complex protein found in plasma which, in combination with the enzyme thrombin, forms fibrin
fibrinolysin: enzyme present in the blood that liquefies fibrin, thus dissolving blood clots
fibroid: *see* tumor, fibroid
fibroma: benign tumor composed of fibrous connective tissue
fibula: the outer of the two bones of the lower leg
field block: form of local anesthesia in which the anesthetic is injected into the tissue area in which surgery is to be performed
filariasis: tropical disease transmitted by mosquitoes and caused by a parasitic worm that invades the lymphatic system, producing edema and elephantiasis
fistula: abnormal channel leading from a hollow organ or cavity to another part or to the surface of the body
flaccidity: lack of firmness or elasticity; limpness
flatulence: accumulation of gas in the stomach and bowels
flexion: state of being bent or flexed
flexor: muscle whose function is to flex or bend a part of the body
flexure: bend or fold, as in the colon sigmoid
floss: *see* dental floss
flu: *see* influenza
fluke: *see* schistosoma
fluoridation: the addition of sodium fluoride to drinking water as a means of preventing tooth decay
fluoride: compound of fluorine, often added to public water supplies or toothpastes to retard or prevent tooth decay in children
fluoroscope: device for directly observing internal body structures by passing X rays through the patient and projecting shadows on a screen coated with a fluorescent substance
fluoroscopy: examination conducted by means of a fluoroscope
flu shots: influenza inoculation
focal convulsion: epileptic convulsion that affects only one part of the body
follicle: small cavity or saclike structure that secretes or excretes body fluids
follicle, hair: tiny sac within the dermis from which hair grows and is nourished
follicle-stimulating hormone/FSH: hormone secreted at the start of puberty by the pituitary gland, causing maturation of ovaries in girls and formation of sperm in boys
follicular cyst: *see* cyst, follicular
fontanel: either of two soft places at juncture points of the skull of a baby, the *anterior fontanel,* near the front, and the *posterior fontanel,* near the back
food chain: the relationship of organisms considered as food sources or consumers or both, as the relationship of a flowering plant to a bee or to a bird
food poisoning: digestive disorder marked by nausea and vomiting, caused by bacteria found in decaying or rancid food
food tube: esophagus
foot doctor: podiatrist
foot drop: condition in which the foot drops when extended in stepping forward, as caused by paralysis of a leg muscle
foramen: natural aperture or passage, as in a bone
forceps: two-bladed instrument for grasping and compressing or pulling, various types of which are used by dentists and surgeons
forces, balance of: *see* Yin; Yang
forensic medicine/forensic pathology: subspecialty of pathology dealing with the various aspects of medicine and the law
forensic pathology: forensic medicine
foreskin: the loose skin (prepuce) covering the head of the penis
fossa: pit or depression in a surface
fovea: shallow rounded depression in the retina, directly in the line of vision at a point where vision is most acute
fracture: break in a bone; *see* closed fracture; complete fracture; incomplete fracture

fraternal twins: twins who are not identical, derived from separately fertilized ova
freckle: small, brownish or dark-colored spot on the skin
free association: psychoanalytic technique in which the patient talks freely about anything that comes to mind
freezing of skin: cryosurgery
Freud, Sigmund: Austrian neurologist (1856–1939) who founded psychoanalysis and shaped the course of modern psychiatry
frigidity: sexual unresponsiveness in women
Froehlich's syndrome: failure of secondary sex characteristics to develop in males because of anterior pituitary disease
frontal lobe: the front portion of each cerebral hemisphere of the brain, whose functions are uncertain
frontal lobotomy: rarely performed surgical operation of cutting into the frontal lobes of the brain to alter behavior
frostbite partial freezing of a part of the body, especially of the extremities or ears
fructose/levulose: very sweet crystalline sugar
FSH: follicle-stimulating hormone
fulguration: destruction of tissue, especially malignant growths, by electric cautery
functional: 1. able to function, especially in spite of structural defect 2. affecting performance, as in illness, but lacking any verifiable physical basis
functional hypertension: hypertension, essential
fundus: the rounded base or bottom of any hollow organ
fungus (*pl., fungi*): any of a group of plants including the mushrooms, molds, yeasts, and various microorganisms, some of which cause diseases in human beings
funnel chest/pectus excavatum: congenital deformity in which the sternum is depressed
furuncle: *see* boil
fusion of spinal joints: *see* spondylitis, rheumatoid

galactosemia: hereditary condition affecting infants who lack an enzyme that converts galactose (a sugar) into glucose in the blood
gallbladder/cholecyst: small pear-shaped pouch situated beneath the liver that serves as a reservoir for bile
gallstone(s): solid substance formed in the gall bladder that can obstruct the flow of bile and prevent the digestion of fats
gamete: either of two mature reproductive cells, an ovum or sperm cell
gamma globulin: component of blood serum which contains various antibodies
ganglion (*pl., ganglia*): 1. cluster of nerve cells outside of the central nervous system 2. cyst of a tendon, as on the wrist
gangrene: death of tissues in a part of the body, caused by lack of adequate blood supply
gastrectomy: surgical removal of all or part of the stomach
gastric analysis: extraction and study of gastric juices
gastric juice: the acid fluid secreted by the glands lining the stomach, containing several enzymes
gastric ulcer: ulcer of the mucous membrane of the stomach
gastritis: inflammation of the stomach
gastrocnemius: the large muscle at the back of the calf of the leg
gastroenteritis: inflammation of the mucous membrane that lines the stomach and intestines
gastroenterologist: physician specializing in the diagnosis and treatment of gastrointestinal disorders
gastroenterology: the branch of medical science dealing with the study of the stomach and intestines and the disorders affecting them
gastroscope: device that allows inspection of the interior of the stomach
gastroscopy: examination of the stomach with a gastroscope
GC: *see* gonorrhea
gene: hereditary unit contained within a chromosome and associated with specific physical characteristics transmitted from parents to offspring
general practitioner/GP: physician whose training is not specialized and includes some preparation in pediatrics, surgery, and obstetrics and gynecology, thus enabling him or her to care for an entire family
genetic counselor: specialist, usually a physician, who counsels couples on the probability of genetic disorders occurring in their offspring
genitalia: genitals
genitals/genitalia: the reproductive organs
genitourinary tract: urinogenital tract
genus: class or category of plants and animals ranking next above the species, as the genus *Homo* in *Homo sapiens*
geriatrics: branch of medicine dealing with diseases and physiological changes associated with aging and old people
German measles: *see* rubella
germicide: disinfectant or other agent capable of killing disease germs
gerontology: scientific study of the processes and phenomena of aging
gestation: the total period of pregnancy, from conception to birth
GI: gastrointestinal

gifted: having ability or intelligence above the normal range
gigantism/giantism: disorder resulting from oversecretion of somatotrophin by the pituitary gland and resulting in excessive growth
gingiva: mucous membrane and soft tissue of the gums surrounding the teeth
gingival: pertaining to the gums
gingivitis: inflammation of the gum tissues
gingivitis, necrotizing ulcerative: *see* trench mouth
GI series/gastrointestinal series: X rays of the esophagus, stomach, and intestines utilizing an opaque substance swallowed by the patient
glabrous: without hair
gland(s): any of various organs that secrete substances essential to the body or for the elimination of waste products
glandular fever: mononucleosis, infectious
glaucoma: disease of the eye characterized by increased pressure on the eyeball and leading to the loss of vision if untreated
glomeruli (*sing., glomerulus*): tiny tufts of capillaries in the kidneys through which the blood passes in the filtering of wastes
glomerulonephritis: inflammation of the glomeruli
glossitis: inflammation of the tongue, characterized by a bright red or glazed appearance
glossopharyngeal nerve: the nerve that supplies sensation to the throat and rear of the tongue
glottis: the passage between the vocal cords at the upper opening of the larynx
glucagon: hormone produced by the islets of Langerhans in the pancreas
glucose/blood sugar: sugar found normally in blood and abnormally in urine, as in the case of diabetes mellitus
glucose tolerance test/GTT: test that determines the rate at which glucose in the blood is reduced, or metabolized, used as an indicator of chemical diabetes or a prediabetic condition
glucosuria: condition, as diabetes mellitus, in which the urine contains glucose
gluten: protein component of wheat and rye
gluteus: any of the three muscles that form each buttock
glycerol/glycerin: sweet, oily alcohol, one of the components of natural fat
glycogen: animal starch usually stored in the liver for conversion to glucose when the body needs energy
glycosuria: glucosuria
goiter: enlargement of the thyroid gland, often because of a lack of iodine in the diet
gonad(s): male or female sex gland; ovary or testicle
gonadotrophic hormone/gonadotrophin/gonadotropin: any of three hormones that stimulate the gonads and are secreted by the anterior pituitary gland
gonioscope: specialized ophthalmoscope for examining the angle between the cornea and the iris
gonococcus: parasitic bacterium that can cause gonorrhea
gonorrhea/clap/GC: contagious venereal disease transmitted by sexual contact
goof balls (*slang*): barbiturates
gout: metabolic disease characterized by painful inflammation of a joint, as of the big toe, and an excess of uric acid in the blood
gouty arthritis, chronic: form of gout characterized by urate deposits and consequent joint stiffness
GP: general practitioner
Graafian follicles: small sacs in the ovaries that contain the developing ova
graft: piece of tissue removed from one organism and inserted in a new site in the same organism or in a different organism
grain alcohol: ethyl alcohol
grand mal: major epileptic seizure, characterized by falling, loss of consciousness, and spasmodic jerking of the arms and legs
granulation: process of forming new tissue in the healing of wounds
granulation tissue/proud flesh: new, temporary, vascular tissue formed in a wound as a stage in the healing process, usually soft and moist
granulocyte: *see* neutrophil
granulocytic leukemia: *see* leukemia, granulocytic
granuloma: small tumor composed mainly of granulation tissue
granuloma inguinale/granuloma venereum: chronic venereal disease that produces lesions in the genital or anal regions
grass (*slang*): marihuana
gravid: pregnant
Grawitz's tumor/hypernephroma: malignant tumor of the kidney, found chiefly among men
gray matter: cortex
greenstick fracture: incomplete fracture, with the bone bending on the unbroken side, more common in children than adults
grippe: influenza
groin: the fold or depressed area where the thigh joins the abdomen
group therapy/group psychotherapy: psychotherapy in which interactions within a group under the direction of a therapist are intended to provoke therapeutic insights and lead to improved social adjustment

growth hormone/growth-stimulating hormone/somatotrophin: hormone secreted by the posterior lobe of the pituitary gland that stimulates growth
GTT: glucose tolerance test
"guard hairs": vibrissae, nasal
gullet: *see* esophagus
gum disease: *see* periodontal disease
gumma: rubbery tumor that develops within organs in the late stages of syphilis
gums: *see* gingiva
gurney: stretcher mounted on wheels, commonly used to move nonambulatory patients in hospitals
gynecologist: physician specializing in gynecology, often an obstetrician as well
gynecology: the branch of medical science that deals with the care and treatment of women and their diseases, especially of the reproductive system

H (*slang*): heroin
hair transplant: the surgical grafting of hair-bearing skin from the back or sides of the scalp onto bald areas of the head
halitosis: offensive mouth odor, usually caused by poor oral hygiene
hallucinate: have hallucinations
hallucination: apparent perception without any corresponding external stimulus
hallucinogen: drug or chemical capable of inducing hallucinations
hallucinogenic: capable of producing hallucinations
halothane: a general anesthetic taken by inhalation
hammer/malleus: the outermost of the three ossicles of the middle ear, the bone between the eardrum and the anvil
hammer toe: clawlike deformity of a toe
hamstrings: any of several tendons at the back of the thigh and controlling the flexing of the knee
hangnail: piece of skin partially torn loose from the root or side of a fingernail
hangover: headache, nausea, dizziness, and other after-effects of excessive alcoholic consumption, an allergic reaction to alcohol, or emotional stress while drinking
Hansen's disease: *see* leprosy
hard palate: *see* palate, hard
hashish: hallucinogenic substance more potent than marihuana, obtained from the leaves and flowers of the Indian hemp plant
hatter's disease: chronic mercury poisoning, common among hatters in former times because of their use of mercury in preparing felt
hay fever: allergic rhinitis
headache: pain or ache across the forehead or within the head
heart: hollow muscular structure which maintains the circulation of the blood by alternate contraction and dilation
heart block: lack of coordination in the heartbeat of the atria and ventricles, often causing unconsciousness and other symptoms (Stokes-Adams syndrome)
heartburn: burning sensation in the lower esophagus caused by a flow of gastric juices from the stomach back into the esophagus
heart failure: inability of the heart to pump enough blood to maintain normal circulation
heart-lung machine: pumping machine used to divert a patient's blood from the heart during heart surgery and to keep it oxygenated and in circulation
heart murmur: abnormal sound heard in the region of the heart
heat cramps: muscle spasms resulting from loss of salt due to excessive sweating
heat exhaustion/heat prostration: weakness or fainting as a result of prolonged exposure to heat, caused by a decreased blood supply to the heart and brain and an increased supply to the skin
heat prostration: heat exhaustion
heat rash: prickly heat
heatstroke: sunstroke
hebephrenic schizophrenia: *see* schizophrenia, hebephrenic
Heimlich maneuver: emergency treatment for obstruction of the windpipe in which sharp pressure is applied just below the rib cage so that the air in the lungs ejects the obstruction
Heine-Medin disease: *see* poliomyelitis
helminth: parasitic worm that invades the intestines, most often via food or water
hemal: of or relating to blood
hemangioma: reddish, usually raised birthmark consisting of a cluster of small blood vessels near the surface of the skin
hematocrit: 1. instrument for measuring the relative amount of plasma and red corpuscles of the blood by centrifuging it (whirling it around to separate parts having different densities) 2. measurement of relative amounts of plasma and red corpuscles by a hematocrit
hematologist: physician specializing in the study of the blood and in the diagnosis and treatment of blood diseases
hematology: the branch of medical science dealing with the blood, including its formation, functions, and diseases
hematoma: blood tumor
hematoma, subdural: mass of blood clots or partially clotted blood in the space beneath the outermost (dura mater) and middle (arachnoid) membranes covering the brain
hematuria: blood in the urine
hemiplegia: paralysis of one side of the body, involving both the arm and leg

hemiplegic: one affected by hemiplegia
hemodialysis: *see* dialysis
hemoglobin: pigment of red blood corpuscles serving as the carrier of oxygen and carbon dioxide
hemophilia: inherited disorder characterized by an incapacity of the blood to clot normally, thus resulting in profuse bleeding even from slight cuts, typically affecting males only
hemophiliac/bleeder: one afflicted with hemophilia
hemorrhage: discharge of blood from a ruptured blood vessel
hemorrhoidal: 1. of or pertaining to the blood vessels in the rectal area 2. of or pertaining to hemorrhoids
hemorrhoidectomy: surgical removal of hemorrhoids
hemorrhoids/piles: swollen varicose veins in the rectal mucous membrane
hemorrhoids, prolapsed: hemorrhoids that protrude from the anus
hemotoxic: (of certain poisonous snakes) transmitting venom that is carried by the bloodstream of the toxified animal
Henle's loop: U-shaped part of a tubule of the kidney
heparin: chemical compound that prevents coagulation of the blood
hepatic: of or relating to the liver
hepaticologist: physician specializing in the diagnosis and treatment of liver diseases
hepaticology: branch of medical science concerned with the study, diagnosis, and treatment of diseases of the liver
hepatitis: inflammation of the liver
hepatitis, infectious: inflammation of the liver caused by a viral infection usually transmitted by food and water contaminated by feces from an infected person
hepatitis, serum: form of infectious hepatitis usually spread by blood transfusions or by infected hypodermic needles
hereditary: acquired through one's genetic makeup by inheritance, as physical characteristics, disease, etc.
hernia/rupture: protrusion of an organ or part, as the intestine, through the wall or body cavity that normally contains it
hernia, hiatus/diaphragmatic hernia: hernia in which the lower end of the esophagus or stomach protrudes through the diaphragm
hernia, inguinal: protuberance of part of the intestine into the inguinal region (near the groin)
hernia, strangulated: hernia that has become tightly constricted, thus cutting off blood supply
hernia, umbilical: hernia in which an abdominal part protrudes through the abdominal wall at the navel
herniate: slip away from its proper position as an organ or part to form a hernia
herniating disk: slipped disk
herniation: forming of a hernia
heroic: extraordinary or extreme, as measures undertaken when life is in immediate danger
heroin/diacetylmorphine: addictive narcotic drug derived from morphine, illegal in the United States
herpes: any of various acute viral diseases characterized by the eruption of small blisters on the skin and mucous membranes
herpes simplex: virus that causes cold sores and other skin conditions in humans
herpes simplex, Type 1/HSV-1: variety of herpes simplex that causes cold sores
herpes simplex, Type 2/HSV-2: variety of herpes simplex that often affects the genital region and can result in congenital damage to the baby of an infected mother
heterograft/xenograft: tissue graft taken for transplanting from a donor of a different species from that of the patient receiving it
hexachlorophene: antibacterial agent used in some soaps
hiatus hernia: *see* hernia
hiccup/hiccough: involuntary, spasmodic grunt caused by spasms of the diaphragm and the abrupt closure of the glottis
high (*slang*): amphetamine
high blood pressure: *see* hypertension
hip bone: ilium
hip joint: acetabulum
hirsutism: abnormal or excessive hairiness, especially in women
histamine: substance found in animal tissues that can cause allergic symptoms when allergens stimulate the body to produce it in large amounts
histoincompatibility: incompatibility between tissues, as between the tissues of a patient and the tissues of a transplanted organ or part
histoplasma: fungus that can cause histoplasmosis
histoplasmosis: chronic fungus disease of the lungs
hives/urticaria: skin condition marked by large, irregularly shaped swellings that burn and itch
Hodgkin's disease: disease of the lymph system, characterized by chronic, progressive enlargement of the lymph nodes, lymphoid tissue, and spleen
homeopathy: system of medicine in which disease is treated by administering minute doses of medicine that would in a healthy person produce the symptoms of the disease treated
homeostasis: maintenance of uniform physiological stability within an organism and between its parts

homograft/allograft: tissue graft taken for transplanting from a donor of the same species as the patient receiving it
hookworm: parasitic intestinal worm whose larvae usually enter the body by penetrating the skin of the feet of people who go barefooted
hormone: internal secretion released in minute amounts into the bloodstream by one of the endocrine glands or other tissue and stimulating a specific physiological activity
horny layer of epidermis: stratum corneum
horse (*slang*)**:** heroin
housemaid's knee: chronic inflammation of the bursa in front of the knee resulting from pressure from constant kneeling or injury
HSV-1: *see* herpes simplex, Type 1
HSV-2: *see* herpes simplex, Type 2
HTLV-3: *see* human T-cell leukemia virus (HTLV)
Hubbard tank: large, specially designed tub in which a patient may be immersed in water for exercises as a means of physical therapy
humerus: the long bone of the arm from elbow to shoulder
humpback, hunchback: kyphosis
hyaline membrane disease/respiratory distress syndrome: disease of newborn babies characterized by severe respiratory distress caused by the presence of a membrane lining the alveoli of the lungs
hydatidiform mole: benign tumor formed from a placenta that has degenerated into a mass of grapelike cysts
hydrocele: localized accumulation of fluid, especially surrounding the testicles in the scrotum
hydrocephalus: accumulation of cerebrospinal fluid within the brain
hydrochloric acid: colorless, corrosive acid which in dilute form is present in gastric juice
hydrogenation: the subjection of a material to hydrogen, as the process by which unsaturated fats are solidified
hydronephrosis: enlargement of the kidneys with urine because of an obstruction of the ureter
hydrophilic: having an affinity for water, as the soft contact lens
hydrophilic lenses: contact lenses, soft plastic
hydrophobia: rabies
hydrotherapy: treatment of disease by the use of water
hymen: thin membrane usually partially covering the entrance of the vagina in virgins
hyperactive child: *see* hyperkinesis
hyperacusis: abnormal and sometimes painful acuteness of hearing
hyperaldosteronism: syndrome of muscle weakness, hypertension, and excessive excretion of urine, because of oversecretion of an adrenal hormone
hyperbaric: of or using pressures in excess of the usual pressure of the atmosphere, as a chamber for treating one suffering from decompression sickness
hyperfunction: disorder of an endocrine gland, characterized by excess secretion of a hormone
hyperglycemia: abnormally high amount of sugar in the blood
hyperkinesis: behavioral disorder of children marked by overactivity, excitability, and inability to concentrate
hyperkinetic: suffering from or pertaining to hyperkinesis
hypermetropia: *see* farsightedness
hypermetropic: farsighted
hypernephroma: *see* Grawitz's tumor
hyperopia: *see* farsightedness
hyperopic: farsighted
hyperplasia: excessive production of cells, resulting in enlargement of tissue or of an organ
hyperplastic: characterized by hyperplasia
hypersensitivity: unusual sensitivity or allergic response to a particular substance
hypertension/high blood pressure: excessively high blood pressure, sometimes caused by a disease (secondary hypertension) and sometimes not (essential hypertension)
hypertension, chronic: essential hypertension
hypertension, essential/chronic/functional: hypertension that is not a symptom of disease and has no known cause
hypertension, malignant: form of essential hypertension with an acute onset and rapid rise in pressure
hypertension, secondary: hypertension arising as a consequence of another known disorder
hypertensive heart disease: *see* heart disease, hypertensive
hyperthyroidism: abnormal and excess activity of the thyroid gland, resulting in oversecretion of thyroxin and an abnormally high metabolism, characterized by fatigue, weight loss, rapid pulse, intolerance to heat, and sometimes by protruding eyes (in which case the disorder is called *exophthalmic goiter*)
hypertonic: characterized by an abnormally high degree of tension, as muscle
hypertrophic: characterized by hypertrophy
hypertrophic arthritis: *see* osteoarthritis
hypertrophy: excessive development of an organ or tissue because of enlargement of the size of its constituent cells
hyperventilation: abnormally fast or deep breathing, resulting in loss of carbon dioxide from the blood and sometimes causing dizziness and muscle spasms
hypnotic: tending to produce sleep
hypoallergenic: less likely to produce an allergic reaction

hypochondria: extreme anxiety about one's health, usually associated with a particular part of the body and accompanied by imagined symptoms of illness
hypochondriac: 1. (*n.*) one suffering from hypochondria 2. (*adj.*) pertaining to the upper right or left parts of the abdomen
hypodermic: pertaining to the tissue just under the skin or to an injection made under the skin
hypofunction: disorder of an endocrine gland, characterized by too little secretion of a hormone
hypogastric: pertaining to the lower middle part of the abdomen
hypogastrium: the lower middle (hypogastric) part of the abdomen
hypoglycemia/low blood sugar: abnormally small amount of glucose in the blood, which can lead to insulin shock
hypoglycemic drug: drug intended to reduce the amount of glucose in the blood by stimulating the release of insulin from the pancreas
hypophysis: *see* pituitary gland
hypophysis cerebri: pituitary gland
hyposensitization: program for desensitizing allergy patients by injecting them with progressively larger doses of pollen or other allergens to build tolerance levels
hypotension: excessively low blood pressure
hypothalamus: region of the brain below the thalamus, important in regulating the internal organs and associated with the functioning of the pituitary gland
hypothermia: artificially low body temperature produced by gradually cooling blood, used to slow metabolism and reduce tissue oxygen need so that heart and brain can withstand short periods of interrupted blood flow during surgery
hypothyroidism: deficient functioning of the thyroid gland, resulting in undersecretion of thyroxin and an abnormally low metabolism, characterized by lack of energy, thick skin, and intolerance to cold
hypotonic: characterized by an abnormally low degree of tension, as muscle
hysterectomy: surgical procedure in which the uterus is completely removed
hysterectomy, radical: surgical removal of the uterus, cervix, ovaries, and Fallopian tubes
hysterectomy, total: surgical removal of the uterus and cervix
hysteria: neurotic condition characterized by impulsive, demonstrative, and attention-getting behavior and sometimes by symptoms of organic disorders
hysteria, conversion: *see* conversion reaction
hysterogram: X-ray examination of the uterus and surrounding areas
id: the concealed, inaccessible part of the mind, the seat of impulses that tend to fulfill instinctual needs
identical twins: twins having the same genetic makeup, derived from a single fertilized egg
identification: mental process, often unconscious, by which a person associates with himself the attributes of another with whom he has formed an emotional tie
idiopathic: (of diseases) originating spontaneously or of unknown cause
ileitis: inflammation of the ileum of the small intestine
ileocecal valve: the valve between the ileum of the small intestine and the cecum, the first section of the large intestine
ileum: the last section of the small intestine, following the jejunum and leading to the large intestine
iliac: pertaining to or near the ilium
ilium: the large upper portion of the hip bone
immune: protected from a communicable or allergic disease by the presence of antibodies in the blood
immunity: resistance to infection or lack of susceptibility of an organism to a disease or poison to which its species is usually subject, either by means of antibodies produced by the organism itself (*active immunity*) or by another and subsequently introduced into its body (*passive immunity*), as by injection
immunization: act or process of making immune, especially by inoculation
immunize: make immune, as by inoculation
immunoglobulin: any of various proteins of the body that are active as antigens or otherwise contribute to the formation of antibodies
immunologist: physician or specialist in the study of immunity
immunology: the branch of medical science concerned with the phenomena and techniques of immunity from disease
immunosuppressive: acting to suppress natural immune responses, as to foreign tissue in an organ transplant
immunotherapy: therapy to relieve allergic response consisting of a series of injections of a dilute allergen, gradually increased in strength
impacted tooth: tooth wedged between the jawbone and another tooth so as to prevent its eruption
impaction: state of being firmly packed or tightly wedged, as feces in the rectum or a tooth in the jaw; *see* impacted tooth
imperforate: lacking a normal opening
impetigo: contagious bacterial skin infection characterized by blisters that break and form yellow encrusted areas
impotence: in men, the inability to have sexual intercourse

incision: 1. cut or gash, as of a wound 2. cut or slit made in a surgical operation
incisor: one of the four upper and four lower cutting teeth near the front of the mouth
incompetence: inadequate performance, as of the heart valves
incomplete fracture: partial fracture of a bone in which continuity of the bone is not destroyed
incontinence: inability to control the flow of urine or the evacuation of the bowels
incubation period: the period between the entry of a disease-causing organism in the body and the onset of the symptoms of that disease
incus: anvil
indomethacin: analgesic and anti-inflammatory drug used for arthritic disorders, often as a substitute for aspirin
infantile paralysis: *see* poliomyelitis
infantile sexuality: the sexual interest and pleasure that infants and young children take in their genitals and other body parts
infarct: tissue rendered necrotic (dead) by an obstructed blood supply, as because of a thrombus (clot) or an embolus
infarction: death of tissue because of deprivation of blood caused by an obstruction, as in a coronary thrombosis (heart attack)
infection(s): communication of disease by entrance into the body of disease-causing organisms
infectious: (of a disease) transmitted by organisms, as bacteria
infectious mononucleosis/glandular fever/kissing disease: acute communicable disease marked by fever, malaise, and swollen lymph nodes, especially in the throat
inferior vena cava: the large vein that brings blood from the lower part of the body to the heart
infertility: inability to conceive or to produce offspring
inflammation: localized reaction to infection, injury, etc., characterized by heat, redness, swelling, and pain
inflammation of arterial walls: arteritis
inflammation of bladder: cystitis
inflammation of bone: osteomyelitis
inflammation of brain: encephalitis
inflammation of brain coverings: meningitis
inflammation of bursa: bursitis
inflammation of femoral head: Legg-Perthes' disease
inflammation of glomeruli: nephritis
inflammation of gums: gingivitis
inflammation of joints: arthritis
inflammation of larynx: laryngitis
inflammation of liver: hepatitis
inflammation of mucous membrane: laryngitis
inflammation of prostate: prostatitis
inflammation of skin: dermatitis
inflammation of spinal joints: spondylitis, rheumatoid
inflammation of stomach lining: gastritis
inflammation of tendons: tendinitis
inflammation of tendon sheath: tenosynovitis
inflammation of tongue: glossitis
inflammation of veins: phlebitis
inflammation of vertebrae: osteomyelitis, spinal
influenza/flu/grippe: acute, contagious, sometimes epidemic disease caused by a virus and characterized by inflammation of the upper respiratory tract, fever, chills, muscle ache, and fatigue
ingrown toenail: toenail that has grown into the surrounding flesh
inguinal: pertaining to or near the groin
inguinal hernia: *see* hernia
inner ear: the innermost part of the ear, containing the essential organs of hearing within the cochlea, the auditory nerve, and the semicircular canals that govern equilibrium
innervation: distribution or supply of nerves to a part
inoculate: immunize by administering a serum or vaccine to 2. introduce microorganisms into (a culture medium)
inoculation: act or process of inoculating
inoperable: characterized by a condition that excludes surgery as a course of treatment
in situ: in its original site or position
insomnia: chronic inability to sleep
insufficiency: inability to function adequately, as the heart (cardiac insufficiency)
insufflation: tubal insufflation
insulin: protein hormone secreted by the islets of Langerhans in the pancreas that checks the accumulation of glucose in the blood and promotes the utilization of sugar in the treatment of diabetes
insulin shock: condition caused by too low a level of blood sugar, and characterized by sweating, dizziness, palpitation, shallow breathing, confusion, and ultimately loss of consciousness
insulin shock therapy: former method of treating psychotic patients involving large injections of insulin, inducing coma
insult: injury to tissue caused by stress or trauma
integument: skin
intelligence quotient/IQ: a score obtained from standardized tests indicating the level of a person's intelligence
intensive care unit (ICU): section of a hospital specially equipped and staffed to monitor the vital systems of patients and provide close, round-the-clock care for a relatively brief pe-

riod, as for patients just removed from surgery or for those in an unstable or critical condition

intercostal muscles: the muscles between each of the ribs that contract when air is exhaled

intercourse: sexual intercourse

intermittent claudication: vascular disease associated with aging and marked by muscle fatigue and pain, especially in the legs, due to atherosclerosis

intern: advanced medical student or graduate (M.D.) undergoing resident training in a hospital

internal medicine: the branch of medical science that deals with the study, diagnosis, and nonsurgical treatment of diseases of the internal organs

internist: physician specializing in internal medicine

interstitial calcinosis: condition characterized by deposits of calcium salts in the skin and subcutaneous tissue

intestine(s): tubular part of the alimentary canal, linking the stomach to the anus

intestine, large: the lower part of the intestine, of greater diameter than the small intestine and divided into the cecum, colon, and rectum

intestine, small: the convoluted upper and narrower part of the intestines, where most nutrients are absorbed by the bloodstream, between the pylorus and the cecum, divided into three parts, the duodenum, jejunum, and ileum

intoxicated: in legal use, having more than 0.10% alcohol in the bloodstream

intracutaneous: within the dermis

intramuscular: situated within or injected into a muscle or muscular tissue

intrauterine device/IUD: contraceptive device consisting usually of a plastic coil, spiral, or loop that is inserted and left within the uterus for as long as contraception is desired

intravenous: into or within a vein, as an injection

intrinsic: originating or situated within an organ or part, as a disease

introitus: entrance into a body cavity, especially into the vagina

intussusception: the turning inward or inversion of a portion of the intestine into an adjacent part, thus obstructing it, found especially in male infants

in utero: in the uterus, prior to birth

invasive: invading or spreading to tissues other than at the place of origin: said of malignant growths

involutional melancholia: *see* depressive reaction

IQ: intelligence quotient

iris: colored, circular, contractile membrane between the cornea and the lens of the eye, whose central perforation is occupied by the pupil

irradiation: process of exposing a part of the body to radiant energy, as X rays

irrigate: wash out or cleanse, as a body cavity or a wound, with a flow of water or other liquid

irrigation: act or process of irrigating a body cavity, wound, etc.

ischemia: localized deficiency of blood, as from a contracted blood vessel

ischium: the part of the hip bone on which the body rests when sitting

islands of Langerhans: islets of Langerhans

islets of Langerhans/islands of Langerhans: small, cellular masses in the pancreas which produce and secrete insulin

isomer: compound with the same molecular weight and formula as another, but with a different arrangement of its atoms, resulting in different properties

isometrics: means of strengthening muscles by forcefully contracting them against immovable resistance

isoniazid/INH: isonicotinic acid hydrazide, a chemical compound used in the treatment of tuberculosis

isopropyl: chemical in the family of methyl alcohol, used as a rubbing alcohol

itch, the: scabies

IUD: intrauterine device

Jacksonian epilepsy: form of epilepsy characterized by recurrent focal seizures, spasmodic movements or tingling or burning sensations, as of an arm, leg, or facial area, caused by a condition affecting a motor area of the brain

Jacksonian seizure: form of focal seizure that characterizes Jacksonian epilepsy

jaundice: yellowish tint to the skin and tissues, as the whites of the eyes, caused by excessive bile in the blood, a symptom of certain disorders

jejunum: the middle section of the small intestine, between the duodenum and the ileum

joint(s): place where two or more bones or separate parts of the skeleton meet

junk (slang): heroin

juvenile rheumatoid arthritis: *see* rheumatoid arthritis, juvenile

kala-azar/black fever/dumdum fever/visceral leishmaniasis: form of leishmaniasis that is usually fatal if not treated

keratin: horny substance that is the main constituent of nails and hair, and in nonhuman animals of claws and horns

keratosis: disease of the skin characterized by an outer layer of horny tissue

ketone bodies: organic compounds that are a by-product of fat metabolism
kidney: one of a pair of organs located at the rear of the abdomen near the base of the spine, whose function is to filter the fluid portion of the blood in regulating the composition and volume of body fluids, and to dispose of waste in the form of urine
kidney failure, acute: sudden loss of kidney function, characterized by decreased amount of urine, passage of bloody urine, edema, fatigue, and loss of appetite
kidney stone/renal calculus: mass of hard material, such as crystallized salt, that may collect within the kidney and obstruct the flow of urine
kissing disease: infectious mononucleosis
kyphosis: backward curvature of the spine characterized as a humpback or hunchback

labia: 1. *pl.* of labium 2. the folds of skin and mucous membrane of the vulva, consisting of the outer folds (*labia majora*) and the inner folds (*labia minora*)
labium: 1. *sing.* of labia 2. lip or liplike part or organ
labor: process of giving birth, during which the uterus undergoes periodic contractions in moving the fetus through the birth canal
labyrinth: the winding passages of the inner ear
labyrinthitis: inflammation of the labyrinth of the inner ear, usually disturbing the sense of equilibrium
laceration: wound made by tearing or ripping
lacrimal gland: tear-producing gland over the eye
lactation: formation or secretion of milk from the breast
lactic acid: bitter, syrupy acid found in sour milk and collected in muscle tissues during anaerobic exercise
lactogenic hormone/LTH/luteotrophic hormone/luteotrophin/luteotropin/prolactin: hormone secreted by the anterior lobe of the pituitary gland that stimulates the production of milk in the mammary glands
Lamaze, Dr. Ferdinand: French physician who pioneered in the development of a natural childbirth technique
Langerhans: islets of Langerhans
laparotomy: surgical procedure for examining or treating the female reproductive organs within the abdominal cavity
lapse attack or seizure: *see* petit mal
laryngectomy: surgical removal of all or part of the larynx
laryngitis: inflammation of the mucous membranes of the larynx, causing the voice to become hoarse or disappear altogether
laryngitis, chronic: permanently hoarse voice resulting from thickened, toughened mucous membrane in the larynx, resulting from too many attacks of laryngitis
laryngologist: physician specializing in the diagnosis and treatment of disorders of the throat
laryngology: the branch of medical science concerned with the study and treatment of the throat and related areas
laryngoscope: instrument for inspecting the larynx
larynx/voice box: the organ of voice in humans and most other vertebrates, consisting of a cartilaginous box in the upper part of the trachea across which are stretched vocal cords whose vibrations produce sound
latent: not visible or apparent, as symptoms of a disease at an early stage
lateral: 1. relating to or directed toward the side 2. more distant from the midline of the body, as compared to a nearer (medial) position
lavage: cleansing or washing out of an organ, as the stomach
laxative: substance that has the power to loosen the bowels, as milk of magnesia
L-dopa/levodopa: medicine used in treating the symptoms of Parkinson's disease
leaflet: flap of a heart valve
learning disability: condition in which a child cannot acquire certain skills or assimilate certain kinds of knowledge at or near the normal rate
Legg-Perthes' disease: inflammation of the bone and cartilage in the head of the femur (thigh bone)
leiomyoma: benign tumor consisting of smooth muscle tissue
leishmaniasis: tropical disease resembling malaria in which an animal parasite is transmitted by the sandfly
leishmaniasis, visceral: *see* kala-azar
lens: biconvex transparent body behind the iris of the eye that focuses entering light rays on the retina
lepromatous: characterized by nodular skin lesions, as a form of leprosy
leprosy/Hansen's disease: chronic bacterial disease characterized by skin lesions, nerve paralysis, and physical deformity
lesion: any abnormal change in an organ or tissue caused by disease or injury
leukemia: form of cancer involving the blood and blood-making tissues, characterized by a marked and persistent excess of leukocytes
leukemia, granulocytic: form of leukemia characterized by predominance of granulocytes (or neutrophils)
leukemia, lymphocytic: form of leukemia characterized by uncontrolled over-activity of the lymphoid tissue

leukemic: of or characteristic of leukemia

leukocyte/white blood cell/white corpuscle: white or colorless cell found in the bloodstream important in providing protection against infection

leukopenia: abnormal reduction in the number of leukocytes in the blood

leukorrhea: whitish, viscid discharge from the vagina

levodopa: medicine used in treating the symptoms of Parkinson's disease

levulose: fructose

LGV: *see* lymphogranuloma venereum

LH: luteinizing hormone

libido: the instinctual craving or drive behind all human activities, especially sexual, the repression of which leads to neurosis

Librium: chlordiazepoxide

lidocaine: chemical used as a local anesthetic

ligament(s): band of tough, fibrous connective tissue that binds together bones and provides support for organs

ligate: tie or close off with a ligature

ligation: the act of tying or binding up, as an artery

ligature: thread, wire, etc., used to close off or tie a vessel

lightening: during the last few weeks of pregnancy, a shift in fetal pressure from the upper abdomen to the pelvic region as the head of the fetus moves toward the birth canal

lipase: enzyme that breaks down fats

lipid: fatty substance essential to living cells

lipid storage disease: any of various usually fatal diseases, typically occurring in childhood, caused by the lack of a particular enzyme

lip reading/speech reading: interpretation of speech by watching the position of the lips and mouth of the speaker, practiced especially by the deaf

lithium salts: salts of lithium (a metal), used as a medication in the treatment of manic-depressive psychosis

lithotomy position: position used in gynecological examinations in which the patient lies on her back and the legs are drawn back and apart at the thighs

liver: large, glandular organ situated just under the diaphragm on the right side, that processes blood and regulates its composition, as by storing sugar and releasing it in assimilable form (glucose), and that secretes bile

liver spots/chloasma: yellowish brown patches that appear on the skin

lobe(s): rounded or protruding section or subdivision, as of an organ

lobotomy: *see* frontal lobotomy

lockjaw: *see* tetanus

locomotor ataxia: *see* tabes dorsalis

loiasis: form of filariasis transmitted by a biting fly from monkey to man or vice versa

loins: the part of the body between the lower rib and the hip bone

lordosis: abnormal inward curvature of the spine

lordotic posture: posture characteristic of some women in late pregnancy, in which the shoulders are slumped, the neck bent, and the lower spine curved forward to bear the weight of the fetus

Lou Gehrig's disease: sclerosis, amyotrophic lateral

low blood sugar: hypoglycemia

LSD/lysergic acid diethylamide: colorless, odorless, tasteless drug produced synthetically that causes the user to experience hallucinations

LTH: lactogenic hormone

lumbago: pain in the lower back

lumbar: pertaining to or situated near the loins

lumbar puncture: *see* spinal tap

lumen: space enclosed by the walls of a blood vessel, duct, etc.

lung: either of two porous organs of respiration in the chest cavity of humans, having the function of absorbing oxygen and discharging carbon dioxide

lunula: the living part of the nail, the pale, half-moon shape at the nail base

luteinizing hormone/LH: a hormone secreted by the anterior lobe of the pituitary gland that stimulates a Graafian follicle to release an ovum during each menstrual cycle and converts the follicle into corpus luteum

luteotrophic hormone: lactogenic hormone

luteotrophin: lactogenic hormone

lymph: transparent fluid resembling blood plasma that is conveyed through vessels (lymphatic vessels) and lubricates the tissues

lymphangiogram: the visualization by X ray of lymph nodes after injection of an opaque fluid

lymphatic: pertaining to or conveying lymph

lymph gland: *see* lymph node

lymph node/lymph gland: one of the rounded bodies about the size of a pea, found in the course of the lymphatic vessels, that produces lymphocytes

lymphoblast: young cell that matures into a lymphocyte

lymphocyte: variety of leukocyte formed in the lymphoid tissue

lymphogranuloma inguinale: *see* lymphogranuloma venereum

lymphogranuloma venereum/LGV/lymphogranuloma inguinale: venereal disease affecting the lymph nodes

lymphoid: pertaining to lymph or to the tissue of lymph nodes

lymphoma: abnormal (neoplastic) growth of lymphoid tissue, symptomatic of various diseases, as lymphocytic leukemia or Hodgkin's disease

lymphosarcoma: malignant growth of the lymphatic system
lysergic acid diethylamide: LSD
lysozyme: enzyme present in tears that is destructive to bacteria
lyssophobia: fear of becoming insane

M (*slang*): morphine
macrobiotic: of or pertaining to macrobiotics
macrobiotics: the idea, Oriental in origin, that an equilibrium should be maintained between foods that make one active (Yang) and foods that make one relax (Yin)
macrocephalic: individual with macrocephaly
macrocephaly: excessive head size
macula: spot or discoloration
macula lutea: yellowish area in the retina related to color perception and marked by most acute vision
mainlining: injection of heroin directly into a vein
malabsorption syndrome/celiac disease: syndrome characterized by bulky, foul-smelling stools and other symptoms resulting from the inability of the body to absorb certain nutrients from the intestinal tract
malaise: feeling of being run-down, listless, uncomfortable, weary, and generally unwell
malaria: disease caused by certain animal parasites transmitted by the bite of the infected Anopheles mosquito, causing intermittent chills, and fever
malignancy: 1. malignant tumor 2. state of being malignant
malignant: so aggravated as to threaten life, usually resistant to treatment, and often having the property of uncontrolled growth, as a cancer
malleus: hammer
malnutrition: nutritional deficiency, as of essential proteins, vitamins, or minerals, causing impairment of health and certain specific diseases
malocclusion: faulty closure of the upper and lower teeth
Malta fever: *see* brucellosis
mammogram: X-ray picture of the breast by the technique of mammography
mammography: specialized X-ray examination of the breasts
mammoplasty: surgical procedure to augment the size of the breasts
mandible: the lower jawbone
mania: psychotic condition characterized by excessive activity, elation, extreme talkativeness, and agitation
manic-depressive reaction/affective reaction: psychosis characterized by mania or depression or by the alternation of both
marihuana: the dried leaves and flowers of the hemp plant (*Cannabis sativa*), which if smoked in cigarettes or otherwise ingested can produce distorted perception and other hallucinogenic effects
marrow: either of two types of soft, vascular tissue found in the central cavities of bones—*red marrow*, which produces red blood cells, and *yellow marrow*, composed mainly of fat cells
mastectomy: surgical removal of the breast
mastectomy, radical: surgical removal of the breast, underlying chest muscles, and lymph glands in the armpit
mastectomy, simple: surgical removal of the breast only
master gland: pituitary gland
mastitis: inflammation of the breast
mastoiditis: inflammation of the air cells in the mastoid process
mastoid process: process of the temporal bone behind the ear
mastoplasty: surgical procedure to reduce the size of the breasts
masturbation: the touching or rubbing of the genitals for sexual pleasure and usually orgasm
materia alba: white, viscous mixture of mucus, molds, tissue cells, and bacteria adhering to teeth or to the spaces between teeth and gums, a potential source of disease
maxilla: the upper jawbone
maxillary sinus: *see* paranasal sinus
MBD: *see* minimal brain dysfunction
MD: *see* muscular dystrophy
M.D.: Doctor of Medicine
measles/rubeola: contagious viral disease, especially of children, marked by rash, fever, and conjunctivitis, sometimes having severe complications
measles, German: *see* rubella
meatus: passage or canal in the human body, especially one with an external opening such as the anterior urethra of the penis
medial: 1. middle, or relatively near the middle 2. nearer to the midline of the body, as compared to a more distant (lateral) position
medical: 1. of or relating to medicine 2. of or relating to the treatment of disease by nonsurgical means
medical history: the questions asked by a doctor of a patient that are designed to give an outline of the patient's state of health
medicine: 1. the profession dealing with the maintenance of health and the treatment of physical and psychological disorders 2. the treatment of disease by nonsurgical means
medulla: 1. medulla oblongata: the lower part of the brain continuous with the spinal cord that controls certain involuntary processes such as

breathing, swallowing, and blood circulation 2. the inner portion of an organ or part, as of the kidneys or the adrenal glands

melancholia, involutional: *see* depressive reaction

melanin: dark brown or black pigment of the skin

melanin cell clusters: *see* moles

melanoma/black cancer: malignant tumor formed of cells that produce melanin

menarche: the first menstrual period of a girl

Ménière's disease/Ménière's syndrome: symptoms including vertigo, ringing or buzzing sensations (tinnitus), nausea, and vomiting, associated with disease of the inner ear and often leading to progressive deafness of one ear

Ménière's syndrome: *see* Ménière's disease

meninges: the membranes that cover the brain and spinal cord

meningioma: uncontrolled new cell growth in one of the membranes (arachnoid) covering the brain and spinal cord

meningitis: inflammation of the membranes that cover the brain and spinal cord

meningitis, aseptic/viral: meningitis thought to be caused by a virus instead of a bacterium

meningococcal: pertaining to meningococcus, a bacterium

meningococcus: bacterium that causes a form of meningitis

menopausal: of or occurring during the menopause

menopause/change of life/climacteric: the cessation of menstruation and the end of a woman's capacity to bear children, normally occurring between 40–50 years of age and often marked by hot flashes, dizzy spells, and other physical and emotional symptoms

menopause, surgical: abrupt onset of menopause in women resulting from the surgical removal of the uterus and ovaries

menses: menstruation

menstrual: of or relating to menstruation

menstruation/the menses: periodic bloody discharge of the unfertilized ovum and tissue from the uterus of a female of child-bearing age

mental retardation: failure in mental development that is severe enough to prevent normal participation in everyday life

mentoplasty: plastic surgery of the chin, especially a procedure to build up an underdeveloped chin

meperidine/pethidine/Demerol: medicine used as an analgesic and sedative

meprobamate/Equanil/Miltown: tranquilizer used as a sedative and muscle relaxant

mescaline: chemical extracted from the peyote cactus that induces hallucinations in its users

mesentery: the fan-shaped fold of the membrane (peritoneum) that enfolds the small intestine and connects it with the abdominal wall

mesoderm: middle layer of tissue

metabolic: of or relating to metabolism

metabolism: aggregate of all physical and chemical processes continuously taking place in living organisms, including those which build up and break down assimilated materials

metacarpal: any of the five bones of the metacarpus

metacarpus: the five bones of the hand connecting the wrist to the fingers (phalanges)

metastasis: the transfer of a disease or its manifestations, as a malignant tumor, from one part of the body to another

metatarsalgia: painful inflammation of the nerves in the region of the metatarsus of the foot

metatarsals: the bones of the metatarsus

metatarsus: the fine bones of the foot connecting the ankle to the toes (phalanges)

methadone/Dolophine: synthetic opiate used as an analgesic and experimentally as a substitute for heroin in the treatment of addicts

methamphetamine/Methedrine/Desoxyn: chemical compound that allays hunger and has a more stimulating effect on the central nervous system than does amphetamine or dextroamphetamine

methanol: methyl alcohol

Methedrine: methamphetamine (meth-head)

methotrexate: drug used in the treatment of psoriasis and leukemia

methylalcohol/woodalcohol/methanol: flammable liquid obtained through the distillation of wood or made synthetically, poisonous if taken internally

metorrhagia: erratic or unpredictable menstrual bleeding

microcephalic: individual with microcephaly

microcephaly: abnormal smallness of the head, with imperfect development of the cranium

micrographia: very minute handwriting, a symptom of some nervous disorders

micron: 1/1000th of a millimeter (symbol *mu*, Greek letter *mu*)

microsurgery: surgery or dissection of minute parts, as of individual cells, with the aid of a microscope and especially precise instruments

micturate: urinate

micturition: urination

middle ear: the part of the ear between the eardrum and the inner ear, including the tympanum and the ossicles—hammer, anvil, and stirrup

migraine/sick headache: recurrent severe form of headache, temporarily disabling, usually affecting one side of the head and often accompanied by nausea, dizziness, and sensitivity to light

miliaria: prickly heat
milk teeth: baby teeth
Miltown: meprobamate
mineral(s): naturally occurring, homogeneous, inorganic material, some of which, as salt and iron, are required by the body
minimal brain dysfunction/minimal brain damage: condition of children who suffer from a motor or perceptual impairment because of slight brain damage
miscarriage/spontaneous abortion: the involuntary expulsion of a nonviable fetus after the first three months of pregnancy
Miss Emma (*slang*): morphine
mitral valve: the membranous valve between the left atrium and left ventricle of the heart that prevents the backflow of blood into the atrium
mittelschmerz: pain during ovulation about midway between menstrual periods
modality: 1. method of treatment or its application, especially a physical procedure 2. any form of sensation, as touch or taste
molar: any of the three upper and three lower grinding teeth with flattened crowns at both sides of the rear of the mouth, making 12 in all
mole: permanent pigmented spot on the skin, usually brown and often raised
molluscum contagiosum: contagious viral disease marked by raised lesions containing waxy material
Mongolism: congenital disorder characterized by mental retardation
moniliasis/candidiasis: fungus infection involving the skin or mucous membranes of various parts of the body, such as the mouth, especially in babies (when it is called thrush) or the vagina
monocyte: relatively large leukocyte
mononucleosis: infectious mononucleosis
monovalent: pertaining to a form of the Sabin polio vaccine in which each dose gives protection against a different strain of polio
morning sickness: nausea and vomiting experienced by some pregnant women in the morning hours, especially in early pregnancy
morphine: addictive narcotic drug derived from opium, used medically to relieve pain
morphinism: abnormal condition of the body system caused by an excessive dose or habitual use of morphine
Morton's toe: painful inflammation of the nerves in the region of the metatarsus of the foot (metatarsalgia) between the third and fourth toes
motion sickness: nausea and sometimes vomiting caused by the effect of certain complex movements on the organ of balance in the inner ear, typically experienced in a moving vehicle, ship, or airplane
motor nerve/efferent nerve: nerve that conveys information from the central nervous system to a muscle with a directive for action
mouth-to-mouth respiration/mouth-to-mouth resuscitation: form of artificial respiration in which the rescuer places his or her mouth over the victim's mouth and breathes rhythmically and forcefully to inflate the victim's lungs and start respiration
MS: multiple sclerosis
mu: micron
mucosa: mucous membrane
mucosal: of or pertaining to the mucous membrane
mucous: pertaining to, producing, or resembling mucus
mucous membrane/mucosa: membrane that lines many of the body's inner surfaces, kept moist by glandular secretions
mucus: viscous substance secreted by the mucous membranes
multipara: woman who has borne more than one child
multiphasic: having many phases or aspects; said especially of testing performed in the course of a comprehensive physical examination
multiple myeloma: malignant tumor of the bone marrow occurring at numerous sites
multiple sclerosis/MS: chronic disease in which patches of nerve tissue thicken (sclerose), causing failure of coordination and other nervous and mental symptoms
mumps: contagious, viral disease marked by fever and swelling of the facial glands
muscular dystrophy/MD: any of various diseases of unknown cause characterized by the progressive wasting away (atrophy) of the muscles
musculoskeletal system: the human body's network of muscles and bones
myasthenia gravis: chronic disease characterized by muscular weakness and general and progressive exhaustion
mycobacterium: kind of rod-shaped, aerobic bacterium
myelin: semisolid fatlike sheath that surrounds the axon of a neuron
myelitis: 1. inflammation of the spinal cord 2. inflammation of the bone marrow
myelogram: X ray of the spinal cord obtained by the injection of a radioopaque liquid material into the spinal cord area
myelography: technique of recording myelograms and the science of interpreting them
myeloma: malignant tumor of the bone marrow
myocardial infarction: the process of congestion and tissue death (necrosis) in the heart muscle caused by an interruption of the blood supply to the heart

myocardium: the muscular tissue of the heart
myomectomy: surgical excision of a type of uterine fibroid tumor
myopathy: any abnormality or disease of the muscles
myopia: nearsightedness
myopic: nearsighted
myotonia: disorder characterized by increased rigidity or spasms of muscle
myotonia, congenita: congenital disease characterized by temporary muscle spasms and muscle rigidity
myotonic dystrophy: chronic, progressive disease characterized by weakness and wasting of muscles, cataracts, and heart abnormality
myringotomy: surgical incision of the eardrum
mysophobia: fear of dirt and contamination

naprapathy: the treatment of disease by the manipulative correction of ligaments and connective tissues
narcolepsy: disease in which the patient is overcome by drowsiness or an uncontrollable desire for sleep
narcosis: stupor or unconsciousness produced by a narcotic drug
narcotic: 1. any of various substances, such as morphine, codeine, and opium, that in medicinal doses relieve pain, induce sleep, and in excessive or uncontrolled doses may produce convulsions, coma, and death 2. inducing sleep, in anesthesia
nares: the nasal passages or nostrils
nasopharyngeal: pertaining to the nasopharynx
nasopharynx: the upper part of the pharynx above and behind the soft palate
Natulan: procarbazine
natural foods: foods processed minimally, although not necessarily organically grown
nausea: feeling of sickness or dizziness usually accompanied by the impulse to vomit
navel/umbilicus: the depression at the middle of the abdomen where the umbilical cord of the fetus was attached
nearsightedness/myopia: inability to see distant objects clearly
neck vertebra: vertebra, cervical
necrosis: death of a group of cells, tissue, or a part of the body
necrotizing ulcerative gingivitis: *see* trench mouth
needle biopsy: the excising of a tissue sample for biopsy by means of a long needle
nematode: any of a class of roundworms, many of which, such as the hookworm or pinworm, are intestinal parasites in man and other animals
neonate: newborn baby
neoplasm: any abnormal growth of new tissue, as a tumor, which may be benign or malignant
neoplastic: of or characteristic of neoplasms
nephrectomy: surgical removal of a kidney
nephric: renal
nephritis/Bright's disease: inflammation of the kidneys
nephroblastoma: *see* Wilm's tumor
nephrologist: physician specializing in the diagnosis and treatment of diseases of the kidney
nephrology: branch of medical science dealing with the structure, function, and diseases of the kidney
nephron: one of the basic filtration units of the kidney, consisting of Bowman's capsule, a glomerulus, and tubules
nephrosis/nephrotic syndrome: disease of the kidneys characterized by degenerative lesions of the renal tubules and loss of protein (albumin) through the urine
nerve block/plexus block: form of local anesthesia in which the anesthetic is injected into nerve trunks leading to the area in which surgery is to be performed
nerve bundle, master: *see* spinal cord
nerve cell: 1. one of the cells of the nervous system 2. the cell body of a neuron
nerve, lingual: nerve beneath the floor of the mouth that conveys taste sensations to the brain motor
nerve, olfactory: the special nerve of smell
nerve, optic: the special nerve of vision connecting the retina with the occipital lobe of the brain
nerve, sensory/afferent: nerve that conveys information and stimuli from the outside world to the central nervous system
nerve, spinal: the thirty-one pairs of nerves that originate in the spinal cord
nervous breakdown: popular, nontechnical term for any debilitating or incapacitating emotional disorder
neural: of or relating to a nerve
neuralgia: acute pain along the course of a nerve
neuralgia, facial: *see* trigeminal neuralgia
neuralgia, trigeminal/facial tic douloureux: acutely painful neuralgia of a region of the face, with paroxysmal muscular twitchings, associated with branches of the trigeminal (cranial) nerve in the affected area
neuritis: inflammation of a nerve
neuroblastoma: malignant tumor of the nerve tissue of the adrenal glands, found especially in children
neurofibroma: tumor on a nerve fiber
neurogenic shock: shock resulting from impairment of the regulatory capacity of the nervous system because of pain, fright, or other stimulus
neurologist: physician specializing in the care and treatment of the nervous system

neurology: the branch of medical science that deals with the nervous system
neuron: nerve cell with all its processes and extensions, such as the axon and dendrites
neuropathologist: physician specializing in neuropathology
neuropathology: the branch of medical science that deals with the study, diagnosis, and treatment of diseases of the nervous system
neurosis/psychoneurosis (*pl., neuroses*): mental disorder having no organic cause and less severe than psychosis
neurosurgeon: physician specializing in surgery of the nervous system
neurosurgery: the branch of medical science that deals with the treatment of disease of the nervous system by means of surgery
neurosyphilis: syphilis of the brain and spinal cord
neurotic: 1. one who has a neurosis 2. of or relating to neurosis
neurotoxic: 1. (of certain poisonous snakes) transmitting venom that directly affects the nervous system and brain of the toxified animal 2. causing destruction or damage to nerve tissue
neutrophil/granulocyte/polymorphonuclear leukocyte: granular leukocyte that can be stained with dyes that are neither acid nor alkaline (i.e., neutral)
nevus: birthmark or congenital mole junction
nicotine: poisonous chemical with acrid taste contained in tobacco leaves
night terrors: childhood nightmares which occur in deep sleep and in which the child cries out in terror
nit(s): the egg of a louse or other parasitic insect
nitrogen dioxide: suffocating gas that is poisonous when inhaled
nitroglycerin: colorless or pale yellow oily liquid used to treat angina pectoris
nocturia: frequent urination during the night
node: 1. swelling or enlargement, as in an arthritic joint, or a firm, flattened tumor on a bone or tendon 2. any knoblike part, as a lymph gland
nodule: little node
Noludar: methprylon
norepinephrine: hormone manufactured by the adrenal medulla that affects heart action and sympathetic nerve impulses
"nose brain": rhinencephalon
nostril: one of the outer openings in the nose
no-take: absence of any reaction to a vaccination, indicating that the person vaccinated has not developed an immunity and should be revaccinated
nutrient: substance that gives nourishment
nutriment: substance that nourishes or promotes development
nutrition: all of the processes by which food is consumed, digested, absorbed, and assimilated by the body
nutritionist: specialist in the study of nutrition
nyctophobia: fear of the dark
nystagmus: spasmodic, involuntary movement of the eyes, symptomatic of certain diseases, as of the inner ear

obesity: excessive accumulation of body fat
ob-gyn specialist: physician trained as an obstetrician and gynecologist
objective: (of symptoms) of a kind that can be observed or measured by the examining physician through diagnostic techniques
obsession: persistent, unwanted idea or feeling, a symptom of certain neuroses
obsessive-compulsive reaction: neurosis characterized by obsessions that are relieved temporarily by the compulsive performance of certain acts
obstetrician: physician specializing in obstetrics, often a gynecologist as well
obstetrics: the branch of medical science dealing with pregnancy and childbirth
obstructive-airway disease: condition characterized by the presence of chronic bronchitis and pulmonary emphysema, and involving damage to lung tissue and the bronchi
obturator: special device inserted into a cleft palate to close it against the flow of air
occipital: of or relating to the lower back part of the skull (occiput)
occipital lobe: the rear portion of each cerebral hemisphere which receives messages from the optic nerve
occlusion: 1. the act of closing or shutting off so as to block a passage, as a blood vessel 2. the manner of being shut, as the teeth of the upper and lower jaws
occupational disease: disease resulting from exposure in one's occupation to toxic substances or other hazards to health
ocular: of or relating to the eye
oculist: ophthalmologist
Oedipal complex: repressed sexual attachment of son to mother, analogous to the Electra complex involving the daughter and father
oil glands: glands, sebaceous
olfaction: the act, sense, or process of smelling
olfactory: pertaining to the sense of smell or the capacity to smell
olfactory lobe: the portion of each cerebral hemisphere of the brain on the underside of the frontal lobes, the centers for smelling
olfactory nerve: *see* nerve, olfactory
oliguria: decreased production of urine
onchocerciasis: form of filariasis transmitted by a blackfly and sometimes leading to blindness

oncologist: physician specializing in the diagnosis and treatment of tumors
oncology: the branch of medical science concerned with the study of tumors
Oncovin: vincristine
oophorectomy: *see* ovariectomy
open bite: form of malocclusion in which incisors of the upper and lower jaws do not meet when the jaws are together
open fracture: compound fracture
open surgery: surgery involving an incision and opening of the skin
ophthalmic: of or pertaining to the eye
ophthalmologist/oculist: physician specializing in the care and treatment of the eyes
ophthalmology: the branch of medical science dealing with the structure, function, and diseases of the eye
ophthalmoscope: optical instrument for examining the interior of the eye
opiate: drug derived from opium, as morphine
opium: narcotic drug obtained from the opium poppy from which morphine, codeine, heroin, and other drugs are derived
optic/optical: pertaining to the eye or to vision
optician: one who makes or sells eyeglasses and other optical equipment
optic nerve: special nerve of vision, conveying sensations from the retina to the brain
optometrist: one who practices optometry
optometry: profession of measuring the power of vision and prescribing corrective lenses
oral: pertaining to or situated near the mouth
oral cancer: *see* mouth
oral surgeon/dental surgeon: dentist who specializes in oral surgery
oral surgery: the diagnosis and surgical treatment of diseases, injuries, and defects of the mouth and jaw
orbit: either of the bony sockets of the eyes
orchidopexy/orchiopexy: surgical correction of an undescended testicle
orchiectomy: surgical removal of one or both testicles
orchiopexy: *see* orchidopexy
orchitis: inflammation of the testicles
organic: 1. of or pertaining to an organ of the body 2. having a physical basis, as a disorder 3. of or pertaining to animals or plants 4. pertaining to foods grown only with natural fertilizers of animal or plant origin
organic foods: foods grown with the use of organic fertilizers only, such as compost or animal (not human) manure, and without the use of pesticides or herbicides
organ of Corti: the true center of hearing within the cochlea of the inner ear, a complex spiral structure of hair cells
orgasm: the climax of the sexual act, normally marked by the male's ejaculation of semen and by relaxation of tension of both male and female
orifice: opening into a body cavity
orthodontia: orthodontics
orthodontics/orthodontia: the care and treatment of irregularities and faulty positions of the teeth, including the fitting of braces
orthodontist: dentist specializing in orthodontics
orthopedics: the branch of surgery dealing with the treatment and correction of deformities, injuries, and diseases of the skeletal system and its associated structures, as muscles and joints
orthopedic surgeon: orthopedist
orthopedist/orthopedic surgeon/orthopod: surgeon specializing in orthopedics
orthopod: orthopedist
orthoptist: medical technician trained to diagnose defects of the eye muscles and to provide corrective exercises
oscilloscope: instrument for visibly representing electrical activity on a fluorescent screen
osseous: osteal
ossicle: one of the three small connecting bones of the middle ear, the hammer (or malleus), the anvil (or incus), and the stirrup (or stapes), that transmit sound from the eardrum to the cochlea
ossification: conversion into bone
ossify: to convert or be converted into bone
osteal/osseous: of or relating to bone
osteitis: inflammation of a bone
osteitis deformans: *see* Paget's disease
osteoarthritis/degenerative joint disease/hypertrophic arthritis: chronic degenerative disease that affects the joints
osteogenesis: formation and growth of bones
osteogenesis, imperfecta: condition in which bones are abnormally brittle and liable to fracture because of a deficiency of calcium
osteogenic: pertaining to osteogenesis
osteomyelitis: inflammation of the bone tissue or marrow
osteopath: physician trained in osteopathy
osteopathy: system of healing based on a theory that most diseases are caused by structural abnormalities that may best be corrected by manipulation
osteophyte(s): abnormal bony outgrowth
osteoporosis: reduction in bone mass and increase in interior space, porosity, and fragility of bone
otitis media: inflammation of the middle ear
otitis media, nonsuppurative: inflammation of the middle ear resulting from a blocked Eustachian tube and fluid collection in the middle ear, causing hearing damage

otolaryngologist: physician specializing in the diagnosis and treatment of the ear, nose, and throat
otolaryngology: the branch of medicine dealing with the study and diseases of the ear, nose, and throat
otologist: one who specializes in the ear and its diseases
otology: the branch of medical science dealing with the functions and diseases of the ear
otoplasty: surgical technique to correct protruding or overlarge ears or to build up or replace a missing ear
otosclerosis: ear disorder resulting in hearing loss caused by the formation of spongy bone in the middle ear
otoscope: instrument used for examining the interior of the ear
outer ear: the external, fleshy part of the ear, including the auditory canal leading to the eardrum (tympanic membrane)
outpatient: patient who is not an inmate of a hospital or clinic at which treatment or diagnosis is received
ova: plural of *ovum*
ovarian: of or relating to the ovaries
ovarian dysgenesis: defective development of ovaries
ovariectomy/oophorectomy: surgical removal of an ovary
ovaries (*sing., ovary*): pair of female reproductive glands (gonads) that produce eggs (ova) and female sex hormones
overbite: extent to which upper teeth extend over lower teeth when the jaws are in closed position
overweight: *see* obesity
ovoid: egg-shaped
ovulation: the discharge of a mature egg cell (ovum) from the ovaries, occurring about once every 28 days at about the middle of the menstrual cycle
ovum/egg cell (*pl. ova*): female reproductive cell or gamete from which an embryo might develop if fertilized
oxytocin: hormone secreted by the pituitary gland to help the muscles of the uterus contract during labor
ozone: blue gas with a pungent odor that can be formed by the passage of electricity through the air

pacemaker, artificial: electrically activited, battery- or nuclear-powered device used to stimulate normal heartbeat if the natural cardiac pacemaker fails to function
pacemaker, cardiac: object or substance in the heart that regulates contraction of the heart muscle, or heartbeat
Paget's disease: 1. (osteitis deformans) chronic disease characterized by the softening and enlargement of the bones and usually the bowing of the long, weight-bearing bones 2. cancerous disease of the breast marked by the inflammation of the areola and nipple
palate: the roof of the mouth
palate, hard: the bony part of the roof of the mouth
palate, soft/velum: the soft, muscular tissue at the rear of the roof of the mouth
palpation: diagnostic procedure of feeling, pressing, or manipulating the body
palpitation: rapid or fluttering heartbeat
palsy/paralysis: Bell's palsy, cerebral palsy
PAN: peroxyacl nitrate
pancreas: large gland situated behind the stomach and containing the islets of Langerhans that produce insulin and glucagon, and secreting pancreatic juice via small ducts to the duodenum
pancreatic juice: secretion of the pancreas containing digestive enzymes
pancreatitis: inflammation of the pancreas
pandemic: epidemic occurring over a very large area or worldwide
Papanicolaou, Dr. George N.: developer of a test, called the *Pap smear* or *Pap test,* for detecting cancer of the cervix
Papanicolaou smear: Pap smear
papillae (*sing., papilla*)**:** tiny, nipple-shaped projections that cover the inner layer (dermis) of the skin and the surface of the tongue
papillary tumor: 1. papilloma: benign tumor of the papillae of the skin, as a wart or corn 2. malignant tumor of the bladder, so called because it is nipplelike in shape (Latin *papilla* means nipple)
Pap smear/Papanicolaou smear/Pap test: method of early detection of cervical cancer consisting of painless removal of cervical cell samples, which are stained and examined
Pap test: Pap smear
papule: pimple
paralysis agitans: Parkinson's disease
paralysis, infantile: *see* poliomyelitis
paranasal sinus: air cavity in one of the cranial bones communicating with the nostrils
paranoid: describing a personality disorder in which the individual is extraordinarily sensitive to praise or criticism and subject to suspicions and feelings of persecution
paranoid reaction/paranoia: psychosis characterized by invariable delusion, usually of persecution, sometimes of grandeur
paranoid schizophrenia: *see* schizophrenia, paranoid
paraplegia: paralysis of the lower half of the body
paraplegic: one who is paralyzed in the lower half of the body, including both legs

parasite(s): animal or plant that lives in or on another organism (called the host), at whose expense it obtains nourishment
parasiticide: medication designed to destroy parasites such as body lice
parasympathetic nervous system: the part of the autonomic nervous system that controls such involuntary actions as the constriction of pupils, dilation of blood vessels and salivary glands, and slowing of heartbeat
parathormone/parathyroid hormone: hormone secreted by the parathyroid glands, important in regulating the amount of calcium in the body
parathyroid glands: four small endocrine glands near or embedded within the thyroid gland, usually two per side, that regulate blood calcium and phosphorus levels
parathyroid hormone: *see* parathormone
paresis: 1. partial paralysis 2. general paralysis (*general paresis*) caused by degeneration of the brain as a result of syphilis
parkinsonism: Parkinson's disease
Parkinson's disease/paralysis agitans/ parkinsonism: chronic, progressive nervous disease characterized by muscle tremor when at rest, stiffness, and a rigid facial expression
parotid gland: either of two large salivary glands located below and in front of the ear
paroxysm: sudden onset of acute symptoms, as an attack or convulsions
parrot fever: psittacosis
particulate matter: fine particles in smoke that are dispersed by the wind and fall back to earth
parturition: act or process of giving birth
passive-dependent: describing a personality disorder in which the individual needs excessive emotional support from an authority figure
patch test: skin test for determining hypersensitivity by applying small pads of possibly allergy-producing substances to the skin's surface
patchy baldness: alopecia areata
patella: the kneecap
pathogen: disease-causing bacterium or microorganism
pathogenic: disease-causing
pathologic: caused by or relating to disease
pathologic fracture: fracture that occurs spontaneously, as because of pre-existing disease, without external cause
pathologist: physician or expert specializing in pathology
pathology: the branch of medical science dealing with the causes, nature, and effects of diseases, especially disease-induced changes in organs, tissues, and body chemistry
PCBs/polychlorinated biphenyls: chemicals related to DDT and having many industrial uses, posing a potential threat to health as a water pollutant from industrial wastes
pectus carinatum: *see* pigeon breast
pectus excavatum: *see* funnel chest
pedal: of or relating to the foot
pediatric dentist: dentist specializing in the care and treatment of the teeth of children
pediatrician: physician specializing in the care and treatment of children
pediatrics: the branch of medicine dealing with the care and treatment of children and their diseases
pedodontics: branch of dentistry specializing in the care of children
pedodontist: dentist specializing in pedodontics
pellagra: disease caused by a vitamin deficiency and characterized by gastric disturbance, skin eruptions, and nervous symptoms
pelvic girdle: the part of the human skeleton to which the lower limbs are attached
pelvis: 1. the part of the skeleton that forms a bony girdle or basin joining the lower limbs to the body, and consisting of the two hip bones and the sacrum 2. the central area of the kidney from which urine drains into the ureter
penicillin: powerful antibacterial substance found in a mold fungus and prepared in several forms for the treatment of a wide variety of infections
penis: tubular male organ of sexual intercourse and excretion of urine, located at the front of the pelvis
Pentothal/sodium Pentothal/thiopental: trademark for an ultra-short-acting barbiturate used as an anesthetic, as in dentistry
pep pills: *see* amphetamines
pepsin: enzyme secreted by the gastric juices of the stomach
peptic ulcer: ulcer of the mucous membrane of the stomach (gastric ulcer) or small intestine (duodenal ulcer) caused by the action of acid juices
percussion: diagnostic procedure of striking or tapping the body with instruments or with the fingers
perianal: situated around the anus
pericarditis: inflammation of the pericardium
pericardium: the membrane that surrounds and protects the heart
peridental: periodontal
perimeter: device for determining peripheral vision
perineal: of or pertaining to the perineum
perineum: region of the body at the lower end of the trunk, between the genital organs and the anus
periodontal/peridental: situated around a tooth

periodontal membrane: membrane, periodontal
periodontia: periodontics
periodontics/periodontia: the branch of dentistry dealing with the diagnosis and treatment of periodontal (gum) diseases
periodontist: dentist who specializes in periodontics
periodontitis: inflammation of the tissues around a tooth, leading to destruction of the alveolar bone
periodontium: the supporting structures of the teeth, comprised of the gingiva, alveolar bone, and periodontal ligaments
periosteum: the tough, fibrous membrane that surrounds and nourishes bones
peripheral nervous system: the nerves and ganglia outside the brain and spinal cord
peristalsis: wavelike muscular contractions of the alimentary canal that move the contents along in the processes of digestion and excretion
peristaltic wave: the alternate contraction and relaxation of muscles in the alimentary canal in peristalsis
peritoneoscopy: technique for examining the female reproductive organs within the abdominal cavity
peritoneoscope/laparoscope: instrument used for examining the organs within the abdominal cavity, especially the female reproductive organs
peritoneum: the serous membrane that lines the abdominal cavity enclosing the abdominal organs
peritonitis: inflammation of the lining (peritoneum) of the abdominal cavity
peritonsillar abscess/quinsy: abscess in the tissues adjoining a tonsil as a complication of tonsillitis
pernicious: severe, destructive, and often fatal
pernicious anemia: severe, progressive anemia caused by lack of vitamin B_{12}, formerly fatal but now controllable
personality disorder/character disorder: any of a group of mental illnesses that apparently stem from an arrested development of the personality
perspiration: *see* sweat
pertussis: *see* whooping cough
pessary: 1. device worn inside the vagina as a contraceptive or to support uterine prolapse 2. medicated suppository for use in the vagina
petit mal: minor epileptic seizure, with very brief loss of consciousness
Peyer's patches: oval areas of lymphoid tissue in the intestine that manufacture lymphocytes
peyote: the mescal cactus of Mexico or the powerful hallucinogenic drug obtained from its dried upper part (called buttons)
phalanges (*sing., phalanx*): the bones of the fingers or toes
pharmacist: one skilled in the compounding and dispensing of medicines
pharmacologist: expert in pharmacology
pharmacology: the science of the action of medicines, their nature, preparation, administration, and effects
pharyngitis: inflammation of the pharynx, commonly called a sore throat
pharynx: the part of the alimentary canal between the palate and the esophagus, serving as a passage for air and food
phenformin: *see* DBI
phenol: *see* carbolic acid
phenylketonuria/PKU: inherited metabolic disorder that can cause mental retardation if not treated by a special diet soon after birth
phlebitis: inflammation of the inner membrane of a vein
phlebotomy/bloodletting/venesection: the opening of a vein for letting blood
phlegm: viscid, stringy mucus secreted in abnormally large amounts, as in the air passages
phobia: intense anxiety irrationally felt for any of a variety of things or situations, such as closed or open places, animals of a particular kind, heights, etc., a manifestation of the phobic reaction
phobic reaction: neurosis characterized by displacement of anxiety of a conflict to a substitute, such as a particular domestic animal, closed places, etc.
phonocardiogram: graph recording the sounds produced by the heart, used to evaluate heart murmurs and other abnormal sounds
physical dependence: accommodation of the body to continued use of a drug, such that withdrawing the drug causes pronounced physical reactions (withdrawal symptoms)
physical fitness: *see* fitness
physical medicine: branch of medicine utilizing physical procedures, such as heat, cold, massage, or mechanical devices, to diagnose disease or treat disabled patients
physical therapist: specialist in physical therapy
physical therapy/physiotherapy: the treatment of disability, injury, or disease by external physical means, such as heat, massage, planned exercises, electricity, or mechanical devices, to restore function or aid rehabilitation
physician(s): 1. any authorized practitioner of medicine 2. one trained in medicine, as distinguished from surgery
physiotherapy: *see* physical therapy
pia mater: the delicate, vascular, innermost membrane of the three membranes that envelop the brain and spinal cord
pica: appetite for substances unfit to eat

piebald skin: vitiligo
pigeon breast/pectus carinatum: congenital deformity in which the sternum protrudes
pigment: substance that imparts coloring to tissue
piles: *see* hemorrhoids
"pill, the": contraceptives, oral
pimple/papule: small, usually inflamed swelling on the skin
pineal body: *see* pineal gland
pineal gland/pineal body: small, cone-shaped body of rudimentary glandular structure located at the base of the brain and having no known function
pinkeye: acute, contagious conjunctivitis, marked by redness of the eyeball
pinworm: parasitic worm of the lower intestines and rectum, especially of children, causing intense itching in the anal area
pituitary body: *see* pituitary gland
pituitary gland/hypophysis cerebri/pituitary body: small endocrine gland situated at the base of the brain, consisting of anterior and posterior lobes whose hormonal secretions stimulate the production of hormones in other glands and regulate vital body functions such as growth and metabolism
pityriasis rosea: skin disease, especially of children, marked by a rash
PKU: *see* phenylketonuria
placebo: any harmless substance given to humor a patient or as a test in controlled experiments on the effects of drugs
placenta: the vascular structure in pregnant women that unites the fetus with the uterus, and through which the fetus is nourished via the umbilical cord, usually expelled naturally immediately following birth (when it is called the *afterbirth*)
Placidyl: ethchlorvynol
plague: 1. any epidemic disease that is contagious and often deadly 2. contagious, often fatal disease caused by a bacterium transmitted by fleas from infected rats, and characterized by fever, chills, prostration, and often by buboes (hence the name *bubonic plague*)
plantar warts: warts on the soles of the feet, caused by a virus
plaque: mucus containing bacteria that collects on teeth
plasma: the clear fluid portion of the blood
plastic surgeon: physician specializing in plastic or cosmetic surgery
plastic surgery: surgery that deals with the restoration or healing of lost, injured, or deformed parts of the body, mainly by the transfer of tissue, and with the improvement of appearance (cosmetic surgery)
platelet/thrombocyte: small, disk-shaped body found in blood that aids in clotting
play therapy: psychotherapy, especially for patients who are children, in which toys or other playthings are made available for the patient to play with in the presence of the therapist
playthings: *see* toys
pleura: serous membrane that enfolds the lungs and lines the chest cavity
pleural cavity: the space between the two pleuras lining the lungs and chest cavity
pleurisy: inflammation of the pleura, characterized by fever, chest pain, and difficulty in breathing
plexus: interlacement of cordlike body structures, such as blood vessels or nerves
plexus block: *see* nerve block
pneumococcus: bacterium that can cause pneumonia
pneumoconiosis: any of various lung disorders, such as silicosis or black lung disease, resulting from the inhalation of dust or other minute particles
pneumoencephalogram: X-ray picture of the brain taken after air or gas has been injected to partially replace the cerebrospinal fluid
pneumoencephalography: technique of producing pneumoencephalograms and interpreting them
pneumonia: inflammation of the lungs, usually bacterial in origin and acute in course, characterized by high fever, chills, breathing difficulty, and cough
pneumothorax: accumulation of air or gas in the pleural cavity, causing the lung to collapse, as from injury or disease, or by injection (artificial pneumothorax) in the treatment of tuberculosis
podiatrist/chiropodist: one who specializes in the treatment of the foot
podiatry/chiropody: the study and treatment of disorders of the feet
polio: *see* poliomyelitis
poliomyelitis/infantile paralysis/Heine-Medin disease: acute viral disease of the central nervous system characterized by fever, headache, sore throat, stiffness of the neck and back, and sometimes by paralysis and eventual atrophy of muscles
pollutant: something that pollutes the air, water, or soil
polycystic: characterized by numerous cysts
polycythemia: condition characterized by too many red blood corpuscles
polycythemia vera/erythremia: condition characterized by abnormally high number and proportion of red blood corpuscles
polymenorrhea: abnormally frequent menstruation
polymorphonuclear leukocyte: *see* neutrophil
polymyositis: inflammation of a number of muscles and connective tissue, characterized by pain, swelling, and weakness

polyp: smooth growth or tumor found in the mucous membranes, as of the nose, bladder, uterus, or rectum
polyunsaturated: (of fats) tending to lower the cholesterol content of the blood
polyuria: excessive urination
pons: mass in the brain containing fibers that connect the medulla oblongata, the cerebellum, and the cerebrum
pontic: in dentistry, a part of a bridge serving as a substitute for a missing tooth
popliteal: pertaining to the back part of the leg behind the knee
portal vein: vein that conveys blood from the intestines and stomach to the liver
"port wine stain": hemangioma
positive pressure breathing: breathing of air or other gas mixture at pressure greater than the surrounding atmospheric pressure
posterior: toward the rear
posterior lobe hypophysis: the posterior part of the pituitary gland that produces hormones regulating kidney function and other vital processes
posterior urethra: prostatic urethra
postmenopausal: being or occurring after menopause
postpartum: after childbirth
postural drainage: the loosening and draining of lung secretions by assuming a prone position with the head lower than the feet
pot (*slang*): marihuana
Pott's disease: tuberculosis or tissue destruction of the spinal vertebrae, causing angular, spinal curvature
PPD: purified protein derivative
prediabetic condition: diabetes, chemical
pre-eclampsia: disorder of late pregnancy or following childbirth
preemie/premie: premature infant
pregnancy: condition or time of being pregnant
pregnant: carrying developing offspring in the uterus
preinvasive: before spreading to other tissues: said of malignant growths
Preludin: phenmetrazine
premature: of a newborn baby, weighing less than 5 pounds
premature ejaculation: ejaculation of semen during sexual intercourse before the female has had time to respond
premenopausal: being or occurring before menopause
premolar: *see* bicuspid
prenatal: before birth
prenatal diagnosis: amniocentesis
preop: *see* preoperative
preoperative/preop: performed or occurring before a surgical operation, as shaving of the affected area, administration of certain drugs, etc.
prep: preparation of a patient for surgery, usually including cleansing and shaving of the affected area
prepuce: the loose skin covering the head of the penis or the clitoris
presbyopia: farsightedness caused by aging of the lens or the muscles that expand and contract it
pressor: tending to raise blood pressure, as certain hormones
preventive medicine: the branch of medical science concerned with preventing disease, as through immunological methods
prickly heat/heat rash/miliaria: itchy rash of small red pimples caused by excessive sweating in hot weather
primary: 1. not produced as a secondary effect or complication of another condition 2. original and not resulting from metastasis or other means of transmission, as a tumor or infection
primary teeth: *see* baby teeth
primipara: woman who is pregnant for the first time or who has borne one child
process: in anatomy, any outgrowth or projecting part of a larger structure, as the knobby portion of a vertebra
proctologist: physician specializing in proctology
proctology: the branch of medicine that deals with the diagnosis and treatment of diseases of the lower colon, rectum, and anus
proctoscope: surgical instrument for examining the interior of the rectum and part of the colon
proctoscopy: examination of the rectum and colon with the aid of a proctoscope
proctosigmoidoscopy: examination of the rectum and a portion of the colon (sigmoid) with the aid of a sigmoidoscope
prodrome: symptom resembling a premonition that signals the onset of a disease or of an epileptic seizure
profibrinolysin: the inactive precursor of fibrinolysin, an agent in the process of dissolving blood clots
progesterone: hormone of the ovary that prepares the uterus for receiving the fertilized ovum
prognathism: the condition of having a protruding jaw, especially the lower
prognosis: prediction made by a doctor as to the probable course of a disease
prolactin: lactogenic hormone
prolapse: move or slip forward or downward, as a displaced organ
prolapsed: slipped or moved from the usual place
pronate: turn, as the hand or foot, in a movement of pronation
pronation: 1. rotation of the hand or forearm so that the palm of the hand faces downward or backward 2. movement of the foot, as in im-

proper walking, in which the sole is raised along the outer side and the toes turned out, often with an inward leaning of the ankle
prone: lying on the chest, with the face downward
proof: strength of alcohol in an alcoholic beverage, indicated by a proof number equal to twice the percentage of alcohol by volume (100 proof = 50% alcohol)
prophylactic: tending to ward off or prevent, as disease or conception
prophylaxis: treatment intended to prevent disease, as the cleaning of teeth
propranolol: drug that causes blood vessels to dilate, used in the treatment of angina pectoris
prostate: partly muscular gland in males at the base of the bladder around the urethra that releases a fluid to convey spermatozoa
prostate, enlarged benign: enlargement of the prostate gland resulting in difficulty in voiding and retention of urine in the bladder
prostate, inflammation of: prostatitis
prostatectomy: surgical removal of all or part of the prostate gland
prostatic urethra/posterior urethra: the part of the male urethra that passes across the prostate gland
prostatitis: inflammation of the prostate gland, characterized by painful and excessive urination
prostatitis, acute: severe, relatively uncommon form of prostatitis, marked by painful and excessive urination, high fever, and a discharge of pus from the penis
prosthesis (*pl., prostheses*)/**prosthetic device:** artificial substitute for a missing or amputated part, as an arm or leg
prosthetic device: prosthesis
protein(s): any of a class of highly complex organic compounds, composed principally of amino acids, that occur in all living things and form an essential part of animal food requirements
proteinuria: excretion of protein through the urine
prothrombin: the inactive precursor of thrombin, an agent in the process of forming blood clots
protozoa (*sing., protozoon*): microscopic animal organisms that exist in countless numbers, including one-celled organisms and parasitic forms that cause malaria, sleeping sickness, and other diseases
proud flesh: *see* granulation tissue
proximal: relatively near the center of the body or near a point considered as central
proximal muscles: those muscles closest to the trunk of the body, such as the shoulder-arm and hip-thigh muscles
pruritus: localized or general itching
pruritus, anal: intense itching in the area of the anus
pseudohypertrophic muscular dystrophy/Duchenne's muscular dystrophy: disease characterized by the enlargement and apparent overdevelopment (hypertrophy) of certain muscles, especially of the shoulder girdle, which subsequently atrophy
pseudoneoplasm: *see* pseudotumor
pseudotumor/pseudoneoplasm: condition that has the appearance of a tumor but is not a tumor, such as an inflammation
psilocybin: derivative of the mushroom *Psilocybe mexicana,* which produces hallucinations in the user
psittacosis/parrot fever: infectious disease of parrots and other birds that can be transmitted to humans and cause symptoms like those of influenza
psoralen: chemical derived from a plant that is used in the treatment of psoriasis
psoriasis: a noncontagious chronic condition of the skin, marked by bright red patches covered by silvery scales
psychiatrist: physician specializing in psychiatry
psychiatry: the branch of medicine that treats disorders of the mind (or psyche), including psychoses and neuroses
psychoanalysis: system of psychotherapy originated by Sigmund Freud for treating emotional disorders by bringing to the attention of the conscious mind the repressed conflicts of the unconscious
psychoanalyst: one who practices psychoanalysis
psychodrama: psychotherapy in which a patient or group of patients act out situations centered about their personal conflicts in the presence of the therapist
psychogenic: caused by or contributed to by psychological factors
psychological dependence: emotional desire or need to continue using a drug
psychologist: specialist in psychology
psychology: the science dealing with the mind, mental phenomena, consciousness, and behavior
psychomimetic: having properties capable of producing changes in behavior that mimic psychoses
psychomotor: having to do with muscular movements resulting from mental processes
psychomotor convulsion/temporal lobe convulsion: epileptic convulsion characterized by compulsive and often repetitious behavior of which the patient later has no memory
psychoneurosis: neurosis
psychopathic: *see* sociopathic

psychophysiological/psychosomatic: pertaining to a class of disorders in which psychological factors contribute substantially to the physiological condition
psychosis (*pl., psychoses*)**:** severe mental disorder often involving disorganization of the total personality, with or without organic disease
psychosomatic: pertaining to the effects of the emotions on body processes, especially with respect to initiating or aggravating disease
psychotherapist: specialist in psychotherapy
psychotherapy: the treatment of emotional and mental disorders by psychological methods, such as psychoanalysis
psychotic: one suffering from a psychosis
psychotropic: affecting the mind: said of certain drugs
ptomaine: substance derived from decomposing or putrefying animal or vegetable protein, rarely the cause of food poisoning, which is usually caused by bacteria such as Salmonella
ptosis: dropping of the upper eyelid
ptyalin: enzyme in saliva that begins the chemical breakdown of starch
puberty: period during which a person reaches sexual maturity and becomes functionally capable of reproduction
puberty, precocious: early menarche (first occurrence of menstruation), before the age of eight or nine
pubic: in the region of the lower abdomen
pubis: the lower anterior part of the hip bone
pulmonary: of or relating to the lungs
pulmonary artery: artery, pulmonary
pulmonary emphysema: emphysema of the lungs; *see* emphysema
pulmonary tuberculosis: *see* tuberculosis
pulmonary vein: *see* vein, pulmonary
pulp: (of teeth) the soft tissue of blood vessels and nerves that fills the central cavity of a tooth
pulpotomy: surgical removal of the pulp of a tooth
pulse: rhythmic pressure in the arteries resulting from the beating of the heart
puncture wound: wound caused by an object that pierces the skin, as a nail or tack, involving increased danger of tetanus
pupil: contractile opening in the iris of the eye through which light reaches the retina
purine: one of a group of chemicals occurring naturally in certain foods and formerly implicated as a contributing cause of gout
purpura: blood disease characterized by hemorrhaging into the skin and mucous membranes
purulent: consisting of or secreting pus
pus: secretion from inflamed and healing tissues, usually viscid or creamy, and containing decaying leukocytes, bacteria, and other tissue debris
pustule: pus-filled bump on the skin, inflamed at the base
pyelitis: pyelonephritis
pyelogram: visualization of the kidney and ureter by X ray
pyelonephritis/pyelitis: infection and inflammation of the kidneys
pyloric sphincter: the ring of muscle surrounding the pylorus that acts as a valve, allowing food to pass from the stomach to the duodenum
pyloric stenosis: congenital condition in which the pylorus is too narrow to allow the stomach's contents to empty normally
pylorus: the opening between the stomach and the duodenum
pyorrhea: discharge of pus, especially when applied to the progressive inflammation of the gingival (gum) tissue, which may lead to loosening and loss of teeth
pyrexia: *see* fever
pyrogenic: causing or inducing fever

Q fever: infectious disease (rickettsial disease) transmitted by sheep and cattle and characterized by high fever, chills, and muscle pains
quadriplegia: paralysis of both arms and both legs
quadriplegic: one suffering from paralysis of both arms and both legs
quinine: bitter substance obtained from the bark of the cinchona tree, used to treat malaria and myotonia
quinsy: *see* peritonsillar abscess

rabies/hydrophobia: acute viral disease of the central nervous system transmitted to humans by the bite or saliva of an infected animal, as a dog, bat, or squirrel, invariably fatal unless treated before symptoms appear
radiation sickness: illness caused by the body's absorption of excess radiation, marked by fatigue, nausea, vomiting, and sometimes internal hemorrhage and tissue breakdown
radiation therapy/radiotherapy: treatment of disease by radiation, as by X rays or other radioactive substances
radical: of or involving procedures or treatment intended to go to the root of a disease and thereby eliminate it, as by excising an entire organ or part that is diseased
radiograph: X-ray photograph
radiography: X-ray photography
radiologist: physician specializing in radiology
radiology: the branch of medical science that deals with radiant energy, such as X rays and energy produced by radium, cobalt, and other radioactive substances, especially in the diagnosis and treatment of disease
radiopaque: impervious to X rays
radiotherapy: *see* radiation therapy

radius (*pl., radii*): the bone of the forearm on the same side as the thumb, thicker and shorter than the ulna bone
rale: abnormal sound heard in the chest with the aid of a stethoscope, indicating the presence of disease
Raynaud's disease: Raynaud's syndrome
Raynaud's syndrome/Raynaud's disease: condition characterized by spasms of small blood vessels when exposed to cold, especially the fingers and toes, which become cyanotic (bluish) and then red
RBC: red blood cell
recovery room: hospital room or section for patients immediately following surgery, where their post-operative conditions can be closely monitored
rectocele: hernia in which part of the rectum protrudes through the wall of the vagina
rectum: the terminal portion of the large intestine, extending from the sigmoid bend of the colon to the anus
red corpuscle: *see* erythroctye
red marrow: marrow
reduce: move back into proper position, as a herniating bowel or the fragments of a broken bone
reducing: *see* weight reduction
reduction: manipulation back into proper position to restore normal function, as a fracture, dislocation, or herniated part
referred pain: pain felt in one part of the body though originating in another part, as pain of the left shoulder and arm caused by a heart attack
reflex: involuntary response to a stimulus
reflux: a flowing back, as of urine from the bladder up into the ureter
refraction: the change of direction of a ray of light as it passes from one medium to another of different density
regional enteritis: enteritis in a chronic state
regurgitation: the act of rushing or surging back, as in vomiting, or the backward rush of blood in the heart because of defective valves or leaflets
Reiter's syndrome: form of arthritis characterized by occurrence of conjunctivitis of the eye and inflammation of the urethra
relaxant: drug or other agent that reduces tension, especially of the muscles
remission: period with less severe symptoms or without symptoms during the course of a disease
renal/nephric: of or relating to the kidneys
renal calculus: kidney stone
renal colic: pain that results from the passage of a kidney stone through the ureter
renal diabetes: renal glucosuria
renal glucosuria/renal diabetes: glucose in the urine in conjunction with normal blood sugar levels, due to failure of the renal tubules to reabsorb glucose
rennin: milk-curdling enzyme present in gastric juice
repression: exclusion from consciousness of painful desires, memories, etc., and consequent manifestation through the unconscious
resect: perform a resection on
resection: surgical removal of a part of a bone, organ, etc.
resectoscope: surgical instrument used especially for resection of the prostate gland by insertion into the urethra
residency: period of training in a hospital, usually in a medical specialty, for physicians preparing for private practice
resident: physician working and undergoing training (residency) in a hospital in preparation for private practice in a specialty
resorb: to reabsorb
respiration: the process by which an animal or plant takes in oxygen from the air and gives off carbon dioxide and other products of oxidation
respiratory arrest: *see* breathing, cessation of
respiratory distress syndrome: *see* hyaline membrane disease
resuscitation: mouth-to-mouth respiration
retardation, mental: *see* mental retardation
retention cyst: *see* cyst, follicular
reticulum: network of cells or cellular tissue
retina: the inner membrane at the back of the eyeball, containing light-sensitive rods and cones which receive the optical image
retinoblastoma: tumor of the eye, found especially in children
retinopathy: diseased condition of the retina of the eye
retinopathy, diabetic: *see* diabetic retinopathy
retinoscope: special device for examining the retina
rhesus factor: Rh factor
rheumatic fever: acute infectious disease chiefly affecting children and young adults, characterized by painful inflammation around the joints, intermittent fever, and inflammation of the pericardium and valves of the heart
rheumatic heart disease: impairment of heart function as a result of rheumatic fever
rheumatism: painful inflammation and stiffness of muscles, joints, or connective tissue
rheumatoid arthritis: chronic disease characterized by swelling and inflammation of one or more joints, often resulting in stiffness and eventual impairment of mobility
rheumatoid arthritis, juvenile/Still's disease: form of rheumatoid arthritis affecting children, often characterized by fever, rash, pleurisy, and enlargement of the spleen as well as rheumatoid joint symptoms

rheumatoid spondylitis: *see* spondylitis, rheumatoid
rheumatologist: physician specializing in rheumatology
rheumatology: subspecialty of internal medicine concerned with the study, diagnosis, and treatment of rheumatism and other diseases of the joints and muscles
Rh factor/rhesus factor: protein present in the blood of most people (called Rh-positive) and absent from others (called Rh-negative). Under certain conditions the blood of a pregnant Rh-negative woman may be incompatible with the blood of her fetus
rhinecephalon/"nose brain": the part of the brain controlling the sense of smell
rhinitis: inflammation of the mucous membranes of the nose
rhinoplasty: plastic surgery of the nose
Rh negative: *see* Rh factor
Rh positive: *see* Rh factor
rhythm method: birth control method whereby sexual intercourse is avoided during the period of ovulation in the menstrual cycle
rhytidoplasty/face lift/facial plasty: plastic surgery to eliminate facial wrinkles
rib(s): one of the series of curved bones attached to the spine and enclosing the chest cavity
rib cage/thoracic cage: the part of the skeleton that encloses the chest, bound by the ribs and the spinal vertebrae
riboflavin/vitamin B_2: member of the vitamin B complex, found in milk, green leafy vegetables, eggs and meats
rickets: early childhood disease characterized by softening of bones and consequent deformity, caused by deficiency of vitamin D
rickettsiae (*sing., rickettsia*)**:** parasitic microorganisms transmitted to humans by the bites of infected ticks, lice, and fleas, and causing Rocky Mountain spotted fever, Q fever, rickettsial pox, and typhus
rickettsial: caused by or pertaining to rickettsiae
rickettsial disease: any of the diseases, as typhus or Rocky Mountain spotted fever, caused by rickettsiae
rickettsial pox: infectious disease, rickettsial disease, transmitted by mites which infest mice, and characterized by fever, chills, rash, headache, and backache
ringworm/tinea: contagious fungus disease of the skin, hair, or nails marked by ring-shaped, scaly, reddish patches of skin
Ritalin: methylphenidate
Rocky Mountain spotted fever: infectious disease (rickettsial disease) transmitted by the bite of certain ticks and characterized by fever, chills, rash, headache, and muscular pain
rod: one of many rod-shaped bodies in the retina of the eye, sensitive to faint light and peripheral objects and movements
roentgenogram: X-ray photograph
roentgenologist: physician specializing in the diagnosis and treatment of diseases with the application of X rays
roentgenology: the branch of medical science dealing with the properties and effects of X rays
root canal: the passageway of nerves and blood vessels in the root of a tooth leading into the pulp
roseola infantum: childhood illness characterized by high fever followed by a body rash
roughage: food material containing a high percentage of indigestible constituents
roundworm/ascaris: parasitic nematode worm, as the hookworm and pinworm, whose eggs hatch in the small intestines
rubella/German measles: contagious viral disease benign in children but linked to birth defects of children born of women infected in early pregnancy
rubeola: measles
Rubin's test: tubal insufflation
rupture: 1. any breaking apart, as of a blood vessel 2. hernia

Sabin vaccine: live polio vaccine taken orally to immunize against polio
sacral: pertaining to the sacrum
sacroiliac: pertaining to the sacrum or the ilium, or to the places on either side of the lower back where they are joined
sacrum: bone in the lower spine formed by the fusing of five vertebrae, constituting the rear part of the pelvis
saddle block: form of anesthesia used especially for childbirth, in which the patient is injected in the lower spinal cord while in a sitting position
safety glass: glass strengthened by any of various methods to reduce the likelihood of the glass shattering upon impact
St. Vitus dance: chorea
saline amniocentesis/salting out: technique of inducing abortion by injecting a saline solution into the amniotic fluid
saliva: fluid secreted by the salivary glands in the mouth that lubricates food and contains an enzyme (ptyalin) that begins to break down starch
salivary glands: glands located in the mouth which secrete saliva
Salk vaccine: dead polio virus taken by injection to immunize against polio
Salmonella: genus of aerobic bacteria that cause food poisoning and other diseases, including typhoid fever

Salmonella typhosa: rod-shaped bacteria that cause typhoid fever
salpingitis: 1. inflammation of a Fallopian tube, a potential cause of sterility 2. inflammation of a Eustachian tube
salt: sodium chloride
salting out: the injection of a saline solution into the amniotic fluid to induce labor and thus terminate a pregnancy
salt, table: *see* sodium chloride
saphenous vein: either of two large, superficial veins of the leg, a common site of varicosity
sarcoid: *see* sarcoidosis
sarcoidosis/Boeck's sarcoid/sarcoid: disease of unknown cause with symptoms resembling those of tuberculosis, marked by the formation of nodules, especially on the skin, lungs, and lymph nodes
sarcoma: malignant tumor that arises in the connective tissue (bones, cartilage, tendons)
saturated: (of fats) tending to increase the cholesterol content of the blood
saucerization: procedure of forming a shallow depression by scraping away tissue to assist healing
scabies/the itch: contagious inflammation of the skin caused by a mite and characterized by a rash and intense itching
scag (*slang*): heroin
scan: to measure for diagnostic purposes the concentration in a particular area of a radioactive material that has been introduced into the body
scapula: shoulder blade
scarlet fever: contagious disease caused by streptococci and characterized by a scarlet rash and high fever
schistosomiasis/bilharziasis: tropical disease caused by a fluke worm (trematode) whose larvae penetrate the skin and invade the circulatory system
schizoid: 1. describing a personality disorder in which the individual is withdrawn from and indifferent to other people 2. pertaining to or resembling schizophrenia
schizophrenia, catatonic: schizophrenia marked by motor disturbances, such as maintenance of fixed, often awkward, position with muscles rigid
schizophrenia, hebephrenic: schizophrenia marked by delusions, hallucinations, and regressed or childish behavior
schizophrenia, paranoid: schizophrenia marked by variable delusions of persecution or grandeur, often with hallucinations and behavioral deterioration
schizophrenic: of or pertaining to schizophrenia
schizophrenic reaction/schizophrenia: psychosis characterized by withdrawal from external reality and a retreat into a fantasy life, with deterioration of behavior
schoolboy (*slang*): codeine
sciatica: pain along the sciatic nerve
sciatic nerve: nerve of the lower spine that traverses the hips and runs down the back of the thigh of each leg
sclera: the firm outer coat of the eye continuous with the cornea, visible as the white of the eye
sclerose: to harden and thicken, as tissue
sclerosis: abnormal thickening and hardening of tissue, as of the lining of arteries
sclerosis, amyotrophic lateral/Lou Gehrig's disease: disease characterized by increasing muscle weakness (atrophy) or paralysis, caused by the progressive degeneration of motor nerve cells in the brain and spinal cord
scoliosis: spine, lateral curvature
scratch test: skin test for allergic response to different substances by applying suspected allergens in diluted form to scratches
scrofula: tuberculosis of the lymph nodes, especially of the neck
scrotum: pouch that contains the testicles
scrub nurse: operating room nurse authorized to handle sterilized equipment in assisting the surgeon
scurvy: disease characterized by livid spots under the skin, swollen and bleeding gums, and prostration, caused by lack of vitamin C
seasickness: motion sickness
sebaceous cyst: hard, round, movable mass contained in a sac, resulting from accumulated oil from a blocked sebaceous gland duct
sebaceous gland: gland within the dermis that secretes oil (sebum) for lubricating the skin and hair
seborrhea: abnormal increase of secretion from the sebaceous skin glands
sebum: fatty lubricating substance secreted by the sebaceous glands
secondary: produced as an effect or complication of another condition, as distinguished from *primary*.
secondary disease: disorder of a target gland caused by an excess or deficiency of a stimulating hormone supplied by the anterior pituitary gland
sedation: reduction of sensitivity to pain, stress, etc., by administering a sedative
sedative: medicine for allaying irritation or nervousness
seizure: *see* convulsion
semen: thick, whitish fluid containing spermatozoa that is ejaculated by the male at orgasm
semicircular canals: three fluid-filled tubes of the inner ear that govern the sense of balance and communicate with the vestibular nerve

seminal fluid: *see* semen
seminal vesicle: one of two small pouches on either side of the prostate gland that serve to store spermatozoa temporarily
senile macula degeneration: visual defect affecting the elderly
senile psychosis/senile dementia: mental disorder of the aged characterized by progressive deterioration of the personality, irritability, loss of memory, etc.
senile purpura: small hemorrhages in the skin of older people
senility: state of being senile
separated retina: detached retina
sepsis: infection of the blood by disease-causing microorganisms
septicemia: blood poisoning
septic shock: shock resulting from infection of the blood by disease-causing microorganisms
septum: dividing wall between two cavities, as in the nose
serous: pertaining to, producing, or resembling serum
serous membrane: membrane producing serum
serratus muscles: muscles that run vertically along the ribs
serum: the watery, clear portion of blood or lymph
serum analysis: laboratory analysis of blood serum as a diagnostic aid
serum sickness: acute illness caused by reaction to serum, such as that used in inoculations
sex act: *see* sexual intercourse
sex glands: *see* ovaries; testicles
sexual intercourse/coitus: male's ejaculation of semen into a female's vagina
sexuality: sexual interest or activity
shingles/herpes zoster: acute viral infection and inflammation of a sensory nerve, characterized by pain and small blisters on the skin along the path of the nerve
shock, allergic: allergic shock
shock, cardiac: shock resulting from diminished heart function
shock, circulatory: emergency condition in which the circulation of the blood is so disrupted that all bodily functions are affected
sick headache: *see* migraine
sickle-cell anemia: hereditary disease occurring most commonly among black men and women, in which many or a majority of the red blood cells are sickle-shaped, producing chronic anemia
sickle-cell trait/sicklemia: trait in the genetic make-up of an individual that could cause sickle-cell anemia in his or her offspring if the other parent also has the trait
sigmoid: 1. (*adj.*) shaped like the letter S 2. (*n.*) (sigmoid colon/sigmoid flexure) S-shaped fold in the colon of the large intestine just above the rectum
sigmoid colon: *see* sigmoid 2
sigmoid flexure: *see* sigmoid 2
sigmoidoscope: surgical instrument for examining the interior of the sigmoid
sign: (of disease) observable or objective manifestation, as distinguished from symptoms reported by the patient
silica: extremely hard mineral, the chief constituent of quartz and sand
silicosis: lung disorder, a form of pneumoconiosis, caused by inhaling silica dust, as of stone or sand
simple fracture: closed fracture
sinoatrial node: sinus node
sinus: opening or cavity, as in bone, or a channel or passageway, as for blood
sinusitis: inflammation of a sinus
sinus node/sinoatrial node: small mass of nerve tissue in the right atrium of the heart that triggers heart contractions and regulates heartbeat, thus serving as cardiac pacemaker
sitz bath: hot bath taken in a sitting position
skeletal muscle/voluntary muscle: striated muscle attached to bones and joints, used chiefly in voluntary action
skeleton, appendicular: the bones of the arms, hands, legs, and feet
skeleton, axial: the bones of the head and the trunk
skin/integument: the outer, membranous covering of the body, consisting of an outer layer (epidermis) and inner layer (dermis)
skin-popping (*slang*)**:** subcutaneous injection of heroin
sleep disorders: *see* insomnia; narcolepsy
sleeping pill: sedative, especially one of the barbiturates taken to relieve insomnia
sleeping sickness/trypanosomiasis: tropical African disease caused by certain protozoa and spread by the bite of the tsetse fly, characterized by lethargy, recurrent fever, and oppressive drowsiness, often fatal
sleepwalking/somnambulism: act of walking in one's sleep
slip lamp microscope/biomicroscope: microscope for examining the eye, as the cornea, with the aid of an intense beam of light
smack (*slang*)**:** heroin
smallpox/variola: acute, highly contagious viral disease characterized by high fever and the eruption of deep-seated pustules that leave scars upon healing
smegma: cheesy secretion that may collect under the prepuce of the uncircumcised penis or of the clitoris

smooth muscle/involuntary muscle: nonstriated muscle, used chiefly in involuntary action, such as that of the stomach and intestines
social worker(s): person trained to work in a clinical, social, or recreational service for improving community welfare or aiding the rehabilitation or emotional adjustment of individuals
sociopathic/psychopathic: describing a personality disorder in which the individual characteristically lacks a sense of personal responsibility or morality and may be disposed to aggressive and violent behavior, to self-destructive behavior, or to sexual deviation
sodium amytal: chemical used as sedative for soldiers in World War I
sodium cyclamate: *see* cyclamate
sodium Pentothal: *see* Pentothal
soft spots: fontanels
soldier's disease: morphinism
somnambulism: *see* sleepwalking
soot-wart: name for cancer of the scrotum that afflicted 18th-century chimney sweeps
sore throat: *see* pharyngitis
spasm: involuntary convulsive contraction of muscles, called *clonic* when alternately contracted and relaxed, and *tonic* when persistently contracted
spastic: of or characteristic of spasms
spasticity: the condition of having spasms
specimen: sample, as of blood, sputum, etc., for laboratory analysis
speculum: instrument that dilates a passage of the body, as for examination
speech reading: lip reading
speed (*slang*): methamphetamine
speed freak (*slang*): heavy user of methamphetamine (speed), especially by intravenous injection, to induce altered mental state
sperm: spermatozoa
spermatozoa (*sing., spermatozoon*)/**sperm/ sperm cells:** male reproductive cells or gametes, one of which must fertilize an ovum to produce an embryo
sperm cell: the male reproductive cell, one of the spermatozoa
sperm cells: spermatozoa
sperm ducts: vas deferens
spermicide: contraceptive substance that destroys sperm
sphincter(s): ringlike muscles surrounding an opening or tube that serves to narrow or close it
sphygmomanometer: device for measuring arterial blood pressure
spinal: *see* spinal anesthesia
spinal anesthesia/spinal: form of anesthesia in which the patient is injected in the region of the spinal cord
spinal arthritis: arthritis of the spine, found especially in the elderly
spinal column/backbone/spine: the series of segmented bones (vertebrae) which enclose the spinal cord and provide support for the ribs
spinal cord: the part of the central nervous system within the spinal column
spinal fluid: *see* cerebrospinal fluid
spinal fluid exam: spinal tap
spinal puncture: spinal tap
spinal reflex: reaction to an outside stimulus that originates in the spinal cord and bypasses the brain
spinal tap/lumbar puncture/spinal fluid exam/spinal puncture: needle puncture and withdrawal of cerebrospinal fluid from the lower spinal column for diagnostic examination
spine: *see* spinal column
spirochete: any of various spiral-shaped bacteria, some of which cause syphilis and yaws
spleen: vascular, ductless organ located near the stomach that produces red blood cells in infancy and modifies blood composition
splint: appliance for supporting or immobilizing a part of the body, as a fractured bone
spondylitis: inflammation of the vertebrae of the spine
spondylitis, rheumatoid/ankylosing: chronic disease characterized by inflammation of the spine and resulting in the fusing (ankylosing) of the spinal joints
spondylolisthesis: forward displacement of one of the lower vertebrae over the vertebra below it or over the sacrum, causing severe pain in the lower back
spontaneous abortion: miscarriage
sporadic: characterized by scattered cases, as of a disease, rather than by concentration in one area
spore: single-celled reproductive body of a flowerless plant, capable of developing into an independent organism
sprain: the stretching or rupturing of ligaments, usually accompanied by damage to blood vessels
sputum: expectorated matter, as saliva, sometimes mixed with mucus
sputum exam: bacteriological, chemical, and microscopic testing of sputum for presence of disease
stapedius: small muscle in the tympanum of the middle ear whose function is to dampen loud sounds
stapes: stirrup
staph: *see* staphylococcus
staphylococcus (*pl., staphylococci*)/ **staph:** parasitic bacterium that can cause boils and other infections
staphylococcus aureus: bacterium that causes food poisoning
startle reflex: *see* startle response

startle response/startle reflex: complex involuntary reaction to sudden noise occurring especially in infancy, where it is marked by a sudden jerk of the arms and legs
static exercises: isometrics
status epilepticus: series of epileptic seizures, occurring virtually without interruption
stenosis: the narrowing of a duct or canal in the body
sterile: 1. being incapable of producing offspring 2. being free of germs
sterility: 1. condition of being incapable of producing offspring 2. condition of being free of germs
sterilization: the process of destroying reproductive capacity by surgical means, as by tying the Fallopian tubes of a woman (tubal ligation) or by tying the seminal duct of a man (vasectomy)
steroid(s): any of a group of organic compounds occurring naturally and produced synthetically, including the sex hormones, the bile acids, oral contraceptives, and many drugs
stethoscope: diagnostic device that conducts sounds produced within the body, as the heartbeat, to the ear of the examiner
stiff toe: pain and stiffness in the joint of the big toe
stilbestrol: *see* diethylstilbestrol
Still's disease: *see* rheumatoid arthritis, juvenile
stimulant: drug or other substance that increases or agitates the physiological processes of body or mind
stimulus (*pl., stimuli*): that which initiates an impulse or affects the activity of an organism
stirrup/stapes: the innermost of the three ossicles of the middle ear, the bone between the anvil and the cochlea
Stokes-Adams syndrome: sudden unconsciousness and sometimes convulsions caused by heart block
stoma: small opening in a surface, as in a membrane or wall of a blood vessel
stomach, ulcers of: *see* peptic ulcer
stool exam: laboratory analysis of feces, as for presence of blood or parasitic organisms
STP: DOM
strabismus/squint: disorder of the eye muscles in which one eye drifts so that its position is not parallel with the other
strain: excessive stretching of a muscle, tendon, or ligament
stratum corneum: the outermost layer of the epidermis, consisting of horny, lifeless cells
strep throat: streptococcal infection of the throat
streptococcal: of or relating to the streptococcus bacterium
streptococcus: kind of bacteria including some forms that cause diseases, as pneumonia and scarlet fever
stress fracture: tiny crack in a bone caused by repeated stress
striated: striped, as certain muscle
striated muscle: *see* skeletal muscle
striped muscle: *see* skeletal muscle
stripping: surgical removal of lengths of varicosed veins, especially one of the saphenous veins of the leg
stroke/apoplexy: attack of paralysis caused by the rupture of an artery and hemorrhage into the brain, or by an obstruction of an artery, as from a blood clot
stupor: condition in which the senses and faculties are suspended or greatly dulled, as from shock, drugs, etc.
sty: small, inflamed swelling of a sebaceous gland on the edge of the eyelid
subacute: intermediate between *acute* and *chronic:* said of a disease
subarachnoid: situated or occurring between the middle layer (arachnoid) and the innermost layer (pia mater) of the brain
subcutaneous: situated or applied beneath the skin
subcutaneous injection: an injection given in the subcutaneous tissue beneath the skin
subcutaneous tissue: layer of fatty tissue below the skin (dermis) which acts as an insulator against heat and cold and as a shock absorber against injury
subdural: situated or occurring between the outermost layer (dura mater) and the middle layer (arachnoid) of the brain
subdural hematoma: *see* hematoma, subdural
subjective: (of symptoms) of a kind that only the patient is aware of
sublingual gland: either of a pair of salivary glands located beneath the tongue
submandibular gland: submaxillary gland
submaxillary gland/submandibular gland: either of a pair of salivary glands located under each side of the lower jaw
subtotal: less than total, as a surgical procedure involving the excision of an organ or part
sudden infant death syndrome/crib death/SIDS: death of an infant, usually between one and six months of age, without any preceding sign of distress and of undetermined cause
sudoriferous glands: *see* sweat gland
sulfa drug: any of a group of organic compounds used in the treatment of a variety of bacterial infections
sulfonamide(s): any of a group of chemical compounds including the sulfa drugs, used in the treatment of bacterial infections
sulfonylurea: drug used to treat diabetes

sunstroke/heatstroke: condition marked by an acutely high fever and the cessation of perspiration, caused by prolonged exposure to heat and sometimes leading to convulsions and coma
superego/conscience: largely unconscious element of the personality, regarded as dominating the ego, for which it acts principally in the role of conscience and critic
superficial: of, situated near, or on the surface
superior vena cava: the large vein that brings blood from the upper part of the body to the heart
supination: rotation of the hand or forearm so that the palm of the hand faces upward or forward
supine: lying on the back, with the face upward
suppository: solid, usually cylindrical medicated preparation that liquefies from heat after insertion in a body cavity, as the rectum or the vagina
suppuration: the formation of pus
suppurative: characterized by the formation of pus; pussy
surgeon: physician who specializes in the diagnosis and treatment of disease by means of surgery
surgery: the branch of medicine dealing with the correction of disorders or other physical change by operation or manipulation
surgical: of or relating to surgery
surgical diathermy: electrosurgery
suture: 1. to sew together cut or separated edges, as of a wound, to promote healing 2. the thread, wire, gut, etc., used in this process
suture line: line formed by the edges of the separate bones of a baby's skull
sweat gland/sudoriferous gland: any of numerous glands that secrete sweat, found almost everywhere in the skin except for the lips and a few other areas
swimmer's itch: mild form of schistosomiasis in which parasitic fluke worm larvae invade the skin of swimmers, causing dermatitis
sycosis/barber's itch: bacterial infection of hair follicles, marked by inflammation, itching, and the formation of pus-filled pimples
sympathetic nervous system: the part of the autonomic nervous system that controls such involuntary actions as the dilation of pupils, constriction of blood vessels and salivary glands, and increase of heartbeat
symptom: change in one's normal feeling or condition of well-being, indicating the presence of disease
symptomatic: having observable symptoms of a disease or condition
symptomatology: the combined symptoms of a disease
Synanon: organized live-in community of drug addicts in which group psychotherapy is used to encourage rehabilitation
synapse: the junction point between two neurons, across which a nerve impulse passes from the axon of one neuron to the dendrite of another
syncope: temporary loss of consciousness; fainting
syndrome: set of symptoms occurring at the same period and indicating the presence or nature of a disease
synovia/synovial fluid: viscid, transparent fluid secreted as a lubricating agent in the interior of joints and elsewhere
synovial aspiration/synovial fluid exam: laboratory analysis of synovia, withdrawn from joints by needle, in order to diagnose gout or certain forms of arthritis
synovial fluid: synovia
synovial fluid exam: synovial aspiration
syphilis: contagious venereal disease transmitted by sexual contact and congenitally to offspring of infected mothers
systemic: pertaining to or affecting the body as a whole
systole: the instant of peak pumping action of the heart, when the ventricles contract and blood is impelled outward into the arteries, followed immediately by relaxation (diastole)
systolic pressure: measure of blood pressure taken when the heart is contracting; the higher of the two figures in a reading

tabes dorsalis/locomotor ataxia: form of syphilis involving demyelination of spinal nerves and other destructive changes in the spinal cord
tachycardia: abnormally rapid heartbeat
tachycardia, paroxysmal: attacks of abnormally rapid heartbeat (tachycardia) that begin and end abruptly
Tagamet: cimetidine
tampon: plug of absorbent material for insertion in a body cavity or wound to stop bleeding or absorb secretions
T and A operation: *see* adenotonsillectomy
tapeworm/cestode: any of various worms with segmented, ribbonlike bodies, often of considerable length, that are parasitic on the intestines of humans and other vertebrates
target gland: any of the endocrine glands that function when stimulated by hormones secreted by the anterior pituitary, as the thyroid adrenal cortex, testicles, or ovaries
tarsal: any of the bones of the tarsus, or ankle
tarsus: ankle
taste bud: one of the clusters of cells in the tongue that contain receptors for discriminating salt, sweet, sour, or bitter tastes

teething: process by which new teeth break (erupt) through the gums in infants and young children
tempered glass: safety glass that has high resistance to blunt objects and breaks by crumbling into small fragments instead of shattering
temporal lobe: the portion of each cerebral hemisphere of the brain in back of and partly below the frontal lobes, the centers for hearing
temporal lobe convulsions: convulsions, psychomotor
tendinitis: inflammation of a tendon
tendon: band of tough, fibrous connective tissue that binds a muscle to another part, as a bone, and by means of which muscular force can be exerted on other parts of the body
tendon sheath, inflammation of: tenosynovitis
tennis elbow: pain in the outer side of the elbow joint, usually caused by a too vigorous twisting motion of the hand that strains a tendon or inflames a bursa
tenosynovitis: inflammation of the sheath that covers a tendon
tension headache: severe headache induced by tension, which causes unconscious constriction of head and neck muscles
Terramycin: trade name for the antibiotic tetracycline
testes: testicles
testicle(s)/testis(*pl., testes*): one of a pair of male reproductive glands (gonads) that produce spermatozoa and male sex hormones, situated in a pouch (scrotum) at the base of the penis
testis: *see* testicle
testosterone: male sex hormone manufactured in the testicles
tetanus/lockjaw: acute bacterial infection usually introduced through a puncture wound leading to muscle spasms, especially of the jaw muscles, and often fatal
tetany: nerve disorder characterized by muscle spasms and sometimes convulsions, caused by too little calcium in the blood
tetracycline: crystalline powder isolated from a soil bacillus that forms the base of several antibiotics, including Aureomycin and Terramycin
tetrahydrocannabinol/THC: principal compound of cannabis (hashish or marihuana), believed to be the active ingredient
thalamus: round mass of gray matter at the base of the brain that transmits sensory impulses to the cerebral cortex
thalassemia/Cooley's anemia: form of anemia caused by inherited abnormality of red blood cells, often fatal in utero
THC: tetrahydrocannabinol
therapeutic: designed or tending to heal or to cure disease
therapist: *see* psychotherapist
therapy: treatment of a disease by prescribed method or medicine
thermogram: measurement of the surface temperature of a region of the body, such as the breast, with an infrared sensing device
thermography: technique of measuring the surface temperature of a region of the body, such as the breast, with an infrared sensing device
thiamine/vitamin B_1: vitamin found in cereal grains, green peas, liver, egg yolk, and other sources, and also made synthetically, that protects against beriberi
thoracic: of or relating to the thorax, or chest cavity
thoracic cage: *see* rib cage
thoracic cavity: *see* chest cavity
thoracic spine: *see* vertebrae, thoracic
thoracic surgeon: surgeon specializing in thoracic surgery, having to do with the chest cavity
thoracic surgery: branch of surgery having to do with the chest cavity and its organs, the heart and lungs, and large blood vessels
thorax: chest
Thorazine/chlorpromazine: trademark for a commonly used tranquilizer
throat: *see* pharynx
throat, sore: *see* pharyngitis
thrombin: enzyme present in the blood that reacts with fibrinogen to form fibrin in the process of clotting
thrombocytes: platelets
thromboembolism: obstruction of a blood vessel by a blood clot (thrombus) that has broken away from the place where it was formed
thrombophlebitis: formation of a blood clot (thrombus) in the wall of an inflamed vein (phlebitis)
thromboplastin: substance found in blood platelets that helps to convert pro-thrombin into thrombin in the clotting process
thrombosis: formation of a blood clot (thrombus) in a blood vessel, resulting in the partial or complete blocking of circulation
thrombus: stationary blood clot within a blood vessel
thrush: fungus infection in the mouth, especially of infants, characterized by white patches that become sores
thymectomy: surgical removal of the thymus
thymus: glandlike, lymphoid organ located near the base of the neck, believed to play a role in the body's immunological responses
thyroid gland: endocrine gland located at the neck just below the larynx, extending around the front and to either side of the trachea (windpipe), and secreting the hormone thyroxin, which is vital to growth and metabolism

thyroid hormone: *see* thyroxin
thyroid-stimulating hormone/TSH: hormone secreted by the anterior lobe of the pituitary gland which stimulates the production of hormones in the thyroid gland
thyroxin: hormone secreted by the thyroid gland, vital to growth and metabolism
tibia: the shin bone, the inner and larger of the two bones of the lower leg
tic: involuntary, recurrent muscle twitch or spasm
tic douloureux: *see* trigeminal neuralgia
tick fever: *see* Rocky Mountain spotted fever
tinea: ringworm
tinnitus: ringing, buzzing, hissing, or clicking sound in the ears, not caused by external stimuli
tissue, death of: *see* gangrene
tolerance: the ability of the body to adjust to increasingly larger doses of a drug through habitual use
tomography: radiography of a section of the body
tomography, computerized axial: *see* CT scanning
tone/tonicity: the normal tension of muscle tissue
tonic: of or characteristic of tonus
tonicity: *see* tone
tonic phase: the period during a grand mal epileptic convulsion when the body is rigid
tonic spasm: *see* spasm
tonometer: device for measuring pressure, as of the eyeball
tonsil: either of two small round, lymphoid organs at each side of the back of the throat
tonsillectomy: surgical removal of the tonsils
tonsillitis: inflammation of the tonsils
tonus: muscular spasm characterized by persistent contraction
tophus (*pl. tophi*): deposit of urate in the joints, a cause of gout
tourniquet: bandage or other material tied tightly to constrict an artery to stop bleeding
toxemia of pregnancy: metabolic disorder of pregnant women, characterized by a rise in blood pressure, swelling of tissue, weight gain, and headaches (pre-eclampsia) and sometimes by convulsions and loss of consciousness (eclampsia)
toxic: 1. caused by or having to do with a toxin or poison 2. poisonous
toxic psychosis: psychosis caused by a toxic agent, such as lead or alcohol
toxin(s): any of a group of poisonous compounds produced by animal, vegetable, or bacterial organisms
trabecula (*pl., trabeculae*): strand of connective tissue, as in a bone
trachea/windpipe: the passageway for air from the larynx to the lungs
tracheostomy/tracheotomy: emergency surgical procedure of cutting into the trachea
tracheotomy: *see* tracheostomy
traction: subjection of muscle or a fractured part to a pulling force, as by a system of weights and pulleys
tranquilizer: drug with a calming or sedative effect
transference: in psychoanalysis, the redirection of repressed childhood emotions to the analyst
transplant: tissue or organ transferred from its original site to another part of the body or to another individual
transsexual: person who is genetically and physically of one sex but who identifies psychologically with the other and may seek treatment by surgery or with hormones to bring the physical sexual characteristics into conformity with the psychological preference
transudate: fluid passing through pores or tissues, as of a membrane
transverse colon: the section of the colon leading from the ascending colon and extending horizontally across the abdomen beneath the liver and stomach
transvestism: practice of wearing the clothes of the opposite sex
transvestite: one who wears the clothes of the opposite sex
trauma: 1. any injury or wound to the body 2. severe emotional shock
trematode: any of a class of parasitic flatworms, as the flukes, causing various diseases such as schistosomiasis
tremor: any involuntary quivering or trembling, as of a muscle
trench foot: foot condition resembling frostbite resulting from exposure to continued dampness and cold
trench mouth/Vincent's angina/Vincent's disease: painful infection of the gums (called necrotizing ulcerative gingivitis) and sometimes of the pharynx and palate, characterized by the formation of ulcers and necrosis
trichina: Trichinella spiralis
Trichinella spiralis/trichina: the parasitic worm that causes trichinosis
trichinosis: disease caused by a parasitic worm (Trichinella spiralis) that enters the body via under-cooked or raw meat, especially pork, invading the intestines and muscles and provoking gastrointestinal symptoms initially and muscle stiffness and pain later
trichomonas: genus of protozoa that cause vaginal infections in women
trichomoniasis: vaginal infection by the trichomonas organism
triglyceride: glycerol compound containing one to three acids

trimester: period of three months, used to identify the progress of a pregnancy which consists of three such periods
trip (*slang*): hallucinogenic experience
trivalent: pertaining to a form of the Sabin polio vaccine in which each dose gives protection against three strains of polio
trophoblast: layer of cells developing around a fertilized ovum and contributing to the formation of the placenta
trophoblastic disease: disease of the trophoblast in a pregnant woman, marked by the degeneration of the placenta into a mass of grapelike cysts (*hydatidiform mole*)
true skin: dermis
trypanosomiasis: sleeping sickness
tropanosomiasis, African: *see* sleeping sickness
tropanosomiasis, American: *see* Chagas' disease
trypsin: enzyme in the pancreatic juice that breaks up proteins for digestion
TSH: thyroid-stimulating hormone
tubal insufflation/Rubin's test: the injection of carbon dioxide gas, or sometimes ordinary air into the uterus to check for obstructions in the Fallopian tubes
tubal ligation: the tying or binding of a tube, especially of the Fallopian tubes as a method of sterilization
tubercle: small nodule or tumor formed within an organ, as that produced by the bacillus causing tuberculosis
tubercle bacillus: rod-shaped bacterium that causes tuberculosis
tuberculin: liquid containing substances extracted from weakened (attenuated) tubercle bacilli, used as a test for tuberculosis
tuberculin test: skin test for determining whether tuberculosis bacteria are present, used especially for children
tuberculoid: of or resembling a tubercle or tuberculosis
tuberculosis: infectious, communicable disease caused by the tubercle bacillus and characterized by the formation of tubercles within some organ or tissue, often the lungs (pulmonary tuberculosis)
tubule(s): very narrow, minute tube or duct of kidney
tularemia: acute bacterial infection that can be transmitted to humans from infected rabbits, squirrels, or other animals, by the bite of certain flies, or by direct contact
tumor: mass of tissue growing independently of surrounding tissue and having no physiological function, sometimes confined to the area of origin (benign) and sometimes invading other cells and tissue and causing their degeneration (malignant)
tumor, fibroid: benign tumor composed of fibrous tissue, usually attached to the wall of the uterus
turbinate: one of the thin, curved bones on the walls of the nasal passages
tympanum: 1. the cavity in the middle ear lined with the tympanic membrane (eardrum) and containing the ossicles 2. eardrum
tympanic membrane: *see* eardrum
typhoid fever/enteric fever: acute infectious disease caused by a Salmonella bacterium and characterized by diarrhea, fever, eruption of bright red spots on the chest and abdomen, and physical prostration
typhus: acute disease caused by a rickettsial microorganism that is transmitted to humans by the bite of certain lice and fleas, and is characterized by high fever, severe headaches, and a red rash

ulcer(s): open sore with an inflamed base on an external or internal body surface
ulcer(s) of gastrointestinal tract: *see* peptic ulcers
ulcerative colitis: colitis accompanied by ulcerated lesions on the colon, characterized by bloody diarrhea and abdominal pain
ulna: the bone of the forearm on the same side as the little finger, longer and thinner than the radius bone
umbilical: pertaining to the middle part of the abdomen
umbilical cord: the ropelike tissue connecting the navel of the fetus with the placenta
umbilicus: navel
unconsciousness: loss of consciousness, having the appearance of sleep, usually caused by injury, shock, or serious physical disturbance
underskin: tissue, subcutaneous
undulant fever: *see* brucellosis
unsaturated: (of fats) not tending to increase the cholesterol content of the blood
ups/uppers/pep pills (*slang*): drugs or compounds that have a stimulating effect on the central nervous system, such as amphetamines
urate: salt of uric acid
urea: soluble compound containing nitrogen, found in urine and in small amounts in the blood
uremia: toxic condition of the blood caused by the failure of the kidneys to function normally in filtering and excreting waste products, such as urea
ureter: either of two narrow, muscular ducts which convey urine from the kidneys to the bladder
urethra: duct from the bladder by which urine is discharged and which in males carries seminal fluid
urethritis: inflammation of the urethra

urinalysis (UA): chemical and microscopic analysis of the urine to determine for diagnostic purposes whether it is normally constituted
urination: the excretion of urine
urine: waste products and excess water separated in the kidneys and stored in the bladder for eventual elimination from the body
urinogenital tract/genitourinary tract/urogenital tract: the urinary and genital systems, including the kidneys, ureters, bladder, urethra, vagina and associated parts
urogenital tract: urinogenital tract
urologist: physician specializing in urology
urology: the branch of medical science that deals with the diagnosis and treatment of diseases of the kidneys, bladder, ureters, urethra, and of the male reproductive organs
urticaria: *see* hives
uterine: of or pertaining to the uterus
uterus/womb: muscular, glandular organ in women in which the developing fetus is protected until birth
uvula: fleshy, teardrop-shaped appendage of the soft palate at the back of the mouth

vaccinate: inoculate with a vaccine as a preventive or therapeutic measure
vaccination: 1. act or process of vaccinating 2. scar produced at the site of inoculation with a vaccine
vaccine: preparation of live, attenuated, or dead microorganisms injected or administered orally to create immunity against a specific disease
vacuum aspiration: technique of inducing abortion in early pregnancy by utilizing suction to draw out embryo tissue
vagina: canal in the female leading from the external genital orifice below the pubis to the uterus
vaginal sponge: contraceptive device made of polyurethane permeated with spermicide nonoxynol-9
vaginitis: inflammation of the vagina
vagotomy: surgical procedure of cutting the vagus nerves
vagus: the tenth cranial nerve, which originates in the brain and extends branches to the lungs, heart, stomach, and intestines
Valium/diazepam: trademark for commonly used tranquilizer
Valmid: ethinamate
valve: membranous structure inside a vessel or other organ, as the heart, allowing fluid to flow in one direction only
valve, disease of: endocarditis
vaporizers: *see* steam inhalators
varicose: abnormally dilated, as veins
varicose ulcer: ulcer resulting from varicose veins, usually on the inner side of the leg above the ankle
varicose vein/varix: swollen and contorted vein, often in the leg
varicosity: 1. condition of being varicose 2. *see* varicose vein
variola: smallpox
varix (*pl., varices*)**:** varicose vein
vascular: of, involving, or supplied with vessels, as blood vessels
vascularization: process of becoming vascular
vascular surgeon: surgeon specializing in vascular surgery, having to do with the blood vessels
vascular surgery: branch of surgery having to do with the operative treatment of diseases of the blood vessels
vas deferens: duct in males that conveys semen from the testicles to the seminal vesicles
vasectomy: surgical removal of part of the vas deferens or sperm duct of the male, thus rendering him sterile by preventing semen from reaching the seminal vesicles
vasoconstrictor: medicine that causes the blood vessels to contract, thus restricting blood flow
vasodilator: medicine that causes the blood vessels to dilate, thus producing greater blood flow
vasomotor: producing contraction or dilation of the blood vessels
vasopressin: hormone secreted by the posterior lobe of the pituitary gland that raises blood pressure and increases peristalsis, known also as antidiuretic hormone because of its action on the kidneys to stimulate the reabsorption of water
VD: *see* venereal disease
vector cardiogram: graph indicating the magnitude and direction of the electrical currents of the heart
vein(s): any of a large number of muscular, tubular vessels conveying blood from all parts of the body to the heart
vein, pulmonary: vein that delivers oxygen-rich blood from the lungs to the heart
velum: soft palate
vena cava: either of two large veins that bring blood to the heart from the upper part of the body (superior vena cava) and lower part of the body (inferior vena cava)
venereal disease: any of those diseases transmitted by sexual intercourse, such as syphilis and gonorrhea
venereal wart/condyloma acuminatum: wart caused by a virus and occurring in the anal and genital areas, transmitted by sexual contact and by other means
venesection: *see* phlebotomy
venom: poison secreted by certain reptiles, insects, etc., transferred to a victim by a bite or sting

venous: having to do with or carried by the veins
ventral: toward, near, or in the abdomen
ventricle(s): any of various body cavities, as of the brain, or chambers, especially either of the two lower chambers of the heart, which receive blood from the atria and pump it into the arteries
ventriculography: technique of X raying the brain after the removal of cerebrospinal fluid and the injection of air into the ventricles
venule: small vein continuous with a capillary
vermiform appendix/appendix vermiformis: the worm-shaped appendage attached to the cecum of the large intestine
vermifuge: any drug or remedy that destroys intestinal worms
vernix caseosa: cheesy substance sometimes covering a newborn baby's skin
vertebra (*pl., vertebrae*)**:** one of the segmented bones that make up the spinal column
vertebra, thoracic/thoracic spine: the vertebra to which the ribs are attached
vertebrate: any animal having a backbone
vertigo: disorder in which a person feels as if self or surroundings are whirling around
vesical: of or pertaining to the bladder
vesicle: small bladderlike cavity, or a small sac containing fluid
vestibular nerve: the part of the auditory nerve leading from the vestibule of the inner ear to the brain, controlling equilibrium
vestibule: space or cavity, as within the labyrinth of the inner ear
vestigial: of the nature of a remnant of an organ that is no longer functional
viable: capable of living and developing normally, as a newborn infant
vibrissae (*sing., vibrissa*)**:** hairs that grow in the nasal cavity
villi (*sing., villus*)**:** minute, hairlike structures on the mucous membrane of the small intestine that absorb nutrients
Vincent's angina: *see* trench mouth
Vincent's disease: *see* trench mouth
virulent: 1. severe and rapid in its progress, as a disease 2. highly infectious, as a disease-causing microorganism
virus (*pl., viruses*)**:** any of a large group of particles too small to be seen by an ordinary microscope, that are typically inert except when in contact with certain living cells, and that can cause a variety of infectious diseases
viscera: 1. the internal organs of the body, as the stomach, lungs, heart, etc. 2. the intestines
visceral: pertaining to the viscera
viscid: sticky or adhesive
viscous: semifluid or gluelike in texture
visual purple: reddish purple protein found in the rods of the retina, especially important to night vision
visual radiations: smaller nerve bundles that split off from the optic nerve and enter the occipital lobes of the brain
vitalometer: device for measuring sensitivity of a tooth
vital signs: measurement of body temperature, pulse rate, and respiration
vitamin(s): any of a group of complex organic substances found in minute quantities in most natural foods and closely associated with the maintenance of normal physiological functions
vitamin A: vitamin found in green and yellow vegetables, dairy products, liver and fish liver oils, that prevents atrophy of epithelial tissue and protects against night blindness
vitamin B_1: thiamine
vitamin B_2: riboflavin
vitamin B_{12}: vitamin extracted from liver and believed to protect against pernicious anemia
vitamin B complex: group of water-soluble vitamins including thiamine and riboflavin
vitamin C: *see* ascorbic acid
vitamin D: vitamin that protects against rickets, found in fish liver oils, butter, egg yolks, and specially treated cow's milk, and also produced in the body on exposure to sunlight
vitamin E: vitamin found in whole grain cereals, legume seeds, corn oil, egg yolks, meat, and milk, sometimes called the anti-sterility vitamin because its absence in rats causes sterility
vitamin K: vitamin that promotes the clotting of blood and is found in green leafy vegetables
vitiligo: An autoimmune disease in which the body's white cells attack its pigment cells, causing loss of pigment in small to large patches of skin. The nose, hands, feet, and genital area are the areas most often affected. About 1 percent of the U.S. population suffers from vitiligo, which can appear any time up to middle age and is believed to be inherited.

No cure exists for vitiligo, but treatments include drugs and exposure to ultraviolet A radiation. The condition is not painful physically but many vitiligo sufferers, particularly dark-skinned persons, often experience emotional pain and embarrassment.
vitreous humor: the transparent, jellylike tissue that fills the posterior chamber or ball of the eye and is enclosed by the hyaloid membrane
vocal cords/vocal folds: two bands of ligaments extending across the larynx which, when tense, are made to vibrate by the passage of air, thereby producing voice
vocal folds: *see* vocal cords
voice box: larynx
void: excrete waste, especially urine
voluntary muscle: *see* skeletal muscle
volvulus: obstruction of the intestines caused by twisting
vomitus: vomited substance
vulva: the external genitals of the female, located beneath the front part of the pelvis

walking pneumonia: mild viral pneumonia that does not confine the patient to bed
walleye: strabismus characterized by a tendency of the eyes to turn outward, away from the nose
wart: small, usually hard, benign growth formed on and rooted in the skin, caused by a virus
Wasserman test: blood test for the presence of the organism causing syphilis
water blister: blister beneath the epidermis that contains lymph
"water pills": diuretics
wet dream/nocturnal emission: male's involuntary expulsion of semen while asleep
wheal: raised area on the skin, as from hives or an insect bite, usually transitory and characterized by itching
whiplash: injury to neck ligaments, usually caused by a sudden jolt to the neck, as in automobile accidents
white blood cells: *see* leukocytes
white corpuscle: *see* leukocyte
white of eye: *see* sclera
white lung disease: byssinosis
WHO: World Health Organization
whooping cough/pertussis: respiratory, bacterial disease of children marked by paroxysms of coughing ending with a sharp sound (or "whoop") upon intake of breath
whooping cough/pertussis, immunization against: *see* DPT injections
Wilms' tumor/nephroblastoma: malignant tumor of the kidney, found especially in children
windpipe: *see* trachea
wisdom tooth: the last tooth, or third molar on either side of the upper and lower jaws
withdrawal symptom: any of the symptoms caused by the withdrawal of a physically addictive drug from an addict, as tremors, sweating, chills, vomiting, and diarrhea
womb: *see* uterus
wood alcohol: methyl alcohol
writer's cramp: spasmodic contraction of the muscles of the fingers and hand, caused by excessive writing

xenograft: *see* heterograft
xenophobia: fear of strangers
xerography: method of reproducing an image of electrostatic attraction, used experimentally as a diagnostic tool
xeroradiogram: picture developed by xeroradiography
xeroradiography: diagnostic procedure utilizing xerography to develop X-ray pictures
X ray: 1. to examine, diagnose, or treat with X rays 2. photograph made with X rays
X rays: electromagnetic radiations of extremely short wavelengths, used to reproduce on photosensitive film images of the internal organs and the skeleton as an aid in the detection, diagnosis, and treatment of certain disorders
Yang: in the Chinese philosophy underlying acupuncture, the masculine principle, identified with activity
yaws: infectious tropical disease that is not venereal but is caused by the syphilis bacterium (spirochete), characterized by rheumatic pains and ulcerating sores of the skin
yellow fever: acute, infectious, intestinal disease of tropical and semi-tropical regions, caused by a virus transmitted by the bite of a mosquito, and characterized by jaundice and hemorrhages
yellow marrow: marrow
Yin: in the Chinese philosophy underlying acupuncture, the female principle, identified with passivity
zymase: enzyme, obtained principally from yeast, important in fermentation